Become a better
and a
BETTER NURSE

MW00846203

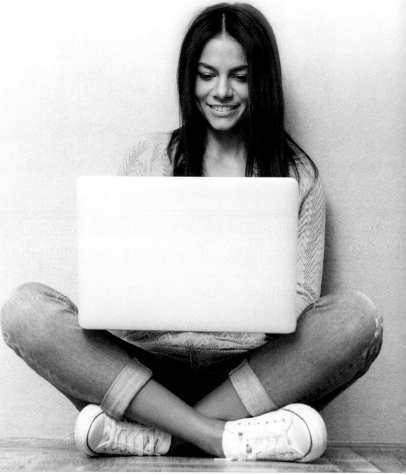

Davis Advantage
offers a personalized, interactive learning platform with proven results to help you succeed in your course.

94%
of students said Advantage improved their test scores.

"My grades have improved; my understanding about topics is much clearer; and overall, it has been the total package for what a nursing student needs to succeed."

— Hannah, Student, Judson University

Your journey to success
BEGINS HERE!

Redeem your access code on the inside front cover of your text to access the tools you need to succeed in your course. Need a code? Visit FADavis.com to purchase access.

TEXT

STEP #1
Build a solid foundation.

Evidence-Based Practice boxes focus on research-based care.

SAFE AND EFFECTIVE NURSING CARE:
Understanding Medication

Rh₀(D) Immune Globulin (RhoGAM)

Laboratory screening during an initial prenatal visit includes blood type and Rh factor with antibody screening to identify isoimmunization. Patients found to be $Rh_0(D)$-negative should be rescreened in the second trimester and given RhoGAM at 26 to 28 weeks and again after delivery if the infant is $Rh_0(D)$-positive.

- Indication: Administered to $Rh_0(D)$-negative women prophylactically at 26 to 28 weeks' gestation to prevent isoimmunization from potential exposure to $Rh_0(D)$-positive fetal blood during the normal course of pregnancy. Also administered [...]

SAFE AND EFFECTIVE NURSING CARE:
Cultural Competence

How Cultural Beliefs Impact Postpartum Care

Cultural beliefs influence the ways parents relate to and care for infants, including the role of fathers during the postpartum period and care of infants. Awareness of [...] practices is an important component i[...] care. Cultural beliefs can influence:

- The degree of the father's involvement
- The role extended family members hav[...] infant and new mother
- The method of infant feeding
- Foods that are eaten and foods that ar[...] postpartum period
- When a woman can bathe and wash he[...]
- When the baby is named and who nan[...]

SAFE AND EFFECTIVE NURSING CARE:
Patient Education

Induction of Lactation

Several methods can be used to induce lactation for non-birthing mothers. These include hormonal therapy, manual or electric pumping of the breast, use of an at-breast supplementation device, or a combination of these methods. The non-birthing mother should begin preparing her breasts for lactation several months before the birth of the baby. The La Leche League International Web site provides additional information for non-birthing women who desire to breastfeed.

Evidence-Based Practice

Maternal Adaptation During the Early Postpartum Period

In the 1960s, Reba Rubin conducted qualitative research studies focusing on maternal adaptation during the early postpartum weeks. Her research is the foundation of our understanding of the psychosocial experience of women during the postpartum period. Two concepts identified through her research are "maternal phases" and "maternal touch." Rubin (1984) refined and modified the process as more evidence was linked to maternal adjustments and behaviors and identified areas of development that women progress through to "becoming a mother."

Ramona Mercer, a student and colleague of Rubin, added to and expanded this body of nursing knowledge through numerous research studies that focused on the maternal role. Based on these studies, Mercer (1995) developed the theory of "maternal role attainment," which describes and explains the process women progress through as they become a mother. Based on her previous research and the research of others, Mercer (2004) supports replacing the term *maternal role attainment* with *becoming a mother*. The term *becoming a mother* reflects that the process is not stagnant but continually evolving as the woman and her child are changing and growing.

The theories generated by Rubin's and Mercer's research agendas are the cornerstone of evidence-based knowledge used in establishing nursing guidelines for the care of postpartum women and families.

Safe and Effective Nursing Care boxes summarize important safety concepts, focusing on Patient Education, Cultural Competence, and Understanding Medication.

Case Study

As the nurse in the postpartum unit, you are caring for the Sanchez family. Margarite gave birth to a healthy boy 5 hours ago. Both she and her son are stable. She breastfed her son for 15 minutes after the birth.

You notice that she is lightly touching the top of her infant's head with her fingertips. She comments that she does not feel comfortable holding her baby close to her body for breastfeeding.

Discuss your nursing actions that are based on your knowledge of maternal touch.

List the maternal phase and expected maternal behaviors for this period of time.

List five expected bonding behaviors for this period of time.

The next day you are again assigned to care for the Sanchez family. Mom and baby are stable. José, Margarite's husband, is present during the shift. Margarite and José voice concern about integrating their infant into the family.

Discuss your nursing actions that reflect an understanding of the couple's tra[...]

Discuss specific str[...]

Margarite tells [...] tum depression wi[...] lot during the first[...] and her infant.

Discuss the approp[...] concerns.

CLINICAL JUDGMENT

The Nurse Role During the Taking-In Phase

Women in the taking-in phase are in a more dependent state and may have difficulty making decisions and initiating self-care and infant care. The nurse needs to be more directive in her patient care (i.e., remind the woman to take a shower or to change her newborn's diapers and then assist her in initiating the action).

NEW! Clinical Judgment boxes provide tips for applying critical thinking in clinical settings.

Case Studies ask you to apply your knowledge in clinical contexts.

Clinical Pathway for Transition to Parenthood

Focus of Care	Postpartum Admission	Postpartum 4 to 24 Hours	Postpartum 24 to 48 Hours	Discharge Criteria
Emotional status	Taking-in phase	Progressing toward the taking-hold phase	Taking-hold phase. The woman shows more independence in managing her own and the infant's care.	The woman is able to provide self-care. The woman demonstrates increased confidence in infant care.
Nursing action	Provide care and comfort to the woman. Provide positive reinforcement of appropriate behaviors. Discuss the infant's unique capabilities. Provide early and consistent contact with the infant to facilitate bonding.	Encourage the woman and her family to participate in self- and infant care. Encourage extended infant contact. Observe for bonding and attachment behaviors. Begin discharge education.	Observe for bonding and attachment behaviors, noting any signs of maladaptive behaviors. Provide written or visual information on infant behaviors and characteristics. Teach methods for comforting the infant.	Positive bonding and attachment behaviors are noted. Parents express understanding of infant behaviors and cues. Parents express positive understanding of how to care for the infant. Provide resources for parents to call as needed.
Family dynamics	Parents demonstrate beginning bonding behaviors. Parents begin introducing the infant to the extended family.	Parents demonstrate positive bonding and attachment behaviors. Extended family demonstrate positive and supportive behaviors toward the infant.	Parents continue to demonstrate bonding and attachment behaviors. Extended family demonstrates positive behaviors toward infant and parents.	Parents demonstrate positive adaptive behaviors.

Clinical Pathways detail the steps in a course of treatment or care plan and summarize important chapter elements.

CRITICAL COMPONENT

Assisting Parents With a Sensory Impairment

Nurses can best assist parents who have sensory impairments by exploring, identifying, and implementing techniques, tools, and alternative ways to:

- Facilitate bonding and attachment.
- Teach parents about infant care.
- Promote a safe environment for the infant.
- Enhance the family dynamics.

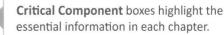

Critical Component boxes highlight the essential information in each chapter.

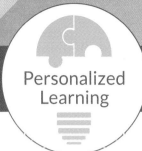

LEARN

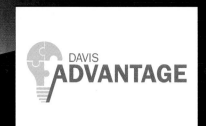

STEP #2

Make the connections to key topics.

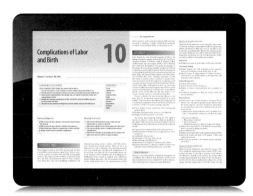

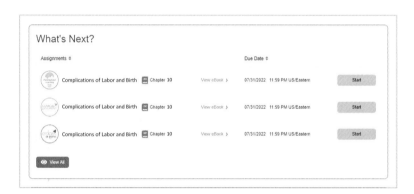

Assignments in Davis Advantage correspond to key topics in your book. Begin by reading from your printed text or click the eBook button to be taken to the **FREE, integrated eBook.**

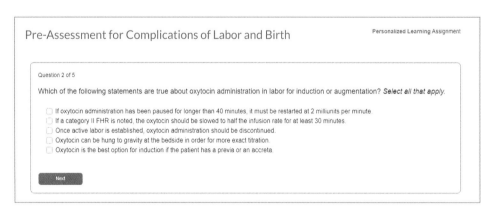

You'll receive **immediate feedback** that identifies your strengths and weaknesses using a thumbs up, thumbs down approach. *Thumbs up* indicates competency, while *thumbs down* signals an area of weakness that requires further study.

Following your reading, take the **Pre-Assessment** quiz to evaluate your understanding of the content. Questions feature single answer, multiple-choice, and select-all-that-apply formats.

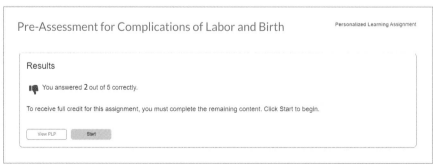

Online content subject to change upon publication.

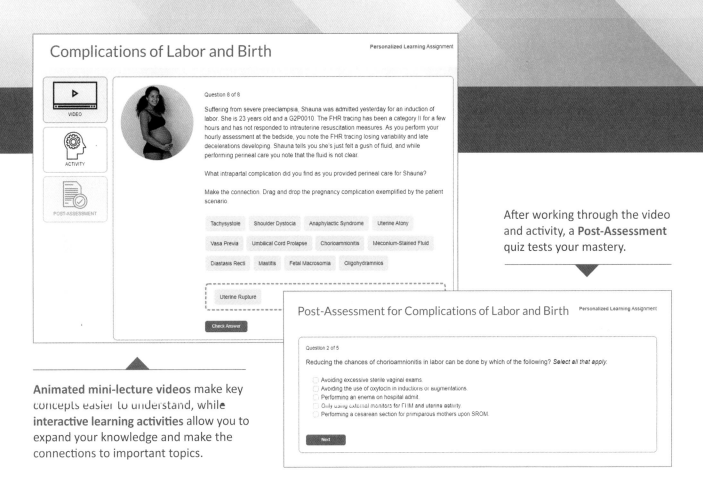

After working through the video and activity, a **Post-Assessment** quiz tests your mastery.

Animated mini-lecture videos make key concepts easier to understand, while **interactive learning activities** allow you to expand your knowledge and make the connections to important topics.

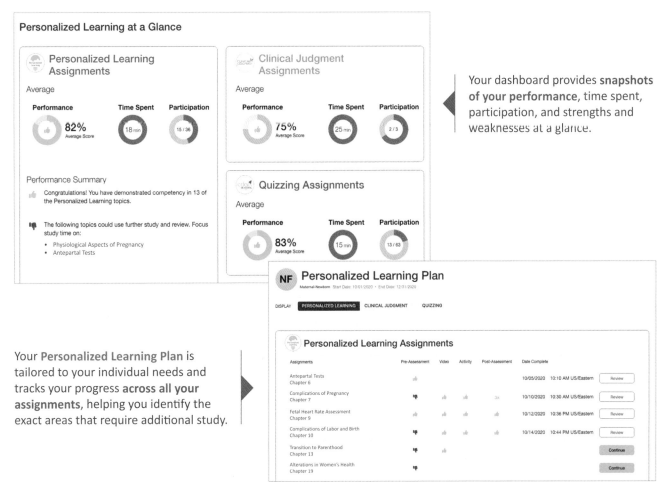

Your dashboard provides **snapshots of your performance**, time spent, participation, and strengths and weaknesses at a glance.

Your **Personalized Learning Plan** is tailored to your individual needs and tracks your progress **across all your assignments**, helping you identify the exact areas that require additional study.

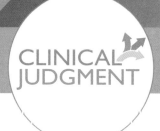
STEP #3

Develop critical-thinking skills & prepare for the Next Gen NCLEX.®

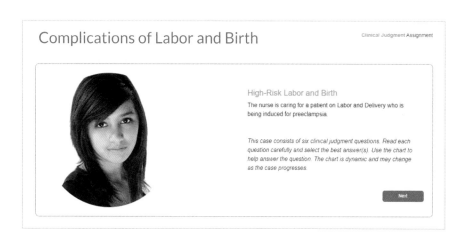

Complications of Labor and Birth

Clinical Judgment Assignment

High-Risk Labor and Birth

The nurse is caring for a patient on Labor and Delivery who is being induced for preeclampsia.

This case consists of six clinical judgment questions. Read each question carefully and select the best answer(s). Use the chart to help answer the question. The chart is dynamic and may change as the case progresses.

Next

Real-world cases mirror the complex clinical challenges you will encounter in a variety of health care settings. Each **case study** begins with a patient photograph and a brief introduction to the scenario.

The Patient Chart displays tabs for History & Physical Assessment, Nurses' Notes, Vital Signs, and Laboratory Results. As you progress through the case, the chart expands and populates with additional data.

Scenario

The nurse is caring for a patient on Labor and Delivery who is being induced for preeclampsia. Use the chart to answer the questions. *The chart may update as the scenario progresses.*

History and Physical Assessment	Nurses' Notes	Vital Signs	Laboratory Results

Obstetric history: Patient is a 17-year-old Hispanic female, G1P0, at 37.2. EDD is June 25, XX based on LMP. Late to prenatal care, first visit at 24.5 weeks, now consistent with scheduled appointments.

Social history: Senior in high school. Smoker, reduced from one pack a day to less than half a pack when she realized she was pregnant. Denies alcohol and illicit drug use. Lives at home with parents who are supportive. Father of the baby uninvolved.

Family history: Maternal history of DM, hypertension, preeclampsia. Father has no medical concerns.

Physical assessment: Pre-pregnancy—height 5'8", weight 138 lb, BMI 21. Weight at appointment 4 days ago 158 lb. Weight on hospital admit 169 lb. Fundal height 32 cm above umbilicus. NST is nonreactive, FHR baseline of 125 bpm. BPP score is 4/10, points deducted for nonreactive NST, fetal movement, and low amniotic fluid volume indicative of

Complications of Labor and Birth

Scenario

The nurse is caring for a patient on Labor and Delivery who is being induced for preeclampsia. Use the chart to answer the questions. *The chart may update as the scenario progresses.*

| History and Physical Assessment | Nurses' Notes | Vital Signs | Laboratory Results |

Obstetric history: Patient is a 17-year-old Hispanic female, G1P0, at 37.2. EDD is June 25, XX based on LMP. Late to prenatal care, first visit at 24.5 weeks, now consistent with scheduled appointments.
Social history: Senior in high school. Smoker, reduced from one pack a day to less than half a pack when she realized she was pregnant. Denies alcohol and illicit drug use. Lives at home with parents who are supportive. Father of the baby uninvolved.
Family history: Maternal history of DM, hypertension, preeclampsia. Father has no medical concerns.
Physical assessment: Pre-pregnancy—height 5'8", weight 138 lb, BMI 21. Weight at appointment 4 days ago 158 lb. Weight on hospital admit 169 lb. Fundal height 32 cm above umbilicus. NST is nonreactive, FHR baseline of 125 bpm. BPP score is 4/10, points deducted for nonreactive NST, fetal movement, and low amniotic fluid volume indicative of...

Question 6 of 6

Determine whether the patient concern is a result of preeclampsia, magnesium toxicity, or oxytocin induction of labor. *Select all that apply in each row.*

	Preeclampsia	Magnesium Toxicity	Oxytocin Induction
Periodic FHR decelerations	✔	☐	☐
Respiratory depression	☐	✔	☐
Pulmonary edema	☐	☐	✔
Tachysystole	☐	✔	☐
Oliguria	✔	✔	☐
Altered DTRs	☐	✔	☐
Thrombocytopenia	☐	☐	✔
Circulatory collapse	✔	✔	☐

Complex questions that mirror the format of the Next Gen NCLEX® require careful analysis, synthesis of the data, and multi-step thinking.

Complications of Labor and Birth

Results

👎 **You answered 3 out of 6 questions correctly.**

Review the questions, answers and rationales below to improve your understanding. Identify which questions you answered correctly (indicated by a green check mark) and incorrectly (identified by a red x). Remember, you must choose all correct options and only the correct options to get a question correct. Expand the questions to review your individual answer choices, the correct answers (indicated by green shading), and complete rationales.

[Hide All Details ▲] [Return to Assignments]

❌ **Question 1 of 6**   Hide ▲

The nurse is reviewing the patient's chart. *Select to highlight the information and findings that would indicate a predisposition and the development of preeclampsia. Select all that apply.*

Patient is a 17-year-old Hispanic female, G1P0, at 37.2. EDD is June 25, XX based on LMP. Late to prenatal care, first visit at 24.5 weeks, now consistent with scheduled appointments. Smoker. Denies alcohol and illicit drug use. Maternal history of DM, hypertension, preeclampsia. Father has no medical concerns. Pre pregnancy height 5'8", weight 138 lb, BMI 21. Weight at appointment 4 days ago 158 lb. Weight on hospital admit 169 lb. Fundal height 32 cm. NST is nonreactive, FHR baseline of 125 bpm. BPP score is 4/10, with points deducted for fetal movement, nonreactive NST and low amniotic fluid volume, +3 pitting edema lower extremities, nonpitting edema upper extremities. Patient complaining of a headache ranking 6 on a scale from 1 to 10 and hip pain of 4 out of 10. No upper right quadrant pain or vision changes. DTRs +3 negative for clonus.

Rationale

Because the patient is under the age of 20 and is Hispanic, her risk of developing preeclampsia is increased. Primiparas and those with a family history of maternal diabetes, hypertension, and preeclampsia are also at greater risk of developing the disease. A sudden weight gain, edema, and pitting indicate fluid retention and possible renal impairment, which is a risk in preeclampsia. Fundal height measurement is lower than expected, indicating possible IUGR. A nonreactive NST and a 4/10 BPP can both indicate fetal compromise due to preeclampsia. Headache and hyperreflexia can indicate worsening preeclampsia.
Being late to prenatal care is a concern but is not a factor for her developing preeclampsia at 37.2 weeks. Smoking, alcohol use, and illicit drug use are not factors for developing preeclampsia. Pre-pregnancy weight and BMI along with her weight gain, until 4 days ago, are in a healthy range. FHR baseline is within normal limits. Hip pain is a normal discomfort of pregnancy. No right upper quadrant pain, lack of vision changes, negative clonus indicate the disease process has not impacted hepatic or neurological systems to the point of being symptomatic.

Clinical Judgment Cognitive Skill: Recognize Cues   Page Reference: pp. 142–143, 145–147, 172–180

 Test-Taking Tip   Determining the cause of a specific finding involves clustering data and then recognizing how those data apply to the current patient situation.

Immediate feedback with **detailed rationales** encourages you to consider what data is important and how to prioritize the information, to ensure safe and effective nursing care.

Test-taking tips provide important context and strategies for how to consider the structure of each question type when answering.

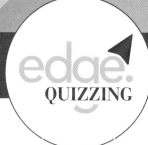

ASSESS

STEP #4
Improve comprehension & retention.

High-quality questions, including more difficult question types like **select-all-that-apply**, assess your understanding and challenge you to think at a higher cognitive level.

PLUS! Brand-new Next Gen NCLEX® stand-alone questions provide you with even more practice answering the new item types and help build your confidence.

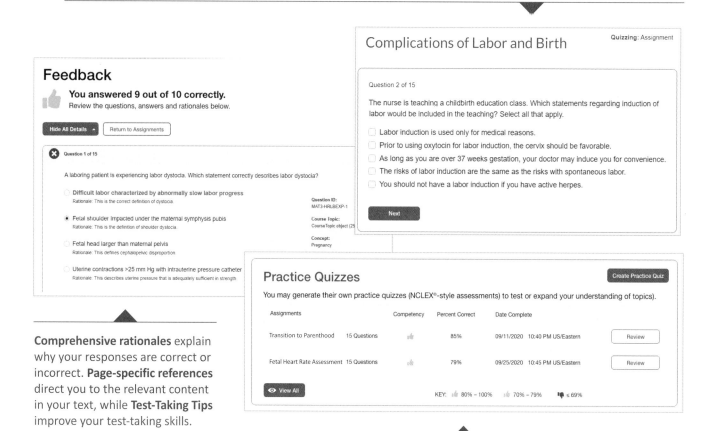

Comprehensive rationales explain why your responses are correct or incorrect. **Page-specific references** direct you to the relevant content in your text, while **Test-Taking Tips** improve your test-taking skills.

Create your own **practice quizzes** to focus on topic areas where you are struggling, or to use as a study tool to review for an upcoming exam.

GET STARTED TODAY!
Use the access code on the inside front cover to unlock
Davis Advantage for **Maternal-Newborn Nursing!**

DAVIS ADVANTAGE for
Maternal-Newborn
Nursing

Critical Components of Nursing Care

DAVIS ADVANTAGE for
Maternal-Newborn
Nursing

Critical Components of Nursing Care

FOURTH EDITION

Roberta F. Durham, RN, PhD

Professor Emeritus
California State University, East Bay
Hayward, California
Professor Alumnus
Fulbright Scholar
Trinidad and Tobago
Samuel Merritt University
Oakland, California

Linda L. Chapman, RN, PhD

Professor Emeritus
Samuel Merritt University
Oakland, California

Connie S. Miller, DNP, RNC-OB, CNE

Clinical Professor
Chair, General Nursing and Health Education Division
The University of Arizona College of Nursing
Tucson, Arizona

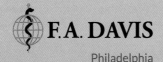

F.A. DAVIS

Philadelphia

F.A. Davis Company
1915 Arch Street
Philadelphia, PA 19103
www.fadavis.com

Printed in the United States of America

Last digit indicates print number: 10 9 8 7 6 5 4 3 2 1

Acquisitions Editor: Jacalyn Sharp
Developmental Editor: Andrea Miller
Manager of Project and eProject Development: Catherine Carroll
Content Project Manager: Amanda Minutola
Design and Illustration Manager: Carolyn O'Brien

As new scientific information becomes available through basic and clinical research, recommended treatments and drug therapies undergo changes. The author(s) and publisher have done everything possible to make this book accurate, up to date, and in accord with accepted standards at the time of publication. The author(s), editors, and publisher are not responsible for errors or omissions or for consequences from application of the book, and make no warranty, expressed or implied, in regard to the contents of the book. Any practice described in this book should be applied by the reader in accordance with professional standards of care used in regard to the unique circumstances that may apply in each situation. The reader is advised always to check product information (package inserts) for changes and new information regarding dose and contraindications before administering any drug. Caution is especially urged when using new or infrequently ordered drugs.

Library of Congress Cataloging-in-Publication Data
Names: Durham, Roberta F. author. | Chapman, Linda, 1949–author. | Miller,
   Connie (Clinical professor) author.
Title: Davis advantage for maternal-newborn nursing: critical components
   of nursing care / Roberta F. Durham, Linda L. Chapman, Connie Miller.
Other titles: Maternal-newborn nursing | Advantage for maternal-newborn nursing
Description: Fourth edition. | Philadelphia, PA: F.A. Davis Company,
   [2023] | Preceded by: Maternal-newborn nursing / Roberta F. Durham,
   Linda L. Chapman. Third edition. [2019] | Includes bibliographical references and index.
Identifiers: LCCN 2022004799 (print) | LCCN 2022004800 (ebook) | ISBN
   9781719645737 (paperback) | ISBN 9781719648288 (ebook)
Subjects: MESH: Maternal-Child Nursing | Perinatal Care
Classification: LCC RG951 (print) | LCC RG951 (ebook) | NLM WY157.3 |
   DDC 618.2/0231--dc23/eng/20220325
LC record available at https://lccn.loc.gov/2022004799
LC ebook record available at https://lccn.loc.gov/2022004800

The authors are grateful more than ever for the tireless work of all nurses and faculty for their role in ensuring every patient receives the care and dignity they deserve regardless of race, sexual orientation, status, or illness.

To my parents, Raymond and Virginia "Ducky" Durham; husband, Douglas Fredebaugh; and sisters, Ginny Durham and Dr. Patricia Durham Taylor, as well as friends and family in the Bay Area and Hawaii. Thank you for your love and support. Aloha

To my husband and best friend, Chuck: Thank-you for a lifetime of love, happiness, and fun adventures. You were and are there to love and support me through my many educational and academic endeavors, and life events. I love you.

To my mother, Lena Winter; husband and love of my life, Mike; sons Colin and Ross; daughter, Aubrey; and grandchildren, Bray and Dakota. Thank you all for your constant love and support while allowing me to follow my dreams! Love, Connie, Mom, and Mimi.

Preface

FOCUS

In this fourth edition of *Davis Advantage for Maternal-Newborn Nursing: Critical Components of Nursing Care,* we continue to emphasize the basics of maternity nursing, focusing on evidence-based practice for all levels of nursing programs. Because we realize that today's students lead complex lives and must juggle multiple roles as student, parent, employee, and partner, we developed this textbook, with its accompanying electronic ancillaries, to present the critical components of maternity nursing in a clear and concise format that lends itself to ease of comprehension while maintaining the integrity of the substantive content. It may be particularly useful for programs designed to present the subject of maternity in an accelerated or condensed way.

We revised the textbook based on the recommendations of those who have used it—faculty from various states and students in all types of programs—and our own experiences. Revisions include enhanced rationales for nursing actions in all chapters, increased content in pathophysiology in many areas, and expanded high-risk content. We have updated content to keep current in standards in practice, including new guidelines for management of pregnancy complications, management of postpartum hemorrhage, management of intrapartal fetal heart rate abnormalities, assessment and care of the late preterm infant, and assessment and care of the newborn. We have expanded sections on patient education, patient teaching resources, and complementary and alternative therapies. Professional standards of care for maternity nurses are based on current practice guidelines and research. We have also expanded the discussion of social determinates of health.

Although the words *woman* and *women* are used herein, the authors recognize the existence of diverse gender identities. To provide culturally appropriate, respectful, and sensitive care, the maternity care provider should always ask individuals what words they use to describe themselves, their bodies, and their health-care practices.

CRITICAL COMPONENTS

This textbook focuses on the critical components of maternity nursing. Critical components are the major areas of knowledge essential for a basic understanding of maternity nursing. The critical components were determined from the authors' combined 60 years of teaching maternity nursing in both traditional and accelerated programs and years of clinical practice in the maternity setting. Current guidelines and standards are integrated and summarized for a pragmatic approach to patient- and family-focused care. This focus is especially evident when discussing complications.

The focus of the text is on normal pregnancy and childbirth. Chapters on low-risk antenatal, intrapartal, postpartum, and neonate conditions are followed by chapters on high-risk events and complications in each area. Complications germane to the nursing domain and childbearing population focus on understanding and synthesizing the critical elements for nursing care.

CLINICAL JUDGMENT

Highlighting clinical judgment is a new feature of the book. The term *clinical judgment* is based on Tanner's definition to mean an interpretation or conclusion about a patient's needs, concerns, or health problems, or the decision to take action (or not), use or modify standard approaches, or improvise new ones as deemed appropriate by the patient's response. Because students need help to gain clinical knowledge related to key factors that impact patient outcomes, we have highlighted specific information to help the student in recognizing the practical manifestations of signs and symptoms, recognizing quantitative and qualitative changes in particular patient conditions, and learning qualitative distinctions among a range of possible manifestations, common meanings, and experiences.

ORGANIZATION

This evidence-based text utilizes theory and clinical knowledge of maternity nursing. The conceptual framework is based on family developmental theory and presents substantive theory that forms the foundation for maternity care. The book is organized according to the natural sequence of the perinatal cycle: pregnancy, labor and birth, postpartum, and neonate. We have taken a biopsychosocial approach dealing with the physiological and psychological adaptation, and the social, political, and cultural influences impacting childbearing families, with emphasis on nursing actions and care of women and families. We believe childbirth is a natural, developmental process.

Nursing is an ever-changing science. New research and clinical knowledge expand knowledge and change clinical practice. *Davis Advantage for Maternal-Newborn Nursing: Critical Components of Nursing Care* reflects current knowledge, standards, and trends in maternity services, including the trend toward higher levels of intervention in maternity care. These standards and trends are reflected in our chapter on tests during the antepartal period, as well as a chapter devoted to fetal assessment and electronic fetal monitoring. We have devoted a chapter to the care of cesarean birth families, as nearly one-third of births in the United States are via cesarean.

This textbook clusters physiological changes, nursing assessment, and nursing care content in each chapter. Typically, a chapter is divided into systems in which the physiology; nursing care, including assessment and interventions; expected outcomes; and common variations of one subsystem are presented. Psychosocial and cultural dimensions of nursing care are highlighted in each chapter with an increased focus on social determinants of perinatal outcomes. The authors and contributors recognized childbirth, and becoming a mother, is a liminal and transformative life experience, a psychological and social experience with impacts for women, infants, and family members. Becoming a parent can bring overwhelming joy and life fulfillment for some, whereas for others it can lead to the onset, continuation, or exacerbation of stressors, adversity, and complications. We have attempted to present a balanced and nurse-centered approach to issues in the care of perinatal families. It is important to state here that there are people in the country who do not identify as women but who desire to have a child or are currently pregnant or in the postpartum period. While we use the term *mother* in this textbook, we must reiterate that all birthing people are equally deserving of patient-centered care that helps them attain their full potential and live authentic, healthy lives. For care to be successful, nurses, providers, and health-care institutions must work toward more inclusivity and best practices that are free of judgment and predetermined norms.

Nurses are uniquely positioned to lead evidence-based health equity efforts specific to the improvement of perinatal health disparities. The power of nursing and our priorities in improving outcomes is aligned with strategies, bundles, and tool kits developed to improve perinatal outcomes in partnership with the most impacted communities. Ethical care of all persons in the perinatal, prenatal, postpartum, and preconception periods requires a well-educated and diverse workforce with foundational knowledge of social determinants of health, health disparities, health inequity, and community engagement. This edition makes an effort to highlight that information and strategies to improve outcomes.

FEATURES

This textbook presents the critical components of maternal-newborn nursing in a pragmatic, condensed format by using the following features:

- Bulleted format: For easy-to-read content
- Figures, tables, boxes, concept maps, and clinical pathways: Summarize information in a visual way
- Learning Outcomes: Identify what the reader will know and be able to do by the end of the chapter
- Concepts: Identify the key concept areas discussed in the chapter
- Critical Components: Highlight critical information in maternal-newborn nursing
- Evidence-Based Practice: Highlights current research and practice guidelines related to nursing care
- Case Studies: Tie it all together by applying critical components in clinical context

- Clinical Judgment: Provides tips on applying critical thinking in a clinical setting
- Safe and Effective Nursing Care (SENC): Highlights SENC concepts as they apply to the chapter content:
  - Cultural Competence: Stresses the importance of cultural factors in nursing care
  - Understanding Medication: Highlights commonly administered medications used during pregnancy, labor and birth, postpartum, and neonatal periods
  - Patient Education: Reflects current evidence-based practice guidelines and recommendations
- Evidence-based health equity efforts specific to the improvement of perinatal health disparities for all persons are presented.

APPENDICES

The appendices include:

- Laboratory Values
- Preeclampsia Early Recognition Tool (PERT)
- Cervical Dilation Chart
- Temperature and Weight Conversion Charts

THE TEACHING AND LEARNING PACKAGE

How students learn is evolving. In this digital age, we consume information in new ways. The possibilities to interact and connect with content in new, dynamic ways are enhancing students' understanding and retention of complex concepts.

In order to meet the needs of today's learners, how faculty teach is also evolving. Classroom (traditional or online) time is valuable for active learning. This approach makes students responsible for the key concepts, allowing faculty to focus on clinical application. Relying on the textbook alone to support an active classroom leaves a gap. *Davis Advantage* is designed to fill that gap and help students and faculty succeed in core courses. It is comprised of the following:

- **A Strong Core Textbook** that provides the foundation of knowledge that today's nursing students need to pass the NCLEX® and enter practice prepared for success.
- **An Online Solution** that provides resources for each step of the learning cycle: learn, apply, assess.
  - **Personalized Learning** assignments are the core of the product and are designed to prepare students for classroom (live or online) discussion. They provide directed learning based on needs. After completing text reading assignments, students take a preassessment for each *topic*. Their results feed into their *Personalized Learning Plan*. If students do not pass the preassessment, they are required to complete further work within the topic: watch an animated mini-lecture, work through an activity, and take the postassessment. The personalized learning content is designed to connect

students with the foundational information about a given topic or concept. It provides the gateway to help make the content accessible to all students and complements different learning styles.

- **Clinical Judgment** assignments are case-based and build off key Personalized Learning topics. These cases help students develop Clinical Judgment skills through exploratory learning. Students will link their knowledge base (developed through the text and Personalized Learning) to new data and patient situations. Cases include dynamic charts that expand as the case progresses and use complex question types that require students to analyze data, synthesize conclusions, and make judgments. Each case will end with comprehensive feedback, which provides detailed rationales for the correct and incorrect answers.

- **Quizzing** assignments build off Personalized Learning topics (and are included for every topic) and help assess students' understanding of the broader scope and increased depth of that topic. The quizzes use NCLEX-style questions to assess understanding and synthesis of content. Quiz results include comprehensive feedback for correct and incorrect answers to help students understand why their answer choices were right or wrong.

- **Online Instructor Resources** are aimed at creating a dynamic learning experience that relies heavily on interactive participation and is tailored to students' needs. Results from the postassessments are available to faculty, in aggregate or by student, and inform a **Personalized Teaching Plan** that faculty can use to deliver a targeted classroom experience. Faculty will know students' strengths and weaknesses *before* they come to class and can spend class time focusing on where students are struggling. Suggested in-class activities are provided to help create an interactive, hands-on learning environment that helps students connect more deeply with the content. NCLEX-style questions from the **Instructor Test Bank** and **PowerPoint** slides that correspond to the textbook chapters are referenced in the Personalized Teaching Plans.

Authors

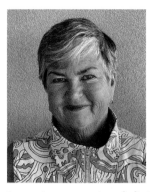

Roberta Durham

Roberta Durham, RN, PhD, is professor emeritus at California State University, East Bay, in Hayward, California, and a professor alumnus at Samuel Merritt University in Oakland, California. She received her bachelor's degree in nursing from the University of Rhode Island and her master's degree in nursing as a perinatal clinical specialist from the University of California, San Francisco. Dr. Durham received her PhD in nursing from the University of California, San Francisco, where she studied grounded theory method with Drs. Anselm Strauss and Leonard Schatzman. Her program of research has been on the management of premature labor and the prevention of premature birth. She has conducted international research and published her substantive and methodological work widely. She was previously a visiting professor at the University of Glasgow and was a Fulbright Specialist at the University of Jordan in Amman, Jordan. She is a Fulbright Scholar for 2022–2023 to Trinidad and Tobago. She is currently involved in international research in Central America to improve perinatal outcomes. She is a founding member of Hands for Global Health and served as the vice chair on the board of directors and director of research. She has worked for over 25 years in labor and delivery units in the San Francisco Bay Area and has taught maternity nursing for over 30 years.

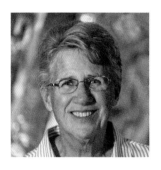

Linda Chapman

Linda Chapman, RN, PhD, is professor emeritus at Samuel Merritt University in Oakland, California. She received her diploma in nursing from Samuel Merritt Hospital School of Nursing, her bachelor's degree in nursing from University of Utah, and her master's degree in nursing from the University of California, San Francisco. Dr. Chapman received her PhD from the University of California, San Francisco, where she studied with Drs. Ramona Mercer and Katharyn May. Her program of research has been on the experience of men during the perinatal period. She has conducted research and published her substantive work in practice and research journals. She worked for 25 years in nursery, postpartum, and labor and birthing units at Samuel Merritt Hospital/Summit Medical Center in the San Francisco Bay Area.

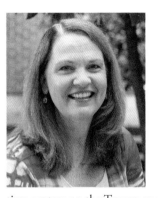

Connie Miller

Connie Miller, DNP, RNC-OB, CNE, is a clinical professor at the University of Arizona College of Nursing in Tucson, Arizona. She is a certified nurse educator and the division chair for the General Nursing and Health Education Division, responsible for three prelicensure nursing programs and simulation centers on the Tucson and Gilbert, Arizona, campuses. Dr. Miller began her nursing career by earning her BSN from Mankato State University in Minnesota. Upon graduation, she was commissioned in the U.S. Air Force Nurse Corps where she enjoyed serving in various stateside and international assignments and retired as a colonel after 24 years of combined active duty and reserve military experience. She received her master's degree in nursing from the University of Arizona, and her doctor of nursing practice in innovation leadership from Arizona State University. She was a fellow in both the University of Arizona Academic Leadership Institute and in the first cohort of the Integrative Nursing Faculty Fellowship at the University of Arizona College of Nursing. She subsequently led the design and development of a new hybrid BSN pathway with an integrative health focus. Her clinical area of focus is maternal-newborn nursing, and she is a nationally certified inpatient obstetrical nurse. She has experience working in a variety of military and civilian health-care settings including acute and primary care, as well as teaching childbirth classes. She loves caring for women during pregnancy and childbirth, and once she transitioned from the bedside to academia full time, she volunteered as a labor support doula with Operation Special Delivery to provide labor support for members in the military separated from their family members at the time of delivery. She is passionate about preparing the next generation of new nurses and is thrilled to participate as an author for this textbook. In her free time, she loves to spend time with her friends and family, and especially enjoys time with her grandchildren.

Contributors

Cecilia Urbina Carrasco RN, BSN
Staff Nurse
Alta Bates Summit Medical Center
Berkeley, California

Liujing Chen RN, BSN
Stanford Health Care
Staff Nurse
Palo Alto, California

Diana Cortez, BSN, RN, PCCN
Clinical Nurse 2
University of California Davis Health
Sacramento, California

Susan Redman Forsyth, PhD, RN
Assistant Professor
California State University, East Bay
Hayward, California

LaShea Haynes, MEd, MSN, APRN, AGCNS-BC, RNC
Clinical Nurse Specialist, Perinatal
Perinatal Potpourri
Powder Springs, Georgia

Scout Emersen Hebnick, RNC-OB, MSN
Lecturer, Nurse Educator
California State University, East Bay
Hayward, California

Sharon C. Hitchcock, DNP, RNC-MN
Assistant Clinical Professor
University of Arizona College of Nursing
Tucson, Arizona

Lisa Kiser, DNP, CNM, WHNP
Assistant Clinical Professor
University of Arizona College of Nursing
Tucson, Arizona

Caroline Lambton, MSN, RN
Staff Nurse II
University of California, San Francisco
San Francisco, California

Tara Leigh Loghry, MSN-Ed, RNC-OB
Faculty
University of Arizona College of Nursing
Gilbert, Arizona

Carolyn Mahaffey, RN, MSN, RNC-NIC
Staff Nurse IV
Alta Bates Summit Medical Center
Berkeley, California

Rachael Miller, RN, BSN
Labor and Delivery Staff Nurse
University of California San Diego Health
San Diego, California

Lyrae D. Perini, MSN, RN, IBCLC, RLC
Lactation Consultant/IBCLC
Banner Health
Gilbert, Arizona

Marissa H. Rafael, DNP, RN, CMSRN
Assistant Professor
California State University East Bay
Staff Nurse
Alta Bates Summit Medical Center
Berkeley, California

Janice J. Stinson, RNC, PhD
Labor and Delivery Staff Nurse
Alta Bates Summit Medical Center
Berkeley, California

Hallie Kay Taylor, DO
Neurology Resident
Mayo Clinic–Arizona Campus
Phoenix, Arizona

Paulina Van, PhD, RN, CNE
Professor
Samuel Merritt University
Oakland, California

Reviewers

Tammy Bryant, MSN, RN
Program Chair for the Associate of Science in Nursing
Southern Regional Technical College
Thomasville, Georgia

Julie Duff, DNP, APRN, WHNP-BC, CNE
Associate Professor
Resurrection University
Chicago, Illinois

Leah Elliot, DNP, MSN-ED, RNC-OB, C-EFM, IBCLC
Professor of Nursing, Maternal Child Health
Bakersfield College
Bakersfield, California

Lisa C. Engel, DNP, RN, CNE
Associate Professor
Harding University Carr College of Nursing
Searcy, Arkansas

Catherine Folker-Maglaya, DNP, APRN-CNM, IBCLC
Associate Professor
City Colleges of Chicago School of Nursing—
    Malcolm X College
Chicago, Illinois

Carolyn Godfrey, PhD
Professor
St. Louis Community College at Forest Park
St. Louis, Missouri

Sarah Harkness, BSN, RNC-OB, MSN, FNP
Faculty Maternal Child Health
    California State University, East Bay, CA
Sutter Health
Berkeley, California

LaShea Haynes, Med, MSN, APRN, AGCNS-BC, RNC
Clinical Nurse Specialist, Perinatal
Wellstar Healthy System
Douglasville, Georgia

Amy M. Hobbs, MSN, RN, IBCLC
Assistant Professor, Lead Obstetric Instructor
Riverside College of Health Careers
Newport News, Virginia

Samantha Iyer, RN, BSN
RNC-OB
Sutter Alta Bates
Berkeley, California

Mary Ann Kelley, PhD, RN
Assistant Professor, Retired
University of Alabama, Capstone College of Nursing
Tuscaloosa, Alabama

Jordan Kilbourn, RNC-OB, BSN
Labor & Delivery RN, OR Lead
Alta Bates Summit Medical Center, Ashby
Berkeley, California

Lisa Kiser, DNP, CNM, WHNP
Assistant Clinical Professor
University of Arizona College of Nursing
Tucson, Arizona

Amy Lee, DNP, ARNP, WHNP-BC
Clinical Associate Professor
The University of Alabama
Tuscaloosa, Alabama

Jeanne M. Leifheit, MSN, RN
Associate Professor
Harper College
Palatine, Illinois

Barbara McClaskey, PhD, APRN, RNC
University Professor
Pittsburg State University
Pittsburg, Kansas

Tamara Mette, RN, DNP
Nursing Faculty
Great Basin College
Elko, Nevada

Rita J. Nutt, DNP, RN
Assistant Professor
Salisbury University
Salisbury, Maryland

Sylvia P. Ross, PhD, CNM
Associate Professor
Rhode Island College School of Nursing
Providence, Rhode Island

Martha C. Ruder, DNP, NP-C, APRN
ADN Program Coordinator
Gulf Coast State College
Panama City, Florida

Donna Shambley-Ebron, PhD, RN
Associate Professor, Emerita
University of Cincinnati College of Nursing
Cincinnati, Ohio

Jamie M. Vincent, MSN, APRN-CNS, RNC-OB
Perinatal CNS
John Muir Health
Walnut Creek, California

Acknowledgments

We are grateful to the following people, who helped us turn an idea into reality:

- Our husbands—Douglas Fredebaugh, Chuck Chapman, and Michael Miller—for their ongoing support and love
- Our colleagues at Samuel Merritt University, and the University of Arizona, who helped us develop from novice to expert teachers
- Our colleagues at the California State University, East Bay, and the University of Arizona College of Nursing for their suggestions and support

- Our teachers and mentors—Katharyn A. May, RN, DNSc, FAAN, Ramona T. Mercer, RN, PhD, FAAN, and Melissa Goldsmith, PhD, RNC-MN
- Our F.A. Davis team—Jacalyn Sharp, Amanda Minutola, and Andrea Miller—for their guidance
- Our contributors for sharing their expertise

Contents in Brief

Table of Contents

Chapter 6

Antepartal Tests 133

Chapter 7

Complications of Pregnancy 153

Chapter 11

Intrapartum and Postpartum Care of Cesarean Birth Families

UNIT 4

The Postpartal Period   397

Chapter 12

Postpartum Physiological Assessments and Nursing Care   399

Maternity Nursing Overview

Trends and Issues

1

Lisa Kiser, DNP, CNM, WHNP

LEARNING OUTCOMES

Upon completion of this chapter, the student will be able to:

1. Discuss evidence-based nursing care that promotes optimal outcomes in labor and birth.
2. Examine maternal and infant health outcomes in the United States and analyze how the social determinants of health impact outcomes and lead to health disparities.
3. Identify leading causes of maternal and infant morbidity and mortality in the United States.
4. Create a framework for the provision of women's health and gender health services that are representative, comprehensive, and holistic.
5. Identify the primary maternal and infant goals of *Healthy People 2030*.

CONCEPTS

Addiction
Behaviors
Caring
Clinical Judgment
Collaboration
Communication
Evidence-Based Practice
Health Policy
Health Promotion
Leadership and Management
Mood and Affect
Population Health
Professionalism
Reproduction and Sexuality
Self-Care
Stress and Coping

WELCOMING AND INCLUSIVE CARE

"Health is a state of complete physical, social and mental well-being and not merely the absence of disease or infirmity. The enjoyment of the highest attainable standard of health is one of the fundamental rights of every human being, without distinction of race, religion, political beliefs or economic and social conditions" (World Health Organization [WHO], 2006).

Welcome to the newest edition of *Maternal-Newborn Nursing*. This textbook introduces the fundamental principles of maternal-newborn nursing and women's health. Recognition exists on both the national and global levels that a more comprehensive understanding of health—one that recognizes the intersection between the social determinants of health and health outcomes—is critical to promoting optimal health and eliminating health disparities (American College of Obstetricians and Gynecologists [ACOG], 2018; U.S Department of Health and Human Services, 2021; WHO, 2021b).

Nowhere is this truer than in the promotion of health and wellness for women, infants, and childbearing families in the presence of significant health disparities that exist in the United States due to differences in the social determinants of health (Fig. 1–1). These include:

● Housing and neighborhood environment
● Economic stability

Social Determinants of Health

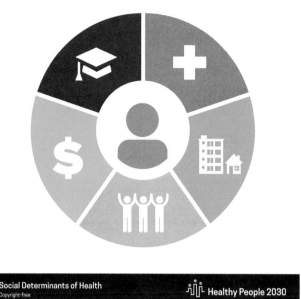

FIGURE 1-1 Social Determinants of Health.

- Access to health care and quality of care
- Access and quality of education
- Community and social context, including the impact of racism
  (U.S. Department of Health and Human Services, 2021).

Obesity, for example, can lead to significant morbidity and mortality for both women and infants, including increased risk of gestational diabetes, gestational hypertension, miscarriage, stillbirth, and birth defects (Mahutte et al., 2018; Pickett-Blakely et al., 2016). To address these risks, nurses must prepare to assess every person for access to healthy food, safe environments to exercise, and affordable prenatal care, then work with the health-care team and community partners to optimize a patient's resources and outcomes.

In discussing the social model of health, we recognize the importance of the medical model of health. This text incorporates the best evidence both models offer to current nursing practice.

Nurses must also be prepared to serve as change leaders and advocates for improved health-care systems and evidence-based health policies that make health outcomes more equitable at a societal level. For example, nurses endorsed the *Protecting Moms That Serve Act* that was introduced in 2021 to improve maternal outcomes for veterans (American Association of Birth Centers [AABC], 2021). Thus, this chapter will explore the urgent health issues in maternal-newborn health from both an individual and societal context and will introduce the *Healthy People 2030* goals to guide the conversation.

Finally, this chapter will examine what it means to provide welcoming and inclusive care to everyone. Welcoming and inclusive care in this context means gender-affirming care to all people, including gender-diverse and transgender individuals. Some people do not identify as women but desire to have a child or are currently pregnant or in the postpartum period. Although we use the term *mother* in this textbook, we advocate for all birthing people to receive patient-centered care that helps them attain their full potential and live authentic, healthy lives.

Welcoming and inclusive care is also provided to all childbearing people and families who identify as LGBTQIA+ (Lesbian, Gay, Bisexual, Transgender, Queer/Questioning, Intersex, Asexual) in recognition that health-care provider attitudes and practices significantly impact health outcomes for members of the LGBTQIA+ communities (Fenway Institute, 2016). Currently, 12% of the U.S. population identifies as LGBTQIA+. That number is significantly higher (20%) for the Millennial generation (Gay and Lesbian Alliance Against Defamation [GLAAD], 2017).

New nurses must face many challenges and opportunities. The COVID-19 pandemic has clarified that issues such as racism, violence, and climate change significantly impact health outcomes. This chapter is an introduction to these issues as they affect maternal, newborn, and gender health and prepare students to address these issues in nursing practice.

ISSUES IN MATERNAL-NEWBORN AND GENDER HEALTH

Childbirth in the United States

During the past 100 years, care of the childbearing family has undergone profound changes as childbirth moved from the comfortable setting of the home to the unfamiliar setting of the hospital. This change was driven by the medicalization of birth and the systemic discreditation of Indigenous midwives and midwives of color, who were responsible for the health and well-being of not just women in labor but also their communities (Davison & Joseph, 2020). This loss of the traditional healers and health providers in communities of color is recognized as one of the key factors that has resulted in ongoing health disparities for communities of color in the United States, especially for Black, Hispanic, and Indigenous communities (Davison & Joseph, 2020).

As noted in Table 1-1, less than 5% of births in 1900 took place in the hospital. By the late 1930s, this had increased to 75% of births (Wertz & Wertz, 1979). Women and childbearing families began to advocate for a return to physiological labor and birth and less medical intervention in the 1950s, and by the 1960s childbirth education became formalized (Lothian, 2016). The birth center movement developed in the early 1970s to provide safe and effective care to families seeking a birthing environment that supported normal physiological birth (AABC, 2016). The past 60 years have seen nurses take a leadership role in evaluating the evidence that supports appropriate medical interventions while also using evidence to support non-intervention in uncomplicated physiological or normal birth (American College of Nurse-Midwives [ACNM], n.d.).

TABLE 1-1   Past and Present Trends

PAST TRENDS	PRESENT TRENDS
Nursing: Focus on physiological changes and needs of the mother and infant	Family-centered maternity nursing: Focus on both the physiological and psychosocial changes and needs of the childbearing family
Primarily home births	Primarily hospital births, with increasing home and birth center births
Women labored in one room and delivered in another room	Women labor, give birth, and recover in the same room
Delivery rooms cold and sterile	Birthing rooms warm and homelike
Expectant fathers and family excluded from the labor and birth experience	Expectant partner, family, and friends involved in the labor and birth experience
Expectant fathers or family members excluded from cesarean births	Expectant partner or family members in the operating room during cesarean births
Labor pain interventions: natural childbirth, amnesia, or "twilight sleep"	Labor pain interventions: natural childbirth, labor support techniques, analgesics, epidurals, nitrous oxide
Hospital postpartum stay of 10 days	Hospital postpartum stay of 48 hours or fewer, birth center stay of 6 hours, in-home birth
Infant mortality rate of 50.1 per 1,000 live births in 1915 (Bureau of the Census, 1917)	Infant mortality rate of 5.7 per 1,000 live births in 2020 (OECD, 2021)
Diarrhea and enteritis: Number one cause of infant death in 1915 (Bureau of the Census, 1917)	Birth defects, prematurity, and low birth weight (LBW) are the leading causes of infant mortality in 2018 (March of Dimes, 2021e)
Maternal mortality rate of 607.9 per 100,000 live births in 1915 (Bureau of the Census, 1917)	Maternal mortality rate of 17.4 per 100,000 live births in 2018 (CDC, 2020b)
Induction of labor rate of 9.5% in 1990 (Martin et al., 2006)	Induction of labor rate of 24.5% in 2016 (Maternal Safety Foundation, 2021)
Cesarean section rate of 20.7% in 1996 (Martin et al., 2006)	Cesarean section rate of 31.7% in 2019 (CDC, 2021a)
Low probability of survival for infants born at or before 28 weeks of gestation	Increased survival rates for infants born between 24 weeks and 28 weeks of gestation

Nurses have been change leaders in these key developments in childbirth practices:

- Electronic fetal monitoring (EFM) during labor, which began in the 1970s. Nurses, nurse-midwives, and nurse researchers helped establish that EFM is effective for confirming fetal well-being for high-risk births and that intermittent fetal monitoring with auscultation is safe and effective for monitoring low-risk births.
- La Leche League International (LLI), started in 1956 by a group of women who wanted to promote breastfeeding during a time when bottle-feeding was recommended by medical practitioners over breastfeeding (LLI, 2021). Nurses helped lead the movement to reestablish breastfeeding as the best method of infant feeding when possible. All nurses working with childbearing patients and families must be trained to provide "equitable, culturally sensitive, gender-affirming breastfeeding support" (Association of Women's Health, Obstetric and Neonatal Nurses [AWHONN], 2021b) and address the cultural concerns related to breastfeeding for patients and families in their care.

- The AWHONN, established in 1969 to "empower and support nurses caring for women, newborns, and their families through research, education, and advocacy" (AWHONN, 2021a). For more than 50 years, AWHONN has helped transform maternal-newborn care, establishing best practices on critical issues such as postpartum depression screening and prevention of complications such as postpartum hemorrhage (AWHONN, 2021a).
- The Baby-Friendly Hospital Initiative, developed by the WHO and the United Nations Children's Fund (UNICEF) in 1991. This initiative focuses on hospital and birth center practices that protect, promote, and support breastfeeding and nurses and has been instrumental in helping organizations receive the Baby-Friendly Center accreditation (see Chapter 16).
- The Back to Sleep campaign, initiated by the National Institute of Child Health and Human Development (NICHD) in 1996 to educate parents about the importance of placing infants on their backs to sleep to reduce the risk of sudden infant death syndrome (SIDS).

- In 2012, the NICHD's Safe to Sleep campaign, which built on the Back to Sleep campaign (see Chapter 15).
- An increase in collaboration over the past decade among professional organizations that care for women in recognition of the urgency to address maternal and infant morbidity and mortality in the United States. This has led to multiple consensus statements and bundles to standardize best practices for all care providers, uniting educators, researchers, physicians, nurse-midwives, and maternal-newborn nurses to improve outcomes (AWHONN, 2021a).
- Community-led initiatives by people of color and national organizational initiatives such as those of the ACNM to address the severe disparities in health outcomes for women and infants of color. These programs seek to mitigate racism in maternal health care and increase the number of maternal-newborn health-care providers who are people of color (American College of Nurse-Midwives, Black Mamas Matter Alliance, and International Confederation of Midwives [ACNM, BMMA, & ICM], 2020).

Advances in science and health care have tremendously impacted the number of maternal and infant deaths in the past century, with maternal mortality rates declining from 607.9 per 100,000 live births in 1915 to 17.4 per 100,000 live births in 2018 (Centers for Disease Control and Prevention [CDC], 2020b) and infant mortality rates declining from 50.1 per 1,000 live births in 1915 to 5.7 per 1,000 live births in 2020 (Organisation for Economic Co-Operation and Development [OECD], 2021). In contrast, cesarean births increased from 20.7% in 1996 to a rate of 31.7% in 2019 (CDC, 2021a). Induction of labor rates increased from a low of 5% in 1970 to a rate of 24.5% in 2016 (Maternal Safety Foundation, 2021).

It is critical to understand that while maternal and infant outcomes have significantly improved in the United States compared with the previous century, the nation still has the highest maternal mortality rate of any high-resource country in the world, and is the only country in the world, other than Afghanistan and the Sudan, where the maternal mortality rate is rising (Center for the Study of Social Policy, 2019). Women in the United States are more likely to die during pregnancy and the first year after birth than women in 48 other high-resource countries (ACNM, 2021). Similarly, despite the 14% decrease in infant mortality from 2007 to 2017, the United States is experiencing slower improvements than in other high-resource countries and has wide disparities in mortality based on race, ethnicity, and geographic location (Drexel University, 2020). Causes and potential solutions to these concerning outcomes will be discussed in the text that follows.

Fertility and Birth Rates

Total fertility rate (TFR) is "the average number of children that would be born per woman if all women lived to the end of their childbearing years and bore children according to a given fertility rate at each age" (Central Intelligence Agency [CIA], 2022). TFR is an indicator of population change; greater than 2 indicates that the country's population is growing, whereas lower than 2 indicates a population decreasing in size. The 2020 U.S. TFR is 1.64. In 2010, it was 1.98, and in 2018 it was 1.73 (CDC, 2019b). TFR decreased significantly in 2020 during the COVID-19 pandemic, with a 4% decrease from 2019 to 2020 (CDC, 2021a). Recent TFR indicates that the U.S. population is decreasing in size and that its members are growing older.

Birth rate is the number of live births per 1,000 people. Since 1960, U.S. birth rates have significantly declined (Table 1-2). In 1960, the birth rate was 23.7. In 1970, it was 18.4, and in 2020, it was 10.9. The United States saw decreases in both the fertility rate and the birth rate between 1960 and 2020, which accelerated in 2019 and 2020 (CDC, 2021a). During this period, the TFR decreased 54%, from 3.7 to 1.7 children born/woman. The birth rate during this same period decreased 58%, from 23.7 to 10.9 live births per 1,000. This decline is attributed to:

- Availability of a variety of highly effective contraceptive methods
- More women delaying reproduction to pursue careers, having fewer children, or remaining child-free
- Legalization and availability of elective abortions
- The rising cost of raising children, leading to smaller families

An interesting trend is noted regarding birth rate and the mother's age for the 30-year period from 1990 to 2020. Birth rates decreased for women aged 15 to 29 but increased for women aged 30 to 45 and older. The greatest increase was seen in women aged 40 and older. The greatest decrease was in women aged 15 to 19. This trend is influenced by the increasing number of women who have delayed childbirth due to career choices or socioeconomic reasons and the increased availability of contraceptives for younger women.

The United States had a total of 3,605,201 births in 2020 (women ages 15–44) (CDC, 2021a). The percentages of these births by race are:

- American Indian or Alaska Native: 0.747%
- Asian: 6.07%
- Native Hawaiian or other Pacific Islanders: 0.266%
- Hispanic: 23.96%
- Black: 14.66%
- White: 51.02% (CDC, 2021a)

TABLE 1-2 Birth Rates, United States of America, 1960–2017

	1960	1970	1980	1990	2000	2010	2015	2017
Birth rate	23.7	18.4	15.9	16.7	14.4	13	12.5	12.5

CIA, 2018a; Hamilton et al., 2007, 2009, 2011, 2016.

These percentages reflect the multicultural population of the United States and present an important challenge to health-care workers, who must provide culturally appropriate care to a wide variety of childbearing families while working to eliminate health disparities among populations.

Preterm Births

Preterm births are divided into three classifications:

- Very premature: Neonates born at less than 32 weeks of gestation
- Moderately premature: Neonates born between 32 and 33 completed weeks of gestation
- Late premature: Neonates born between 34 and 36 completed weeks of gestation

Globally, it is estimated that 15 million premature births occur each year, with a global preterm birth rate of 10.6% (WHO, 2018b). Complications related to preterm birth are the leading cause of death for children younger than 5 (WHO, 2018a). In the United States from 2000 to 2015, preterm births decreased by 24% to a total preterm birth rate of 9.62; however, the preterm birth rate has begun to increase since 2015 and saw a 2% increase from 2018 to 2019 to a rate of 10.23% (CDC, 2021a).

Despite widespread advances in perinatal care, the preterm birth rate remains high in the United States compared with that of other high-income countries, such as Canada, Japan, Australia, Israel, and Norway. The effect of social determinants of health is stark when looking at preterm birth by race: Black, non-Hispanic women have a 50% higher rate of preterm birth (14.35%) than Hispanic women (9.83%) or non-Hispanic White women (9.10%) (CDC, 2021a) (Table 1-3).

These rates substantially contribute to racial and ethnic disparities in maternal and infant health outcomes, discussed later in this chapter. Premature birth impacts the well-being of parents, the childbearing family, and the community as well as the length and quality of life for the preterm infant. A shorter gestational period increases the risk of complications related to immature body organs and systems that have lifelong negative effects, including but not limited to:

- Respiratory disorders
- Cerebral palsy
- Vision and hearing disorders
- Developmental delays

Of all infant deaths, 36% are related to preterm birth (CDC, 2016). Parents of preterm infants also face economic, social, and educational challenges in caring for a premature infant.

Neonatal Birth Weight Rates

Neonatal birth weight rates are reported by the CDC in three major categories: low, normal, and high. Normal birth weight is between 2,500 and 3,999 grams; high birth weight is 4,000 grams or greater; low birth weight (LBW) is below 2,500 grams. LBW is divided into two categories:

- LBW is defined as birth weight that is lower than 2,500 grams but greater than 1,500 grams. The percentage of LBW neonates has increased from 8% in 2014 to 8.3% in 2019 (CDC, 2021a; March of Dimes, 2021).
- Very low birth weight (VLBW) is defined as a birth weight of lower than 1,500 grams. The percentage of VLBW neonates has remained stable at 1.4% in 2014 and decreased slightly in 2019 to 1.38% (CDC, 2021a).

The weight of neonates at birth is an important predictor of future morbidity and mortality rates, including increased lifetime risk of diabetes and heart disease (March of Dimes, 2021a). Neonates with birth weights between 4,000 and 4,999 grams have the lowest mortality rate during the first year of life. VLBW neonates are 100 times more likely to die during the first year of life than are neonates with birth weights greater than 2,500 grams.

Infant Mortality Rates

Infant mortality is defined as a death before age 1. Globally, infant mortality has decreased from 65 deaths per 1,000 live births in 1990 to 29 deaths per 1,000 live births in 2016 (WHO, 2021a). Infant mortality rates in the United States decreased from 26 per 1,000 live births in 1960 to 5.7 in 2018 (CDC, 2021a). This decrease is related to improvement and advances in knowledge and care of high-risk neonates, notably:

- Advances in medical technology such as extracorporeal membrane oxygenation therapy (ECMO), used for respiratory distress in preterm infants (see Chapter 17)
- Advances in medical treatment such as exogenous pulmonary surfactant (see Chapter 17)
- Improved prenatal care
- Increased infant sleep safety education

Although this is a significant decrease, the infant mortality rate remains too high for a nation with the available wealth and health-care resources of the United States. The leading causes of infant deaths are listed in Table 1-4. Infant deaths related to SIDS significantly decreased between 1995 and 2018. The decrease can

TABLE 1-3	Premature Births by Race: United States, Provisional 2020				
AMERICAN INDIAN OR ALASKA NATIVE	ASIAN	BLACK	HISPANIC	NATIVE HAWAIIAN OR OTHER PACIFIC ISLANDERS	WHITE
11.57	8.51	14.35	9.83	11.98	9.10

CDC, 2021a.

TABLE 1-4   Leading Causes of Infant Deaths and Mortality Rates (Rates per 100,000 Live Births)

CAUSE OF DEATH	1995 RATE	CAUSE OF DEATH	2015 RATE	CAUSE OF DEATH	2020 RATE
Congenital malformations and chromosomal abnormalities	168.1	Congenital malformations and chromosomal abnormalities	121.3	Congenital malformations and chromosomal abnormalities	111.9
Disorders related to short gestation and LBW	100.9	Disorders related to short gestation and LBW	102.7	Disorders related to short gestation and LBW	86.9
Sudden infant death syndrome	87.1	Sudden infant death syndrome	39.4	Sudden infant death syndrome	38.4
Respiratory distress of newborns	37.3	Newborns affected by maternal complications of pregnancy	38.3	Accidents	33.0
Newborns affected by maternal complications of pregnancy	33.6	Accidents	32.4	Newborns affected by maternal complications of pregnancy	30.9

Anderson et al., 1997; Kochanek et al., 2016; Murphy et al., 2012; Murphy et al., 2021

be attributed to Safe to Sleep, a public education program led by NICHD and other initiatives to teach parents safe newborn sleep habits, such as placing the child in the crib on their back.

In 1995, infant death from respiratory syndrome (RDS) was the fourth leading cause of death in newborns. In 2018, it was the ninth leading cause of infant death (CDC, 2020a). The decrease in RDS-related death rates reflects advances in medical and nursing care of preterm infants.

Maternal Death and Mortality Rates

The Department of Health and Human Services uses several definitions of maternal death:

- Maternal death is defined by the WHO as the death of a woman during pregnancy or within 42 days of pregnancy termination caused by conditions aggravated by the pregnancy or associated medical treatments. This category excludes death from accidents or injuries.
- Direct obstetric death results from complications during pregnancy, labor, birth, or the postpartum period, including deaths caused by interventions, omission of interventions, or incorrect treatment. An example of this category is death caused by postpartum hemorrhage.
- Indirect obstetric death is caused by a preexisting disease or a disease that develops during pregnancy without direct obstetrical cause but is aggravated by the pregnancy. One example is death related to complications of systemic lupus erythematosus worsened by pregnancy.
- Late maternal death occurs more than 42 days after termination of pregnancy from a direct or indirect obstetrical cause.
- Pregnancy-related death is the death of a woman during pregnancy or within 1 year of the end of pregnancy from a pregnancy complication, a chain of events initiated by pregnancy, or the aggravation of an unrelated condition by the physiological effects of pregnancy (Hoyert, 2007). An example

is a pulmonary embolism related to deep vein thrombosis that leads to death during or after pregnancy.

Maternal mortality ratio (MMR) is defined as the number of maternal deaths per 100,000 live births. In the United States, MMR had significantly decreased from 607.9 in 1915 to 12 in 1990 (Hoyert, 2007); however, MMR has risen significantly since 2015 to a current rate of 17.4 (Commonwealth Fund, 2020). The United States ranks last among all high-resource countries in maternal mortality rates (Commonwealth Fund, 2020). Most concerning are differences in mortality rates based on race: The MMR for Black women (37.1) is 2.5 times higher than in White women (14.7) and three times higher than for Hispanic women (11.8) in the United States (Commonwealth Fund, 2020). Inconsistency in reporting by the states resulted in a lack of thorough official data from the National Vital Statistics System (NVSS) on maternal mortality rates from 2007 to 2017, so the full scope of the problem may be lacking (Hoyert et al., 2020). Maternal morbidity has also increased significantly in the United States in the past decade: 700 women will die every year due to conditions related to their pregnancy, and 500,000 more will experience severe complications during pregnancy, birth, and the postpartum period (ACNM, 2021).

Research has clearly demonstrated that social determinants of health, which include systemic racism and health-care biases toward people of color, have significantly contributed to the health disparities in maternal-infant health in the United States (ACNM, BMMA, & ICM, 2020). A Black mother with a college education has a 60% greater risk of maternal death than a White or Hispanic mother without a high school education (Commonwealth Fund, 2020). Black women are also twice as likely to experience severe maternal complications such as cardiomyopathy, eclampsia, and embolism (CDC, 2019d). Similarly, American Indian and Alaska Native women also have three to four times higher maternal mortality rates and two times higher rates of maternal morbidity, including postpartum hemorrhage and preterm birth (National Partnership for Women and Families, 2019). Behind all these statistics are real people and families who experience the devastating effects when poor outcomes occur for women and infants. Addressing racism and health care to improve outcomes will be discussed in the next section of the chapter.

Globally, the decrease in maternal mortality in developing countries is attributed to increased female education, increased contraception use, improved antenatal care, and increased number of births attended by skilled health personnel (WHO, UNICEF, UNFPA, World Bank Group and United Nations Population Division, 2015). Primary causes of maternal deaths worldwide are:

- Severe hemorrhage
- Infections
- Eclampsia
- Obstructed labor
- Complications of abortions
- Other causes, such as anemia, HIV/AIDS, and cardiovascular disease (WHO, UNICEF, UNFPA, World Bank Group and United Nations Population Division, 2015)

ISSUES

Primary issues affecting the health of people, mothers, and infants in the United States include teen pregnancy, tobacco and electronic cigarette use, substance abuse during pregnancy, medications use during pregnancy, obesity, violence, sexually transmitted infections, climate change, depression and perinatal mood disorders, racism, and health disparities.

Teen Pregnancy

As shown in Table 1-5, the birth rate for teenagers in the United States has been declining since 1990:

- The birth rate for teenagers aged 15 to 17 has decreased 83.2% from 1990 to 2020, with a decrease of 36% from 2010 to 2020.
- The greatest percentage of change occurred in ages 10 to 14, with a decrease of 85.7% from 1990 to 2020.

TABLE 1-5 Birth Rates for Teen Females: Births per 1,000 Live Births

AGE	1990	2005	2010	2015	2020
10–14	1.4	0.7	0.4	0.2	0.2
15–17	37.5	21.4	17.3	9.9	6.3
18–19	88.6	69.9	58.3	40.7	28.8

CDC, 2021a; Hamilton et al., 2011, 2016.

- The introduction of long-acting reversible contraceptives (LARCs), including the contraceptive implant and intrauterine devices (IUDs) for teens, has been key to reducing unintended pregnancy rates in this population.
- The teen birth rate in the United States in 2020 was higher than in other developed countries, with 17 births per 1,000 females aged 15 to 19 compared with Switzerland's rate of 3 and Canada's rate of 9.

Implications of Teen Pregnancy and Birth

Teen births can have adverse long-term effects on both the mothers and children, presenting challenges to teen parents and society. These include:

- Educational issues:
  - 50% of teen mothers receive a high school diploma compared with 90% of women who did not give birth during adolescence (CDC, 2019a).
  - Only half of teen mothers earn a high school diploma by age 22 and less than 2% finish college by age 30 (National Conference of State Legislators, 2016).
- Poverty and income disparities:
  - 66% of teen mothers are poor and 25% begin receiving welfare within 3 years of the birth of their first child (National Conference of State Legislators, 2016).
  - 17% of teen mothers will have a second child before age 20, which further decreases their ability to complete school and qualify for well-paying jobs (National Campaign to Prevent Teen Pregnancy, 2016a).
- Risk of sexually transmitted illnesses, including HIV, which can impact neonatal and maternal outcomes, including prematurity
- Increased risk for hypertensive disorders of pregnancy

Children born to teen mothers are at increased risk for:

- Health problems related to prematurity or LBW, including infant death, respiratory distress syndrome, intraventricular bleeding, vision problems, and intestinal problems
- A higher mortality rate for infants of women younger than 15 compared with infants born to women of all ages
- Behavioral problems
- Placement in foster homes
- Lower school achievement and dropping out of school
- Incarceration during adolescence (Youth.gov, 2016)
- Increased risk of becoming a teen mother themselves

Teen fathers have a 30% lower probability of graduating from high school than boys who are not fathers (Youth.gov, 2016). In addition, teenage males without an involved father are at higher risk for being incarcerated, dropping out of school, and abusing drugs or alcohol.

Tobacco and Electronic Cigarette Use During Pregnancy

Tobacco use during pregnancy is associated with increased risk of LBW, intrauterine growth restriction, miscarriage, abruptio placenta, premature birth, SIDS, and respiratory problems in the newborn.

- Cigarette smoking during pregnancy declined from 19.5% in 1989 to 7.2% in 2016 (CDC, National Center for Health Statistics, 2017).
- Women who smoke during pregnancy are less likely to breastfeed their infants.
- Of women who smoked before pregnancy, 20.6% quit during pregnancy (Curtain & Mathews, 2016).
- Based on age, the highest smoking prevalence rate is among women aged 20 to 24 (Curtain & Mathews, 2016).
- Based on race, the highest percentage of female smokers is among American Indians and Alaska Natives (Curtain & Mathews, 2016).
- Based on educational level, the highest percentage of female smokers are women with less than a high school education (Curtain & Mathews, 2016).

Electronic cigarettes (e-cigarettes) are increasingly prevalent in the United States, but they are not considered safe in pregnancy and the CDC has advised against all e-cigarette use, including in pregnancy (CDC, 2019c). E-cigarettes are not controlled by the Food and Drug Administration (FDA) and contain carcinogenic and toxic compounds (healthychildren .org, 2019). Nicotine, which is present in e-cigarettes, is a health danger to both the pregnant woman and her fetus and can adversely affect the developing fetal brain and lungs. E-cigarettes have not been demonstrated to be effective in helping women quit smoking, so nurses should advise against all e-cigarette use in pregnancy (ACOG, 2020; healthychildren .org, 2019).

CRITICAL COMPONENT

Tobacco and E-Cigarettes

Nicotine is a health danger for pregnant women and their developing fetuses. Pregnant women should not use any tobacco product or e-cigarettes because nicotine is toxic to developing fetuses and impairs fetal brain and lung development (CDC, 2018).

Substance Abuse During Pregnancy

In the general U.S. population, the use of illegal drugs and cannabis is greatest in women aged 18 to 25, and the use of alcohol is greatest for women aged 26 to 34. With the rapidly changing regulatory status of cannabis in many states, the rate of use has more than doubled in pregnant women from 2010 to 2017, with 12.1% of women reporting use in the first trimester and 7.0% reporting use overall in pregnancy (National Institute on Drug Abuse, 2020). Evidence shows that regular cannabis use can affect fetal growth and cause LBW. The current recommendation is to discontinue marijuana use during pregnancy and in women considering pregnancy until more data is available on safety in pregnancy (National Institute on Drug Abuse, 2020). Substantial evidence shows that use of illegal drugs such as heroin, cocaine, methamphetamine, and MDMA can cause stillbirth, preterm birth, and birth defects. All women should be screened in pregnancy for drug use and abuse, with 5% of women in the United States reporting illegal street drug use (AWHONN, 2018; March of Dimes, 2021b).

Use of alcohol and illegal drugs during pregnancy can have a profound effect on the developing fetus and the health of the neonate. Fourteen percent of women report use of alcohol during pregnancy and 5% of women report binge drinking during pregnancy (CDC, 2022). Exposure to alcohol during pregnancy places the developing fetus at risk for fetal death; LBW; intrauterine growth retardation; mental retardation; and fetal alcohol spectrum disorders (FASDs), "a group of conditions that can occur in a person whose mother drank alcohol during pregnancy" (CDC, 2017). The impact of substance use on pregnancy and neonates is addressed in relevant chapters. For more information on FASDs, which have physical, behavioral, and cognitive effects, see Chapter 17.

Exposure to illegal drugs during pregnancy is associated with preterm birth, abruptio placenta, drug withdrawal for the neonate, and congenital defects. Cocaine use during pregnancy can cause strokes and seizure in the developing fetus and affect cognitive performance, information processing, and attention to tasks in children (March of Dimes, 2021b). Marijuana use during pregnancy may cause preterm birth, LBW, and neural tube defects (March of Dimes, 2021d).

Medication Use During Pregnancy

Although much focus is given to the use of tobacco, alcohol, cannabis, and illegal substances, it is equally important to assess women for use of prescription and over-the-counter (OTC) medications, including prescription medications that may belong to another person. Of the six million pregnancies in the United States each year, 9 in 10 women will use an OTC or prescribed medication in pregnancy (National Institute on Drug Abuse, 2020). Most drug trials do not include pregnant women due to ethical considerations and potential risk of harm to the fetus, so the majority of OTC and prescribed medications have not been tested in pregnant women; thus, all substances including supplements and herbal preparations should be discussed with a health-care provider before use in pregnancy (National Institute on Drug Abuse, 2020). In keeping with the opioid crisis in the United States, the number of women who had a use disorder at the time of birth quadrupled between 1999 and 2014 (CDC, 2018b).

Nursing Actions

Nurses can help reduce the negative outcomes from cigarette, alcohol, substance abuse, and improper medication use with preconception counseling for all women considering pregnancy in addition to routine screenings for substance use and abuse throughout pregnancy, the postpartum period, and for breast-feeding women.

Overweight and Obesity

Overweight is defined as a body mass index (BMI) of 25 to 29, obesity is defined as a BMI greater than or equal to 30, and severe obesity is defined as a BMI greater than 40. In the United States, the percentage of adults and youth who are overweight and obese is increasing exponentially. In 2000, 30.5% of adults and 13.9% of youth were obese compared with the current rate of 42.4% of adults, with the rate of severe obesity increasing from 4.7% to 9.2% in 2018 (CDC, 2021c). Maternal and infant health are among the areas most impacted by the obesity epidemic: overall, 28% of pregnant women meet the criteria for obesity and 75% of pregnant Black women meet the criteria for being overweight or obese (Pickett-Blakely et al., 2016). The impacts of obesity on pregnancy, labor, birth, and postpartum are addressed in relevant chapters.

CRITICAL COMPONENT

Obesity

In the United States, obesity is a major health concern for both adults and youth. Pregnant women who are overweight or obese are at higher risk for complications such as diabetes and cesarean birth. Infants born to women who are overweight or obese are at higher risk for complications such as intrauterine fetal death and birth injuries related to macrosomia.

Obesity in childbearing women has adverse effects on both the women and their children. Pregnant women who are overweight or obese are at higher risk for:

- Infertility (two times greater risk)
- Spontaneous abortion (miscarriage)
- Gestational hypertension
- Preeclampsia (two to three times greater risk)
- Gestational diabetes (two to three times greater risk)
- Thromboembolism
- Cesarean birth
- Wound infection
- Shoulder dystocia related to macrosomia (birth weight more than 4,000 grams)

- Sleep apnea
- Anesthesia complications
- Maternal death (Mahuette et al., 2018; Pickett-Blakely et al., 2016)

Fetuses and infants of overweight and obese pregnant women are at higher risk for:

- Fetal abnormalities, including spina bifida, heart defects, anorectal atresia, and hypospadias
- 20% increased risk for oral cleft defects, 39% increase in neural tube defects, and 50% increase in spina bifida (Mahuette et al., 2018; Pickett-Blakely et al., 2016)
- 20% increase in stillbirth
- Intrauterine fetal death
- Birth injuries related to macrosomia
- Childhood obesity and diabetes
- Increased lifetime risk of obesity, hypertension, and diabetes

Nursing Actions

Addressing the obesity epidemic is a national priority and evidence has demonstrated that change must occur at the population level.

- Addressing the social determinants of health that lead to obesity, including funding for access to healthy foods, safe living and play environments, equal access to affordable and effective health care, and increased educational and employment opportunities (National Partnership for Women and Families, 2019)
- Preventing lifetime risks for infants by addressing maternal obesity
- Providing preconception counseling and care with targeted weight loss before pregnancy
- Referral for specialized care if failure to lose weight with lifestyle modifications
- Preventing excessive weight gain in the first pregnancy through education regarding diet, exercise, and danger of being overweight

Violence

Intimate partner violence (IPV), sexual assault, and trauma are also key factors that impact maternal and child health, as well as the health of women and LGBTQIA+ communities in the United States. The scope of the problem is profound:

- More than one in three women will experience IPV, rape, physical violence, verbal abuse, and stalking in their lifetime. Ten million incidences (both women and men) of IPV occur in the United States each year (ACOG, 2012; National Coalition Against Domestic Violence [NCADV], 2021a).
- One in six pregnant women experience IPV before and during pregnancy (Agency for Healthcare Research and Quality [AHRQ], 2015; March of Dimes, 2021a), and more than 320,000 pregnant women experience abuse each year (ACOG, 2012; March of Dimes, 2021a). Women who experience abuse during pregnancy are at higher risk for inadequate

weight gain, substance abuse, depression, posttraumatic stress disorder (PTSD), suicide, and homicide, whereas infants are at risk for LBW, preterm birth, small for gestational age (SGA), and neonatal death (ACOG, 2012; March of Dimes, 2021a).

- One in five adolescents who identifies as female reports having experienced dating violence and 1.5 million teens will experience IPV in dating relationships each year (NCADV, 2021b).
- Older women who are dependent on caregivers are also at increased risk, with an estimated 1 in 10 older adults experiencing elder abuse each year (ACOG, 2021).
- Immigrant women are at increased risk and health-care providers must be aware of the cultural, linguistic, economic, and legal barriers for immigrant women and people to report IPV and assault, especially when there is a fear of deportation (ACOG, 2021).
- Women with disabilities are a population at increased risk as well, and health-care providers' lack of education and biases against women with disabilities leads to low screening rates. Women with disabilities experience sexual assault and abuse at three times the rate of the general population. In fact, 83% of women with disabilities will be sexually assaulted in their lifetime, and half of women with developmental disabilities who have been sexually assaulted are assaulted more than 10 times in their lifetime (Disability Justice, 2021).

Nursing Actions

- Screen all women (especially pregnant women) for IPV and assault at the initiation of prenatal care, in each trimester, and at the postpartum visit (ACNM, 2021; ACOG, 2012).
- Provide counseling, home visits, and mentoring support to pregnant women experiencing IPV (AHRQ, 2015).
- Provide routine screening for PTSD, depression, and suicide risk during prenatal care, postpartum visits, and well-woman examinations (ACNM, 2021).
- Make IPV screening an integral part of all health visits, inclusive of all women, including older women and women with disabilities (ACOG, 2012).
- Screen for adverse childhood experiences (ACE) and history of trauma as part of all prenatal care and well-infant care (Mersky & Lee, 2019; Olsen, 2018).
- Know the risk for homicide increases five times if IPV is occurring and there is a gun in the home. Screen for the presence of guns in the home (Everytown for Gun Safety, 2020).

Perinatal Depression and Mood Disorders

Depression, anxiety, and other perinatal mood disorders create a significant patient safety issue for women and infants:

- One in seven women experience postpartum depression.
- Between 13% and 21% of women experience perinatal anxiety.
- Two of three young pregnant women report one or more mental health issues.

- Around 20% of postpartum deaths are from suicide (Kendig et al., 2017; Slomain et al., 2017).

Maternal outcomes from perinatal mood disorders can include decreased participation on care, smoking and substance abuse, decrease in self-care and care of infant, discontinuation of breastfeeding, and suicide (Kendig et al., 2017).

Infant outcomes include poor weight gain; increased illnesses; decreased mother–infant bonding; sleep disorders; delays in motor, cognitive, language, and social development; and infanticide (Kendig et al., 2017; Slomain et al., 2017). The impact of depression and mood disorders on pregnancy and postpartum is addressed in relevant chapters.

Nursing Actions

- Implement the Consensus Bundle on Maternal Mental Health (Kendig et al., 2017):
  - Readiness
  - Recognition and Prevention
  - Response
  - Reporting and Systems Learning
- Screen for mood disorders in all three trimesters and for 1 year after birth.
- Initiate earlier and more frequent postpartum visits.
- Perform universal screening and education for postpartum depression (PPD) and mood disorders before every discharge.
- Create and support community services for treatment of PPD and perinatal mood disorders.

Sexually Transmitted Infections

The onset of COVID-19 created "pandemics within pandemics" with significant increases in the number of drug overdoses, rates of IPV, and the transmission of sexually transmitted infections (STIs). Here are the key findings on STIs from the latest data:

- Reportable STIs increased 30% between 2015 and 2019.
- The most significant increase was in congenital syphilis, which quadrupled from 2015 to 2019.
- Congenital syphilis neonatal deaths have increased by 22%.
- Health disparities exist among different population groups, with a five to eight times higher rate of STIs in 2019 for Black Americans; three to five times higher rate for American Indian, Alaska Native, and Pacific Islander women; and one to two times higher rate for Hispanic women (CDC, 2021d).
- Emerging data shows that HPV infection may increase the risk of preterm birth and maternal complications (Niyabizi et al., 2020).

Nursing Actions

Health-care providers must take the lead in preventing, screening, diagnosing, and treating STIs to reduce maternal and neonatal morbidity and mortality. Nurses should lead in health promotion and STI prevention through education on vaccination, safe sex practices, informed consent, and violence reduction.

Climate Change

Climate change is a significant and increasing threat to maternal and neonatal health, as well as global health, and nurses need to be educated on how to assess this threat and effectively respond (Kincaid, 2017; Public Health Institute, 2016; U.S. Global Change Research Program, 2016). Low-resource countries and communities are at increased risk for the negative health effects of climate change, and both globally and nationally these nations and communities are advocating for recognition of the specific harms to their communities and a reduction in global warming (Public Health Institute, 2016; U.S. Global Change Research Program, 2016). The six areas of climate change that impact maternal and child health are:

- Extreme heat
- Outdoor air quality
- Flooding
- Vector-borne infection
- Water quality, drought, and water-related illnesses
- Mental health and well-being (Public Health Institute, 2016; U.S. Global Change Research Program, 2016)

Although the exact causes of COVID-19 are not yet fully determined, significant evidence shows that climate change increases the risk of the emergence and transmission of new infectious diseases, mostly through deforestation and loss of habitat that brings animals and humans in closer contact (Harvard School of Public Health, n.d.; The Lancet, 2021). Data has demonstrated that people living in areas with poorer air quality are more likely to die from COVID-19, and future outbreaks of novel diseases will be prevented in part by addressing climate change, protecting the environment, and preserving biodiversity and natural habitats (Harvard School of Public Health, n.d.; The Lancet, 2021).

Nursing Actions

- Educate patients on climate change and how to mitigate the effects on maternal and child health.
- Know the specific threats in your communities and participate in disaster planning.
- Advocate for policies that address climate change and global warming.
- Advise pregnant women and childbearing families to monitor heat exposure and hydration during periods of extreme heat.
- Monitor the Air Quality Index and avoid being outside when critical.
- Create an emergency response plan.
- Reduce exposure and limit travel to avoid vector-borne illnesses (Public Health Institute, 2016; U.S. Global Change Research Program, 2016).

CRITICAL COMPONENT

Extreme Temperatures
Pregnant women are vulnerable to temperature extremes and susceptible to dehydration, which releases labor-inducing hormones.

Health Disparities, Racism, and Discrimination

In any discussion of health disparities in the United States, it is critical to name and address the role that racism and discrimination play in adverse outcomes. Although it is essential to identify these disparities to prepare nurses to provide effective care to all people, it is also imperative to create nursing interventions that systemically address inequities, starting by partnering with communities as they create their own solutions to the urgent health-care issues affecting them.

LGBTQIA+ Care

Health-care disparities and discrimination based on sexual orientation, gender identity, and sexual practices are routinely experienced by LGBTQIA+ individuals (Fenway Institute, 2016). Although data shows that LGBTQIA+ individuals are at higher risk for smoking, substance abuse, violence, and obesity, research demonstrates that these disparities do not result from individual vulnerabilities but from societal discrimination and abuse, which extends to health-care biases and discrimination (Fenway Institute, 2016). Comprehensive reform at the societal level as well as in health-care policy and practices is needed to support LGBTQIA+ individuals and communities in optimal wellness.

Extensive disparities in health outcomes exist for the LGBTQIA+ communities, and it is imperative that nurses and health-care professionals proactively screen for these disparities using the social determinants of health framework, avoiding actions or statements that confer individual blame or judgment (Healthy People.gov, 2021). Examples of disparities include:

- In a study that focused on sexual minority birth outcomes, 59% of women who identified as bisexual and 31% of women who identified as lesbian reported giving birth. However, study findings demonstrated higher rates of miscarriage, preterm birth, LBW, and stillbirth for bisexual and lesbian women (Everett et al., 2019).
- LGBTQIA+ youth have a two to three times higher rate of suicide than non-LGBTQIA+ youth (HealthyPeople.gov, 2021).
- LGBTQIA+ individuals have the highest rates of tobacco, alcohol, and drug use in the United States (Healthy People.gov, 2021).
- LGBTQIA+ individuals have higher incidences of asthma (21% of adult population), diabetes (20% of adult population), and uninsured status (17% of adult population) as compared with the non-LGBTQIA+ population. These conditions have led to worse health outcomes overall, including increased risk of severe COVID-19 infection (Fields, 2021).
- One in two transgender people report discrimination by health-care providers, which has led to 40% postponing or avoiding preventive health care (Medina, 2021).

Nursing Actions

- Advocate for policy changes that remove legal discrimination against LGBTQIA+ people at the local, state, and national level.

- Create LGBTQIA+ welcoming and gender-affirming environments, which include inclusive forms, signage, and office practices.
- Revise electronic health records (EHRs) to be inclusive of all people and collect data on gender identity and sexual orientation.
- Publicize nondiscrimination policies in patient materials, Web sites, and waiting areas.
- Provide training to all health-care staff to treat LGBTQIA+ patients in a caring and respectful manner, including using preferred names and pronouns.
- Recognize that facilities that participate in Medicare or Medicaid are required to let patients choose who can visit them and make medical decisions on their behalf, irrespective of sexual orientation, gender identity, or marital status (Fenway Institute, 2016).

Racism and Discrimination

The purpose of evidence-based care is to identify root causes of health disparities and systemically address these causes to achieve health equity. This discussion of racism and discrimination as it applies to maternal and infant health outcomes is based on decades of research and evidence that have demonstrated that systemic racism and discrimination in the United States is a key contributor to worsening maternal and infant outcomes for women of color (ACNM, BMMA, & ICM, 2020; ACOG, 2018; California Maternal Quality Care Collaborative, 2020).

At a physiological level, systemic racism and ongoing discrimination create persistent stressors in the body that cause biological weathering, including elevated cortisol levels, increased blood pressure, and shortening of telomeres in women of color—especially Black women—in the United States (Martin & Montagne, 2017). These impacts contribute to maternal complications such as hypertension, preterm birth, and earlier onset of chronic diseases that affect birth outcomes.

Similarly, women of color, specifically Black women in the United States, experience racism and discrimination that directly impact social determinants of health and, thus, negatively affect maternal and infant health outcomes. Seventy-four percent of Black women in the United States, for example, give birth in hospitals that care for predominantly Black patients. These hospitals are often in areas of historical segregation, score lower on maternal outcomes, and have higher levels of maternal morbidity and mortality (Creanga et al., 2014; Howell et al., 2016; Martin & Montagne, 2017).

Finally, research has clearly demonstrated that health-care providers, including nurses, are affected by systemic racism in the United States and exhibit biases against women of color while providing health care that causes harm and leads to poorer outcomes. Examples of biases against women of color that lead to health disparities include reduced rates of screening for diabetes in the postpartum period, significantly less pain medication given during labor and postpartum, and lower rates of epidural administration for women of color (Choo, 2017).

It is difficult to overstate the severity of racism's impact on maternal and newborn outcomes in the United States. These statistics are included to clarify that this is an ongoing and worsening national crisis, but similar to the disparities seen with LGBTQIA+ communities, these statistics must be seen as a call to action—led by communities of color—and not as a criticism of the people and communities experiencing these outcomes.

- Black women have three to four times higher maternal mortality rates and two times higher rates of severe maternal complications, including cardiomyopathy, embolism, and eclampsia (ACNM, BMMA, & ICM, 2020).
- Black infants have two times the rate of infant death of White infants (Taylor et al., 2019).
- American Indian and Alaska Native women have three to four times higher maternal mortality rates and two times higher rates of severe maternal morbidity, including postpartum hemorrhage and preterm birth (National Partnership for Women and Families, 2019).
- Maternal morbidity and mortality rates for Black women are independent of education, income, or other socioeconomic factors (ACNM, BMMA, & ICM, 2020).
- A college-educated Black woman is three times more likely to experience severe maternal complications than a White woman without a high school education (Choo, 2017).

Communities and organizations composed of people of color are leading the effort to address the racial disparities and inequities in maternal and infant health outcomes in the United States, and health-care and governmental organizations are joining the effort to prioritize equitable health outcomes for all women of childbearing age, especially women of color (ACNM, BMMA, & ICM, 2020).

Nursing Actions

1. Increasing the number of maternal health-care providers that are people of color significantly improves maternal outcomes (ACNM, BMMA, & ICM, 2020).
2. Community-led initiatives significantly improve maternal outcomes (California Maternity Care Collaborative, 2020; Choo, 2017).
3. Leadership by people of color significantly improves maternal outcomes (ACNM, BMMA, & ICM, 2020).
4. Addressing racism in practice is critical (ACNM, BMMA, & ICM, 2020).
5. Racial equity trainings that focus on addressing racism at both an interpersonal and institutional level help to improve maternal outcomes (National Birth Equity Collaborative, 2021).

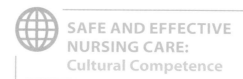

SAFE AND EFFECTIVE NURSING CARE:
Cultural Competence

Community Resources

Organizations such as the Black Mamas Matter Alliance and Sister Song: Women of Color Reproduction Collaborative are instrumental in creating community-led initiatives to improve infant and maternal health for people of color at a local, state, and national level (Black Mamas Matter Alliance, 2021).

TABLE 1-6 *Healthy People 2030* Maternal and Infant Health Goals

OBJECTIVES	BASELINE	2030 TARGET
Reduce rate of fetal deaths at 20 or more weeks of gestation	5.9 per 1,000 live births and fetal deaths	5.7 per 1,000 live births and fetal deaths
Reduce maternal deaths	17.4 maternal deaths per 100,000 live births	15.7
Reduce cesarean births among low-risk women with no prior cesarean births	25.6%	23.6%
Reduce total preterm births	10.2% of live births	9.4%
Increase proportion of pregnant women who receive early and adequate prenatal care	76.7%	80.5%
Increase abstinence from alcohol among pregnant women	89.3% past 30 days	92.2%
Increase abstinence from cigarette smoking among pregnant women	94%	95.7%
Increase abstinence from illicit drugs among pregnant women	93%	95.3%
Increase the proportion of women of childbearing age who get enough folic acid	82.6%	86.2%
Increase the proportion of women delivering a live birth who had a healthy weight before pregnancy	41%	47.1%
Increase the proportion of infants who are put to sleep on their backs	78.7%	88.9%
Increase the proportion of infants who are breastfed exclusively through age 6 months	24.9%	42.4%

U.S. Department of Health and Human Services, Office of Disease Prevention and Health Promotion. Healthy People 2030. https://health.gov/healthypeople

MATERNAL AND CHILD HEALTH GOALS

The health of a nation is reflected in the health of pregnant women and their infants. Identifying interventions to improve social determinants of health, reduce health disparities, and improve maternal and infant outcomes are all integral to the *Healthy People 2030* goals for the nation. The CDC and Health Resources and Services have set national maternal and child health goals in *Healthy People 2030* (Table 1-6). Reviewing these goals helps nurses focus their nursing care and advocacy to achieve health outcomes at the population level, and improving the health of mothers and children will have lifelong effects on the health of the nation.

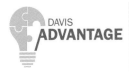

Go to Davis Advantage to complete your learning: strengthen understanding, apply your knowledge, and prepare for the Next Gen NCLEX®.

REFERENCES

Agency for Healthcare Research and Quality. (2015). *Intimate partner violence screening.* https://www.ahrq.gov/ncepcr/tools/healthier-pregnancy/fact-sheets/partner-violence.html

American Association of Birth Centers. (2016). *History.* https://www.birthcenters.org/page/history

American Association of Birth Centers. (2021). *Legislation endorsed by AABC.* https://www.birthcenters.org/page/history

American College of Nurse-Midwives. (2021). *Disparities in maternal mortality in the United States.* Quickening [online journal]. https://quickening.midwife.org/roundtable/clinical/disparities-in-maternal-morality-in-the-u-s/

American College of Nurse-Midwives. (n.d.). *Our philosophy of care.* https://www.midwife.org/our-philosophy-of-care

American College of Nurse-Midwives, Black Mamas Matter Alliance, and International Confederation of Midwives. (2020). *Eliminating the racial disparities contributing to the rise in U.S. maternal mortality: Perspectives from the American College of Nurse-Midwives (ACNM), Black Mamas Matter Alliance (BMMA), and International Confederation of Midwives (ICM).* https://quickening.midwife.org/roundtable/eliminating-racial-disparities-contributing-to-the-rise-in-u-s-maternal-mortality-perspectives-from-acnm-bmma-and-icm/

American College of Obstetricians and Gynecologists. (2012). *Intimate partner violence.* Committee Opinion 518. https://www.acog.org/clinical/clinical-guidance/committee-opinion/articles/2012/02/intimate-partner-violence

American College of Obstetricians and Gynecologists. (2018). Importance of social determinants of health and cultural awareness in the delivery of reproductive health care. Committee Opinion No. 729. *Obstetrics and Gynecology, 131*(1), e43–e48. https://doi.org/10.1097/AOG.0000000000002459

American College of Obstetricians and Gynecologists. (2020). Tobacco and nicotine cessation during pregnancy. ACOG Committee Opinion No. 807. *Obstetrics & Gynecology, 135,* e221–e229.

American College of Obstetricians and Gynecologists. (2021). *Elder abuse and women's health.* https://www.acog.org/clinical/clinical-guidance/committee-opinion/articles/2021/03/elder-abuse-and-womens-health

Anderson, R., Kochanek, K., & Murphy, S. (1997). Report of final mortality statistic, 1995. *Monthly Vital Statistics Reports, 45*(suppl 2), 11. National Center for Health Statistics. https://www.cdc.gov/nchs/data/mvsr/supp/mv45_11s2.pdf

Association of Women's Health, Obstetric and Neonatal Nurses. (2018, September 1). Marijuana use during pregnancy. *AWHONN Position Statement, 47*(5), 719–721.

Association of Women's Health, Obstetric, and Neonatal Nurses. (2021a). *About us.* https://www.awhonn.org/about-us/

Association of Women's Health, Obstetric and Neonatal Nurses. (2021b). *Breastfeeding and the use of human milk.* AWHONN Position Paper. https://www.jognn.org/article/S0884-2175(21)00116-7/fulltext

Black Mamas Matter Alliance. (2021). *About Black Mamas Matter Alliance* https://blackmammasmatter.org

Bureau of the Census. (1917). *Statistical abstract of the United States: 1917.* https://www.census.gov/library/publications/1918/compendia/statab/40ed.html

California Maternal Quality Care Collaborative. (2020). *Birth equity.* https://www.cmqcc.org/content/birth-equity

Center for the Study of Social Policy. (2019). *Reversing current terms in Black maternal and infant outcomes.* https://cssp.org/2019/05/trends-in-black-maternal-and-infant-health-outcomes/

Centers for Disease Control and Prevention. (2016). *Preterm birth.* www.cdc.gov/reproductivehealth/maternalinfanthealth/pretermbirth.htm

Centers for Disease Control and Prevention. (2017). *Basics of FASDs.* https://www.cdc.gov/ncbddd/fasd/facts.html

Centers for Disease Control and Prevention. (2018a). *E-cigarette information.* https://www.cdc.gov/tobacco/basic_information/e-cigarettes/

Centers of Disease Control and Prevention (2018b). *The number of women with opioid disorder at labor and delivery have quadrupled from 1999–2014.* https://www.cdc.gov/media/release/2018/p0809-women-opioid-use.html

Centers for Disease Control and Prevention. (2019a). *About teen pregnancy.* https://www.cdc.gov/teenpregnancy/about/index.htm

Centers for Disease Control and Prevention. (2019b). *Births: Provisional data for 2018.* https://www.cdc.gov/nchs/data/vsrr/vsrr-007-508.pdf

Centers for Disease Control and Prevention. (2019c). *E-cigarettes and pregnancy.* https://www.cdc.gov/reproductivehealth/maternalinfanthealth/substance-abuse/e-cigarettes-pregnancy.htm

Centers for Disease Control and Prevention. (2019d). Racial/Ethnic disparities in pregnancy-related deaths—United States, 2007–2016. *Morbidity and Mortality Weekly Report; 68*(35); 767–765. https://www.cdc.gov/mmwr/volumes/68/wr/mm6835a3.htm

Centers for Disease Control and Prevention. (2021a). *Adult obesity facts.* https://www.cdc.gov/obesity/data/adult.html

Centers for Disease Control and Prevention. (2021b). *Births: Provisional data for 2020.* https://www.cdc.gov/nchs/data/vsrr/vsrr012-508.pdf

Centers for Disease Control and Prevention. (2021c). *Fetal alcohol spectrum disorders: Data & statistics.* https://www.cdc.gov/ncbddd/fasd/data.html#:~:text=Among%20pregnant%20women%2C%201%20in%2010%20reported%20any,reported%20an%20average%20of%204.6%20binge%20drinking%20episodes

Centers for Disease Control and Prevention, (2021d). *Reported STD's reach all time high for sixth consecutive year.* https://www.cdc.gov/nchhstp/newsroom/2021/2019-STD-surveillance-report.html#:~:text=Reported%20STDs%20reach%20all-time%20high%20for%206th%20consecutive,an%20all-time%20high%20for%20the%20sixth%20consecutive%20year.

Centers for Disease Control and Prevention. (2021e). *STD's during pregnancy—CDC fact sheet.* http://www.cdc.gov/std/pregnancy/stdfact-pregnancy/.htm

Centers for Disease Control and Prevention (2022). Alcohol use and binge drinking among pregnant people in the United States. Cdc/gov/ncbddd/fasd/data.html

Centers for Disease Control and Prevention, National Center for Health Statistics. (2018). *Cigarette smoking during pregnancy: United States, 2016.* https://www.cdc.gov/nchs/data/databriefs/db305.pdf#:~:text=One%20in%202014%20women%20who%20gave%20birth%20in,states%20and%20D.C.%2C%20and%20higher%20in%2031%20states.

Centers for Disease Control and Prevention, National Center for Health Statistics. (2020a). *Births in the United States, 2019.* https://www.cdc.gov/nchs/products/databriefs/db387.htm

Centers for Disease Control and Prevention, National Center for Health Statistics. (2020b). *First data released on maternal mortality in over a decade.* https://www.cdc.gov/nchs/pressroom/nchs_press_releases/2020/202001_MMR.htm

Central Intelligence Agency. (2018a). *Birth rates.* https://www.cia.gov/library/publications/resources/the-world-factbook/rankorder/2054rank.html

CIA Central Intelligence Agency. (2022). *Total fertility rates.* https://www.cia.gov/the-world-factbook/field/total-fertility-rate/

Choo, E. (2017). *The elephant in the delivery room: How doctor bias hurts Black and Brown mothers.* NBC News. http://www.nbcnews.com/think/opinion/elephant-delivery-room-doctor-bias-hurts-black-brown-mothers-ncna832616

Commonwealth Fund. (2020). *Maternal mortality in the United States: A primer.* https://www.commonwealthfund.org/publications/issue-brief-report/2020/dec/maternal-mortality-united-states-primer

Creanga, A., Bateman, B., Mhyre, J., Kuklina, E., Shilkrut, A., & Callaghan, W. (2014). Performance of racial and ethnic minority-serving hospitals on delivery-related indicators. *American Journal of Obstetrics & Gynecology, 211,* 647.e 641–661. https://doi.org/10.1016/j.ajog.2014.06.006

Curtain, M., & Mathews, M. (2016). Smoking prevalence and cessation before and during pregnancy: Data from birth certificate, 2014. *National Vital Statistics, 65,* 1.

Davison, A., & Joseph, L. (2020). *An open letter from two Black midwives to our community.* California Nurse Midwives Association [online newsletter]. https://www.cnma.org/post/an-open-letter-from-two-black-midwives-to-our-community

Disability Justice. (2021). *Sexual abuse.* https://disabilityjustice.org/sexual-abuse/

Drexel University. (2020). *Infant mortality in the U.S. remains high: A new Drexel study shows how to best spend money to save lives.* https://drexel.edu/now/archive/2020/June/Infant-Mortality-in-the-US-Remains-High-Heres-How-to-Best-Spend-Money-to-Save-Lives/

Everett, B. G., Kominiarek, M. A., Mollborn, S., Adkins, D. E., & Hughes, T. L. (2019). Sexual orientation disparities in pregnancy and infant outcomes. *Maternal and Child Health Journal, 23*(1), 72–81. https://doi.org/10.1007/s10995-018-2595-x

Everytown for Gun Safety. (2020). *Domestic violence.* https://www.everytown.org/issues/domestic-violence/#what-are-the-solutions

Fenway Institute. (2016). *Improving the health care of lesbian, gay, bisexual, and transgender people (LGBT): Understanding and eliminating health disparities.* https://www.lgbtqiahealtheducation.org/publication/improving-the-health-care-of-lesbian-gay-and-transgender-lgbt-people-understanding-and-eliminating-health-disparities/

Fields, A. (2021). *CDC releases report confirming lesbian, gay and bisexual people at greater risk of COVID-19 illness, calls for more data collection.* https://www.hrc.org/press-releases/cdc-releases-report-confirming-lesbian-gay-and-bisexual-people-at-greater-risk-of-covid-19-illness-calls-for-more-data-collection

Gay and Lesbian Alliance Against Defamation. (2017). *Accelerating Acceptance 2017.* https://www.glaad.org/files/aa/2017_GLAAD_Accelerating_Acceptance.pdf

Hamilton, B., Martin, J., & Osterman, J. (2016). Births: Preliminary data for 2015. *National Vital Statistics Reports, 65*(3).

Hamilton, B., Martin, J., & Ventura, S. (2007). Births: Preliminary data for 2005. *National Vital Statistics Reports, 55*(11).

Hamilton, B., Martin, J., & Ventura, S. (2009). Births: Preliminary data for 2006. *National Vital Statistics Reports, 56*(7). https://www.cdc.gov/nchs/data/nvsr/nvsr56/nvsr56_07.pdf

Hamilton, B., Martin, J., & Ventura, S. (2011). Preliminary data for 2010. *National Vital Statistics Reports, 60,* 1–25. https://www.cdc.gov/nchs/data/nvsr/nvsr60/nvsr60_02.pdf

Harvard School of Public Health. (n.d.). *Coronavirus, climate change, and the environment: A conversation on COVID-19 with Dr. Aaron Bernstein, Director of Harvard Chan C-CHANGE.* https://www.hsph.harvard.edu/c-change/subtopics/coronavirus-and-climate-change/

Healthychildren.org. (2021). *E-cigarette use during pregnancy and breastfeeding FAQ's.* https://www.healthychildren.org/English/ages-stages/prenatal/Pages/E-Cigarette-Use-During-Pregnancy-Breastfeeding.aspx

HealthyPeople.gov. (2021). *Lesbian, gay, bisexual, and transgender health.* https://www.healthypeople.gov/2020/topics-objectives/topic/lesbian-gay-bisexual-and-transgender-health#25

Howell, E., Egorova, N., Balbierz, A., Zeitlin, J., & Hebert, P. (2016). Black-white differences in severe maternal morbidity and site care. *American Journal of Obstetrics & Gynecology, 214*(1), 122.e121–127. https://doi.org/10.1016/j.ajog.2015.08.019

Hoyert, D. (2007). Maternal mortality and related concepts. *National Center for Human Statistics. Vital Health Stats, 3*(33), 2–10.

Hoyert, D., Uddin, S., & Minino, A. (2020). *Evaluation of the pregnancy status checkbox on the identification of maternal deaths.* https://www.cdc.gov/nchs/data/nvsr/nvsr69/nvsr69_01-508.pdf

Kendig, S., Keats, J., Hoffman, M., Kay, L., Miller, E., Moore, S., . . . Bsla, L. (2017). Consensus bundle on maternal mental health: Perinatal depression and anxiety. *Journal of Midwifery and Women's Health, 62*(2), 232–239. https://doi.org/10.1111/jmwh.12603

Kincaid, E. (2017). Global warming may be especially dangerous for pregnant women. *The Atlantic.* https://www.theatlantic.com/health/archive/2017/11/pregnancy-heat-outcomes/546362/

Kochanek, M., Murphy, S., Xu, J., & Tejada, B. (2016). Deaths: Final data for 2014. *National Vital Statistics Reports, 65*(4), 1–121. Hyattsville, MD: National Center for Health Statistics. https://www.cdc.gov/nchs/data/nvsr/nvsr65/nvsr65_04.pdf

La Leche League International. (2021). *A brief history of La Leche League International.* https://www.llli.org/about/history/

Lancet. (2021). *Climate change and COVID 19: Converging crises.* https://www.thelancet.com/journals/lancet/article/PIIS0140-6736(20)32579-4/fulltext

Lothian. (2016). *Childbirth education: Does it make a difference?* https://www.ncbi.nlm.nih.gov/pmc/articles/PMC6265608/

Mahutte, N., Kamga-Ngande, C., Sharma, A., & Sylvestre, C. (2018). *Obesity and reproduction.* https://pubmed.ncbi.nlm.nih.gov/29921431/

March of Dimes. (2021a). *Abuse during pregnancy.* https://www.marchofdimes.org/pregnancy/abuse-during-pregnancy.aspx

March of Dimes. (2021b). *Cocaine and pregnancy.* https://www.marchofdimes.org/pregnancy/cocaine.aspx

March of Dimes. (2021c). *Low birthweight.* https://www.marchofdimes.org/complications/low-birthweight.aspx

March of Dimes. (2021d). *Marijuana and pregnancy.* https://www.marchofdimes.org/pregnancy/marijuana.aspx

March of Dimes. (2021e). *Quick facts: Birthweight.* https://www.marchofdimes.org/peristats/ViewTopic.aspx?reg=99&top=4&lev=0&slev=1#:~:text=Quick%20Facts%3A%20Birthweight&text=Babies%20born%20too%20small%20are,birthweight%20in%20the%20United%20States

Martin, J., Hamilton, B., Sutton, P., Ventura, S., Menacker, F., & Kirmeyer, S. (2006). Birth: Final data for 2004. *National Vital Statistic Report, 55* (1) 1–114. https://www.cdc.gov/nchs/data/nvsr/nvsr55/nvsr545_11.pdf

Martin, J., Osterman, M., Driscoll, A., & Drake, P. (2018). Births: Final data for 2016. *National Vital Statistics Reports, 67*(1), 1–54.

Martin, N., & Montagne, R. (2017). *Nothing protects Black women from dying in pregnancy and childbirth.* ProPublica. https://www.propublica.org/article/nothing-protects-black-women-from-dying-in-pregnancy-and-childbirth

Maternal Safety Foundation. (2021). *Labor induction, percent by state, 2016.* https://www.cesareanrates.org/labor-induction-by-state

Medina, C. (2021). *Fact sheet: Protecting and advancing health care for transgender adult communities.* https://www.americanprogress.org/issues/lgbtq-rights/reports/2021/08/25/503048/fact-sheet-protecting-advancing-health-care-transgender-adult-communities/

Mersky, J., & Lee, C. (2019). *Adverse childhood experiences and poor birth outcomes in a diverse, low income sample.* https://www.ncbi.nlm.nih.gov/pmc/articles/PMC6819344/

Murphy, S., Kochanel, K., Xu, J., & Arias, E. (2021). Mortality in the United States, 2020, 1–8.

Murphy, S., Xu, J., & Kochanek, K. (2012). Deaths: Preliminary data for 2010. *National Vital Statistics Report, 60*(4), 1–8.

Murphy, S., Xu, J., Kochanek, K., Curtin, M., & Arias, E. (2017). Deaths: Final data for 2015. *National Vital Statistics Reports, 66*(6), 1–8.

National Birth Equity Collaborative. (2021). *Racial equity training.* https://birthequity.org/what-we-do/racial-equity-training/

National Campaign to Prevent Teen Pregnancy. (2016a). *Counting it up: The public costs of teen childbearing.* https://www.thenationalcampaign.org

National Center for Health Statistics. (2017). *Health, United States, 2015.* https://www.cdc.gov/nchs/data/hus/hus15.pdf#050

National Coalition Against Domestic Violence. (2021a). *Domestic violence.* https://assets.speakcdn.com/assets/2497/domestic_violence-2020080709350855.pdf?1596828650457

National Coalition Against Domestic Violence. (2021b). *Teen, campus, and dating violence.* https://assets.speakcdn.com/assets/2497/dating_abuse_and_teen_violence_ncadv.pdf

National Conference of State Legislatures. (2016). *Teen pregnancy prevention.* https://www.ncsl.org/research/health/teen-pregnancy-prevention.aspx#proverty

National Institute on Drug Abuse. (2020). *Substance use in women research report: Substance use while pregnant and breastfeeding.* https://www.drugabuse.gov/publications/research-reports/substance-use-in-women/substance-use-while-pregnant-breastfeeding

National Partnership for Women and Families. (2019). *American Indian and Alaska Native women's maternal health: Addressing the crisis.* https://www.nationalpartnership.org/our-work/resources/health-care/maternity/american-indian-and-alaska.pdf

Niyibizi, J., Zanré, N., Mayrand, M. H., & Trottier, H. (2020). Association between maternal human papillomavirus infection and adverse pregnancy outcomes: Systematic review and meta-analysis. *Journal of Infectious Diseases, 221*, 1925–1937. https://doi.org/10.1093/infdis/jiaa054

Olsen, J. (2018). Integrative review of pregnancy health risks and outcomes associated with adverse childhood experiences. *Journal of Obstetrics & Gynecology Neonatal Nursing, 47*(6), 783–794. https://doi.org/10.1016/j.jogn.2018.09.005

Organisation for Economic Co-Operation and Development. (2021). *Health status: Maternal and infant mortality.* https://stats.oecd.org/index.aspx?queryid=30116

Pickett-Blakely, O., Uwakwe, L., & Rashid, F. (2016). *Obesity in women: The clinical impact on gastrointestinal and reproductive health and disease management.* https://pubmed.ncbi.nlm.nih.gov/27261901/

Public Health Institute. (2016). *Special focus: Climate change and pregnant women.* https://climatehealthconnect.org/wp-content/uploads/2016/09/Pregnant Women.pdf

Taylor, J., Novoa, C., Hamm, K., & Phadke, S. (2019). *Eliminating racial disparities in maternal and infant mortality.* https://www.americanprogress.org/issues/women/reports/2019/05/02/469186/eliminating-racial-disparities-maternal-infant-mortality/

U.S. Department of Health and Human Services. (2021). *Social determinants of health.* https://health.gov/healthypeople/objectives-and-data/social-determinants-health

U.S. Department of Health and Human Services, Office of Disease Prevention and Health Promotion. (2022). *Healthy People 2030.* https://health.gov/healthypeople

U.S. Global Change Research Program. (2016). *The impacts of climate change on human health in the United States: A scientific assessment.* https://health2016.globalchange.gov/

Wertz, R., & Wertz, D. (1979). *Lying-in: A history of childbirth in America.* Schocken Books.

World Health Organization. (2006). *Basic documents, forty-fifth edition, supplement October 2006.* https://www.who.int/governance/eb/who_constitution_en.pdf

World Health Organization. (2018a). *Infant mortality.* http://www.who.int/gho/child_health/mortality/neonatal_infant_text/en/

World Health Organization. (2018b). *Key facts.* https://www.who.int/en/news-room/fact-sheets/detail/preterm-birth

World Health Organization. (2021a). *Social determinants of health.* https://www.who.int/health-topics/social-determinants-of-health#tab=tab_1

World Health Organization. (2021b). *Infant mortality.* https://www.who.int/data/gho/data/themes/topics/indicator-groups/indicator-group-details/GHO/infant-mortality

World Health Organization, United Nations Children's Fund, United Nations Population Fund, World Bank Group and United Nations Population Division. (2015). *Trends in maternal mortality: 1990 to 2015: Estimates by WHO, UNICEF, UNFPA, World Bank Group and the United Population Division.* WHO Document Production Services.

Youth.gov. (2016). *Adverse effects of teen pregnancy.* http://www.youth.gov/youth-topics/teen-pregnancy-prevention/adverse-effects-teen-pregnancy

Ethics and Standards of Practice Issues

2

Roberta F. Durham, RN, PhD

LEARNING OUTCOMES

Upon completion of this chapter, the student will be able to:
1. Debate ethical issues in maternity nursing.
2. Explore standards of practice in maternity nursing.
3. Describe legal issues in maternity nursing.
4. Analyze concepts related to evidence-based practice.

CONCEPTS

Caring
Clinical Judgment
Collaboration
Comfort
Communication
Evidence-Based Practice
Family
Grief and Loss
Health Policy
Health-Care Systems
Leadership and
　Management
Professionalism
Quality Improvement
Safety
Self

INTRODUCTION

Maternity nursing is an exciting, dynamic area of nursing practice. There are unique ethical challenges in maternity nursing, with an obligation to practice safe, evidence-based nursing care that is responsive to the needs of women and their families. This chapter presents the foundational principles set forth by the American Nurses Association (ANA, 2015a) Code of Ethics and addresses specialty practice standards from the Association of Women's Health, Obstetric and Neonatal Nurses (AWHONN, 2019), which outline duties and obligations of obstetric and neonatal nurses. The chapter reviews ethical principles within the context of perinatal dilemmas and ethical decision making and presents common issues in maternity nursing litigation. Finally, the chapter explores evidence-based practice (EBP) and challenges in research utilization in the perinatal setting.

ETHICS IN NURSING PRACTICE

The terms *ethics* and *morality* are often used interchangeably, but they have different meanings. Morality is very personal and can be adaptable over time; in a pluralistic society, there are many different standards of morality. Ethics, however, are the results of a disciplined study of morality expressed in systemic norms (Stephenson, 2016). In nursing, current professional ethical standards are codified in the ANA Code of Ethics (2015a). These standards are based on universal ethical principles (Stephenson, 2016) and are binding to nurses, regardless of whether they agree with a nurse's personal morality.

TABLE 2-1 Overview of American Nurses Association Code of Ethics

Provision 1	The nurse practices with compassion and respect for the inherent dignity, worth, and uniqueness of every person.
Provision 2	The nurse's primary commitment is to the patient, whether an individual, family, group, or community.
Provision 3	The nurse promotes, advocates for, and strives to protect the health, safety, and rights of all patients.
Provision 4	The nurse has authority, accountability, and responsibility for nursing practice, decisions, and actions consistent with the nurse's obligation to promote health and provide optimum care.
Provision 5	The nurse owes the same duties to self as to others, including the responsibility to promote health and safety, to preserve wholeness of character and integrity, to maintain competence, and to continue personal and professional growth.
Provision 6	The nurse, through individual and collective effort, establishes, maintains, and improves the ethical environment of the work setting and provides quality health care.
Provision 7	The nurse, in all roles and settings, advances the profession through research and scholarly inquiry development of professional standards and policy.
Provision 8	The nurse collaborates with other health professionals and the public to promote human rights and health diplomacy and to decrease health disparities.
Provision 9	The profession of nursing, collectively through its professional organizations, articulates nursing values, maintains the integrity of the profession, and integrates the principle of social justice into nursing and health policy.

©2015a by American Nurses Association. Reprinted with permission. All rights reserved.

ANA Code of Ethics

The ANA Code of Ethics describes the goals, values, and obligations of nursing. This code applies to all nurses and is intended to be adaptable to areas of specialty nursing. The purpose of the Code of Ethics is to be a:

- Nonnegotiable ethical standard for the profession;
- Reflection of the profession's own understanding of its commitment to society;
- Statement on the ethical duties and obligations of every nurse;
- Resource for nurses confronted with ethical dilemmas.

Table 2-1 lists the fundamental values and ethical principles of the nursing profession as described in the ANA's 2015 Code of Ethics. The ANA offers interpretive statements to further clarify the nine basic provisions outlined in the table and how they should be applied.

Ethical Principles

In addition to medically sound care, nurses are called on to provide compassionate and ethically sound care. This is not always an easy task. Maternity nursing is unique in that the nurse is caring for two patients at the same time, the woman and fetus, and decisions are often complicated by the timeline of fetal development. Medical decisions that were ethical in the 12th week of gestation may no longer be ethical at 35 weeks' gestation and vice versa. Technological advances in the neonatal intensive care unit (NICU) blur the line of viability, defined as the moment when a fetus is developed enough to survive outside of the uterus with a reasonable probability of growing and developing as a human being; this definition adds another dimension of complexity (Stephenson, 2016).

Understanding the ethical principles that form the basis of a code of ethics can help guide nurses confronted with ethically complex situations (ANA, 2015a). Although the principles are not difficult to define, they can become complicated and mutually contradictory in some circumstances:

- **Beneficence:** The obligation to do good. In maternity nursing, this applies to both the woman and the fetus and is usually uncomplicated. Educating your patient about interventions and behaviors that benefit both her and her fetus is an example of beneficence.
- **Nonmaleficence:** The obligation to do no harm to either the woman or the fetus. For example, helping a mother understand the potential consequences of drug abuse or alcohol ingestion during pregnancy is an act of nonmaleficence.
- **Fidelity:** Being accountable for your responsibilities and loyal to your commitments, such as ensuring your patient has appropriate care from your relief nurse before going off shift.
- **Veracity:** Being truthful. This can mean being honest with your patient about risks and benefits of a cesarean or admitting that you need assistance to give appropriate care.
- **Autonomy:** The right to self-determination. It is related to free choice and personal decisions and is the basis for informed consent in health care. This applies only to the pregnant woman, as the fetus is not able to conceive of or express preferences.
- **Justice:** This is related to allocation of resources and ensures that resources are used equitably. What is considered equitable,

however, may be subjective and cause conflict. For example, at the societal level justice relates to which initiatives or programs are funded, whereas at the individual level justice may influence who receives an organ transplant.

Ethical Approaches

Ethical principles can compete in every area of nursing. In maternity nursing, this is compounded by the nurse's responsibilities to both the woman and the fetus. A woman's autonomy can include her right to make decisions that are not in the best interest of the fetus. In contrast, she may forgo necessary therapies for herself until after her delivery despite her own best interests, such as chemotherapy treatment for malignant cancer that would harm the fetus. A nurse is not in a position to voice approval or disapproval of the decisions the woman makes but should advocate for a woman to make informed decisions.

When considering the best approach to managing limited resources, there are three primary philosophies to consider (ANA, 2015a): utilitarianism, libertarianism, and egalitarianism. Each has its own strengths and weaknesses, and they can all be effective decision-making strategies in various situations:

- **Utilitarianism:** This is the principle of distributing resources to produce the greatest good for the most people and opposes using large amounts of resources for the benefit of a few.
- **Libertarianism:** This philosophy promotes the idea that some people are more valuable to society than others and thus need to be given the resources they require to survive. To do otherwise is to waste resources.
- **Egalitarianism:** This moral principle focuses on the belief that all people are equal. This principle emphasizes distributing resources according to need to protect those in society who are marginalized and vulnerable.

Consider the situation of a premature but healthy infant who needs extensive and expensive technological support to survive for the first few weeks. Should the infant's access to lifesaving support be dependent on the family's ability to pay? What if the infant is not healthy and will likely be severely disabled even if the child survives, requiring lifelong care and intensive resources? Does that change the decision to provide resources for the child to survive infancy? Should it change the decision? These situations can be very challenging to nurses as they advocate for both mothers and infants and navigate ethical dilemmas.

Ethical Dilemmas

Ethical dilemmas occur in all areas of life. Although they can be addressed in many ways, nurses must consider their clear obligations and duties to their patients. Because maternity nurses must advocate for both maternal and fetal well-being, it may not be possible to "do the right thing" for both. Ethical dilemma refers to when there is difficulty in deciding which action takes precedence over the other. A dilemma has been described as a situation requiring a choice between what appears to be equally desirable or undesirable alternatives (Aderemi, 2016). It can also be described as a situation in which the patient's rights and the professional's obligations conflict.

Ethical dilemmas occur in maternal and child health nursing as they do in other areas of nursing. Such situations are common in perinatal and neonatal care because the well-being of both the mother and her neonate must be considered. Most believe pregnancy is not an exception to the principle that a patient capable of making decisions has the right to refuse treatment, even treatment needed to maintain life. Therefore, a capable pregnant woman's decision to refuse recommended medical or surgical interventions should be respected (American College of Obstetricians and Gynecologists [ACOG], 2016). The most suitable ethical approach for medical decision making in obstetrics is one that recognizes the pregnant woman's freedom to make decisions within caring relationships, incorporates a commitment to informed consent and refusal within a commitment to provide medical benefit to patients, and respects patients as individuals. This ethical approach recognizes that the primary duty is to the pregnant woman. This duty most often also benefits the fetus. However, circumstances may arise in which the interests of the pregnant woman and those of the fetus diverge, demonstrating the primacy of the provider's duties to the woman (ACOG, 2016).

Some ethical dilemmas may be more easily avoided. Implementing safe practices according to evidence-based practice (EBP) guidelines, helping to establish a culture of safety and professionalism in your workplace, and reporting both individual and system errors can prevent many ethically challenging situations. Consider the example from earlier in which the mother requires chemotherapy that may harm the fetus or the ethics of deciding to terminate a severely abnormally developed fetus. Is it ethical to delay treatment for a pregnant woman with cancer, potentially shortening her life? Or, in the other situation, is it ethical to continue a pregnancy with a nonviable fetus that results in a painful, short life for the newborn? How does one balance advocating for the mother and the fetus if the mother insists on continuing with high-risk behaviors during her pregnancy? There are no simple answers to such situations, yet maternity nurses must help mothers and families navigate these and other ethical dilemmas. Practice dictates that the primary advocacy role of maternity nurses is on behalf of the mother. Obligations to the fetus are tempered by the context of the mother's decisions, and that can be complicated. As individuals with their own ideas of morality, maternity nurses may not agree with the mother's choices, yet their duty to respect her autonomy will help guide them in managing the consequences. Adding to the challenge is the fact that while caring for women and their families, nurses encounter diverse cultural practices, spiritual beliefs, and attitudes toward health and health care. Patterns of communication and decision making are influenced by culture, so cultural awareness and cultural humility can help nurses navigate decision making with patients and families. Striving to support women's choices is a fundamental moral responsibility for nurses. Awareness of the broader context that influences health supports patient-centered care and can help reduce health inequities (ACOG, Committee on Health Care for Underserved Women, 2018).

Other issues in which maternity nurses will be required to help educate, guide, and ultimately advocate for patients include:

- Court-ordered treatments that infringe on the pregnant woman's right to autonomy.
- Criminalization of pregnant women with substance use disorders.
- The difficult decision to withdraw life support from the infant or the mother.
- Treatment of genetic disorders or fetal abnormalities.
- Systemic inequities that prevent or delay pregnancy care during the previable period.
- Equal access to prenatal care.
- Genetic engineering, cloning, and surrogacy.
- Navigating decisions such as sanctity of life versus quality of life for extremely premature or severely disabled infants, including whether to resuscitate borderline-viable infants.
- Fetal reduction and preconception gender selection.

An ethics committee in hospitals is an advisory group appointed by the hospital medical executive board. The multidisciplinary ethics committee represents the hospital and the community it serves. Most hospitals have an ethics committee, made up of doctors, nurses, lawyers, and clergy, which can get together to help families or health-care workers when difficult ethical questions arise. Staff and family members can request an ethics committee consultation at many hospitals.

CLINICAL JUDGMENT

Evidence shows that nurses who understand and internalize professional nursing ethics are less likely to suffer from a loss of confidence and self-esteem as a result of facing these difficult situations (Aderemi, 2016; Iacobucci et al., 2013). Nurses can experience moral distress from situations in which their core beliefs conflict with providing care. Moral distress occurs in the day-to-day setting and involves situations in which one acts against one's better judgment due to internal or external constraints. Putting aside one's values and carrying out an action one believes is wrong threatens the authenticity of the moral self. Unfortunately, situations of moral distress are common in health care, and damage to providers' moral integrity occurs with alarming frequency (Tessman, 2020) (Box 2-1). This negotiation between individual conscience and patient responsibility arises in many circumstances (e.g., abortion, near viability infant resuscitation, end-of-life care, informed refusals, and withdrawal of treatment and medical assistance in dying). The opportunity to develop these skills in relationship to an individual's own moral conscience is an important part of nursing and nursing education (Swartz et al., 2020). A nurse who demonstrates moral courage speaks up and asks questions when discussing decisions about care with patients and with colleagues. She practices self-reflection about personal, health-related values and beliefs to increase the capacity to respect the same in others (Ruhl et al., 2016). The goal is to preserve moral sensitivity and integrity by recognizing, valuing, and hearing staff.

BOX 2-1 | Clinical Examples of Perinatal Ethical Dilemmas

Ethical dilemmas occur in all areas of nursing. However, because maternity nurses must advocate for both maternal and fetal well-being, there is not always a clear path for doing the right thing for both the mother and the fetus. Examples include:

- Court-ordered treatment
- Withdrawal of life support
- Harvesting of fetal organs or tissue
- In vitro fertilization and decisions for disposal of remaining fertilized ova
- Allocation of resources in pregnancy care during the previable period
- Fetal surgery
- Treatment of genetic disorders or fetal abnormalities found on prenatal screening
- Equal access to prenatal care
- Maternal rights versus fetal rights
- Extraordinary medical treatment for pregnancy complications
- Using organs from an anencephalic infant
- Genetic engineering
- Cloning
- Surrogacy
- Drug testing in pregnancy
- Sanctity of life versus quality of life for extremely premature or severely disabled infants
- Substance abuse in pregnancy
- Borderline viability: to resuscitate or not
- Fetal reduction
- Preconception gender selection
- Sex selection

Ethics in Neonatal Care

Care of extremely sick infants is especially challenging. Maternity and NICU nurses have an ethical obligation to care for the infant and respect parental decisions regarding the infant, but also have a duty to do no harm (Fig. 2–1). Categories for neonates in the NICU may include:

- Infants for whom aggressive care would probably be futile, where prognosis for a meaningful life is extremely poor or hopeless.
- Infants for whom aggressive care would probably result in clear benefit to overall well-being, where prevailing knowledge and evidence indicate excellent chances for beneficial outcomes and meaningful interactions.
- Infants for whom the effect of aggressive care is mostly uncertain.

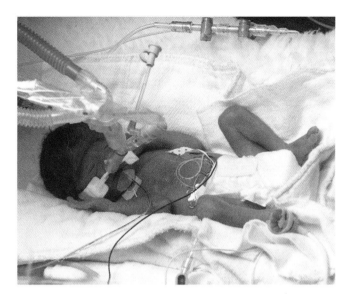

FIGURE 2–1 Extremely premature baby in the NICU.

An especially important related ethical issue concerns futility (Chervenak et al., 2013). Families sometimes request inappropriate or futile care for their newborns. However, this does not relieve nurses of their ethical duty to advocate for appropriate care. Identifying the neonate's status will help guide the perinatal nurse's parental counseling and decision making. It is critical to remember that veracity is one of the ethical principles binding the nurse; keeping parents fully informed supports their ability to make the best choices for themselves. Withholding information, even to protect the parents from emotional pain and disappointment, may be well-intentioned, but makes assumptions about what is best for the mother and her family without giving them a chance to participate in that decision. This represents a form of paternalism, in which an authority figure, in this case health-care personnel, makes choices for others; this is considered disrespectful and inappropriate (Chervenak et al., 2013; Stephenson, 2016).

Parents often lack the expertise to make fully informed decisions regarding the care of their neonate, so communication and collaboration are critical. The parents are the ones who must manage the long-term consequences of decisions, whether that means grieving over the death of their child or adapting to the difficult realities of having a child who may require lifelong care. Developing a consensus for the plan of care that incorporates parental wishes, ethical standards, and realistic assessments of available resources requires a team approach between the appropriate health-care professionals and parents, in which parental concerns are acknowledged and validated. Such a plan will minimize needless harm or suffering for the neonate and ethical dilemmas for the NICU nurse, as well as give parents a sense of participation and control.

Nurses must keep parents fully informed of all developments and respect parental decisions, but they also have a duty to the neonate. This may require counseling the parents, offering support, and referring them to additional resources. At times, balancing these obligations can lead to an ethical dilemma. Nurses are the primary link between neonates in the ICU and their parents, and they interact more with families than any other health-care professional, putting them in a unique position to help identify

and ensure the best possible outcome (Mattson & Smith, 2016). Sensitivity to the ethical contexts and being receptive to parental concerns can help the nurse navigate these situations. A common goal in neonatal units is to increase parents' participation in daily care and decisions regarding the health care of their infants and empowerment of parents. This improves the quality of health care for newborns and parents and is conducive to successful development of the parental role (Wisner et al., 2019).

Additionally, moral distress is prevalent in the NICU, where decisions regarding end-of-life care, periviable resuscitation, and medical futility are common. Advances in medical technology have allowed the smallest, sickest neonates to survive. The treatment for critically ill infants is no longer simply limited by the capability of medical technology but also by moral and ethical boundaries of what is right for a given child and family. Shared decision making and the zone of parental discretion can inform and challenge the NICU team to balance the complexities of patient autonomy against harm and suffering. Limited ability to prognosticate and uncertainty in outcomes add to the challenges faced with ethical dilemmas. Subjective views of quality of life and personal values in these situations can lead to moral distress if the plans of care and the validity of each path are not fully explored. Differences in opinions and approaches between members of the medical team can strain relationships and affect each individual differently (Mills & Cortezzo, 2020).

In the NICU, disagreements about whether life-sustaining treatment can ethically be withheld or withdrawn are not uncommon. Usually, the dilemma comes down to questions about the value of life with severe physical or cognitive impairments. Disagreements can go in both directions. Sometimes providers recommend treatments and parents refuse. Sometimes parents request continued treatment that providers think is inappropriate (Lantos, 2019). These disagreements can cause moral distress among physicians and nurses and debates about the ethical justifiability of unilateral decisions that treatment is futile and should be withdrawn. Usually, disagreements are resolved by ongoing discussion between the NICU team and parents, by bringing in other family members, or by consulting an ethics committee.

From an ethics perspective, traditionally when treatment is clearly beneficial, the baby's right to treatment outweighs parents' rights to make medical decisions for their baby. When benefits of treatment are less clear, ethicists (and courts) defer to parental choices (Lantos, 2018).

Decision making in the NICU has recently shifted to focus on the process rather than the results. A newer approach recommends that care providers help parents discern their own values and ethical commitments as they face an unanticipated situation and a series of life-altering decisions (Lantos, 2018). The goal is to help parents understand their child's clinical situation and prognosis as well as the meaning of the choices they face in light of that clinical situation.

Ethical Decision-Making Models

Clinical situations that raise ethical questions are a challenge to navigate, with multiple clinical facts to consider. In addition, patient and family values, concerns, and preferences must be considered. In some cases, a decision is needed quickly. When faced with these difficult clinical situations, a systematic approach can help health-care providers reach an ethical decision or recommendation (Schumann & Alfandre, 2008). One common approach for ethical decision making in clinical settings is the Jonsen model, widely referred to as the "four topics method" (Jonsen et al., 2002).

The four topics method was developed to provide clinicians with a framework for sorting through and focusing on specific aspects of clinical ethics cases and connecting the circumstances of a case to their underlying ethical principles. Each topic—medical indications, patient preferences, quality of life, and contextual features—represents a set of specific questions to be considered in working through the ethical conflict or case. The purpose of the four topics method is to sort out data to determine what is central to the discussion (Jonsen et al., 2002). The boxes do not give us an answer, but point us to areas of confusion or contention. When you finish sorting the data, ask, "In which quadrant does the problem seem to lie?" This provides guidance for physicians and nurses on where to gather more resources and how to intervene. The next sections review the four topics, relate them to ethical concepts, and present relevant questions.

Medical Indications

Clinical ethics case analysis using the four topics method begins with an articulation of the medical facts of the case, including the diagnosis, prognosis, treatment options, and how the patient can benefit, if at all, from treatment (Schumann & Alfandre, 2008). This topic relates to the ethical principles of and consideration of beneficence and nonmaleficence. Relevant questions include:

- What is the patient's medical problem? History? Diagnosis? Prognosis?
- Is the problem acute? Chronic? Critical? Emergent? Reversible?
- What are the goals of treatment?
- What are the probabilities of success?
- In sum, how can this patient benefit from medical and nursing care, and how can harm be avoided?

Patient Preferences

This topic focuses on the expressed or presumed wishes and values of the patient, including respect for patient autonomy. Although the United States prioritizes the autonomy of the individual, most cultures value the family, the community, and the overall population in concert with the individual. Relevant questions include:

- Has the patient been informed of benefits and risks, understood this information, and given consent?
- Has the patient expressed prior preferences, such as advance directives?
- Is the patient unwilling or unable to cooperate with medical treatment? If so, why?
- In sum, is the patient's right to choose being respected to the extent possible in ethics and law?

Since the women's health movement (WHM) of the 1960s, a primary goal has been to improve health care for all women at all reproductive stages of their lives. Despite challenges and setbacks in reproductive rights, significant gains were made in women's health at the federal policy level during the 1980s and 1990s (Nichols, 2000). For example, women gained more control over their reproductive rights. Abortion was legalized, although restrictions remain, and new contraceptive technology became available. Gender-based research emerged as an important area of biomedicine. Violence and discrimination against women have been recognized as a significant problem worldwide. Progress has been made, but we still have much to accomplish. Nursing has always led in the development of needed and effective programs for women's health during the 20th century and play an important role as political activists in promoting the WHM and gender equity, empowering women to be active in their own care (Nichols, 2000).

Many "traditional" but outdated ways of providing care to childbearing women have been replaced with partnerships. The patriarchal culture that tells women what to do, expecting them to follow without questions and treating them disrespectfully when they are unable or unwilling to comply, is being slowly transformed to include women and their families as true partners in care. Nurses are in an ideal position to take a leadership role in improving maternity care in the United States and reducing risk of preventable adverse outcomes (Simpson, 2021).

Quality of Life

In clinical ethics case analysis, it is important to consider what effect the indicated treatment will have on the patient's quality of life (Schumann & Alfandre, 2008). However, how does one define quality of life? Clearly, this is a question of perspective as perceptions of quality vary significantly from one person to the next. To honor a patient's idea of quality of life, the principles of beneficence, nonmaleficence, and respect for autonomy should be considered. Relevant questions include:

- What are the prospects, with or without treatment, for a return to normal life?
- What physical, mental, and social deficits will the patient likely experience if treatment succeeds?
- Do biases exist that might prejudice the provider's evaluation of the patient's quality of life?
- Is the patient's present or future condition such that continued life might be judged as undesirable?
- Are there plans for comfort and palliative care?

Contextual Features

The final step in the four topics method is consideration of the larger context in which the case is occurring and determining whether any contextual features are relevant to the case and its ethical analysis (Schumann & Alfandre, 2008). The context of a case is determined by multiple social factors including (among others) the dynamics of the family, the living situation of the patient, and the cultural and religious beliefs of the patient and the family. This includes consideration of the concepts of loyalty and fairness.

Health Disparities

Awareness of the contexts that influence health supports respectful, patient-centered care that incorporates lived experiences, optimizes health outcomes, improves communication, and helps reduce health and health-care inequities. Although genetics and lifestyle play an important role in shaping the overall health of individuals, researchers have demonstrated how the conditions in the environment in which people are born, live, work, and age are equally important in shaping health outcomes. These factors, referred to as social determinants of health, are shaped by historical, social, political, and economic forces and help explain the relationship between environmental conditions and individual health. Recognizing the importance of social determinants of health can help health-care providers better understand patients, effectively communicate about health-related conditions and behavior, and improve health outcomes (ACOG, Committee on Health Care for Underserved Women, 2018).

Health equity requires addressing equity not only in health care but in all human-made and modifiable determinants of health. Justice and fairness as the foundations of equity demand correcting injustices. Injustices may occur among marginalized or excluded groups of people based on their multiple and intersectional identities or other characteristics closely linked with social exclusion, marginalization, and social disadvantage (Jackson et al., 2020).

Nurses are uniquely positioned to lead health equity efforts specific to the resolution of perinatal health disparities. The power of nursing including our code of ethics is aligned with strategies, bundles, and tool kits developed to improve perinatal outcomes in partnership with the most impacted communities. Specifically, the ANA Code of Ethics (2015a) outlines the role of the professional nurse and includes the concept that nurses practice with compassion and respect for the inherent dignity, worth, and uniqueness of every individual, without exceptions for socioeconomic status, personal attributes, or the nature of the individual's health problem.

Data clearly show disparities in perinatal outcomes for Black women (Scott et al., 2019). The ANA Code of Ethics guides practice for all nurses and is one of many documents to inform ethical principles in the care of Black women. Ethical perinatal care for all pregnant women is clearly outlined in the ANA Code of Ethics; however, social determinants of health, including structural racism and discrimination, are not equally experienced by pregnant women. According to the Centers for Disease Control and Prevention (CDC), health equity is when everyone has the opportunity to be as healthy as possible (CDC, 2020). By extension, birth equity is "the assurance of the conditions of optimal births for all people with a willingness to address racial and social inequalities in a sustained effort" (National Birth Equity Collaborative, 2019, p. 1).

Multiple determinants underlying inequities in health and health care result in worse health outcomes and lower quality of health care for marginalized populations. Population health disparities are rooted in interconnected systems and interactions that occur on multiple levels. Individual population health disparities include socioeconomic status, race and ethnicity, gender, behaviors, beliefs, biology, and genetics. Intermediate factors include neighborhoods, communities, and social networks, whereas distal or structural factors comprise social and political policies and health-care institutions (Howell et al., 2018).

Relevant questions include:

- Are there family issues that might influence treatment decisions?
- Are there financial and economic factors?
- Are there religious or cultural factors?
- Are there problems of allocation of resources?
- How does the law affect treatment decisions?

Cultural Humility

A core value of nursing is cultural humility. This principle informs the ways in which people build trusting and intentional relationships with each other. Cultural humility governs language, behavior, and interactions with our partners within the health-care system. Tervalon and Murray-Garcia (1998) first defined cultural humility, which requires a commitment to four core tenets:

- Critical self-reflection and lifelong learning
- Recognizing and mitigating inherent power imbalances
- Developing mutually beneficial nonhierarchical clinical and advocacy partnerships with community members, amplifying the expertise of the residents in the community
- Creating institutional alignment and accountability

We challenge nurses to reflect on these four tenets as they engage in the care of women and their families in the childbearing period.

In summary, the four topics approach helps to highlight areas of controversy and clarify the principles underlying the circumstances of a clinical ethics case, which in turn guides discussion among care team members, patients, and families toward achieving a resolution that respects the patient's values and preferences.

Ethics and Practice: Nurses' Rights and Responsibilities

The AWHONN is the professional nursing association representing nurses in neonatal nursing. AWHONN supports the protection of an individual nurse's right to choose to participate in any reproductive health-care service or research activity. Nurses have the right under federal law to refuse to assist in the performance of any health-care procedure in keeping with personal moral, ethical, or religious beliefs (AWHONN, 2016b).

However, as AWHONN considers access to affordable and acceptable health-care services a basic human right (AWHONN, 2016a), it also advocates that nurses adhere to these principles:

- Nurses should not abandon a patient nor refuse to provide care based on prejudice or bias.
- Nurses have the professional responsibility to provide high-quality, impartial nursing care to all patients in emergency situations, regardless of the nurses' personal beliefs.
- Nurses have a professional obligation to inform their employers of any attitudes and beliefs that may interfere with essential job functions.

The core values defined by AWHONN (2019), aligned with the Code of Ethics, are as follows:

- **C**ommitment to professional and social responsibility
- **A**ccountability for personal and professional contribution
- **R**espect for diversity of and among colleagues and clients
- **I**ntegrity in exemplifying the highest standards in personal and professional behavior
- **N**ursing excellence for quality outcomes in practice, education, research, advocacy, and management
- **G**eneration of knowledge to enhance the science and practice of nursing to improve the health of women and newborns

These core values, denoted by the acronym CARING, are foundational to excellence in nursing practice and support environments that promote optimal patient outcomes and staff engagement.

STANDARDS OF PRACTICE

The ANA is charged with maintaining the scope of practice statement and standards that apply to the practice of all professional nurses. The ANA defines nursing as: "the protection, promotion, and optimization of health and abilities, prevention of illness and injury, facilitation of healing, alleviation of suffering through the diagnosis and treatment of human response, and advocacy in the care of individuals, families, groups, communities, and populations" (ANA, 2015b, p. 1). In addition to the Scope and Standards of Practice general practice standards and the Code of Ethics from the ANA (2015a, 2015b), practice standards from AWHONN help to guide professional nursing practice.

The standards summarize what AWHONN believes is the nursing profession's best judgment and optimal protocol based on current research and clinical practice (Box 2-2). AWHONN believes that these standards are helpful for all nurses engaged in the functions described.

As with most or all such standards, certain qualifications should be considered:

- These standards articulate general guidelines; additional considerations or procedures may be warranted for particular patients or settings. The best interest of an individual patient is always the touchstone of practice.
- These standards are but one source of guidance. Nurses also must act in accordance with applicable law, institutional rules and procedures, and established interprofessional arrangements concerning the division of duties.
- These standards represent optimal practice. Full compliance may not be possible at all times with all patients in all settings.
- These standards serve as a guide for optimal practice. They do not define standards of practice for employment, licensure, discipline, reimbursement, legal, or other purposes.
- These standards may change in response to changes in research and practice.

- The standards define the nurse's responsibility to the patient and the roles and behaviors to which the nurse is accountable. The definition of terms delimits the scope of the standards (Table 2-2).

The standards of practice for women and newborns describe a competent level of nursing care and consist of the six components of the nursing process: assessment, diagnosis, outcomes, planning, implementation, and evaluation (ANA, 2015b). Standard 5: Implementation has additional subcomponents—5a: Coordination of Care and 5b: Health Teaching and Health Promotion—that are new to this edition and consistent with ANA's Standards, Third Edition. Each component and subcomponent is presented with a goal statement and a list of competencies specific to the health care of women and newborns in the context of woman-, newborn-, and family-centered care. The goals and corresponding competencies reflect the values and priorities of AWHONN and relate broadly to the nurse's responsibility to the health-care consumer (AWHONN, 2019). The standards of practice are set forth to define the roles, functions, and competencies of the nurse who strives to provide high-quality service to patients. The Standards of Professional Performance delineate the various roles and behaviors for which the professional nurse is accountable. The standards are enduring and should remain largely stable over time because they reflect the philosophical values of the profession (ANA, 2015b).

LEGAL ISSUES IN DELIVERY OF CARE

Because of an ever-changing practice care environment and ethical and legal dilemmas inherent in the profession, nurses have an increased risk of being named in a malpractice litigation process. Current trends in medical malpractice lawsuits suggest that the gold standard is evidence-based practice (EBP).

The charge of "failure to communicate" is a major issue in most malpractice suits against nurses. Nurses have been found negligent for placing patients in harm's way by failing to communicate issues and concerns to colleagues, charge nurses, and physicians (Brown, 2016).

Despite increased awareness in the health-care community about preventable errors, reports indicate they still occur at alarming rates. Communication issues, most notably between providers, have been identified in nearly half of cases and include lack of timely acknowledgment and effective communication. Other factors were lack of appreciation for clinical significance or decline, variation in willingness to escalate concerns about care, and poor communication due to lack of team structure and function that often led to delays in care management and effective response (CRICO Comparative Benchmarking Report, 2018). Recent trends indicate a substantial decline in medical malpractice cases on OB, indicating multidisciplinary initiatives on communication and electronic fetal monitoring (EFM) are reducing medical malpractice claims.

BOX 2-2 | Standards for Professional Nursing Practice in the Care of Women and Newborns

Standards of Care

Standard 1. Assessment
The nurse collects pertinent health data in the context of woman-, newborn-, and family-centered care.

Standard 2. Diagnosis
The nurse analyzes assessment data to determine actual or potential diagnoses, problems, and issues relevant to the health of women and newborns.

Standard 3. Outcome Identification
The nurse identifies expected outcomes for the patient and creates an individualized plan of care in the context of woman-, newborn-, and family-centered care.

Standard 4. Planning
The nurse develops a plan of care that includes interventions and alternatives to attain expected, quantifiable outcomes for women and newborns in the context of woman-, newborn-, and family-centered care.

Standard 5. Implementation
The nurse implements the identified plan to promote woman-, newborn-, and family-centered care in a safe and timely manner.

Standard 5(a). Coordination of Care
The nurse coordinates care delivery within their scope of practice.

Standard 5(b). Health Teaching and Health Promotion
The nurse employs health teaching strategies that promote, maintain, or restore health within the context of a safe environment.

Standard 6. Evaluation
The nurse evaluates the progress toward attainment of expected outcomes in the context of woman-, newborn-, and family-centered care.

Standards of Professional Performance

Standard 7 Ethics
The nurse's decisions and actions on behalf of women, fetuses, and newborns are determined in an ethical manner and guided by a sound framework for ethical decision making.

Standard 8. Culturally Congruent Practice
The nurse practices in a manner that is congruent with cultural diversity and inclusion principles when caring for women, newborns, and families.

Standard 9. Communication
The nurse communicates with women, families, health-care providers, and the community in providing safe and holistic care.

Standard 10. Collaboration
The registered nurse collaborates with women, families, health-care providers, and the community in providing safe and holistic care.

Standard 11. Leadership
The nurse should serve as a role model, change agent, consultant, and mentor to women, families, health-care consumers, and other health-care professionals.

Standard 12. Education
The nurse acquires and maintains knowledge and competencies that reflect current evidence-based nursing practice for women, newborns, and families.

Standard 13. Evidence-Based Practice and Research
The nurse generates or integrates evidence to identify, examine, validate, and evaluate interprofessional knowledge, theories, and varied approaches in providing care to women and newborns.

Standard 14. Quality of Practice
The nurse systematically practices, evaluates, and, if indicated, implements new measures to improve the quality of nursing practice for women and newborns.

Standard 15. Professional Practice Evaluation
The nurse evaluates their own nursing practice and participates in the evaluation of others in relation to current evidence-based consumer care information, professional practice standards and guidelines, statutes, rules, and regulations.

Standard 16. Resource Utilization
The nurse studies resource factors related to safety, effectiveness, technological advances, and fiscal responsibility when planning and delivering care to women and newborns.

Standard 17. Environmental Health
The nurse practices in an environmentally safe and healthy manner when planning and delivering care.

Association of Women's Health, Obstetric and Neonatal Nurses (2019).

Because intrapartum care is inherently dynamic and nuanced, crucial evidence gaps exist. Therefore, road signs may be unclear or change quickly, leading providers to have completely different interpretations of the right course of action. Conflicting approaches are easily exacerbated by the dynamic nature of labor. Differences of opinion and prioritization are bound to occur. Data suggest that despite encouraging progress in developing cultures of safety in individual centers and systems, significant

and necessary work will be required to reverse overt disruptive behaviors in labor and delivery and to correct more subtle forms of systemic disrespect. It has been suggested that hospitals need to transparently address deficiencies in interpersonal interaction and clinical performance to achieve optimal care of childbearing women (Lyndon et al., 2014).

Maternity nursing is the most litigious of all practice areas. Contributing to this is the complexity of caring for two patients

TABLE 2-2   Terms Related to Standards

TERM	DEFINITION
Assessment	A systematic, dynamic process by which the nurse, through interaction with women, newborns, families, significant others, and health-care providers, collects, monitors, and analyzes data. Data may include the following dimensions: psychological, biotechnological, physical, sociocultural, spiritual, cognitive, developmental, and economic, as well as functional abilities and lifestyle.
Cultural consciousness	The acceptance of and respect for the attributes of diversity; this includes the acknowledgment of both similarities and differences. Culturally competent care includes recognition and awareness of the cultural perspective of those who are served. Within the scope of law and institutional policies, providers should consider how best to adapt their treatment approach in light of the values and cultural preferences of the client.
Childbearing and newborn health care	A model of care addressing health promotion, maintenance, and restoration needs of women from preconception through the postpartum period, and low-risk, high-risk, and critically ill newborns from birth through discharge and follow-up, within the social, political, economic, and environmental context of the mother's, her newborn's, and the family's lives.
Cultural congruence	The application of evidence-based nursing that is in agreement with the preferred cultural values, beliefs, worldviews, and practices of the health-care consumer and other stakeholders.
Cultural sensitivity	The ability to be appropriately responsive to the attitudes, feelings, or circumstances of groups of people that share a common and distinctive racial, national, religious, linguistic, or cultural heritage.
Diagnosis	A clinical judgment about the patient's response to actual or potential health conditions or needs. Diagnoses provide the basis for determination of a plan of nursing care to achieve expected outcomes.
Diversity	A quality that encompasses acceptance and respect related to but not limited to age, class, culture, people with special health-care needs, education level, ethnicity, family structure, gender, ideologies, political beliefs, race, religion, sexual orientation, style, and values.
Equity	The absence of unnecessary or remediable differences among groups of people, whether those groups are defined socially, demographically, or geographically. Equitable health care is accessible health care for all individuals that is affordable, high in quality, culturally sensitive, timely, and linguistically appropriate.
Evaluation	The process of determining the patient's progress toward attainment of expected outcomes and the effectiveness of nursing care.
Expected outcomes	Response to nursing interventions that is measurable, desirable, and observable.
Family-centered maternity care	A model of care based on the philosophy that the physical, sociocultural, psychological, spiritual, and economic needs of the woman and her family, however the family may be defined, should be integrated, and considered collectively. Provisions of family-centered care (FCC) require mutual trust and collaboration between the woman, her family, and health-care professionals.
Guideline	A framework developed through experts' consensus and review of literature, which guides patient-focused activities that affect provisions of care.
Implementation	The process of taking action by intervening, delegating, or coordinating. Women, newborns, families, significant others, or health-care providers may direct implementation of interventions within the plan of care.
Oppression	When a dominant group develops a series of norms and regards outsiders as inferior, oppression may be characterized by unfair behavior, ignoring others' rights, or disrespecting their dignity. Oppression of practice is when registered nurses and APRNs are not allowed to practice to the fullest extent of their education and license.
Outcome	A measurable individual, family, or community state, behavior, or perception that is responsive to nursing interventions.
Social justice	The fair and proper administration of laws conforming to the natural law that all persons, irrespective of diversity (e.g., ethnic origin, gender, economic status, race, religion, sexual orientation, age, language, literacy), are to be treated equitably and without prejudice.

TABLE 2-2   Terms Related to Standards—cont'd

TERM	DEFINITION
Standard	Authoritative statement defined and promoted by the profession and by which the quality of practice, service, or education can be evaluated.
Standards of practice	Authoritative statements that describe competent clinical nursing practice for women and newborns demonstrated through assessment, diagnosis, outcome identification, planning, implementation, and evaluation.
Standards of professional performance	Authoritative statements that describe competent behavior in the professional role, including activities related to quality of practice, education, professional practice evaluation, ethics, collegiality, collaboration, communication, research, resources and technology, and leadership.
Women's health care	A model of care addressing women's health promotion, maintenance, and restoration needs occurring across the life span and relating to one or more life strategies: adolescence, young adulthood, middle years, and older within the social, political, economic, and environmental context of their lives (AWHONN, 2019).

Association of Women's Health, Obstetric and Neonatal Nurses (2019).

at once. Five clinical situations account for most fetal and neonatal injuries and litigation in obstetrics (Simpson, 2014):

● Inability to recognize or inability to appropriately respond to intrapartum fetal compromise
● Inability to perform a timely cesarean birth (30 minutes from decision to incision) when indicated by fetal or maternal condition
● Inability to appropriately initiate resuscitation of a depressed neonate
● Inappropriate use of oxytocin or misoprostol, leading to uterine tachysystole, uterine rupture, and fetal intolerance of labor or fetal death
● Inappropriate use of forceps/vacuum or preventable shoulder dystocia

The expectation of obstetrics is a perfect outcome. Obstetrics malpractice can cause morbidity and mortality that may lead to litigation (Adinima, 2016). The number of obstetric malpractice claims represents only about 5% of all malpractice claims, but the dollar amount for the claims represents up to 35% of the total financial liability of a hospital or health-care system (Simpson, 2014). The literature indicates that patients who are more dissatisfied with the interpersonal interaction with health-care providers are more likely to pursue litigation (Hoffman, 2021; Lagana, 2000). It has also been suggested that increased use of technology may interfere with a nurse's ability to engage with women and families in a therapeutic and caring interaction.

Fetal Monitoring

Interpretation of fetal heart rate (FHR) monitoring is often a key element of litigation; this clinical issue relates to the nurse's ability to recognize and appropriately respond to intrapartal fetal compromise. For that reason, this example will serve to illustrate how nursing standards, guidelines, and policies should be the foundation of safe practice. Common allegations related to fetal monitoring are:

● Failure to accurately assess maternal and fetal status.
● Failure to appreciate a deteriorating fetal status
● Failure to treat an abnormal or indeterminate FHR
● Failure to reduce or discontinue oxytocin with an abnormal or indeterminate FHR
● Failure to correctly communicate maternal and fetal status to the care provider
● Failure to institute the chain of command in a clinical disagreement

Nurses are accountable for safe and effective FHR assessment, and failure to do so contributes to claims of nursing negligence (Gilbert, 2007; Mahlmeister, 2000; Pearson, 2011; Simpson, 2014, 2021). AWHONN (2015) provides a position statement on fetal assessment that states:

● AWHONN strongly advises that nurses complete a course of study that includes physiological interpretation of EFM and its implications for care in labor.
● Each facility should develop a policy that defines when to use EFM and auscultation of FHR and specifies frequency and documentation based on best available evidence, professional association guidelines, and expert consensus.

Effective, timely communication and collaboration among health-care professionals is central to providing quality care and optimizing patient outcomes and to ensuring Category II (indeterminate) or Category III (abnormal) FHR patterns are managed appropriately. Organizational resources and systems should be in place to support timely interventions when FHR is indeterminate or abnormal (Simpson, 2014; 2021; Simpson & Knox, 2003). Uniform FHR terminology and interpretation are necessary to facilitate appropriate communication and legally defensible documentation (Lyndon & Ali, 2015).

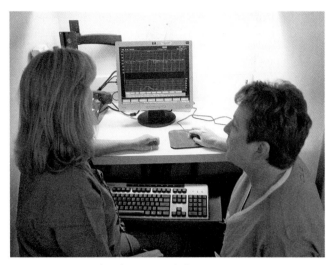

FIGURE 2-2 Together the nurse and physician review an EFM strip.

Interpretation of FHR data can sometimes result in conflict. There may be agreement about ominous patterns and normal patterns, but often care providers encounter patterns that fall between extremes (Freeman, 2002; O'Brien-Abel & Simpson, 2021). Conflicts in the clinical setting must be resolved quickly but sometimes cannot be resolved between caregivers immediately involved. When this occurs:

● The nurse must initiate the course of action when the clinical situation is a matter of maternal or fetal well-being.
● In a case of a primary care provider not responding to an abnormal FHR or a deteriorating clinical situation, the nurse should use the chain of command to resolve the situation, advocate for the patient's safety, and seek necessary interventions to avoid a potentially adverse outcome.
● At the first level, notify the immediate supervisor for assistance. Further steps are defined by the structure of the institution, and a policy outlining communication for the chain of command should exist (Fig. 2–2).

Risk Management

Risk management is a systems approach to litigation prevention that involves the identification of systems problems, analysis, and treatment of risks before a suit is brought. There are two key components of a successful risk-management program:

● Avoiding preventable adverse outcomes to the fetus during labor requires competent care providers who use consistent and current FHR-monitoring language in practice environments with systems in place that permit timely clinical intervention.
● Decreasing risk of liability exposure includes methods to demonstrate evidence that the provision of appropriate, timely care accurately reflects maternal-fetal status before, during, and after interventions occurred.

Not all adverse or unexpected outcomes are preventable or result from poor care. Some suggest the risk of liability can be reduced, and injuries to mothers and neonates can be reduced when all members of the perinatal team follow two basic tenets (Simpson, 2014; Simpson & Knox, 2003):

1. Use applicable evidence or published standards and guidelines as the foundation of care.
2. Make patient safety a priority over convenience, productivity, and costs.

All nurses need to bear in mind that the most—and sometimes the only—defensible nursing actions are those whose sole focus is on the health and well-being of the patient. AWHONN provides guidelines and recommendations for safe staffing of perinatal units to promote safe and effective perinatal nursing care (AWHONN, 2010).

EVIDENCE-BASED PRACTICE

EBP is widely recognized as the key to improving health-care quality and patient outcomes. EBP is defined as "Integrate best current evidence with clinical expertise and patient/family preferences and values for delivery of optimal health care" (Cronenwett et al., 2007, p. 126). EBP reflects a very important global paradigm shift in how to view health-care outcomes, how the discipline is taught, how practice is conducted, and how health-care practices are evaluated for quality. EBP and conduct of research have distinct purposes, questions, approaches, and evaluation methods. Conduct of research is typically defined as the systematic investigation of a phenomenon that addresses research questions or hypotheses to create generalizable knowledge and advance the state of the science.

In contrast, EBP is the conscientious and judicious use of current best evidence in conjunction with clinical expertise, patient values, and circumstances to guide health-care decisions. EBP is the actual application of evidence in practice (the "doing of" EBP), whereas translation science is the study of implementation interventions, factors, and contextual variables that effect knowledge uptake and use in practices and communities. Translation science is research; various research designs and methods are used to address the research questions or hypotheses. Advancements in translation science expedite and sustain the successful integration of evidence in practice to improve care delivery, population health, and health outcomes (Titler, 2018).

In the early 1990s, agencies were established with interdisciplinary teams to gather and assess available research literature and develop evidence-based clinical guidelines. Previously the Agency for Healthcare Research and Quality (AHRQ) served as a clearinghouse for clinical guidelines (www.guidelines.gov). Since that agency was defunded in 2018, other resources for clinical guidelines are presented in Box 2-3.

Most have adopted the definition of EBP to include the integration of best *research evidence, clinical expertise,* and *patient values* in making decisions about patient care. Clinical expertise comes from knowledge and experience over time and includes professional practice opinions and professional position statements. Patient values are the unique circumstances of each patient and should include individual preferences. Best research evidence includes current findings from both quantitative and qualitative research methods.

BOX 2-3 | Resources for Clinical Guidelines

Guideline Central has a Web site and mobile app that includes thousands of other guideline summaries and clinical resources. Examples of the freely available resources include:

2,000 guideline summaries syndicated from the National Guideline Clearinghouse

MEDLINE/PubMed ClinicalTrials.gov search access

Quality measures from NGC's sister site, the National Quality Measures Clearinghouse (NQMC)

Read more at https://www.guidelinecentral.com/alternatives-to-ahrqs-national-guidelines-clearinghouse/

CRITICAL COMPONENT

Evidence-Based Practice in Nursing

EBP definition: Integrate best current evidence with clinical expertise and patient/family preferences and values for delivery of optimal health care.

Nurses are in a unique position to explore a woman's preferences and advocate for the use of best current evidence and clinical expertise for delivery of optimal health care. Some suggestions to foster EBP in clinical settings include the following:

- Describe and locate reliable sources for evidence reports and clinical practice guidelines.
- Question rationale for routine approaches to care that result in less-than-desired outcomes or adverse events.
- Base individualized care plan on patient values, clinical expertise, and evidence.

Evidence-Based Practice: Cochrane Reviews

An important resource for EBP is systematic reviews. One such source is Cochrane Reviews (www.cochrane.org). The Cochrane Review is an international consortium of experts who perform systematic reviews and meta-analysis on all available data, evaluating the body of evidence on a clinical topic for quality of study design and study results. These reviews look at randomized clinical trials of interventions related to a specific clinical problem and, after assessing the findings from rigorous studies, make recommendations for clinical practice. They consider the randomized controlled trial (RCT) the gold standard of research evidence.

Although not absolute, a hierarchy can be helpful when evaluating research evidence. When considering potential interventions, nurses should look for the highest level of evidence (LOE) relevant to the clinical problem. A hierarchy of strength of evidence for treatment decisions is presented in Figure 2–3, indicating unsystematic clinical observations as the lowest level and systematic reviews of RCTs as the highest level of evidence. There are many levels of evidence hierarchies, and they have continued to evolve and change with time (Hokanson Hawks, 2016).

Utilization of Research in Clinical Practice

Professional nursing practice is grounded in the translation of current evidence into practice (American Association of Colleges of Nursing [AACN], 2008). Although EBP is central to the knowledge base for nursing (Fain, 2017; O'Brien-Abel & Simpson, 2021), its critics dislike the central role of RCTs in providing evidence for nursing, claiming that the context and experience of nursing care are removed from evaluation of evidence. The principles of evidence-based health care have been driven by requirements to deliver quality care within economically constrained conditions. Some nurses have adopted a predominantly medical model of evidence, with RCTs as the central, methodological approach to defining good evidence. EBN has been criticized for this stance, citing the lack of relevance of RCTs for some important areas of nursing practice. Criticisms stem from the fact that RCTs are given an illusionary stance of credibility when there may not be credible evidence relevant to nursing practice and theory (Fawcett & Garity, 2009). Most experts now believe both quantitative and qualitative research findings are relevant to inform the practice of nursing.

To enhance EBP and support the choices of childbearing women and families, we must utilize quantitative *and* qualitative research findings in practice (Durham, 2002). Although nursing has developed models for assisting practitioners in applying research findings in practice (Cronenwett, 1995; Stetler, 1994; Titler & Goode, 1995), these models only assist in applying quantitative research findings for utilization in practice.

Qualitative research is increasingly recognized as an integral part of EBP. Qualitative researchers investigate naturally occurring phenomena and describe, analyze, and sometimes theorize on these occurrences. They also describe context and relationships of key factors related to the phenomena. This work is conducted in the "real world," not in a controlled situation, and yields important findings for practice. Reports of qualitative research are conveyed in language that may be more understandable to practitioners. Story lines from qualitative research are often a more compelling and culturally resonant way to communicate research findings, particularly to staff, affected groups, and policy makers (Sandelowski, 1996). Guidelines for utilization of qualitative research findings are outlined by Swanson, Durham, and Albright (1997) and include evaluating the findings or proposed theory for its context, generalizability, and fit with one's own practice; evaluating concepts, conditions, and variation explained in findings; and evaluating findings for enhancing and informing one's practice.

In the current era of cost containment, nurses must know what is going on in their patients' lives, because practitioners are limited to interacting with clients within an ever-smaller window of time and space. Qualitative research can assist in bringing practitioners an awareness of that larger world and its implications for

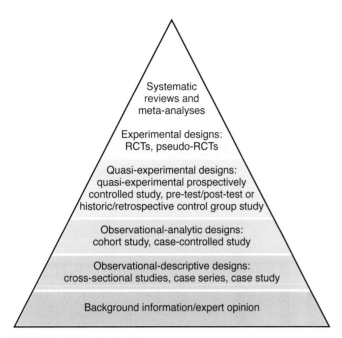

FIGURE 2–3 Levels of evidence.

their scope of practice (Swanson et al., 1997). Qualitative research describes and analyzes our patients' realities. The research findings have the capacity to influence conceptual thinking and cause practitioners to question assumptions about a phenomenon in practice (Cronenwett, 1995). Incorporating qualitative research as evidence to support research-based practice can enhance nursing practice and can resolve some of the tensions between art and science with which nurses sometimes find themselves struggling (Durham, 2002). Experts have presented guidelines for utilizing qualitative research in practice that can enhance clinicians' ability to use qualitative findings for EBP (Miller, 2010; Sandelowski, 1996; Sandelowski & Barroso, 2003; Thorne, 2009).

Research Utilization Challenges

Health care often falls short in translating research into practice and improvement of care. Although adopting EBP has resulted in improvements in patient outcome, large gaps remain between what we know and what we do. Failing to use the latest health-care research is costly and harmful, and can lead to ineffective care. Many innovations have become common practice in perinatal nursing, such as EFM and family-centered care. These changes in care were influenced by factors such as medical and technological innovations and social context of the time and families' preferences.

The increasing use of technology during birth, threats of litigation, and providing the best care under time and cost constraints are the realities facing perinatal nurses today. Continuous EFM in labor is one of the most common interventions during labor. However, there is little evidence to support the use of continuous EFM, especially with low-risk patients. One Cochrane Review compared the efficacy and safety of routine continuous EFM of labor with intermittent auscultation (Alfirevic et al., 2017). The reviewers concluded that use of routine EFM

has no measurable impact on infant morbidity and mortality. In the latest review, the authors concluded continuous EFM during labor is associated with a reduction in neonatal seizures but no significant differences in cerebral palsy, infant mortality, or other standard measures of neonatal well-being. However, continuous EFM was associated with an increase in cesarean births and operative vaginal births. They noted the real challenge is how to convey this uncertainty to women to enable them to make an informed choice without compromising normal labor.

Additionally, an example of an evidence-based clinical practice in the perinatal setting is the limited use of intermittent fetal monitoring (IFM). IFM is a "high touch, low tech" obstetric procedure used to monitor the fetus during labor. Utilization of IFM is recommended by professional organizations as a safe and reasonable method to evaluate fetal well-being in low-risk pregnancies during labor and birth (AWHONN, 2015; Wisner et al 2019). Use of IFM is associated with fewer cesarean deliveries with no difference in newborn health outcomes when compared with other fetal monitoring methods (Alfirevic et al., 2017). IFM allows more freedom of movement, associated with decreased pain and expedited fetal descent. It may also lead to more favorable birth experiences. Despite these benefits, IFM is rarely used in intrapartum settings. A recent study examined labor and delivery nurses' perceptions of barriers to research utilization in the work setting. The issue of time has consistently been reported as a barrier to translating research into practice. This study confirms this finding. Specifically, if nurses reported nurse-to-patient ratios as a problem in providing IFM, then their perception of barriers to research utilization increased (Heelan-Fancher et al., 2019).

Although EBP is the goal of nursing care and has become the standard of care in the United States, the evidence about EFM has not been used in practice. Research evidence does not support the use of continuous EFM. Use can instead be attributed to habit, convenience, liability, staffing, and economics. It is no longer acceptable for nurses to continue doing things the way they have always been done without questioning if it is the best approach. Nurses can support EBP by participating in multidisciplinary teams that generate research-based practice guidelines.

Barriers to Evidence-Based Practice

Despite concerns that the rise of EBP threatens to transform nursing practice into a performative exercise disciplined by scientific knowledge, others have found that scientific knowledge is by no means the preeminent source of knowledge within the dynamic settings of health care (Angus et al., 2003). Nurses face challenges in translating research into practice because of several factors, including a lack of time, training, and mentoring (Johnston et al., 2016; Mazurek Melnyk et al., 2016; Simpson, 2014). Barriers commonly cited focus on areas of knowledge, skills, and attitudes:

- Inadequate knowledge and skills in EBP by nurses and other health-care professionals
- Lack of cultures and environments that support EBP
- Misperceptions that EBP takes too much time

- Outdated organizational politics and policies
- Limited resources and tools available for point-of-care providers, including budgetary investment in EBP by chief nurse executives
- Resistance from colleagues, nurse managers, and nurse leaders
- Inadequate numbers of EBP mentors in health-care systems
- Academic programs that continue to teach baccalaureate, master's, and doctor of nursing practice students the rigorous process of how to conduct research instead of taking an evidence-based approach to care

A current systematic review of nursing literature on barriers to research utilization reported lack of awareness about research, lack of authority to change practice, overwhelming publications, and lack of compiled literature were the most identified barriers to research utilization (Tuppal et al., 2019). On the other hand, the reviewers note organizational and colleague support, and continuing education as both personal and professional commitment can further facilitate research utilization.

Strategies to Enhance Evidence-Based Practice

Authors describe a strategic approach to engaging, empowering, and supporting a nursing workforce to participate in EBP (McKeever et al., 2016). This can be facilitated through the formation of a committee dedicated to developing and implementing evidence-based clinical guidelines that support nursing practice. Other strategies to improve EBP in clinical practice include initiatives driven by an organizational desire to reduce variation in nursing care delivered to patients and families. Recognizing that some nurses do not possess requisite skills to conduct a literature search, critically appraise pertinent literature, and synthesize evidence into a clinical guideline, the Nursing Clinical Effectiveness Committee established processes to support nurses in activities to foster the development, implementation, and evaluation of clinical guidelines. Support provided to the staff should include identifying areas of practice requiring clinical guidance, evidence identification and evaluation, clinical guideline development, and strategic development of an education-based implementation plan to promote guideline adoption into practice (McKeever et al., 2016).

Social determinants of health are conditions in which people are born, grow, work, live, and age that affect health and quality of life. These factors are strongly associated with disparities in reproductive health status and outcomes. Nurses require a comprehensive understanding of social determinants and their associations with health outcomes to provide patient-centered and evidence-based care (Lathrop, 2020). Nurses can advance health equity by screening for social determinants that affect women and collaborating to address complex social needs.

Resistance to change can be difficult to overcome. Therefore, strategies that target knowledge, skills, and attitudes must be utilized for successful implementation of EBP clinical guidelines. These can include:

- Grand rounds
- Simulation training
- Learning and skills fairs
- Posters
- One-on-one meetings
- Case conferences

Tools have been developed to guide nurses and students through the basic steps to locate and critically appraise online scientific literature while linking users to quality electronic resources to support EBP. As the world becomes increasingly digital, advances in technology have changed how students access evidence-based information, yet some research suggests a limited ability to locate quality online research and a lack of skills needed to evaluate the scientific literature (Long et al., 2016). Earlier publications outline a general attitude and offer specific suggestions to promote EBP (Melnyk & Fineout-Overholt, 2011). They include:

- Cultivating a spirit of inquiry within an EBP culture and environment
- Asking the burning clinical question in PICOT (i.e., **P**atient population, **I**ntervention or **I**ssue of interest, **C**omparison intervention or group, **O**utcome, and **T**ime frame) format
- Searching for and collecting the most relevant best evidence
- Critically appraising the evidence (i.e., rapid critical appraisal, evaluation, synthesis, and recommendations)
- Integrating the best evidence with one's clinical expertise and patient preferences and values in making a practice decision or change
- Evaluating outcomes of the practice decision or change based on evidence
- Disseminating the outcomes of the EBP decision or change

AWHONN Perinatal Quality Measures

AWHONN advances the nursing profession by providing evidence-based education and practice resources, legislative programs, research, and interprofessional collaboration to help them deliver the highest quality care for women and newborns. Because actions of nurses have a significant impact on patient outcomes, measuring the quality of care provided by registered nurses is a vital component of health-care improvement. Nurses' expert knowledge can and should shape the care environment and influence the decisions of patients. Since 2012, AWHONN has developed an introductory set of nursing care quality measures. These measures, also referred to as *nurse-sensitive measures,* align with The Joint Commission's Perinatal Care Core Measures Set. This is one of many steps AWHONN is taking to lead and support efforts to improve the quality of health care provided to women and newborns (2014). Initiatives reflect current priorities and EBP and are listed in Box 2-4.

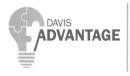

BOX 2-4 | AWHONN Nursing Care Quality Measures

Examples of AWHONN Nursing Care Quality Measures

Triage of a Pregnant Woman and Her Fetus(es)

The purpose of this measure is to increase the percentage of pregnant women who present to the labor and birth unit with a report of a real or perceived problem or an emergency condition who are triaged by a registered nurse or nurse-midwife within 10 minutes of arrival.

Second Stage of Labor: Mother-Initiated, Spontaneous Pushing

The purpose of this measure is to support mother-initiated, spontaneous pushing in the second stage of labor.

Skin-to-Skin Is Initiated Immediately Following Birth

The purpose of this measure is to increase the percentage of healthy, term newborns who are placed in skin-to-skin contact with their mothers within the first 5 minutes following birth.

Duration of Uninterrupted Skin-to-Skin Contact

The purpose of this measure is to increase the percentage of healthy, term newborns of stable mothers who receive uninterrupted skin-to-skin contact for at least 60 minutes.

Eliminating Supplementation of Breast Milk-Fed, Healthy, Term Newborns

The purpose of this measure is to reduce the percentage of healthy, term newborns fed any breast milk who also receive supplementation with water, glucose water, or formula without medical indication during their hospital stays.

Protect Maternal Milk Volume for Premature Infants Admitted to the NICU

The purpose of this measure is to increase the percentage of mothers of premature newborns admitted to the NICU who receive a breast pump, receive the appropriate instruction and support from a registered nurse, and have the nurse remain with them throughout the first pumping session within 6 hours postbirth.

Initial Contact With Parents Following a Neonatal Transport

The purpose of this measure is to increase the percentage of mothers who receive a phone call from the referral hospital's NICU nurse within 4 hours of infant arrival to the referral hospital.

Perinatal Grief Support

The purpose of this measure is to increase the percentage of women who are offered support for grief responses after perinatal loss.

Women's Health and Wellness Coordination Throughout the Life Span

The purpose of this measure is to increase the percentage of women who are offered annual health and wellness screening in the ambulatory care setting.

Continuous Labor Support

The purpose of this measure is to increase the percentage of women in labor who receive continuous, nonpharmacological labor support customized to meet their physical and emotional needs provided by a registered nurse (RN) or by a certified doula who follows the guidance of the RN.

Partial Labor Support

The purpose of this measure is to increase the percentage of women who receive nonpharmacological labor support from an RN at least once every hour during intrapartum labor care.

Freedom of Movement During Labor

The purpose of this measure is to increase the percentage of women with term pregnancies who experience freedom of movement during labor.

Association of Women's Health, Obstetric and Neonatal Nurses (2014).

REFERENCES

Aderemi, R. A. (2016). Ethical issues in maternal and child health nursing: Challenges faced by maternal and child health nurses and strategies for decision making. *International Journal of Medicine and Biomedical Research, 5,* 67–76. https://doi.org/10.14194/ijmbr.5.2.3

Adinima, J. (2016). Litigations and the obstetrician in clinical practice. *Annals of Medical and Health Sciences, 6*(2), 74–79.

Alfirevic, Z., Devane, D., Gyte, G. M., & Cuthbert, A. (2017). Continuous cardiotocography (CTG) as a form of electronic fetal monitoring (EFM) for fetal assessment during labor. *Cochrane Database of Systematic Reviews,* CD006066. https://doi.org/10.1002/14651858 CD006066.pub3

American Association of Colleges of Nursing. (2008). *The essentials of baccalaureate education for professional nursing practice.* American Association of Colleges of Nursing.

American College of Obstetricians and Gynecologists. (2016). Refusal of medically recommended treatment during pregnancy. Committee Opinion No. 664. *Obstetric Gynecology, 2016*(127), e175–e182.

American College of Obstetricians and Gynecologists, Committee on Health Care for Underserved Women. (2018). ACOG Committee Opinion No. 729: Importance of social determinants of health and cultural awareness in the delivery of reproductive health care. *Obstetrics and Gynecology, 131*(1), e43–e48. https://doi.org/10.1097/AOG.0000000000002459

American Nurses Association. (2015a). *Code of ethics for nurses with interpretive statements.* American Nurses Publishing.

American Nurses Association. (2015b). *Nursing: Scope and standards of practice* (3rd ed.). Author.

Angus, J., Hodnett, E., & O'Brien-Pallas, L. (2003). Implementing evidence-based nursing practice: A tale of two intrapartum nursing units. *Nursing Inquiry, 10*(4), 218–228.

Association of Women's Health, Obstetric and Neonatal Nurses. (2010). *Guidelines for professional registered nurse staffing for perinatal units.* Author.

Association of Women's Health, Obstetric and Neonatal Nurses. (2014). *Women's health and perinatal nursing care quality refined draft measures specifications.* Author.

Association of Women's Health, Obstetric and Neonatal Nurses. (2015). *AWHONN position statement: Fetal heart monitoring.* Author.

Association of Women's Health, Obstetric and Neonatal Nurses. (2016a). *AWHONN position statement: Ethical decision making in the clinical setting.* Author.

Association of Women's Health, Obstetric and Neonatal Nurses. (2016b). *Rights and responsibilities of nurses related to reproductive health care.* Author.

Association of Women's Health, Obstetric and Neonatal Nurses. (2019). *Standards for professional nursing practice in the care of women and newborns* (8th ed.). Author.

Brown, G. (2016). Averting malpractice issues in today's nursing practice. *ABNF Journal, 27*(2), 25–27.

Centers for Disease Control and Prevention. (2020). *Health equity.* https://www.cdc.gov/healthequity/inclusion

Chervenak, F., McCullough, L., & Burke Sosa, M. E. (2013). Ethical challenges. In N. Troirano, C. Harvey, & B. Flood Chez (Eds.), *High-risk & critical care obstetrics* (3rd ed.). Lippincott, Williams & Wilkens.

CRICO Comparative Benchmarking Report. (2018). *Medical malpractice in America.* CRICO Strategies Boston, MA.

Cronenwett, L. (1995). Effective methods for disseminating research findings to nurses in practice. *Nursing Clinics of North America, 30*(3), 429–438.

Cronenwett, L., Sherwood, G., Barnsteiner, J., Disch, J., Johnson, J., Mitchell, P., . . . Warren, J. (2007). Quality and safety education for nurses. Nursing Outlook, 55(3), 122–131. https//doi.org/10.1016/j.outlook.2007.02.006

Durham, R. (2002). Women, work and midwifery. In R. Mander & V. Flemming (Eds.), *Failure to progress* (pp. 122–132). Routledge.

Fain, J. (2017). *Reading, understanding and applying nursing research* (5th ed.). F.A. Davis Co.

Fawcett, J., & Garity, J. (2009). *Evaluating research for evidence-based nursing practice.* F.A. Davis.

Freeman, R. (2002). Problems with intrapartal fetal heart rate monitoring interpretation and patient management. *American Journal of Obstetrics and Gynecology, 100*(4), 813–816.

Gilbert, E. (2007). *Manual of high-risk pregnancy and delivery.* C. V. Mosby.

Heelan-Fancher, L., Edmonds, J. K., & Jones, E. J. (2019). Decreasing barriers to research utilization among labor and delivery nurses. *Nursing Research, 68*(6), E1–E7. https://doi.org/10.1097/NNR.0000000000000388

Hoffman, J. (2021). *In the name of respect.* CRICO Strategies Boston, MA.

Hokanson Hawks, J. (2016). Changing the level of evidence. *Urologic Nursing, 36*(6), 265–281. https://doi.org/10.7257/1053-816X.2016.36.6.265

Howell, E. A., Brown, H., Brumley, J., Bryant, A. S., Caughey, A. B., Cornell, A. M., . . . Grobman, W. A. (2018). Reduction of peripartum racial and ethnic disparities: A conceptual framework and maternal safety consensus bundle. *Obstetrics and Gynecology, 131*(5), 770–782. https://doi.org/10.1097/AOG.0000000000002475

Iacobucci, T. A., Daly, B. J., Lindell, D., & Griffin, M. Q. (2013). Professional values, self-esteem, and ethical confidence of baccalaureate nursing students. *Nursing Ethics, 20*(4), 479–490. https://doi.org/10.1177/0969733012458608

Jackson, F., Rashied-Henry, K., Braveman, P., Dominguez, T., Ramos, D., Maseru, N., . . . James, A. (2020). A prematurity collaborative birth equity consensus statement for mothers and babies. *Maternal Child Health Journal, 24,* 1231–1237. https://doi.org/10.1007/s10995-020-02960-0

Johnston, B., Coole, C., Feakes, R., Whitworth, G., Tyrell, T., & Hardy, B. (2016). Exploring the barriers to and facilitators of implementing research into practice. *British Journal of Community Nursing, 21*(8), 392–398.

Jonsen, A. R., Siegler, M., & Winslade, W. J. (2002). *Clinical ethics: A practical approach to ethical decision in clinical medicine* (5th ed.). McGraw-Hill.

Lagana, K. (2000). The "right" to a caring relationship: The law and ethic of care. *Journal of Perinatal & Neonatal Nursing, 14*(2), 12–24.

Lantos, J. D. (2018). Ethical problems in decision making in the neonatal ICU. *New England Journal of Medicine, 379*(19), 1851–1860. https://doi.org/10.1056/NEJMra1801063. PMID: 30403936

Lantos, J. D. (2019, March). Ethical problems in decision making in the neonatal ICU. *Obstetric Anesthesia Digest, 39*(1), 44. https://doi.org/10.1097/01.aoa.0000552919.43448.d2

Lathrop, B. (2020). Moving toward health equity by addressing social determinants of health. *Nursing for Women's Health, 24*(1), 36–44.

Long, J., Gannaway, P., Ford, C., Doumit, R., Zeeni, N., Sukkarieh-Haraty, O., & Song, H. (2016). Effectiveness of a technology-based intervention to teach evidence-based practice: The EBR tool. *Worldviews on Evidence-Based Nursing, 13*(1), 59–65.

Lyndon, A., & Ali, L. U. (2015). *Fetal heart monitoring: Principles and practices* (5th ed.). Kendall Hunt Publishing.

Lyndon, A., Zlatnik, M. G., Maxfield, D. G., Lewis, A., McMillan, C., & Kennedy, H. P. (2014). Contributions of clinical disconnections and unresolved conflict to failures in intrapartum safety. *Journal of Obstetric, Gynecologic & Neonatal Nursing, 43*(1), 2–12.

Mahlmeister, L. (2000). Legal implications of fetal heart rate assessment. *Journal of Obstetric, Gynecologic, & Neonatal Nursing, 29,* 517–526.

Mattson, L., & Smith, J. (2016). *Core curriculum for maternal-newborn nursing* (5th ed.). Elsevier.

Mazurek Melnyk, B., Gallagher-Ford, L., & Fineout-Overholt, E. (2016). Improving healthcare quality, patient outcomes, and costs with evidence-based practice. *Reflections on Nursing Leadership, 42*(3), 1–8.

McKeever, S., Twomey, B., Hawley, M., Lima, S., Kinney, S., & Newall, F. (2016). Engaging a nursing workforce in evidence-based practice: Introduction of a nursing clinical effectiveness committee. *Worldviews on Evidence-Based Nursing, 13*(1), 85–88. https://doi.org/10.1111/wvn.12119

Melnyk, B. M., & Fineout-Overholt, E. (2011). *Evidence-based practice in nursing & healthcare. A guide to best practice* (pp. 1–24). Wolters Kluwer/Lippincott Williams & Wilkins.

Miller, W. R. (2010). Qualitative research findings as evidence: Utility in nursing practice. *Clinical Nurse Specialist, 24*(4), 191–193. https://doi.org/10.1097/NUR.0b013e3181e36087

Mills, M., & Cortezzo, D. E. (2020). Moral distress in the neonatal intensive care unit: What is it, why it happens, and how we can address it. *Frontiers in Pediatrics, 8,* 581. https://doi.org/10.3389/fped.2020.00581

National Birth Equity Collaborative. (2019). *Solutions.* https://birthequity.org/about/birth-equity

Nichols, F. H. (2000). History of the women's health movement in the 20th century. *Journal of Obstetric, Gynecologic, & Neonatal Nursing, 29,* 56–64. https://doi.org/10.1111/j.1552-6909.2000.tb02756.x

O'Brien-Abel, N., & Simpson, K. R. (2021). Fetal assessment during labor. In K. Simpson, P. Creehan, N. Obrien-Abel, C. Roth, & A. Rohan (Eds.), *Perinatal nursing* (5th ed.). Wolters Kluwer.

Pearson, N. (2011). Oxytocin safety. *Nursing for Women's Health, 15*(2), 110–117.

Ruhl, C., Golub, Z., Santa-Donato, A., Cockey, C., Davis, C. & Bingham, D., (2016). Providing nursing care women and babies deserve. *Nursing for Women's Health, 20*(2), 129–133.

Sandelowski, M. (1996). Using qualitative methods in intervention studies. *Research in Nursing and Health, 19,* 359–364.

Sandelowski, M., & Barroso, J. (2003). Classifying the findings in qualitative studies. *Qualitative Health Research, 13,* 905–923.

Schumann, J. H., & Alfandre, D. (2008). Clinical ethical decision making: The four topics approach. *Seminars Medical Practice, 11,* 36–42.

Scott, K. A., Britton, L., & McLemore, M. R. (2019, April/June). The ethics of perinatal care for Black women. *The Journal of Perinatal & Neonatal Nursing, 33*(2), 108–115. https://doi.org/10.1097/JPN.0000000000000394

Simpson, K. R. (2014). Perinatal patient safety and professional liability issues. In K. Simpson, P. Creehan, & AWHONN (Eds.), *Perinatal nursing* (4th ed.). Lippincott Williams & Wilkins.

Simpson, K. R. (2021). Perinatal patient safety and quality. In K. Simpson, P. Creehan, N. Obrien-Abel, C. Roth, & A. Rohan (Eds.), *Perinatal nursing* (5th ed.). Wolters Kluwer.

Simpson, K. R., & Knox, G. E. (2003). Common area of litigation related to care during labor and birth: Recommendations to promote patient safety and decrease risk exposure. *Journal of Perinatal and Neonatal Nursing, 17*(2), 110–125.

Stelwagen M. A., van Kempen A. A. M. W., Westmaas A., Blees Y. J., & Scheele F. (2020). Integration of maternity and neonatal care to empower parents. *Journal of Obstetric, Gynecologic, and Neonatal Nursing, 49*(1), 65–77.

Stephenson, C. (2016). Ethics. In S. Mattson & J. Smith (Eds.), *Core curriculum for maternal-newborn nursing* (5th ed.). Elsevier.

Stetler, C. (1994). Refinement of the Stetler/Marram model for application of research findings to practice. *Nursing Outlook, 42,* 15–25.

Swanson, J., Durham, R., & Albright, J. (1997). Clinical utilization/application of qualitative research. In J. Morse (Ed.), *Completing a qualitative project: Details and dialogue* (pp. 253–282). Sage.

Swartz, A., Hoffmann, T. J., Cretti, E., Burton, C. W., Eagen-Torkko, M., Levi, A. J., . . . McLemore, M. R. (2020). Attitudes of California registered nurses about abortion. *Journal of Obstetric, Gynecologic & Neonatal Nursing, 49*(5), 475–486. https://doi.org/10.1016/j.jogn.2020.06.005

Tervalon, M., & Murray-Garcia, J. (1998). Cultural humility versus cultural competence: A critical distinction in defining physician training outcomes in multicultural education. *Journal of Health Care for the Poor and Underserved, 9*(2), 111–125.

Tessman, L. (2020). Moral distress in health care: When is it fitting? *Medicine, Health Care, and Philosophy, 23*(2), 165–177. https://doi.org/10.1007/s11019-020-09942-7

Thorne, S. (2009). The role of qualitative research within an evidence-based context: Can metasynthesis be the answer? *International Journal of Nursing Studies, 46*(4), 569–575.

Titler, M. G. (2018, May 31). Translation research in practice: An introduction. *The Online Journal of Issues in Nursing, 23*(2), Manuscript 1.

Titler, M. G., & Goode, C. (1995). Research utilization. *Nursing Clinics of North America, 30*(3), xv.

Tuppal, C. P., Vega, P. D., Ninobla, M. M. G., Reñosa, M. D., Al-Battashi, A., Arquiza, G., & Baua, E. P. (2019). Revisiting the barriers to and facilitators of research utilization in nursing: A systematic review. *Nurse Media Journal of Nursing, 9*(1), 90–102. https://doi.org/proxylib.csueastbay.edu/10.14710/nmjn.v9i1.20827

The Antepartal Period

Genetics, Conception, Fetal Development, and Reproductive Technology

3

Linda L. Chapman, RN, PhD

LEARNING OUTCOMES

Upon completion of this chapter, the student will be able to:

1. Discuss the relevance of genetics within the context of the care of the childbearing family.
2. Identify critical components of conception, embryonic development, and fetal development.
3. Describe the development and function of the placenta and amniotic fluid.
4. List the common causes of infertility.
5. Describe the common diagnostic tests used to identify causes of infertility.
6. Describe the most common methods used in assisted fertility.
7. Discuss the ethical and emotional implications of assisted reproductive therapies (ART).

CONCEPTS

Cellular Regulation
Growth and Development
Health Promotion
Oxygenation
Reproduction and Sexuality
Stress and Coping

GENETICS AND THE CHILDBEARING FAMILY

Genes, the basic functional and physical units of heredity, are composed of DNA and protein. The human genome—the complete set of an organism's DNA—contains approximately 30,000 genes. Each human cell contains 46 chromosomes, including 22 homologous pairs of chromosomes and one pair of sex chromosomes designated as either XX (female) or XY (male). Each chromosome contains numerous genes. Genotype is a person's genetic makeup, whereas phenotype is the way in which these genes are outwardly expressed, such as eye color, hair color, or height.

Advances in genetics (the study of heredity) and genomics (the study of genes and their function and related technology) are providing better methods for:

● Preventing diseases and abnormalities
● Diagnosing diseases
● Predicting health risks
● Personalizing treatment plans

CRITICAL COMPONENT

Genetics and Genomics

"The main difference between genomics and genetics is that genetics scrutinizes the functioning and composition of the single gene whereas genomics addresses all genes and their interrelationships in order to identify their combined influence on the growth and development of the organism" (World Health Organization [WHO], 2012).

Dominant and Recessive Inheritance

Genes are either dominant or recessive. When dominant and recessive genes are paired, such as a gene for brown eyes and a gene for blue eyes, the traits of the dominant gene (brown eyes) will be present. If both genes in a pair are recessive, the recessive trait will be present.

Genetic diseases and disorders are often related to a defective recessive gene. They are present at birth when a person has a pair of genes with the same defect on both (Fig. 3–1). People

Autosomal Recessive-Cystic Fibrosis

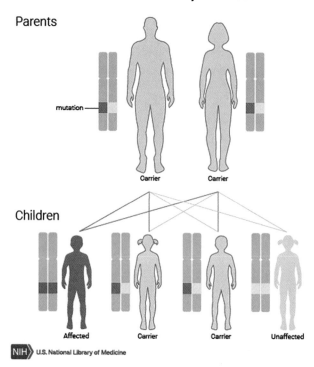

FIGURE 3–1 Two unaffected parents each carry one copy of the mutation for cystic fibrosis. They have one affected child and three unaffected (two of which carry one copy of the affected gene).

who have just one defective gene carry the disorder and can pass it on to a child but do not have it themselves. Examples of these autosomal-recessive disorders include cystic fibrosis, sickle cell anemia, thalassemia, and Tay-Sachs disease (Table 3-1). Autosomal-dominant disorders such as Huntington's disease (Fig. 3–2), familial hypercholesterolemia, and xeroderma pigmentation present when one or both genes in a pair carry the defect.

Sex-Linked Inheritance

Conditions can be either X-linked inheritance or Y-linked inheritance. With X-linked inheritance:

- The mutated gene is located only on the X chromosome.
- The gene can be either recessive or dominant.
- Male children who receive an X chromosome with a mutated gene present with the disorder when the Y chromosome does not carry that gene; the gene, even though it may be recessive, becomes dominant.
- Female children who have one X chromosome with a sex-linked trait disorder do not present with the trait but are carriers of the trait.
- Hemophilia is an example of an X-linked inheritance disorder (Fig. 3–3).
- With Y-linked inheritance, the mutation is located only on the Y chromosome. This means the disease can be passed only from father to son.

TABLE 3-1   Genetic Diseases

DISEASE (PATTERN OF INHERITANCE)	DESCRIPTION
Sickle-cell anemia (R)	The most common genetic disease among people of African ancestry. Sickle-cell hemoglobin forms rigid crystals that distort and disrupt red blood cells; oxygen-carrying capacity of the blood is diminished.
Cystic fibrosis (R)	The most common genetic disease among people of European ancestry. Production of thick mucus clogs in the bronchial tree and pancreatic ducts. Most severe effects are chronic respiratory infections and pulmonary failure.
Tay-Sachs disease (R)	The most common genetic disease among people of Jewish ancestry. Degeneration of neurons and the nervous system results in death by the age of 2 years.
Phenylketonuria (PKU) (R)	Lack of an enzyme to metabolize the amino acid phenylalanine leads to severe mental and physical retardation. These effects may be prevented by the use of a diet (beginning at birth) that limits phenylalanine.
Huntington's disease (D)	Uncontrollable muscle contractions between the ages of 30 and 50 years, followed by loss of memory and personality.
Hemophilia (X-linked)	Lack of factor VIII impairs chemical clotting; may be controlled with factor VIII from donated blood.
Duchenne's muscular dystrophy (X-linked)	Replacement of muscle by adipose or scar tissue, with progressive loss of muscle function; often fatal before age 20 years due to involvement of cardiac muscle.

R = recessive; D = dominant.
Scanlon & Sanders, 2019.

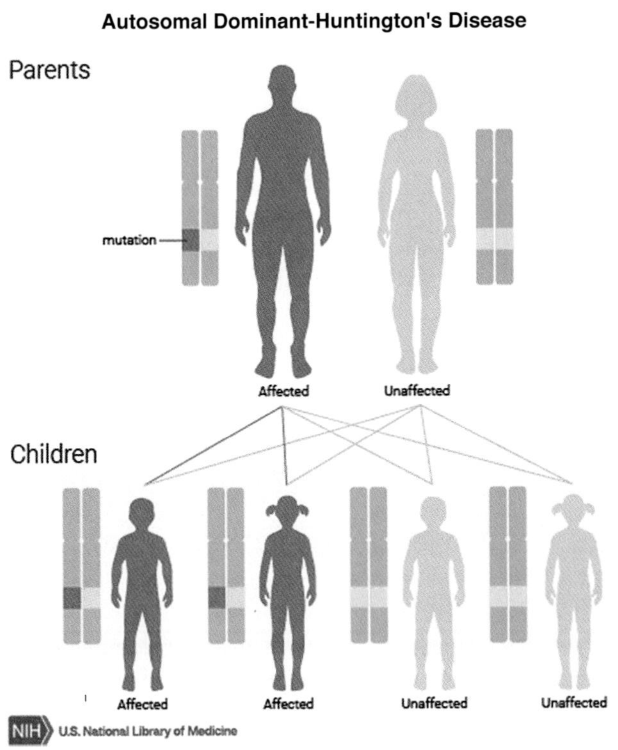

Autosomal Dominant-Huntington's Disease

Parents

Children

Affected   Affected   Unaffected   Unaffected

NIH U.S. National Library of Medicine

FIGURE 3-2 A man with Huntington's disease has two affected children and two unaffected children.

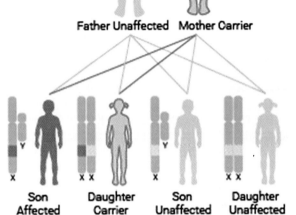

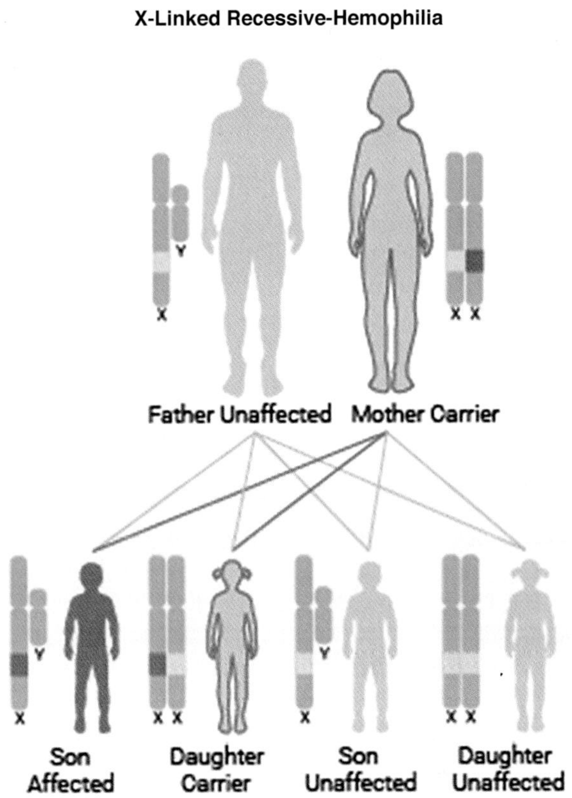

X-Linked Recessive-Hemophilia

Father Unaffected   Mother Carrier

Son Affected   Daughter Carrier   Son Unaffected   Daughter Unaffected

FIGURE 3-3 A woman who is a carrier of hemophilia has one affected son, one daughter who is a carrier, and one son and one daughter who are unaffected.

Genomic Medicine

The Human Genome Project, a 13-year international, collaborative research program completed in 2003, has provided the scientific community with valuable information used in the diagnosis, treatment, and prevention of genetically linked disorders. Current genomic medicine is building upon and expanding the knowledge gained from the Human Genome Project. The National Human Genome Research Institute (NHGRI) defines *genomic medicine* as an emerging medical discipline that involves using genomic information about an individual as part of their clinical care (e.g., for diagnostic or therapeutic decision making) and the health outcomes and policy implications of that clinical use (NHGRI, 2020). Examples of genomic medicine include:

● Newborn screening for inherited, treatable genetic diseases
● Cell-free circulating DNA as a biomarker for cancer
● Pharmacogenomics to determine whether a therapy will be effective for an individual
● Development drugs that can treat genetic diseases such as ivacaftor, which treats a specific mutation for one form of cystic fibrosis

Genetic Testing

Several genetic tests are selectively used in the care of childbearing families. These include:

● Carrier testing is used to identify individuals who carry one copy of a gene mutation when there is a family history of a genetic disorder. When both prospective parents are tested, the test can provide information about their risk of having a child with a genetic condition.
● Preimplantation testing, also known as preimplantation genetic diagnosis, is used to detect genetic changes in embryos created using assisted reproductive techniques. Before transferring an in vitro embryo into the woman's uterus, a cell from the developing fetus is removed for genetic testing.
● Prenatal testing allows for the early detection of genetic disorders such as trisomy 21, hemophilia, and Tay-Sachs disease.
● Newborn screening is used to detect genetic disorders that can be treated early in life.

Couples who have a higher risk for conceiving a child with a genetic disorder include those with:

● A maternal age older than 35
● A history of previous pregnancy resulting in a genetic disorder or newborn abnormalities
● One or both partners having a genetic disorder
● A family history of a genetic disorder

Diagnosis of genetic disorders during pregnancy allows parents to use gene therapy when available, prepare to raise a child with the specific genetic disorder, or seek genetic counseling to make the decision to continue or terminate the pregnancy.

Nursing Actions

Nursing actions for couples who elect to continue pregnancy based on information of a genetic disorder include:

- Providing additional information about the genetic disorder
- Referring them to support groups for parents who have children with the same genetic disorder
- Providing a list of websites that contain accurate information about the disorder
- Explaining that they will experience grief over the loss of the "dream child" and that this is normal
- Encouraging them to talk openly to each other about their feelings and concerns

Nursing actions for couples who elect to terminate the pregnancy based on information from genetic testing are as follows:

- Explaining the stages of grief they will experience
- Informing the couple that grief is a normal process
- Encouraging the couple to communicate with each other and share their emotions
- Referring the couple to a support group if available in their community

Nurses, especially those practicing in the obstetrical or pediatric areas, need a general understanding of genetics and the possible effects on the developing human. They may be required to explain diagnostic procedures used in genetic testing, including purpose, findings, and possible side effects. Nurses may also need to clarify or reinforce information couples receive from their health-care providers or genetic counselors. Maternal-child nurses should be able to provide information regarding:

- Genetic counseling services available in the parents' community
- Access to genetic services
- Procedure for referral to the different services
- The information or services these agencies provide

CRITICAL COMPONENT

Teratogens

The developing human is most vulnerable to the effects of teratogens during the period of organogenesis, the first 8 weeks of gestation. An example of a teratogen is toxoplasmosis.

Toxoplasma is a protozoan parasite found in cat feces and uncooked or rare beef and lamb. When an embryo is exposed to *Toxoplasma*, fetal demise, mental retardation, or blindness can result. Women who are pregnant or attempting to conceive should:

- Avoid contact with cat feces, such as through cleaning or changing a litter box.
- Avoid eating rare beef or lamb.

TERATOGENS

Birth defects can occur from genetic disorders or result from teratogen exposure. Teratogens are drugs, viruses, infections, or other exposures that have the potential to cause embryonic or fetal developmental abnormality (Table 3-2). The degree or types of malformation caused by teratogen exposure vary based on length of exposure, amount of exposure, and when it occurs during human development. Developing humans are most vulnerable to the effects of teratogens during organogenesis, which occurs during the first 8 weeks of gestation. Exposure during this time can cause gross structural defects. Exposure to teratogens after 13 weeks of gestation may cause fetal growth restriction or reduction of organ size.

ANATOMY AND PHYSIOLOGY REVIEW

Knowledge of the male and female reproductive systems is essential for the maternity nurse.

Male

The major structures and functions of the male reproductive system are pictured in Figure 3–4 and Figure 3–5.

They include the following:

- The scrotum is a loose bag of skin and connective tissue in which the two testes are suspended. The temperature inside the scrotum is approximately 96°F (35.6°C) lower than body temperature. This environment facilitates the production of viable sperm (Scanlon & Sanders, 2019).
- In the fetus, the testes develop near the kidney and normally descend into the scrotum before birth. Each of the two testes is divided into lobes that contain several seminiferous tubules in which spermatogenesis takes place. Sperm travel from the seminiferous tubules and through the rete testis (a tubular network) and enter the epididymis.
- The epididymis is a coiled, tube-like structure on the posterior surface of each testis, inside which sperm complete their maturation.
- The ductus deferens, also called the vas deferens, extends from the epididymis into the abdominal cavity. In the abdominal cavity, it extends over the urinary bladder and down the posterior side of the bladder, where it joins with the ejaculatory duct.
- Two ejaculatory ducts receive sperm from the ductus deferens and secretions from the seminal vesicles. The ducts empty into the urethra.
- Located posterior to the urinary bladder, the seminal vesicles produce secretions that contain fructose, an energy source for sperm. These secretions are alkaline, which increases sperm motility.
- The prostate gland is a muscular gland located beneath the urinary bladder that surrounds the first inch of the urethra as it extends from the bladder. It secretes an alkaline fluid that further increases sperm motility.
- Bulbourethral glands, also referred to as Cowper's glands, are located below the prostate gland. They secrete an alkaline solution that coats the interior of the urethra to neutralize the acidic urine that is present.
- Located within the penis, the urethra is the final duct through which semen passes as it exits the body.

TABLE 3-2   Teratogenic Agents

AGENT	EFFECT
Drugs and Chemicals	
Alcohol	Increased risk of fetal alcohol syndrome when the pregnant woman ingests six or more alcoholic drinks a day. No amount of alcohol is considered safe during pregnancy. Newborn characteristics of fetal alcohol syndrome include low birth weight, microcephaly, mental retardation, unusual facial features caused by midfacial hypoplasia, and cardiac defects.
Angiotensin-converting enzyme (ACE) inhibitors	Increased risk for renal tubular dysplasia that can lead to renal failure and fetal or neonatal death; intrauterine growth restriction.
Carbamazepine (anticonvulsant)	Increased risk for neural tubal defects; craniofacial defects, including cleft lip and palate; intrauterine growth restriction
Cocaine	Increased risk for heart, limbs, face, gastrointestinal tract, and genitourinary tract defects; cerebral infarctions; placental abnormalities
Warfarin (Coumadin)	Increased risk for spontaneous abortion, fetal demise, fetal or newborn hemorrhage, and central nervous system abnormalities.
Infections and Viruses	
Cytomegalovirus	Increased risk for hydrocephaly, microcephaly, cerebral calcification, mental retardation, hearing loss
Herpes varicella (chicken pox)	Increased risk for hypoplasia of hands and feet, blindness or cataracts, mental retardation
Rubella	Increased risk for heart defects, deafness or blindness, mental retardation, fetal demise
Syphilis	Increased risk for skin, bone, or teeth defects; fetal demise
Toxoplasmosis	Increased risk for fetal demise, blindness, mental retardation
Zika	Increased risk for microcephaly, blindness, hearing defects, impaired growth

American College of Obstetricians and Gynecologists, 1997; CDC, 2019; Scanlon & Sanders, 2019.

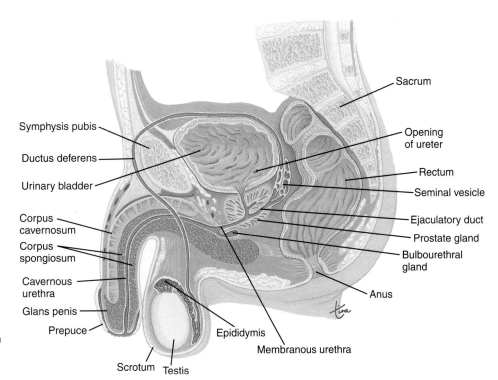

FIGURE 3–4 Male reproductive system shown in a midsagittal section through the pelvic cavity.

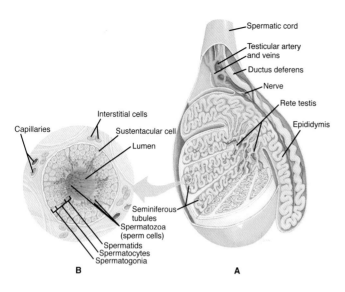

FIGURE 3-5 (A) Midsagittal section of the testis; the epididymis is on the posterior side of the testis. (B) Cross section through a seminiferous tubule showing development of the sperm.

● The penis is the external male genital organ, consisting of smooth muscle, connective tissue, and blood sinuses. The penis is flaccid when blood flow to the area is minimal and becomes erect when its arteries dilate and the sinuses fill with blood.

Female

The major structures and functions of the female reproductive system, pictured in Figure 3–6 and Figure 3–7, include the following:

● The ovaries are two oval-shaped organs, each about 4 centimeters long, located on either side of the uterus and held in place by the ovarian ligament and broad ligament. Several thousand primary follicles are present in the ovaries at birth, each containing an oocyte. The follicle cells secrete estrogen. A mature follicle is known as a graafian follicle.

● Fertilization occurs within one of the two fallopian tubes, also called oviducts. The lateral end of these tubes partially surrounds the ovary. Fringe-like projections called fimbriae protrude from the lateral end to create a current that pulls the ovum into the tube. Peristaltic waves created by the fallopian tubes' smooth muscle contractions move the ovum through the tube and into the uterus, where the medial end of the tube lies (Scanlon & Sanders, 2019).

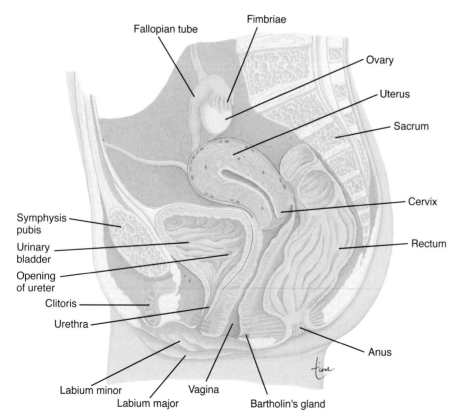

FIGURE 3-6 Female reproductive system shown in a midsagittal section through the pelvic cavity.

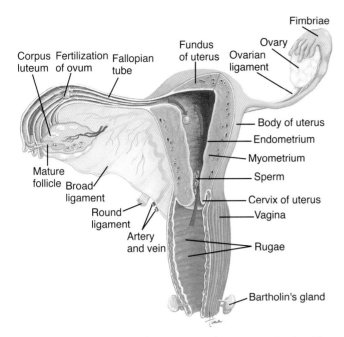

FIGURE 3-7 Female reproductive system shown in anterior view. The ovary on the left side of the illustration has been sectioned to show the developing follicles. The fallopian tube on the left side of the illustration has been sectioned to show fertilization. The uterus and vagina have been sectioned to show internal structures. Arrows indicate the movement of the ovum toward the uterus and the movement of sperm from the vagina toward the fallopian tube.

- The uterus is the site of implantation and expands during pregnancy to accommodate the developing embryo or fetus and its placenta. This organ is shaped like an upside-down pear and is about 3 inches wide, 2 inches long, and 1 inch deep. The upper portion of the uterus is known as the fundus, whereas the large central portion is called the body. The narrow, lower end that opens to the vagina is called the cervix. The inner lining of the uterus, called the endometrium, consists of a permanent layer (the basilar layer) and a regenerative layer (the functional layer). Each month, estrogen and progesterone stimulate the functional layer to thicken in preparation for egg implantation. If implantation occurs, the endometrium continues to thicken. If implantation does not occur, the functional layer is shed during the menstrual cycle.
- The vagina is a muscular tube approximately 4 inches long, extending from the cervix to the perineum. It has multiple functions: receiving sperm during sexual intercourse, providing exit for menstrual blood flow, and serving as the birth canal during the second stage of labor.
- The external genitalia, also known as the vulva, comprise the clitoris, labia majora and minora, and Bartholin's glands.
- The clitoris, a small mass of erectile tissue anterior to the urethral orifice, responds to sexual stimulus.
- The labia majora and minora are paired folds of skin that cover the urethral and vaginal openings and prevent drying of their mucous membranes.

- Bartholin's glands, located in the floor of the vestibule, have ducts that open onto the mucus of the vaginal orifice. Their secretions keep the mucous membranes moist and lubricate the vagina during sexual intercourse.

MENSTRUAL CYCLE

A woman's menstrual cycle is influenced by the ovarian cycle and endometrial cycle (Fig. 3–8).

Ovarian Cycle

The ovarian cycle pertains to the maturation of ova and consists of three phases:

1. The follicular phase begins the first day of menstruation and lasts 12 to 14 days. During this phase, the graafian follicle matures under the influence of two pituitary hormones: luteinizing hormone (LH) and follicle-stimulating hormone (FSH). The maturing graafian follicle produces estrogen.
2. The ovulatory phase begins when estrogen levels peak and ends with the release of the oocyte (egg) from the mature graafian follicle. The release of the oocyte is referred to as ovulation. LH levels surge 12 to 36 hours before ovulation. Before this surge, estrogen levels decrease and progesterone levels increase.

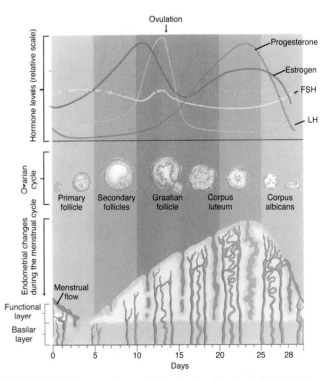

FIGURE 3-8 The menstrual cycle. The levels of the major hormones are shown in relationship to one another throughout the cycle. Changes in the ovarian follicle are depicted. The relative thickness of the endometrium is also shown.

3. The luteal phase begins after ovulation and lasts approximately 14 days. During this phase, the cells of the empty follicle morph to form the corpus luteum, which produces high levels of progesterone and low levels of estrogen. If pregnancy occurs, the corpus luteum releases progesterone and estrogen until the placenta matures enough to assume this function. If pregnancy does not occur, the corpus luteum degenerates, resulting in a decrease in progesterone and the beginning of menstruation.

Endometrial Cycle

The endometrial cycle pertains to the changes in the endometrium of the uterus in response to the hormonal changes that occur during the ovarian cycle. This cycle consists of three phases:

1. The proliferative phase occurs following menstruation and ends with ovulation. During this phase, the endometrium prepares for implantation by becoming thicker and more vascular. These changes are in response to the increasing levels of estrogen produced by the graafian follicle.
2. The secretory phase begins after ovulation and ends with the onset of menstruation. During this phase, the endometrium continues to thicken. The primary hormone during this phase is progesterone secreted from the corpus luteum. If pregnancy occurs, the endometrium continues to develop and begins to secrete glycogen, the energy source for the blastocyst during implantation. If pregnancy does not occur, the corpus luteum begins to degrade and the endometrial tissue degenerates.
3. The menstrual phase occurs in response to hormonal changes and results in the sloughing off and expulsion of the endometrial tissue.

OOGENESIS

Oogenesis is the formation of a mature ovum (egg). This process is regulated by two primary hormones:

- FSH: Secreted from the anterior pituitary gland, FSH stimulates growth of the ovarian follicles and stimulates the follicles to secrete estrogen.
- Estrogen: Secreted from the follicle cells, estrogen promotes the maturation of the ovum.

The process of oogenesis includes the following steps:

- FSH stimulates the growth of the ovarian follicle, which contains an oogonium (stem cell).
- Through mitosis, the oogonium within the ovary forms into two daughter cells: the primary oocyte and a new stem cell (Fig. 3–9). *Mitosis* is the process by which a cell divides and forms two genetically identical cells (daughter cells), each containing the diploid number of chromosomes.
- Through meiosis, the primary oocyte forms into the secondary oocyte and a polar body. The polar body forms into two polar bodies. The secondary oocyte forms into a polar body

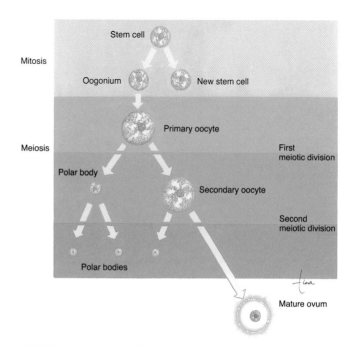

FIGURE 3–9 Oogenesis. The process of mitosis and meiosis are shown. For each primary oocyte that undergoes meiosis, only one functional ovum is formed.

and a mature ovum. *Meiosis* is a process of two successive cell divisions that produce cells that contain half the number of chromosomes (haploid).

SPERMATOGENESIS

Spermatogenesis is the formation of mature spermatozoa (sperm), a process regulated by three primary hormones:

- FSH: Secreted from the anterior pituitary gland, FSH stimulates sperm production.
- LH: Secreted from the anterior pituitary gland, LH stimulates testosterone production.
- Testosterone: Secreted by the testes, testosterone promotes the maturation of the sperm.

Through mitosis, the spermatogonium (stem cell) within the seminiferous tubules of the testes forms into two daughter cells: a new spermatogonia and a spermatogonium. The latter differentiates and is referred to as the primary spermatocyte. Through meiosis, it forms two secondary spermatocytes, each of which forms two spermatids with the haploid number of chromosomes (Fig. 3–10). Mature spermatids are called spermatozoa.

CONCEPTION

Conception, also known as fertilization, occurs when a sperm nucleus enters the nucleus of the oocyte (Fig. 3–11). Fertilization normally occurs in the outer third of the fallopian tube. The

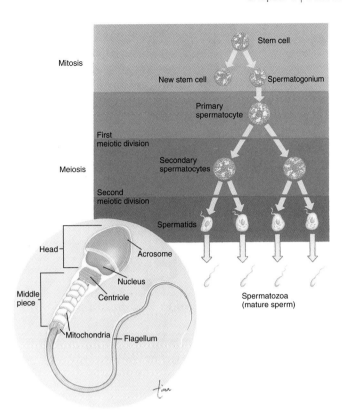

FIGURE 3-10 Spermatogenesis. The process of mitosis and meiosis are shown. For each primary spermatocyte that undergoes meiosis, four functional sperm cells are formed. The structure of the sperm cell is also shown.

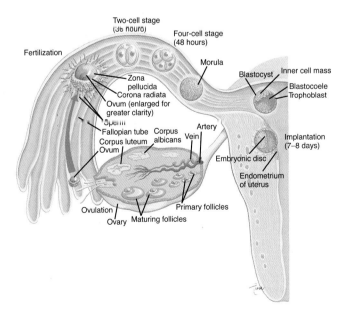

FIGURE 3-11 Ovulation, fertilization, and early embryonic development. Fertilization takes place in the fallopian tube, and the embryo reaches the blastocyst stage when it becomes implanted in the endometrium of the uterus.

fertilized oocyte is called a zygote and contains the diploid number of chromosomes (46). The following conditions are needed for fertilization to occur:

- Ovulation occurs and the mature ovum enters the fallopian tube.
- Sperm cells are deposited in the vagina and travel to the fallopian tube.
- One sperm cell is able to penetrate the mature ovum.

Cell Division

The single-cell zygote undergoes mitotic cell division known as cleavage. By the third day after fertilization, the zygote has morphed into a 16-cell, solid sphere called a morula. Mitosis continues; around day 5, the developing human enters the uterus and becomes a *blastocyst.* The blastocyst consists of an inner cell mass; the *embryoblast,* which will develop into the embryo; and an outer cell mass, the *trophoblast,* which assists in implantation and will become part of the placenta.

Multiple gestation refers to more than one developing embryo, such as in the case of twins. Twins can be either monozygotic or dizygotic. *Monozygotic twins,* also called identical twins, result from a fertilized ovum that splits during the early stages of cell division to form two identical embryos that are genetically the same. *Dizygotic twins,* also called fraternal twins, result from two separate ova fertilized by two separate sperm; they are not genetically identical.

Implantation

Implantation, the embedding of the blastocyst into the endometrium of the uterus, begins around day 5 or 6. To prepare for implantation, progesterone stimulates the endometrium to become thicker and more vascular whereas enzymes secreted by the trophoblast, now referred to as the chorion, digest the surface of the endometrium. Implantation normally occurs in the upper part of the posterior wall of the uterus.

EMBRYONIC AND FETAL DEVELOPMENT

The developing human is referred to as an embryo from the time of implantation through 8 weeks of gestation.

Embryo

Organogenesis, the formation and development of body organs, occurs during this critical time of human development. Primary germ layers known as the ectoderm, mesoderm, and endoderm form the organs, tissues, and body structures of the developing human. The ectoderm is the outer germ layer, the mesoderm is the middle layer, and the endoderm is the inner layer. These primary germ layers begin to develop around day 14 (Table 3-3). The heart forms during the third week of gestation and begins to beat and circulate blood during the fourth week. By the end of the eighth

TABLE 3-3   Structures Derived From the Primary Germ Layers

LAYER	STRUCTURES DERIVED*
Ectoderm	Epidermis; hair and nail follicles; sweat glands Nervous system; pituitary gland; adrenal medulla Lens and cornea; internal ear Mucosa of oral and nasal cavities; salivary glands
Mesoderm	Dermis; bone and cartilage Skeletal muscles; cardiac muscles; most smooth muscles Kidneys; adrenal cortex Bone marrow and blood; lymphatic tissue; lining of blood vessels
Endoderm	Mucosa of esophagus, stomach, and intestines Epithelium of respiratory tract, including lungs Liver and mucosa of gallbladder Thyroid gland; pancreas

*These are representative lists, not all-inclusive ones. Most organs are combinations of tissues from each of the three germ layers.
Scanlon & Sanders, 2019.

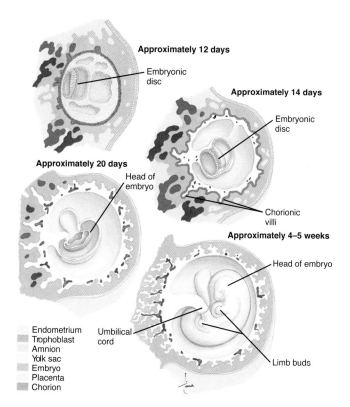

FIGURE 3–12 Embryonic development at 12 days (after fertilization), 14 days, 20 days, and 4 to 5 weeks. By 5 weeks, the embryo has distinct parts but does not yet look definitely human.

gestational week, the primary germ layers have transformed into a clearly defined human about 3 centimeters long with all organ systems formed (Fig. 3–12).

Fetus

The developing human is referred to as a fetus from week 9 to birth. During this stage of development, organ systems grow and mature (Table 3-4).

Fetal Circulation

The cardiovascular system begins to develop within the first few weeks after conception. The heart begins to beat during the third week after conception. Fetal circulation (Fig. 3–13) has several unique features:

● High levels of oxygenated blood enter the fetal circulatory system from the placenta via the umbilical vein.
● The *ductus venosus* connects the umbilical vein to the inferior vena cava. This allows the majority of the highly oxygenated blood to enter the right atrium.
● The *foramen ovale* is an opening between the right and left atria. Blood high in oxygen is shunted to the left atrium via the foramen ovale. After delivery, the foramen ovale closes in response to increased blood returning to the left atrium. It may take up to 3 months for full closure.
● The *ductus arteriosus* connects the pulmonary artery with the descending aorta. The majority of the oxygenated blood is shunted to the aorta via the ductus arteriosus with smaller amounts going to the lungs. After delivery, the ductus arteriosus constricts in response to the higher blood oxygen levels and prostaglandins.

PLACENTA, MEMBRANES, AMNIOTIC FLUID, AND UMBILICAL CORD

These structures provide a range of functions for the mother and developing fetus.

Placenta

● The placenta is formed from both fetal and maternal tissue (Fig. 3–14).
● The chorionic membrane that develops from the trophoblast, along with the chorionic villi, forms the fetal side of the placenta. The *chorionic villi* are projections from the chorion that embed into the decidua basalis and later form the fetal blood vessels of the placenta.
● The endometrium is referred to as the decidua and consists of three layers: decidua basalis, decidua capsularis, and decidua vera. The decidua basalis, the portion directly beneath the blastocyst, forms the maternal portion of the placenta.

TABLE 3-4   Summary of Fetal Development

GESTATIONAL WEEK	LENGTH*/ WEIGHT	FETAL DEVELOPMENT/CHARACTERISTICS
12	9 cm/45 grams	Red blood cells are produced in the liver. Fusion of the palate is completed. External genitalia are developed to the point that sex of fetus can be noted with ultrasound. Eyelids are fused closed. Fetal heart tone can be heard by Doppler device.
16	14 cm/200 grams	Lanugo is present on head. Meconium is formed in the intestines. Teeth begin to form. Sucking motions are made with the mouth. Skin is transparent.
20	20 cm/450 grams	Lanugo covers the entire body. Vernix caseosa covers the body. Nails are formed. Brown fat begins to develop.
24	30 cm/820 grams	Alveoli form in the lungs and begin to produce surfactant. Footprints and fingerprints are forming. Respiratory movement can be detected.
28	37 cm/1,300 grams	Eyelids are open. Adipose tissue develops rapidly. The respiratory system has developed to a point where gas exchange is possible, but lungs are not fully mature.
32	42 cm/2,100 grams	Bones are fully developed. Lungs are maturing. Increased amounts of adipose tissue are present.
36	47 cm/2,900 grams	Lanugo begins to disappear. Labia majora and minora are equally prominent. Testes are in upper portion of scrotum.
40	51 cm/3,400 grams	Fetus is considered full term at 38 weeks. All organs and systems are fully developed.

*Length is measured from the crown (top of head) to the rump (buttock). This is referred to as the crown-rump length (CRL).
Scanlon & Sanders, 2019; Thompson, 2020.

- The maternal side of the placenta is divided into compartments or lobes known as cotyledons.
- The placental membrane separates the maternal and fetal blood and prevents fetal blood from mixing with maternal blood, but it allows for the exchange of gases, nutrients, and electrolytes.

The placenta serves several critical functions for the mother and developing fetus. These include:

- Metabolic and gas exchange: In the placenta, fetal waste products and CO_2 are transferred from the fetal blood into the maternal blood sinuses by diffusion. Nutrients such as glucose and amino acids and O_2 are transferred from the maternal blood sinuses to the fetal blood through the mechanisms of diffuse and active transport.
- Hormone production: The major hormones the placenta produces are progesterone; estrogen; human chorionic gonadotropin (hCG); and human placental lactogen (hPL), also known as human chorionic somatomammotropin.
- Progesterone facilitates implantation and decreases uterine contractility.
- Estrogen stimulates the enlargement of the breasts and uterus.
- hCG stimulates the corpus luteum so that it will continue to secrete estrogen and progesterone until the placenta is mature enough to do so. This is the hormone assessed in pregnancy tests. hCG rises rapidly during the first trimester and then rapidly declines.
- hPL promotes fetal growth by regulating available glucose and stimulates breast development in preparation for lactation.

Viruses such as rubella and cytomegalovirus can cross the placental membrane and enter the fetal system, potentially causing fetal death or defects. Drugs can also cross the placental membrane. Women should consult their health-care

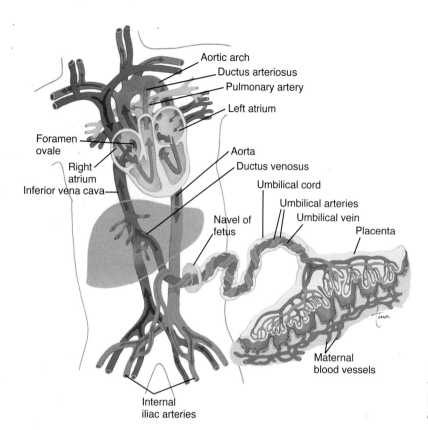

Aortic arch
Ductus arteriosus
Pulmonary artery
Left atrium
Foramen ovale
Aorta
Ductus venosus
Right atrium
Umbilical cord
Inferior vena cava
Umbilical arteries
Umbilical vein
Navel of fetus
Placenta
Maternal blood vessels
Internal iliac arteries

FIGURE 3–13 Fetal circulation. Fetal heart and blood vessels are shown on the left. Arrows depict direction of blood flow. The placenta and umbilical vessels are shown on the right.

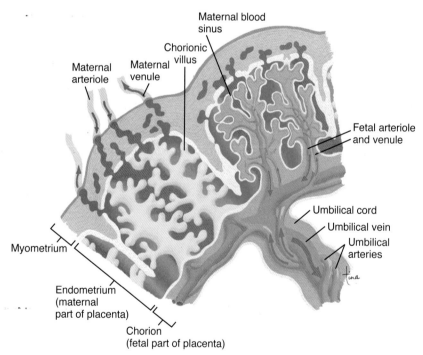

Maternal blood sinus
Chorionic villus
Maternal arteriole
Maternal venule
Fetal arteriole and venule
Umbilical cord
Umbilical vein
Umbilical arteries
Myometrium
Endometrium (maternal part of placenta)
Chorion (fetal part of placenta)

FIGURE 3–14 Placenta and umbilical cord. The fetal capillaries in the chorionic villi are within the maternal blood sinuses. Arrows indicate the direction of blood flow in the maternal and fetal vessels.

providers before taking any medications or vaccines during pregnancy. Drugs with an FDA pregnancy category of C, D, or X should be avoided during pregnancy or when attempting to conceive.

The placenta becomes fully functional between the eighth and tenth weeks of gestation. By the ninth month, it measures between 15 and 25 cm in diameter, is 3 cm thick, and weighs approximately 600 grams.

CRITICAL COMPONENT

Medications

Women who are pregnant or attempting pregnancy should consult with their health-care provider before taking any prescribed or over-the-counter medications, as these can cross the placental membrane.

Embryonic Membranes

The *amniotic sac,* also called the bag of waters, is formed by the amniotic and chorionic membranes. The amniotic membrane is the inner membrane and develops from the embryoblast, whereas the chorionic or outer membrane develops from the trophoblast. The amniotic sac contains the embryo and amniotic fluid. Both membranes stretch to accommodate the growth of the developing fetus and subsequent increase in amniotic fluid. The intact membranes help maintain a sterile environment by forming a barrier that prevents bacteria from entering the amniotic fluid through the vagina.

Amniotic Fluid

Contained within the amniotic sac (Fig. 3–15), amniotic fluid is clear and is mainly composed of water. It also contains proteins, carbohydrates, lipids, electrolytes, fetal cells, lanugo, and vernix caseosa. During the first trimester, the amniotic membrane produces amniotic fluid; during the second and third trimesters, it is produced by the fetal kidneys. The amount of amniotic fluid peaks at 800 to 1,000 mL around 34 weeks' gestation and decreases to 500 to 600 mL at term.

Amniotic fluid:

- Cushions the fetus from sudden maternal movements
- Prevents the developing human from adhering to the amniotic membranes
- Allows freedom of fetal movement, which aids in symmetrical musculoskeletal development and prevents adhesions to self or the amniotic membrane
- Provides a consistent thermal environment

Abnormalities of the amniotic fluid may be related to fetal anomalies or decreased placental function. Two such abnormalities are:

- *Polyhydramnios* or hydramnios, which refers to an excess amount of amniotic fluid (1,500–2,000 mL). Newborns of mothers who experience polyhydramnios have an increased incidence of chromosomal disorders and gastrointestinal, cardiac, and neural tube disorders.
- *Oligohydramnios,* which refers to a decreased amount of amniotic fluid (less than 500 mL at term or 50% reduction of normal amount). This is generally related to a decrease in placental function. Newborns of mothers who experienced oligohydramnios have an increased incidence of congenital renal problems.

Umbilical Cord

The umbilical cord connects the fetus to the placenta and consists of two umbilical arteries and one umbilical vein. The arteries carry deoxygenated blood whereas the vein carries oxygenated blood. These vessels are surrounded by Wharton's jelly, a collagenous substance that protects the vessels from compression. The umbilical cord is usually inserted in the center of the placenta and is about 55 cm long.

CRITICAL COMPONENT

Umbilical Vessels

After delivery of the newborn, assess the number of vessels in the cord. Newborns with only two vessels (one artery and one vein) have a 20% chance of having a cardiac or vascular defect. Document the number of vessels present in the newborn. Record and report abnormalities to the pediatric care provider.

INFERTILITY AND REPRODUCTIVE TECHNOLOGY

Infertility is defined as the inability to conceive after 12 months (6 months for woman older than age 35) of unprotected sexual intercourse. Infertility affects the physical, social, psychological, sexual, and economic dimensions of the couple's lives. Percentages of infertile women are:

- Women aged 15-29: 12.6%
- Women aged 30-39: 22.1%
- Women aged 40-49: 26.8%
  (Centers for Disease Control and Prevention [CDC], 2021)

Causes of Infertility

A cause can be identified in approximately 80% of couples who experience infertility. According to the CDC, in 35% of couples with infertility, a male factor is found with or without a female factor. In 8% of couples with infertility, a male factor is the only cause found (CDC, 2021).

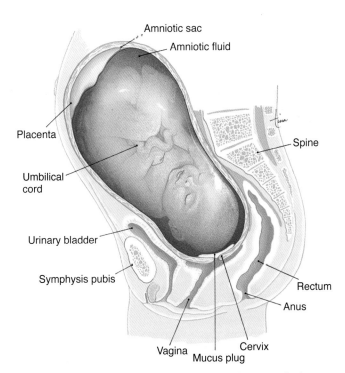

FIGURE 3–15 Fetus, placenta, umbilical cord, and amniotic fluid.

Male causative factors are classified into five categories:

1. Endocrine causes include pituitary diseases, pituitary tumors, and hypothalamic diseases that may interfere with male fertility. Low levels of LH, FSH, or testosterone can also decrease sperm production.
2. Spermatogenesis is the process in which mature functional sperm are formed. Several factors can affect the development of mature sperm. These factors are referred to as *gonadotoxins* and include:
   - Drugs (e.g., chemotherapeutics, calcium channel blockers, heroin, and alcohol)
   - Infections and viruses (e.g., prostatitis, sexually transmitted infections [STIs], and contracting mumps after puberty)
   - Systemic illness
   - Prolonged heat exposure to the testicles (e.g., use of hot tubs, wearing tight underwear, and frequent bicycle riding)
   - Pesticide exposure
   - Radiation to the pelvic region
3. Sperm antibodies are an immunological reaction against the sperm that causes a decrease in sperm motility. This is seen mainly in men who have had either a vasectomy reversal or who experienced testicular trauma.
4. Sperm transport factor includes missing or blocked structures in the male reproductive anatomy that interfere with sperm transport (e.g., vasectomy, prostatectomy, inguinal hernia, and congenital absence of the vas deferens).
5. Disorders of intercourse include erectile dysfunction (inability to achieve or maintain an erection), ejaculatory dysfunctions (retrograde ejaculation), anatomical abnormalities (hypospadias), and psychosocial factors that can interfere with fertility.

Female causative factors are classified into three major categories:

1. Ovulatory dysfunction includes anovulation or inconsistent ovulation. These factors have a very high success rate with appropriate treatment. Causes of ovulatory dysfunction are:
   - Hormonal imbalances
   - Hyperthyroidism and hypothyroidism
   - High prolactin levels
   - Premature ovarian failure (menopause before age 40)
   - Polycystic ovarian syndrome (see Chapter 19)
2. Tubal and pelvic pathology factors include damage to the fallopian tubes and uterine fibroids. Damage to the fallopian tubes is commonly related to previous pelvic inflammatory disease or endometriosis. Uterine fibroids, benign growths of the muscular wall of the uterus, can cause a narrowing of the uterine cavity and interfere with embryonic and fetal development, causing a spontaneous abortion.
3. Cervical mucus factors include infection and cervical surgeries such as cryotherapy, a medical intervention used to treat cervical dysplasia. These factors may interfere with the ability of sperm to enter or survive in the uterus.

CRITICAL COMPONENT

Risk Factors for Infertility
Women
Autoimmune disorders
Diabetes
Eating disorders or poor nutrition
Excessive alcohol use
Excessive exercising
History of cancer treated with gonadotoxic therapy or pelvic irradiation
Obesity
Older age
STIs

Men
Environmental pollutants
Heavy use of alcohol, marijuana, or cocaine
Impotence
Older age
STIs
Smoking

Diagnosis of Infertility

When a couple has difficulty conceiving, both the man and the woman need to be evaluated. The woman is evaluated by her gynecologist or reproductive endocrinologist. The man is evaluated by a urologist. Common diagnostic tests to determine the underlying cause of infertility include:

- Screening for STIs
- Laboratory tests to assess hormonal levels (thyroid-stimulating hormone [TSH], FSH, LH, anti-Müllerian hormone [AMH], and testosterone)
- Semen analysis, which entails the following:
  - The man abstains for 2 to 3 days before providing a masturbated sample of his semen.
  - Specimens are either collected at the site of testing or brought to the site within an hour of collection.
  - The semen analysis includes volume, sperm concentration, motility, morphology, white blood cell count, immunobead, and mixed agglutination reaction test.
  - Several semen analyses may be required because sperm production normally fluctuates.
- Detecting LH surge: A rapid increase in LH 36 hours before ovulation can be tested with urine or serum. The urine test (ovulation predictor test) can be performed at home to assist in identifying the ideal time for intercourse when pregnancy is desired.
- Ovarian reserve testing: Used to determine size of the remaining egg reserve. On day 3 of the menstrual cycle, blood is drawn to evaluate the levels of FSH, estradiol, and AMH. The same day, a transvaginal ultrasound is performed to assess ovarian volume and antral follicle count.

- Sonohysterogram or hysteroscopy: Used to evaluate the uterus (Kallen & Carson, 2020)
- Hysterosalpingogram, a radiological examination that provides information about the endocervical canal, uterine cavity, and fallopian tubes. Under fluoroscopic observation, dye is slowly injected through the cervical canal into the uterus. This examination can detect tubal problems such as adhesions or occlusions and uterine abnormalities such as fibroids, bicornate uterus, and uterine fistulas.

Treatment

Treatment depends on the cause of infertility and can range from lifestyle changes to surgery. For male infertility patients, treatment options may include:

- Hormonal therapy for endocrine factors
- Lifestyle changes to correct abnormal sperm count, such as stress reduction, improved nutrition, smoking cessation, and elimination of drugs that have an adverse effect on fertility
- Corticosteroids to decrease the production of sperm antibodies
- Antibiotics to clear infections of the genitourinary tract
- Repair of varicocele or inguinal hernia to facilitate sperm transport
- Transurethral resection of ejaculatory ducts to treat disorders related to intercourse

Treatments for female infertility may include:

- Treatments for anovulation, such as:
  - Lifestyle changes that include stress reduction, improved nutrition, smoking cessation, and elimination of drugs that have an adverse effect on fertility
  - Drug therapy to stimulate ovulation: clomiphene citrate, which has a very high success rate; letrozole; injectable gonadotropins; the gonadotropin-releasing hormone [GnRH] pump; and bromocriptine

SAFE AND EFFECTIVE NURSING CARE: Understanding Medication

Clomiphene Citrate (Clomid)

- Indication: Anovulatory infertility
- Action: Stimulates release of FSH and LH, which stimulates ovulation
- Common side effects: Hot flashes, breast discomfort, headaches, insomnia, bloating, blurry vision, nausea, vaginal dryness
- Route and dose: PO; 50 to 200 mg/day from cycle day 3 to 7
- Nursing actions:
  - Provide information on use of medication and its side effects.
  - Instruct woman not to drive if she is experiencing blurry vision.

- Surgery to open the fallopian tubes if tubal abnormalities are present
- Removal of uterine fibroids through a surgical procedure called *myomectomy*
- Antibiotics to treat cervical infection

When the previously mentioned treatments are not successful, the couple is usually referred to an obstetrician who has specialized training in infertility. Additional testing is done, and based on the outcome, various procedures can be used to assist in fertility (Table 3-5).

Emotional Implications

Couples who are infertile experience a "roller coaster" effect during diagnosis and treatment. Each month they become excited and hopeful that they will conceive. When the woman has a period, their excitement and hopes turn to sadness and possibly depression. Infertility can cause a crisis in the couple's lives and relationship. Diagnosis and treatment of infertility can cause:

- Stress, anxiety, and depression for both the female and male partner
- Guilt for one or both partners if they blame themselves for the inability to conceive
- Marital strain if one partner blames the other for the infertility
- Sexual dysfunction caused by the stress of prescribed sexual activity in infertility treatment
- Strain within the extended family, as the couple may avoid events that include children and may even isolate socially if they find it too painful to be around children
- Lack of support network, particularly for those who do not share information about their fertility problems with family members and friends
- Self-esteem issues, including the feeling of being "less of a man" or "less of a woman" because conception does not occur, or shame associated with the feeling of having a "defective" body

Most couples can benefit from counseling during the time of diagnosis and treatment, as well as after treatment ends. Ideally, counseling should start before treatment begins. Couples may have high expectations of reproductive technology and fail to recognize that treatment may not be successful. Counseling includes discussion about:

- The effects treatment may have on them as a couple, as individuals, and as a family
- Information about different treatment methods and ethical dilemmas they may encounter
- Information about the effects, consequences, and resolution of treatment
- The decision on when to stop treatment
- Adoption
- The use of a gestational surrogate, an option for a woman with unhealthy or no eggs in which another woman is impregnated with the partner's sperm and carries the baby on behalf of the couple

TABLE 3-5   Common Assisted Fertility Technologies

TECHNOLOGY	PROCEDURE
Artificial insemination (AI): Intracervical Intrauterine Partner's sperm Donor sperm	Sperm that has been removed from semen is deposited directly into the cervix or uterus using a plastic catheter. The sample is collected by masturbation, and the sperm are separated from the semen and prepared for insemination. Sperm can be from the partner or from a donor when the male partner does not produce sperm. Examples of fertility conditions where this procedure is used include (1) poor cervical mucus production due to previous surgery of the cervix, (2) anti-sperm antibodies, (3) diminished amount of sperm, and (4) diminished sperm motility.
Testicular sperm aspiration	Sperm are aspirated or extracted directly from the testicles. Sperm are then microinjected into the harvested eggs of the female partner. This is also referred to as intra-cytoplasmic injection. This procedure is used with men who (1) had an unsuccessful vasectomy reversal, (2) have an absence of vas deferens, or (3) have an extremely low sperm count or no sperm in their ejaculated semen.
In vitro fertilization (IVF)	IVF is a procedure in which oocytes are harvested and fertilization occurs outside the female body in a laboratory.
Zygote intrafallopian transfer (ZIFT)	In ZIFT, a zygote is placed into the fallopian tube via laparoscopy 1 day after the oocyte is retrieved from the woman and IVF is used.
Gamete intrafallopian transfer (GIFT)	In GIFT, sperm and oocytes are mixed outside the woman's body and then placed into the fallopian tube via laparoscopy. Fertilization takes place inside the fallopian tube. This procedure is used when there has been (1) a history of failed infertility treatment for anovulation, (2) unexplained infertility, and (3) low sperm count.
Embryo transfer (ET)	ET is when, through IVF, an embryo is placed in the uterine cavity via a catheter. Example of fertility condition in which this procedure is used is when the fallopian tubes are blocked.

● The use of a gestational surrogate in which a woman's own egg is fertilized by her partner's sperm and placed inside the uterus of the surrogate, who agrees to carry the baby on behalf of the couple

Evidence-Based Practice

Infertile Mother's Vulnerability to Depression

Olshansky, E. (2003). A theoretical explanation for previously infertile mothers' vulnerability to depression. *Journal of Nursing Scholarship, 35,* 263–268.

Since the 1980s, Ellen Olshansky, PhD, RN, FAAN, has researched the psychosocial effects of infertility. She synthesized the results of several grounded theory studies on the experience of infertility and summarized her theory of identity as infertility. According to her theory:

• Women who are distressed by their infertility become consumed with concerns about the infertility and often neglect their relationships with friends, spouse, or family members. This can lead to social isolation.

• Infertility becomes the focus of the couple's relationship, and other aspects of the relationship are often ignored. This can lead to a dysfunctional marriage or couple relationship.

• Career women may experience a sense of loss of self, due to the shift of focus from career to infertility. This also contributes to social isolation.

• Once pregnancy has been achieved, women often have difficulty perceiving themselves as pregnant women.

Ethical Implications

Assisted reproductive technologies (ART) are treatments that involve the surgical removal of the oocytes and their combination with sperm in a laboratory setting. These treatments include in vitro fertilization (IVF), zygote intrafallopian transfer (ZIFT), gamete intrafallopian transfer (GIFT), and embryo transfer (ET). ART has created numerous ethical dilemmas. The primary one is "surplus" embryos, those produced from hyperstimulation of the ovaries that occurs when IVF technologies are being used. Several eggs from the woman may be harvested and fertilized using IVF, but only two or three are returned to the woman's body. These surplus embryos are either frozen for future use or allowed to perish. This has raised the question of when life begins and the rights of the embryo. Other ethical questions that arise are:

● Who owns the embryos—the woman or the man?
● Who decides what will happen to the surplus embryos?
● Who has access to ART, which has substantial costs that are often not covered by health insurance providers?
● At what point should the health-care provider recommend that the couple stop using ART?
● When artificial insemination with donor sperm or surrogacy is used, do you tell the child? If so, when?
● Does the sperm donor have any rights or responsibilities regarding the child produced from his donation?
● What are the rights of the gestational surrogate?

The Nurse's Role

The role of the nurse varies based on where they interface with the couple who is experiencing infertility. Nurses who work in an infertility clinic take on various roles, including counseling, teaching, supporting, and assisting in the procedures. Nurses who work in acute care, clinics, or other settings must be aware of the emotional impact infertility has on the individual and on the couple.

CRITICAL COMPONENT

Infertility

The experience of infertility affects the individual's and the couple's emotional well-being.

Nurses' awareness of how infertility affects all aspects of the individual's and of the couple's relationship will enhance the effectiveness of the nursing care provided to these couples or individuals.

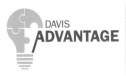

Go to Davis Advantage to complete your learning: strengthen understanding, apply your knowledge, and prepare for the Next Gen NCLEX®.

REFERENCES

American College of Obstetricians and Gynecologists. (1997). *Teratology* (educational bulletin no. 236). Author.

Centers for Disease Control and Prevention. (2019). *Zika virus.* http://www.cdc.gov/zika/about/overview.html

Kallen, A., & Carson, S. (2020). The diagnosis of the infertile couple. *OB/GYN, 65,* 26–30.

National Human Genome Research Institute. (2020). *Genomics and medicine.* http://www.genome.gov/health/genomics-and-medicine

Olshansky, E. (2003). A theoretical explanation of previously infertile mothers' vulnerability to depression. *Journal of Nursing Scholarship, 35,* 236–268.

Scanlon, S., & Sanders, T. (2019). *Essentials of anatomy and physiology* (8th ed.). F.A. Davis.

Thompson, G. (2020). *Understanding anatomy & physiology* (3rd ed.). F.A. Davis.

World Health Organization. (2012). *Human Genetics Programme.* http://www.who.int/genomics/geneticsVSgenomics/en

Physiological Aspects of Pregnancy

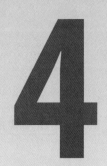

Connie Miller, DNP, RNC-OB, CNE

LEARNING OUTCOMES

Upon completion of this chapter, the student will be able to:

1. Identify the major components of preconception health care.
2. Describe methods to diagnose pregnancy and determine estimated date of delivery (EDD).
3. Explain progression of anatomical and physiological changes during pregnancy.
4. Link the anatomical and physiological changes of pregnancy to signs, symptoms, and common discomforts of pregnancy.
5. Discuss appropriate interventions to relieve common discomforts of pregnancy.
6. Compare critical elements of assessment and nursing care during initial and subsequent prenatal visits.
7. Outline the elements of patient education and anticipatory guidance appropriate for each trimester of pregnancy.

CONCEPTS

Comfort
Family
Growth and Development
Health Promotion
Nutrition
Reproduction and Sexuality

Nursing Diagnosis

- Readiness for enhanced knowledge related to physiological changes of pregnancy
- Readiness for enhanced knowledge related to nutritional requirements during pregnancy
- Altered health maintenance related to knowledge deficit regarding self-care measures during pregnancy
- Readiness for enhanced knowledge of warning signs of pregnancy
- Sleep pattern disturbance related to discomforts of late pregnancy
- Constipation related to changes in the gastrointestinal (GI) tract during pregnancy

Nursing Outcomes

- The pregnant woman will demonstrate knowledge of expected anatomical and physiological changes of pregnancy.
- The pregnant woman will report eating a diet following healthy eating practices and MyPlate guidelines with the recommended calorie intake.
- The pregnant woman will verbalize understanding of self-care needs in pregnancy such as posture and body mechanics, rest and relaxation, personal hygiene, and activity and exercise.
- The pregnant woman will report use of measures for relieving discomforts associated with normal physical changes. For example, she will verbalize an understanding of strategies for constipation management in pregnancy.
- The pregnant woman will identify warning signs of pregnancy that should be reported to the health-care provider (HCP).
- The pregnant woman will explain appropriate strategies to foster sleep during pregnancy.

INTRODUCTION

The scope of this chapter is nursing care and interventions before conception and throughout a normal pregnancy based on an understanding of the physiological aspects of pregnancy. During pregnancy, the woman undergoes significant anatomical and physiological changes to nurture and accommodate the developing fetus. These changes begin after conception and affect every organ system. However, for women experiencing an uncomplicated pregnancy, these changes resolve after pregnancy with minimal residual effects. It is important to understand the normal physiological changes occurring in pregnancy to help differentiate adaptations that are abnormal.

The second half of the chapter presents preconception and prenatal care (PNC). Within the continuum of reproductive health care, preconception care and PNC provide a platform for important health-care functions, including health promotion, screening and diagnosis, and disease prevention. It has been established that by implementing timely and appropriate evidence-based practices, preconception and PNC can improve maternal and fetal outcomes and save lives. It also provides the opportunity to communicate with and support women, families, and communities at a critical time in a woman's life. Chapter 5 addresses the psychosocial and cultural components of the antepartum period.

Before pregnancy, nursing care focuses on assessment of the woman's health and potential risk factors, as well as education on health promotion and disease prevention. During pregnancy, nursing care shifts to regular assessment of the health of the pregnancy, including assessment and screening of risk factors for potential complications, education on health promotion, and disease prevention. The focus is on implementation of appropriate interventions based on risk status or actual complications and inclusion of significant others and family in care and education to promote pregnancy adaptation.

PHYSIOLOGICAL PROGRESSION OF PREGNANCY

Pregnancy results in maternal physiological adaptations involving every body system, with each change meant to protect the woman and the fetus and based in the maintenance of the pregnancy, the development of the fetus, and the preparation for labor and birth. To both understand a woman's experience of normal pregnancy and be effective in identifying deviations from normal, the nurse must have a foundation in the physiology of pregnancy.

This understanding is critical not only for risk assessment and implementation of appropriate nursing interventions to reduce risk, but also for providing effective patient education and anticipatory guidance grounded in knowledge of the normal physical changes in pregnancy and their resulting common, normal discomforts. The next sections present the changes that occur in each system, and Table 4-1 summarizes the major physiological changes and factors that influence these changes.

Reproductive System

Maternal physiological adaptations to pregnancy are most profound in the reproductive system. The uterus undergoes phenomenal growth, breasts prepare for lactation, and the vagina changes to accommodate the birthing process.

Breasts

Breast changes begin early in pregnancy and continue throughout gestation and into the postpartum period. These changes are primarily influenced by increases in hormone levels and occur in preparation for lactation (see Table 4-1).

Uterus

The uterus is described in three parts (Fig. 4–1):

- Fundus or upper portion
- Isthmus or lower segment
- Cervix, the lower narrow part, or neck; the external part of the cervix interfaces with the vagina. The cervical os is the opening of the cervix that dilates (opens) during labor to allow passage of the fetus through the vagina.

Uterine changes over the course of pregnancy are profound (see Table 4-1).

- Before pregnancy, this elastic, muscular organ is the size and shape of a small pear and weighs 40 to 50 g.
- During pregnancy, the uterine wall progressively thins as the uterus expands to accommodate the developing fetus.
- By mid-pregnancy, the uterine fundus reaches the level of the umbilicus abdominally.
- Toward the end of pregnancy, the enlarged uterus, containing a full-term fetus, fills the abdominal cavity, altering placement of the lungs, rib cage, and abdominal organs (Fig. 4–2).
- Intermittent, painless, and physiological uterine contractions, referred to as *Braxton-Hicks contractions,* begin in the second trimester, but some women do not feel them until the third trimester. These contractions are irregular and more noticeable as the uterus grows.
- At term, the uterus weighs 1,100 to 1,200 g.

Vagina

The vagina is an elastic muscular canal. As pregnancy progresses, various changes take place in the vasculature and tone (see Table 4-1):

- An increase of vascularity due to expanded circulatory needs
- An increase of vaginal discharge (leukorrhea) in response to the estrogen-induced hypertrophy of the vaginal glands
- Relaxation of the vaginal wall and perineal body, which allows stretching to accommodate the birthing process
- Acid pH of the vagina, which inhibits growth of bacteria but allows overgrowth of *Candida albicans.* This places the pregnant woman at risk for candidiasis (yeast infection).

TABLE 4-1   Physiological Changes in Pregnancy

PHYSIOLOGICAL CHANGES	CLINICAL SIGNS AND SYMPTOMS
Reproductive System—Breasts	
Increased estrogen and progesterone levels: Initially produced by the corpus luteum and then by the placenta Increased blood supply to breasts to prepare for lactation	Tenderness, feeling of fullness, and tingling sensation Increase in weight of breast by 400 g Enlargement of breasts, nipples, areola, and Montgomery follicles (small glands on the areola around the nipple) Darkening of the areola and nipple Striae: Caused by stretching of skin with enlarging breast tissue Prominent veins caused by a twofold increase in blood flow
Increased prolactin: Produced by the anterior pituitary	Increased growth of mammary glands Increase in lactiferous ducts and alveolar system Colostrum, a yellow secretion rich in antibodies, begins to be produced as early as 16 weeks
Reproductive System—Uterus, Cervix, and Vagina	
Increased levels of estrogen and progesterone	Hypertrophy of uterine wall Softening of vaginal muscle and connective tissue in preparation for expansion of tissue to accommodate passage of fetus through the birth canal Uterus contractibility increases in response to increased estrogen levels, leading to Braxton-Hicks contractions. Hypertrophy of cervical glands leads to formation of mucus plug, the protective barrier between uterus or fetus and vagina. Increased vascularity and hypertrophy of vaginal and cervical glands leads to increase in leukorrhea. Cessation of menstrual cycle (amenorrhea) and ovulation
Enlargement and stretching of uterus to accommodate developing fetus and placenta	Increase in uterine size to 20 times that of nonpregnant uterus Weight of uterus increases from 70 g to 1,100 g. Capacity increases from 10 mL to 5,000 mL.
Expanded circulatory volume leads to increased vascular congestion.	Blood flow to the uterus is 500–600 mL/min at term. Goodell's sign: Softening of the cervix Hegar's sign: Softening of the lower uterine segment Chadwick's sign: Bluish coloration of cervix, vaginal mucosa, and vulva
Acid pH of vagina	Acid environment inhibits growth of bacteria. Acid environment allows growth of *Candida albicans,* leading to increased risk of candidiasis (yeast infection).
Cardiovascular System	
Decrease in peripheral vascular resistance	Decrease in blood pressure (first trimester)
Increase in blood volume by 30%–50%	Hypervolemia of pregnancy
Increase in cardiac output by 30%-50%	Increased resting heart rate of 10–20 bpm
BMR increased 15% by third trimester	Increased stroke volume of 25%–30%
Increase in peripheral dilation	Systolic murmurs, loud and wide S1 split, loud S2, obvious audible S3

Continued

TABLE 4-1   Physiological Changes in Pregnancy—cont'd

PHYSIOLOGICAL CHANGES	CLINICAL SIGNS AND SYMPTOMS
Increase in RBC count by 30% Increase in RBC volume by 20%–30% Increase in plasma volume by 40%–60%	Physiological anemia of pregnancy due to hemodilution caused by the increase in plasma volume being relatively larger than the increase in RBCs. This results in decreased hemoglobin and hematocrit values (see Appendix A for pregnancy laboratory values).
Increase in WBC count	Values up to 16,000 mm^3 in the absence of infection
Increased demand for iron in fetal development	Iron-deficiency anemia: Hemoglobin <11 g/dL, hematocrit <33%
Plasma fibrin increase of 40% Fibrinogen increase of 50% Decrease in coagulation-inhibiting factors Protective of inevitable blood loss during birth	Hypercoagulability
Increased venous pressure and decreased blood flow to extremities due to compression of iliac veins and inferior vena cava	Edema of lower extremities Varicosities in legs and vulva Hemorrhoids
In supine position, the enlarged uterus compresses the inferior vena cava, causing reduced blood flow back to the right atrium and a drop in cardiac output and blood pressure.	Supine hypotensive syndrome
Respiratory System	
Hormones of pregnancy stimulate the respiratory center and act on lung tissue to increase and enhance respiratory function. Increase of oxygen consumption by 20%–40%	Increase in tidal volume by 30%–40% Slight increase in respiratory rate Increase in inspiratory capacity Decrease in expiratory volume Slight hyperventilation Slight respiratory alkalosis
Estrogen, progesterone, and prostaglandins cause vascular engorgement and smooth muscle relaxation.	Dyspnea Nasal and sinus congestion Epistaxis
Upward displacement of diaphragm by enlarging uterus Estrogen causes a relaxation of the ligaments and joints of the ribs. Slight decrease in lung capacity	Shift from abdominal to thoracic breathing Chest and thorax expand to accommodate thoracic breathing and upward displacement of diaphragm.
Renal System	
Alterations in cardiovascular system (increased cardiac output and increased blood and plasma volume) lead to increased renal blood flow of 60%–80% in first trimester and then decreases. Increased progesterone levels, which cause a relaxation of smooth muscles	Urinary frequency and incontinence and increased risk of UTI
Dilation of renal pelvis and ureters Ureters become elongated with decreased motility Decreased bladder tone	Increased risk of UTI
Pressure of enlarging uterus on renal structures Displacement of bladder in third trimester	Urinary frequency and nocturia Some degree of incontinence common in third trimester
Increased GFR	Increased urinary output

TABLE 4-1   Physiological Changes in Pregnancy—cont'd

PHYSIOLOGICAL CHANGES	CLINICAL SIGNS AND SYMPTOMS
Increased renal excretion of glucose and protein	Glucosuria and proteinuria
Decreased renal flow in third trimester	Dependent edema
Gastrointestinal System	
Increased levels of hCG and altered carbohydrate metabolism	Nausea and vomiting during early pregnancy
Esophageal sphincter tone decreased	Reflux of acidic secretions into lower esophagus resulting in heartburn
Increased progesterone levels relax smooth muscle to slow the digestive process and movement of stool	Bloating, flatulence, and constipation
Decreased contractility of gallbladder results in prolonged emptying time	Increased risk of gallstone formation and cholestasis
Changes in senses of taste and smell	Increase or decrease in appetite Nausea Pica: Abnormal; craving for and ingestion of nonfood substances such as clay or starch
Displacement of intestines by uterus	Flatulence, abdominal distention, abdominal cramping, and pelvic heaviness
Increased estrogen levels increase vascular congestion of mucosa	Gingivitis, bleeding gums, increased risk of periodontal disease
Musculoskeletal System	
Increased progesterone and relaxin levels lead to softening of ligaments and increased joint mobility, resulting in widening and increased mobility of the sacroiliac and symphysis pubis.	Facilitates birthing process Low back pain or pelvic discomfort Pelvis tilts forward, leading to shifting of center of gravity that results in change in posture (increasing lordosis) and "waddle" gait. Increased risk of falls due to shift in center of gravity and change in gait and posture
Distention of abdomen related to expanding uterus, reduced abdominal tone, and increased breast size	Round ligament spasm
Increased estrogen and relaxin levels lead to increased elasticity and relaxation of ligaments.	Increased risk of joint pain and injury
Abdominal muscles stretch due to enlarging uterus	Diastasis recti
Integumentary System	
Estrogen and progesterone levels stimulate increased melanin deposition, causing light brown to dark brown pigmentation.	Linea nigra Melasma (chloasma) Increased pigmentation of nipples, areola, vulva, scars, and moles
Increased blood flow, increased BMR, progesterone-induced increase in body temperature, and vasomotor instability	Hot flashes, facial flushing, alternating sensation of hot and cold Increased perspiration
Increased action of adrenocorticosteroids leads to cutaneous elastic tissues becoming fragile	Striae gravidarum (stretch marks) on abdomen, thighs, breast, and buttocks
Increased estrogen levels lead to color and vascular changes	Angiomas (spider nevi) Palmar erythema: Pinkish-red mottling over palms of hands and redness of fingers
Increased androgens lead to increase in sebaceous gland secretions	Increased oiliness of skin and increase of acne

Continued

TABLE 4-1   Physiological Changes in Pregnancy—cont'd

PHYSIOLOGICAL CHANGES	CLINICAL SIGNS AND SYMPTOMS
Endocrine System	
Decreased follicle-stimulating hormone	Amenorrhea
Increased progesterone	Maintains pregnancy by relaxation of smooth muscles, leading to decreased uterine activity, which results in decreased risk of spontaneous abortions
	Decreases GI motility and slows digestive processes
Increased estrogen	Facilitates uterine and breast development
	Facilitates increases in vascularity
	Facilitates hyperpigmentation
	Alters metabolic processes and fluid and electrolyte balance
Increased prolactin	Facilitates lactation
Increased oxytocin	Stimulates uterine contractions
	Stimulates the milk let-down or ejection reflex in breastfeeding
Increased hCG	Maintenance of corpus luteum until placenta becomes fully functional
Human placental lactogen or human chorionic somatomammotropin	Facilitates breast development
	Alters carbohydrate, protein, and fat metabolism
	Facilitates fetal growth by altering maternal metabolism; acts as an insulin antagonist
Hyperplasia and increased vascularity of thyroid	Enlargement of thyroid
	Heat intolerance and fatigue
Increased BMR related to fetal metabolic activity	Depletion of maternal glucose stores leads to increased risk of maternal hypoglycemia
Increased need for glucose due to developing fetus	Increased production of insulin
Increase in circulating cortisol	Increase in maternal resistance to insulin leads to increased risk of hyperglycemia
Neurological System	
	Headache
	Syncope

Blackburn, 2021; Cunningham, 2018.

Ovaries

The corpus luteum, which normally degrades after ovulation when the egg is not fertilized, is maintained during the first couple months of pregnancy by high levels of human chorionic gonadotropin (hCG). In early pregnancy, the corpus luteum produces progesterone to maintain the endometrium, the thick uterine lining. This allows implantation and establishment of the pregnancy. There is subsequently no endometrial shedding that would result in menstruation. Ovulation ceases as the hormones of pregnancy inhibit follicle maturation and release. By 6 to 7 weeks' gestation, the placenta begins producing progesterone and the corpus luteum degenerates.

Cardiovascular System

The cardiovascular system undergoes significant adaptations during pregnancy to support the maintenance and development of the fetus while also meeting maternal physiological needs during both the pregnancy and the postpartum period. Changes in the cardiovascular system in pregnancy are profound and begin early in pregnancy as maternal blood volume begins to increase. The most rapid increase in blood volume occurs in the second trimester and continues slower during the third trimester, with maternal blood volume peaking in the final weeks of pregnancy (Cunningham, 2018). The hemodynamic changes help to support the rapidly growing fetus and placenta and are

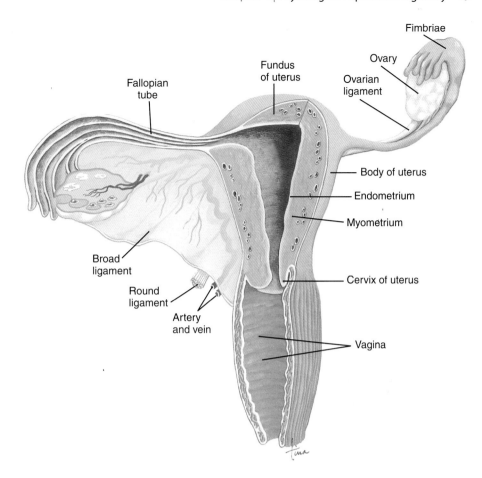

FIGURE 4-1 Reproductive system.

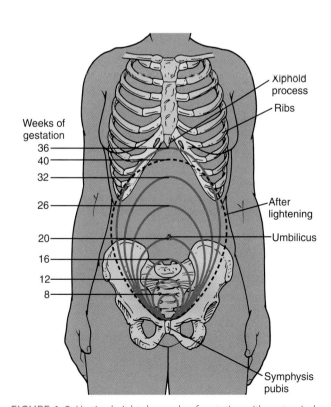

FIGURE 4-2 Uterine heights by weeks of gestation with anatomical landmarks.

also a protective mechanism for the inevitable maternal blood loss during the intrapartum period (see Table 4-1). Cardiovascular system changes include the following:

- Cardiac output increases 30% to 50% and peaks at 25 to 30 weeks.
- The resting heart rate increases 10 to 20 beats per minute (bpm).
- Stroke volume increases by 25% to 30%.
- Basal metabolic rate (BMR) increases 10% to 20% by the third trimester.
- The white blood cell (WBC) count increases, with values up to 16,000 mm³ without infection.
  - The increase is hormonally induced and similar to elevations seen in physiological stress such as exercise.
- Plasma volume increases 40% to 60% during pregnancy until reaching a peak at about 32 to 34 weeks and remaining there until term.
- In response to increased oxygen requirements of pregnancy, the red blood cell (RBC) count increases 30% and RBC volume increases up to 20% to 30% with iron supplementation (up to 18% without supplementation).
  - The increase in plasma volume is relatively larger than the increase in RBCs. This hemodilution is evidenced by decreased hemoglobin and hematocrit values and is known as physiological anemia of pregnancy or pseudo anemia of

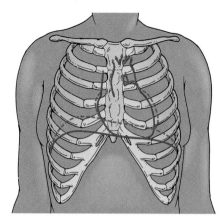

FIGURE 4–3 Dotted lines indicate displacement of the heart and lungs as pregnancy progresses and the uterus enlarges.

pregnancy. See Appendix A for laboratory values during pregnancy.

- Cardiac work is eased as the decrease in blood viscosity facilitates placental perfusion.
- Iron-deficiency anemia is defined as hemoglobin less than 11 g/dL and hematocrit less than 33%.
  - Maternal iron stores cannot meet the demands for iron in fetal development.
- Blood volume increases by 1,200 to 1,600 mL or by 30% to 50% to support uteroplacental demands and maintenance of pregnancy. This is referred to as hypervolemia of pregnancy.
- Heart enlarges slightly due to hypervolemia and increased cardiac output.
- Heart shifts upward and laterally as the growing uterus displaces the diaphragm (Fig. 4–3).
- Hypercoagulation occurs during pregnancy to decrease the risk of postpartum hemorrhage. These changes place the woman at increased risk for thrombosis and coagulopathies.
  - Plasma fibrin increase of 40%
  - Fibrinogen increase of 50%
  - Coagulation inhibiting factors decrease
- In most women, a systolic heart murmur or a third heart sound (gallop) may be heard by mid-pregnancy.
- Peripheral dilation is increased.
- Varicosities may develop in the legs or vulva due to increased venous pressure below the level of the uterus.
- Dependent edema in the lower extremities is caused by increased venous pressure from the enlarging uterus.
- Blood pressure decreases in the first trimester due to a decrease in peripheral vascular resistance. The blood pressure returns to normal by term.
- Supine hypotension can occur when the woman is in the supine position, as the enlarging uterus can compress the inferior vena cava.

Respiratory System

Throughout the course of pregnancy, the respiratory system adapts in response to physiological and anatomical demands related to fetal growth and development and maternal metabolic

CRITICAL COMPONENT

Supine Hypotensive Syndrome

Supine hypotensive syndrome is a hypotensive condition resulting from a woman lying on her back in mid- to late pregnancy (Fig. 4–4). In a supine position, the enlarged uterus compresses the inferior vena cava, leading to a significant drop in cardiac output and blood pressure that results in the woman feeling dizzy and faint.

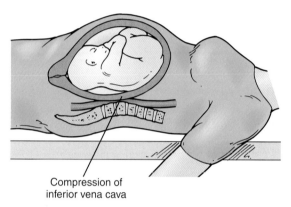

Compression of
inferior vena cava

FIGURE 4–4 Supine hypotension compression of the inferior vena cava by the gravid uterus while in the supine position reduces venous blood return to the heart, causing maternal hypotension.

needs (see Table 4-1). There is a significant increase in oxygen demand during normal pregnancy due to a 15% increase in metabolic rate and a 20% to 40% increased consumption of oxygen. There is a 30% to 50% increase in minute ventilation, mostly due to an increase in tidal volume rather than in respiratory rate. Pulmonary function is not compromised in normal pregnancy.

Physiological changes occur to accommodate the additional requirements for oxygen delivery and carbon dioxide removal in mother and fetus during pregnancy. These include the following:

- Tidal volume increases 30% to 40%.
- Slight respiratory alkalosis occurs.
  - Decrease in P_{CO_2} leads to an increase in pH (more alkaline) and a decrease in bicarbonate.
  - This change promotes transport of carbon dioxide away from the fetus.
- Increases in estrogen, progesterone, and prostaglandins cause vascular engorgement and smooth muscle relaxation resulting in edema and tissue congestion, which can lead to:
  - Dyspnea
  - Nasal and sinus congestion
  - Epistaxis (nosebleeds)

Anatomical changes include the following:

- Diaphragm is displaced upward approximately 4 cm.
- Increase in chest circumference of 6 cm occurs with an increase in costal angle greater than 90 degrees.

- Shift from abdominal to thoracic breathing occurs as the pregnancy progresses (see Fig. 4–3).
- These anatomical changes may contribute to the physiological dyspnea that is common during pregnancy.

Renal System

The kidneys undergo change during pregnancy as they adapt to perform their basic functions of regulating fluid and electrolyte balance, eliminating metabolic waste products, and helping to regulate blood pressure (see Table 4-1). Physiological changes include the following:

- Renal plasma flow increases.
- Glomerular filtration rate (GFR) increases.
- Renal tubular reabsorption increases.
- Proteinuria and glucosuria can normally occur in small amounts related to an exceeded tubal reabsorption threshold of protein and glucose due to increased volume.
  - Even though a small amount of proteinuria and glucosuria can be normal, it is important to assess and monitor for pathology.
- Shift occurs in fluid and electrolyte balance.
  - The need for increased fluid and electrolytes results in alteration of regulating mechanisms, including the renin–angiotensin–aldosterone system and antidiuretic hormone.
- Positional variation occurs in renal function.
  - In the supine and upright maternal position, blood pools in the lower body, causing a decrease in cardiac output, GFR, and urine output; it also causes excess sodium and fluid retention.
  - A left lateral recumbent maternal position can:
    - Maximize cardiac output, renal plasma volume, and urine output.
    - Stabilize fluid and electrolyte balance.
    - Minimize dependent edema.
    - Maintain optimal blood pressure.

These changes support increased circulatory and metabolic demands of pregnancy because the renal system secretes maternal and fetal waste products. Anatomical changes include the following:

- Renal pelvis dilation occurs with increased renal plasma flow.
- Ureters become elongated, tortuous, and dilated.
- Bladder pressure increases from the enlarging uterus.
- Urinary stasis promotes bacterial growth and increases the risk for urinary tract infections (UTIs) and pyelonephritis.
- Hyperemia of the bladder and urethra relate to increased vascularity that results in pelvic congestion; edematous mucosa is easily traumatized.
- Urinary incontinence is experienced by 20% of women in their first trimester and at least 40% of women in their third trimester.
- Most women experience urinary symptoms of frequency, urgency, and nocturia beginning early in pregnancy and continuing to varying degrees throughout the pregnancy. These symptoms are primarily a result of the systemic hormonal changes of pregnancy and may also be attributed to anatomical changes in the renal system and other body system changes during pregnancy but are not generally indicative of infection. Physiological changes that occur in the renal system during pregnancy predispose pregnant women to UTIs.
- UTIs are common in pregnancy and may be asymptomatic. Symptoms of a UTI include urinary frequency, dysuria, urgency, and sometimes pus or blood in the urine. Treatment includes anti-infective medication for a 7- to 10-day period. If untreated, the infection can lead to pyelonephritis or premature labor.

Gastrointestinal System

The gastrointestinal (GI) system adapts in its anatomy and physiology during pregnancy in support of maternal and fetal nutritional requirements (see Table 4-1). The adaptations are related to hormonal influences and the impact of the enlarging uterus on the GI system as pregnancy progresses.

Most pregnant women experience some degree of nausea and vomiting in pregnancy (NVP). For most, the symptoms are an expected part of pregnancy and tolerated well; however, about a third of affected women experience significant distress. As the pregnancy progresses, NVP symptoms usually diminish; most experience significant symptom improvement by 16 weeks. It is important to identify women with significant NVP so they can be successfully treated.

Additional alterations in nutritional patterns commonly seen in pregnancy include:

- Increase in appetite and food intake
- Cravings for specific foods
  - Pica is a craving for and consumption of nonfood substances such as starch and clay. It can result in toxicity due to ingested substances or malnutrition from replacing nutritious foods with nonfood substances.
- Avoidance of specific foods

Anatomical and physiological changes include the following:

- Uterine enlargement displaces the stomach, liver, and intestines as the pregnancy progresses.
- By the end of pregnancy, the appendix is high and to the right along the costal margin.
- The GI tract experiences a general relaxation and slowing of its digestive processes during pregnancy, contributing to heartburn, abdominal bloating, and constipation.
- Hemorrhoids (varicosities in the anal canal) are common in pregnancy due to increased venous pressure and are exacerbated by constipation; 30% to 40% of pregnant women experience hemorrhoidal discomfort, pruritus, or bleeding.
- Gallstones: Relaxation of smooth muscle slows gallbladder emptying of bile; bile stasis and elevated levels of cholesterol contribute to formation of gallstones.
- Pruritus: Abdominal pruritus may be an early sign of cholestasis.
- Profuse salivation (ptyalism) may be experienced by some pregnant women.

● Bleeding gums and periodontal disease may occur.
  ● Increased vascularity of the gums can result in gingivitis.

Musculoskeletal System

Significant adaptation occurs in the musculoskeletal system due to pregnancy (see Table 4-1). Hormonal shifts are responsible for many of these changes. Mechanical factors attributable to the growing uterus also contribute to musculoskeletal adaptation. Anatomical and physiological changes include the following:

● Altered posture and center of gravity related to distention of the abdomen by the expanding uterus and reduced abdominal tone that shifts the center of gravity forward.
● Lordosis: Abnormal anterior curvature of the lumbar spine. The body compensates for the shift in the center of gravity by developing an increased curvature of the spine.
  ● A shift in the center of gravity places the woman at higher risk for falls.
● Altered gait ("pregnant waddle"): Hormonal influences of progesterone and relaxin soften ligaments and increase joint mobility.
● Round ligament spasm: Abdominal distention stretches round ligaments, causing spasm and pain.
● Diastasis recti: This is the separation of the rectus abdominis muscle in the midline caused by the abdominal distention. It is a benign condition that can occur in the third trimester.

The impact of the musculoskeletal adaptations in pregnancy, which result in numerous common discomforts, can sometimes be reduced if the woman maintains a normal body weight and exercises regularly before and throughout her pregnancy.

Integumentary System

The integumentary system includes the skin, hair, nails, and glands. Hormonal influences are primary factors in integumentary system adaptations during pregnancy (see Table 4-1). Anatomical and physiological changes include:

● Hyperpigmentation: Estrogen and progesterone stimulate increased melanin deposition of light brown to dark brown pigmentation.
  ● Linea nigra: Darkened line in midline of abdomen (Fig. 4–5A)
  ● Melasma (chloasma), also referred to as *mask of pregnancy:* This brownish pigmentation of the skin appears over the cheeks, nose, and forehead. This occurs in 50% to 70% of pregnant women and is more common in darker-skinned women. It usually occurs after the 16th week of pregnancy and is exacerbated by sun exposure.
● Striae gravidarum (i.e., stretch marks): Skin stretching that is caused by the growth of breasts, hips, abdomen, and buttocks, which may tear subcutaneous connective tissue and collagen (Fig. 4–5B).
● Varicosities, spider nevi, and palmer erythema: Vascular changes that are related to a hormonally induced increase in elasticity of vessels and increase in venous pressure from an enlarged uterus.

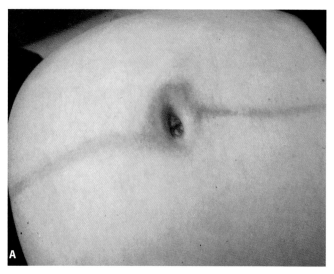

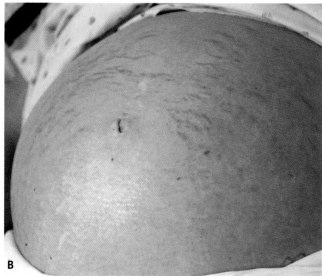

FIGURE 4–5 Pregnant abdomen with linea nigra (A) and striae (B).

● Hot flashes and facial flushing: Caused by increased blood supply to the skin, increase in BMR, progesterone-induced increased body temperature, and vasomotor instability.
● Oily skin and acne: These are effects of an increase in androgens.
● Sweating: The thermoregulation process at the level of skin increases in response to increases in thyroid activity, BMR, metabolic activity of the fetus, and increased maternal body weight.
● Although none of these integumentary system adaptations is seen universally, each alteration is seen commonly, is not of pathological significance, and typically resolves or regresses significantly after pregnancy.

Endocrine System

Endocrine system adaptations are essential for maintaining the stability of both the woman and her pregnancy and for promoting fetal growth and development. Endocrine glands mediate the many metabolic process adaptations in pregnancy. General endocrine system alterations occur due to pregnancy, and pregnancy-specific endocrine adaptations related to the placenta develop after conception (see Table 4-1).

Physiological changes during pregnancy include significant alterations in pituitary, adrenal, thyroid, parathyroid, and pancreatic functioning. For example, the hormonal production activity and size of the thyroid gland increase during pregnancy in support of maternal and fetal physiological needs, and pancreatic activity increases during pregnancy to meet both maternal and fetal needs related to carbohydrate metabolism.

Hormones of pregnancy are responsible for most of its physiological adaptations and physical changes. The placental hormones are initially produced by the corpus luteum of pregnancy. Once implantation occurs, the fertilized ovum and chorionic villi produce hCG.

● The high hCG level in early pregnancy maintains the corpus luteum and its production of progesterone and, to a lesser extent, estrogen until the placenta develops and takes over this function.
● After the development of a functioning placenta, the placenta produces most of the hormones of pregnancy, including estrogen, progesterone, human placental lactogen, and relaxin.
● Each of these hormones plays a role in the physiology of pregnancy, resulting in specific alterations in nearly all body systems, as described in this chapter, to support maternal physiological needs, maintenance and progression of the pregnancy, and fetal growth and development. Table 4-1 provides additional details on pregnancy hormones.

Immune System

Every aspect of the body's very complicated immune system undergoes adaptation during pregnancy to maintain a tenuous balance between preserving maternal-fetal well-being through normal immune responses and making the necessary alterations of the maternal immune system required to maintain the pregnancy. This adaptive process involves the maternal immune system becoming tolerant of the "foreign" fetal system so that the fetus is not rejected and is protected from infection. Immune function changes in pregnancy are far-reaching and beyond the scope of this chapter. This is also a relatively new body of science that is not fully understood.

PRECONCEPTION HEALTH CARE

Preconception health care is a broad term for the process of identifying social, behavioral, environmental, and biomedical risks and the medical care a woman or man receives to optimize health and wellness and reduce risks through education, counseling, and appropriate intervention when possible, to increase

SAFE AND EFFECTIVE NURSING CARE: Patient Education

Education about common pregnancy-related changes and comfort measures:

● Importance of wearing a properly fitted supportive bra
● Possibility of breasts leaking colostrum
● Braxton-Hicks contractions and contraction patterns that should be reported to the woman's health-care provider (HCP)
● Causes of supine and orthostatic hypotension and self-care measures to prevent
● Iron-rich foods and iron supplementation to prevent anemia
● Prevention and relief measures for dependent edema and varicosities
● Stand, stretch, and take a deep breath periodically throughout the day
● Reasons for increased frequency of urination during the first and third trimesters
● Signs and symptoms of a UTI with advice to seek prompt treatment
● UTI-prevention measures such as emptying the bladder frequently, wiping front to back, washing hands before and after urination, urinating before and after intercourse, and maintaining adequate hydration with at least eight glasses of liquid a day
● Kegel exercises and wearing a perineal pad if needed
● Normalcy and self-limiting nature of nausea and vomiting along with prevention and relief measures
● Importance of good oral hygiene and routine preventive dental care
● Importance of high-fiber diet with adequate hydration and physical activity to prevent constipation and hemorrhoids
● Prevention and relief measures for heartburn, flatulence, constipation, and hemorrhoids
● Musculoskeletal system changes during pregnancy and symptom relief measures for back or ligament pain
● Gentle abdominal strengthening exercises
● Reassurance as skin pigmentation or other changes occur
● Normalcy of striae in pregnancy and encourage good weight control
● Maintaining skin comfort with daily bathing, lotions, nonbinding clothing
● Limit sun exposure and wear sunscreen

the chances of having a healthy baby. Preconception care is not limited to a single visit to a health professional but is a process of care that is designed to meet the needs and improve the health of women during the different stages of their reproductive life. All women and men of reproductive age are candidates for preconception care.

The aim of preconception care is to optimize health and wellness by identifying and managing medical, behavioral, social, environmental, or biomedical potential risk to a woman's health or fertility before conception to increase the chances of a healthy baby. Preconception care is important because risk behaviors (e.g., smoking) and environmental exposures (e.g., Zika) can negatively affect fetal development and pregnancy outcomes. In addition, because almost half of pregnancies in the United States are unintended (Finer & Zolna, 2016), preconception care provides an opportunity to educate on modifiable risks, such as obesity or smoking, and intervene through motivational counseling or referrals to specialists as needed to reduce risks and optimize health before conception. If pregnancy occurs, preconception care can reduce such complications as congenital disorders or fetal growth abnormalities (Sackey & Blazey-Martin, 2020).

CRITICAL COMPONENT

Zika Virus Infection

The Zika virus is spread primarily through infected mosquitoes, but it can also be sexually transmitted from a person infected by the virus even without symptoms. A pregnant woman can spread the virus to her fetus, causing birth defects such as microcephaly, impaired growth, and visual abnormalities or hearing deficits.

Currently there is no vaccine to prevent the virus. Symptoms such as conjunctivitis, fever, joint pain, muscle pain, rash, or headache are generally mild and can last up to a week. Treatment consists of rest, fluids to prevent dehydration, and medications such as acetaminophen to reduce fever and pain. If a woman has symptoms of Zika virus before conceiving, she should be advised to wait at least 8 weeks from her first symptom before trying to conceive. If a woman's partner has been exposed or has symptoms, pregnancy should be avoided for at least 3 months to ensure he is not infected. Pregnant women and those wishing to conceive should avoid travel to areas known to have active mosquito transmissions of Zika. While pregnant, women should protect themselves from mosquitoes, use protection throughout pregnancy against sexual transmission from a partner who may be infected, and adhere to recommendations for standard infection precautions (March of Dimes, 2019).

Routine Physical Examination and Screening

Primary components of a preconception health-care visit are the physical examination, risk factor assessment, and relevant health screenings in the form of laboratory or diagnostic testing (Table 4-2).

- The physical examination includes:
  - Height and weight measurements to calculate body mass index (BMI) and assess for healthy weight
  - Comprehensive physical examination, including breast and pelvic examination
- Laboratory and diagnostic tests include:
  - Serum blood tests to determine blood type and Rh factor, complete blood count (CBC), cholesterol, glucose, IgG Rubella, HIV, and syphilis
  - Urinalysis
  - Cultures for sexually transmitted infections (STIs)
  - Papanicolaou smear (Pap smear), a screening test for cervical cancer
  - Tuberculin skin test
- Additional testing may be ordered based on history and physical examination findings.

Nursing Actions in Preconception Care

- Provide comfort and privacy.
- Use therapeutic communication techniques.
- Obtain the health history and conduct a review of systems.
- Provide teaching about procedures.
- Assist with physical and pelvic examinations and obtaining specimens.
- Provide anticipatory guidance and education related to the plan of care and appropriate follow-up and assess the patient's understanding.
- Provide education, recommendations, and referrals to help women make appropriate behavioral, lifestyle, or medical changes based on history or physical examination.

Preconception Anticipatory Guidance and Education

Anticipatory guidance is the provision of information and guidance to women and their families that enables them to be knowledgeable and prepared as the process of pregnancy and childbirth unfolds. Anticipatory guidance and education in the childbearing-aged population spans topics from health maintenance, self-care, and lifestyle choices to contraception and safety behaviors. The nurse is key in providing this aspect of care (Fig. 4–6). It is imperative that a woman's age, sexual orientation, culture, religion, and additional values and beliefs are acknowledged and respected and information incorporated appropriately into the nurse's teaching plan.

Preconception Education

The goal of preconception education is to provide a woman information she can use to enhance her health before becoming pregnant. When a woman seeks care specifically because she is planning for a future pregnancy, more emphasis is placed on counseling and anticipatory guidance related to preparation and planning for a pregnancy. Preconception anticipatory guidance and education topics include nutrition, vitamin supplements such as folic acid, exercise, self-care, contraception cessation, timing of conception, and modifying behaviors to reduce risks.

TABLE 4-2   Preconception Health History and Risk Factor Assessment

COMPONENT	PURPOSE AND ACTIONS
Identifying Information	
Age, gravida or para, address, race or ethnicity, religion, marital or family status, occupation, education	To determine specific risks based on sociodemographic characteristics: • Provide education and anticipatory guidance. • Identify psychosocial resources and available sources of support (see Chapter 5 for psychosocial and cultural assessment). • Refer for social services, counseling services, and spiritual support.
Health Promotion	
Prior and present health status Family planning and reproductive life plan Vaccination status Use of prenatal vitamins and folic acid	To determine past and present health status: • Provide education and anticipatory guidance. • Refer for additional testing and procedures. • Refer to a physician specialist, counseling services, genetic counseling, dietitian, or social services as indicated. • Administer rubella or hepatitis and flu vaccines as indicated. • Follow CDC guidelines for COVID-19 vaccinations while pregnant. • Advise on folic acid supplementation.
Disease and Complications	
History of or current medical conditions and diseases Surgeries (including blood transfusions) Medication use (prescription, over the counter, complementary) Allergies	To identify any components in medical history that may increase risk: • Initiate actions to minimize risks.
Family Medical	
Family history and current health status Medical conditions and diseases Known genetic conditions	To determine both modifiable and nonmodifiable risk factors related to family and genetic history: • Initiate actions to minimize risks.
Reproductive	
Menstrual Obstetric Gynecological Contraceptive Sexual History of physical or sexual abuse	To ascertain details about menstrual cycles; past pregnancies and their outcomes; prior preterm births or cesarean deliveries; any gynecological disorders, including infertility; past or present contraceptive use; history of STIs; sexual orientation; past or present sexuality issues; or use of safe sex practices
Self-care, Lifestyle, and Safety Behaviors	

	To determine:
	• Frequency of health maintenance visits (well-woman and dental)
	• Bowel patterns
	• Sleep patterns
	• Stress management
	• Nutrition, BMI, and exercise patterns:
	  • Counsel on the importance of achieving a normal BMI before conception
	• Safety practices such as use of seat belts, sunscreen, smoke alarms, and carbon monoxide detectors, as well as gun safety:
	  • Initiate actions to minimize risks.
	• Tobacco, alcohol, and substance use or abuse, as well as caffeine use:
	  • Refer to smoking cessation programs or substance abuse treatment as appropriate.
	• Use of complementary and alternative medicine modalities
	• Spiritual or religious practices

Continued

TABLE 4-2 Preconception Health History and Risk Factor Assessment—cont'd

COMPONENT	PURPOSE AND ACTIONS
Psychosocial	
Mental health Social	To ascertain past and present psychological and emotional health, barriers to care, communication obstacles, desire for pregnancy, stress, depression, intimate partner violence, and to identify sources of emotional and social support in family and friends: • Refer to mental health providers as needed.
Cultural	
Beliefs and values Practices Primary language	To identify cultural practices and beliefs or values impacting health and pregnancy: • Incorporate knowledge of beliefs and practices in care. To determine need for translation: • Obtain translation assistance as needed. • Provide educational materials in woman's primary language.
Environmental	
Home Workplace	To identify past and current exposure to environmental or occupational hazards or toxins: • Refer for environmental exposure counseling or genetic counseling when indicated.
Financial	
Basic needs related to food and housing Resources Health insurance	To determine access to care and adequacy of resources to meet basic ongoing needs: • Refer for social services or economic support services as indicated.

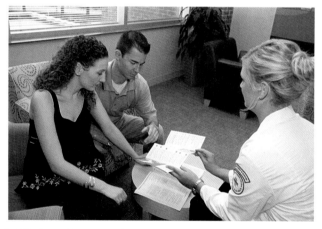

FIGURE 4–6 Nurse providing anticipatory guidance and education on self-care.

Nutrition

Maintaining a healthy weight is especially important for women planning a pregnancy. BMI is a number calculated based on a person's height and weight and represents a measure of body fat. The BMI can be used as an easy method of screening the nutritional status of women and to identify weight categories that may lead to health problems. The number of women of childbearing age who are overweight or obese has grown over the last three decades.

According to 2019 data, 31.6% of women aged 18 to 44 in the United States were obese (March of Dimes Peristats, 2021). Obesity increases a woman's risk for infertility and is associated with increased perinatal morbidity and mortality from a variety of causes:

● Complications such as spontaneous abortions, congenital anomalies, gestational diabetes, macrosomia, and fetal growth restriction
● Delivery complications such as preterm delivery, failed trial of labor, cesarean delivery, or shoulder dystocia
● Risks to her child include birth defects; metabolic abnormalities such as diabetes or childhood obesity; allergy or immunological issues such as asthma; behavioral and cognition abnormalities such as attention-deficit disorder; and long-term cardiovascular morbidity (Dow & Szymanski, 2020; Kahn et al., 2020)
● Postpartum obese women are at increased risk of endometritis, wound rupture or dehiscence, venous thrombosis, and postpartum hemorrhage (American College of Obstetricians and Gynecologists [ACOG], 2015).

Considering the lifelong health consequences associated with obesity, the Institute of Medicine (IOM) published guidelines in 2009 recommending that women achieve their normal BMI before conceiving, and this remains the current recommendation (IOM, 2009).

CLINICAL JUDGMENT

Pre-Pregnancy Weight

An overweight or obese pre-pregnancy weight increases the risk for poor maternal and neonatal outcomes and may have far-reaching implications for long-term health and development of chronic disease. At the other end of the spectrum, underweight pre-pregnancy weight or inadequate weight gain increases the risk for poor fetal growth and low birth weight. Women who are either significantly overweight or underweight should be counseled about potential issues with infertility and associated risks during and after pregnancy. Referral for dietary counseling and planning is recommended as needed to achieve a healthier weight before conception to decrease the risk of adverse pregnancy outcome (ACOG, 2015; Hanprasertpong, 2020).

World Health Organization Body Mass Index Categories

Underweight: Lower than 18.5

Normal weight: 18.5 to 24.9

Pre-obesity: 25 to 29.9

Obesity class I: 30 to 34.9

Obesity class II: 35 to 39.9

Obesity class III: 40 or greater

World Health Organization (WHO), 2021.

Given the detrimental influence of maternal overweight and obesity on reproductive and pregnancy outcomes for the mother and child, nutrition education and counseling are recommended before pregnancy, during pregnancy, and in the interconceptional period.

Nutritional education for women of childbearing years should include:

- Education on diet and physical activity and their role in reproductive health
- Advice on the importance of achieving and maintaining a healthy weight before conception
- Encouragement to make nutritious food choices emphasizing fresh fruits and vegetables, lean protein sources, low-fat or nonfat dairy foods, whole grains, and small amounts of healthy fats
- Choosing appropriate foods and serving sizes
- Appropriate vitamin and mineral supplementation

Certain foods and drinks should be avoided or limited during pregnancy. Those to avoid include highly caffeinated drinks; fish high in mercury (king mackerel, marlin, orange roughy, shark, or swordfish); undercooked fish, meat, or eggs; unpasteurized milk, cheese, or juices; and unwashed fruits and vegetables. Alcohol should be avoided as even small amounts can be harmful. Herbal supplements and medicines should generally be avoided, as they are not regulated for strength and purity and can interact with other prescribed medications.

One exception is ginger, which has been shown to improve nausea when prescribed at dosages of 1 to 1.5 g divided over a 24-hour period.

Prenatal Vitamins

Many women planning to conceive begin taking prenatal vitamin supplements. These contain a wide range of vitamins and minerals important for good health during pregnancy:

- Folic acid supplementation decreases risk of neural tube defects (NTDs). Folic acid supplementation of 0.4 mg daily for childbearing-aged women reduces the incidence of NTDs such as spina bifida. The beneficial impact of folic acid supplementation is greatest between 1 month before pregnancy and through the first trimester, the period of neural tube development. Due to the large percentage of unplanned pregnancies and the fact that the neural tube closes very early in pregnancy, before many women know they are pregnant, all women of childbearing potential are recommended to take a daily folic acid supplement containing 0.4 mg. Prenatal vitamins contain at least 0.4 mg of folic acid.
  - Women with a higher risk of offspring with NTD should consult their provider about recommendations for a higher daily dose (1 to 4 mg) and preferably initiated 1 to 3 months before conceiving and maintaining this dosage throughout the first trimester; after that, 0.4 mg/day for the remainder of the pregnancy is recommended.
- Calcium, magnesium, and vitamin D contribute to bone health and osteoporosis prevention throughout the life span, including during the childbearing years.
- Iron supplementation is commonly prescribed during pregnancy, although there is some controversy about the benefit of this practice as a routine recommendation.
  - A woman who is anticipating a short time between pregnancies is at risk for iron-deficiency anemia. Iron supplementation may be prescribed, and she is encouraged to include iron-rich foods in her diet in between pregnancies because she is likely to have reduced iron stores and may also be anemic from the previous recent pregnancy.
- Megadoses—doses many times the usual amount—of vitamins and minerals are not advised, as they may be toxic to the developing fetus.

Exercise

A program of regular physical activity positively impacts a woman's health and may generally be continued once she has conceived. If the woman is healthy and her pregnancy is normal, exercise will not increase her risks for early delivery or other complications and physical activity is safe when practiced according to recommendations (Michalek et al., 2020). It is best to implement such a program several months in advance of conception so that when pregnancy occurs, regular exercise is already comfortable and routine. Women embarking on a new exercise regime are advised to discuss this with their provider during their prenatal visits.

- Aerobic activity, including regular weight-bearing exercise such as walking or running, combined with stretching exercises and some type of weight work or muscle strengthening provides overall body conditioning, helps with weight management, and can enhance psychological well-being.

- The weight-bearing exercise and weight or strengthening work also enhance bone health and help prevent osteoporosis.
- Swimming and water workouts exercise many muscles while avoiding muscle strain.
- Riding a stationary bicycle is safer than a standard bicycle.
- Pregnant women should avoid the following:
  - Yoga poses that require lying on the back for long periods
  - "Hot" yoga or Pilates which could cause overheating
  - Contact sports, scuba diving, skydiving, or activities that could result in injury or a fall, such as horseback riding or downhill snow skiing

Exercise may be contraindicated in certain conditions such as:

- Women with significant pulmonary or cardiovascular disease
- Pregnancy complications: preeclampsia, placenta previa, anemia, morbid obesity, fetal growth restriction, poorly controlled diabetes
- High risk for preterm labor: multifetal gestation, premature rupture of membranes, cerclage.

CRITICAL COMPONENT

When to Stop Exercising and Notify the Health-Care Provider

A pregnant woman should stop exercising and call her HCP if she experiences:

- Abdominal pain with or without nausea
- Calf pain or swelling
- Chest pain
- Dizziness, syncope
- Headache
- Muscle weakness affecting balance
- New dyspnea before exercising
- Regular, painful uterine contractions
- Vaginal bleeding or leaking fluid from the vagina

ACOG, 2020.

Self-Care

Most women are pregnant for at least 1 to 2 weeks before becoming aware of their pregnancy. For this reason, it is helpful to counsel all those interested in becoming pregnant to decrease risk behaviors and eliminate exposure to substances that are known or suspected to be harmful during gestation as soon as contraception is stopped, or she begins trying to become pregnant. The following should be avoided if planning to conceive:

- Illicit drugs, cannabis, alcohol, tobacco (even secondhand smoke), and excessive caffeine
- Medications contraindicated in pregnancy (prescription, over-the-counter, and herbal supplements)
- Environmental toxins. Exposure to some toxic substances—including lead, mercury, arsenic, cadmium, pesticides,

solvents, and household chemicals—can increase the risk of miscarriage, preterm birth, and other pregnancy complications.

Encourage the following self-care activities:

- Engage in safe-sex practices to prevent STIs.
- Wear seat belts whenever driving or riding in a car.
- Ensure that smoke alarms and carbon monoxide detectors are in working order.
- Apply sunscreen when outdoors.
- Maintain adequate relaxation and sleep.
- Take good care of teeth and gums and treat periodontal disease before pregnancy.
- Discuss the use of complementary or alternative medicine modalities, such as acupuncture, herbal supplements, homeopathy, and massage, with her primary HCP. Some of these interventions may need to be discontinued before a pregnancy for safety reasons.

Contraception Cessation

Before conception, it is ideal for a woman to have at least two or three normal menstrual periods. For all women planning a pregnancy, discontinuing contraception and tracking menstrual cycles will aid in facilitating conception and in dating the pregnancy once conception is achieved.

- Women using hormonal contraception should stop and begin using a barrier method of birth control or fertility awareness family planning techniques for the few months before conception.
- Women using Depo-Provera for contraception should be informed that it may take several months to more than a year to conceive after discontinuing injections.
- Women using an intrauterine device will need to have the device removed.

Timing of Conception

Many women are interested in learning more about their menstrual cycles to gain more control over their ability to conceive.

- Preconception counseling can include basic information about the menstrual cycle, when in the cycle a woman can conceive, signs of ovulation, the life span of ovum and sperm, and how to time sexual intercourse to increase the likelihood of conception.
- Women who used fertility awareness family planning principles are familiar with these concepts and can reverse behaviors they practiced when using the method to avoid conception.

Preconception Care for Men

Preconception care for men offers an opportunity for disease prevention and health promotion and is an important factor in improving family planning and pregnancy outcomes for women, enhancing the reproductive health and health behaviors of men and their partners, and preparing men for fatherhood. When a couple is planning to conceive, the man should have a medical evaluation to identify and manage poorly controlled disease states such as diabetes or hypertension. Preconception education and counseling for healthy behaviors (such as reproductive life planning, proper nutrition, and healthy weight maintenance) and avoidance of certain risks, such as tobacco use and exposure to toxic substances, is recommended.

Access to Care

Various institutional, cultural, and economic barriers make it challenging for some groups of people to access the health care they need. Because perinatal nurses provide care to women and infants, we are especially concerned with eliminating the barriers to care for these populations. Nurses are members of one of the most trusted professions and thus play an invaluable role in leading and supporting efforts to increase access to care for all women, regardless of their race, socioeconomic status, or environment. Nurses should be aware of barriers that affect access to health care and strive to reduce health disparities through advocacy work with organizations such as the Association of Women's Health, Obstetric and Neonatal Nurses (AWHONN); with state and federal legislators; and within their communities. In addition to providing support, information, and referrals to women from underserved communities, nurses can improve health care and further narrow the health disparities gap by following these actionable steps:

- Enhance communication between the patient and provider with language aides, interpreter services, or teach-back methods.
- Practice shared decision making with all clients.
- Address implicit bias or unconscious bias and enhance cultural sensitivity through training.
- Monitor data related to quality metrics stratified according to race, ethnicity, language, poverty, and literacy.
- Use continuous quality improvement strategies to address disparities identified.
- Promote culture of equity with equal standards of care for patients of all races and ethnic groups.
- Develop new models of care promoting women's health across the life span.
- Engage key stakeholders such as state agencies, public health-care systems, patient advocacy groups, and organizations dedicated to improving health care for all women (Howell & Ahmed, 2019)

DIAGNOSIS OF PREGNANCY

The diagnostic confirmation of pregnancy is based on a combination of the presumptive, probable, and positive changes and signs of pregnancy. This information is obtained through history, physical and pelvic examinations, and laboratory and diagnostic studies.

Presumptive Signs of Pregnancy

The presumptive signs of pregnancy include all subjective signs of pregnancy (i.e., physiological changes perceived by the woman). These changes could have causes outside of pregnancy and are not considered diagnostic:

- Amenorrhea: Absence of menstruation
- Nausea and vomiting: Common from week 2 through 12
- Breast changes: Changes begin to appear at 2 to 3 weeks
  - Enlargement, tenderness, and tingling
  - Increased vascularity
- Fatigue: Common during the first trimester
- Urination frequency: Related to pressure of enlarging uterus on bladder; decreases as uterus moves upward and out of pelvis
- Quickening: A woman's first awareness of fetal movement; occurs around 18 to 20 weeks' gestation in primigravidas (between 14 and 16 weeks in multigravidas)

Probable Signs of Pregnancy

The probable signs of pregnancy are objective signs of pregnancy and include all physiological and anatomical changes that can be perceived by the HCP. These changes could also have causes other than pregnancy and are not considered diagnostic:

- Chadwick's sign: Bluish-purple coloration of the vaginal mucosa, cervix, and vulva seen at 6 to 8 weeks
- Goodell's sign: Softening of the cervix and vagina with increased leukorrheal discharge; palpated at 8 weeks
- Hegar's sign: Softening of the lower uterine segment; palpated at 6 weeks
- Uterine growth and abdominal growth
- Skin hyperpigmentation
  - Melasma (chloasma), also referred to as the *mask of pregnancy:* Brownish pigmentation over the forehead, temples, cheek, or upper lip
  - Linea nigra: Dark line that runs from the umbilicus to the pubis
  - Nipples and areola: Become darker; more evident in primigravidas and dark-haired women
- Ballottement: A light tap of the examining finger on the cervix causes the fetus to rise in the amniotic fluid and then rebound to its original position; occurs at 16 to 18 weeks
- Positive pregnancy test results
  - Laboratory tests are based on detection of the presence of hCG in maternal urine or blood.
  - The tests are extremely accurate but not 100%. There can be both false-positive and false-negative results. Due to this, a positive pregnancy test is considered a probable rather than a positive sign of pregnancy.
  - A maternal blood pregnancy test can detect hCG levels before a missed period.
  - A urine pregnancy test is best performed using a first morning urine specimen, which has the highest concentration of hCG and becomes positive about 4 weeks after conception.
  - Home pregnancy tests are accurate (but not 100%) and simple to perform. These urine tests use enzymes and rely on a color change when agglutination occurs, indicating a pregnancy. The home tests can be performed at the time of a missed menstrual period or as early as 1 week before a missed period. If a negative result occurs, the instructions

suggest that the test be repeated in 1 week if a menstrual period has not begun.

The presumptive and probable signs of pregnancy are important components of assessment in confirming a pregnancy. Early in gestation, before positive signs of pregnancy, a combination of presumptive and probable signs is used to make a practical diagnosis of pregnancy.

Positive Signs of Pregnancy

The positive signs of pregnancy are the objective signs of pregnancy (noted by the examiner) that can only be attributed to the fetus:

- Auscultation of the fetal heart by 10 to 12 weeks' gestation with a Doppler
- Observation and palpation of fetal movement by the examiner after about 20 weeks' gestation
- Sonographic visualization of the fetus: Cardiac movement noted at 4 to 8 weeks

Sonographic Diagnosis of Pregnancy

Ultrasound using a vaginal probe can confirm a pregnancy slightly earlier than with the transabdominal method. With a transvaginal ultrasound, the gestational sac is visible by 4.5 to 5 weeks' gestation and fetal cardiac movement can be observed as early as 4 weeks' gestation. Ultrasound has increasingly become a routine and expected part of PNC. Indications for ultrasound examination of an early pregnancy for purposes of diagnosis include:

- Pelvic pain or vaginal bleeding in the first trimester
- History of repeated pregnancy loss or ectopic pregnancy (the implantation of a fertilized ovum outside the uterus)
- Uncertain menstrual history
- Discrepancy between actual size and expected size of pregnancy based on history

PREGNANCY

The antepartum (antepartal) period, also referred to as the prenatal period, begins with the first day of the last menstrual period (LMP) and ends with the onset of labor (the intrapartal period). Pregnancy is also counted in terms of trimesters, each roughly 3 months in length.

Due Date Calculation

An important piece of information to share with a newly pregnant woman and her family is her "due date," or estimated date of birth, more commonly known as estimated date of delivery (EDD). This date represents a best estimation as to when a full-term infant will be born. The original term used for this date was estimated date of confinement.

Calculation of the EDD is best accomplished with a known and certain LMP. If the LMP is unknown, other tools are used to determine the most accurate EDD possible:

- Physical examination to determine uterine size
- First auscultation of fetal heart rate with a Doppler or a fetoscope (stethoscope for auscultation of fetal heart tones)
- Date of quickening
- Ultrasound examination
- History of assisted reproduction

Naegele's Rule

Naegele's rule is the standard formula for determining an EDD based on the LMP: First day of LMP − 3 months + 7 days.

LMP	September 7
	− 3 months
	June 7
	+ 7 days
EDD	June 14

It is important to remember that the EDD as determined by Naegele's rule is only a best guess of when a baby is likely to be born. Two factors influence the accuracy of Naegele's rule:

- Regularity of a woman's menstrual cycles
- Length of a woman's menstrual cycles
- Results may be inaccurate if menstrual cycles are irregular or are greater than 28 days apart.

Most women give birth within 3 weeks before to 2 weeks after their EDD. The length of pregnancy is approximately 280 days, or 40 weeks from the first day of the LMP. In recent years, there has been conflicting or inconsistent information on the definition of a "term" pregnancy. The window for full-term gestation is between 38 and 42 weeks from the LMP; however, in 2012, a workgroup of experts met to review the definition of term gestation. Based on evidence that infant mortality is lowest for deliveries between 39 weeks 0 days and 41 weeks 6 days, the workgroup recommended that "early term" be used to refer to births between 37 weeks 0 days and 38 weeks 6 days and "late term" be used to refer to births between 41 weeks 0 days and 41 weeks 6 days (Spong, 2013).

CRITICAL COMPONENT

Classification of Deliveries From 37 Weeks of Gestation

Early term: 37 0/7 weeks through 38 6/7 weeks

Full term: 39 0/7 weeks through 40 6/7 weeks

Late term: 41 0/7 weeks through 41 6/7 weeks

Post term: 42 0/7 weeks and beyond

ACOG, 2017; Spong, 2013.

Weeks of Gestation

Once an EDD has been determined, a pregnancy is counted in terms of weeks of gestation, beginning with the first day of the LMP and ending with 40 completed weeks (the EDD). A useful tool for quickly and easily calculating the EDD is the gestational wheel (Fig. 4–7), but it is less reliable than Naegele's rule due to variations of up to a few days between wheels. It is best to calculate a due date initially using Naegele's rule and then employ a gestational wheel to determine a woman's current gestational age (Box 4-1).

To use the gestational wheel, place the arrow labeled "first day of last period" from the inner circle on the date of the LMP on the outer circle. The EDD is then read as the date on the outside circle that lines up with the arrow at 40 completed weeks on the inside circle. With the example, the LMP is September 7 and the EDD is June 14.

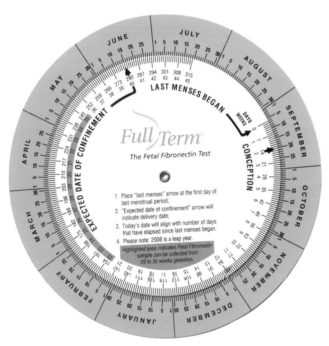

FIGURE 4–7 Gestational wheel. To use the gestational wheel, place the arrow labeled "first day of last period" from the inner circle on the date of the LMP on the outer circle. The EDD is then read as the date on the outside circle that lines up with the arrow at 40 completed weeks on the inside circle. Here the LMP is September 7 and the EDD is June 14.

BOX 4-1 | Gestational Age

What Is Gestational Age?

Gestational age refers to the number of completed weeks of fetal development, calculated from the first day of the last normal menstrual period. Embryologists date fetal age and development from the time of conception (known as *conceptual* or *embryological age*), which is usually 2 weeks later. Unless otherwise specified, all references to dating or fetal age in this textbook will be gestational ages (based on time since the LMP and not time since conception).

Prenatal Assessment Terminology

An important shorthand system for explaining a woman's obstetrical history uses the terms *gravida* and *para* (G/P) in describing numbers of pregnancies and births.

- G/P is a two-digit system used to denote pregnancy and birth history.
- Gravida refers to the total number of times a woman has been pregnant, without reference to how many fetuses there were with each pregnancy or when the pregnancy ended. It is simply how many times a woman has been pregnant, including the current pregnancy.
- Para refers to the number of births after 20 weeks' gestation whether live births or stillbirths. There is no reference to the number of fetuses delivered with this system, so twins count as one delivery, similar to a singleton birth. A pregnancy that ends before the end of 20 weeks' gestation is considered an abortion, whether it is spontaneous (miscarriage) or induced (elective or therapeutic) and is not counted using the G/P system.
- GTPAL (gravida, term, preterm, abortion, living) is a more comprehensive system that gives more information than gravida and para alone. This system designates numbers as follows:
  - **G** = total number of times pregnant (same as G/P system)
  - **T** = number of Term pregnancies
  - **P** = number of Preterm pregnancies
  - **A** = number of Abortions (either spontaneous or induced) before 20 weeks' gestation
  - **L** = the number of children currently Living
- Because GTPAL can be used by some organizations to designate the number of infants rather than pregnancies, it can be a bit confusing if not used consistently. For more clarity, GTPALM may be used as previously noted with the addition of *M* representing pregnancies with multiple gestations.
- Nulligravida is a woman who has never been pregnant or given birth.
- Primigravida is a woman who is pregnant for the first time.
- Multigravida is a woman who is pregnant for at least the second (or more) time.

ANTEPARTAL NURSING CARE: PHYSIOLOGY-BASED NURSING ASSESSMENT AND NURSING ACTIONS

Nurse actions have significant impact on patient outcomes; the care nurses provide to women before, during, and after birth is fundamental to the well-being of them and their newborns. The nurse's expert knowledge confers the authority to shape the care environment and influence patient decisions. Therefore, understanding the physiological and psychosocial adaptations and changes of pregnancy improves the overall quality of health care provided to women.

Prenatal Assessment

The prenatal period is the entire period a woman is pregnant, through the birth of the baby. It is a time of transition in a family's life as they prepare for the birth of a child, affording an opportunity for positive change in all aspects of health and health maintenance behaviors. PNC is health care related to pregnancy, also referred to as antenatal care.

During ongoing interactions, the nurse places emphasis on health education and health promotion involving the woman in her care. The integrative view of health inherent in nursing care for the childbearing woman and her family contributes to a unique situation in which the antepartal patient has ready access to health information, individualized woman-centered support, and guidance to help achieve the healthiest possible pregnancy and the best possible outcome for the woman and baby. The impact of health care related to pregnancy and the possibility for positive change can extend well beyond the antepartal period for the new family.

Early, adequate PNC has long been associated with improved pregnancy outcomes including reduced maternal and perinatal morbidity and mortality both directly through detection and treatment of pregnancy-related complications and indirectly through the identification of women and girls at increased risk of developing complications during labor and delivery. Three basic components of adequate PNC are early and continuing risk assessment, health promotion, and medical and psychosocial intervention with follow-up. The goal of PNC is to detect potential problems early, prevent them if possible, and direct women to appropriate specialists or hospitals if necessary. PNC also provides an important opportunity to prevent and manage concurrent diseases through integrated service delivery. In addition, PNC can provide reassurance of well-being to a pregnant woman and her family while providing education and information.

Assessment during the initial prenatal visit parallels a preconception health-care visit (see Tables 4-2 and 4-3) and includes a general physical assessment including a pelvic examination. The focus of patient education and anticipatory guidance shifts toward pregnancy-related health concerns, but the basic components of the visit and the emphasis on health maintenance and health promotion remain the same.

Prenatal visits also include specific assessment of the pregnancy and fetal status. Some components are uniform across prenatal visits, and others are specific to one or more trimesters.

Assessment during prenatal visits also includes information about the health and health history of the father of the baby (i.e., age, blood type and Rh status, current health status, history of any chronic or past medical problems, genetic history, occupation, lifestyle factors impacting health, and his involvement in the woman's life and with her pregnancy).

Subsequent prenatal visits are more abbreviated than the initial visit, with nursing care and interventions focused on current pregnancy status and patient needs, always with an emphasis on patient education and anticipatory guidance (see Table 4-3 and the Clinical Pathway for Routine Prenatal Care).

With each prenatal visit, maternal weight and blood pressure are evaluated and fetal heart rate, activity, growth, and amniotic fluid volume are assessed. In late pregnancy, vaginal examinations may be done as indicated. Current guidelines on the frequency of prenatal visits are monthly up to 28 weeks of gestation, then every 2 weeks between 28 and 36 weeks' gestation, and then weekly from 36 weeks' gestation until delivery (American Academy of Pediatrics [AAP]/ACOG, 2017).

Prenatal nursing care and interventions also contribute to the woman's and family's ability to make informed choices about the health of the entire family throughout the childbearing cycle, based on information provided by the nurse and integrated with the family's personal values, preferences, and beliefs. One *Healthy People 2030* objective is to increase the proportion of pregnant women who receive early and adequate PNC from 76.4% to 80.5% (U.S. Department of Health and Human Services, 2020). Family-centered maternity care is based on a view that pregnancy and childbirth are normal life events, a life transition that is not primarily medical but rather developmental.

Evidence-Based Practice

Screening and Counseling Reduces Alcohol Use in Pregnancy

O'Connor, E. A., Perdue, L. A., Senger, C. A., Rushkin, M., Patnode, C. D., Bean, S. I., & Jonas, D. E. (2018). Screening and behavioral counseling interventions to reduce unhealthy alcohol use in adolescents and adults: Updated evidence report and systematic review for the US Preventive Services Task Force. *Journal of the American Medical Association. 320*(18), 1910–1928. https://doi.org/10.1001/jama.2018.12086

Pregnant women or those trying to get pregnant should abstain from all alcohol use as it has been associated with fetal alcohol spectrum disorders (FASDs). There is no known amount or type of alcohol that is considered safe to drink during pregnancy, and no safe time during pregnancy to drink alcohol. In this systematic review, researchers found that validated screening tools for alcohol use are available and can quickly identify those with unhealthy alcohol use, including women who are pregnant or of reproductive age. For pregnant women screening positive for alcohol use, brief counseling intervention sessions were found to be associated with more reporting abstinence as compared with those in the control group. Screening and counseling may further prevent progression of alcohol consumption to more serious forms of unhealthy use.

Goals of Prenatal Care

- Maintenance of maternal fetal health
- Accurate determination of gestational age
- Ongoing assessment of risk status and implementation of risk-appropriate intervention
- Rapport built with the childbearing family
- Referrals to appropriate resources

At every PNC appointment, it is imperative that the nurse provides a relaxed environment for the woman and her family

TABLE 4-3 Prenatal Care: Content and Timing of Routine Prenatal Visits

	HISTORY AND PHYSICAL ASSESSMENT	LABORATORY AND DIAGNOSTIC STUDIES IN NORMAL PREGNANCY (RECOMMENDED TIMING)
First Trimester		

Initial visit at 6 to 8 weeks	Comprehensive health and risk assessment (see Table 4-1)
	
	Height and weight or BMI
	
	Current pregnancy history
	
	Complete physical and pelvic examination
	
	EDD evaluation
	
	Psychosocial assessment (see Chapter 5) including depression screen
	
	Assessment for IPV
		• Blood type and Rh factor
		• Antibody screen
		• CBC, including:
		  • Hemoglobin
		  • Hematocrit
		  • RBC count
		  • WBC count
		  • Platelet count
		• RPR, VDRL (syphilis)
		• HIV screen
		• Hepatitis B screen (surface antigen)
		• Genetic screening may be done between 10 0/7 weeks and 13 6/7 weeks.
		• Rubella titer
		• PPD (tuberculosis screen)
		• Urinalysis
		• Urine culture and sensitivity
		• Pap smear
		• Gonorrhea and chlamydia cultures
		• Ultrasound

Visit 2 at 10 to 12 weeks (4 weeks after initial visit)	Chart review Interval history Focused physical assessment: Vital signs, urine, weight, fundal height Fetal heart tones EDD evaluation Clinical pelvimetry	
Second Trimester		
Visit 3 at 16 to 18 weeks Visit 4 at 22 weeks	Chart review Interval history Nutrition follow-up Focused physical assessment: Vital signs, urine dipstick for glucose, albumin, ketones, weight, fundal height, FHR, fetal movement, Leopold's maneuver, edema Pelvic examination or sterile vaginal examination if indicated Confirm established due date Depression screen	• Triple screen, quad screen, or penta screen • Ultrasound • Screening for gestational diabetes at 24–28 weeks • Hemoglobin and hematocrit • Antibody screen if Rh negative • Administration of RhoGAM if Rh negative and antibody screen negative
Third Trimester		
Visits 5 to 12 are every 2 to 3 weeks until 36 weeks, then weekly until 40 weeks; typically, twice weekly after 40 weeks)	Chart review Interval history Nutrition follow-up Focused physical assessment: Vital signs, urine dipstick for glucose, albumin, ketones, weight, fundal height, FHR, fetal movement (i.e., kick counts), Leopold's maneuver, edema Cervix examination starting at visit around 36 weeks Confirm fetal position	Screenings: • H&H if not done in second trimester • Repeat GC, chlamydia, RPR, HIV, HBsAg (if indicated and not done in late second trimester) • 1-hour glucose challenge test at 24–28 weeks • Group B streptococcus culture done at 35–37 weeks' gestation to determine presence of GBS bacterial colonization before the onset of labor in order to anticipate intrapartum antibiotic treatment needs

where they feel comfortable asking questions and sharing details about their lives related to the health of the woman, her fetus, and the developing family. For some, pregnancy is the only time they come into frequent contact with an HCP, and due to the increased prevalence of intimate partner violence (IPV) during pregnancy, all women should be screened at each encounter (see Critical Component: Intimate Partner Violence [Abuse]). Early identification of IPV is necessary to minimize its serious physical and mental effects, as well as its adverse health outcomes for the fetus.

CRITICAL COMPONENT

Intimate Partner Violence (Abuse)

IPV against women consists of actual or threatened physical or sexual violence, as well as psychological and emotional abuse, by a current or former partner or spouse. IVP affects women of every age, race, religion, socioeconomic status, and educational level and is the most common form of violence against women. Pregnant women are at a higher risk for IPV, especially those who have unplanned pregnancies, and the highest risk for IPV is among pregnant adolescents. According to the National Perinatal Association (2020), 20% to 30% of women in the United States have experienced IPV; however, the true prevalence may be unknown due to fear of disclosure by the victim or failure on the part of the provider to screen adequately. The U.S. Preventive Services Task Force (USPSTF) (2018) recommends that all women of reproductive age be screened for IPV and women who disclose abuse or screen positive should be referred to ongoing support services. The following are effective screening tools recommended by the USPSTF for detecting IPV in the past year: Humiliation, Afraid, Rape, Kick (HARK); Hurt/Insult/Threaten/Scream (HITS); Extended-Hurt/Insult/Threaten/Scream (E-HITS); Partner Violence Screen (PVS); and Woman Abuse Screening Tool (WAST).

Any woman who screens positive for IPV should have further screening to determine her risk for serious harm or femicide and receive ongoing support services including counseling and home visits to address multiple risk factors in addition to IPV.

National Perinatal Association, 2020; USPSTF, 2018.

Nursing Actions

- Provide for comfort and privacy and use therapeutic communication techniques during the interview and conversation.
  - Demonstrate sensitivity toward the patient related to the personal nature of the interview and conversation.
  - To maintain patient confidentiality and protection, some assessment questions should always be asked in private such as those related to gravida/para status or IPV.
- Obtain the woman's identifying information (initial prenatal visit).
- Obtain a complete health history (initial prenatal visit) or an interval history (subsequent visits) (see Tables 4-2, 4-3, and the Clinical Pathway feature).

- Conduct a review of systems (initial prenatal visit).
- Obtain blood pressure, temperature, pulse, respirations, weight, height, and BMI (initial prenatal visit).
- Assess for absence or presence of edema.
- Provide anticipatory guidance for the patient before and during the physical examination (initial prenatal visit and subsequent visits when indicated).
- Assist with physical and pelvic examination as needed (initial prenatal visit and subsequent visits when indicated).
- Assist with obtaining specimens for laboratory or diagnostic studies as ordered (initial prenatal visit and subsequent visits when indicated) and assess urine specimen for protein, glucose, and ketones.
- Provide teaching about procedures as needed (initial prenatal visit and subsequent visits when indicated).
- Provide anticipatory guidance related to the plan of care and appropriate follow-up, including how and when to contact a care provider with warning signs or symptoms.
- Provide teaching appropriate for the woman, her family, and her gestational age; assess the woman's understanding of the teaching provided; and allow time for the woman to ask questions.
- Document, according to agency protocol, all findings, interventions, and education provided.

Cultural assessment is an important part of PNC. To plan culture-specific care, the nurse should assess the woman's beliefs, values, and behaviors that relate to pregnancy and childbearing. This includes information about ethnic background, religious preferences, language, communication style, common etiquette practices, and expectations of the health-care system (see further discussion in Chapter 5).

First Trimester

Another *Healthy People 2030* objective is to increase the proportion of pregnant women who receive early and adequate PNC, with a target goal of 80.5% (U.S. Department of Health and Human Services, 2020). The baseline report from the National Center for Health Statistics indicated that 76.4% of pregnant females received early and adequate PNC in 2018.

During the initial prenatal visit, the woman learns the frequency of follow-up visits and what to expect from her prenatal visits as the pregnancy progresses (see Table 4-3 and the Clinical Pathway feature). If the patient is seen for her initial prenatal visit early in the first trimester, she may have more than one visit during that trimester. Subsequent visits are similar to those described for the second trimester. If the woman presents late for PNC and is in her second or third trimester at her initial prenatal visit, the nurse may need to modify typical patient education content to meet the current needs of the patient and her family.

Components of Initial Prenatal Assessment

- History of current pregnancy:
  - First day of LMP and degree of certainty about the date
  - Regularity, frequency, and length of menstrual cycles

- Recent use or cessation of contraception
- Woman's knowledge of conception date
- Signs and symptoms of pregnancy
- Whether the pregnancy was intended
- The woman's response to being pregnant
- Obstetrical history, detail about all previous pregnancies:
  - GTPAL
  - Whether abortions, if any, were spontaneous or induced
  - Dates of pregnancies
  - Length of gestation
  - Type of birth experiences (e.g., induced or spontaneous labors, vaginal or cesarean births, use of forceps or vacuum-assist, type of pain management)
  - Complications with pregnancy, labor, or birth
  - Neonatal outcomes, including Apgar scores, birth weight, neonatal complications, feeding method, health and development since birth
  - Pregnancy loss and grieving status
- Physical and pelvic examinations:
  - The bimanual component of the pelvic examination enables the examiner to internally palpate the dimensions of the enlarging uterus. This information assists with dating the pregnancy, either confirming an LMP-based EDD or providing information in the absence of a certain LMP. When gestational age is uncertain, a decision may be made to perform an ultrasound examination of the pregnancy to determine an EDD. It is important to determine an accurate EDD as early as possible because numerous decisions related to timing of interventions and management of pregnancy are based on gestational age as determined by the EDD.
  - Clinical pelvimetry (measurement of the dimensions of the bony pelvis through palpation during an internal pelvic examination) may be performed during the initial pelvic examination; however, it is not routinely done.
- Assessment of uterine growth:
  - Uterine growth after 10 to 12 weeks' gestation is assessed by measuring the height of the fundus with the use of a centimeter measuring tape. The zero point of the tape is placed on the symphysis pubis, and the tape is then extended to the top of the fundus. The measurement should approximately equal the number of weeks pregnant. Instruct the woman to empty her bladder before the measurement because a full bladder can displace the uterus (Fig. 4–8).
  - Maternal position and examiner uniformity are variables that render this evaluation somewhat imprecise, but it is useful as a gross measure of progressive fetal growth as well as to help identify a pregnancy that is growing outside the optimal or normal range, either too large or too small for its gestational age. This serves as a screening tool for fetal growth.
- Assessment of fetal heart tones is performed with an ultrasound Doppler in the first trimester, initially heard by 10 and 12 weeks' gestation. The normal fetal heart rate (FHR) baseline is between 110 and 160 beats per minute.

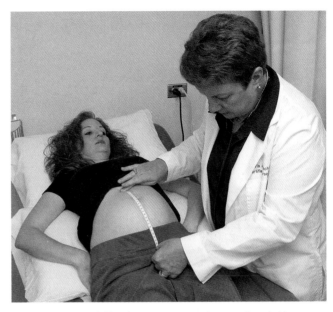

FIGURE 4–8 Fundal height measurement during prenatal visit.

- Comprehensive laboratory and diagnostic studies:
  - Laboratory studies are ordered or obtained at the initial prenatal visit to establish baseline values for follow-up and comparison as the pregnancy progresses.
  - Ultrasound might be performed during the first trimester to confirm intrauterine pregnancy, viability, and gestational age.

CRITICAL COMPONENT

Warning or Danger Signs of the First Trimester
Educate pregnant women in the first trimester to contact their HCP immediately if they experience any of the following symptoms:

- Abdominal cramping or pain indicates possible threatened abortion, UTI, or appendicitis.
- Vaginal spotting or bleeding indicates possible threatened abortion.
- Absence of fetal heart tone indicates possible missed abortion.
- Dysuria, frequency, and urgency indicate possible UTI.
- Fever or chills indicate possible infection.
- Prolonged nausea and vomiting indicate possible hyperemesis gravidarum; increased risk of dehydration.

Nutritional Assessment and Education

Obesity, defined as a pre-pregnancy BMI of 30 kg/m^2 or more, is the most prevalent medical condition for women of childbearing age. Maternal obesity during pregnancy has been linked to adverse outcomes such as early pregnancy loss, stillbirth, congenital anomalies, preterm and post-term birth, gestational diabetes, pregnancy-associated hypertension, postpartum depression, and venous thromboembolism (Ramsey & Schenken, 2021). Pregnancy is a time when women are open to nutritional

BOX 4-2 | Recommendations for Total and Rate of Weight Gain During Pregnancy, by Pre-Pregnancy BMI

The impact of pre-pregnancy weight and gestational weight gain on perinatal outcomes is significant and is directly related to infant birth weight, morbidity, and mortality. The current evidence suggests that inadequate weight gain or an underweight pre-pregnancy weight increases risk for poor fetal growth and low birth weight. At the other end of the spectrum, excessive weight gain or an overweight or obese pre-pregnancy weight increases the risk for poor maternal and neonatal outcomes and may have far-reaching implications for long-term health and development of chronic disease. Pre-pregnancy weight and BMI, as well as gestational weight gain, have increased nationally. The recommendations for maternal weight gain in a singleton pregnancy are individualized based on pre-pregnancy BMI.

PRE-PREGNANCY BMI	TOTAL WEIGHT GAIN RECOMMENDED IN POUNDS	RATES OF WEIGHT GAIN,* SECOND AND THIRD TRIMESTER MEAN (RANGE) IN LB/WEEK
Underweight (<18.5)	28–40	1 (1–1.3)
Normal weight (18.5–24.9)	25–35	1 (0.8–1)
	37–54 for twin pregnancies	
Overweight (25–29.9)	15–25	0.6 (0.5–0.7)
	31–50 for twin pregnancies	
Obese (≥30)	11–20	0.5 (0.4–0.6)
	25–42 for twin pregnancies	

*Calculations assume a 1.1 to 4.4 lb weight gain in the first trimester.
AAP & ACOG, 2017; Institute of Medicine, 2009.

and lifestyle education, so it is an optimal time for needed behavioral changes in overweight and obese women. Nutrition should be discussed at all prenatal visits to reinforce the importance of appropriate weight gain, as both excessive and inadequate weight gain in pregnancy are associated with poor perinatal outcomes.

- Discuss appetite, cravings, or food aversions.
- Obtain a 24-hour diet recall and review for obvious deficiencies.
- Based on the woman's pre-pregnancy BMI and National Academy of Medicine (formerly the IOM guidelines [Box 4-2]):
  - Assist the woman to set weight-gain goals with a recommended weight gain of between 1 and 5 pounds during the first trimester.
  - Discuss distribution of weight gain during pregnancy (Box 4-3).
  - Encourage the woman to eat a variety of unprocessed foods from all food groups, including fresh fruits, vegetables, whole grains, lean meats or beans, and low-fat dairy products.
  - For more detailed information on nutritional needs during each trimester of pregnancy or to design a personalized daily food plan tailored to personal life circumstances, refer the patient to www.myplate.gov.
- Encourage the woman to drink 8 to 10 glasses of fluid per day and limit caffeine to 200 mg per day.
- Certain types of fish (king mackerel, orange roughy, marlin, shark, swordfish, and tilefish) should be avoided due to high levels of mercury; most other fish and seafood are safe as long as fully cooked. Tuna is safe but limit white (albacore) tuna to 6 ounces per week.

BOX 4-3 | Maternal Weight Gain Distribution

Baby: 7 to 8 lb

Placenta: 1.5 lb

Amniotic fluid: 2 lb

Breasts: 1 to 3 lb

Uterus: 2 lb

Increased fluid volume: 2 to 3 lb

Increased blood volume: 3 to 4 lb

Maternal fat stores: 6 to 8 lb

Poston, 2021.

- Advise on prevention of food-borne illnesses:
  - Wash hands frequently, before and after handling food. Use warm water and soap.
  - Thoroughly rinse all raw vegetables and fruits before eating.
  - Cook eggs and all meats, poultry, or fish thoroughly, and sanitize all dishes, utensils, cutting boards, or areas that contact these during food preparation.
  - Discard cooked food left out at room temperature for more than 2 hours.
  - Foods to avoid:
    - Unpasteurized juices or dairy products
    - Raw sprouts of any kind

- Unpasteurized soft cheeses such as Brie, Camembert, or feta
- Refrigerated, smoked seafood
- Unheated deli meats or hot dogs
- Raw eggs
- Raw fish and shellfish
- Teas with chamomile, peppermint, licorice, or raspberry leaf

---

CRITICAL COMPONENT

Initial Prenatal Laboratory Tests With Rationale
Laboratory screening includes:

- ABO and Rh type with antibody screening to identify isoimmunization. Patients who are Rh negative should be rescreened in the second trimester and given RhoGAM at 26 to 28 weeks and again after delivery if the infant is Rh positive.
- Either Hct or Hgb levels should be monitored for signs of anemia. Blood volume in pregnancy increases more than red cell volume and hematocrit typically falls. Anemia is often caused by iron deficiency and should be treated with supplemental iron taken in addition to routine prenatal vitamins.
- Serological screening for rubella is used to determine if the mother is susceptible or immune. If susceptible, she should receive vaccination postpartum.
- Varicella is used to determine if the mother is susceptible or immune. If susceptible, she should receive vaccination postpartum.
- Syphilis using venereal disease research laboratory (VDRL) or rapid plasma reagin (RPR) is used to check for serological evidence of syphilis so treatment can be initiated as soon as possible to avoid vertical transmission and the sequelae of congenital syphilis.
- Gonorrhea and chlamydia tests are used to identify and treat infection.
- Urine protein as a baseline and urine culture are used to identify and treat UTI, including asymptomatic bacteriuria, which is associated with a 25% risk of pyelonephritis if left untreated.
- Hepatitis B surface antigen is used to identify women whose infants need immunoprophylaxis postdelivery to minimize the risk of congenital infection and carrier status.
- Regarding human immunodeficiency virus (HIV), antiretroviral therapy during gestation and around the time of delivery can decrease the risk of vertical transmission to lower than 2%. HIV-positive women should be counseled on the risks and benefits of treatment and mode of delivery.
- Women aged 21 to 29 years should have cytology screening every 3 years. Women aged 30 to 65 years should have human papillomavirus (HPV) and cytology co-screening every 5 years or cytology alone every 3 years.
- Tuberculosis skin tests are performed for patients at risk—for example, recent immigrants from developing countries, inmates, and residents of mental institutions or group homes.
- Discussion of prenatal screening for chromosome abnormalities, genetic disease, and birth defects should be performed and documented in the patient's medical record (see Chapter 6 for details related to screening and diagnostic tests).
- Other selective screening tests may be performed as indicated based on the patient's history or symptoms (Lockwood & Magriples, 2021)

Migrant Women

Women of reproductive age constitute a large proportion of new immigrants to the United States and are among the most vulnerable members of the population. Pregnancy can be an entry point into the health-care system for immigrant women, though they are less likely to access maternal care services than their nonimmigrant counterparts. In a systematic review, Heaman et al. (2013) reported that immigrants were more likely to receive inadequate PNC, initiate PNC late in pregnancy, and have less than the recommended number of prenatal appointments.

A systematic review of qualitative research indicates migrant women had pregnancy expectations strongly rooted in home beliefs, values, and practices that were supported by family, husband, and friends. However, when women lacked support, they experienced several challenges in navigating the HCS. Furthermore, the overall experience of a woman's pregnancy is negatively affected when she believes that her HCPs are unsupportive, insensitive, and disrespectful to her wishes (Winn et al., 2017). The author recommends strategies be implemented to increase cultural sensitivity within the HCS and recognize a need for awareness that immigrant women may be isolated in their new country and need additional assistance to navigate an unfamiliar system. For example, women with support from the community and from providers were more likely to be receptive to the care and accept new practices if they understood their benefit or if the practice was supported by someone they knew. Women reported that to feel comfortable asking questions, they must feel practices from their country of origin were respected. Understanding that a woman's expectations of pregnancy are rooted in home practices, values, and beliefs can help providers support women. Working with immigrant support groups can help identify potential cultural advisors to help new immigrants navigate the HCS (Winn et al., 2017).

Second Trimester

Subsequent or return prenatal visits begin with a chart review from the previous visit(s) and an interval history. This history includes information about the pregnancy since the previous prenatal visit (see Table 4-3 and the Clinical Pathway feature).

SAFE AND EFFECTIVE NURSING CARE:
Patient Education

Patient education topics for women in the first trimester of pregnancy should include general information on the following:

- Physical changes and common discomforts of pregnancy may occur (see Table 4-1).
  - Relief measures for normal discomforts in early pregnancy are discussed based on patient need (Table 4-4).
- Fetal development: By the end of the first trimester, the fetus is 3 inches in length and weighs 1 to 2 ounces, all organ systems are present, the head is large, and the heartbeat is audible with Doppler.
- Health maintenance and health promotion information:
  - Avoid exposure to tobacco, alcohol, and recreational drugs.
  - Avoid exposure to environment hazards with teratogenic effects.
  - Obtain input from the care provider before using medications, complementary and alternative medicine, and nutritional supplements.
  - Reinforce safety behaviors (e.g., seat belt, sunscreen).
  - Recognize the need for additional rest.
  - Maintain daily hygiene.
  - Decrease risk for UTIs and vaginal infections by wiping from front to back, wearing cotton underwear, maintaining adequate hydration, voiding after intercourse, and not douching.
  - Maintain good oral hygiene: Perform gentle brushing of teeth and flossing, and continue routine preventive dental care.
  - Exercise 30 minutes each day: Avoid risk for trauma to abdomen, avoid overheating, and maintain adequate hydration while exercising.
  - Establish a daily Kegel exercise routine to maintain pelvic floor muscle strength and decrease the risk of urinary incontinence and uterine prolapse.
  - Travel is safe in low-risk pregnancy; however, the woman may need to stop more frequently to stretch and walk to decrease the risk of thrombophlebitis; take a copy of the prenatal record.
  - Use coping strategies for stress, such as relaxation exercises and meditation.
  - Communicate with the partner regarding changes in sexual responses: Sexual responses and desires change throughout pregnancy. Couples need to talk openly about these changes and explore different sexual positions that accommodate the changes of pregnancy.
- Warning and danger signs need to be reported to the care provider.

Components of Second-Trimester Prenatal Assessments

- Focused physical assessment
- Vital signs
  - Vital signs within normal limits; slight decrease in blood pressure toward end of second trimester
- Weight
  - Average weight gain per week depending on pre-pregnancy BMI (see Box 4-2)
- Urine dipstick for glucose, albumin, and ketones
  - Mild proteinuria and glucosuria are normal.
- FHR
  - Able to auscultate FHR with Doppler; rate 110 to 160 bpm (Fig. 4–9)
- Fetal movement
  - Assess for quickening (when the woman feels her baby move for the first time).
- Leopold's maneuvers (palpation of the abdomen) to identify the position of the fetus in utero (Chapter 8)
  - Examiner able to palpate fetal parts.
- Fundal height measurement
  - Fundal height should equal weeks of gestation.
- Confirm established due date
  - Quickening occurs around 18 weeks' gestation (usually between 18 and 20 weeks of gestation, but sometimes as early as 14 to 16 weeks of gestation in a multigravida and occasionally as late as 22 weeks of gestation in some primigravidas).
  - Ultrasound around 20 weeks' gestation to confirm EDD and scan fetal anatomy

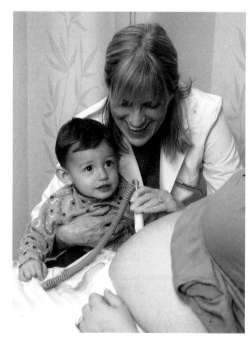

FIGURE 4–9 A nurse practitioner listening to fetal heart tone with a pregnant mom and her toddler.

TABLE 4-4   Self-Care and Relief Measures for Physical Changes and Common Discomforts of Pregnancy

BODY SYSTEM	PHYSICAL CHANGES AND COMMON DISCOMFORTS OF PREGNANCY (COMMON TIMING)	NURSING ACTIONS FOR PATIENT EDUCATION FOR SELF-CARE AND RELIEF MEASURES
Generalized or multisystem	Fatigue (first and third trimesters)	Reassure the woman of the normalcy of her response. Encourage the woman to plan for extra rest during the day and at night; focus on the "work" of growing a healthy baby. Enlist support and assistance from friends and family. Encourage the woman to eat an optimal diet with adequate caloric intake and iron-rich foods and iron supplementation if anemic.
	Insomnia (throughout pregnancy)	Instruct the woman to implement sleep hygiene measures (regular bedtime, relaxing or low-key activities pre-bedtime). Encourage the woman to create a comfortable sleep environment (body pillow, additional pillows). Teach breathing exercises and relaxation techniques or measures (progressive relaxation, effleurage [a massage technique using a very light touch of the fingers in two repetitive circular patterns over the gravid abdomen], warm bath, or warm beverage before bed). Evaluate caffeine use.
	Emotional lability (throughout pregnancy)	Reassure the woman of the normalcy of response. Encourage adequate rest and optimal nutrition. Encourage communication with partner or significant support people. Refer to a pregnancy support group.
Reproductive		
Breasts	Tenderness, enlargement, upper back pain (throughout pregnancy; tenderness mostly in the first trimester)	Encourage the woman to wear a well-fitting, supportive bra. Instruct woman in correct use of good body mechanics.
	Leaking of colostrum from nipples (starting second trimester onward)	Reassure the woman of the normalcy. Recommend soft cotton breast pads if leaking is troublesome.
Uterus	Braxton-Hicks contractions (mid-pregnancy onward)	Reassure the woman that occasional contractions are normal. Instruct the woman to call her provider if contractions become regular and persist before 37 weeks. Ensure adequate fluid intake. Recommend a maternity girdle for uterus support.
Cervix and vagina	Increased secretions Yeast infections (throughout pregnancy)	Encourage daily bathing. Recommend cotton underwear. Recommend wearing panty liner and changing the pad frequently. Instruct the woman to avoid douching or using feminine hygiene sprays. Inform the provider if discharge changes in color or is accompanied by foul odor or pruritus.
	Dyspareunia (throughout pregnancy)	Reassure the woman or couple of normalcy of response, and provide information. Suggest alternative positions for sexual intercourse and alternative sexual activity to sexual intercourse.

Continued

TABLE 4-4   Self-Care and Relief Measures for Physical Changes and Common Discomforts of Pregnancy—cont'd

BODY SYSTEM	PHYSICAL CHANGES AND COMMON DISCOMFORTS OF PREGNANCY (COMMON TIMING)	NURSING ACTIONS FOR PATIENT EDUCATION FOR SELF-CARE AND RELIEF MEASURES
Cardiovascular		
	Supine hypotension (mid-pregnancy onward)	Instruct the woman to avoid the supine position from mid-pregnancy onward.
		Advise her to lie on her side and rise slowly to decrease the risk of a hypotensive event.
	Orthostatic hypotension	Advise the woman to keep her feet moving when standing and avoid standing for prolonged periods.
		Instruct the woman to rise slowly from a lying position to sitting or standing to decrease the risk of a hypotensive event.
	Anemia (throughout pregnancy; more common in late second trimester)	Encourage the woman to include iron-rich foods in daily dietary intake and take iron supplementation.
	Dependent edema in lower extremities or vulva (late pregnancy)	Instruct the woman to: • Wear loose clothing • Use a maternity girdle (abdominal support), which may help reduce venous pressure in the pelvis and lower extremities and enhance circulation • Avoid prolonged standing or sitting • Dorsiflex feet periodically when standing or sitting • Elevate legs when sitting • Position on side when lying down
	Varicosities (later pregnancy)	Instruct the woman in all measures for dependent edema (see earlier).
		Suggest the woman wear support hose (put on before rising in the morning, before legs have been in dependent position).
		Instruct the woman to lie on her back with legs propped against a wall in an approximately 45-degree angle to spine periodically throughout the day.
		Instruct the woman to avoid crossing her legs when sitting.
Respiratory		
	Hyperventilation and dyspnea (throughout pregnancy; may worsen in later pregnancy)	Reassure the woman of the normalcy of her response and provide information.
		Instruct the woman to slow down respiration rate and depth when hyperventilating.
		Encourage good posture.
		Instruct the woman to stand and stretch, taking a deep breath periodically throughout the day; also stretch and take a deep breath periodically throughout the night.
		Suggest sleeping semi-sitting with additional pillows for support.
	Nasal and sinus congestion and epistaxis (throughout pregnancy)	Suggest the woman try a cool-air humidifier.
		Instruct the woman to avoid use of decongestants and nasal sprays and instead to use normal saline drops.

TABLE 4-4   Self-Care and Relief Measures for Physical Changes and Common Discomforts of Pregnancy—cont'd

BODY SYSTEM	PHYSICAL CHANGES AND COMMON DISCOMFORTS OF PREGNANCY (COMMON TIMING)	NURSING ACTIONS FOR PATIENT EDUCATION FOR SELF-CARE AND RELIEF MEASURES
Renal		
	Frequency and urgency or nocturia (may be throughout pregnancy; most common in first and third trimesters)	Reassure the woman of the normalcy of response. Encourage the woman to empty her bladder frequently, always wiping front to back. Stress the importance of maintaining adequate hydration and reducing fluid intake only near bedtime. Instruct her to urinate after intercourse. Teach the woman to notify her provider if there is pain or blood with urination. Encourage Kegel exercises; wear perineal pad if needed.
Gastrointestinal		
	Nausea or vomiting in pregnancy (NVP) (first trimester and sometimes into the second trimester)	Reassure the woman of normalcy and self-limiting nature. Avoid causative factors (e.g., strong odors, spicy or greasy foods, large meals, stuffy rooms, hot places, loud noises). Encourage women to experiment with alleviating factors: • Eat small, frequent meals as soon as, or before, feeling hungry. • Eat at a slow pace. • Eat crackers or dry toast before rising or whenever nauseous. • Drink cold, clear carbonated beverages such as ginger ale, or sour beverages such as lemonade. • Avoid fluid intake with meals. • Eat ginger-flavored lollipops or peppermint candies. • Brush teeth after eating. • Wear P6 acupressure wrist bands. • Take vitamins at bedtime with a snack (not in the morning). • Suggest vitamin B_6, 25 mg by mouth three times daily or ginger, 250 mg by mouth four times daily Oral or rectal medications may be prescribed for management of troublesome symptoms. Identify, acknowledge, and support women with significant NVP to offer additional treatment options.
	Increase or sense of increase in salivation (mostly first trimester if associated with nausea)	Suggest use of gum or hard candy or use astringent mouthwash.
	Bleeding gums (throughout pregnancy)	• Encourage the woman to maintain good oral hygiene (brush gently with soft toothbrush, perform daily flossing). • Maintain optimal nutrition.
	Flatulence (throughout pregnancy)	Encourage the woman to: • Maintain regular bowel habits. • Engage in regular exercise. • Avoid gas-producing foods. • Chew food slowly and thoroughly. • Use the knee–chest position during periods of discomfort.

Continued

TABLE 4-4   Self-Care and Relief Measures for Physical Changes and Common Discomforts of Pregnancy—cont'd

BODY SYSTEM	PHYSICAL CHANGES AND COMMON DISCOMFORTS OF PREGNANCY (COMMON TIMING)	NURSING ACTIONS FOR PATIENT EDUCATION FOR SELF-CARE AND RELIEF MEASURES
	Heartburn (later pregnancy)	Suggest the following: • Eat small, frequent meals. • Maintain good posture. • Maintain adequate fluid intake but avoid fluid intake with meals. • Avoid fatty or fried foods. • Remain upright for 30–45 minutes after eating. • Refrain from eating at least 3 hours before bedtime.
	Constipation (throughout pregnancy; see Concept Map feature)	Encourage the woman to: • Maintain adequate fluid intake. • Engage in regular exercise such as walking. • Increase fiber in diet through vegetables, fruits, and whole grains. • Maintain regular bowel habits. • Maintain good posture and body mechanics.
	Hemorrhoids (later pregnancy)	Avoid constipation (see earlier). Instruct the woman to avoid bearing down with bowel movements. Instruct the woman in comfort measures (e.g., ice packs, warm baths or sitz baths, witch hazel compresses). Elevate the hips and lower extremities during rest periods throughout the day. Gently reinsert hemorrhoid into the rectum while doing Kegel exercises.
Musculoskeletal		
	Low back pain, joint discomfort, or difficulty walking (later pregnancy)	Instruct the woman to: • Utilize proper body mechanics (e.g., stoop using knees vs. bend for lifting). • Maintain good posture. • Do pelvic rock and pelvic tilt exercises. • Wear supportive shoes with low heels. • Apply warmth or ice to the painful area. • Use a maternity girdle. • Use massage. • Use relaxation techniques. • Sleep on a firm mattress with pillows for additional support of extremities, abdomen, and back.
	Diastasis recti (later pregnancy)	Instruct the woman to do gentle abdominal strengthening exercises (e.g., tiny abdominal crunches, may cross arms over abdomen to opposite sides for splinting, no sit-ups). Teach proper technique for sitting up from lying down (i.e., roll to side, lift torso up using arms until in sitting position).
	Round ligament spasm and pain (late second and third trimester)	Instruct the woman to: • Lie on her side and flex the knees up to the abdomen. • Bend toward pain. • Do pelvic tilt and pelvic rock exercises. • Use warm baths or compresses. • Use side-lying in exaggerated Sim's position with pillows for additional support of the abdomen and in between legs. • Use a maternity belt.

TABLE 4-4 Self-Care and Relief Measures for Physical Changes and Common Discomforts of Pregnancy—cont'd

BODY SYSTEM	PHYSICAL CHANGES AND COMMON DISCOMFORTS OF PREGNANCY (COMMON TIMING)	NURSING ACTIONS FOR PATIENT EDUCATION FOR SELF-CARE AND RELIEF MEASURES
	Leg cramps (throughout pregnancy)	Instruct the woman to: • Dorsiflex the foot to stretch the calf muscle. • Apply warm baths or compresses to the affected area. • Change position slowly. • Massage the affected area. • Engage in regular exercise and muscle conditioning.
Integumentary	Striae (stretch marks) (later pregnancy)	Reassure the woman that there is no method to prevent them. Suggest maintaining skin comfort (e.g., lotions, oatmeal baths, nonbinding clothing). Encourage good weight control.
	Dry skin or pruritus (itching) (later pregnancy)	Suggestions for maintaining skin comfort: Use tepid water for baths and showers and rinse with cooler water. Avoid hot water (drying effect may increase itching). Use moisturizing soaps or body wash. Avoid exfoliating scrubs or deodorant soaps (has drying effect and may increase itching). Use of lotions, oatmeal baths, and nonbinding clothing may lessen itching.
	Skin hyperpigmentation	Limit sun exposure. Wear sunscreen regularly.
	Acne	Use products developed for the face only (e.g., cleansers, sunscreen), avoid body soaps and facial scrubs (both have drying effects), as well as body lotions and creams (clog pores); use tepid water when washing the face and always follow with a cold rinse to close pores before applying moisturizers (if needed) or sunscreen.
Neurological	Headaches Syncope	Maintain adequate hydration. Rise slowly from sitting to standing. Instruct the woman to avoid the supine position from mid-pregnancy onward. Advise the woman to lie on her side and rise slowly to decrease the risk of a hypotensive event.

- Presence of edema
  - Slight lower-body edema is normal due to decreased venous return.
  - Upper-body edema, especially of the face, is abnormal and needs further evaluation.
- Laboratory and diagnostic studies
  - Screening tests for NTD and trisomy 21 (Chapter 6)
  - Screening for gestational diabetes: 1-hour glucose challenge test recommended between 24 and 28 weeks; 3-hour glucose tolerance test (GTT) is ordered if 1-hour screen is elevated.
  - Hemoglobin and hematocrit between 28 and 32 weeks to identify anemia and the need for an iron supplement. This is the time in pregnancy when the hemoglobin and hematocrit are likely to be at their lowest, so the result provides the care provider with valuable information for management of late pregnancy.
  - Syphilis serology if prevalent or as indicated
  - Antibody screen for Rh-negative women

- Administer anti-D immunoglobulin (i.e., RhoGAM) to Rh-negative women with negative antibody screen results.
  - Anti-D immunoglobulin is administered at 28 weeks' gestation to help prevent isoimmunization and the resulting risk of hemolytic disease in fetuses in subsequent pregnancies.

SAFE AND EFFECTIVE NURSING CARE: Understanding Medication

Rh$_o$(D) Immune Globulin (RhoGAM)

Laboratory screening during an initial prenatal visit includes blood type and Rh factor with antibody screening to identify isoimmunization. Patients found to be Rh$_o$(D)-negative should be rescreened in the second trimester and given RhoGAM at 26 to 28 weeks and again after delivery if the infant is Rh$_o$(D)-positive.

- Indication: Administered to Rh$_o$(D)-negative women prophylactically at 26 to 28 weeks' gestation to prevent isoimmunization from potential exposure to Rh$_o$(D)-positive fetal blood during the normal course of pregnancy. Also administered with likely exposure to Rh$_o$(D)-positive blood, such as with pregnancy loss, amniocentesis, or abdominal trauma. If the infant is Rh$_o$(D)-positive, another dose is given within 72 hours after delivery.
- Action: Prevents production of anti-Rh$_o$(D) antibodies in Rh$_o$(D)-negative women exposed to Rh$_o$(D)-positive blood. Prevention of antibody response and hemolytic diseases of the newborn (erythroblastosis fetalis) in future pregnancies of women who have conceived an Rh$_o$(D)-positive fetus.
- Adverse reactions: Pain at intramuscular (IM) site; fever
- Route/dosage: One vial standard dose (300 mcg) IM at 26 to 28 weeks' gestation. Use cautiously in patients with preexisting idiopathic thrombocytopenic purpura (ITP) anemia (decrease dose if Hgb is lower than10 g/dL) (Vallerand & Sanoski, 2021).

CRITICAL COMPONENT

Warning and Danger Signs of the Second Trimester

- Abdominal or pelvic pain indicates possible preterm labor (PTL), UTI, pyelonephritis, or appendicitis.
- Absence of fetal movement once the woman has been feeling daily movement indicates possible fetal distress or death.
- Prolonged nausea and vomiting indicates possible hyperemesis gravidarum; this woman is at risk for dehydration.
- Fever and chills indicate possible infection.
- Dysuria, frequency, and urgency indicate possible UTI.
- Vaginal bleeding indicates possible infection, friable cervix caused by pregnancy changes, placenta previa, abruptio placenta, or PTL.

SAFE AND EFFECTIVE NURSING CARE: Patient Education

Patient education topics during the second trimester should include information on:

- Fetal development during the second trimester
  - At 20 weeks' gestation, the fetus is 8 inches long, weighs 1 pound, and is relatively long and skinny.
- General health maintenance and health promotion topics
- Nutritional follow-up and reinforcement
  - Consume recommended daily caloric intake during the second trimester.
  - Offer counseling and guidance on dietary intake or physical activity as needed.
- Physical changes during the second trimester (see Table 4-1)
- Relief measures for normal discomforts commonly experienced during the second trimester (see Table 4-4)
- Warning signs of pregnancy complications
  - Signs and symptoms of PTL
  - Rhythmic lower abdominal cramping or pain
  - Low backache
  - Pelvic pressure
  - Leaking of amniotic fluid
  - Increased vaginal discharge
  - Vaginal spotting or bleeding
- Signs and symptoms of hypertensive disorders
  - Severe headache that does not respond to usual relief measures
  - Visual changes
  - Facial or generalized edema
- Benefits and risks of procedures and tests with the goal of enabling the woman to make informed decisions about what procedures she will choose based on her knowledge of the available options coupled with her and her family's values and beliefs.

Third Trimester

The focused assessment includes all aspects of the second trimester assessment and may also include a pelvic examination to identify cervical change, depending on weeks of gestation and maternal symptoms. Assessment of pregnancy in the third trimester becomes more frequent and involved than in previous return visits as the pregnancy advances and the fetus nears term (see Table 4-3 and the Clinical Pathway feature).

Components of Third-Trimester Assessments

- Chart review
- Interval history
- Focused assessment (e.g., fundal height)
- Assessment of fetal well-being
  - Auscultation of FHR

- Record woman's assessment of "kick counts"
  - Daily fetal movement count (kick counts) is a maternal assessment of fetal movement by counting fetal movements in a period of time to identify potentially hypoxic fetuses. Maternal perception of fetal movement was one of the earliest tests of fetal well-being and remains an essential assessment of fetal health. The pregnant woman is instructed to palpate the abdomen and track fetal movements daily by tracking fetal movements for 1 or 2 hours.
  - In the 2-hour approach recommended by the ACOG, maternal perception of at least 10 distinct fetal movements within 2 hours is considered reassuring; once movement is achieved, counts can be discontinued for the day.
  - In the 1-hour approach, the count is considered reassuring if it equals or exceeds the established baseline; in general, four movements in 1 hour is reassuring.
  - Define fetal movements or kick counts to include kicks, flutters, swishes, or rolls.
  - Instruct the mother to keep a journal or documentation of the time it takes to feel fetal movement.
  - Instruct the mother to perform counts at the same time every day.
  - Instruct the mother to monitor the time intervals it takes and to contact HCP immediately if there are deviations from normal (i.e., no movements or decreased movements).
  - Decreased fetal activity should be reported to the provider, as further evaluation of the fetus, such as a non-stress test or biophysical profile, is indicated.
- Pelvic examination to identify cervical change, depending on weeks of gestation and maternal symptoms
- Leopold's maneuvers to identify the position of the fetus in utero (Chapter 8)
- Screening for Group B streptococcus (GBS)
  - One-quarter to one-third of women are colonized with GBS in the lower GI or urogenital tract (typically asymptomatic).
  - GBS infection in a newborn, either early onset (first week of life) or late onset (after first week of life), can be invasive and severe, with potential long-term neurological sequelae.
  - Vaginal and rectal swab cultures are done at 35 to 37 weeks' gestation to determine the presence of GBS bacterial colonization before the onset of labor to anticipate intrapartum antibiotic treatment needs.
- Laboratory tests and screening
  - Conduct 1-hour glucose test at 24 to 28 weeks' gestation (may have already been done in the second trimester).
  - Perform hemoglobin and hematocrit (H&H) (if not recently done in the second trimester).
  - Repeat gonorrhea culture (GC), chlamydia, syphilis test by RPR if indicated and not screened in second trimester, HIV, and hepatitis B surface antigen (HBsAg) tests as indicated.
- Travel limitations regarding the last month
- Discussion of preparation for labor and birth
  - Attend childbirth classes.
  - Discuss the method of labor pain management.
  - Develop a birth plan; list preferences for routine procedures.

- Signs of impending labor
  - Discussion of true versus false labor
  - Instruction on when to contact the doctor or midwife
  - Instructions on when to go to the birthing unit
- Discussion on parenting and infant care
  - Attend parenting classes.
  - Select the method of infant feeding.
  - Select the infant's HCP.
  - Prepare siblings.

CRITICAL COMPONENT

Warning and Danger Signs of the Third Trimester
- Abdominal or pelvic pain (PTL, UTI, pyelonephritis, appendicitis)
- Decreased or absent fetal movement (fetal hypoxia or death)
- Prolonged nausea and vomiting (dehydration, hyperemesis gravidarum)
- Fever, chills (infection)
- Dysuria, frequency, urgency (UTI)
- Vaginal bleeding (infection, friable cervix caused by pregnancy changes or pathology, placenta previa, placenta abruptio, PTL)
- Signs and symptoms of PTL: Rhythmic lower abdominal cramping or pain, low backache, pelvic pressure, leaking of amniotic fluid, increased vaginal discharge
- Signs and symptoms of hypertensive disorders: Severe headache that does not respond to usual relief measures, visual changes, facial or generalized edema

---

SAFE AND EFFECTIVE NURSING CARE:
Patient Education

Patient education for women in the third trimester should include information on the following:

- Fetal growth during the third trimester
- At term fetus is about 17 to 20 inches in length, weighs between 6 and 8 pounds, has increased deposits of subcutaneous fat, and has established sleep and activity cycles.
- Offer general health maintenance and health promotion topics.
- Provide nutritional follow-up and reinforcement.
- Recommend daily caloric intake during third trimester.
- Offer counseling and guidance on dietary intake or physical activity as needed.
- Review physical changes during the third trimester (Table 4-4).
- Explain relief measures for normal discomforts commonly experienced during the third trimester (Table 4-4).
- Prepare for childbirth.
- Review the warning signs of pregnancy complications.

Clinical Pathway for Routine Prenatal Care

Focus of Care	Initial Prenatal Visit	First Trimester	Second Trimester	Third Trimester
Frequency of Prenatal Visits	Initial visit	Return visit (4 weeks after initial visit) and then every 4 weeks	Return visit every 4 weeks	Return visits every 2 to 3 weeks until 36 weeks, then weekly until 40 weeks; twice weekly after 40 weeks
Assessments	Comprehensive health and risk assessment Current pregnancy • First day of LMP • Regularity, frequency, and length of menstrual cycles • Recent use or cessation of contraception • Woman's knowledge of conception date • Determine EDD • Signs and symptoms of pregnancy • Inquire whether the pregnancy was intended • Assess the woman's response to being pregnant • Obstetrical history GTPAL • Date of pregnancies • Length of gestation • Type of birth experiences • Complications with previous pregnancies • Prior pregnancy losses • Neonatal outcomes, including Apgar scores • Medical history • Family history • Social history • Smoking • Alcohol • Substance use Sexual history and practices Complete physical assessment • Vital signs • Urine • Pelvic examination	Chart review Interval history since last visit Focused physical assessment: • Weeks, gestation • Blood pressure • Urine dipstick for glucose, albumin, ketones • Weight, including cumulative weight gain or loss • Fundal height measurement • Fetal heart tones • Clinical pelvimetry	Chart review Interval history Nutrition follow-up Focused physical assessment: • Blood pressure and vital signs • Urine dipstick for glucose, albumin, ketones • Weight • Fundal height measurement • Fetal heart tones • Fetal movement—note beginning of fetal movement (quickening) • Leopold's maneuver • Edema Pelvic examination or sterile vaginal examination if indicated Reevaluate pregnancy risk status	Chart review Interval history Nutrition follow-up Focused physical assessment: • Vital signs • Urine dipstick for glucose, albumin, ketones • Weight • Fundal height measurement • Leopold's maneuver • Edema • Pelvic examination or sterile vaginal examination if indicated • Assessment of fetal well-being • FHR • Fetal movement (i.e., kick counts)

Clinical Pathway for Routine Prenatal Care—cont'd

Focus of Care	Initial Prenatal Visit	First Trimester	Second Trimester	Third Trimester
	Nutrition assessment • Height and weight to calculate BMI • 24-hour diet recall Physical activity level Psychosocial and cultural assessment (see Chapter 5) Depression evaluation Assessment for IPV			
Laboratory and Diagnostic Studies	Blood type and Rh factor Antibody screen CBC, including: • Hemoglobin • Hematocrit • RBC count • WBC count • Platelet count (see Appendix A for normal laboratory values in pregnancy) RPR, VDRL (syphilis serology) HIV screen Hepatitis B screen (surface antigen) Offer genetic screening Rubella titer purified protein derivative (PPD) (tuberculosis screen) Urinalysis Urine culture and sensitivity Pap smear Gonorrhea and chlamydia cultures Ultrasound	Review laboratory tests	Triple screen or quad screen at 15 to 20 weeks Ultrasound as indicated Screening for gestational diabetes with 1-hour glucose challenge test at 24 to 28 weeks Hemoglobin and hematocrit (see Appendix A for normal laboratory values in pregnancy) Antibody screen if Rh-negative around 26 to 28 weeks • Administration of RhoGAM at 28 weeks if Rh-negative and antibody-screen negative	Group B streptococcus screening: • Vaginal and rectal swab cultures done at 35 to 37 weeks on all pregnant women Additional screening testing: H&H if not done recently in second trimester (see Appendix A for normal laboratory values in pregnancy) Repeat if indicated (and not done in late second trimester): • GC • Chlamydia • RPR • HIV • HBsAg 1-hour glucose challenge test 24 to 28 weeks Ultrasound as indicated
Prenatal Education and Anticipatory Guidance	Provide information to the woman and her support person on the following: • Physical changes and common discomforts to expect during first trimester	Same as for initial visit	Provide information to the woman and her support person on the following: • Physical changes and common discomforts to expect during second trimester	Provide information to the woman and her support person on the following: • Physical changes and common discomforts to expect during third trimester

Continued

Clinical Pathway for Routine Prenatal Care—cont'd

Focus of Care	Initial Prenatal Visit	First Trimester	Second Trimester	Third Trimester
	• Relief measures for common discomforts • Fetal development • General health maintenance and health promotion • Warning and danger signs to report to care provider • Nutrition, prenatal vitamins, and folic acid • Exercise • Self-care and modifying behaviors to reduce risks • Physiology of pregnancy • Course of care		• Relief measures for common discomforts • Fetal development and growth during second trimester • Reinforce warning and danger signs to report to care provider • Nutritional follow-up and recommendation of increase in daily caloric intake by 340 kcal/day • Follow up on physical activity as needed • Follow up on modifiable risk patterns • Begin teaching on preparing for birth	• Relief measures for normal and common discomforts • Fetal development and growth during third trimester • Reinforce warning and danger signs to report to care provider • Nutritional follow-up and recommendation of increase in daily caloric intake by 452 kcal/day • Follow up on modifiable risk patterns Teach fetal movement kick counts Continue teaching and preparing the couple for delivery • Discussion on attending childbirth preparation classes • Teach signs of impending labor • Discuss true vs. false labor • Instruction on when to contact the care provider or go to birthing unit • Discussion on attending parenting classes • Select the method of infant feeding • Select the infant HCP • Preparation of siblings

CONCEPT MAP

Constipation

Altered Pattern of Elimination
- Decrease in normal frequency of defecation
- Bowel movement every 3 days
- Bloated abdominal sensation

Altered Fluid Intake Related to Occasional Nausea and Vomiting
- Reports of nausea once or twice a week
- Occasional vomiting
- Decreased oral intake

Constipation
Alteration in elimination related to physiologic and anatomic changes in pregnancy including alteration in gastrointestinal tone by relaxation of smooth muscle, increased nausea and vomiting, and displacement of small and large intestine by gravid uterus.

Decrease GI Motility Related to Effect of Prostaglandin on Smooth Muscle of Intestines
- Passage of hard and dry stool
- Increase reabsorption of water from the intestines

Hemorrhoids
- Visually apparent varicosities in rectum on anal inspection
- Woman reports pain in rectum on defecation

CARE PLANS

Problem No. 1: Altered pattern of elimination

Goal: Resumption of typical bowel patterns

Outcome: Patient will resume her normal bowel patterns.

Nursing Actions

1. Assess prior bowel patterns before pregnancy, including frequency, consistency, shape, and color.
2. Auscultate bowel sounds.
3. Assess prior experiences with constipation.
4. Explore prior successful strategies for constipation.
5. Explain contributing factors to constipation in pregnancy.
6. Teach strategies for dealing with constipation, including dietary modifications, exercise, and adequate fluid intake.
7. Encourage high-fiber foods and fresh fruits and vegetables.
8. Encourage dietary experimentation to evaluate what works for her.
9. Establish regular time for bowel movement.
10. Discuss rationale for strategies.
11. Explore with the woman and discuss with care provider use of stool softener or bulk laxative.
12. Encourage patient to discuss concerns about constipation by asking open-ended questions.

Problem No. 2: Altered fluid intake related to nausea and vomiting

Goal: Normal fluid intake

Outcome: Normal fluid intake and decreased nausea and vomiting are achieved.

Continued

Nursing Actions

1. Assess factors that increase nausea and vomiting.
2. Suggest small, frequent meals.
3. Decrease fluid intake with meals.
4. Avoid high-fat and spicy food.
5. Explore contributing factors to nausea in pregnancy.
6. Teach strategies for dealing with nausea in pregnancy.
7. Encourage the woman to experiment with strategies to alleviate nausea.
8. Suggest vitamin B_6 or ginger to decrease nausea.

Problem 3: Decreased gastric motility
Goal: Increased motility
Outcome: Patient has normal bowel movement.

Nursing Actions

1. Provide dietary information to increase fiber and roughage in diet.
2. Review high-fiber foods, such as pears, apples, prunes, kiwis, and dried fruits.
3. Suggest bran cereal in the morning and instruct woman to check labels for at least 4 to 5 grams of fiber per serving.

4. Discuss strategies to increase fluid intake.
5. Drink warm liquid upon rising.
6. Encourage exercise to promote peristalsis.
7. Reinforce relationship of diet, exercise, and fluid intake on constipation.

Problem 4: Discomfort with defecation due to hemorrhoids
Goal: Decreased pain with bowel movement
Outcome: Patient will have decreased pain and maintain adequate bowel function.

Nursing Actions

1. Reinforce strategies to avoid constipation.
2. Encourage the woman to not avoid defecation.
3. Instruct the woman to avoid straining on evacuation.
4. Discuss care of hemorrhoids, including witch hazel pads and hemorrhoid creams.
5. Discuss use of stool softeners.
6. Recommend that the woman support a foot on a footstool to facilitate bowel evacuation.
7. Reinforce relationship of diet, exercise, and fluid intake on constipation.

Case Study

As a nurse in an antenatal clinic, you are part of an interdisciplinary team that is caring for Margarite Sanchez during her pregnancy. Margarite is a 28-year-old G3 P1 Latina woman here for her first PNC appointment. By her LMP she is at 8 weeks' gestation. She is 5 feet, 7 inches tall and her weight today is 140 pounds (states pre-pregnancy weight was 137 pounds, BMI = 21.5). Margarite reports some spotting 2 weeks ago that prompted her to do a home pregnancy test that was positive. The spotting has stopped. She tells you that she is very tired throughout the day and has some nausea in the morning, as well as breast tenderness. She is happy but a bit surprised.

Outline the aspects of your initial assessment.

Outline for Margarite what laboratory tests are done during this first prenatal visit and rationale for the tests.

Detail the prenatal education and anticipatory guidance appropriate for the first trimester of pregnancy.

What teaching would you do for Margarite's discomforts of pregnancy?

Discuss nursing diagnosis, nursing activities, and expected outcomes related to this woman.

At 18 weeks' gestation, Margarite comes to the clinic for a prenatal visit. She states she thinks she felt her baby move for the first time last week and that the pregnancy now feels real to her. She states, "I feel great! The nausea and fatigue are gone." She is concerned she is not eating enough protein, as she has little interest in red meat but eats beans and rice at dinner. She remembers discussing with you at her first visit some screening tests for

problems with the baby but now is unsure how they are done and what they are for.

Outline for Margarite nutritional needs during pregnancy, highlighting protein requirements.

Outline for Margarite screening tests that are done in the second trimester and their purposes.

Detail prenatal education and anticipatory guidance appropriate for the second trimester of pregnancy.

Discuss nursing diagnosis, nursing activities, and expected outcomes related to Margarite.

Margarite comes to your clinic for a prenatal visit and is now at 34 weeks' gestation. She states she feels well but has some swelling in her legs at the end of the day, a backache at the end of the day, and difficulty getting comfortable enough to fall asleep. She is also having difficulty sleeping, as she gets up to go to the bathroom two or three times a night.

She remembers from her first pregnancy some things she should be aware of that indicate a problem at the end of pregnancy but is not sure what they are.

Detail prenatal education and anticipatory guidance appropriate for the third trimester of pregnancy.

What teaching would you do for Margarite's discomforts of pregnancy?

What warning signs would you reinforce with Margarite at this point in her pregnancy?

Discuss nursing diagnosis, nursing activities, and expected outcomes specific to Margarite.

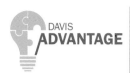

Go to Davis Advantage to complete your learning: strengthen understanding, apply your knowledge, and prepare for the Next Gen NCLEX®.

REFERENCES

American Academy of Pediatrics/American College of Obstetricians and Gynecologists. (2017). *Guidelines for perinatal care* (8th ed.). American Academy of Pediatrics; American College of Obstetricians and Gynecologists.

American College of Obstetricians and Gynecologists. (2015). Practice bulletin no. 156: Obesity in pregnancy. *Obstetrics & Gynecology, 126*(6), e112–e126.

American College of Obstetricians and Gynecologists. (2017). Definition of term pregnancy. Committee Opinion No. 579. *Obstetrics & Gynecology, 122,* 1139–1140.

American College of Obstetricians and Gynecologists. (2020). Committee Opinion no. 804: Physical activity and exercise during pregnancy and the postpartum period. *Obstetrics & Gynecology, 135*(4), e178.

American College of Obstetricians and Gynecologists' Committee on Practice Bulletins-Obstetrics. (2021). Practice bulletin no. 230: Obesity in pregnancy. *Obstetrics & Gynecology, 137*(6), e128–e144. https://doi.org/10.1097/AOG.0000000000004395. PMID: 34011890.

Blackburn, S. T. (2021). Physiologic changes of pregnancy. In K. Simpson & P. Creehan (Eds.), *Perinatal nursing* (5th ed., pp. 47–64.). Wolters Kluwer.

Cunningham, F. (2018). *Williams obstetrics* (25th ed.). McGraw-Hill Medical.

Dow, M. L., & Szymanski, L. M. (2020). Effects of overweight and obesity in pregnancy on health of the offspring. *Endocrinology and Metabolism Clinics, 49*(2), 251–263.

Finer, L. B., & Zolna, M. R. (2016). Declines in unintended pregnancy in the United States, 2008–2011. *New England Journal of Medicine, 374*(9), 843–852. https://doi.org/10.1056/NEJMsa1506575

Hanprasertpong, T. (2020). Overweight and obesity in pregnancy. *Thai Journal of Obstetrics and Gynaecology, 28*(1) (January-March) 2–5. https://doi.org/10.14456/tjog.2020.1

Heaman, M., Bayrampour, H., Kingston, D., Blondel, B., Gissler, M., Roth, C., . . . Gagnon, A. (2013). Migrant women's utilization of prenatal care: A systematic review. *Maternal Child Health Journal, 17,* 816. https://doi.org/10.1007/s10995-012-1058-z

Howell, D. E. A., & Ahmed, M. Z. N. (2019). Eight steps for narrowing the maternal health disparity gap: Step-by-step plan to reduce racial and ethnic disparities in care. *Contemporary Ob/Gyn, 64*(1), 30. PMID: 31673195; PMCID: PMC6822100.

Institute of Medicine. (2009). *Weight gain during pregnancy: Reexamining the guidelines.* National Academies Press.

Kahn, S., Wainstock, T., & Sheiner, E. (2020). Maternal obesity and offspring's cardiovascular morbidity–Results from a population based cohort study. *Early Human Development, 151,* 105221.

Lockwood, C. J., & Magriples, U. (2021). *Prenatal care: Initial assessment.* www-uptodate-com/contents/prenatal-care-initial-assessment

March of Dimes. (2019). *Zika virus and pregnancy.* https://www.marchofdimes.org/complications/zika-virus-and-pregnancy.aspx

March of Dimes Peristats. (2021). *Obesity among women of childbearing age: United States, 2009–2019.* www.marchofdimes.org/Peristats

Michalek, I. M., Comte, C., & Desseauve, D. (2020). Impact of maternal physical activity during an uncomplicated pregnancy on fetal and neonatal well-being parameters: A systematic review of the literature. *European Journal of Obstetrics & Gynecology and Reproductive Biology, 252,* 265. https://doi.org/10.1016/j.ejogrb.2020.06.061

National Perinatal Association. (2020). *Intimate partner violence.* https://www.nationalperinatal.org/what-we-do

O'Connor, E. A., Perdue, L. A., Senger, C. A., Rushkin, M., Patnode, C. D., Bean, S. I., & Jonas, D. E. (2018). Screening and behavioral counseling interventions to reduce unhealthy alcohol use in adolescents and adults: Updated evidence report and systematic review for the US Preventive Services Task Force. *Journal of the American Medical Association. 320*(18), 1910–1928. https://doi.org/10.1001/jama.2018.12086

Postin, L. (2021). *Gestational weight gain.* https://www-uptodate-com.ezproxy4.library.arizona.edu/contents/gestational-weight-gain

Ramsey, P. S., & Schenken, R. S. (2021). *Obesity in pregnancy: Complication and maternal management.* http://www-uptodate-com/contents/obesity-in-pregnancy-complications-and-maternal-management

Sackey, J. A., & Blazey-Martin, D. (2020). *The preconception office visit.* www.uptodate.com/contents/the-preconception-office-visit

Spong, C. Y. (2013). Defining "term" pregnancy: Recommendations from the Defining "Term" Pregnancy Workgroup. *Journal of the American Medical Association, 309*(23), 2445–2446.

U.S. Department of Health and Human Services. (2020). *Healthy People 2030.* Office of Disease Prevention and Health Promotion. https://health.gov/healthypeople/objectives-and-data/browse-objectives/pregnancy-and-childbirth/increase-proportion-pregnant-women-who-receive-early-and-adequate-prenatal-care-mich-08

U.S. Preventive Services Task Force. (2018). Screening for intimate partner violence, elder abuse, and abuse of vulnerable adults: Recommendation statement. *American Family Physician, 99*(10), 648A–648F.

Vallerand, A. H., & Sanoski, C. A. (2021). *Davis's drug guide for nurses* (17th ed.). F.A. Davis.

Winn, A., Hetherington, E., & Tough, S. (2017). Systematic review of immigrant women's experiences with perinatal care in North America. *Journal of Obstetric, Gynecologic & Neonatal Nursing, 46*(5), 764–775. https://doi.org/10.1016/j.jogn.2017.05.002

World Health Organization. (2021). *Body mass index—BMI.* https://www.euro.who.int/en/health-topics/disease-prevention/nutrition/a-healthy-lifestyle/body-mass-index-bmi

The Psycho-Social-Cultural Aspects of Pregnancy

5

Scout Hebinck, RNC OB, MSN

Roberta F. Durham, RN, PhD

LEARNING OUTCOMES

Upon completion of this chapter, the student will be able to:

1. Describe expected emotional changes of the pregnant woman and appropriate nursing responses to these changes.
2. Identify the major developmental tasks of pregnancy as they relate to maternal, paternal, and family adaptation.
3. Identify critical variables that influence adaptation to pregnancy, including age, parity, and social, cultural, and sexual orientation.
4. Identify nursing assessments and interventions that promote positive psycho-social-cultural adaptations for the pregnant woman and her family.
5. Analyze critical factors in preparing for birth, including choosing a provider and birth setting and creating a birth plan.
6. Identify key components of childbirth preparation education for expectant families.
7. Analyze and critique current evidence-based research regarding psycho-social-cultural adaptation to pregnancy.
8. Identify awareness of one's own assumptions and biases that may contribute to health disparities.
9. Identify and create a safe environment to provide informed, respectful, and inclusive care.
10. Describe and identify the difference between cultural competence and cultural humility.

CONCEPTS

Addiction
Behaviors
Caring
Clinical Judgment
Cognition
Collaboration
Comfort
Communication
Evidence-Based Practice
Family
Health Promotion
Health Care Systems
Grief and Loss
Professionalism
Reproduction and Sexuality
Safety
Self
Stress and Coping
Teaching and Learning

Nursing Diagnosis

- Risk for anxiety and fear related to unknown processes of pregnancy and birth
- Risk for anxiety and fear related to issues around race, sexual orientation, and immigration status
- Deficient knowledge related to pregnancy psychosocial and emotional changes

Nursing Outcomes

- The pregnant woman and her family will be able to communicate effectively with health-care providers.
- The pregnant woman and her family will verbalize fears related to anxiety.
- The pregnant woman and her family will verbalize appropriate family dynamics.

Continued

Nursing Diagnosis—cont'd

- Risk for interrupted family processes related to role changes and developmental stressors in pregnancy
- Risk for ineffective communication related to cultural differences between family and health-care providers
- Risk for increased stress and ineffective coping related to inadequate social support during pregnancy
- Risk for inadequate prenatal care related to inaccessible health care second to race, immigration status, and sexual orientation
- Risk for ineffective coping
- Deficient knowledge related to psychosocial and emotional changes in pregnancy
- Readiness for enhanced family processes

Nursing Outcomes—cont'd

- The pregnant woman and her family will report increasing acceptance of changes in body image.
- The pregnant woman and her family will seek clarification of information about pregnancy and birth.
- The pregnant woman and her family will demonstrate knowledge regarding expected changes of pregnancy.
- The pregnant woman and her family will develop a realistic birth plan and be open to possible changes.
- The pregnant woman and her family will exhibit acceptance of their roles as parents.
- The pregnant woman and her family will identify appropriate support systems.
- The pregnant woman and her family will receive positive and effective social support.
- The pregnant woman and her family will express satisfaction with health-care providers' sensitivity to traditional beliefs and practices of her culture, race, immigration status, or sexual orientation.

INTRODUCTION

This chapter explores the influence of culture on values and beliefs, the effects of pregnancy on the woman and on members of the immediate and extended family, and variables that influence the woman's adaptation to pregnancy. We explore topics related to patient and family empowerment, along with barriers to culturally competent care and strategies to remove those barriers. We describe how diverse cultural, ethnic, and social backgrounds function as sources of patient, family, and community values, and we explore patient-centered care with sensitivity and respect for the diversity of the human experience. Nursing actions focus on supporting and encouraging the patient's autonomy and choices based on the respect for the woman's preferences, values, and needs. Health promotion, individualized care, and a family-centered approach are all crucial components of nursing care. Details on prenatal care are included in Chapter 4.

Patient-centered respectful care is a central concept in maternity nursing. It recognizes the patient or designee as the source of control and full partner in providing compassionate and coordinated care based on respect for the patient's preferences, values, and needs. Because all women deserve and desire respectful care that affirms their cultural beliefs and practices, strategies to accomplish these objectives are outlined.

MATERNAL ADAPTATION TO PREGNANCY

The news of pregnancy confers profound and irrevocable changes in a woman's life and the lives of those around her. With this news, the woman begins her journey to becoming a mother. Less visible than the physical adaptations of pregnancy but just as profound are the woman's psychological adaptations and development of her identity as a mother, crucial aspects of the childbearing cycle. Psychological, cultural, and social variables all significantly influence this process. Psychosocial support for the pregnant woman and her family is a distinct and major nursing responsibility during the antepartum period. This chapter presents the expected emotional changes a woman and her family must navigate to achieve a positive adaptation to pregnancy. Factors influencing these changes are also described.

Successful adaptation to the maternal role requires important psychological work. Although becoming a mother occurs on a long-term continuum, the psychological groundwork is laid during the course of each woman's individual experience during pregnancy. The pregnant woman can use the 9 months before the child's birth to restructure her psychological and cognitive self toward motherhood. Motherhood, an irrevocable change in a woman's life, progressively becomes part of a woman's total identity (Koniak-Griffin et al., 2006; Mercer, 1995, 2004).

MATERNAL TASKS OF PREGNANCY

Maternal tasks of pregnancy were first identified in the psychoanalytic literature (Bibring et al., 1961), then explored and outlined by classic maternity nurse researchers Reva Rubin, Ramona Mercer, and Regina Lederman. Rubin's research has provided a framework and core knowledge base for researchers and clinicians. She identified these significant maternal tasks women undergo during pregnancy (Rubin, 1975, 1984):

- Ensuring a safe passage for herself and her child: the mother's knowledge and care-seeking behaviors to ensure that both she and the newborn emerge from pregnancy healthy.

- Ensuring social acceptance of the child by significant others: the woman's engagement of her family and social network in the pregnancy.
- Attaching or "binding-in" to the child: the development of maternal-fetal attachment.
- Giving of oneself to the demands of motherhood: the mother's willingness and efforts to make personal sacrifices for the child.

Building on Rubin's work, Regina Lederman (1996; Lederman & Weis, 2009) identified seven dimensions of maternal role development: acceptance of the pregnancy, identification with the motherhood role, relationship to her mother, reordering partner relationships, preparation for labor, prenatal fear of losing control in labor, and prenatal fear of losing self-esteem in labor.

Acceptance of the Pregnancy

This task focuses on the woman's adaptive responses to the changes related to pregnancy growth and development (Lederman, 1996):

- Responding to mood changes
- Responding to ambivalent feelings
- Responding to nausea, fatigue, and other physical discomforts of the early months of pregnancy
- Responding to financial concerns
- Responding to increased dependency needs

Expected findings include:

- Desire for and acceptance of pregnancy
- Predominately happy feelings during pregnancy
- Little physical discomfort or a high tolerance for the discomfort
- Acceptance of body changes
- Minimal ambivalent feelings and conflict regarding pregnancy by the end of her pregnancy
- A dislike of being pregnant but a feeling of love for the unborn child

---

CRITICAL COMPONENT

Ambivalent Feelings Toward Pregnancy
It is common for women to experience ambivalent feelings toward pregnancy during the first trimester. These feelings decrease as pregnancy progresses. Ambivalence that continues into the third trimester may indicate unresolved conflict. When evaluating ambivalence, it is important to assess the reason for the ambivalence and its intensity.

Identification With the Motherhood Role

Accomplishment of this task is influenced by the woman's acceptance of pregnancy and the relationship she has with her own mother. Women who have accepted their pregnancy and who have a positive relationship with their own mothers more easily accomplish this task (Lederman, 1996). Accomplishment of this task is also influenced by the woman's degree of fears about labor, such as helplessness, pain, loss of control, and loss of self-esteem (Lederman, 1996). Vivid dreams are common during pregnancy, allowing the woman to envision herself as a mother in various situations. A woman often rehearses or pictures herself in her new role in different scenarios (Rubin, 1975). The motherhood role is progressively strengthened as she attaches to the fetus. Fetal attachment influences the woman's sense of her child and her sense of being competent as a mother.

Events that facilitate fetal attachment include:

- Hearing the fetal heartbeat
- Seeing the fetus move during an ultrasound examination
- Feeling the fetus kick or move

Expected findings:

- Moves from viewing herself as a woman-without-child to a woman-with-child
- Anticipates changes motherhood will bring to her life
- Seeks company of other pregnant women
- Is highly motivated to assume the motherhood role
- Actively prepares for the motherhood role

Transmasculine individuals who are pregnant should keep in mind that pregnancy is a gendered experience that may trigger feelings of dysphoria or isolation for some patients. In addition, some transgender individuals may not identify as "mothers"; thus, all health-care professionals should be mindful of the language they use (American College of Obstetricians and Gynecologists [ACOG], 2021b). It may be appropriate to use a more neutral term such as "parent."

Relationship to Her Mother

A woman's relationship with her mother is an important determinant of adaptation to motherhood. Unresolved mother–daughter conflicts may emerge and confront women during pregnancy (Lederman, 1996). Important components of the woman's relationship with her own mother are:

- Availability of the woman's mother to her in the past and in the present
- The mother's reaction to her daughter's pregnancy
- The mother's relationship with her daughter
- The mother's willingness to reminisce with her daughter about her own childbirth and child-rearing experiences

Expected findings:

- The woman's mother was available to her in the past and continues to be available during the pregnancy (Fig. 5–1).
- The woman's mother accepts the pregnancy, respects her autonomy, and acknowledges her daughter becoming a mother.
- The woman's mother relates to her daughter as an adult versus as a child.
- The woman's mother reminisces with her daughter about her own childbearing and child-rearing experiences.

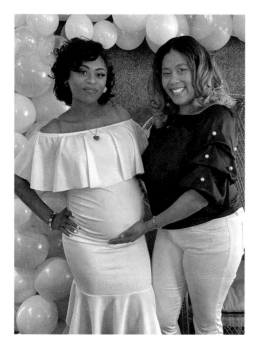

FIGURE 5-1 Pregnant woman and her mother.

Reordering Partner Relationships

Pregnancy has a dramatic effect on a couple's relationship. Some couples view pregnancy and childbirth as a growth experience and an expression of deep commitment to their bond, whereas others see it as an added stressor to a relationship already in conflict. The partner's support during pregnancy enhances the woman's feelings of well-being and is associated with earlier and continuous prenatal care (Lederman, 1996; Lederman & Weis, 2009). A woman's partner is the fundamental and natural source of social support, favorably influencing the emotional state of pregnancy. This emotional support is manifested by caring, understanding, empathy, and generation of positive feelings in the supported person (Skurzak, 2015). Evidence shows that fathers and partners are influential in maternal psychological variables and smoking behavior during pregnancy (Cheng et al., 2016).

Assessment of the couple's relationship includes:

- The partner's concern for the woman's needs during pregnancy
- The woman's concerns for her partner's needs during pregnancy
- The varying desire for sexual activity among pregnant women
- The effect pregnancy has on the relationship (e.g., whether it brings them closer together or causes conflict)
- The partner's adjustment to the new role

Expected findings include the following:

- The partner is understanding and supportive of the woman.
- The partner is thoughtful and "pampers" the woman during pregnancy.
- The partner is involved in the pregnancy.
- The woman perceives that her partner is supportive.

- The woman is concerned about her partner's needs of making emotional adjustments to the pregnancy and new role.
- Women in relationships with established open communication about sexuality are likely to have less difficulty with changes in sexual activity.
- Couples indicate that they are growing closer to each other during pregnancy.
- The partner is happy and excited about the pregnancy and prepares for the new role.

Preparation for Labor

Preparation for labor means preparing for the physiological processes of labor as well as the psychological processes of separating from the fetus and becoming a mother to the child. Preparation for labor and birth occur through taking classes, reading, fantasizing, and dreaming about labor and birth (Lederman, 1996; Lederman & Weis, 2009). The degree of preparation affects the woman's level of anxiety and fear, with more preparation lessening fear.

Expected findings include:

- The woman attends childbirth classes and reads books and online resources about labor and birth.
- The woman uses smartphone applications to track her pregnancy and growing fetus.
- The woman mentally rehearses (fantasizes) the labor and birthing process and may dream about labor and birth.
- The woman develops realistic expectations of labor and birth and works with her partner or birthing coach to develop a birth plan.
- The pregnant woman may engage in a flurry of activity known as "nesting behavior," hurrying to finish preparing for the newborn's arrival.

Prenatal Fear of Losing Control in Labor

Loss of control includes two factors (Lederman, 1996; Lederman & Weis, 2009): loss of control over the body and loss of control over emotions. The degree of fear is related to:

- The woman's degree of trust with medical and nursing staff, partner, and other support persons
- The woman's attitude regarding use of medication and anesthesia for labor pain management

Expected findings include:

- The woman perceives individual attention from medical staff.
- The woman perceives that she is being treated as an adult and her questions and concerns are addressed by the medical staff.
- The woman perceives that the nursing staff is compassionate, empathetic, and available.
- The woman perceives that she is being supported by her partner, family, and friends.
- The woman has realistic expectations regarding management of labor pain and these expectations are met.
- The woman perceives that she is receiving unbiased care for her and her unborn child.

Prenatal Fear of Losing Self-Esteem in Labor

Some women fear they will lose self-esteem and "fail" during labor. When a woman feels a threat to her self-esteem, it is important to assess the following areas (Lederman & Weis, 2009):

- The source of the threat
- The response to the threat
- The intensity of the reaction to the threat

Behaviors that reflect self-esteem are:

- Tolerance of self
- Value of self and assertiveness, and decisions about her labor process
- Positive attitude regarding body image and appearance

Expected findings include the ability to:

- Develop realistic expectations of self during labor and birth and have an awareness of risks and potential complications.
- Identify and respect her own feelings.
- Assert herself in acquiring information needed to make decisions.
- Recognize her own needs and limitations.
- Adjust to the unexpected and unknown.
- Recover from threats quickly.
- Verbalize fears and concerns without feeling judged negatively for those fears and concerns.

As the woman prepares to experience labor, give birth, and take on the maternal role, the process of maternal adaptation to pregnancy is potentially completed. With the dominating physical discomforts of the third trimester, most women become impatient for labor to begin. There is relief and excitement about going into labor. The mother is ready and eager to deliver and hold her baby. She has prepared for her future as a mother (Rubin, 1984).

Nursing Actions

During the antepartal period, the nurse can take on a variety of roles: teacher, advocate, counselor, clinician, resource person, and role model. Nursing actions should be focused on health promotion, individualized care, and prevention of individual and family crises and are highlighted in the critical component nursing actions that facilitate adaptation to pregnancy (Lederman & Weis, 2009; Mattson & Smith, 2016).

FACTORS THAT INFLUENCE MATERNAL ADAPTATION

The ability of the woman to adapt to the maternal role is influenced by various factors, including parity, maternal age, sexual orientation, single parenting, planned versus unplanned pregnancy, multiple gestation (twins, triples), socioeconomic factors, cultural beliefs, and history of abuse.

Multiparity

Multigravidas may have the benefit of experience, but it should not be assumed that they need less help than a first-time mother. They know more of what to expect in terms of pain during labor, postpartum adaptation, and the many added responsibilities of motherhood, but they may need time to process and develop strategies for integrating a new member into the family.

Pregnancy tasks may be more complex. Giving adequate attention to all her children and supporting sibling adaptation are unique challenges faced by the multigravida. She may spend a great deal of time working out a new relationship with the first child and grieve for the loss of their special relationship. She also must consider the financial issues associated with feeding, clothing, and providing for another child while at the same time maintaining a relationship with her partner and continuing her career, whether inside or outside the home (Jordan, 1989).

Maternal Age

Mothers who give birth at an older or younger than average age face unique circumstances and challenges.

Adolescent Mothers

Adolescence is a period of accelerated growth and change that bridges the complex transition from childhood to adulthood. The second decade of life is often a turbulent period in which adolescents experience hormonal changes, physical maturation, and, frequently, opportunities to engage in risk behaviors. The patterns of behavior they adopt may have long-term consequences for their health and quality of life. Because of the rapid physical, cognitive, and emotional developments that take place during this age period, adolescence is also a time when many health problems may first emerge. Moreover, adolescents also experience special vulnerabilities, health concerns, and barriers to accessing health care (MacKay & Duran, 2007).

Definitions of adolescence and the years encompassed vary. Adolescence is generally regarded as the period of life from puberty to maturity, the meanings of which are often debated by health professionals. Many children begin puberty by the age of 10, although the developmental and maturation timeline varies significantly by individual. During their teenage years, adolescents are learning financial, social, and personal independence, and they are expected to become capable of adult behaviors and responses.

In 2019, the birth rate for teenagers aged 15 to 19 declined in 21 states, but rates were essentially unchanged in the remaining 29 states (Martin et al., 2021). Although birth rates for adolescents are decreasing in some areas and the reasons for the declines are not totally clear, evidence suggests these declines are due to more teens abstaining from sexual activity, and more teens who are sexually active using birth control than in previous years (Lindberg et al., 2016). Less favorable socioeconomic conditions, such as low education and low-income levels of a teen's family, may contribute to high teen birth rates. Teens in child welfare systems are at higher risk of teen pregnancy and birth than other groups. For example, young women living in foster care are more than twice as likely to become pregnant than those not in foster care (Centers for Disease Control and Prevention [CDC], 2019).

Teen pregnancy and childbearing bring substantial social and economic costs through immediate- and long-term impacts on teen parents and their children. Adolescents who have an unintended pregnancy face a number of challenges, including abandonment by their partners, increased adverse pregnancy outcomes, and inability to complete school education, which may ultimately limit their future social and economic opportunities (CDC, 2017b; CDC, 2019). For example, pregnancy and birth are significant contributors to high school dropout rates among girls. Only about 50% of teen mothers receive a high school diploma by 22 years of age, whereas approximately 90% of women who do not give birth during adolescence graduate from high school. The children of teenage mothers are more likely to have lower school achievement and to drop out of high school, have more health problems, be incarcerated at some time during adolescence, give birth as a teenager, and face unemployment as a young adult (CDC, 2019).

The major developmental task of adolescence is to form and become comfortable with a sense of self. Pregnancy presents a challenge for teenagers who must cope with the conflicting developmental tasks of pregnancy and adolescence at the same time. Achieving a maternal identity is very difficult for an adolescent who is in the throes of evolving her own identity as an adult capable of psychosocial independence from her family. Although she may achieve the maternal role, research indicates that she may function at a lower level of competence than would an older woman (Mercer, 2004).

Adolescents face considerable potential harms to their health from mental health disorders, interpersonal violence, substance use, and unprotected sexual activity. As adolescents navigate this important developmental period, care providers should engage with them and promote best practices that protect adolescents' vulnerability and assist them in developing autonomy (ACOG, 2020). Providing alone time, apart from a parent or guardian, for discussion between the adolescent patient and health-care provider is an important aspect of the prenatal care visit. Adolescents are beginning to take responsibility for their health care, and this should be encouraged and supported as they transition to adult patients.

In addition, the younger the adolescent is, the more difficulty she will have with body image changes, as well as acknowledging the pregnancy, seeking health care, and planning for the changes that pregnancy and parenting will bring. Delayed entry into prenatal care is common.

Complications common in pregnant adolescents include low birth weight, preeclampsia and pregnancy-induced hypertension, intrauterine growth restriction (IUGR), and preterm labor. In younger mothers, socioeconomic factors largely explain increased neonatal mortality risk (Adams, 2021). One contributor to a successful outcome of adolescent pregnancy is assured confidentiality with health-care providers. The Association of Women's Health, Obstetric and Neonatal Nurses (AWHONN) encourages the establishment of interdisciplinary educational initiatives that will increase health-care providers' competency in delivering effective and confidential adolescent health care (AWHONN, 2009).

Partner support is another important factor in maternal and infant health for adolescents. Studies show lack of partner

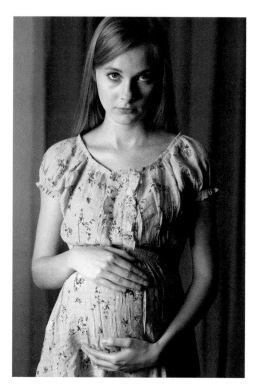

FIGURE 5–2 Pregnant adolescent.

support and poor relationships with partners during pregnancy and postpartum are associated with negative maternal behaviors, adverse emotional health, and low birth weight (Smith et al., 2016). In a national sample of women and girls ages 10 to 19 who experienced pregnancy, lack of partner support was associated with adverse birth outcomes. Even after adjusting for key confounding factors, pregnancy loss and low birth weight remained lower in the group with higher partner support. Teens with partner support were less likely to have a preterm birth than those without support from the partner, although this difference was not statistically significant (Shah et al., 2014).

Successful adaptation to pregnancy and parenthood may depend on an adolescent's age (Fig. 5–2).

- Comprehensive and community-based health-care programs for adolescents are effective in improving outcomes for the teen mother and her infant (CDC, 2017b, 2019). Examples include programs that have been implemented in schools, clinics, community agencies, or home visitation programs. In addition to evidence-based prevention programs, teens need access to youth-friendly contraceptive and reproductive health services and support from parents and other trusted adults who can play an important role in helping teens make healthy choices about relationships, sex, and birth control (CDC, 2019).
- Early adolescence is defined as the period between ages 11 and 13 years. Adolescents in this phase of life are self-centered and oriented toward the present. Additionally, there is a greater likelihood that pregnancy at this age is a result of abuse or coercion. Moving into the maternal role is a difficult challenge for this age group. Grandmothers will play a significant role in caring for the infant as well as providing guidance

to their daughter regarding mothering skills (Mercer, 1995; Pinazo-Hernandis & Tompkins, 2009).

- Middle adolescence is defined as the period between 14 and 18 years. During this time, the adolescent will be more capable of abstract thinking and understanding consequences of current behaviors.
- The young adolescent has fewer coping mechanisms, less experience to draw on, incomplete cognitive development, fewer problem-solving capabilities, and an ego identity that is more easily threatened by the stress and discomfort of pregnancy and birth. Interventions that support pregnancy adaptation should be age- and developmentally appropriate for adolescents (AWHONN, 2009). By age 19 to 20, as adolescents mature into late adolescence, abstract thinking and understanding consequences are further developed and eventually mastered. The older pregnant adolescent is more likely to be a capable and active participant in health-care decisions.

Older Mothers

In North America, an increasing number of women have delayed childbearing until after age 35. Most women in this age group deliver at term without adverse outcomes. However, even with good prenatal care, they have an increased incidence of adverse perinatal outcomes. For example, maternal age of 35 years or older is associated with an increased risk of poor fetal outcomes, obstetrical complications, and perinatal morbidity and mortality (Adams, 2021). The association between Down syndrome and advanced maternal age has been long documented. Chronic diseases such as hypertension that are more common in women over 35 may affect the pregnancy. Older mothers are also more likely to have miscarriages, fetal chromosomal abnormalities, low birth weight infants, premature births, and multiple births.

In women older than 40, the risk increases for placenta previa, placenta abruptio, cesarean deliveries, preeclampsia, and gestational diabetes. In fact, 47.4% of babies born from women older than 40 of all races are delivered via cesarean section (Martin et al., 2019).

The more mature woman may be better equipped psychosocially to assume the maternal role than women in younger age groups. However, she also might have increased difficulty with the changing roles in her life, experiencing heightened ambivalence. She might have difficulty balancing a career with the physical and psychological demands of pregnancy. The unpredictable nature of pregnancy, labor, and life with a newborn may challenge a woman who has developed a predictable, controlled life (Carolan, 2005; Dobrzykowski & Stern, 2003; Schardt, 2005). The stress and concerns related to increased risk may impact the pregnancy experience.

CRITICAL COMPONENT

Nursing Actions That Facilitate Adaptation to Pregnancy

First Trimester
- Begin psychosocial assessment at initial contact; assess woman's response to pregnancy; assess stressors in woman's life. This allows the nurse to identify issues that may require referrals and begin developing the plan of care.
- Promote pregnancy and birth as a family experience; encourage family and father or partner participation in prenatal visits; encourage questions from father and family members about the pregnancy. It is important to offer an inclusive model of care that acknowledges the needs of the family as well as the individual. Pregnancy significantly affects all family members. Meeting with family members provides additional information to the nurse and helps complete the family assessment. Positive family support is associated with positive maternal adaptation.
- Assess learning needs. This allows the nurse to provide individualized information.
- Offer anticipatory guidance regarding normal developmental stressors of pregnancy, such as ambivalence during early pregnancy, feelings of vulnerability, mood changes, and an active dream and fantasy life. This allows the nurse to emphasize normalcy, health, universality, strengths, and developmental concepts, to decrease anxiety.
- Assess for increased anxieties and fear; if anxieties seem greater than normal, refer to a psych care provider. Excessive anxiety, stress, and prenatal depression have a negative impact on a woman's pregnancy and affect the physiology of the developing fetus. Specialized intervention is needed.
- Listen, validate, provide reassurance, and teach expected emotional changes. Educate partner and family members, and stress normalcy of feelings to decrease anxiety and ensure the woman feels "heard" and validated.
- If appropriate, discuss common phases through which expectant fathers progress through pregnancy. Be aware of phases of paternal adaptation when counseling parents about expected changes of pregnancy; provide anticipatory guidance regarding potential communication conflicts. This acknowledges the partner as a significant participant in the pregnancy and assists in improving communication and decreasing relationship stress.

Second Trimester
- Encourage verbalization of a possible grief process during pregnancy related to body image changes, loss of old life, and changing relationships with family and friends. The woman may be more anxious about body changes in the second trimester. She may begin to have fears or phobias. The nurse needs to acknowledge and validate the woman's feelings and help her work toward resolving any conflicting feelings.
- Discuss normal changes in sexual activity and provide information and acknowledge the woman's sexuality.
- Encourage "tuning in" to fetal movements; discuss fetal capacities for hearing, responding to interaction, and maternal activity. This will encourage the attachment process and help empower the woman with increased involvement in care.
- Reinforce to partner and family the importance of giving the expectant mother extra support; give specific examples of ways to help (e.g., helping her eat well, helping with heavy work, giving extra attention). This will encourage family and partner participation in the pregnancy process and promote

support for the woman. A well-supported woman will likely have a more positive adaptation to pregnancy.

Third Trimester

- Encourage attendance at childbirth classes to promote knowledge and decrease fears. Childbirth education can give women the information they need to make informed decisions, such as educational information on the risks and benefits of vaginal delivery and cesarean delivery. Further, childbirth education can ensure that women from all population groups understand the relative risks and benefits of their choices, empowering them to make informed decisions regarding birthing options.
- Discuss preparations for birth and parenthood; explore expectations of labor. The woman will begin to focus on impending birth during the third trimester, and her learning needs emphasize this area. It is important to provide anticipatory information and guidance.
- Assess the partner's comfort level with the labor coach role and reassure as needed; stress that help in labor will be available; encourage the presence of a second support person if appropriate. The woman's partner may not feel comfortable providing labor support, and it is important to discuss before the onset of labor so all roles can be clarified.
- Refer to appropriate educational materials on parenthood. Encourage discussions of plans and expectations with the partner. Give anticipatory guidance regarding the realities of infant care, breastfeeding, and so on. Breastfeeding benefits are presented and classes are encouraged. This will promote communication and planning with the expectant parents, as well as a positive transition to parenthood.
- If psychosocial complications develop, plan for appropriate referrals to coordinate with social workers, a nutritionist, and community agencies to ensure continuity of psychosocial assessment and provide appropriate support during the woman's pregnancy.
- Help the expectant mother identify and use support systems to promote positive adaptation to pregnancy, birth, and postpartum; anticipate the need for postpartum support; and decrease the risk of postpartum depression (Callister, 2021; Lederman & Weis, 2009; Mattson & Smith, 2016; McCants & Greiner, 2016).

Lesbian Mothers

Despite advances in equality for the lesbian, gay, bisexual, transgender, and queer (LGBTQ) population, lesbian women face unique challenges in accessing health care, including social, political, and economic barriers. Documented social and political barriers to care include fear of or experiences of homophobia, discrimination, and stigmatization. Homophobic or heterosexist attitudes, heteronormative assumptions, and lack of knowledge regarding health needs for this population also pose significant barriers that may affect lesbian women's experiences and interactions with their maternity care providers.

Currently, most health-care communication tends toward heterosexist language that may marginalize same-sex couples and their families. Negative experiences with providers and the health system have discouraged many LGBTQ women from obtaining necessary health care, including preventive care (ACOG, 2012). The emotional cost and lack of community and family support compared with their heterosexual counterparts can impede lesbian women on their journeys to becoming mothers. Mercer's classic model of becoming a mother explains the process of beginning motherhood as a period of significant transition (Mercer, 2004). The process—now termed maternal role attainment to better account for the constantly evolving nature of motherhood—consists of repeated instances of adaptation as the demands of a woman shift. It also involves a reformation of a woman's identity, as her relationships to others and to oneself change (Mercer, 2004). This is especially true of LGBTQ women, as the transition to motherhood may involve struggles such as lack of acceptance from families, feelings of isolation from support groups, social stigma, and issues related to seeking care as a sexual minority. A recent review of research on lesbian women's experiences with pregnancy and birth found that:

- In all studies reviewed, researchers reported that lesbian women seeking maternity care experienced some heteronormativity or homophobia in their health-care encounters.
- Finding sensitive, nonjudgmental, and culturally competent care was a challenge for many women. Most women expressed that they wanted a focus on woman-centered care. However, many women experienced instances of stigma.

This review of research emphasizes the importance of nurses to promote open and welcoming environments, to use and foster health language that is inclusive for all types of families, and to ensure that all families can thrive to promote optimal transitions to motherhood for all women (Gregg, 2018).

Lesbian women may be more likely to lack social support, particularly from their families of origin. They may be exposed to additional stress due to homophobic attitudes, particularly from the health-care system. The journey of lesbians to parenthood may consist of several unique steps (Gregg, 2018; Wojnar & Katzenmeyer, 2014). Lesbian women considering parenting face unique challenges: finding a caregiver, options for conception, involvement of their partner, and legal implications of same-sex parenthood (Gregg, 2018; McManus et al., 2006).

Finding supportive health-care providers with whom they are comfortable disclosing sexual orientation is an important need identified by lesbian women (Fig. 5–3). Heteronormative health-care environments in which parents are assumed to be a man and a woman can present barriers to care for all same-sex couples. The role of the woman's partner and legal considerations of the growing family will also affect the lesbian experience of pregnancy (Gregg, 2018; McManus et al., 2006; Rondahl et al., 2009; Ross, 2005).

Lesbian mothers most commonly plan their pregnancies, conceiving through donor insemination. In addition, it has been observed that many lesbian couples participate in a relatively equal division of childcare. These factors can combine to help decrease the stress a lesbian mother might experience and act as protection from perinatal depression (Ross, 2005).

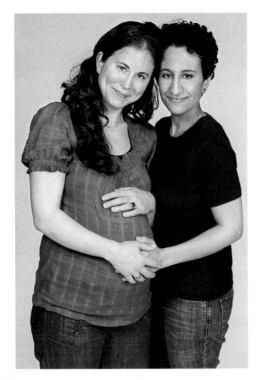

FIGURE 5–3 Lesbian pregnant couple.

Nursing assessments of lesbian women should be adapted accordingly. Nurses need to strive toward using inclusive language and avoid making assumptions about a woman's gender orientation without further information. Birth partners who are not the biological fathers experience the same fears, questions, and concerns. Birth partners need to be kept informed, supported, and included in all activities in which the mother desires their participation. To date, researchers who explored the roles of lesbian nonbiological mothers (also known as lesbian comothers, social mothers, or other mother) focused on how these women sought to legitimize and formalize their roles and positions within the family (Wojnar & Katzenmeyer, 2014). Researchers have identified some similarities between lesbian nonbiological mothers and new fathers; however, they noted that lesbian nonbiological mothers did not receive the same level of societal support and recognition as fathers (Goldberg & Sayer, 2006; Wojnar & Katzenmeyer, 2014). They also reported feelings of jealousy related to perceptions of unequal ties to the children and desire to carry children themselves.

Single Parenting

The literature reports a higher degree of stress for pregnant single women, such as greater anxiety and less tangible reliable support from family and friends (Simpson & Creehan, 2014). The reasons surrounding the pregnancy and the presence or absence of strong support persons can significantly influence the woman's adaptation (Beeber & Canuso, 2005). Initial assessments are crucial for providing appropriate care and possible resources she may or may not need:

● Is the woman single by choice? Did she decide later in her life that she wanted a family unit or wanted to raise a baby herself?

● Is she a single mother by unintended circumstance (e.g., death of partner following conception, separation, divorce)?
● Did she get pregnant by a casual acquaintance? Or a partner they are not married to and do not live with?

Single mothers may live at or below the poverty level, facing greater financial challenges, resulting in a higher risk of depression. However, some single mothers are financially stable and have well-established careers. Solo mothers—those who are raising at least one child with no spouse or partner in the home—parent about 20% of children in the United States. Among solo parents, the vast majority (81%) are mothers; only 19% are fathers (Pew Research Center, 2018). A much larger percentage of solo parents live in poverty compared with cohabiting parents (27% vs. 16%) (Pew Research Center, 2018). With the initial news, many women must decide whether to proceed with the pregnancy. Single women engage in the maternal tasks of pregnancy while facing more complex tasks and challenges such as:

● Telling the family, which may cause concern
● Considering issues about legal guardianship in the event she is incapacitated
● Deciding whether to put the father's name on the birth certificate

Multigestational Pregnancy

The incidence of multifetal gestations in the United States has increased dramatically over the past several decades. The long-term changes in the incidence of multifetal gestations have been attributed to two main factors: (1) a shift toward an older maternal age at conception, when multifetal gestations are more likely to occur naturally and (2) an increased use of assisted reproductive technology (ART), which is more likely to result in a multifetal gestation (ACOG, 2021c). A multiple gestation pregnancy (twins, triples, etc.) places added psychosocial stressors on the family unit. The diagnosis shocks many expectant parents, who may need additional support and education to help them cope with the changes they face. The very nature of a high-risk pregnancy increases stress and anxiety for expectant mothers and may be intensified by the unknowns of a multiple pregnancy. The increased risk for adverse outcomes for both the mother and her babies results in increased fears and anxieties for the pregnant woman.

Parents expecting multiples have unique perinatal educational needs. The high-risk nature and extraordinary aspects of their pregnancy, along with the unknowns of parenting multiple infants, present a need for specialized education. Providing education about their condition and health-care options allows women expecting multiples to make informed decisions concerning care (Bowers, 2021). Preparation for multiple infants requires significant adjustments for families even before the babies are born, which can be impacted by pregnancy complications.

Nurses play an integral role in providing psychosocial support for families expecting multiples. Anticipatory guidance includes the expected physical and emotional changes of a multiple pregnancy; the need for contingency planning at home for children and household management; nutritional assessment and counseling; expected plans for testing, interventions, and treatment options; referrals to support organizations such as local parents of multiples groups; and information about multiple birth prenatal education classes (Bowers, 2021).

If the woman is carrying more than three fetuses, the parents may receive counseling regarding selective reduction of the pregnancies to reduce the incidence of premature birth and allow the remaining fetuses to grow to term gestation. This poses an ethical dilemma and emotional strain for many parents, particularly if they have been attempting to achieve pregnancy for a long time (ACOG, 2021c; Maifeld et al., 2003).

Women Who Are Abused

Intimate partner violence, also called domestic violence, is a serious, sometimes fatal, preventable public health problem. The term *intimate partner violence* is used to describe physical violence, sexual violence, stalking, and psychological aggression by a current or former intimate partner, to include current or former spouses, boyfriends or girlfriends, dating partners, or sexual partners (AWHONN, 2018). Pregnancy is often a trigger for beginning or increased abuse or intimate partner violence (see Chapters 4 and 7).

Abuse, whether emotional or physical, crosses all racial, ethnic, and economic lines. Although IPV can occur against men, 74% of all IPV is directed toward women and is perpetrated by current or former partners. Approximately one in three women in the United States experience rape, physical violence, or stalking by intimate partners during their lifetimes (Smith et al., 2017). However, the true prevalence of IPV is difficult to determine because many survivors do not disclose their experiences. Current and past experiences with IPV can have profound effects on women's physical and emotional health.

Abuse often gets worse during pregnancy. According to the March of Dimes, almost one in six pregnant women have been abused by a partner (March of Dimes, 2017). Pregnancy offers a unique opportunity for health-care providers to recognize abuse and to intervene appropriately. Nurses are ideally situated to screen, assess, and counsel women and should be aware of populations at greater risk for IPV, such as immigrant women and adolescents. A recent Cochrane Review concluded that training care providers on IPV, including how to respond to survivors of IPV, is an important intervention to improve providers' knowledge, attitudes, and practice, and subsequently the care and health outcomes for IPV survivors (Kalra et al., 2021). This is further addressed in Chapters 4 and 7.

Military Deployment and Spousal Military Deployment

Military deployment can significantly influence adaptation to pregnancy. Thousands of women of childbearing age are serving in the U.S. military and are deployed. Overall, 15% of Department of Defense active-duty military personnel are women, up from 11% in 1990. In 2015, 17% of active-duty officers were female, up from their share of 12% in 1990. In addition, 15% of enlisted personnel were female in 2015, up from 11% in 1990 (Parker et al., 2017).

Although women have traditionally been excluded from serving in direct combat roles in the military, they have positions that put them in the direct line of fire and may cause significant stress (e.g., convoy driver, patrol). Military life presents many challenging obstacles, including deployments, moves, separation from family, and possibly life as a single parent. These events can create added stressors on soon-to-be mothers (Recame, 2013). Women with deployed spouses have more frequent diagnoses of depressive disorders, sleep disorders, anxiety, acute stress reaction, and adjustment disorders compared with women with no spouse deployed. Deployment effects vary by maternal age and the number of children in the household. These findings may help inform military support programs including autogenic training to reduce anxiety during pregnancy, and other mind–body interventions may be effective at managing stress and anxiety during delivery and in the postpartum period (Spieker et al., 2016).

- For veterans, pregnancy can exacerbate mental health conditions (Mattocks et al., 2010).
- Women with deployed spouses during pregnancy have a 2.8-fold increased risk of depression and 1.9-fold increased risk of self-reported stress compared with women who do not have deployed spouses. This is true at different stages of pregnancy and in the postpartum period. Women with two or more children had a higher risk of small gestation age if a spouse was deployed. Mothers younger than 20 were at increased risk of cesarean delivery when their spouse was deployed. An increased risk of stress or depression may explain adverse birth outcomes among women with deployed spouses (Spieker et al., 2016).
- Women with deployed partners may have more difficulty accepting the pregnancy and experience greater conflict. Evidence shows on-base community support can have a positive effect on pregnancy acceptance for these women (Weis et al., 2008; Weis & Ryan, 2012).
- The Centering Pregnancy model of care, implemented at various military treatment facilities, also shows promise for offering effective group support for military women and their spouses (Foster et al., 2012).

Little is known about mental health problems or treatment among pregnant women veterans. Veterans may experience significant stress during military service that can have lingering effects. A quality improvement project was conducted in a single Veterans Administration (VA) health-care system between 2012 and 2015. It included a screen for depressive symptoms (using the Edinburgh Postnatal Depression Scale [EPDS] three times during the perinatal period), a dedicated maternity care coordinator, an on-site clinical social worker, and an on-site OB/GYN. Information on prior mental health diagnosis was collected. The prevalence of perinatal depressive symptoms and receipt of mental health care among those with such symptoms are reported by the presence of a pre-pregnancy mental health diagnosis.

Of the 199 women who used VA maternity benefits between 2012 and 2015, 56% had at least one pre-pregnancy mental health diagnosis. Compared with those without a pre-pregnancy mental health diagnosis, those with such a diagnosis were more likely to be screened for perinatal depressive symptoms at least once (61.5% vs. 46.8%). Prevalence of depressive symptoms was 46.7% among those with a pre-pregnancy mental health diagnosis and 19.2% among those without. Improving perinatal mental health care for women veterans requires a multidisciplinary approach, including on-site integrated mental health care (Katon et al., 2017).

Nursing Actions

- Assess adaptation to pregnancy at every prenatal visit. Early assessment and intervention may prevent or greatly reduce later problems for the pregnant woman and her family.
- Identify areas of concern, validate major issues, and offer suggestions and resources for possible changes.
- Refer to and follow up with the appropriate member of the health-care team.
- Establish a trusting relationship and rapport, as women may be reluctant to share information until one has been formed (e.g., questions asked at the first prenatal visit bear repeating with ongoing prenatal care).
- Assess need for psychotropic medications and determine effective use in the past.
- Use psychosocial health assessment screening tools to assess adaptation to pregnancy and to identify risk factors. Psychosocial assessment reported in the literature ranges from a few questions asked by the health-care provider to questionnaires and risk screening tools focusing on a specific area such as depression or abuse (Beck, 2002; Carroll et al., 2005; Midmer et al., 2002; Priest et al., 2006).
- The Antenatal Psychosocial Health Assessment (ALPHA) form, developed in Ontario, Canada, is a useful evidence-based prenatal tool that can identify women who would benefit from additional support and intervention (Box 5-1) (Carroll et al., 2005; Midmer et al., 2002). Other validated tools such as the Antenatal Risk Questionnaire (ANRQ) can be used to assess psychosocial risk (Austin et al., 2017).

BOX 5-1 | Antenatal Psychosocial Health Assessment

The ALPHA is an evidence-based prenatal tool to help providers identify women who would benefit from additional support and intervention. This tool assesses the following areas:

- Social support
- Recent stressful life events
- Couple's relationship
- Onset of prenatal care
- Plans for prenatal education
- Feelings toward pregnancy after 20 weeks
- Relationship with parents in childhood
- Self-esteem
- History or psychiatric/emotional problems
- Depression in this pregnancy
- Alcohol/drug use
- Family violence

Source: Carroll et al., 2005.

CLINICAL JUDGMENT

Psychosocial Screening in Prenatal Care

Psychosocial screening of every woman presenting for prenatal care is an important step toward improving health and birth outcomes (Adams, 2021). Psychosocial screening allows the nurse to identify areas of concern, validate major issues, and suggest possible changes. Depending on the nature of the problem, a referral may be made to an appropriate member of the health-care team. Remember that women may be reluctant to share information before forming a trusting relationship with the provider. Repeat questions asked at the first prenatal visit during ongoing prenatal care. The woman may need reassurance that information will remain confidential.

SOCIAL AND STRUCTURAL DETERMINANTS OF HEALTH

Social and structural determinants of health describe conditions, both physical and social, that influence health outcomes. Physical conditions such as lack of access to safe housing, clean drinking water, nutritious food, and safe neighborhoods contribute to poor health. Sociopolitical conditions such as institutional racism, police violence targeting people of color, gender inequity, discrimination against LGBTQ individuals, poverty, lack of access to quality education and jobs that pay a livable wage, and mass incarceration all shape behavior and biological processes that ultimately influence individuals' health and the health of communities (ACOG, 2018a). Such social conditions not only influence individual health but also work to create cycles that can perpetuate intergenerational disadvantage.

The resources of the family to meet the needs for food, shelter, and health care play a crucial role in how its members respond to pregnancy. Health equity is achieved when everyone has an equal opportunity to reach their health potential regardless of social position or characteristics such as race, ethnicity, gender, religion, sexual identity, or disability. Health inequities are closely linked with social determinants of health (SDOH)—conditions in the environments in which people are born, live, learn, work, play, worship, and age. SDOHs affect a wide range of health, functioning, and quality-of-life outcomes and risks. Certain social determinants, such as high unemployment, low education, and low income, have been associated with higher teen birth rates. Interventions that address SDOH play a critical role in reducing disparities observed in U.S. birth rates and outcomes (CDC, 2017b).

Underlying factors in racial and ethnic disparities in health care include knowing the full scope of the problem. Many issues involving health-care disparities are not well studied. There has been a lack of recognition or awareness of inequitable care; a lack of appreciation of the SDOH, poverty, and long-standing disadvantages; fragmented care through pregnancy, birth, and postpartum; miscommunication; poor communication; language and cultural barriers to understanding health information; and general misconception of etiologies and potentially successful strategies for improvement (Howell et al., 2018).

Experts propose that eliminating racism in the health-care system may reduce the disparities and promote healthier outcomes (Simpson, 2021). Bundle workgroup experts offer suggestions for improvement including learning about personal, institutional, and system implicit biases and ways to address each of these problems (Howell et al., 2018). Mindfulness may be beneficial. Advocating for processes to identify, report, and remedy instances of bias and inequitable health care has merit. Implicit bias can be addressed with self-awareness, a focus on concern for others (a characteristic of the majority of caregivers in all disciplines), and leadership support from the top of the organization (Council on Patient Safety in Women's Health Care, 2016).

- Financial barriers have been identified as among the most important factors contributing to maternal inability to receive adequate prenatal care.
- Homelessness plays a vital role in accessibility of prenatal health care, consistency in attending scheduled appointments, and care after birth and beyond.
- Immigrant women face significant economic barriers. Women in this group are often marginalized, and many work in low-income service-oriented jobs. Access to health care is often limited (Callister, 2021; Jentsch et al., 2007; Meleis, 2003).
- Lack of awareness, knowledge, and sensitivity along with bias from health-care professionals leads to inadequate access to, underuse of, and inequities within the health-care system for transgender patients (ACOG, 2021b).

Racial and Ethnic Disparities

Significant racial and ethnic disparities persist in women's health and health care. Women of racial and ethnic minority populations in the United States experience more maternal deaths, comorbid illnesses, and adverse perinatal outcomes than White women (Lowe, 2018). Black women are three to four times more likely to die from pregnancy-related causes and have more than a twofold greater risk of severe maternal morbidity than White women (Howell et al., 2018). Socioeconomic status accounts for some of these disparities, but factors at the patient, practitioner, and health-care system levels also contribute to existing and evolving disparities in women's health outcomes.

Although race and ethnicity are primarily social constructs, the effect of common ancestral lineage on the segregation and frequency of genetic variations in combination with the influence of cultural factors on environmental exposures cannot be ignored and should be considered a potential contributor to health disparities. Subtle ambiguities in practitioners' and patients' interpretations of medical information because of cultural and language differences also contribute to disparities in care. Studies suggest that race and language concordance between patients and practitioners may improve communication and outcomes. Providers must acknowledge the role they play in perpetuating health-care disparities and must advocate for a system more culturally and linguistically appropriate for all (ACOG, 2015; AWHONN, 2021, 2022).

Nursing Actions

- Raise awareness among colleagues and hospital administration about the prevalence of racial and ethnic disparities and the effect on health outcomes.
- Understand the role that care provider bias plays in health outcomes and care.
- Support and assist in the recruitment of other nurses from racial and ethnic minorities into academic and community health-care fields.
- Encourage health system leadership to advocate for local, state, and national policies to improve women's health care and reduce disparities.

Implicit Bias

Implicit bias refers to attitudes or stereotypes that unconsciously affect our understanding, actions, and decisions, resulting in attitudes about other people based on personal characteristics including but not limited to age, race and ethnicity, body, disability, gender, or sexual orientation. The potential influence of implicit bias is especially relevant in settings prone to cognitive overload or high stress, such as emergency department and labor and delivery environments. These settings frequently require reliance on automatic or unconscious processes, when stereotypes and unconscious beliefs are often activated (Byrne & Tanesini, 2015).

After many decades of study and exposition in the medical and sociological literature, policy makers and health-care providers have finally turned their attention to SDOH and their effects on health outcomes. In addition to demographic characteristics such as race, SDOH include economic characteristics such as education, income, housing, transportation, food insecurity, and many others according to the World Health Organization (WHO, 2011). In addition to the long overdue focus on SDOH, a groundbreaking 2003 report by the National Academy of Medicine confronted the uncomfortable truth about the scope of bias within the health-care system—about the uneven access, poor quality, and at times nonexistent care experienced by racial minorities (Institute of Medicine [IOM], 2003). This report clarified that medical care can exacerbate the impact of social factors outside the health-care system that led to poor health, contributing to even worse outcomes and experiences by minority patients. Individuals and communities interacting with the health-care system are subjected to disparate treatment at the hands of clinicians, with particular focus on disparities in maternal and child health. Implicit bias, by contrast, is "internally" driven and must be addressed by the delivery system.

The term *respectful maternity care (RMC)* has emerged as both a description of a basic human right and an optimal strategy to ensure that all women receive equitable maternity care, free from abuse and disrespect (AWHONN, 2022). Because organizational culture and the availability of resources have been shown to influence a nurse's ability to deliver respectful care, the health-care environment and policies should be structured to support all clinicians in providing RMC. Maternity care should maintain dignity, privacy, and confidentiality; ensure freedom from harm and mistreatment; and enable informed choice and continuous support during labor and childbirth.

Acknowledging that interactions within the health-care system can drive poor outcomes is no easy task and has no readily available solutions (ACOG, 2018a; AWHONN, 2021). Investigators suggest that implicit biases are malleable, remediable traits that can be improved through increased personal awareness and concerns about the effect of bias. Nurses and health-care providers must receive training about how to acknowledge and address internal bias. A diverse health-care team can improve patients' overall access and experience with care, feelings of being understood, and, consequently, adherence to improve health outcomes.

Nursing Actions

Nurses should ensure that women from varied backgrounds, races, and ethnicities receive quality health care free from racism and bias (AWHONN, 2021). They make these recommendations:

- That knowledge matters. Nurses would learn about the role and impact of racism and ways to overcome its effects on the provision of care. Health-care providers should demonstrate cultural competency in listening and communicating effectively with patients.
- That language matters. The way nurses communicate with patients, their families and communities, other health-care professionals, and each other is vitally important. Written materials, toolkits and bundles, and educational documents should be evaluated to ensure that they reflect the patient population served.
- That action matters. Nurses need to advocate for change in maternity and perinatal care settings to achieve nondiscriminatory, quality health services for all patients.
- That nurses need to challenge themselves, their colleagues, and nurse leaders to promote clear and directive actions with built-in accountability measures.

PATERNAL AND PARTNER ADAPTATION DURING PREGNANCY

The news of a pregnancy has a profound effect on the woman's partner. Partners have fears, questions, and concerns regarding the pregnancy, their partner, and the transition to parenthood. Each partner has a unique childhood and history that informs his own parenthood experience. Some relish the role and look forward to actively nurturing a child. Others may be detached or even hostile to the idea of parenthood.

Partners' Participation

Changing cultural and professional attitudes encourage the partner's participation in the birth experience. Some partners and fathers respond well to this expectation and want to explore every aspect of pregnancy, childbirth, and parenting (May, 1980).

Others are more task-oriented and view themselves as managers. They may direct the woman's diet and rest periods and act as coaches during childbirth but remain detached from the emotional aspects of the experience. Some are more comfortable as observers and prefer not to participate. In some cultures, pregnancy and childbirth are viewed as a woman's domain, and partners may be removed from the experience completely. In high-risk populations, increased partner involvement can improve birth outcomes, reduce health-care disparities, and increase positive maternal behaviors. Parenthood initiatives and employment assistance are examples of programs that can promote partner involvement (Alio et al., 2011; Alio et al., 2010; Callister, 2021; Misra et al., 2010).

Effect of Pregnancy on Partners

An expectant partner may have increased concern about his partner's well-being and worry about whether they will be good parents. A metasynthesis of research into parenthood revealed common themes, including reports that all expectant partners voiced some anxiety or worry in response to their partner's pregnancy; this was the single most powerfully shared experience (Kowlessar et al., 2015). Worry appeared to be a normal cognitive process, with many men expressing concern over the health of their partner and unborn baby. Partners talked about conflicting feelings in response to finding out they were going to become parents, spanning the entire spectrum of emotions from joy to disappointment.

Partners and men enter the unknown realm of pregnancy with expectations of how they should think and feel, imposed by oneself and by societal attitudes of male hegemony. Internal conflict arises when there is a discrepancy between how men and partners are expected to feel and how they actually feel. During the pregnancy, men and partners can feel their needs are neglected and their role underutilized.

Unintentional stress may result from how antenatal services are delivered and the attitudes of health professionals. Research on fathers and partners in the second trimester revealed expectant partners started to accept the pregnancy as real when they noticed evidence of the pregnancy in their partner's body, catalyzed by seeing and feeling the movements of their unborn baby. Consequently, they were able to relate to their unborn baby and pregnancy experience in a different way and started to develop an emotional attachment to their unborn baby. Toward the end stages of the pregnancy, partners can move away, both socially and psychologically, from their lives as nonparents and redefine themselves as fathers and parents (Kowlessar et al., 2015). Characteristics of this process may include the following:

- Increased emphasis on provider role causes reevaluation of lifestyle and job or career status.
- He may have anxiety about providing financial stability for their growing family.
- Changes in relationships and roles challenge expectant parents, creating the potential for distancing from their partners.
- Abuse may begin or escalate with the news of pregnancy. The risk of infidelity also increases (Kowlessar et al., 2015).

● With the focus of prenatal care on the woman and the growing fetus, the man may struggle to feel that he is relevant in the pregnancy (Widarsson et al., 2012).

● Some partners are without models to assist them in taking on the role of active and involved parent (Genesoni & Tallandini, 2009; Hanson et al., 2009).

● Some partners experience pregnancy-like symptoms and discomforts similar to those of their pregnant partner, such as nausea, weight gain, or abdominal pains. This is referred to as Couvade syndrome (Brennan et al., 2007) or sympathetic pregnancy. The partner may experience minor weight gain, altered hormone levels, morning nausea, and disturbed sleep.

Paternal Developmental Tasks

Paternal adaptation involves unique developmental tasks for fathers (Table 5-1). May's classic research (1982) on men identified three phases that expectant fathers experience as pregnancy progresses:

1. The announcement phase: Partners may react to the news of pregnancy with joy, distress, or a combination of emotions, depending on whether the pregnancy is planned or unwanted.

2. The moratorium phase: During this phase, many partners appear to put conscious thought of the pregnancy aside, even as their partners undergo dramatic physical and emotional changes before their eyes.

3. The focusing phase: This phase begins in the last trimester. Men will be actively involved in the pregnancy and their relationship with the child. These experiences unfold concurrently but in a distinctly different manner than the pregnant woman's adaptive experience.

Nursing Actions

● Explore the partner's response to news of pregnancy.

● Reassure that ambivalence is common in the early months of pregnancy and postpartum.

● Reassure normalcy of pregnancy-like symptoms (Couvade syndrome).

● Encourage and state the importance of attendance and involvement with childbirth education (i.e., provide resources for classes, electronic resources, and smartphone applications and discuss advantages of attending classes and utilizing a father's or parents group).

● Encourage the partner to negotiate their role in labor with their partner.

● Explore their attitudes, expectations, and inquiries of pregnancy, childbirth, and parenting.

● Encourage and explore options and resources for paternity or maternity time and bonding time for the partner.

TABLE 5-1   Paternal Adaptation to Pregnancy

ANNOUNCEMENT PHASE

Men may react to the news of pregnancy with joy, distress, or a combination of emotions, depending on whether the pregnancy is planned or unwanted.	Occurs as the news of the pregnancy is revealed. It may last from a few hours to several weeks. It is very common at this phase for men to feel ambivalence. The main developmental task is to accept the biological fact of pregnancy. Men will begin to attempt to take on the expectant father role.

MORATORIUM PHASE

During this phase, many men appear to put conscious thought of the pregnancy aside for some time, even as their partners are undergoing dramatic physical and emotional changes right before their eyes.	This can cause potential conflict when women attempt to communicate with their partners about the pregnancy. Sexual adaptation will be necessary as well; men may fear hurting the fetus during intercourse. Feelings of rivalry may surface as the fetus grows larger and the woman becomes more preoccupied with her own thoughts of impending motherhood. Men's main developmental task during this phase is to accept the pregnancy. This includes accepting the changing body and emotional state of his partner, as well as accepting the reality of the fetus, especially when fetal movement is felt.

FOCUSING PHASE

The focusing phase begins in the last trimester. Men will be actively involved in the pregnancy and their relationship with the child.	Men begin to think of themselves as fathers. Men participate in planning for labor and delivery, and the newborn. Men's main developmental task is to negotiate with their partner the role they are to play in labor and to prepare for parenthood.

May, 1982.

SEXUALITY IN PREGNANCY

Sexuality is one of the least understood and most superficially discussed topics by health-care providers. Sexuality encompasses physical capacity for sexual arousal and pleasure (i.e., libido), personalized and shared social meanings attached to sexual behavior, and formation of sexual and gender identities. Sexuality and gender attitudes and behaviors carry profound significance for women and men in every society. Sexuality is a vital component of physical and emotional well-being for people (Adams, 2021). Physiological changes during pregnancy affect the body's hormonal milieu as well as a woman's sexual desires, responses, and practices. Sexuality in pregnancy occurs on a wide continuum of responses for women. Some women feel more beautiful and desirable with advancing pregnancy and others feel unattractive and ungainly. The sexual relationship can be significantly affected during this time. Physical, emotional, and interactional factors all play a part in the woman's and her partner's sexual response during pregnancy (Crooks & Baur, 2010). A more open discussion between clinicians and patients about sexual activity during pregnancy is relevant and may help to alleviate women's fears, close knowledge gaps, and reassure those who wish to be sexually active throughout pregnancy (Adams, 2021; Afshar, My-Lin, et al., 2017).

- The desire for sexual activity varies among pregnant women. Sexual desire can vary even in the same woman at different times during the pregnancy. Typically, a woman's sexual interest and frequency declines in the first trimester of pregnancy, shows variable patterns in the second trimester, and decreases sharply in the third trimester (Afshar, My-Lin, et al., 2017).
- During the first trimester, fatigue, nausea, and breast tenderness may affect sexual desire.
- During the second trimester, desire may increase because of increased sense of well-being and the pelvic congestion associated with this time in pregnancy.
- During the third trimester, sexual interest may once again decrease as the enlarging abdomen creates feelings of awkwardness and bulk.
- Many women have some level of apprehension about sexual intercourse during pregnancy.
- Women in relationships with established open communication about sexuality are less likely to have difficulty with changes in sexual activity. For example, it may be necessary for a couple to modify intercourse positions for the pregnant woman's comfort.
- The side-by-side, woman-above, and rear-entry positions are generally more comfortable than the partner-above positions.
- Nonsexual expressions of affection are just as important.

Common concerns related to sexual activity include:

- Fears about hurting the fetus during intercourse or causing permanent anomalies because of sexual activity.
- Fear the birth process will drastically change the woman's genitals.
- Changes in body shape and body image influence both partners' desire for sexual expression.

Nursing Actions

- Discuss fears and concerns related to sexual activity.
- Encourage communication between partners and discuss possible changes with couples.
- Encourage the couple to verbalize fears and to ask questions.
- Use humor and encourage the couple to use humor to relieve anxiety or embarrassment.
- Evidence currently is insufficient to justify recommending against sexual intercourse during pregnancy. Advise pregnant women that there are no contraindications to intercourse or masturbation to orgasm if the woman's membranes are intact, there is no vaginal bleeding, and there are no current problems or history of premature labor (Adams, 2021; Crooks & Baur, 2010).
- During prenatal visits, asking patients whether they continue to be sexually active during pregnancy may make them comfortable asking questions about their sexual health. This can open the door to review sexual positions to increase comfort for the couple with advancing pregnancy.
- Cultural influences can affect forms of sexual contact in some populations, sometimes leading to avoidance during pregnancy because of ethnic or religious beliefs (Afshar, My-Lin, et al., 2017). It may be important to discuss alternative forms of sexual expression.

FAMILY ADAPTATION DURING PREGNANCY

Pregnancy affects the entire family; psychosocial assessment and interventions must be considered from a family-centered perspective (Barron, 2014). The family is a basic structural unit of the community and constitutes one of society's most important institutions. It is a key target for perinatal assessment and intervention. This primary social group assumes major responsibility for the introduction and socialization of children and forms a potent network of support for its members. Understanding of the different family structures and the life cycle of the family and the related developmental tasks can assist the nurse in providing care for pregnant women. Because of the many definitions of "family" and the changing realities of the current times, there is a need to redefine this term. One example is, "People related by marriage, birth, consanguinity or legal adoption, who share a common kitchen and financial resources on a regular basis" (Sharma, 2013, p. 308). The structure of families varies widely among and within cultures. Social scientists now commonly recognize that families exist in a variety of ways and that, during their lives, children may indeed belong to several different family groups.

Changing Familial Structures

U.S. census data indicate major shifts in the configuration of families over the past several decades. Cohabitation and domestic partnerships are on the rise, more adults are delaying or forgoing marriage, a growing share of children live with an

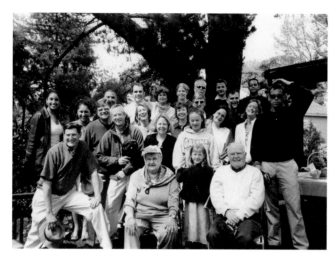

FIGURE 5–4 Multicultural family.

unmarried parent, and same-sex marriage is legal in all 50 states (PEW, 2020). A woman's family is the primary support during the childbearing years and has a direct influence on her emotional and physical health. It is essential that the nurse identify the woman's definition of family and provide care on that basis. Nurses must support all types of families (Fig. 5–4).

The variety of family configurations includes:

- The nuclear family: A father, mother, and child living together but apart from both sets of grandparents.
- The extended family: Three generations, including married siblings and their families.
- Single-parent family: Divorced, never married, separated, or widowed man or woman and at least one child, also now referred to as solo parenting.
- Three-generational families: Any combination of first-, second-, and third-generation members living within a household.
- Dyad family: Couple living alone without children.
- Stepparent family: One or both spouses have been divorced or widowed and have remarried into a family with at least one child.
- Blended or reconstituted family: A combination of two families with children from one or both families and sometimes children of the newly married couple.
- Cohabiting family: An unmarried couple living together.
- Gay or lesbian family: A same-sex couple living together with or without children; children may be adopted, from previous relationships, or conceived via artificial insemination.
- Adoptive family: Single persons or couples who have at least one child who is not biologically related to them and to whom they have legally become parents.

Family theorists have identified eight stages in the life cycle of a family that provide a framework for nurses caring for childbearing families (Duvall, 1985; Friedman et al., 2003): beginning families, childbearing families, families with preschool children, families with school-aged children, families with teenagers, families launching young adults, middle-aged parents, and aging families. Each of these stages has developmental tasks the family must accomplish to successfully move to the next stage.

Developmental Tasks

The events of pregnancy and childbirth are considered a developmental (maturational) crisis in the life of a family, defined as a change associated with normal growth and development. All family members are significantly affected. Previous life patterns may be disturbed, and there may be a sense of disorganization.

Certain developmental tasks have been identified that a family must face and master to successfully incorporate a new member into the family unit and allow the family to be ready for further growth and development. The developmental tasks for the childbearing family are:

- Acquiring knowledge and plans for the needs of pregnancy, childbirth, and early parenthood
- Preparing to provide for the physical care of the newborn
- Adapting financial patterns to meet increasing needs
- Realigning tasks and responsibilities
- Adjusting patterns of sexual expression to accommodate pregnancy
- Expanding communication to meet emotional needs
- Reorienting relationships with relatives
- Adapting relationships with friends and community to take account of the realities of pregnancy and the anticipated newborn

Accomplishment of these tasks during pregnancy lays the groundwork for adaptation required to add the newborn to the family (Duvall, 1985; Friedman et al., 2003).

Nursing Actions

- Assess knowledge related to pregnancy, childbirth, and early parenting.
- Assess cultural family traditions for new family additions.
- Assess progress in developmental tasks of pregnancy.
- Explore communication patterns related to emotional needs, responsibilities, and new roles.
- Include the entire family; assessments and interventions must be considered in a family-centered perspective.
- Provide education and guidance related to pregnancy, childbirth, and early parenting for the entire family.

Sibling Adaptation

Individual children react differently to the infant sibling's birth. Some children experience significant disruption, but others respond positively or with little to no distress. Interestingly, some researchers propose that children's initial reactions in the weeks after the sibling's birth predicted the quality of the relationship between siblings nearly a year later (Beyers-Carlson & Volling, 2017). For some children, sharing the spotlight with a new brother or sister is a major crisis. The older child may experience a sense of loss or jealousy about being "replaced" by the new sibling. During pregnancy, areas of change that impact siblings the most involve maternal appearance, parental behavior, and changes in the home such as sleeping arrangements.

Sibling adaptation is greatly influenced by the child's age and developmental level, as well as by the attitude of the parents.

- Children younger than 2 are usually unaware of the pregnancy and may not understand explanations about the future arrival of the newborn.
- Children from 2 to 4 years of age may respond to the obvious changes in their mother's body. This age group is particularly sensitive to the disruptions of the physical environment. Therefore, if the parents plan to change the sibling's sleeping arrangements to accommodate the new baby, these arrangements should be implemented well in advance of the birth. Children sleeping in a crib should be moved to a bed at least 2 months before the baby is due.
- Children aged 4 to 5 often enjoy listening to the fetal heartbeat and may show interest in the development of the fetus. As pregnancy progresses, however, they may resent the changes in their mother's body that interfere with her ability to lift and hold them or engage in physical play.
- School-age children (6 to 12) are usually enthusiastic and keenly interested in the details of pregnancy and birth. They have many questions and are eager to learn. They often plan elaborate welcomes for the newborn and want to help when their new sibling comes home.
- Adolescent responses to pregnancy vary according to developmental level. They may be uncomfortable with the obvious evidence of their parents' sexuality or embarrassed by the changes in their mother's appearance. They may be fascinated and repelled by the birth process all at once. Older adolescents may be somewhat indifferent to the changes associated with pregnancy but also may respond in a more adult fashion by offering support and help.
- Expectant parents should make a special effort to prepare and include the older child as much as their developmental age allows. Preparation must be carried out at the child's level of understanding and readiness to learn (Box 5-2).
- Some children express interest in being present at the birth. If siblings attend the birth, they should participate in a class that prepares them for the event. During the labor and birth, a familiar person who has no other role should be available to explain what is taking place and comfort or remove children if the situation becomes overwhelming.

Nursing Actions

- Explore with parents strategies for sibling preparation (see Box 5-2).
- Assess adaptation to pregnancy at every prenatal visit. Early assessment and intervention may prevent or greatly reduce later problems for the pregnant woman and her family.
- Discuss strategies to facilitate sibling adaptation based on the child's age and development.
- Facilitate discussion of the birth plan if parents want children present during the sibling's birth and a contingency plan if the labor doesn't go as planned and additional care is needed.
- Providing parents with advice and guidance on how to prepare their firstborn for the arrival of the infant may be beneficial

---

BOX 5-2 | Tips for Sibling Preparation

Pregnancy

- Take the child on a prenatal visit. Let the child listen to the fetal heartbeat and feel the baby move.
- Take the child to the homes of friends who have babies to give the child an opportunity to see babies and their lives firsthand.
- Take the child on a tour of the hospital or birthing center; if available, enroll in a sibling preparation class, if age appropriate.

After the Birth

- Encourage parents to be sensitive to the changes the sibling is experiencing; jealousy and a sense of loss are normal feelings at this time.
- Plan for high-quality, uninterrupted time with the older child.
- Encourage older children to participate in care of their sibling (i.e., bringing a diaper, singing to the baby, sitting with Mom during infant feeding times).
- Teach a parent to be watchful when the older child is with the newborn; natural expressions of sibling jealousy may involve rough handling, slapping or hitting, or throwing toys.
- Reassure parents that regressive behaviors in the very young child may be a normal part of sibling adjustment (i.e., return to diapers, wanting to breastfeed or take a bottle, tantrums), and with consistent attention and patience the behaviors will decrease. This is a transition time for the child.
- Praise the child for age-appropriate behavior; show the child how and where to touch the baby.
- In the hospital: Encourage sibling visitation; call older children on the phone; have visitors greet the older child before focusing on the newborn.
- Give a gift to the new sibling from the newborn; let the sibling select a gift for the baby before delivery to bring to the newborn after the birth.

---

for children and parents as they undergo the potentially stressful transition surrounding the birth of another child.

Grandparent Adaptation

Grandparents are often the first family members to be told about a pregnancy and must make complex adjustments to the news. Most grandparents look forward to the birth of a grandchild, especially the first grandchild, and the pleasure of getting to know the child without the responsibility of being a parent. Grandparents often have fulfilling relationships with their grandchildren, watching them learn and grow and being part of their lives, whereas others find that they are expected to do too much. Some have to bring up their grandchildren when the parents cannot, and some do more childminding than they expected. Some grandparents have less contact than they want, often due to the separation or divorce of the parents. A first pregnancy is also undeniable evidence that they are growing older, and some may respond negatively, indicating that they are not ready to be grandparents.

- New parents recognize that the tie to the future represented by the fetus is of special significance to grandparents.
- Grandparents provide a unique sense of family history to expectant parents that may not be available elsewhere. They can be a valuable resource and can strengthen family systems by widening the circle of support and nurturance.
- Grandparents may be called upon for more long-term help. Teen pregnancy, parents' incarceration, substance abuse, child abuse, and death or mental illnesses of the parents are some situations where grandparents may have to assume care and upbringing of the newborn.
- The demands of helping to raise a grandchild may create stressors in their lives that grandparents did not anticipate. Grandparent caregivers reported higher levels of distress in this role. Predictors of caregiver stress included severity of child behavior problems (Lee & Blitz, 2016).

Nursing Actions

- Assess the grandparents' response to pregnancy.
- Explore grandparents as a resource during pregnancy and early parenting.
- Involve social services, as they may assess the grandparents' financial and community resources for possible parenting.

MENTAL HEALTH DIFFICULTIES WITH PREGNANCY ADAPTATION

The importance of a woman's physical and mental health should be central to every aspect of maternity care. As well as affecting a woman's emotional welfare and happiness, mental health conditions affect her experience of pregnancy and parenting, increase the risk of obstetric and neonatal complications, and impact her ability to bond with her baby (Austin et al., 2017). Studies have reported that up to one in five to ten women experience anxiety and depression during pregnancy (AWHONN, 2015). Anxiety disorders are also prevalent (around one in five women in both the antenatal and postnatal periods) and comorbidity with depression is high. Severe mental illnesses are much less common than depression and anxiety disorders. All these conditions potentially have a negative impact on maternal and infant outcomes, especially when a mental health condition is combined with serious or multiple adverse psychosocial circumstances (Austin et al., 2017).

Women may present with psychosocial issues and concerns beyond the realm of the perinatal nurse. Severe and persistent mental illness (SPMI) refers to complex mood disorders that include major depressive disorder with or without psychosis; severe anxiety disorders resistant to treatment; affective psychotic disorders, including bipolar affective disorder, schizophrenia, and schizoaffective disorder; and other nonaffective subtypes of schizophrenia (McKeever et al., 2016). SPMIs affect 1 in 17 people and are among the leading causes of disability and impaired health-related quality of life in the United States.

Caring for childbearing women with preexisting SPMI can challenge maternal-child health clinicians with issues such as early identification, accuracy of diagnoses, and appropriate management through care coordination with an interdisciplinary team of obstetric providers, psychiatrists, nurses, and others (McKeever et al., 2016). Interventions to support women with mental health conditions in the perinatal period include psychosocial support, structured and systematic psychological interventions, and pharmacological treatment, depending on the severity of a woman's symptoms or condition. The woman and her significant other(s) choose interventions based on risk–benefit analysis, which accounts for the benefit to the woman and the fetus or newborn and the potential for harm (Austin et al., 2017).

Nurses must be aware of community mental health resources and prepared to collaborate with psychiatric or mental health specialties, social services, or community agencies. Mental health issues during pregnancy can create problems for the pregnant woman across several dimensions. Remember, perinatal mood disorders occur on a continuum. Extreme manifestations are life-threatening for women and newborns.

- Difficulty adapting to the maternal role, making the necessary transitions to parenthood, and mourning losses associated with the time before pregnancy are potential areas of concern.
- Perinatal depression often goes unrecognized because changes in sleep, appetite, and libido may be attributed to normal pregnancy (ACOG, 2018b). Several screening instruments have been validated for use during pregnancy and the postpartum period to assist with systematically identifying patients with perinatal depression such as the EPDS.
- Prenatal depression, maternal stress, and anxiety exert biochemical influences that significantly impact the developing fetus and contribute to adverse birth outcomes that have long-term consequences (e.g., low birth weight, shorter gestational age, adverse neonatal behavioral responses) (Lederman & Weis, 2009). Decreased utero-placental blood flow because of high maternal stress levels may affect the onset and duration of labor by interfering with mechanisms that modulate uterine contractions and impact delivery (Stadtlander, 2017).
- When assessing mood, emotional states, and anxiety, the nurse should consider these aspects: frequency, duration, intensity, and source. Screening and treatment interventions should be encouraged during the prenatal period. Early diagnosis and intervention may mitigate potential harm to the mother and child (Phua et al., 2017).
- Rates of serious mental illness during pregnancy, although low, are of concern given their association with adverse outcomes and the effects of psychotropic medication use or discontinuation during pregnancy.

Even in their more common manifestations, perinatal mood and anxiety disorders can affect the woman's health, her ability to connect with her child, her relationship with her partner, and her child's long-term health and development. For example, women with untreated depression during pregnancy are more likely to have trouble sleeping; poor nutrition and inadequate weight gain; missed prenatal visits; and use of harmful substances such as tobacco, alcohol, or illegal drugs. They are also less likely to follow a health-care provider's advice (AWHONN, 2015).

Nursing Actions

- Assess adaptation to pregnancy at every prenatal visit. Early assessment and intervention may prevent or reduce later problems for the woman and her family. Systematic screening in pregnancy can help detect early symptoms of perinatal psychiatric distress (ACOG, 2018b).
- Assess the woman's social support system and coping mechanisms and what has worked for her historically.
- Assess the woman's mood, anxiety, and emotional state and consider frequency, duration, intensity, and source of patients' emotional response.
- Explore other mechanisms that might be helpful.
- Discuss expectations about pregnancy, childbirth, and parenting.
- Identify areas of concern, validate major issues, and offer suggestions or resources for possible changes.
- Refer to the appropriate member of the health-care team and follow up with those team members for an interdisciplinary plan of care.
- Establish a trusting relationship, as women may otherwise be reluctant to share information (e.g., questions asked at the first prenatal visit bear repeating with ongoing prenatal care).
- Make appropriate referrals to other health professionals and follow up as needed. Always act with compassion and openness while keeping the woman at the center of care.

PSYCHOSOCIAL ADAPTATION TO PREGNANCY COMPLICATIONS

Most pregnancies progress with few problems and result in generally positive outcomes. However, with the diagnosis of pregnancy complications, normal concerns and anxieties of pregnancy are exacerbated. Uncertainty of fetal outcome can interfere with parental attachment.

- Response to pregnancy complications depends on:
  - Pregnancy condition
  - Perceived threat to mother or fetus
  - Coping skills
  - Available support and resources
- Disequilibrium, feelings of powerlessness, increased anxiety and fear, and a sense of loss are all responses to the news of a pregnancy complication.
- The pregnant woman may distance herself emotionally from the fetus as she faces varying levels of uncertainty about the pregnancy, impacting attachment (Gilbert, 2010).

- Events such as antepartal hospitalization or activity restrictions may contribute to a greater incidence of depression in the pregnant woman.
- The risk of crisis for the pregnant woman and her family clearly increases due to an unpredictable or uncertain pregnancy outcome (Durham, 1998).
- How a woman and her family respond to this additional stress is crucial in determining whether a crisis will develop along with what support system they have in place.
- Having a realistic perception of the event, adequate situational support, and positive coping mechanisms help a woman maintain her equilibrium and avoid crisis.
- Poor self-esteem, lack of confidence in the mothering role, perception of being judged as at fault, and an inability to communicate concerns to health-care providers and close unsupportive family members are factors that increase the risk of crisis.

The weathering hypothesis states that chronic exposure to social and economic disadvantage leads to accelerated decline in physical health outcomes. This could partially explain racial disparities in perinatal health outcomes (Forde et al., 2019). Prolonged exposure to stress can accelerate cellular aging, disregulating neuroendocrine, cardiovascular, metabolic, and immune systems and resulting in poorer health outcomes (Geronimus et al., 2020).

Research has demonstrated the physical health of mothers with a high-risk pregnancy, demographic and emotional factors, and the health condition of newborns jointly affect mental health. High-risk pregnancy is a potential risk factor for postpartum anxiety and depression and needs follow-up. High-risk pregnancies create additional health problems in both mothers and infants. Research findings indicate that prenatal distress, and to some degree pregnancy complications, may hinder postnatal adaptation and interfere with the early formation of parent–infant relationships. Expecting parents' prenatal distress should be assessed routinely, and especially if pregnancy complications are diagnosed. Furthermore, the findings suggest that psychological intervention should be offered to distressed parents as early as possible, preferably during the perinatal phase, to ameliorate depressive and anxiety symptoms (Dollberg et al., 2016). Pregnant women need emotional support from both providers and family members. Counseling sessions on various aspects of pregnancy and parenthood may reduce the incidence of postpartum depression (Zadeh et al., 2012).

There is growing awareness that a pregnant woman's experiences of childhood and cumulative adversity may have intergenerational effects. While the prenatal period is a window when the consequences of maternal adversity and resulting problems with mental health and stress physiology impact the fetus, it is also a window of opportunity for resilience and intervention. Research provides compelling evidence that the trajectory of fetal development is profoundly influenced by the intrauterine environment, including signals to the fetus that stem from maternal stress and mental health problems. Findings also support the ability of intervention to disrupt this intergenerational transmission of adversity and mental health problems from mothers to infants (Davis & Narayan, 2020).

Nursing Actions

When caring for a pregnant woman with complications, the priority is to reestablish and maintain physiological stability. However, nurses must also be able to intervene to promote psychosocial adaptation to the news of pregnancy complications (Giurgescu et al., 2006; Lederman, 2011; Mattson & Smith, 2016). The following actions can reduce or limit the detrimental effects of complications on individual or family functioning:

- Provide frequent and clear explanations about the problem, planned interventions, and therapy and continue to encourage parents to ask questions and verbalize concerns.
- Account for questions and concerns and individualize resources for compatibility.
- Assess and encourage the use of the woman's support systems and provide knowledge about new support systems and resources.
- Support individual adaptive coping mechanisms and resources more if needed.
- Make appropriate referrals and follow up when additional assistance is needed.

SOCIAL SUPPORT DURING PREGNANCY

Social support is provided by a person with whom the expectant mother has a personal relationship. It involves the primary groups of most importance to the individual woman: her spouse or partner, her mother, and her close friends. Involvement of and support from the baby's partner during pregnancy is associated with improved maternal mental health and may contribute to a less distressed infant temperament (Stapleton et al., 2012). The following have been identified as important types of social support for the pregnant woman.

- Material (instrumental) support consists of practical help such as assistance with chores, meals, finances, and crises that arise.
- Emotional support involves affection, approval, and encouragement as well as feelings of togetherness, acceptance, and inclusivity.
- Informational support consists of sharing resources or helping women investigate new sources of information.
- Comparison support consists of help given by someone in a similar situation. Their shared information is useful and credible because they are experiencing or have experienced the same events in their lives and can help the woman feel included.
- Spiritual support consists of creating a space for the woman to express and explore her pregnancy experience.

Social Support Research

Research from several disciplines provides evidence for the importance of social support for the pregnant woman's health, positive adaptation to pregnancy, and the prevention of pregnancy complications. This naturally occurring resource can prevent health problems and complications and promote health. Receiving adequate help from others enhances self-esteem and feelings of control. Mothers who perceived stronger social support from partners during midpregnancy had lower emotional distress postpartum after controlling for their distress in early pregnancy, and infants were reported to be less distressed in response. Partner support mediated effects of the mothers' interpersonal security and relationship satisfaction on maternal and infant outcomes (Stapleton et al., 2012). Pregnant women need the support of caring family members, friends, and health professionals. A Cochrane Review concluded that although programs that offer social support during pregnancy are unlikely to have a large impact on the proportion of low birth weight babies or birth before 37 weeks' gestation and no impact on stillbirth or neonatal death, they may reduce the risk of cesarean birth and antenatal hospital admission (East et al., 2019).

- Social support benefits the expectant mother most when it matches her expectations, referred to as *perceived social support*. It is important that the woman identify and clarify expectations and needs for support. Perceived support expectations that do not materialize lead to distress and problems with adaptation to pregnancy (Ngai et al., 2010).
- Pregnant women frequently need social support that differs from the support they receive. Nurses can advise the pregnant woman how best to use her existing support networks or how to expand her support network so her needs are met. Nurses have the opportunity and responsibility to help women explore potential sources of support such as childbirth education classes, electronic resources, church, work, school, or the community.
- High-risk populations, including adolescents, women with pregnancy complications, and women with a low income, may need particular direction from nurses in obtaining adequate support (Beeber & Canuso, 2005; Logsdon et al., 2005). Involving disciplines such as social work, psychiatry, legal, and maternal-fetal specialists could be necessary for these populations.
- Recent immigrants face challenges in obtaining needed social support. Disruption of lifelong attachments can cause anxiety and disorientation. Language barriers, socioeconomic struggles, and biases are additional stressors facing immigrant women, increasing risk for depression (Ganann et al., 2016). Their families, experiencing the same difficulties, may not be able to provide sufficient support or any support at all.
- Researchers have recognized that women conceptualize meanings of pregnancy from their homelands and thus have culturally derived pregnancy practices and beliefs that are often different from the practices in their new country (Jentsch et al., 2007). However, having a good formal support system from HCPs amplified the positive experiences of pregnancy in a new country. Satisfaction with care was improved when providers took time to build a rapport and explain the plan of care (Winn et al., 2017).
- Social support is not considered professional support, although professionals can provide supportive actions such as counseling, teaching, role modeling, or problem-solving. When expectant mothers have no other support, some community programs employ paraprofessionals to visit them for

education and social support. Programs that capitalize on the skills of experienced mothers in communities may be less expensive and more culturally sensitive than hospital-based programs led by teams of health-care professionals. Additionally, postdelivery follow-up programs offering home-based social support may also have important benefits for mothers and children who have social disadvantages (Cannella, 2006; Dawley & Beam, 2005; Logsdon et al., 2005).

Assessing Social Support

Assessing social support is a crucial component of prenatal care. The following areas of assessment should be addressed when planning care:

- Who is available to help provide support (material, emotional, informational, comparison, and spiritual)? Is the support adequate in each category?
- With whom does the pregnant woman have the strongest relationships, and what type of support is provided by these individuals?
- Does conflict exist in relationships with support providers? Is the conflict violent or has it resulted in abuse?
- Is there potential for improvement of the woman's support network? Should she remove members who provide more stress than support, or will that cause more stress? Should new members be added?
- Who lives with the pregnant woman?
- Who assists with household chores and finances?
- Who assists with childcare and parenting activities?
- Who does the pregnant woman turn to when problems occur or a crisis arises?
- What is the woman's financial situation?
- If she works outside the home, is she supported at work? What is her work situation once the baby has arrived?
- How many other children does the mother have? Does having another child cause a crisis?

Nursing Actions

The nursing profession plays an important role in promoting patient-centered, individualized, and respectful care (Adams, 2021; Wilson & Leese, 2013). Due to the strong evidence that social support improves pregnancy outcomes, the following nursing actions are recommended:

- Provide opportunities for the woman to ask for support and rehearse with her appropriate language to use. Encourage her to ask for support whenever she needs it. Individualize her support to be compatible for the patient.
- Invite key support providers to attend prenatal and postpartum visits and provide inclusivity during discussions.
- Facilitate supportive functioning and interactions within the family, encouraging them to ask questions and to be involved if the mother permits.
- Encourage the pregnant woman to interact with other pregnant or postpartum women she knows. Provide access if possible to the Centering Pregnancy model of care.

- Suggest worship centers or faith communities, health clubs, work or school, and electronic resources as sites to meet women with similar interests and concerns.
- Provide information regarding community resources, such as mom groups and online networks, that are compatible with the mother's culture and racial preferences.

TRAUMA-INFORMED CARE

Trauma is experienced throughout the life span; it may result from remote events or be current and ongoing. Traumatic events range from sexual abuse to natural disasters to simple encounters, including within the health-care system. These experiences may include intimate partner violence; sexual assault and rape, including military sexual trauma, violence perpetrated based on race or sexual orientation; neglect during childhood; combat and service trauma; repeated exposure to community violence; refugee and immigration status; or family separation.

Specific to obstetrics is the increasing acknowledgment of traumatic birth experiences, which may include unexpected outcomes, procedures, obstetric emergencies, and neonatal complications. The nonmedical term *obstetric violence* is used to refer to situations in which a pregnant or postpartum individual experiences disrespect, indignity, or abuse from health-care practitioners or systems that can stem from and lead to loss of autonomy (ACOG, 2021a). These situations may include, for example, repeated and unnecessary vaginal examinations, unindicated episiotomy, activity and food restrictions during labor, and forced cesarean delivery. More subtle manifestations may include minimization of patient symptoms and differential treatment based on race, substance use, or other characteristics.

Trauma's effects on the brain and body are real, resulting in neurobehavioral, social, emotional, and cognitive changes (ACOG, 2021a). Trauma-informed care practices seek to create physical and emotional safety for survivors and rebuild their sense of control and empowerment during health-care interactions (ACOG, 2021a). The guiding principles of trauma-informed care are safety, choice, collaboration, trustworthiness, and empowerment (Substance Abuse and Mental Health Services Administration [SAMHSA], 2014). Engaging in patient-centered communication and care can be accomplished by seeking patient input on how best to make them comfortable and can be particularly valuable for establishing trust and rapport. Offering options during care that can lessen anxiety, such as seeking permission before initiating contact, providing descriptions before and during examinations and procedures, allowing clothing to be shifted rather than removed, and agreeing to halt the examination at any time upon request, are all beneficial practices.

Trauma-informed care can empower patients by recognizing the significance of power differentials and the historical diminishing of voice and choice in past coercive exchanges. Patients should be offered the choice to be actively involved in all decision making regarding their care. Educating patients about the health effects of trauma and offering patients opportunities to disclose their traumatic events should be common practice. There is no single best way to screen for trauma. A framing statement can be used to preface trauma screening, prepare the patient for potentially difficult questions, and convey the universality of the screening (ACOG, 2021a). The goals of trauma informed care are to **realize** the widespread effect of trauma and understand potential paths for recovery; **recognize** the signs and symptoms of trauma in clients, families, staff, and others involved with the system; **respond** by fully integrating knowledge about trauma into policies, procedures, and practices; and seek to actively resist **re-traumatization.**

Nursing Actions

Maintaining a calm, supportive, nonjudgmental demeanor that is stabilizing and reassuring to patients with a history of trauma can be challenging even for experienced clinicians. It requires a commitment to ongoing self-reflection, practice, and both individual and systems transformation. To understand how to enact practices that support trauma-informed care, the simple 4 Cs paradigm is a concrete and memorable rubric (Kimberg & Wheeler, 2019).

- Calm: Pay attention to your feelings when caring for the patient. Breathe deeply and calm yourself to model and promote calmness for the patient, yourself, and your coworkers.
- Contain: Ask the level of detail of trauma history that will allow the patient to maintain emotional and physical safety.
- Care: Practice self-care and self-compassion while caring for others; practice cultural humility; adopt behaviors, practices, and policies that minimize and mitigate power differentials to reduce trauma and structural violence; and normalize and destigmatize trauma symptoms and harmful coping behaviors.
- Cope: Emphasize coping skills for patients and yourself to build upon strength, resiliency, and hope.

IMMIGRANT AND REFUGEE WOMEN

Migration has been part of human history and an ever-growing phenomenon. The number of displaced people worldwide in 2019 was about 79.5 million and nearly half are estimated to be women (United Nations High Commissioner for Refugees [UNHCR], 2020). Refugee women flee their countries because of war, abuse of human rights, poverty, and other life-threatening conditions. The common themes in millions of stories of refugee experiences include loss and violence: loss of loved ones; loss of freedom, status, and social and cultural identity; loss of physical and mental health; and loss of community and support networks. Refugee and asylum-seeking women and LGBTQ people escape situations of abuse of their human rights (e.g., sexual torture, rape, and other forms of gender-based violence). They are exposed to hardships and different types of extreme violence throughout the migration process and in the context of the destination countries. Although migration for women is more

difficult due to their lack of means and traditional care duties, the number of refugee women is rising.

The trauma generated by such experiences has long-lasting damaging effects on their lives, physical and mental health, and impedes their integration in the destination country.

The so-called refugee crisis is instrumentalized by the media that portray refugees as "illegal," rendering them prey to xenophobic rhetoric. Gender is a central dimension that merits attention. Women and members of the LGBTQ community are more prone to be victims of violent incidents due to patriarchal structures, cultural factors, and their socioeconomic status, while in their countries of origin, as well as during the migration journey and in the postmigration periods. Race, socioeconomic status, and culture intersect with gender and lead to compound discrimination. An intersectionality approach, combined with feminist, trauma, and postcolonial analyses, will help health-care providers understand and capture the multitude of effects traumatic experiences cause for refugee and asylum-seeking women. Health issues are part of the vulnerabilities of migrant populations because of diseases endemic in the countries of origin, inadequate health care, health complications during the migration journey, and often insufficient health facilities in transit camps and accommodation centers (Davaki, 2021).

Global migration is at an all-time high with significant implications for perinatal health. Migrant women, especially asylum seekers and refugees, represent a particularly vulnerable group (Heslehurst et al., 2018). Pregnant migrant and refugee women can face severe marginalization when seeking care. In combination with increasing rates of abuse and higher maternal morbidity, these women live in unsafe conditions. As displaced people, they are likely fleeing severe disasters, crises, or persecution with accompanying trauma from these experiences, or their journey to escape them. Pregnant refugee women may be prohibited by fear of costs or be unable to find transportation to clinics; they may have a general mistrust of the health-care system, a fear of stigma, or lack fluency in the language. As first-generation immigrants, these women often have stronger ties to cultural traditions and customs than second- or third-generation Americans. For instance, they may have given birth previously in their home attended by a traditional midwife and their mother or mother-in-law. The biomedical and highly technologic environment of birthing units in the United States may be foreign and frightening. Limitations in literacy and language make it difficult to enter the health-care system. Feelings of fear and paranoia create circumstances where these women are unwilling to access care (Callister, 2021). Some suggestions to improve services include (Davaki, 2021):

- Prioritizing a holistic approach to addressing refugee women's needs
- Creating interventions that draw on cultural diversity and harness cultural beliefs and attitudes to enhance healing potential

Integrating health and psychological support services with housing, employment and education training, and financial assistance can help refugee women regain their self-esteem, confidence, and optimism to make a new start.

CHILDBEARING AND CULTURE

Childbirth is a time of transition and celebration in all cultures (Callister, 2014, 2021). Culture has a significant influence on a patient's perspective of health. Health-care beliefs and behaviors surrounding pregnancy, childbirth, and parenting are deeply rooted in cultural context. Culture is a set of behaviors, beliefs, and practices, a value system transmitted from one woman in a cultural group to another (Lauderdale, 2011). Culture is more than background, language, or country of origin; it provides a framework within which women think, make decisions, and act. The extent to which a woman adheres to cultural practices, beliefs, and rituals is complex and depends on acculturation and assimilation into the dominant culture within the society, social support, length of time in the United States, generational ties, and linguistic preference (Callister, 2021). Even within individual cultural groups, there is tremendous heterogeneity; although women may share a common birthplace or language, they do not always share the same cultural traditions.

Cultural beliefs and practices affect the health status of pregnant women by influencing use of health-care services and beliefs regarding her body, pregnancy, illness, and her confidence in providers and their recommendations (Barron, 2014). A culturally responsive nurse recognizes these influences and considers them carefully and when planning inclusive care (Amidi-Nouri, 2011; Moore et al., 2010). Box 5-3 lists resources for cultural information.

Each individual woman should be treated as such—an individual who may or may not espouse specific cultural beliefs, practices, and behaviors. Generalizations are made about cultural groups; however, a stereotypical approach to the provision of perinatal nursing care is not appropriate. It is critical that nurses acquire the knowledge and skills to provide quality care to culturally divergent groups. Expectations of nursing practice will increasingly require cultural humility and sensitivity to the cultural needs of families and competence in providing care.

All nursing care is given within the context of many cultures: that of the patient, nurse, health-care system, and the larger society. Childbirth directly involves two bodies in one; it's the only time in life when the care surrounds two (or more) humans contained in one body. The mother's body must adapt to changes associated with accommodating another life, whereas the baby must adapt to life outside the womb after birth (Romano, 2014).

Culturally Sensitive Behavioral Practices

Culturally sensitive practices and patient preferences can be viewed from a variety of dimensions nurses must consider when planning care (Callister, 2021; Moore et al., 2010).

- Decision making: Are decisions made by the woman alone or by others such as her partner, extended family, male elders, spiritual leaders, older adults, or the oldest female relative present?
- Concept of time: Is the culture past, present, or future-oriented? This may affect the woman's understanding about the need for time commitments, such as prenatal care appointments. The dominant U.S. culture is future-oriented, which means people act today with expectations for future rewards. Cultures that are not future-oriented may not seek preventive, prenatal, or well-woman care.
- Communication: Verbal communication may be challenging because of language barriers, meanings of words in different cultures, and willingness to disclose personal information. Cultures may have different practices regarding nonverbal communication practices such as eye contact, personal space, use of gestures, facial expressions, and appropriate touching. A nurse born in the United States might misinterpret a smile as agreement or understanding about something, rather than as confusion about the provided information.
- Religion: One's religious background may have a powerful influence on sexual attitudes and behaviors. It is important to appreciate that all people from one country, one neighborhood, or one faith do not share one culture or a single set of religious beliefs (Moore et al., 2010).
- Worldview: A client's understanding of how human life fits into the larger picture.
- How is illness explained? Examples include ancestral displeasure, body imbalance, breach of taboo, evil eye, germ theory of disease, spirit possession, or karma.
- Modesty and gender: What are the norms for interaction between men and women? What are the norms for undressing in front of someone not in your family?
- Some cultures accept public exposure of the human body, whereas in others women are expected to cover almost all their bodies. The nurse must understand and be open to the mores of the woman and her social group.

BOX 5-3 | Resources for Further Cultural Information

Alliance for Hispanic Health: www.hispanichealth.org

American Civil Liberties Union: www.aclu.org

Arab topics: www.al-bab.com

Asian and Pacific Islander American health forum: www.apiahf.org

AT&T Language Line: www.languageline.com

Gay & Lesbian Medical Association: www.glma.org

Hmong studies Internet resource center: www.hmongstudies.com/HmongStudiesJournal

Indian Health Services: www.ihs.gov

LGBTQ: www.aecf.org

Office of Minority Health: https://minorityhealth.hhs.gov/

Transcultural Nursing Society: www.tcns.org

Common Themes for the Childbearing Family

During the prenatal period, preventing harm to the fetus and ensuring a safe and easy birth are common themes in many cultures. Common aspects influencing labor and delivery include general attitudes toward birth, preferred positions, methods of pain management, and the role of family members and the health-care provider.

- The postpartum period is considered a time of increased vulnerability for both mothers and babies, influencing care of the new mother as well as infant care practices related to bathing, swaddling, feeding, umbilical cord care, and circumcision (Mattson & Smith, 2016).
- Pregnancy and childbirth may elicit customs and beliefs during pregnancy about acceptable and unacceptable practices that have implications for planning nursing care and interventions. These beliefs must be considered when assessing and promoting adaptation to pregnancy (Box 5-4).

BOX 5-4 | Examples of Cultural Prescriptions, Restrictions, and Taboos

Prescriptive Beliefs

- Remain active during pregnancy to aid the baby's circulation.
- Remain happy to bring the baby joy and good fortune.
- Drink chamomile tea to ensure an effective labor.
- Soup with ginseng root is a good general strength tonic.
- Pregnancy cravings need to be satisfied or the baby will be born with a birthmark.
- Sleep flat on your back to protect the fetus from harm.
- Attach a safety pin to an undergarment to protect the fetus from cleft lip or palate.

Restrictive Beliefs

- Do not have your picture taken because it might cause stillbirth.
- Avoid sexual intercourse during the third trimester because it will cause respiratory distress in the newborn.
- Coldness in any form may cause arthritis or other chronic illness.
- Avoid seeing an eclipse of the moon; it will result in a cleft lip or palate.
- Do not reach over your head or the cord will wrap around the baby's neck.

Taboos

- Avoid funerals and visits from widows or women who have lost children because they will bring bad fortune to the baby.
- Avoid hot and spicy foods, as they can cause overexcitement for the pregnant woman.
- An early baby shower will invite the evil eye and should be avoided.

Adapted from Lauderdale, 2011.

- Prescriptive behavior is an expected behavior of the pregnant woman during childbearing.
- Restrictive behavior describes activities during the childbearing period that are limited for the pregnant woman.
- Taboos are cultural restrictions believed to have serious supernatural consequences.

Cultural practices can also be classified as functional (enhances well-being), neutral (does not harm or help), or nonfunctional (potentially harmful). Nurses must be able to differentiate among these beliefs and practices, and respect functional and neutral practices, especially when these patient practices differ from the provider's own beliefs.

Nurses must remember that few cultural customs related to pregnancy are dangerous; although they might cause a woman to limit her activity and exposure to some aspects of life, they rarely harm herself or her fetus. When encountering nonfunctional practices, the nurse should first try to understand the meaning of the practice for the woman and her family and then work carefully to bring about change. An example of a nonfunctional practice would be the ingestion of clay during pregnancy (Lauderdale, 2011; Moore et al., 2010).

Barriers to Culturally Competent Care

Barriers to culturally competent care include values, beliefs, and customs as well as communication challenges and the biomed health-care environment (Callister, 2014, 2021). Cultural health disparities are created when nurses and other care providers fail to understand the importance of client beliefs about health and illness (Moore et al., 2010). Nurses' attitudes can create barriers to culturally competent care. Ethnocentrism, the belief that the customs and values of the dominant culture are preferred or superior in some way, is an obstacle to implementation of culturally sensitive care. Stereotyping, the assumption that everyone in a group is the same as everyone else in the group, also creates barriers. Cultural imposition is the tendency to thrust one's beliefs, values, and patterns of behaviors on another culture (Callister, 2021). Communication barriers include not only language barriers but also lack of knowledge, fear and distrust, racism, and bias. The health-care environment can create barriers through lack of translators, rigid policies, and protocols that do not support cultural diversity. Remember, maternity care may be the first encounter immigrant women have with health-care delivery systems in the United States. Reflect on how difficult it may be for the woman who may be living here without the support of extended family (especially female family members), speaking little or no English, and with limited understanding of the dominant culture and maternity care services. Other barriers to care include the following:

- Lack of diversity and inclusivity among health-care providers contributes to this issue. For example, the RN population is 80.8% White, 6.2% Black, 7.5% Asian, 5.3% Hispanic, 0.4% American Indian/Alaskan Native, 0.5 Native Hawaiian/ Pacific Islander, 1.7% two or more races, and 2.9% other (American Association of Colleges of Nursing [AACN], 2019).

- Strong evidence exists that the quality of health care varies as a function of race, ethnicity, and language (Amidi-Nouri, 2011; Callister, 2021; Meleis, 2003; Moore et al., 2010).
- Mainstream models of obstetric care as practiced in North America may present a strange and confusing picture to women from different ethnic backgrounds. The predominant culture's emphasis on formal prenatal care, technology, hospital deliveries, and a bureaucratic health-care system presents barriers to care for many groups.
- Protocols, an unfamiliar environment, and health-care providers who only speak English may confuse and intimidate patients, resulting in inadequate access to care.
- Health literacy is the capacity to obtain, process, and understand basic health information and services needed to make appropriate health decisions. Approximately half of the adult population lacks the needed literacy skills to use the U.S. health-care system. Low literacy has been linked to poor health outcomes, such as higher rates of hospitalization and less frequent use of preventive services (CDC, 2017a).

These obstacles to health care significantly contribute to health-care disparities, which are differences in care experienced by one population compared with another population. Disparities also occur in gender, age, economic status, religion, cultural background, disability, sexual orientation, and immigration status. For further information on health-care disparities, see Chapters 1 and 2.

Culturally Responsive Nursing Practice

Nurses have an obligation to provide patients and families effective, understandable, and respectful care in a manner compatible with the patient's cultural beliefs, practices, and preferred language. *Cultural assessment* is assessment of shared cultural beliefs, values, and customs related to health behaviors (Callister, 2021; Mattson & Smith, 2016). The goal is to gain knowledge to create an environment for development of a trusting patient relationship.

Mandates from professional health-care accrediting bodies and government agencies provide evidence of increased commitment to providing culturally appropriate health care. Examples of these directives include the following:

- The Joint Commission–mandated plan of patient care includes cultural and spiritual assessments and interventions (The Joint Commission, 2018).
- The AACN has stated that nursing graduates should have the knowledge and skills to provide holistic care that addresses the needs of diverse populations. AACN has also published specific end-of-program cultural competencies for baccalaureate nursing education (AACN, 2008).
- The HHS office of minority health has published national standards for Culturally and Linguistically Appropriate Services (CLAS) (U.S. DHSS, 2017).

Culturally sensitive nursing practice requires the nurse to maintain an open attitude and inclusivity along with sensitivity to differences.

CRITICAL COMPONENT

Strategies for Nurses: Improving Culturally Responsive Care

- Maintain an open, inclusive attitude.
- Recognize yourself as a part of the diversity in society and acknowledge your own belief system.
- Examine and create your own awareness about the biases and assumptions you hold about different cultures.
- Avoid preconceptions and cultural stereotyping.
- Explore and understand historical and current portrayals of racial and ethnic groups in society.
- Develop an understanding of how racial or ethnic differences affect the quality of health care and how it can lead to disparities.
- Acknowledge your power to use professional privilege positively or negatively.
- Recall your commitment to "individualized care," "respect," and "professionalism."
- Identify who the client calls "family."
- Include notes on cultural preferences and family strengths and resources as part of all intake and ongoing assessments, as well as nursing care plans and care maps.
- Use the cultural wisdom (beliefs, values, customs, and habits) of the client to shape their participation in health practices and care plans.
- Seek out client-friendly and compatible teaching and assessment tools.
- Review the literature to generate a culture database.
- Read literature from other cultures. If an ethnic group is well represented in the local population, learn about that culture to provide optimal care.
- Participate in professional development and continuing education programs that address cultural competence and humility, and strive to know the difference.
- Recognize that all care is given within the context of many cultures.
- Develop linguistic and relatable skills related to your client population.
- Learn to use nonverbal communication in an appropriate way.
- Learn about communication patterns of local cultures and use appropriate names and titles.
- Advocate for organizational change on racism, diversity, and inclusiveness.
- Understand and apply the various regulatory standards (CLAS, AACN, etc.).
- Promote cultural practices that are helpful, tolerate practices that are neutral, and work to educate women to renegotiate cultural practices that are potentially harmful (Leininger's Theory of Culture Care and Sunrise Model).
- Understand and develop possible methods of support that are compatible in the culture (Amidi-Nouri, 2011; Barron, 2014; Callister, 2014, 2021; Melo, 2013; Mojaverian & Heejung, 2013; Moore et al., 2010).

Cultural Assessment

To consider and individualize cultural aspects of care (Andrews & Boyle, 2011; Callister, 2021; Moore et al., 2010), the nurse caring for expectant families must answer these questions:

- What is the woman's predominant culture? To what degree does the client identify with the cultural group? Is there anything she wants to observe on her culture's traditions?
- What language does the client speak at home? What are the styles of nonverbal communication (e.g., eye contact, space orientation, touch, decision making)?
- How does the woman's culture influence her beliefs about pregnancy and childbirth? How is childbirth valued? Is pregnancy considered a state of illness or health? How does the culture explain illness? Are there particular attitudes toward age at the time of pregnancy? Marriage? Who would be an acceptable father or partner? What is considered acceptable in terms of pregnancy frequency?
- What does childbirth mean to the woman?
- Are there cultural prescriptions, restrictions, or taboos related to certain activities, dietary practices, or expressions of emotion? What does the pregnant woman consider to be normal practice during pregnancy, birth, and postpartum? Are there dietary, nutritional, pharmacological, and activity-prescribed practices? What maternal precautions or restrictions are necessary during childbearing?
- What support is given during pregnancy, childbirth, and beyond, and who appropriately gives that support?
- How does the woman interpret and respond to experiences of pain? Will she want pain medication?
- Are there culturally defined expectations about male–female relationships and relationships outside the culture?
- What is the client's educational background? Does it affect her knowledge level concerning the health-care delivery system, teaching or learning, written material given, or understanding?
- How does the client relate to persons outside her cultural group? Does she prefer a caregiver with the same cultural background?
- What is the role of religious beliefs related to pregnancy and childbirth?
- How are childbearing decisions made, and who is involved in the decision-making process?
- How does the woman's predominant culture view the concept of time? (Cultures may be past, present, or future-oriented.)
- How does the woman's culture explain illness? (Examples: ancestral displeasure, germ theory, etc.)
- How is the newborn viewed? What are the patterns of infant care? What are the relationships within the nuclear and extended families?

Nursing Actions

With the increasingly diverse patient population, it is imperative that nurses provide culturally sensitive care and act with cultural humility. Cultural humility reflects lifelong commitment to self-evaluation and critique, to redressing power imbalances.

Cultural humility, cultural awareness, and cultural respect all emphasize the nurse being humble about recognizing the limits of their knowledge of a patient's situation, avoiding generalizing assumptions, being aware of their own and patient biases, ensuring mutual understanding through patient-centered communication, and respectfully asking open-ended questions about patients' circumstances and values when appropriate (ACOG, 2018a). Professionals must be aware of belief and value systems different from their own and consider these differences when delivering care to women and their families (Callister, 2014, 2021; Leininger, 1991; Moore et al., 2010).

- Enhance clear effective communication.
- Greet respectfully.
- Establish rapport over time.
- Demonstrate empathy, interest, and inclusion.
- Listen actively and sincerely.
- Emphasize the woman's strengths; consider each woman's individuality regarding how she conforms to traditional values and norms.
- Respect functional and neutral practices.
- If proposed practices are nonfunctional, work with the woman and her support network to bring about negotiation.
- Accommodate or negotiate cultural practices and beliefs as appropriate.
- Identify who the client calls "family."
- Determine who the family decision makers are and involve them in care if the mother permits.
- Provide an interpreter when necessary and when patient requests.
- Recognize that a patient agreeing and nodding yes to the nurse's instruction or questions may not always guarantee comprehension but instead may indicate confusion.
- Use nonverbal communication and visual aids in an applicable way.
- When providing patient education, include family and elicit support from the established caretakers in the family (i.e., grandmother, aunt, etc.), and encourage questions to verbalize concerns.
- Demonstrate how scientific and folk practices can be combined to provide optimal care.

CLINICAL JUDGMENT

Characteristics of Cultural Competence
The culturally competent nurse:

- Demonstrates comfort with cultural differences that exist between oneself and patients
- Knows specifics about the cultural groups they work with and move from cultural unawareness to awareness and sensitivity
- Understands the significance of historic events and sociocultural context for cultural groups
- Understands and respects the diversity that exists within and between cultures
- Endeavors to learn more about cultural communities
- Makes a continuous effort to understand others' points of view

- Demonstrates flexibility and tolerance of ambiguity and is nonjudgmental
- Demonstrates willingness to relinquish control in clinical encounters, to risk failure, and to look within for sources of frustration, anger, and resistance
- Promotes cultural practices that are potentially helpful, tolerates cultural practices that are harmless or neutral, and works to educate women to avoid cultural practices that may be potentially harmful

PLANNING FOR BIRTH

Planning and preparing for childbirth requires many decisions by the woman and her family during pregnancy (i.e., choosing a provider, choosing a place of birth, planning for the birth, preparing for labor through education, and planning for labor support). These choices affect how the woman approaches her pregnancy and can contribute significantly to a positive adaptation and positive fetal outcomes.

Choosing a Provider

One of the first decisions a woman makes is her care provider during pregnancy and birth, which also influences where her birth will take place. Most U.S. births take place in the hospital and are attended by physicians, whereas fewer than 10% are attended by midwives (National Academies of Sciences, Engineering, and Medicine et al., 2020).

Physicians

Obstetricians and family practice physicians attend approximately 91% of births in the United States. Most physicians care for patients in a hospital setting. Physicians providing maternal and newborn care evaluate, diagnose, manage, and treat patients; order and evaluate diagnostic tests; prescribe medications; and attend births. Care often includes pharmacological and medical management of problems as well as use of technological procedures. Physicians care for both low- and high-risk patients.

Midwives

Midwifery is noninterventionist care that emphasizes on the normalcy of the birth process. Midwives facilitate natural birth processes while practicing evidence-based, individualized, holistic care of women within the context of their families and communities. In the United States, 94.6% of births attended by CNMs occurred in hospitals, 2.8% in freestanding birth centers, and 2.6% in homes. Midwives care for women in hospitals, alternative birth centers, or at the family home.

- In many countries, midwives are the primary providers of care for healthy pregnant women, and physicians are consulted when medical or surgical intervention is required. In European countries, more than 75% of births are attended by midwives.

- Certified nurse-midwives (CNM) practice legally and hold prescriptive authority in all 50 states. Nurse-midwives are RNs with advanced training in care of obstetric patients.
- Certified midwives (CMs) also are educated at the graduate level, are authorized to practice in five states, and hold prescriptive authority in three states. Both CNMs and CMs are certified by the American Midwifery Certification Board.
- Certified professional midwives (CPMs) hold high school diplomas or the equivalent and are educated through an apprenticeship model that meets NARM standardized criteria or through the Midwifery Education Accreditation Council. CPMs are authorized to practice in 28 states through mechanisms determined by the states and are certified by NARM. Most CPMs work in home or birth center settings in the United States.
- Credentialed midwives in the United States differ from "lay," "traditional," or "plain" midwives, who practice without having completed formal educational and national certification requirements. Lay midwives manage about 1% of the births in the United States, mostly in the home setting. Although some are self-taught, others have various levels of formal training.
- Direct-entry midwives are trained in midwifery schools or universities as a profession distinct from nursing. Increasing numbers of midwives in the United Kingdom and Ireland fall into this category.

Given the variations in midwifery training and knowledge, pregnant women considering midwifery care may need education and information regarding the experience and credentials of the midwife providing their care to make informed decisions. AWHONN (2016) has a Position Statement on midwifery to guide nurses on midwifery practice and training (Box 5-5).

Choosing a Place of Birth

Pregnant women must decide whether to give birth in a hospital setting, at a birthing center, or at home. In the United States, 98.4% of women give birth in hospitals, 0.99% at home, and 0.52% at freestanding birth centers (National Academies of Sciences, Engineering, and Medicine et al., 2020). Because health professionals attending birth centers and home births do not offer some services during labor (e.g., epidural pain relief, induction, or augmentation with medications) and do not have the capacity to provide certain emergency services (e.g., cesarean capability, neonatal intensive care unit), some women need to transfer to a hospital during or after birth.

Hospitals

Among birth settings, hospitals provide the widest array of medical interventions for pregnant women and newborns. However, significant variation in provider types and practices exists among hospitals, so a woman's experience will also vary depending on such factors as the hospital's level of care, staffing, maternal-fetal status, local values and culture, and resources.

- Hospital maternity services vary greatly, from traditional labor and delivery rooms with separate newborn and postpartum units to in-hospital birth centers.

BOX 5-5 | AWHONN Position Statement on Midwifery

AWHONN supports midwives as independent providers of health-care services for women and newborns. The certified nurse-midwife's practice should include appropriate professional consultation, collaboration, and referral as indicated by the health status of the patient and applicable state and federal laws (AWHONN, 2016).

Background

AWHONN identifies a wide range of disparate educational requirements and certification standards in the United States that fall under the umbrella category of midwifery. The following titles are attributed to midwives without prior nursing credentials who are not graduates of American College of Nurse Midwives (ACNM)–accredited programs: direct entry, lay, licensed, or professional. Direct entry midwives cover the spectrum from the doctoral prepared European midwife to the self-taught, beginning practitioner.

The wide range of what is actually meant by the designation "midwife" can easily confuse consumers, health-care institutions, and legislators. Definitions of various certification levels are:

- CNM: certified nurse-midwife (administered by ACNM) prepared at the graduate level and educated in nursing and midwifery.
- CM: certified midwife (administered by ACNM) educated at the graduate level, authorized to practice in five states, and holds prescriptive authority in three states.
- CPM: certified professional midwife (administered by the North American Registry of Midwives). Also referred to as *direct entry, lay,* or *licensed midwife.* Must hold high school diploma, is educated through an apprenticeship model, and meets standardized criteria.
- Midwives with a state license or permit (administered on a state-by-state basis). Also referred to as *direct entry, lay,* or *licensed midwife.* Certification through the state.
- Midwives without formal credentials (no administrative oversight). Also referred to as *direct entry* or *lay midwife.*

Individual state-by-state laws govern the practice of midwifery in the United States. Certified nurse-midwives and certified midwives often practice in collaboration and consultation with other health-care professionals to provide primary, gynecological, and maternity care to women in the context of the larger health-care system. Certified nurse-midwives may have prescriptive privileges, admitting privileges to hospitals, and may own or manage freestanding practices. The scope of practice for a direct entry, or lay, midwife who is not ACC accredited is typically limited to the practice of home birth or birth center options for women but varies according to state-by-state regulations.

Association of Women's Health, Obstetric and Neonatal Nurses, 2016.

- Labor, delivery, and recovery (LDR) rooms may be available in which the expectant mother is admitted, labors, gives birth, and spends the first 2 hours of recovery.
- In labor, delivery, recovery, postpartum (LDRP) units, the mother remains in the same room for her entire hospital stay.

Birth Centers

Some U.S. hospitals have separate units within or associated with the labor and delivery unit that offer women a more home-like atmosphere. A birth center can also be a freestanding health facility. All birth centers are intended for low-risk women who desire less medical intervention during birth, a home-like atmosphere, and an emphasis on individually tailored care.

- Freestanding birth centers are separate from the hospital but may be located nearby in case transfer of the woman or newborn is needed.
- Only women at low risk for complications are included in care.
- Birth centers are usually staffed by nurse-midwives or physicians who also have privileges at the local hospital.
- They offer home-like accommodations, with emergency equipment available but out of view.

Home Births

Women who plan home births may do so to experience physiological childbirth, create a personalized experience, avoid unneeded medical interventions, or preserve a sense of control. They may lack a community hospital, dislike the hospital atmosphere, or have geographic or financial barriers to accessing hospital care. Home births may also stem from cultural beliefs and practices. Most home births are planned, but about 15% are unplanned. A home birth may be attended by a midwife, physician, or other attendant, or by no medical attendant at all. For planned home births only, about 80% are attended by midwives, 0.7% by physicians, and 19.1% by "other" (National Academies of Sciences, Engineering, and Medicine et al., 2020).

- Home births are popular in European countries such as Sweden and the Netherlands, with rigorous screening policies to ensure that only low-risk women have home births and are attended by trained midwives (Zielinski et al., 2015).
- In developing countries, home births may occur because of the lack of hospitals, adequate birthing facilities, and staff.
- In the North American medical community, many have concluded that home birth exposes the mother and fetus to unnecessary danger. Consequently, a woman seeking a home birth may be unable to find a qualified health-care provider willing to give prenatal care and attend the birth.
- Home births allow the expectant family to control the experience, and the mother may be more relaxed than in the hospital environment. It may be less expensive, and risk of serious infection may be decreased.
- If home birth is the woman's choice, these criteria will promote a safe experience:
  - The woman must be comfortable with her decision.
  - The woman should be in good health; home birth is not for high-risk pregnancy.

- The woman should have access to reliable transportation in case of transfer to a hospital.
- The woman should be attended by a well-trained health-care provider with adequate medical supplies and resuscitation equipment.

Nursing Actions

- Support a woman's access to reliable and unbiased information about care options.
- Understand the factors that influence a woman's choice of birth providers and settings.
- Respect the woman's choice of birth setting.
- Facilitate efficient and respectful transitions of care when a woman in labor changes from one care setting to another.

The Birth Preference Plan

Involving women and families in decisions about perinatal care increases satisfaction and promotes a collaborative relationship with health-care providers. A birth preference plan or birth plan documents what a woman would prefer to happen during her birth and helps individualize the family's care. The preference plan gives the health-care provider information about the family's special needs, concerns, and requests, facilitating and guiding a meaningful discussion with the family about their expectations. Ideally, this discussion occurs during pregnancy with the primary health-care provider and the perinatal nurse on admission to the unit for labor and birth. A birth plan is a tool parents can use to explore their childbirth options and choose those most important to them. A written birth plan can help women clarify desires and expectations and communicate those wishes to their care providers (Callister, 2021; Lothian, 2011).

Birth plans typically emphasize specific requests for labor and immediate postdelivery care. Some involve expectations surrounding postpartum and newborn care as well, including breastfeeding and who is in her room during delivery. The birth plan document can be inserted into the woman's prenatal record or hospital chart as a way of communicating with care providers. It also gives the patient some autonomy in deciding her care while birthing.

Doula Care

The word *doula* comes from ancient Greek and means "woman's servant" (International Childbirth Education Association [ICEA], 1999). The role of doulas is to provide nonclinical support during labor and birth, as well as during the prenatal and postpartum periods. Doulas do not perform clinical tasks such as giving medication or conducting examinations. Being a doula does not require formal education or training, although an individual who has experience working in health care may elect to train as a doula. Certification is not required to practice as a doula (National Academies of Sciences, Engineering, and Medicine et al., 2020).

- Continuous support by a trained doula during labor is associated with shorter labors, decreased need for analgesics and medical interventions, and increased maternal satisfaction Bohren et al., 2017; Campbell et al., 2006; Hodnett et al., 2013; Pascali-Bonaro & Kroeger, 2004).
- Pregnant women should be made aware of the benefits of doula care before coming to the hospital to deliver and given resources as to how to find a doula.
- Many hospitals have implemented doula services that are free or fee-based.

Childbirth Education

Prenatal education began in the early 1900s with classes in maternal hygiene, nutrition, and baby care taught by the American Red Cross in New York City. Childbirth education as we know it today developed as a consumer response to the increasing medical control and technological management of normal labor and birth during the 1950s and 1960s in Europe and North America. Early proponents of childbirth education such as Lamaze, Bradley, and Dick-Read focused primarily on the prevention of pain in childbirth. Methods of "natural childbirth" (Dick-Read), "psychoprophylaxis" (Lamaze), and "husband-coached childbirth" (Bradley) attained great popularity among middle-class groups.

Childbirth education has evolved since that time to a more eclectic approach. The focus has shifted from rigid techniques to embrace a philosophy that advocates for the normalcy of birth, acknowledges women's natural ability to give birth to their babies, and explores the ways that women find strength and well-being during labor and birth (Lamaze International, 2009; Walker et al., 2009). The content of childbirth education classes has greatly expanded, assisting women and their families to make informed decisions about pregnancy and birth based on knowledge of their options and choices.

Antenatal education programs have a range of aims, such as to influence health behavior, build women's confidence in their ability to give birth, prepare women and their partners for childbirth, prepare for parenthood, develop social support networks, promote confident parents, and contribute to reducing perinatal morbidity and mortality. Antenatal education thus comprises a range of educational and supportive measures that help parents and prospective parents understand their own social, psychological, and physical needs during pregnancy, labor, and parenthood. From conception to childbirth, parental education is an important tool to help parents understand the milestones that are necessary for healthy social, emotional, and intellectual growth (CDC, 2018).

Traditionally, prepared childbirth classes are offered during the third trimester when the mother and her partner or support person are intent on learning about what to expect during labor and birth. There is a significant need for information to assist in preparing couples for labor and birth; thus, pregnant women and their partners or support person and family can benefit from a comprehensive educational program. Prenatal education should be designed to meet the needs of the population served and based on the knowledge of what information and skills are useful and relevant to expectant parents at various stages of pregnancy. The education should be presented in a manner that supports women's ability to have the information they need to make informed decisions based on their personal reproductive goals and values. Shared decision making should be the norm, not the exception (James & Suplee, 2021).

● Specialized classes are designed to meet the needs of specific groups, including classes for breastfeeding, sibling preparation, refreshers, prenatal and postpartum exercise, online childbirth preparation, and grandparents' education. Programs have been developed for adolescents, mothers expecting twins, and mothers older than 35. Nurses and childbirth educators have played an important role in the development of these innovative education programs.

● Professional organizations, including the ICEA, Lamaze International, and AWHONN, have published position papers establishing expectations of basic components of prenatal education. Through the development of these papers as well as teacher training and certification programs, these organizations ensure that childbirth educators have a sound knowledge base and specific competencies.

● The goal of childbirth education is to promote competence of expectant parents to meet the challenges of childbirth and early parenting. Programs emphasize healthy pregnancy and birth outcomes, a positive transition to parenting, and decreased anxiety about birth. Attending childbirth education (CBE) class or having a birth plan were associated with increased vaginal delivery rates (Afshar, Wang, et al., 2017).

● Class content typically includes the physical and emotional aspects of pregnancy, childbirth and early parenting, coping skills, and labor support techniques (Box 5-6).

● Values clarification and informed decision making are emphasized along with the promotion of wellness behaviors and healthy birth practices. Pregnant women are encouraged to identify their own goals for childbirth (Callister, 2021; Green & Hotelling, 2009; Lothian, 2011).

● Class formats have evolved to meet the varied needs of expectant families and may include a traditional weekly series, 1-day intensives, or online classes.

Childbirth classes remain a popular and well-established component of care during the childbearing years. However, evidence about effects of antenatal education remains inconclusive. As research on childbirth and childbirth education increases and as more educators use these findings as a basis for teaching, evidence-based practice will be enhanced.

Information via technology is convenient and can be retrieved in seconds, but the results may be inaccurate, inconsistent, or poorly referenced, so trusted sources for evidence-based information should be provided by nurses. Nurses must be aware of powerful influences on the health-related decisions of childbearing women and their families. The quality of information and advice varies widely. For a list of reliable online resources for parent education, see Box 5-7.

BOX 5-6 | Perinatal Education: Sample Content in a Childbirth Preparation Class

Introduction

Introductions

Overview of childbirth education: Rationale and pain theory

Physical and emotional changes of pregnancy; fetal development

Nutrition, exercise, and self-care during pregnancy

Introduction to breathing and relaxation techniques

Labor

Signs of labor

Stages and phases of labor and delivery

Labor support techniques; the role of the support person in labor

Practice of breathing and relaxation techniques

Birth Plans

Labor review, incorporating labor support techniques and nonpharmacological comfort strategies

Birth options and birth plans: developing advocacy skills

Pharmacological interventions

Practice of breathing and relaxation techniques

Hospital tour

Variations in Labor

Variations of labor: back labor, prodromal labor, precipitous labor

Cesarean delivery

Medical procedures (IVs, episiotomy, assisted delivery, electronic fetal monitoring [EFM], Pitocin, epidurals)

Practice of relaxation and breathing techniques

Newborn

Review of labor; practice of relaxation and breathing techniques

Newborn care

Breastfeeding

Postpartum

Postpartum and transition to parenthood

Community resources for new parents

BOX 5-7 | Internet Resources for Expectant Families

American Pregnancy Association: www.americanpregnancy.org

African American Wellness: www.aawellnessproject.com

Centers for Disease Control and Prevention: www.cdc.gov

Healthline: www.healthline.com

Gay Parents to Be: www.gayparentstobe.com

Migrants and Health Care: www.icmc.net

Global Maternal Health: www.everymothercounts.org

Health Affairs: www.caimmigrant.org

Babycenter: www.babycenter.com

Childbirth Connection: www.childbirthconnection.org

Doulas of North America: www.dona.org

Healthy Mothers, Healthy Babies Coalition: www.hmhb.org

ICEA (International Childbirth Education Association): www.icea.org

La Leche League: www.lalecheleague.org

Lamaze International: www.lamaze.org

American College of Nurse-Midwives: www.Mymidwife.org

AWHONN Patient Education: www.Health4women.org

Centers for Disease Control and Prevention (https://www.cdc.gov/pregnancy/index.html), breastfeeding (https://www.cdc.gov/breastfeeding/), and parenting (https://www.cdc.gov/parents/)

SAFE AND EFFECTIVE NURSING CARE:
Patient Education

Mobile Phone Education: Text4Baby

Text4Baby is an innovative educational program offering perinatal education via text messages as well as an app used on smartphones. More than 90% of American households have cell phones, the majority with text messaging capabilities. The program was developed through a collaboration of public and private partnership, including ZERO TO THREE, Voxiva, CTIA Wireless Foundation, the Department of Health and Human Services, White House Office of Science and Technology Policy, and Discovery Fit and Health. These partnerships include government agencies, corporations, academic institutions, professional associations, and nonprofit organizations. Message content was reviewed by an interdisciplinary panel of experts to ensure the information reflected evidence-based practice.

Once signed up for the service, women will receive three free SMS text messages each week timed to their due dates throughout pregnancy until the baby reaches age 1. The program provides vital health information to pregnant women and new mothers in areas such as nutrition, seasonal flu prevention and treatment, mental health, risks of tobacco use, oral health, safe infant sleeping, parenting, and developmental milestones. Women can sign up for the program by texting BABY to 511411 (or by texting BEBE for Spanish) (Hunt, 2015).

Evidence-Based Practice

Effectiveness of Childbirth Education

Afshar, Y., Wang, E., Mai, J., Esakoff, T., Pisarska, M., & Gregory, K. (2017). Childbirth education class and birth plans are associated with a vaginal delivery. *BIRTH, 44*(1), 29–34; Gagnon, A. J. (2011). Individual or group antenatal education for childbirth or parenthood, or both. *Cochrane Database of Systematic Reviews*, (10). https://doi.org/10.1002/14651858.CD002869.pub2

Childbirth education aims to help prospective parents prepare for childbirth and parenthood. Prospective parents often look to childbirth classes or antenatal education to provide important information on issues such as decision making about and during labor, skills for labor, pain relief, infant and postnatal care, breastfeeding, and parenting skills. This antenatal education can be provided in many ways. A retrospective cross-sectional study placed women into four categories: those who attended a CBE class, those with a birth plan, those who attended a CBE class and had a birth plan, and those who neither attended a CBE class nor had a birth plan. In the study, 14,630 deliveries met the inclusion criteria: 31.9% of the women attended CBE, 12% had a birth plan, and 8.8% had both. Women who attended CBE or had a birth plan were older, more likely to be nulliparous, had a lower body mass index, and were less likely to be Black. After adjusting for significant covariates, women who participated in either option or both had higher odds of a vaginal delivery. Attending CBE class and/or having a birth plan were associated with a vaginal delivery. These findings suggest that patient education and birth preparation may influence the mode of delivery. CBE and birth plans could be used as quality improvement tools to potentially decrease cesarean rates (Afshar, Wang, et al., 2017). An older Cochrane Review indicates many varied ways of providing antenatal education, some of which may be more effective than others. The review found nine trials involving 2,284 women. Interventions varied greatly, and no consistent outcomes were measured. The review of trials found a lack of high-quality evidence, so the effects of antenatal education remain largely unknown. Further research is required to ensure that effective ways of helping health professionals support pregnant women and their partners in preparing for birth and parenting are investigated. They concluded the effects of general antenatal education for childbirth or parenthood, or both, remain largely unknown. Individualized prenatal education directed toward avoidance of a repeat cesarean birth does not increase the rate of vaginal birth after cesarean section (Gagnon, 2011).

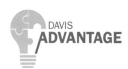

DAVIS ADVANTAGE

Go to Davis Advantage to complete your learning: strengthen understanding, apply your knowledge, and prepare for the Next Gen NCLEX®.

CONCEPT MAP |

Maternal Adaptation to Pregnancy Complications

Frustration
* Woman expresses anger or aggression
* Withdrawal from pregnancy or partner

Fear
* Woman states she is afraid of fetal death
* Woman states she is afraid of newborn disability
* Woman is crying

Pregnancy Complication
Woman diagnosed with high-risk pregnancy

Anxiety
* Unexpected pregnancy complication
* Unanticipated interruption in normal pregnancy

Threat to Self-Esteem
* Woman feels lack of self-confidence related to pregnancy
* Woman reports feeling she has failed as a woman
* Woman feels little confidence to be a mother

CARE PLANS

Problem 1: Anxiety related to uncertain labor processes and fetal outcome
Goal: Decrease anxiety and possess knowledge of processes.
Outcome: Verbalize fears to decrease anxiety and verbalize knowledge of processes.

Nursing Actions
1. Provide time for the patient and family to express their concerns regarding fetal outcome.
2. Encourage the woman to vent apprehension, uncertainty, anger, fear, or worry.
3. Discuss prior pregnancy outcomes if applicable.
4. Explain pregnancy complications, management, and reason for each treatment.
5. Help the woman to obtain needed social support.
6. Refer the family to community or hospital resources such as a social worker, case manager, or chaplain services as needed.
7. Provide resource information for the woman and family as issues arise.

Problem 2: Impaired self-esteem related to pregnancy complication
Goal: Improved self-esteem
Outcome: Patient will express improved self-esteem.

Nursing Actions
1. Encourage verbalization of feelings.
2. Practice active listening.
3. Provide emotional support.
4. Encourage the patient to participate in decision making.
5. Make needed referrals to social services and mental health specialists.

Problem 3: Anxiety related to unexpected pregnancy complication(s)
Goal: Decreased anxiety
Outcome: Patient verbalizes that she feels less anxious and verbalizes a plan of care with complication(s).

Nursing Actions
1. Be calm and reassuring in interactions with the patient and family.

2. Explain all information repeatedly related to complications.
3. Provide autonomy and choices.
4. Encourage the patient and family to verbalize their feelings regarding diagnosis by asking open-ended questions.
5. Explore past coping strategies.
6. Explore spiritual practices and beliefs with the woman.

Problem 4: Frustration related to pregnancy complication
Goal: Positive pregnancy adaptation
Outcome: Patient demonstrates adaptation to pregnancy.

Nursing Actions
1. Allow the woman to express her feelings related to loss of normal pregnancy.
2. Allow the woman to express her feelings related to not having a normal birth.
3. Allow the woman to express her feelings related to uncertainty of fetal outcome.
4. Provide choices related to management when possible.

Case Study

As a nurse in an antenatal clinic, you are part of an interdisciplinary team that is caring for Margarite Sanchez during her pregnancy. Margarite is 10 weeks pregnant and is a 28-year-old G3 P1 Latina woman from Mexico. She began prenatal care at her 8 weeks' gestation visit. She works in a day-care center and has a 2-year-old son. José, her husband, has not accompanied her to her second prenatal appointment, as he is in his busy season as a landscaper. Margarite reports they are pleased about the pregnancy although they planned to wait another year or two before attempting another pregnancy. Margarite was seen for some spotting at 6 weeks' gestation that has resolved. She tells you she has been irritable and short-tempered with her husband and son, particularly at the end of the day when she feels exhausted. She states she is relieved the spotting stopped but is not sure she feels ready to be a mother of two children. Her mother lives four blocks away, and they speak on the phone daily and see each other several times a week. She is very involved in her parish, and the women in her church study group all know she is pregnant and are all certain the baby is a girl.

Detail the aspects of your psychosocial assessment at 10 weeks' gestation.

Discuss the rationale for the assessment.

Discuss the nursing diagnosis, nursing activities, and expected outcomes related to this problem.

Discuss the importance of the pregnant woman's mother during pregnancy.

Suggest two interventions that could help to prepare Margarite's 2-year-old son during the pregnancy.

REFERENCES

Adams, E. D. (2021). Antenatal care. In K. Simpson, P. Creehan, N. Obrien-Abel, C. Roth, & A. Rohan (Eds.), *Perinatal nursing* (5th ed., pp. 65-97). Wolters Kluwer.

Afshar, Y., My-Lin, N., Mei, J., & Grisales, T. (2017). Sexual health and function in pregnancy: Counseling about sexuality in pregnancy and postpartum offers an opportunity to allay fears and increase patient satisfaction during a unique period in a woman's life. *Contemporary OB/GYN, 62*(8), 24–30.

Afshar, Y., Wang, E., Mai, J., Esakoff, T., Pisarska, M., & Gregory, K. (2017). Childbirth education class and birth plans are associated with a vaginal delivery. *BIRTH, 44*(1), 29–34.

Alio, A., Bond, M., Padilla, Y., Heidelbaugh, J., Lu, M., & Parker, W. (2011). Addressing policy barriers to paternal involvement during pregnancy. *Maternal Child Health Journal, 15,* 425–430.

Alio, A., Salihu, H., Komosky, J., Richman, A., & Marty, P. (2010). Feto-infant health and survival: Does paternal involvement matter? *Maternal Child Health Journal, 14,* 931–937.

American Association of Colleges of Nursing. (2008). *The essentials of baccalaureate education for professional nursing practice.* http://aacn.nche.edu/education-resources/BaccEssentials08.pdf

American Association of Colleges of Nursing. (2019). *Fact sheet: Enhancing diversity in the nursing workforce.* American Association of Colleges of Nursing.

American College of Obstetricians and Gynecologists. (2012). Health care for lesbians and bisexual women. Committee Opinion No. 525. *Obstetrics & Gynecology, 119,* 1077–1080.

American College of Obstetricians and Gynecologists. (2015). Racial and ethnic disparities in obstetrics and gynecology. Committee Opinion No. 649. *Obstetrics & Gynecology, 126,* e130–e144.

American College of Obstetricians and Gynecologists. (2018a). Importance of social determinants of health and cultural awareness in the delivery of reproductive health care. ACOG Committee Opinion No. 729. *Obstetrics & Gynecology, 131,* e43–e48.

American College of Obstetricians and Gynecologists. (2018b). Screening for perinatal depression. ACOG Committee Opinion No. 757. *Obstetrics & Gynecology, 132,* e208–e212.

American College of Obstetricians and Gynecologists. (2020). Confidentiality in adolescent health care. ACOG Committee Opinion No. 803. *Obstetrics & Gynecology, 135,* e171–e177.

American College of Obstetricians and Gynecologists. (2021a). Caring for patients who have experienced trauma. ACOG Committee Opinion No. 825. *Obstetrics & Gynecology, 137,* e94–e99.

American College of Obstetricians and Gynecologists. (2021b). Health care for transgender and gender diverse individuals. ACOG Committee Opinion No. 823. *Obstetrics & Gynecology, 137,* e75–e88.

American College of Obstetricians and Gynecologists. (2021c). Multifetal gestations: Twin, triplet, and higher-order multifetal pregnancies. ACOG Practice Bulletin No. 231. *Obstetrics & Gynecology, 137*(6), e145–162.

Amidi-Nouri, A. (2011). Culturally responsive nursing care. In A. Berman & S. Snyder (Eds.), *Kozier & Erb's fundamentals of nursing* (9th ed.). Pearson.

Andrews, M., & Boyle, C. (2011). *Transcultural concepts in nursing care* (6th ed.). Lippincott Williams & Wilkins.

Association of Women's Health, Obstetric and Neonatal Nurses. (2009). *Confidentiality in adolescent health care.* Position statement. Author.

Association of Women's Health, Obstetric and Neonatal Nurses (2022). Respectful maternity care framework and evidence-based clinical practice guideline. *Journal of Obstetric, Gynecologic & Neonatal Nursing, 51*(2), e3–e54.

Association of Women's Health Obstetrics and Neonatal Nursing. (2015). *Mood and anxiety disorders in pregnant and postpartum women.* AWHONN position statement. Author.

Association of Women's Health Obstetrics and Neonatal Nursing. (2016). *Midwifery.* AWHONN position statement. Author.

Association of Women's Health Obstetrics and Neonatal Nursing. (2018). *Intimate partner violence.* AWHONN position statement. Author.

Association of Women's Health Obstetrics and Neonatal Nursing. (2021). *Racism and bias in maternity care settings.* AWHONN position statement. Author.

Austin, M.-P., Highet, N., and the Expert Working Group. (2017). *Mental health care in the perinatal period: Australian clinical practice guideline.* Centre of Perinatal Excellence.

Barron, M. (2014). Antenatal care. In K. Simpson & P. Creehan (Eds.), *AWHONN perinatal nursing* (4th ed., pp. 41–70). Lippincott Williams & Wilkins.

Beck, C. (2002). Revision of the postpartum depression predictors inventory. *Journal of Obstetric, Gynecologic, and Neonatal Nursing, 31*(4), 394–402.

Beeber, L., & Canuso, R. (2005). Strengthening social support for the low-income mother: Five critical questions and a guide for intervention. *Journal of Obstetric, Gynecologic, and Neonatal Nursing, 34*(6), 769–776.

Bohren M. A., Hofmeyr G., Sakala C., Fukuzawa R. K., & Cuthbert, A. (2017). Continuous support for women during childbirth. *Cochrane Database of Systematic Reviews,* (7). https://doi.org/10.1002/14651858.CD003766.pub6

Beyers-Carlson, E., & Volling, B. L. (2017). Efficacy of sibling preparation classes. *Journal of Obstetric, Gynecologic, and Neonatal Nursing, 46*(4), 521–531. https://doi.org/10.1016/j.jogn.2017.03.005

Bibring, G., Dwyer, T., Huntington, D., & Valenstein, D. (1961). A study of the psychological processes in pregnancy and of the early mother–child relationships. *Psychoanalytic Study of the Child, 16*(9), 9–24.

Bowers, N. (2021). Multiple gestation. In K. Simpson, P. Creehan, N. Obrien-Abel, C. Roth, & A. Rohan (Eds.), *Perinatal nursing* (5th ed., pp. 248–294). Wolters Kluwer.

Brennan, A., Ayers, S., Ahmed, H., & Marshall-Lucette, S. (2007). A critical review of the Couvade syndrome: The pregnant male. *Journal of Reproductive and Infant Psychology, 25*(3), 173–189.

Byrne, A., & Tanesini, A. (2015). Instilling new habits: Addressing implicit bias in healthcare professionals. *Advances in Health Sciences Education: Theory and Practice, 20*(5), 1255–1262. https://doi.org/10.1007/s10459-015-9600-6

Callister, L. (2014). Integrating cultural beliefs and practices into the care of childbearing women. In K. Simpson & P. Creehan (Eds.), *AWHONN perinatal nursing* (4th ed., pp. 41–70). Lippincott Williams & Wilkins.

Callister, L. C. (2021). Integrating cultural beliefs and practices when caring for childbearing women and families. In K. Simpson, P. Creehan, N. Obrien-Abel, C. Roth, & A. Rohan (Eds.), *Perinatal nursing* (5th ed., pp. 17-46). Wolters Kluwer.

Campbell, D., Lake, M., Falk, M., & Backstrand, J. (2006). A randomized trial of continuous support in labor by a lay doula. *Journal of Obstetric, Gynecologic, and Neonatal Nursing, 35*(4), 456–464.

Cannella, B. (2006). Mediators of the relationship between social support and positive health practices in pregnant women. *Nursing Research, 55*(6), 437–445.

Carolan, M. (2005). "Doing it properly": The experience of first-time mothering over 35 years. *Health Care for Women International, 26*(9), 764–787.

Carroll, J., Reid, A., Biringer, A., Midmer, D., Glazier, R., Wilson, L., . . . Stewart, D. (2005). Effectiveness of the Antenatal Psychosocial Health Assessment (ALPHA) form in detecting psychosocial concerns: A randomized controlled trial. *Canadian Medical Association Journal, 173*(3), 253–259.

Centers for Disease Control and Prevention. (2017a). *Lead health literacy initiative.* https://www.cdc.gov/nceh/lead/tools/leadliteracy.htm

Centers for Disease Control and Prevention. (2017b). *Teen pregnancy in the United States.* https://www.cdc.gov/teenpregnancy/about/index.htm

Centers for Disease Control and Prevention. (2018). *Child development.* https://www.cdc.gov/ncbddd/childdevelopment/facts.html

Centers for Disease Control and Prevention. (2019). *Reproductive health: Teen pregnancy.* Division of Reproductive Health National Center for Chronic Disease Prevention and Health Promotion.

Cheng, E. R., Rifas-Shiman, S. L., Perkins, M. E., Rich-Edwards, J. W., Gillman, M. W., Wright, R., & Taveras, E. M. (2016). The influence of antenatal partner support on pregnancy outcomes. *Journal of Women's Health, 25*(7), 672–679. https://doi.org/10.1089/jwh.2015.5462

Council on Patient Safety in Women's Health Care. (2016). *Reduction of peripartum racial/ethnic disparities.* American College of Obstetricians and Gynecologists.

Crooks, R., & Baur, K. (2010). *Our sexuality* (11th ed.). Benjamin Cummings Publishing Company.

Davaki, K. (2021). *The traumas endured by refugee women and their consequences for integration and participation in the EU host country.* Policy Department for Citizens' Rights and Constitutional Affairs, European Parliament, Brussels, BE.

Davis, E., & Narayan, A. (2020). Pregnancy as a period of risk, adaptation, and resilience for mothers and infants. *Development and Psychopathology, 32*(5), 1625–1639. https://doi.org/10.1017/S0954579420001121

Dawley, K., & Beam, R. (2005). "My nurse taught me how to have a healthy baby and be a good mother": Nurse home visiting with pregnant women 1888 to 2005. *Nursing Clinics of North America, 40,* 803–815.

Dobrzykowski, T., & Stern, P. (2003). Out of sync: A generation of first-time mothers over 30. *Health Care for Women International, 24*(3), 242–253.

Dollberg, D., Rozenfeld, T., & Kupfermincz, M. (2016, September). Early parental adaptation, prenatal distress, and high-risk pregnancy. *Journal of Pediatric Psychology, 41*(8), 915–929. https://doi.org/10.1093/jpepsy/jsw028

Durham, R. (1998). Strategies women engage in when analyzing preterm labor at home. *Journal of Perinatology, 19,* 61–69.

Duvall, E. (1985). *Marriage and family development.* Harper & Row.

East, C. E., Biro, M. A., Fredericks, S., & Lau, R. (2019). Support during pregnancy for women at increased risk of low birthweight babies. *Cochrane Database of Systematic Reviews, 4,* CD000198. https://doi.org/10.1002/14651858.CD000198.pub3.

Forde, A. T., Crookes, D. M., Suglia, S. F., & Demmer, R. T. (2019). The weathering hypothesis as an explanation for racial disparities in health: A systematic review. *Annals of Epidemiology, 33,* 1–18.e3. https://doi.org/10.1016/j.annepidem.2019.02.011

Foster, G., Alviar, A., Neumeier, R., & Wootten, A. (2012). A tri-service perspective on the implementation of a centering pregnancy model in the military. *Journal of Obstetric, Gynecologic, and Neonatal Nursing, 41*(2), 315–321.

Friedman, M., Bowden, V., & Jones, E. (2003). *Family nursing: Research, theory, and practice* (5th ed.). Prentice Hall.

Gagnon, A. J. (2011). Individual or group antenatal education for childbirth or parenthood, or both. *Cochrane Database of Systematic Reviews,* (10). https://doi.org/10.1002/14651858.CD002869.pub2

Ganann, R., Sword, W., Thabane, L., Newbold, B., & Black, M. (2016). Predictors of postpartum depression among immigrant women in the year after childbirth. *Journal of Women's Health, 25*(2), 155–165.

Genesoni, L., & Tallandini, M. (2009). Men's psychological transition to fatherhood: An analysis of the literature, 1989–2008. *Birth, 36*(4), 305–317.

Geronimus, A. T., Pearson, J. A., Linnenbringer, E., Eisenberg, A. K., Stokes, C., Hughes, L. D., & Schulz, A. J. (2020). Weathering in Detroit: Place, race, ethnicity, and poverty as conceptually fluctuating social constructs shaping variation in allostatic load. *The Milbank Quarterly, 98*(4), 1171–1218. https://doi.org/10.1111/1468-0009.12484

Gilbert, E. (2010). *Manual of high-risk pregnancy and delivery* (5th ed.). C.V. Mosby.

Giurgescu, C., Penckofer, S., Maurer, M., & Bryant, F. (2006). Impact of uncertainty, social support, and prenatal coping on the psychological well-being of high-risk pregnant women. *Nursing Research, 55*(5), 356–365.

Goldberg, A. E., & Sayer, A. G. (2006). Lesbian couples' relationship quality across the transition to parenthood. *Journal of Marriage and Family, 68,* 87–100.

Green, J., & Hotelling, B. A. (2009). *Healthy birth practice #3: Bring a loved one, friend, or doula for continuous support.* Lamaze International.

Gregg, I. (2018). The health care experiences of lesbian women becoming mothers. *Nursing for Women's Health, 22*(1), 40–50. https://doi.org/10.1016/j.nwh.2017.12.003

Hanson, S., Hunter, L., Bormann, J., & Sobo, E. (2009). Paternal fears of childbirth: A literature review. *Journal of Perinatal Education, 18*(4), 12–20.

Heslehurst, N., Brown, H., Pemu, A., Coleman, H., & Rankin, J. (2018). Perinatal health outcomes and care among asylum seekers and refugees: A systematic review of systematic reviews. *BMC Medicine, 16,* 89. https://doi.org/10.1186/s12916-018-1064-0

Hodnett E. D., Gates S, Hofmeyr G. J., & Sakala C. (2013). Continuous support for women during childbirth. *Cochrane Database of Systematic Reviews,* (7). https://doi.org/10.1002/14651858.CD003766.pub5.

Howell, E. A., Brown, H., Brumley, J., Bryant, A. S., Caughey, A. B., Cornell, A., . . . Grobman, W. A. (2018). Reduction of peripartum racial and ethnic disparities: A conceptual framework and maternal safety consensus bundle. *Obstetrics & Gynecology, 131*(5), 770–782. https://doi.org/10.1097/AOG.0000000000002475

Hunt, S. (2015). Text4Baby app. *Nursing for Women's Health, 19*(1), 77–79.

Institute of Medicine. (2003). *Unequal treatment: Confronting racial and ethnic disparities in health care.* National Academies Press. https://doi.org/10.17226/12875

International Childbirth Education Association. (1999). Position paper: The role and scope of the doula. *International Journal of Childbirth Education, 14*(1), 38–45.

James, D., & Suplee, P. (2021). Postpartum care. In K. Simpson, P. Creehan, N. Obrien-Abel, C. Roth, & A. Rohan (Eds.), *Perinatal nursing* (5th ed., pp. 508–562). Wolters Kluwer.

Jentsch, B., Durham, R., Hundley, V., & Hussein, J. (2007). Creating consumer satisfaction in maternity care: The neglected needs of migrants, asylum seekers and refugees. *International Journal of Consumer Studies, 31,* 128–134.

Jordan, P. (1989). Support behaviors identified as helpful and desired by second time parents over the perinatal period. *Maternal Child Nursing Journal, 18*(2), 133–145.

Kalra, N., Hooker, L., Reisenhofer, S., Di Tanna. G. L., & García Moreno, C. (2021). Training healthcare providers to respond to intimate partner violence against women. *Cochrane Database of Systematic Reviews, (5),* CD012423. https://doi.org/10.1002/14651858.CD012423.pub2

Katon, J., Lewis, L., Hercinovic, S., McNab, A., Fortney, J., & Rose, S. (2017). Improving perinatal mental health care for women veterans: Description of a quality improvement program. *Maternal Child Health, 21*(8), 1598–1605.

Kimberg, L., & Wheeler, M. (2019). Four C's—Skills in trauma-informed care trauma and trauma-informed care. In M. R. Gerber (Ed.), *Trauma-informed healthcare approaches: A guide for primary care* (pp. 25–56). Springer.

Koniak-Griffin, D., Logsdon, C., Hines-Martin, V., & Turner, C. (2006). Contemporary mothering in a diverse society. *Journal of Obstetric, Gynecologic, and Neonatal Nursing, 35*(5), 671–678.

Kowlessar, O., Fox, J. R., & Wittkowski, A. (2015). The pregnant male: A meta-synthesis of first-time fathers' experiences of pregnancy. *Journal of Reproductive & Infant Psychology, 33*(2), 106–127. https://doi.org/10.1080/02646838.2014.970153

Lamaze International (2007). Position paper: promoting, supporting, and protecting normal birth. *The Journal of perinatal education, 16*(3), 11–15. https://doi.org/10.1624/105812407X217084

Lauderdale, J. (2011). Transcultural perspectives in childbearing. In M. Andrews & J. Boyle (Eds.), *Transcultural concepts in nursing care* (6th ed., pp. 95–131). Lippincott Williams & Wilkins.

Lederman, R. (1996). *Psychosocial adaptation in pregnancy* (2nd ed.). Springer.

Lederman, R. (2011). Preterm birth prevention: A mandate for psychosocial assessment. *Issues in Mental Health Nursing, 32,* 163–169.

Lederman, R., & Weis, K. (2009). *Psychosocial adaptation in pregnancy: Seven dimensions of maternal role development* (3rd ed.). Springer.

Lee, Y., & Blitz, L. (2016). We're grand: A qualitative design and development pilot project addressing the needs and strengths of grandparents raising grandchildren. *Child & Family Social Work, 21,* 381–390.

Leininger, M. (Ed.). (1991). *Culture care diversity & universality: A theory of nursing.* National League for Nursing Press.

Lindberg, L. D., Santelli, J. S., & Desai, S. (2016). Understanding the decline in adolescent fertility in the United States, 2007–2012. *Journal of Adolescent Health, 59*(5), 577–583.

Logsdon, C., Gagne, P., Hughes, T., Patterson, J., & Rakestraw, V. (2005). Social support during adolescent pregnancy: Piecing together a quilt. *Journal of Obstetric, Gynecologic, & Neonatal Nursing, 34*(5), 606–614.

Lothian, J. (2011). Lamaze breathing: What every pregnant woman needs to know. *Journal of Perinatal Education, 20*(2), 118–120.

Lowe, N. (2018, May 1). Disparities in the health of women and children. Editorial. *Journal of Obstetric, Gynecologic, and Neonatal Nursing, 47*(3), 273–274.

MacKay, A. P., & Duran, C. (2007). *Adolescent health in the United States, 2007.* National Center for Health Statistics.

Maifeld, M., Hahn, S., Titler, M., Marita, G., & Mullen, M. (2003). Decision making regarding multifetal reduction. *Journal of Obstetric, Gynecologic, & Neonatal Nursing, 32*(3), 357–369.

March of Dimes. (2017). *Abuse during pregnancy.* https://www.marchofdimes.org/pregnancy/abuse-during-pregnancy.aspx

Martin, J. A., Hamilton, B. E., Osterman, M. J. K., & Driscoll, A. K. (2021). *Births: Final data for 2019. National Vital Statistics Reports, vol. 70, no. 2.* National Center for Health Statistics. https://doi.org/10.15620/cdc:100472

Mattocks, K., Skanderson, M., Goulet, J., Brandt, C., Womack, J., Krebs, E., & Haskell, S. (2010). Pregnancy and mental health among women veterans returning from Iraq and Afghanistan. *Journal of Women's Health, 19*(12), 2159–2166. https://doi.org/10.1089/jwh.2009.1892

Mattson, S., & Smith, J. (2016). *Core curriculum for maternal newborn nursing* (4th ed.). Elsevier Saunders.

May, K. (1980). A typology of detachment/involvement styles adopted by first time expectant fathers. *Western Journal of Nursing Research, 2,* 443–453.

May, K. (1982). Three phases of father involvement in pregnancy. *Nursing Research, 31*(6), 337–342.

McCants, B. M., & Greiner, J. R. (2016). Prebirth education and childbirth decision making. *International Journal of Childbirth Education, 31*(1), 24–27.

McKeever, A., Alderman, S., Luff, S., & DeJesus, B. (2016). Assessment and care of childbearing women with severe and persistent mental illness. *Nursing for Women's Health, 20*(5), 484–499. https://doi.org/10.1016/j.nwh.2016.08.010

McManus, A., Hunter, L., & Renn, H. (2006). Lesbian experiences and needs during childbirth: Guidance for health care providers. *Journal of Obstetric, Gynecologic, & Neonatal Nursing, 35*(1), 13–23.

Meleis, A. (2003). Theoretical consideration of health care for immigrant and minority women. In P. St. Hill, J. Lipson, & A. Meleis (Eds.), *Caring for women cross culturally.* F.A. Davis.

Lucas Pereira de Melo. (2013) The sunrise model: A contribution to the teaching of nursing consultation in collective health. *American Journal of Nursing Research, 1*(1), 20–23. https://doi.org/10.12691/ajnr-1-1-3

Mercer, R. (1995). *Becoming a mother.* Springer.

Mercer, R. (2004). Becoming a mother versus maternal role attainment. *Journal of Nursing Scholarship, 36*(3), 226–233.

Midmer, D., Carroll, J., Bryanton, J., & Stewart, D. (2002). From research to application: The development of an antenatal psychosocial health assessment tool. *Canadian Journal of Public Health, 93*(4), 291–296.

Misra, D. P., Caldwell, C., Young, A. A., & Abelson, S. (2010). Do fathers matter? Paternal contributions to birth outcomes and racial disparities. *American Journal of Obstetrics and Gynecology, 202,* 99–100.

Mojaverian, T., & Heejung, K. (2013). Interpreting a helping hand: Cultural variation in the effectiveness of solicited and unsolicited social support. *Personality and Social Psychology Bulletin, 39*(1), 88–99.

Moore, M., Moos, M., & Callister, L. (2010). *Cultural competence: An essential journey for perinatal nurses.* March of Dimes Foundation.

National Academies of Sciences, Engineering, and Medicine; Health and Medicine Division; Division of Behavioral and Social Sciences and Education; Board on Children, Youth, and Families; Committee on Assessing Health Outcomes by Birth Settings; (2020). Maternal and newborn care in the United States. In E. P. Backes, & S. C. Scrimshaw (Eds.), *Birth settings in America: Outcomes, quality, access, and choice.* National Academies Press. https://www.ncbi.nlm.nih.gov/books/NBK555484/

Ngai, F., Chan, S., & Ip, W. (2010). Predictors and correlates of maternal role competence and satisfaction. *Nursing Research, 59*(3), 185–193.

Parker, K., Cilluffo, A., & Stepler, R. (2017). 6 facts about the U.S. military and its changing demographics. *PEW Research Reports.* http://www.pewresearch.org/fact-tank/2017/04/13/6-facts-about-the-u-s-military-and-its-changing-demographics/

Pascali-Bonaro, D., & Kroeger, M. (2004). Continuous female companionship during childbirth: A crucial resource in times of stress or calm. *Journal of Midwifery & Women's Health, 49*(4), 19–27.

Pew Research Center. (2018, April). *The changing profile of unmarried parents.* Pew Research Center.

Pew Research Center. (2020, April). As family structures change in U.S., a growing share of Americans say it makes no difference. Pew Research Center. https://www.pewresearch.org/fact-tank/2020/04/10/as-family-structures-change-in-u-s-a-growing-share-of-americans-say-it-makes-no-difference/

Phua, D. Y., Kee, M.K.Z.L., Koh, D.X.P., Rifkin-Graboi, A., Daniels, M., Chen, H., & Meaney, M. J. (2017). Growing up in Singapore towards healthy outcomes study group. Positive maternal mental health during pregnancy associated with specific forms of adaptive development in early childhood: Evidence from a longitudinal study. *Developmental Psychopathology, 29*(5), 1573–1587. https://doi.org/10.1017/S0954579417001249. PubMed PMID: 29162171

Pinazo-Hernandis, S., & Tompkins, C. (2009). Custodial grandparents: The state of the art and the many faces of this contribution. *Journal of Intergenerational Relationships, 7*(2–3), 137–143.

Priest, S., Austin, M., & Sullivan, E. (2006). Antenatal psychosocial screening for prevention of antenatal and postnatal anxiety and depression (Protocol). *Cochrane Library,* 1.

Purnell, L. (2014). *Guide to culturally competent health care* (3rd ed.). F. A. Davis.

Recame, M. A. (2013). Childbirth education and parental support programs within the U.S. military population. *International Journal of Childbirth Education, 28*(1), 67–70.

Romano, A. (2014). Why holistic care for childbirth? *International Journal Childbirth Education, 29,* 4.

Rondahl, G., Bruhner, E., & Lindhe, J. (2009). Heteronormative communication with lesbian families in antenatal care, childbirth and postnatal care. *Journal of Advanced Nursing, 65*(11), 2337–2344.

Ross, L. (2005). Perinatal mental health in lesbian mothers: A review of potential risk and protective factors. *Women & Health, 41*(3), 113–128.

Rubin, R. (1975). Maternal tasks in pregnancy. *Maternal-Child Nursing Journal, 4*(3), 143–153.

Rubin, R. (1984). *Maternal identity and the maternal experience.* Springer.

Schardt, D. (2005). Delayed childbearing: Underestimated psychological implications. *International Journal of Childbirth Education, 20*(3), 34–37.

Shah, M. K., Gee, R. E., & Theall, K. P. (2014). Partner support and impact on birth outcomes among teen pregnancies in the United States. *Journal of Pediatric and Adolescent Gynecology, 27*(1), 14–19. https://doi.org/10.1016/j.jpag.2013.08.002

Sharma, R. (2013). The family and family structure classification redefined for the current times. *Journal of Family Medicine and Primary Care, 2*(4), 306–310.

Simpson, K. (2021). Perinatal patient safety and quality. In K. Simpson, P. Creehan, N. Obrien- Abel, C. Roth, & A. Rohan (Eds.), *Perinatal nursing* (5th ed., pp. 1–15). Wolters Kluwer.

Simpson, K., & Creehan, P. (Eds.). (2014). *AWHONN perinatal nursing* (4th ed.). Lippincott.

Skurzak, A. (2015). Social support for pregnant women. *Polish Journal Public Health, 125*(3), 169–172.

Smith, P., Buzi, R., Kozinetz, C., Peskin, M., & Weimann, C. (2016). Impact of a group prenatal program for pregnant adolescents on perceived partner support. *Child Adolescent Social Work, 33,* 417–428.

Smith, S. G., Chen, J., Basile, K. C., Gilbert, L. K., Merrick, M. T., Patel, N., . . . Jaine, A. (2017). *The National Intimate Partner and Sexual Violence Survey 2010–2012 state report.* https://www.cdc.gov/violenceprevention/pdf/NISVS-StateReportBook.pdf

Spieker, A., Schiff, M., & Davis, B. (2016). Spousal military deployment during pregnancy and adverse birth outcomes. *Military Medicine, 181*(3), 243.

Stadtlander, L. (2017). Anxiety and pregnancy. *International Journal of Childbirth Education, 32*(1), 32–35.

Stapleton, L., Schetter, C., Westling, E., Rini, C., Hobel, C., & Sandman, C. (2012). Perceived partner support in pregnancy predicts lower maternal and infant distress. *National Institute of Health, 26*(3), 453–463.

Substance Abuse and Mental Health Services Administration. (2014). *SAMHSA's concept of trauma and guidance for a trauma-informed approach. HHS Publication No. (SMA).* Substance Abuse and Mental Health Services Administration.

The Joint Commission. (2018). *The Joint Commission standards interpretation.* Author. https://www.jointcommission.org/standards_information/jcfaq.aspx

United Nations High Commissioner for Refugees. (2020). *Global trends: Forced displacement in 2019.* United Nations High Commissioner for Refugees Global Data Service.

U.S. Department of Health and Human Services, Office of Minority Health. (2017). *Cultural competency.* https://www.minorityhealth.hhs.gov/

Walker, D., Visger, J., & Rossie, D. (2009). Contemporary childbirth education models. *Journal of Midwifery and Women's Health, 54*(6), 469–476.

Weis, K., Lederman, R., Lilly, A., & Schaffer, J. (2008). The relationship of military imposed marital separations on maternal acceptance of pregnancy. *Research in Nursing & Health, 31,* 196–207.

Weis, K., & Ryan, T. (2012). Mentors offering maternal support: A support intervention for military mothers. *Journal of Obstetric, Gynecologic, and Neonatal Nursing, 42*(2), 303–314.

Widarsson, M., Kerstis, B., Sundquist, K., Engström, G., & Sarkadi, A. (2012). Support needs of expectant mothers and fathers: A qualitative study. *Journal of Perinatal Education, 21*(1), 36–44.

Wilson, C., & Leese, B. (2013). Do nurses and midwives have a role in promoting the well-being of patients during their fertility journey? *British Fertility Society, 16*(1), 2–7.

Winn, A., Hetherington, E., & Tough, S. (2017) Systematic review of immigrant women's experiences with perinatal care in North America. *Journal of Obstetric, Gynecologic & Neonatal Nursing, 46* (5), 764–775.

Wojnar, D., & Katzenmeyer, A. (2014). Experiences of preconception, pregnancy, and new motherhood for lesbian nonbiological mothers. *Journal of Obstetric, Gynecological & Neonatal Nursing, 43*(1), 50–59.

World Health Organization. (2011). Rio political declaration on social determinants of health. World Health Organization.

Zadeh, M. A., Khajehei, M., Sharif, F., & Hadzic, M. (2012). High-risk pregnancy: Effects on postpartum depression and anxiety. *British Journal of Midwifery, 20*(2), 104–113.

Zielinski, R., Ackerson, K., & Kane-Low, L. (2015). Planned home birth: Benefits, risks and opportunities. *Dove Press, 7,* 361–377. https://doi.org/10.2147/IJWH.S55561

Antepartal Tests

6

Roberta F. Durham, RN, PhD
Hallie K. Taylor, DO

LEARNING OUTCOMES

Upon completion of this chapter, the student will be able to:
1. Define terms used in antenatal tests.
2. Identify the purpose and indication for key antenatal tests.
3. Describe the procedure, interpretation, advantages, and risks of common antenatal tests.
4. Articulate the nursing responsibilities related to key antenatal tests.
5. Identify patient teaching needs related to antenatal tests.

CONCEPTS

Clinical Judgment
Comfort
Communication
Evidence-Based Practice
Family
Health Promotion
Health-Care Technology
Oxygenation
Perfusion
Safety
Teaching and Learning

Nursing Diagnoses

- Deficient knowledge related to antenatal tests
- Anxiety related to antenatal tests
- Grief related to abnormal results from antenatal tests
- Risk for disturbed maternal fetal dyad because of fetal injury or death related to invasive antenatal tests

Nursing Outcomes

- The pregnant woman and her family will understand the purpose, procedure, and results of antenatal tests.
- The pregnant woman will be able to make informed decisions about antenatal tests.
- Complications of antenatal tests will be identified promptly, and appropriate nursing interventions will be initiated.

INTRODUCTION

Care of the pregnant woman in the antenatal period is multifaceted, requiring knowledge of the normal and abnormal pregnancy, risk factors affecting pregnancy outcome, screening and diagnostic tests, and issues surrounding the childbearing continuum and appropriate nursing interventions. This chapter presents various tests offered to pregnant women, focusing on tests for at-risk or high-risk pregnancies. Common maternal conditions indicating a need for antenatal tests are presented in Table 6-1. The purpose, indication, basic procedure, interpretation, advantages, risks, and nursing actions are outlined. Specifics on procedures are not detailed, as they may vary from institution to institution. Routine tests performed during pregnancy are presented

133

TABLE 6-1 Indications for Antepartum Fetal Surveillance: Common Maternal Conditions Indicating Need for Antenatal Tests

Maternal Conditions	Antiphospholipid syndrome
	Hemoglobinopathies
	Hypertensive disorder
	Renal disease
	Cardiac disease
	Systemic lupus erythematosus
	Insulin-treated diabetes mellitus
	Hyperthyroidism
Pregnancy-Related Conditions	Gestational hypertension
	Preeclampsia
	Gestational diabetes
	Decreased fetal movement
	Hydramnios, oligohydramnios, and polyhydramnios
	Fetal growth restriction
	Multiple gestation with growth discrepancy or monochorionic diamniotic multiples
	Post-term pregnancy
	Previous unexplained fetal demise
	Isoimmunization
	Fetal anomalies

and detailed in Chapter 4. Antenatal tests are often performed as outpatient procedures, including ultrasound, amniocentesis, and nonstress tests (NST). Antenatal tests may also be performed during an antenatal hospitalization for a high-risk pregnancy. The nurse's role and responsibility related to antenatal tests may vary based on the inpatient or outpatient setting. Nursing care may be provided before, during, or after a procedure.

ASSESSMENT FOR RISK FACTORS

The nurse needs to assess for factors that place the woman or her fetus at risk for adverse outcomes. The goal of risk assessment is to identify women and fetuses at risk for developing antepartum, intrapartum, postpartum, or neonatal complications and promote risk-appropriate care that will optimize perinatal outcomes (Adams, 2021).

- Biophysical factors originate from the mother or fetus and impact the development or function of the mother or fetus. They include genetic, nutritional, medical, and obstetric issues (see Table 6-1).

- Psychosocial factors include maternal behaviors or lifestyles that have a negative effect on the mother or fetus. Examples include smoking, alcohol or drug use, and psychological status.
- Sociodemographic factors are variables pertaining to the woman and her family that place the mother and the fetus at increased risk. Examples include access to prenatal care, age, parity, marital status, income, and ethnicity.
- Environmental factors are hazards in the workplace or the general environment that impact pregnancy outcomes. Various environmental substances can affect fetal development. Examples include exposure to chemicals, radiation, and pollutants.

The underlying mechanism for how some risk factors impact pregnancy outcomes is not fully understood. Many risk factors appear to have a combined or cumulative effect. Identification of risk factors for poor perinatal outcomes is essential to minimize maternal and neonatal morbidity and mortality. Risk factors are described in more detail in Chapters 7, 10, 14, and 17 as they relate specifically to pregnancy, labor, the postpartum period, and the neonate, respectively.

THE NURSE'S ROLE IN ANTEPARTAL TESTING

The nurse's role during antepartal testing varies based on the specific test. In general, it includes assessing for risk factors and providing information, emotional support, and comfort to women undergoing antenatal tests. Many women having antenatal tests are at high risk for fetal and maternal complications and are anxious and vulnerable. Sometimes, the nurse assists or performs the antenatal test, which may require advanced competencies (i.e., ultrasound).

CRITICAL COMPONENT

Nursing Actions Related to Antenatal Tests

Nurses are involved in antenatal testing in a variety of ways, depending on the test. Regardless of the level of involvement in antenatal testing, nurses must provide appropriate support to families and understand the variety of tests available during pregnancy, the risks and benefits of tests and procedures, the indications for tests and procedures, the interpretation of findings, the nursing care associated with the test or procedure, and the physical and psychological benefits, limitations, and implications of the test or procedure (Adams, 2021). Nurses have a professional and ethical responsibility to facilitate women's informed decision making regarding antenatal testing so that women can make meaningful decisions about their health. Only by having complete information about health problems and treatment can the patient exercise the right to free choice in determining what care is acceptable.

Meeting the ethical obligations of informed consent requires that the primary care provider (medical doctor [MD] or certified nurse-midwife [CMN]) gives the patient adequate, accurate, and understandable information. Thus, the patient has the ability to understand and reason through this information and is free to ask questions and to make an intentional and voluntary choice, which may include refusal of care or treatment (American College of Obstetricians and Gynecologists [ACOG], 2021b). Shared decision making is a patient-centered, individualized approach to the informed consent process that involves discussion of the benefits and risks of available treatment options in the context of a patient's values and priorities.

Although a physician may appoint a nurse to obtain the patient's signature on the consent form, they may not delegate the professional task of educating the patient about the risks and benefits of the proposed procedure, available alternatives to surgery, and the expected outcome. A physician or other independent practitioner performing the procedure alone has the legal duty to obtain informed consent. The nurse's role in obtaining informed consent is limited to the patient advocate role and being a witness to the patient's signature (Rock & Hoebeke, 2014).

After the details of the procedure are explained adequately to the patient and the patient signs the informed consent form, the nurse simply witnesses that (a) the patient is giving consent voluntarily to the treatment or procedure without coercion or undue influence; (b) the patient has sufficient mental capacity to make a decision about the specific treatment under consideration; in other words, the patient appears lucid and is competent to give consent; and (c) all information relevant to the decision has been disclosed to the patient. Nurses should ensure to the degree feasible that the patient understands and appreciates the information (Olsen & Brous, 2018). If the nurse has any concerns, the consent should not be witnessed. Nurses are patient advocates who should protect and preserve their patient's interests by assessing the patient's understanding of presented information and the implications of treatment decisions (American Nurses Association [ANA], 2010).

The nurse, whether in the role of caregiver or acting as patient advocate, can help to ensure that patients receive quality care by explaining medical and nursing procedures. Specific nursing actions for women undergoing antenatal testing include the following:

- Promote informed decisions and prevent uninformed decisions by patients.
- Assess for factors that place the woman or her fetus at risk for adverse outcomes.
- Establish a trusting relationship.
- Provide information regarding the test:
  - Explain how the test or procedure is performed.
  - Explain potential risks and benefits.
  - Explain what the woman can expect during the test or procedure.
  - Explain what the test measures.
  - Encourage questions.
  - Encourage and foster open communication with providers.
  - Provide online resources for further information (Box 6-1).
- Provide comfort:
  - Assist the woman into a comfortable position.
  - Preserve the woman's modesty by closing doors and exposing only the portions of her body necessary for the test or procedure.

- Reassure the woman and her significant other:
  - Address concerns regarding the test or procedure such as the type of discomfort or pain she may experience and effects on her or her unborn child.
  - If she prefers, encourage the woman's significant other to be with her during procedures.
- Provide psychological support to the woman and her significant other (Fig. 6–1):
  - Incorporate understanding of cultural and social issues.
  - Remain with the woman and her significant other during the test or procedure.
  - Assess for anxiety and provide care to reduce the level of anxiety.
  - Allow the client to vent feelings and frustrations with the discomfort, time-consuming demands, and limitations imposed by high-risk pregnancy and antenatal testing.
  - Allow the woman to express feelings related to high-risk pregnancy.
  - Encourage expression and exploration of feelings.
- Document the woman's response and the results of tests.
- Report results of tests to providers.
- Schedule appropriate follow-up.
- Reinforce information given by the woman's provider regarding the results of the tests and need for further testing, treatment, or referral.
- A pregnant woman experiencing pregnancy complications that requires antenatal testing and surveillance during pregnancy may develop additional stress for herself, her partner, and her family.

It is important to remember childbearing women have a vested interest in their pregnancy and outcome. They know their bodies, preferences, concerns, and fears. Provide accurate information to the woman and her family in understandable terms to make sure the woman can be an informed participant in shared decision making. Communication and shared decision making improve outcomes. Establishing a plan of care includes a discussion of the risks and benefits of tests and procedures in the context of the woman's values, preferences, obstetric history, and treatment plan so the woman can make an informed decision about her care. Timely reporting of results is also essential. Delays in communicating test results in obstetric practice have the potential to limit diagnostic and management options for women and their families (ACOG, 2017a). Testing centers and providers should have procedures in place that ensure timely disclosure of test results to patients

BOX 6-1 | Informative Online Resources

American College of Obstetrics and Gynecology (ACOG): http://acog.net

Association of Women's Health, Obstetrics and Neonatal Nursing (AWHONN): http://awhonn.org

Gene testing: http://genetests.org

March of Dimes: http://marchofdimes.com/gyponline

National Society of Genetic Counseling: http://nsgc.org

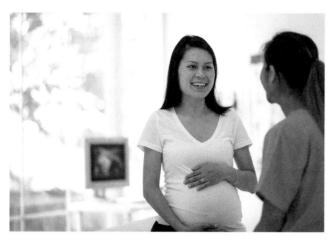

FIGURE 6–1 Nurse counseling a pregnant woman.

SCREENING AND DIAGNOSTIC TESTS

Prenatal detection of abnormalities provides an opportunity for the patient and provider to prepare and intervene. Normal test results can decrease a patient's anxiety; however, screening results are not definite. Screening tests are designed to identify those who are *not* affected by a disease or abnormality. Certain screening tests assess the risk that the fetus has specific common birth defects, but screening tests cannot tell whether the baby actually has a birth defect. These tests carry no risk to the fetus.

Diagnostic tests provide a yes or no answer to whether a fetus is normal or abnormal and can detect many, but not all, birth abnormalities caused by defects in a gene or chromosomes. Diagnostic testing may be done instead of screening if a couple has a family history of a birth defect, belongs to a certain ethnic group, or already has a child with a birth defect. Diagnostic tests also are available as a first choice for all pregnant women, including those who do not have risk factors. Some diagnostic tests carry risks, including a small risk of pregnancy loss.

CLINICAL JUDGMENT

Antepartal Screening and Diagnostic Tests

Screening Test

A screening test is a test designed to identify those who are *not* affected by a disease or abnormality. Some screening tests are offered to all pregnant women, such as multiple marker screening and ultrasound. Other screening tests are reserved for high-risk pregnancies to provide information on fetal status and well-being. If the results of screening tests indicate an abnormality, further testing is indicated. Screening tests include the following:

- Amniotic fluid index (AFI)
- Biophysical profile
- Contraction stress test
- Daily fetal movement count
- Multiple marker screening: alpha-fetoprotein screening, triple marker, and quad marker

- Nonstress test (NST)
- Ultrasonography
- Nuchal translucency
- Umbilical artery Doppler flow
- Vibroacoustic stimulation

Diagnostic Tests

Prenatal diagnosis is the science of identifying structural or functional anomalies or birth defects in the fetus (Cunningham et al., 2018). Diagnostic tests help to identify a disease or provide information that aids in diagnosis. Most fetal diagnostic tests are reserved for high-risk pregnancies in which the fetus is at increased risk for developmental or physical problems.

Diagnostic tests include the following:

- Amniocentesis
- Chorionic villi sampling
- Magnetic resonance imaging (MRI)
- Percutaneous umbilical blood sampling
- Ultrasonography

Historically, diagnostic testing was offered only to patients considered to be high risk because of maternal age or personal or family history. However, given the personal nature of prenatal testing decision making as well as the inefficiency of offering testing only to patients at high risk, the current recommendation from ACOG (2020) is that all patients should be offered both screening and diagnostic testing options.

GENETIC TESTS

The objective of prenatal genetic testing is to detect health problems that could affect the woman, fetus, or newborn and provide the woman and her providers with information to allow a fully informed decision about pregnancy management. Fetal genetic disorders are abnormalities in structure or function caused by differences in the genome (ACOG, 2016a). Chromosomal abnormalities include aberrations in chromosome number or structure. The most common abnormality of chromosome number is aneuploidy, in which there is an extra or missing chromosome or chromosomes. This differs from polyploidy, which is an abnormal number of haploid chromosome sets such as in triploidy (Cunningham et al., 2018). A haploid cell only has one set of chromosomes, typically the sex cells (either eggs or sperm). The critical transition from a diploid cell to a haploid cell allows normal reproduction to occur. When these two haploid cells come together with a single set of genetic information (chromosome), they create a zygote that reconstitutes as a diploid cell, which can then become a new individual. Abnormalities in chromosome number can be mosaic, which means that the abnormal number of chromosomes is not present in all cell lines (ACOG, 2016a).

The leading indication for prenatal diagnostic testing is the possible presence of fetal chromosomal abnormalities. Testing is most commonly done with cells obtained by amniocentesis or

CVS using traditional karyotype analysis, with results available in 7 to 14 days. Analysis of cell-free DNA from maternal plasma has been used for prenatal testing for several DNA abnormalities or traits, such as Rh type, but cell-free DNA testing still is considered to be a screening method and is not sufficiently accurate to be considered diagnostic for any indication (ACOG, 2016a).

Prenatal genetic testing cannot identify all abnormalities or problems in a fetus, and testing should focus on the individual woman's risks, reproductive goals, and preferences. It is important that women understand the benefits and limitations of all prenatal screening and diagnostic testing, including the conditions for which tests are available and the conditions that will not be detected by testing. It also is essential that a woman and her family understand there is a broad range of clinical presentations, or phenotypes, for many genetic disorders and that results of genetic testing cannot predict all outcomes. Prenatal genetic testing has many benefits, including reassuring patients when results are normal, identifying disorders for which prenatal treatment may provide benefit, optimizing neonatal outcomes by ensuring the appropriate location for delivery and the necessary personnel to care for affected infants, and allowing the opportunity for pregnancy termination (ACOG, 2016a).

Preconception and prenatal genetic screening and testing are recommended for a limited number of severe child-onset diseases to give families the chance to pursue assisted reproductive technology to avoid conception of an affected child, consider termination of a pregnancy, or prepare for the birth of a chronically ill child. With advancing genetic technology, however, providers increasingly face requests for testing of fetuses for less severe child-onset conditions, adult-onset conditions, or genetically linked traits (ACOG, 2016a).

Patients with increased risk of a fetal genetic disorder include those in these categories:

- Older maternal age above 35: risk of aneuploidy increases with increasing maternal age.
- Older paternal age, with 40 to 50 years as a definition of advanced paternal age: risk of having a child with a single-gene disorder.
- Parental carrier of chromosome rearrangement—In general, this refers to carriers of chromosome rearrangements that are identified after the birth of a child with an abnormality.
- Parental aneuploidy or aneuploidy mosaicism are concerns.
- Prior child with a structural birth defect—This refers to most birth defects, because these conditions tend to recur in families.
- Parental carrier of a genetic disorder—Parents who are affected by or are carriers of genetic disorders are at increased risk of having an affected child.
- Previous fetus or child with autosomal trisomy or sex chromosome aneuploidy is a concern.
- Structural anomalies identified by ultrasonography—The presence of a fetal structural abnormality increases the likelihood of aneuploidy, copy number variants such as microdeletions, and other genetic syndromes.

Factors associated with the likelihood of chromosomal abnormalities include increasing maternal age, a parental translocation or other chromosomal abnormality, having a previous pregnancy with a chromosomal abnormality, prenatal ultrasonographic abnormalities, or a screen positive test result.

If a diagnosis of a genetic abnormality is made, counseling should include family education and preparation; obstetric management recommendations, including fetal surveillance, intrapartum monitoring, and mode of delivery; referral to pediatric specialists and a tertiary care center for delivery, if appropriate; availability of adoption or pregnancy termination; and perinatal palliative care services and comfort care for delivery of a child with a diagnosis or fetal presentation that is incompatible with long-term survival (ACOG, 2020).

BIOPHYSICAL ASSESSMENT

Since the 1970s, the fetus has become more accessible with the refinement of new technology such as ultrasound. Fetal physiological parameters that can now be assessed and observed include movement, urine production, and structures and blood flow. Tests used in biophysical assessment of the fetus are ultrasonography, umbilical artery Doppler flow, and MRI.

Fetal Ultrasound Imaging

Ultrasonography is the use of high-frequency sound waves to produce an image of an organ or tissue (Fig. 6–2). Ultrasonography is not associated with risk and is the imaging technique of choice for the pregnant patient but should be used prudently to answer a relevant clinical question or otherwise provide medical benefit to the patient (ACOG, 2017b). The principle of ALARA (*as low as reasonably achievable*) should be considered in the use of fetal ultrasound (Cunningham et al., 2018), meaning sonography should only be performed for a valid indication using the lowest possible exposure.

Standard ultrasounds are typically done in the first trimester to confirm pregnancy and calculate gestational age. Additional ultrasounds may be done at other times as needed. The timing and type of ultrasound performed should be such that the clinical question being asked can be answered (American Academy

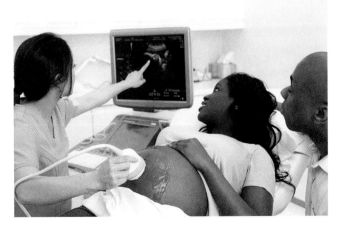

FIGURE 6–2 Nurse explains ultrasound to a pregnant woman having an ultrasound test.

of Pediatrics [AAP] & ACOG, 2017). A standard ultrasound performed in the second or third trimester includes evaluation of fetal presentation, quantification of amniotic fluid volume, documentation of the presence or absence of cardiac activity, placental position in relationship to the cervix, appropriate fetal biometric measurements, and determination of fetal number. In addition, a fetal anatomic survey includes imaging of specific anatomic structures (AWHONN, 2016).

Standard Examination

Standard obstetric ultrasound examination includes evaluation of fetal presentation and number, amniotic fluid volume, cardiac activity, placental position, fetal biometry (gestational age measurements), and fetal anatomic survey (AAP & ACOG, 2017). The maternal cervix and adnexa may be examined as clinically appropriate and when technically feasible (ACOG, 2016b).

Limited Examination

A limited examination is performed when a specific question requires investigation. It does not replace a standard examination. For example, a limited examination in the second trimester or the third trimester could be performed to confirm fetal heart activity to establish fetal presentation in a laboring patient. A limited examination also may be performed in any trimester to estimate amniotic fluid volume, evaluate the cervix, or assess embryonic or fetal viability (ACOG, 2016b).

Specialized Examination

The components of the specialized examination are more extensive than for a standard ultrasound examination and are determined on a case-by-case basis. Also referred to as a "detailed," "targeted," ultrasound examination, the specialized anatomic examination is performed when there is an increased risk of an anomaly based on the history, laboratory abnormalities, or the results of the limited examination or the standard examination. Other specialized examinations include fetal Doppler ultrasonography, biophysical profile, fetal echocardiography, or additional biometric measurements. Indications for specialized examinations include the possibility of fetal growth restriction and multifetal gestation (AAP & ACOG, 2017; ACOG 2016b; AWHONN, 2016). Point-of-care ultrasound is ultrasound imaging performed during a patient encounter to enhance care (AWHONN, 2016).

Ultrasound use varies based on the trimester (Table 6-2) and is commonly used to obtain vital information such as:

- Presence of a gestational sac
- Gestational age

TABLE 6-2   Indications for Ultrasound by Trimester of Pregnancy

FIRST TRIMESTER	SECOND TRIMESTER	THIRD TRIMESTER
Confirm intrauterine pregnancy.	Confirm the gestational age and due date.	Confirm gestational age.
Confirm fetal cardiac activity.	Confirm fetal cardiac activity.	Confirm fetal viability.
Detect multiple gestation (number and size of gestational sacs).	Confirm fetal number, fetal position, fetal size, amnionicity, and chorionicity.	Detect fetal number, fetal position, congenital anomalies, fetal growth, and intrauterine growth restriction (IUGR).
Assessment of amnionicity and chorionicity of multiples.	Confirm placental location.	Detect placental position, abruption, previa, or maturity.
Visualization during chorionic villus sampling.	Confirm fetal weight and gestational age.	Evaluation of fetal condition. Assess biophysical profile and amniotic fluid index. Perform Doppler flow studies.
Estimate gestational age.	Detect fetal anomalies (best after 18 weeks) or IUGR.	Assess fetal growth.
Evaluate uterine structures.	Evaluate uterine and cervical structures.	Evaluate uterine and cervical structures.
Detect missed abortion, tubal, or ectopic pregnancy, or hydatidiform mole.	Evaluate vaginal bleeding.	Evaluate vaginal bleeding
Evaluate vaginal bleeding.		
To screen for aneuploidy (nuchal translucency).	Visualize for diagnostic tests and external version.	Visualize for diagnostic tests and external version.

American Academy of Pediatrics and the American College of Obstetricians and Gynecologists, 2017; American College of Obstetricians and Gynecologists, 2016b; Association of Women's Health, Obstetric and Neonatal Nurses, 2016.

- Fetal growth
- Fetal anatomy and presentation when performed in the second and third trimesters
- Placental location and possible abnormalities
- Fetal activity
- Number of fetuses
- Viability
- Amount of amniotic fluid
- Visual assistance for some invasive procedures, such as amniocentesis

Ultrasound equipment has become more portable, affordable, and efficient and thus easier to utilize at the bedside. Point-of-care sonography is brought to the patient and performed by health-care providers in real time to directly correlate findings to presenting signs and symptoms. These examinations are within the scope of practice for licensed registered nurses (RNs) who have the necessary knowledge, skills, and training in the specific imaging procedure to be performed. Examples in maternity nursing care where nurses may use point-of-care ultrasound are varied and include determining fetal presentation, evaluating fetal well-being (e.g., biophysical profile [BPP]), and assessing amniotic fluid volume. Performing an obstetric ultrasound primarily to produce keepsake images or to determine fetal gender without a medical indication is not recommended.

Procedures

An ultrasound examination may be performed either transabdominally or transvaginally. If a transabdominal examination is inconclusive, a transvaginal scan is recommended. Transvaginal ultrasound is generally performed in the first trimester for earlier visualization of the fetus. With the woman in a lithotomy position, the provider inserts a sterile covered probe or transducer into the vagina.

Abdominal ultrasound requires the woman to be in a supine position. A full bladder is necessary to elevate the uterus out of the pelvis for better visualization when performed during the first half of pregnancy. Transmission gel and transducer are placed on the maternal abdomen.

The transducer is then moved over the maternal abdomen to create an image of the structure being evaluated (see Fig. 6–2).

Interpretation of Results

- Post-procedure interpretation is typically done by a practitioner such as a radiologist, obstetrician, or nurse-midwife. After specialized training, nurses can perform limited obstetrical ultrasound (Box 6-2).
- Ultrasound for gestational age is determined through measurements of fetal-crown rump length, biparietal diameter, and femur length. It is most accurate when performed before 14 weeks to determine gestational age plus or minus 1 week (AAP & ACOG, 2017;).
- Normal findings for the fetus are appropriate gestational age, size, viability, position, and functional capacities (see Fig. 6–3).
- Normal findings for the placenta are expected size, normal position and structure, and an adequate amniotic fluid volume.
- One screening test done by ultrasound in the first trimester is nuchal translucency (NT). The NT refers to the fluid-filled space on the dorsal aspect of the fetal neck. An enlarged NT (often defined as 3.0 mm or more or above the 99th percentile for the crown–rump length) is independently associated with fetal aneuploidy and structural malformations such as cardiac anomalies (ACOG, 2020).
- Abnormal findings should be referred for further testing and management of fetal anomalies (AAP & ACOG, 2017).

BOX 6-2 | AWHONN Ultrasound Guidelines

The AWHONN has developed didactic and clinical preparation guidelines for nurses who perform limited obstetric ultrasound. A minimum of 8 hours of didactic content is recommended in the following areas: (1) ultrasound physics and instrumentation, (2) patient education, (3) nursing accountability, (4) documentation, (5) image archiving, (6) legal and ethical issues, and (7) lines of authority and responsibility (AWHONN, 2016).

Currently there are no certification requirements for nurses performing limited ultrasound. Appropriate institutional policies, didactic and clinical education, and evaluation components are needed to ensure competence for nurses to perform limited ultrasound.

Obstetric first-trimester ultrasound

a. Identification of number and measurement of yolk sac(s), gestational sac(s), embryo(s), and fetus(es)

b. Identification and confirmation of early fetal cardiac activity

c. Determination of uterine versus extrauterine pregnancy

d. Use as an aid for ultrasound-guided procedures

Obstetric second- and third-trimester ultrasound

a. Fetal number and location

b. Fetal cardiac activity

c. Fetal position and presentation

d. Placental location

e. Amniotic fluid volume assessment

f. Biometric measurements to estimate fetal age and weight

g. Cervical length measurement

h. Use as aid for ultrasound-guided procedures

i. Modified BPP (AFI and NST)

j. Biophysical profile including fetal tone, fetal movement, fetal breathing, amniotic fluid, and NST

Association of Women's Health, Obstetric and Neonatal Nurses, 2016.

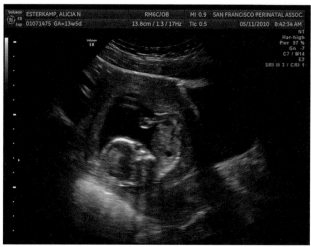

Courtesy of Allbin family

FIGURE 6–3 2D ultrasound picture.

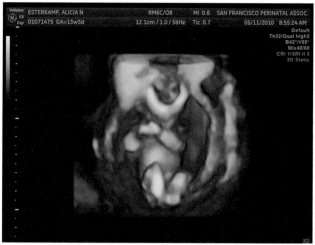

Courtesy of Allbin family

FIGURE 6–4 3D ultrasound picture.

Advantages

● Accurate assessments of gestational age, fetal growth, and detection of fetal and placental abnormalities
● Noninvasive
● Provides information on fetal structures and status

Risks

● None, but controversy exists on the use of routine ultrasound for low-risk pregnant women, as there is no evidence it improves outcomes.
● Ultrasonography is safe for the fetus when used appropriately and should be used when medical information about a pregnancy is needed.

Nursing Actions

● Explain to the woman and her family that ultrasound uses sound waves to produce an image of the baby.
● Assess for latex allergies with transvaginal ultrasound.
● For transvaginal ultrasound, have the patient put on a gown and undress from the waist down. For abdominal ultrasound, only the lower abdomen needs to be exposed.
● For transvaginal ultrasound, inform the woman that a sterile sheathed probe is inserted into the vagina. Inform her that she may feel pressure, but pain is not usually felt.
● Position the patient in a lithotomy position for transvaginal ultrasound and supine for abdominal ultrasound.
● Provide comfort measures to the woman during the procedure, such as a pillow under her head and a warm blanket above and below her abdomen.
● Be sensitive to cultural and social as well as modesty issues.
● Provide emotional support.
● Schedule appropriate follow-up.
● Document the ultrasound examination according to the institutional policy.

Although there is no data indicating harm to fetuses from ultrasound imaging, casual use of ultrasonography should be avoided. Use of ultrasonography without a medical indication and only to

view the fetus, obtain a "keepsake" picture, or determine the fetal sex is inappropriate and contrary to responsible medical practice (ACOG, 2016b).

Three-Dimensional and Four-Dimensional Ultrasound

Three-dimensional (3D) ultrasound and four-dimensional (4D) ultrasound are advanced types of transabdominal ultrasounds that take thousands of images at once to produce a 3D or 4D image. They allow visualization of complex facial movements and features, branching of placental stem vessels, and connection of the umbilical vessels to the chorionic plate of the placenta (Fig. 6–4). Current recommendations are that 3D ultrasound be used only as an adjunct to conventional ultrasonography.

Purpose

● Standard determination is made of gestational age, fetal size, presentation, and volume of amniotic fluid.
● Determination is made of complications such as vaginal bleeding, ventriculomegaly, hydrocephaly, and congenital brain defects.
● Diagnosis is made of fetal malformations, uterine or pelvic abnormalities, hypoxic ischemic brain injury, and inflammatory disorders of the brain (ACOG, 2016b; Cunningham et al., 2018).
● Despite these technical advantages, proof of a clinical advantage of 3D ultrasonography in prenatal diagnosis in general still is lacking.
● Potential areas of promise include fetal facial anomalies, neural tube defects, fetal tumors, and skeletal malformations for which 3D ultrasonography may be helpful in diagnosis (ACOG, 2016b).

Timing

● The 3D and 4D ultrasounds are ordered as needed for further evaluation of possible fetal anomalies such as facial, cardiac, and skeletal.

- The 3D and 4D ultrasounds are most commonly requested by the patient to see a more lifelike picture of their developing baby in utero.

Procedure

- See abdominal ultrasound.

Interpretation of Results

- See abdominal ultrasound.
- Despite these technical advantages, proof of a clinical advantage of 3D ultrasonography in prenatal diagnosis in general still is lacking.

Advantages

- More detailed assessment of fetal structures
- 3D—presentation of placental blood flow
- Measurement of fetal organs
- 4D—allows for evaluation of brain morphology and identification of brain lesions

Risks

- Same as with standard ultrasound

Nursing Actions

- Same as with standard ultrasound

Magnetic Resonance Imaging

MRI is a diagnostic radiological evaluation of tissue and organs from multiple planes. During pregnancy, it is used to visualize maternal or fetal structures for detailed imaging when screening tests indicate possible abnormalities. It is most commonly performed for complex fetal anomalies such as suspected brain abnormality or to further evaluate abnormal placentation (AAP & ACOG, 2017; Cunningham et al., 2018).

Purpose

- Tissue, organs, and vascular structures can be evaluated without the need to inject iodinated contrast.

Procedure

- The woman is instructed to remove all metallic objects before the test.
- The woman is placed in a supine position with left lateral tilt on the MRI table.
- The woman's abdominal area is scanned.

Interpretation

- The study is interpreted by a radiologist.

Advantages

- Provides very detailed images of fetal anatomy; particularly useful for brain abnormalities and complex abnormalities of the thorax, gastrointestinal, and genitourinary systems and to evaluate abnormal placentation.

Risks

- No known harmful effects

Nursing Actions

- Nurses are involved in the pre- and post-procedure.
- Explain the procedure to the woman and her family. The MRI is used to see maternal or fetal structures for detailed pictures.
- Address questions and concerns and provide information and support; some women may experience claustrophobia or fear of equipment.

Doppler Flow Studies (Doppler Velocimetry)

Blood flow velocity measured by Doppler ultrasound reflects downstream impedance. Because more than 40% of the combined fetal ventricular output is directed to the placenta, obliteration of the placental vascular channel increases afterload and leads to fetal hypoxemia. This in turn leads to dilation and redistribution of the middle cerebral artery (MCA) blood flow. Ultimately, pressure rises in the ductus venosus due to afterload in the right side of the fetal heart. In this scheme, placental vascular dysfunction results in increased umbilical artery blood flow resistance, which progresses to decreased MCA impedance followed ultimately by abnormal flow in the ductus venosus (Cunningham et al., 2018). Three fetal vascular circuits—umbilical artery, MCA, and ductus venosus—are currently used to determine fetal health and aid in clinical decision making for growth-restricted fetuses.

Umbilical artery Doppler flow is a noninvasive screening technique that uses advanced ultrasound technology to assess resistance to blood flow in the placenta. It evaluates the rate and volume of blood flow through the placenta and umbilical cord vessels using ultrasound. Increased resistance in the placenta, suggestive of poor function, results in reduced diastolic blood flow (Everett & Peebles, 2015). Evaluating fetal circulation and uteroplacental blood flow with Doppler flow provides critical information regarding fetal reserves and adaptation (Cypher, 2016). Umbilical artery DV plays an important role in the management of a pregnancy complicated by a diagnosis of fetal growth restriction. Once fetal growth restriction is diagnosed, serial umbilical artery assessment should be performed to assess for deterioration. Umbilical artery DV used in conjunction with standard fetal surveillance, such as NSTs, biophysical profiles, or both, is associated with improved outcomes in fetuses in which fetal growth restriction has been diagnosed. Doppler assessment may provide insight into the etiology of fetal growth restriction. Increased impedance in the umbilical artery suggests that the pregnancy is complicated by underlying placental insufficiency. Also, absent or reversed end-diastolic flow in the umbilical artery is associated with an increased frequency of perinatal mortality and can affect decisions regarding timing of delivery in the context of fetal growth restriction (ACOG, 2021a). Doppler ultrasound can also be used in the evaluation of twin–twin transfusion syndrome (Simpson, 2013).

Purpose

- Assesses placental perfusion
- Used in combination with other diagnostic tests to assess fetal status in intrauterine growth restriction (IUGR) fetuses
- Not a useful screening tool for determining fetal compromise and therefore not recommended to the general obstetric population (AAP & ACOG, 2017)

Procedures

- The woman is assisted into a supine position.
- Transmission gel and transducer are placed on the woman's abdomen.
- Images are obtained of blood flow in the umbilical artery.

Interpretation of Results

- The directed blood flow within the umbilical arteries is calculated using the difference between systolic and diastolic flow (Everett & Peebles, 2015).
- As peripheral resistance increases, diastolic flow decreases and the systolic and diastolic increases. Reversed end-diastolic flow can be seen with severe cases of IUGR (AAP & ACOG, 2017).
- Umbilical artery Doppler is considered abnormal if the systolic/diastolic ratio is above the 95th percentile for gestational age, or the end-diastolic flow is absent or reversed (Cunningham et al., 2018).
- When interpreting results, factors such as maternal position, fetal heart rate (FHR), and fetal breathing movements can alter the vessel waveforms. Ideally, the Doppler examination should be conducted during times of fetal apnea (Berkley et al., 2012).

Advantages

- Noninvasive
- Allows for assessment of placental perfusion

Risks

- None

Nursing Actions

- Explain the procedure to the woman and her family. The Doppler test evaluates the blood flow through the placenta and umbilical cord vessels using ultrasound.
- Address questions and concerns.
- Provide comfort measures.
- Provide emotional support.
- Schedule appropriate follow-up.

Additional Doppler Studies

Recent advances in Doppler technology have led to the development of noninvasive methods to assess the degree of fetal anemia. Doppler was used to measure the peak systolic velocity in the fetal MCA in fetuses at risk for fetal anemia. Moderate or severe anemia was predicted by values of peak systolic velocity in the fetal MCA above 1.5 times the median for gestational age (ACOG, 2018a). Correct technique is a critical factor when determining peak systolic velocity in the fetal MCA with Doppler ultrasonography. This procedure should be used only by those with adequate training and clinical experience. The MCA Doppler is an important indicator of fetal anemia. The role of cerebral arteries and the changes that occur in vessels in relation to the concept of "brain sparing" in potentially hypoxic fetuses is under investigation (Everett & Peebles, 2015). In the situation of chronic fetal hypoxemia or nutrient deprivation, the fetus redistributes its cardiac output to maximize oxygen and nutrient supply to the brain, described as a brain-sparing.

Changes in cerebral blood flow associated with brain-sparing can be detected by Doppler sonography (Cohen et al., 2015). The value of MCA Doppler in the prediction of adverse fetal outcomes has been inconsistent. However, the cerebroplacental ratio (CPR), a measure of cerebral centralization of fetal blood flow, provides proposed values for predicting adverse outcomes (less than 1, less than 1.05, 1.08 or lower, less than the 5th percentile) (Conde-Agudelo et al., 2018). The CPR, an important obstetric ultrasound tool used as a predictor of adverse pregnancy outcome in growth restricted fetuses, is calculated by dividing the Doppler pulsatile indices of the MCA by the umbilical artery. The index will reflect mild increases in placental resistance with mild reductions in fetal brain vascular resistance.

The ductus venosus Doppler is DV of the fetal central venous circulation that helps identify fetuses with suspected IUGR at an advanced stage of compromise. Absent or reversed flow in late diastole in the ductus venosus is associated with increased perinatal morbidity, fetal acidemia, and perinatal and neonatal mortality. The value of the DV waveform is in the premature fetus with IUGR. Flow in the ductus venosus also has been measured in an attempt to assess fetal status, but its use has not been shown to improve outcomes (ACOG, 2021b).

BIOCHEMICAL ASSESSMENT

Biochemical assessment involves biological examination and chemical determination. Procedures used to obtain biochemical specimens include chorionic villi sampling, amniocentesis, percutaneous blood sampling, and maternal assays. More than 15% of pregnancies are at sufficient risk to warrant invasive testing (Cypher, 2016).

Chorionic Villus Sampling

Chorionic villus sampling (CVS) is aspiration of a small amount of placental tissue (chorionic villi) for chromosomal, metabolic, or DNA testing (AAP & ACOG, 2017). This test is used for chromosomal analysis between 10 and 13 weeks' gestation to detect fetal abnormalities caused by genetic disorders. There appears to be no significant difference between transcervical and transabdominal CVS (ACOG, 2020). The primary advantage of CVS over amniocentesis is that the procedure can be performed earlier in pregnancy and the viable cells obtained by CVS for analysis allow for shorter specimen processing time (5 to 7 days versus 7 to 14 days), so the results are available earlier in pregnancy. After an abnormal first-trimester ultrasound examination or screening test, the earlier CVS results allow for more management options.

Timing

- Performed during first or second trimester, ideally at 10 to 13 weeks' gestation

Procedure

- The woman is in a supine position or lithotomy position, depending on the route of insertion.
- A catheter is inserted either transvaginally through the cervix or abdominally using a needle. With each route, ultrasonography is used to guide placement. Transabdominally, a needle is inserted through the abdomen and uterus to the placenta.
- A small biopsy of chorionic (placental) tissue is removed with aspiration.
- The villi are harvested and cultured for chromosomal analysis and processed for DNA and enzymatic analysis as indicated (Fig. 6–5).

Interpretation of Results

- Results of chromosomal studies are available within 1 week.
- Detailed information is provided on the specific chromosomal abnormality detected.

Advantages

- Can be performed earlier than amniocentesis but is not recommended before 10 weeks (AAP & ACOG, 2017)
- Examination of fetal chromosomes

Risks

- There is a 0.22% (1 in 455) fetal loss rate due to bleeding, infection, and rupture of membranes (AAP & ACOG, 2017).

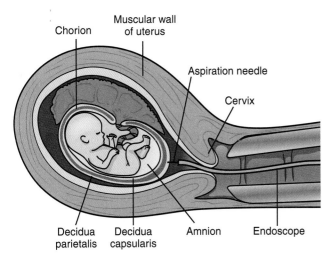

Chorion

Muscular wall of uterus

Aspiration needle

Cervix

Decidua parietalis   Decidua capsularis   Amnion   Endoscope

FIGURE 6–5 Chorionic villi sampling procedure.

- Ten percent of women experience some bleeding after the procedure (AAP & ACOG, 2017).
- Pregnant women who have hepatitis B virus, hepatitis C virus, or HIV should be counseled about the possibility of an increased risk of transmission to the newborn that may come with CVS or amniocentesis.

Nursing Actions

- Review the procedure with the woman and her family. This test obtains amniotic fluid to test for fetal abnormalities caused by genetic problems.
- Instruct the woman in breathing and relaxation techniques she can use during the procedure.
- Assist the woman into the proper position.
  - Lithotomy for transvaginal aspiration
  - Supine for transabdominal aspiration
- Provide comfort measures.
- Provide emotional support.
- Recognize anxiety related to test results.
- Label specimens.
- Assess fetal and maternal well-being post-procedure. Auscultate FHR twice in 30 minutes.
- Instruct the woman to report abdominal pain or cramping, leaking of fluid, bleeding, fever, or chills to the care provider.
- Administer RhoGAM to Rh-negative women post-procedure as per order to prevent antibody formation in Rh-negative women.

Amniocentesis

Amniocentesis is the most common technique used for obtaining fetal cells for genetic testing (AAP & ACOG, 2017). It is a diagnostic procedure in which a needle is inserted through the maternal abdominal wall into the uterine cavity to obtain amniotic fluid. Although commonly performed for genetic testing, it can also be done for assessment of fetal lung maturity, assessment of hemolytic disease, or intrauterine infection and therapy for polyhydramnios.

Timing

- Usually offered between 15 and 20 weeks for genetic testing. For other purposes, it is used as clinically indicated.

Procedure

- A detailed ultrasound is performed to take fetal measurements and locate the placenta to choose a site for needle insertion.
- A needle is inserted transabdominally into the uterine cavity using ultrasonography to guide placement (Fig. 6–6).
- Amniotic fluid is obtained.

Interpretation of Results

- Amniocentesis has an accuracy rate of 99% (AAP & ACOG, 2017).
- An amniotic fluid sample is sent to a laboratory for cell growth, and results of the chromosomal studies are available within 2 weeks.

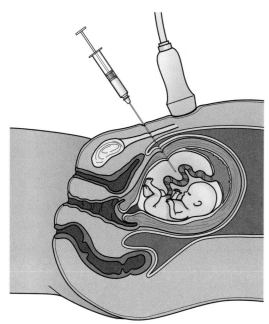

Amniocentesis:
Technique of amniocentesis is illustrated. A pocket of amniotic fluid is located by sonogram. A small amount of fluid is removed by aspiration.

FIGURE 6–6 Amniocentesis procedure.

- Elevated bilirubin levels indicate fetal hemolytic disease.
- A positive culture indicates infection.
- Standards do not recommend amniocentesis be done solely to evaluate the lecithin/sphingomyelin (L/S) ratio or the presence of phosphatidyl glycerol (PG). Although amniotic fluid can be analyzed to evaluate fetal lung maturity, current practice does not recommend this. If the purpose of the test is to determine fetal lung maturity, L/S ratio, PG, and lamellar body count (LBC), results are interpreted as follows (Cypher, 2016):
  - L/S ratio greater than 2:1 indicates fetal lung maturity.
  - L/S ratio less than 2:1 indicates fetal lung immaturity in increased risk of respiratory distress syndrome.
  - Positive PG indicates fetal lung maturity.
  - Negative PG indicates immature fetal lungs.
  - An LBC of 50,000/µL or greater is highly indicative of fetal lung maturity.
  - An LBC of 15,000/µL or lower is highly indicative of fetal lung immaturity.
  - LBC results can be hindered by the presence of meconium, vaginal bleeding, vaginal mucus, or hydramnios.

Advantages

- Examines fetal chromosomes for genetic disorders
- Direct examination of biochemical specimens

Risks

- Studies suggest a loss rate as low as 0.1% to 0.3% (ACOG, 2020).
- Trauma to the fetus or placenta

- Bleeding or leaking of amniotic fluid in 1% to 2% of cases (AAP & ACOG, 2017)
- Preterm labor
- Maternal infection
- Rh sensitization from fetal blood into maternal circulation
- Pregnant women who have hepatitis B virus, hepatitis C virus, or HIV should be counseled about the possibility of an increased risk of transmission to the newborn that may come with CVS or amniocentesis.

Nursing Actions

- Review the procedure with the woman and assure her that precautions are followed during the procedure with ultrasound visualization of the fetus to avoid fetal or placental injury.
- Explain that in the amniocentesis procedure a needle is inserted through the abdomen into the womb to obtain amniotic fluid for testing.
- Explain that discomfort will be minimized during needle aspiration with a local anesthetic.
- Explain that a full bladder may be required for ultrasound visualization if the woman is less than 20 weeks' gestation.
- Instruct the woman in breathing and relaxation techniques she can use during the procedure.
- Provide comfort measures.
- Provide emotional support.
- Recognize anxiety related to test results.
- Prep the abdomen with an antiseptic such as betadine if indicated.
- Label specimens.
- Assess fetal and maternal well-being post-procedure, monitoring and evaluating the FHR.
- Instruct the woman to report abdominal pain or cramping, leaking of fluid, bleeding, decreased fetal movement, fever, or chills to the care provider.
- Instruct the woman not to lift anything heavy for 2 days.
- Administer Rho(D) immune globulin (RhoGAM) to Rh-negative women post-procedure as per order to prevent antibody formation in the Rh-negative woman.

Fetal Blood Sampling and Percutaneous Umbilical Blood Sampling

Fetal blood sampling and percutaneous umbilical blood sampling (FBS/PUBS), or cordocentesis, is the removal of fetal blood from the umbilical cord. The blood is used to test for metabolic and hematological disorders, fetal infection, and fetal karyotyping. It can also be used for fetal therapies such as red blood cell and platelet transfusions.

Timing

- Usually used after ultrasound has detected an anomaly in the fetus.

- Usually performed after 18 weeks' gestation to evaluate results of potential diagnoses and make further recommendations for medical management if necessary (Berry et al., 2013).

Procedure

- A needle is inserted into the umbilical vein at or near the placental origin and a small sample of fetal blood is aspirated (Fig. 6–7).
- Ultrasound is used to guide the needle.

Interpretation of Results

- Results are usually available within 48 hours.
- Interpretation of studies is based on the indication for the procedure.
- Biochemical testing on the blood may include a complete blood count with a differential analysis, anti-1 and anti-I cold agglutinin, ß-hCG, factors IX and VIIIC, and AFP levels (Berry et al., 2013).

Advantages

- Direct examination of fetal blood sample for fetal anomalies

Risks

- Complications are similar to those for amniocentesis and include cord vessel bleeding or hematomas, maternal-fetal hemorrhage, fetal bradycardia, and risk for infection.
- PUBS is typically not indicated when less invasive measures such as evaluation of amniocytes or chorionic villi will provide adequate diagnostic information (Berry et al., 2013).
- The overall procedure-related fetal death rate is 1.4% but varies depending on indication (Cunningham et al., 2018).

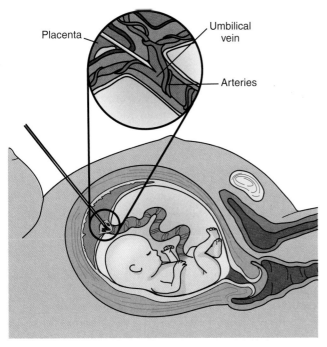

Placenta

Umbilical vein

Arteries

FIGURE 6–7 Percutaneous umbilical blood sampling procedure.

Nursing Actions

- Nurses may be involved in the pre- and post-procedure.
- Explain the procedure to the woman and her family. During PUBS, fetal blood is removed from the umbilical cord.
- Address questions and concerns.
- Position the client in a lateral or wedged position to avoid supine hypotension during fetal monitoring tests.
- Have terbutaline ready as ordered in case uterine contractions (UCs) occur during the procedure.
- Assess fetal well-being post-procedure for 1 to 2 hours via external fetal monitoring.
- Educate the patient on how to count fetal movements for when she goes home.

MATERNAL ASSAYS

Maternal assays are an increasingly common way to screen pregnant women for fetal birth defects or genetic anomalies (Allyse et al., 2015). The choice of screening tests depends on many factors, including timing of entry into prenatal care. The goal is to offer tests with high detection rates and low false-positive rates that provide patients diagnostic options. Ideally, patients are seen in the first trimester and can receive first-trimester aneuploidy screening or integrated or sequential aneuploidy screening that combines first trimester and second trimester testing (see Chapter 4). The following section details a few of the maternal assays used as part of testing.

Cell-Free DNA Screening

Cell-free DNA screens for aneuploidies using the analysis of cell-free DNA fragments in the maternal circulation starting at about 9 to 10 weeks of pregnancy. Cell-free DNA is the most sensitive and specific screening test for the common fetal aneuploidies. Nevertheless, it has the potential for false-positive and false-negative results. Further, cell-free DNA testing is not equivalent to diagnostic testing. Cell-free DNA is the only laboratory screening test to identify fetal sex and sex chromosome aneuploidies (ACOG, 2020).

Alpha-Fetoprotein/₁-Fetoprotein/Maternal Serum Alpha-Fetoprotein

Alpha-fetoprotein (AFP) is a glycoprotein produced in the fetal liver, gastrointestinal tract, and yolk sac in early gestation. Assessing for the levels of AFP in the maternal blood is a screening tool for certain developmental defects in the fetus, such as fetal NTDs and ventral abdominal wall defects. Because 95% of NTDs occur in the absence of risk factors, routine screening is recommended (Cunningham et al., 2018).

Timing

- 15 to 20 weeks' gestation

Procedure

● Maternal blood is drawn and sent to the laboratory for analysis.

Interpretation of Results

● Increased levels are associated with defects such as NTDs, anencephaly, omphalocele, and gastroschisis.
● Decreased levels are associated with trisomy 21 (Down syndrome).
● Abnormal findings require additional testing such as amniocentesis, CVS, or ultrasonography to make a diagnosis.

Advantages

● Between 80% and 85% of all open NTDs and open abdominal wall defects and 90% of anencephalies can be detected early in pregnancy (AAP & ACOG, 2017).

Risks

● The high false-positive rate (meaning the test results indicate an abnormality in a normal fetus) can result in increased anxiety for a woman and her family as they wait for the results of additional testing. High false positives can occur with oligohydramnios, multifetal gestation, decreased maternal weight, and underestimated fetal gestational age. False low levels can also occur as a result of fetal death, increased maternal weight, and overestimated fetal gestational age (Cunningham et al., 2018).

Nursing Actions

● Educate the woman about the screening test. The AFP test is a maternal blood test that evaluates the levels of AFP in the maternal blood to screen for certain fetal abnormalities.
● Support the woman and her family, particularly if results are abnormal.
● Assist in scheduling diagnostic testing when results are abnormal.
● Provide information on support groups if an NTD occurs.

Quadruple Marker Screen

The quadruple marker screen ("quad" screen) is a maternal serum test performed in the second trimester that gives information regarding the risk of open fetal defects in addition to risk assessment for trisomy 21 and 18. The quad screen involves the measurement of four maternal serum analytes—human chorionic gonadotropin (hCG), AFP, dimeric inhibin A (DIA), and unconjugated estriol (uE3)—in combination with maternal factors such as age, weight, race, and the presence of pregestational diabetes to calculate a risk estimate. Second-trimester quad screening has a detection rate for trisomy 21 of 80% with a 5% false-positive rate. A few laboratories offer the penta screen, which adds hyperglycosylated hCG to the quad screen. The triple marker screen measures serum hCG, AFP, and uE3, and provides a lower sensitivity for the detection of trisomy 21 (sensitivity of 69% at a 5% positive screening test result rate) than quad screen and first-trimester screening (ACOG, 2020).

Timing

● 15 to 22 weeks' gestation

Procedure

● Maternal blood is drawn and sent to the laboratory for analysis.

Interpretation

● Low levels of maternal serum alpha-fetoprotein and unconjugated estriol levels suggest an abnormality.
● hCG and inhibin-A levels are twice as high in pregnancies with trisomy 21.
● Decreased estriol levels are an indicator of NTDs.

Advantages

● Between 60% and 80% of cases of Down syndrome can be identified.
● Between 85% and 90% of open NTDs are detected.

Risks

● None

Nursing Actions

● Educate the woman about the test. This is a maternal blood test that assesses for the levels of chemicals in the maternal blood to screen for certain developmental abnormalities.
● Provide emotional support for the woman and her family.
● Assist in scheduling additional testing if needed.
● Provide information on support groups if an NTD occurs.

ANTENATAL FETAL SURVEILLANCE AND FETAL ASSESSMENT

The assessment of fetal status is a key component of perinatal care. FHR pattern, fetal activity, and degree of fetal muscular tone are sensitive to hypoxemia and acidemia (AAP & ACOG, 2017). Therefore, a variety of methods are available for ongoing assessment of fetal well-being during pregnancy, including:

● Fetal movement counting (FMC; kick counts)
● NST
● Vibroacoustic stimulation (VAS)
● Contraction stress test (CST)
● Biophysical profile (BPP)
● Amniotic fluid index (AFI)

The goal of fetal testing is to reduce the number of preventable stillbirths and to avoid unnecessary interventions (Cunningham et al., 2018). The purpose of antenatal testing is to validate fetal well-being or identify fetal hypoxemia and intervene before permanent injury or death occurs (AAP & ACOG, 2017; Cypher, 2016). In most clinical situations, a normal test result indicates that intrauterine fetal death is highly unlikely in the next 7 days and is highly reassuring (AAP & ACOG, 2017).

Antepartum testing is intended for use in pregnancies at high risk for fetal demise; testing begins by 32 to 34 weeks. Because of the risk of a high false positive potentially resulting in unnecessary delivery of a healthy baby, this testing is reserved for high-risk pregnancies. The schedule for antepartal testing for fetal surveillance may vary. For example, a Cochrane Review concluded there is limited evidence from randomized controlled trials to inform best practice for fetal surveillance regimens when caring for women with pregnancies affected by impaired fetal growth (Grivell et al., 2012).

Daily Fetal Movement Count

Women who report decreased fetal movement are at increased risk of adverse perinatal outcome (AAP & ACOG, 2017). In FMC, the pregnant woman counts fetal movements in a specified time period to identify potentially hypoxic fetuses. FMC is based on physiological principles that compromised fetuses reduce activity in response to decreased oxygenation, conserving energy. Maternal perception of fetal movement was one of the earliest and easiest tests of fetal well-being and remains an essential assessment of fetal health. Fetal activity is diminished in the compromised fetus, and cessation of fetal movement has been documented preceding fetal demise. Maternal perception of fetal activity is highly correlated with fetal activity (Adams, 2021; AAP & ACOG, 2017).

Timing

- Kick counts have been proposed as a primary method of fetal surveillance for all pregnancies.

Procedure

- The pregnant woman is instructed to palpate her abdomen and track fetal movements daily for 1 to 2 hours.

Interpretation

- In the 2-hour approach, maternal perception of 10 distinct fetal movements within 2 hours is considered normal and reassuring; once movement is achieved, counts can be discontinued for the day.
- In the 1-hour approach, the count is considered reassuring if it equals or exceeds the established baseline; in general, four movements in 1 hour is reassuring.
- Decreased fetal movement should be reported to the provider and is an indication for further fetal assessment, such as an NST or biophysical profile (AAP & ACOG, 2017).
- Fewer than four fetal movements in 2 hours should be reported to the provider (Adams, 2021).

Advantages

- Done by pregnant women
- Inexpensive, reassuring, and relatively easily taught to pregnant women
- No monitoring devices required

Risks

- None

Nursing Actions

- Teach the woman how to do kick counts and provide a means to record them. Instruct the woman to lie on her side while counting movements. Explain that maternal assessment of counting fetal movements is an important evaluation of fetal well-being.
- If fetal movement is decreased, the woman should be instructed to eat something, rest, and focus on fetal movement for 1 hour. Four movements in 1 hour are considered reassuring, whereas fewer than four movements in 2 hours should be reported.
- Instruct the woman to report decreased fetal movement below normal, as this is an indication for further assessment by care providers.

Nonstress Test

The NST is a screening tool that uses FHR patterns and accelerations as an indicator of fetal well-being (Fig. 6–8). The heart rate of a physiologically normal fetus with adequate oxygenation and an intact autonomic nervous system accelerates in response to movement (AWHONN, 2015; Cunningham et al., 2018). Acceleration in the FHR is a sign of fetal well-being. The NST records accelerations in the FHR in relation to fetal activity. It is the most widely accepted method of evaluating fetal status, particularly for high-risk pregnant women with complications such as hypertension, diabetes, multiple gestation, trauma, or bleeding; woman's report of lack of fetal movement; and placental abnormalities. NST is the most common method of antepartum fetal surveillance.

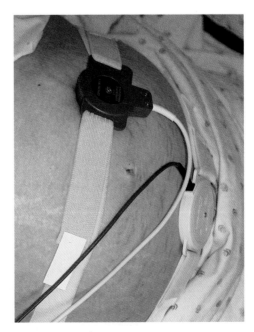

FIGURE 6–8 Monitoring for a nonstress test.

Procedure

- The FHR is monitored with the external FHR transducer until reactive (up to 40 minutes), while running an FHR contraction strip for interpretation.
- Monitor FHR and fetal activity for 20 to 40 minutes (placement of electronic fetal monitoring [EFM] and interpretation of EFM are described in Chapter 9).

Interpretation

- The NST is considered reactive when the FHR increases 15 beats above baseline for 15 seconds twice or more in 20 minutes (Fig. 6–9).
- In fetuses less than 32 weeks' gestation, two accelerations peaking at least 10 bpm above baseline and lasting 10 seconds in a 20-minute period is reactive (AWHONN, 2015).
- Nonreactive NST is one without sufficient FHR accelerations in 40 minutes and should be followed up with further testing such as an ultrasound or biophysical profile (AAP & ACOG, 2017).
- Presence of repetitive variable decelerations that are longer than 30 seconds requires further assessment of amniotic fluid or prolonged monitoring (Cunningham et al., 2018).

Advantages

- Noninvasive, easily performed, and reliable indicator of fetal well-being

Risks

- No indicated risks
- NST has a high false-positive rate of over 50% but a low false-negative rate of less than 1% (AAP & ACOG, 2017; Cypher, 2016).

Nursing Actions

- Explain the procedure to the woman and her family. The NST uses EFM to assess fetal well-being.
- Have the patient void before the procedure and lie in a semi-Fowler's or lateral position to avoid aortocaval compression.
- Provide comfort measures.
- Provide emotional support.

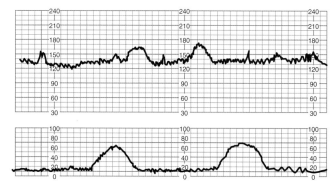

FIGURE 6–9 Fetal heart rate accelerations indicating a reactive nonstress test.

- Interpret FHR and accelerations; report results to the care provider.
- Document the date and time the test was started, the patient's name, the reason for the test, and the maternal vital signs.
- Schedule appropriate follow-up; the typical interval for testing is biweekly or weekly, depending on indication.

Vibroacoustic Stimulation

Vibroacoustic stimulation (VAS, also referred to as *fetal vibroacoustic stimulation*, is a screening tool that uses auditory stimulation (with an artificial larynx) to assess fetal well-being with EFM when NST is nonreactive. Vibroacoustic stimulation may be effective in eliciting a change in fetal behavior, fetal startle movements, and increased FHR variability. VAS is only used when the baseline rate is determined to be within normal limits. When deceleration or bradycardia is present, VAS is not an appropriate intervention (Gilbert, 2011).

Procedure

- VAS is conducted by activating an artificial larynx on the maternal abdomen near the fetal head for 1 second in conjunction with the NST. This can be repeated at 1-minute intervals up to three times.

Interpretation

- The NST using VAS is considered reactive when the FHR increases 15 beats above baseline for 15 seconds twice in 20 minutes.

Advantages

- Using VAS to stimulate the fetus has reduced the incidence of nonreactive NSTs and reduced the time required to conduct NSTs.
- It differentiates nonreactive NSTs caused by hypoxia from those associated with fetal sleep states.
- Using the VAS decreases the incidence of faults and findings of a nonreactive NST (AAP & ACOG, 2017).

Risks

- No adverse effects reported
- Not recommended as a routine procedure in high-risk pregnancies

Nursing Actions

- Explain the procedure to the woman and her family. The test uses a buzzer (in auditory stimulation) to assess fetal well-being.
- Position the patient in a semi-Fowler's or lateral position to avoid aortocaval compression.
- Provide comfort measures.
- Provide emotional support.
- Interpret FHR and accelerations and conduct VAS appropriately. Report results to the physician or midwife and document.
- Schedule appropriate follow-up.

Contraction Stress Test

The contraction stress test (CST is a screening tool to assess the ability of the fetus to maintain a normal FHR in response to UCs in women with a nonreactive NST at term gestation. The purpose of the CST is to identify a fetus that is at risk for compromise through observation of the fetal response to intermittent reduction of in utero placental blood flow associated with stimulated UCs (AAP & ACOG, 2017; Treanor, 2015).

Procedure

- Monitor FHR and fetal activity for 20 minutes.
- If no spontaneous UCs, contractions can be initiated in some women by having them brush the nipples for 10 minutes or with IV oxytocin.

Interpretation

- The CST is considered negative or normal when there are no significant variable decelerations or no late decelerations in a 10-minute strip with three UCs in more than 40 seconds, assessed with moderate variability.
- The CST is positive when there are late decelerations of FHR with 50% of UCs.
- A positive result has been associated with an increased rate of fetal death, fetal growth restriction, lower 5-minute Apgar scores, cesarean section, and the need for neonatal resuscitation due to neonatal depression. This requires further testing such as BPP.
- The CST is equivocal or suspicious when there are intermittent late or significant variable decelerations; further testing may be done, or the test may be repeated in 24 hours.

Advantages

- Negative CSTs are associated with good fetal outcomes.

Risks

- CST has a high false-positive rate, which can result in unnecessary intervention.
- It cannot be used with women who have a contraindication for uterine activity (conditions with an increased risk for preterm labor, bleeding, or uterine rupture).

Nursing Actions

- Explain the procedure to the woman and her family. The CST stimulates contractions to evaluate fetal reaction to the stress of contractions.
- Have patient void before testing.
- Position patient in a semi-Fowler's position.
- Monitor vitals before and every 15 minutes during the test.
- Provide comfort measures.
- Provide emotional support.
- Correctly interpret FHR and contractions.
- Safely administer oxytocin (i.e., avoid uterine tachysystole). Uterine tachysystole is defined as more than five UCs in 10 minutes, fewer than 60 seconds between contractions, or a contraction greater than 90 seconds.
- Recognize adverse effects of oxytocin.
- Schedule appropriate follow-up.

Amniotic Fluid Index

The AFI is a screening tool that measures the volume of amniotic fluid with ultrasound to assess fetal well-being and placental function. The amniotic fluid level is based on fetal urine production, which is the predominant source of amniotic fluid and is directly dependent on renal perfusion (Cypher, 2016). In prolonged fetal hypoxemia, blood is shunted away from the fetal kidneys to other vital organs. Persistent decreased blood flow to the fetal kidneys results in reduction of amniotic fluid production and oligohydramnios (AAP & ACOG, 2017). Used with NST, AFI is a strong indicator of fetal status, as it is accurate in detecting fetal hypoxia.

Procedure

- Ultrasound measurement of pockets of amniotic fluid in four quadrants of the uterine cavity via ultrasound

Interpretation of Results

- Average measurement in pregnancy is 8 cm to 24 cm (Cunningham et al., 2018).
- Abnormal AFI is below 5 cm. An AFI less than 5 cm is indicative of oligohydramnios, which is associated with increased prenatal mortality and a need for close maternal and fetal monitoring.
- Represented graphically: decreased uteroplacental perfusion → decreased fetal renal blood flow → decreased urine production → oligohydramnios
- An AFI above 24 cm is polyhydramnios, which may indicate fetal malformation such as NTDs, obstruction of the fetal gastrointestinal tract, or fetal hydrops.

Advantages

- AFI reflects placental function and perfusion to the fetus as well as overall fetal condition.

Risks

- None

Nursing Actions

- Explain the procedure to the woman and her family. This test uses ultrasound to measure the amount of amniotic fluid to assess fetal well-being and how well the placenta is working.
- Provide comfort measures.
- Provide emotional support.
- Schedule appropriate follow-up.
- Special training in obstetric ultrasound is required for evaluation of amniotic fluid volume (see Box 6-2).

Biophysical Profile

The BPP is an ultrasound assessment of fetal status along with an NST. The BPP was first introduced as an intrauterine Apgar score in response to a high proportion of false-positive NSTs and CSTs. It uses real-time ultrasound with EFM to assess five fetal variables: NST reactive, fetal movement, tone, breathing, and amniotic fluid volume. The combination accounts for acute changes in fetal reserve (NST, breathing, flexion, and extensions) as well as changes influenced over a more chronic time (amniotic fluid volume and fetal tone). If fetal oxygen consumption is reduced, the immediate fetal response is reduction of activity regulated by the CNS. The BPP provides improved prognostic information because physiological parameters associated with chronic and acute hypoxia are evaluated (AAP & ACOG, 2017). It is indicated in pregnancies involving increased risk of fetal hypoxia and placental insufficiency, such as maternal diabetes and hypertension. Some controversy exists related to this test, as a Cochrane Review concluded that available evidence from randomized clinical trials provides no support for the use of BPP as a test of fetal well-being in high-risk pregnancies (Grivell et al., 2012).

Procedure

- BPP consists of an NST with the addition of 30 minutes of ultrasound observation for five indicators: FHR reactivity, fetal breathing movements, fetal movement, fetal tone, and measurement of amniotic fluid.
  - NST reactive
  - Fetal breathing movements: One or more episodes of rhythmic breathing movements of 30 seconds or movement within 30 minutes is expected.
  - Fetal movement: Three or more discrete body or limb movements in 30 minutes are expected.
  - Fetal tone: One or more fetal extremity extensions with return to fetal flexion or opening and closing of the hand is expected within 30 minutes.
  - Amniotic fluid volume: A pocket of amniotic fluid that measures at least 2 cm in two planes perpendicular to each other is expected.

Interpretation

- A score of 2 (present) or 0 (absent) is assigned to each of the five components.
- A total score of 8/10 is reassuring.
- A score of 6/10 is equivocal and may indicate possible fetal asphyxia; may repeat testing in 12 to 24 hours of delivery, depending on gestational age.
- A score of 4/10 is nonreassuring, as it indicates probable fetal asphyxia and warrants further evaluation and consideration of delivery (AAP & ACOG, 2017, Cunningham et al., 2018).
- A score of 2/10 or lower indicates almost certain fetal asphyxia, which prompts immediate delivery.
- Fetal activity decreases or stops to reduce energy and oxygen consumption as fetal hypoxemia worsens. Decreased activity occurs in reverse order of normal development.
- Fetal activities that appear earliest in pregnancy (tone and movement) are usually the last to cease, and activities that are the last to develop are usually the first to be diminished (FHR variability) (Table 6-3).

Advantages

- Lower false-positive rate compared with other tests

Risks

- None

TABLE 6-3 Biophysical Profile Scoring

FETAL BIOPHYSICAL PROFILES	SCORE 2	SCORE 0
Movement	At least three episodes of trunk or limb movement	Fewer than three episodes of trunk or limb movement
Tone	At least one episode of active extension with return to flexion of the fetal limb or trunk; opening and closing of the hand is deemed normal tone	Absent movement or slow extension or flexion
Breathing movement	At least one breathing episode lasting a minimum of 30 seconds	Absent breathing movement or less than 30 seconds of sustained breathing movement
Amniotic fluid	At least one pocket of amniotic fluid that measures at least 2 cm in two perpendicular planes	Absent pockets of amniotic fluid that measure at least 2 cm in two perpendicular planes
Nonstress test (NST)	Reactive	Nonreactive

Cypher, 2016.

Nursing Actions

- Explain the procedure to the woman and her family. The BPP is an ultrasound evaluation of fetal status and involves observation of various fetal reflex activities.
- Provide comfort measures.
- Provide emotional support.
- Special training in obstetric ultrasound is required for interpretation of ultrasound components of the test (see Box 6-2).
- Schedule appropriate follow-up; the typical interval for testing is 1 week but for specific pregnancy complications, it may be biweekly.

Modified Biophysical Profile

The modified BPP combines an NST as an indicator of short-term fetal well-being and AFI as an indicator of long-term placental function to evaluate fetal well-being (AAP & ACOG, 2017). It is indicated in high-risk pregnancy related to maternal conditions or pregnancy-related conditions (see Table 6-1).

Procedure

- A modified BPP combines the use of an NST with an AFI.

Interpretation

- A modified BPP is considered normal when the NST is reactive and the amniotic fluid volume is greater than 2 cm in the deepest vertical pocket or if the AFI is normal.
- A modified BPP is considered abnormal if either the NST is nonreactive or the amniotic fluid volume is less than 2 cm in the deepest vertical pocket or if the AFI is less than 5.0.
- An AFI less than or equal to 5 is indicative of oligohydramnios. Oligohydramnios is associated with increased perinatal mortality, and decreased amniotic fluid may reflect acute or chronic fetal asphyxia (Treanor, 2015). Amniotic fluid volume changes more slowly over time as the fetus preferentially shunts cardiac output to the heart and brain while decreasing renal perfusion and thus fetal urine output, thereby decreasing the volume of amniotic fluid.

Advantages

- Less time to complete
- NST and AFI are considered most predictive of perinatal outcomes.

Risks

- None

Nursing Actions

- Explain the procedure to the woman and her family. A modified BPP is an NST and measurement of the amount of amniotic fluid.
- Provide comfort measures.
- Provide emotional support.

- Special training in ultrasound is required for interpretation of amniotic fluid volume (see Box 6-2).
- Schedule appropriate follow-up; the typical interval for testing is 1 week, but for specific pregnancy complications it may be biweekly.

ISSUES IN ANTEPARTAL TESTS

Responsible translation of reproductive and genetic technologies into prenatal care requires that all health-care professionals ensure women's informed decision making in clinical practice. Nurses have a professional and ethical responsibility to facilitate women's informed decision making regarding antenatal testing so they can make meaningful decisions about their health.

A recent study of women's experiences with prenatal testing indicates health literacy and the ability to actively engage with health-care providers are critical for informed decision making about prenatal testing. The findings highlight the need for woman-centered strategies to promote open and intentional communication about prenatal testing (Shea, 2020).

Interventions are needed to ensure access to comprehensive information about testing with assessment of women's understanding in a prenatal care environment that conveys understanding and nonjudgmental guidance throughout the decision-making process (Shea, 2020). As we continue advances in prenatal diagnosis and fetal therapy and genomic testing, more fetal anomalies will be diagnosed early in pregnancy. Parents will face more complex choices than they do today about terminating pregnancy, trying innovative fetal therapy, or waiting for postnatal treatment options. Many parents choose to terminate pregnancies after severe fetal anomalies have been diagnosed, but others choose to continue their pregnancies. The likely effect of better prenatal diagnosis will be that parents who learn that the fetus has congenital anomalies and choose not to terminate the pregnancy may require individualized treatment plans not only prenatally but during labor and birth, as well as postpartum, and their infants will require treatment in the NICU (Lantos, 2018).

Antenatal forecasts of fetal health have been widely investigated. However, the precision or efficacy of some tests can be limited. Additionally, a wide range of normal biological fetal variation makes interpretation of some tests challenging. In addition, some tests have a high false positive, leading the clinician to use antenatal tests to indicate fetal well-being rather than fetal disorders (Cunningham et al., 2018).

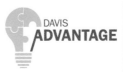

DAVIS ADVANTAGE | Go to Davis Advantage to complete your learning: strengthen understanding, apply your knowledge, and prepare for the Next Gen NCLEX®.

REFERENCES

Adams, E. (2021). Antenatal care. In K. Simpson, P. Creehan, N. O'Brien-Abel, C. Roth, A. J. Rohan, & Association of Women's Health, Obstetrics and Neonatal Nursing. *Perinatal nursing* (pp. 65–97). Wolters Kluwer.

Allyse, M., Minear, M. A., Berson, E., Sridhar, S., Rote, M., Hung, A., & Chandrasekharan, S. (2015). Non-invasive prenatal testing: A review of international implementation and challenges. *International Journal of Women's Health, 7,* 113–126. https://doi.org/10.2147/IJWH.S67124

American Academy of Pediatrics and the American College of Obstetricians and Gynecologists. (2017). *Guidelines for perinatal care* (8th ed.). Author.

American College of Obstetricians and Gynecologists. (2008). Ethical issues in genetic testing. ACOG Committee Opinion No. 410. *Obstetrics & Gynecology, 111,* 1495–1502.

American College of Obstetricians and Gynecologists. (2016a). Prenatal diagnostic testing for genetic disorders. ACOG Practice Bulletin 162. *Obstetrics & Gynecology, 127,* e108–e122.

American College of Obstetricians and Gynecologists. (2016b). Ultrasound in pregnancy. Practice Bulletin No. 175. *Obstetrics & Gynecology, 128,* e241–e256.

American College of Obstetricians and Gynecologists. (2017a). Counseling about genetic testing and communication of genetic test results. Committee Opinion No. 693. *Obstetrics & Gynecology, 129,* e96–e101.

American College of Obstetricians and Gynecologists. (2017b). Guidelines for diagnostic imaging during pregnancy and lactation. Committee Opinion No. 723. *Obstetrics & Gynecology, 130,* e210–e216.

American College of Obstetricians and Gynecologists. (2018a). Management of alloimmunization during pregnancy. ACOG Practice Bulletin No. 192. *Obstetrics & Gynecology, 131,* e82–e90.

American College of Obstetricians and Gynecologists. (2018b). Modern genetics in obstetrics and gynecology. ACOG Technology Assessment in Obstetrics and Gynecology No. 14. *Obstetrics & Gynecology, 132,* e143–e168.

American College of Obstetricians and Gynecologists. (2020). Screening for fetal chromosomal abnormalities. ACOG Practice Bulletin No. 226. *Obstetrics & Gynecology, 136,* e48–e69.

American College of Obstetricians and Gynecologists. (2021a). Fetal growth restriction. ACOG Practice Bulletin No. 227. *Obstetrics & Gynecology, 137,* e16–e28.

American College of Obstetricians and Gynecologists. (2021b). Informed consent and shared decision making in obstetrics and gynecology. ACOG Committee Opinion No. 819. *Obstetrics & Gynecology, 137,* e34–e41.

American Nurses Association. (2010). *Guide to the code of ethics for nurses.* Author.

Association of Women's Health, Obstetric and Neonatal Nurses. (2015). *Fetal heart rate monitoring: Principles and practice* (5th ed.). Author.

Association of Women's Health, Obstetric and Neonatal Nurses. (2016). *Ultrasound examinations performed by nurses in obstetric gynecologic and reproductive medicine settings: Clinical competencies and education guide* (4th ed.). Author.

Berkley, E., Chauhan, S. P., & Abuhamad, A.; with the assistance of Society for Maternal-Fetal Medicine Publications Committee. (2012). Doppler assessment of the fetus with intrauterine growth restriction. *American Journal of Obstertrics and Gynecology, 206,* 300–308. https://doi.org/10.1016/j.ajog.2012.01.022

Berry, S. M., Stone, J., Norton, M. E., Johnson, D., & Berghella, V. (2013). Fetal blood sampling. *Society for Maternal-Fetal Medicine, 209*(3), 170–180.

Cohen, E., Baerts, W., & van Bel, F. (2015). Brain-sparing in intrauterine growth restriction: Considerations for the neonatologist. *Neonatology, 108,* 269–276.

Conde-Agudelo, A., Villar, J., Kennedy, S. H., & Papageorghiou, A. T. (2018). Predictive accuracy of cerebroplacental ratio for adverse perinatal and neurodevelopmental outcomes in suspected fetal growth restriction: Systematic review and meta-analysis. *Ultrasound in Obstetrics and Gynecology, 52*(4). https://doi.org/10.1002/uog.19117

Cunningham, F., Leveno, K., Bloom, S., Dashe, J., Hoffman, B., Casey, B., & Spong, C. (2018). *Williams obstetrics* (25th ed.). McGraw-Hill.

Cypher, R. (2016). Antepartal fetal surveillance and prenatal diagnosis. In S. Mattson & J. Smith (Eds.), *Core curriculum for maternal-newborn nursing* (5th ed., pp. 135–158). Elsevier.

Everett, T., & Peebles, D. (2015). Antenatal tests of fetal wellbeing. *Seminars in Fetal and Neonatal Medicine, 20*(3), 138–143.

Gilbert, E. (2011). *Manual of high risk pregnancy and delivery* (6th ed.). C. V. Mosby.

Grivell, R., Wong, L., & Bhatia, V. (2012). Regimens of fetal surveillance for impaired fetal growth. *Cochrane Database of Systematic Reviews, 13*(6), CD007113. https://doi.org/10.1002/14651858.CD007113.pub3

Lantos, J. D. (2018). Ethical problems in decision making in the neonatal ICU. *New England Journal of Medicine, 379*(19), 1851–1860.

Olsen, D. P., & Brous, E. (2018). The ethical and legal implications of a nurse's arrest in Utah. *American Journal of Nursing, 118*(3), 47–53. https://doi.org/10.1097/01.NAJ.0000530938.88865.7f

Rock, M. J., & Hoebeke, R. (2014). Informed consent: Whose duty to inform? *MEDSURG Nursing, 23*(3), 189–194.

Shea, T. (2020). Informed decision making regarding prenatal aneuploidy screening. *Journal of Obstetric, Gynecologic & Neonatal Nursing, 49*(1), 41–54. https://doi.org/10.1016/j.jogn.2019.11.001

Simpson, L. L. (2013). Twin–twin transfusion syndrome. *American Journal of Obstetrics and Gynecology, 208*(1), 3–18. https://doi.org/10.1016/j.ajog.2012.10.880

Treanor, C. (2015). Antenatal fetal assessment and testing. In *Fetal heart rate monitoring: Principles and practice* (5th ed.). Association of Women's Health, Obstetrics and Neonatal Nursing.

Complications of Pregnancy

7

Roberta F. Durham, RN, PhD
Rachael Miller, RN, BSN

LEARNING OUTCOMES

Upon completion of this chapter, the student will be able to:

1. Describe the primary complications of pregnancy and related nursing and medical care.
2. Delineate clinical features indicative of pregnancy complications and tests to predict, screen for, diagnose, and manage pregnancy complications.
3. Identify potential pregnancy complications for the woman, the fetus, and the newborn.
4. Formulate a plan of care that includes the physical, emotional, and psychosocial needs of women diagnosed with pregnancy complications.
5. Describe the key aspects of teaching for women with antenatal complications.
6. Demonstrate understanding of knowledge related to preexisting medical conditions impacting pregnancy and related management.

CONCEPTS

Addiction
Collaboration
Communication
Evidence-Based Practice
Family
Grief and Loss
Health Promotion
Immunity
Infection
Mood and Affect
Oxygenation
Perfusion
Population Health
Safety
Self-Care
Stress and Coping
Teaching and Learning

Nursing Diagnosis

- Risk for disturbed maternal fetal dyad
- Risk of maternal injury related to pregnancy complications
- Risk for ineffective family coping related to high-risk pregnancy
- Risk of maternal injury related to preexisting medical conditions
- Disturbance in self-esteem or self-identity related to high-risk pregnancy
- Risk of maternal stress related to pregnancy complications

Nursing Outcomes

- The woman will understand warning signs and management of pregnancy complications.
- The family exhibits a pattern of management of adaptive tasks by family involved with the pregnancy challenges.
- The woman and her family will receive adequate support related to high-risk pregnancy and disruption in family functioning.

Continued

Nursing Diagnosis—cont'd

- Interrupted family process
- Powerlessness related to uncertain pregnancy outcome
- Risk of fetal injury related to complications of pregnancy
- Caregiver role strain

Nursing Outcomes—cont'd

- The woman will verbalize acceptance and understanding of pregnancy complications and management of pregnancy complications.
- The family exhibits a pattern of family function that supports the family's well-being.
- The woman reports a perception that her actions do significantly impact outcomes and participates in decisions related to management of pregnancy complications.
- The woman will give birth to a healthy infant without complications.

INTRODUCTION

This chapter presents information on key complications and high-risk conditions that can occur during pregnancy and pre-existing medical conditions that pregnancy may exacerbate. An overview of each complication is presented, including underlying pathophysiology, risk factors, risks posed to the woman and fetus, and typical medical management and nursing actions.

The nature of perinatal nursing is unpredictable, and pregnancy complications can arise abruptly, resulting in rapid deterioration of maternal and fetal status. It is imperative that nurses understand the underlying physiological mechanisms of pregnancy, the impact of complications on maternal and fetal well-being, and current interventions to optimize maternal and fetal outcomes. Pregnancy complications can have profound effects on the physical, emotional, and psychosocial health of women and their newborns both during and beyond pregnancy, ultimately increasing future health risks for women and their children. Nurses have a significant collaborative and direct role in the care of women with pregnancy complications. Nurses can optimize outcomes for women and newborns by providing safe care during the perinatal period and acting as advocates for women and families during the difficult perinatal period. They are the members of the health-care team who are most present with mothers and newborns, and they can provide the ongoing surveillance needed for women with complicated and challenging high-risk pregnancies (Phillips & Boyd, 2016).

GESTATIONAL COMPLICATIONS

Although most pregnant women experience a normal pregnancy, various complications can develop that affect maternal and fetal well-being. When women experience these pregnancy complications, astute assessment, rapid intervention, and a collaborative team approach are essential to optimize maternal and neonatal outcomes. In this section, complications related to pregnancy are presented along with the physiological and pathological basis for the most common complications of pregnancy. Nursing care and appropriate management are discussed.

Risk Assessment

A high-risk pregnancy is one of greater risk to the mother or her fetus than an uncomplicated pregnancy. Pregnancy places additional physical and emotional stress on a woman's body. Health problems that occur before a woman becomes pregnant or during pregnancy may also increase the likelihood for a high-risk pregnancy. The goal of risk assessment is to identify pregnant women at risk for developing complications and promote risk-appropriate care that will enhance maternal and fetal outcomes. These factors include demographic, medical, obstetric, sociocultural, lifestyle, and environmental risks.

Risk assessment tools have poor predictive value but can be helpful in distinguishing between women at high and low risk for complications. However, no cause-and-effect relationship between risk factors and poor outcomes has been established. For example, up to one-third of women who develop complications may not have identifiable risk factors. Additionally, the underlying causes of some complications, such as preterm labor (PTL) and intrauterine growth restriction (IUGR), are not fully understood. Racial and ethnic disparities exist for multiple adverse obstetric outcomes and do not appear to be explained by differences in patient characteristics (Grobman et al., 2015). The prevalence of preterm birth (PTB), fetal growth restriction, fetal demise, maternal mortality, and inadequate receipt of prenatal care all vary by maternal race and ethnicity. These disparities have their roots in maternal health behaviors, genetics, the physical and social environments, and access to and quality of health care (Bryant et al., 2010).

It is well-established that marked racial and ethnic disparities exist in maternal outcomes. These disparities have persisted for years related to a variety of factors, including those within and beyond the day-to-day control of health-care systems and the providers who work within these systems (Howell et al., 2018). The persistent nature and multifactorial, complex origins of these disparities are not beyond the capacity of the health-care system to improve or eliminate; however, we must acknowledge a portion of the disparities arise within and are potentially modifiable by the health system. Nurses can work toward remediation of these disparities.

The Council on Patient Safety in Women's Health Care disseminates patient safety bundles to help reduce variation and facilitate the standardization process. A concept introduced by the Institute for Healthcare Improvement, our patient safety bundles, are built upon established best-practices and designed to be universally implementable. One of the safety bundles on reduction of peripartum racial and ethnic disparities provides excellent resources for further information and strategies to reduce disparities and can be accessed at https://safehealthcareforeverywoman.org /aim/patient-safety-bundles/#core (Council on Patient Safety in Women's Health Care, 2016).

Awareness of broader contexts that influence health supports respectful, patient-centered care that incorporates lived experiences, optimizes health outcomes, improves communication, and can help reduce health and health-care inequities (American College of Obstetricians and Gynecologists [ACOG], Committee on Health Care for Underserved Women, 2018d). Researchers have demonstrated how the environmental conditions in which people are born, live, work, and age play an equally important role in health outcomes. These social determinants of health (SDOH) are shaped by historical, social, political, and economic forces and help explain the relationship between environmental conditions and individual health. Recognizing the importance of SDOH can help nurses better understand patients, effectively communicate about health-related conditions and behavior, and improve health outcomes (ACOG, Committee on Health Care for Underserved Women, 2018d).

Birth Equity

Birth equity advocates focus on redressing structural racism and social determinants through systems-level initiatives to improve maternal and infant health (March of Dimes [MOD], 2018b). They propose we have an incomplete understanding of the role of race, racism, and structural factors in creating disparities in birth outcomes, even sometimes blaming individual mothers for poor birth outcomes. However, evidence suggests social rather than behavioral causes of disparities in birth outcomes, with many social and structural factors contributing to disparities.

Public health researchers have been taking a closer look at birth outcomes to identify the effects of the health environment, which includes factors such as access to quality medical care, housing, transportation, safe neighborhoods, and nutrition. Overall national statistics reveal a troubling picture: America's health environment begins to negatively affect Black children from the earliest stages of life (Sweetland, 2018). For instance, PTB, which comes with serious health risks, is about 50% higher among Blacks than Whites (MOD, 2018b).

Some hypothesize that chronic and severe adversity floods the body with dangerous levels of stress hormones, a condition known as toxic stress. Toxic stress has been proposed as a driving factor behind the higher rates of premature birth in the Black community. Research indicates preventive and supportive group prenatal care can reduce PTB among Black women (MOD, 2018b).

Other suggestions include strategies as first steps in reversing historical patterns of poor sexual and reproductive health outcomes among Black women: (1) ensure strategies focus on culturally and contextually appropriate research and prevention, (2) ensure equal access to effective sexual health information and quality health-care services, (3) support quality education and training for public health professionals, and (4) support policies that promote sexual and reproductive health equity (Prather et al., 2018).

BOX 7-1 | Common Risk Factors

A high-risk pregnancy is one that threatens the health or life of the mother or her fetus. For most women, early and regular prenatal care promotes a healthy pregnancy and delivery without complications. But some women are at an increased risk for complications even before they get pregnant for a variety of reasons. Risk factors for a high-risk pregnancy can include:

- Existing health conditions, such as high blood pressure, diabetes, or being HIV-positive
- A history of prior pregnancy complications
- Complications that arise during pregnancy, such as gestational diabetes or preeclampsia
- Being overweight or obese
- Carrying more than one fetus (twins and higher-order multiples)
- Being 18 or younger, or older than 35
- Advanced maternal age increases the risk due to preexisting health problems and increased risk of preeclampsia and diabetes.

The risk for poor birth outcomes as a consequence of SDOH begins long before pregnancy and childbirth. The accumulation of environmental exposures, starting in utero, may determine differential risks and protection for health outcomes across the life course. In the case of pregnancy and inequity, studies suggest that repeated stress that accumulates over time triggers responses leading to early birth (Jackson et al., 2020). The "weathering" over time from constant assaults of inequity places a woman at risk of an adverse pregnancy outcome (Geronimus, 1992), conferring risk for compromised health upon her infant throughout life. The study of epigenetics builds on these associations by exploring gene expression based on environmental changes and considering the multigenerational impact of these biological changes (National Academies of Sciences, Engineering, and Medicine [NASEM], 2019). Further examination in this growing area is needed.

Common risk factors are presented in Box 7-1. Specific risk factors are discussed related to each complication presented.

CRITICAL COMPONENT

Nursing Activities to Promote Adaptation to Pregnancy Complications

Pregnancy complications represent a threat to both the woman's and fetus's health and to the emotional well-being of the family. Assessment of emotional status and coping of the entire family is necessary to provide comprehensive care. Implementing an individualized plan of care will facilitate the family's transition during an often unexpected and frightening experience. Responses to high-risk pregnancy can include:

- Stress and anxiety about the maternal illness and its effect on the fetus, as well as the disruption to their home- and work-related activities.

Continued

CRITICAL COMPONENT—cont'd

- Threats to self-esteem; the woman may feel she has somehow failed as a woman or is failing as a mother. Self-blaming commonly occurs for real or imagined wrongdoing.
- Disappointment and frustration often occur when goals of having a healthy pregnancy, a normal birth, and a healthy baby are impeded by a pregnancy complication.
- Conflict can occur when competing and opposing goals are present during high-risk pregnancy.
- Crisis occurs when the woman and her family are threatened by a pregnancy complication and an uncertain outcome.

General nursing actions include the following:

- Provide time for the woman and family to express their concerns and feelings, which may include apprehension, fear, anger, disappointment, and frustration. Talking can help them identify, analyze, and understand their experience and fears. Practice active listening.
- Provide information repeatedly with the patient and significant other(s) to facilitate a realistic appraisal of events. That includes explaining high-risk conditions, procedures, diagnostic tests, and treatment plans in layman's terms, providing ongoing updates, and clarifying misconceptions. Discussing the underlying causes of a complication with the woman may help to alleviate feelings of self-blaming and guilt.
- Facilitate referrals related to the condition, which may include social services and chaplain services to enhance family coping and provide resources.
- Encourage the woman and her family to participate in decision making and express preferences to enhance autonomy and patient-centered care.
- Remember childbearing women have a vested interest in their pregnancy and outcome, and they know their bodies, their preferences, their concerns, and their fears. Make efforts to meet their needs and desires. Communication and shared decision making improve outcomes.
- If the patient is hospitalized, have flexible guidelines for the family to minimize separation.
- Be a skilled communicator; take the emotional "temperature" in the room and convey an accurate assessment of the psychological state of the patient and family.
- Be a witness to events, which can help during debriefing and patient processing in high-risk situations.
- Consistently noted as members of one of the most trusted professions, nurses play an invaluable role in leading and supporting efforts to increase access to care for all women, regardless of their race, socioeconomic status, or environment.
- Nurses should be aware of barriers that affect health-care access and strive to reduce disparities through advocacy work with organizations such as the Association of Women's Health, Obstetric and Neonatal Nurses (AWHONN), with state and federal legislators, and within their communities.
- Nurses can also provide support, information, and referrals to women from underserved communities.

Preterm Labor and Birth

Preterm labor (PTL) is defined as regular contractions of the uterus resulting in changes in the cervix before 37 weeks of gestation. In the United States, approximately 10% of all live births occur before term, and PTL preceded approximately 50% of these preterm births (PTB). PTB is defined as birth between 20 0/7 weeks of gestation and 37 0/7 weeks of gestation. Preterm is less than 37 weeks and 0 days and late preterm is 34 weeks and 0 days through 36 weeks and 6 days (American Academy of Pediatrics [AAP] & ACOG, 2017). The U.S. PTB rate rose to 10.02% in 2018, a 1% rise from 2017, and the fourth straight year of increases in this rate (Martin et al., 2019). The increase in the PTB rate among births to White mothers between 2017 and 2018 (9.05% to 9.09%) was not statistically significant, but rates also rose among births to Black (from 13.93% to 14.13%) and Hispanic mothers (9.62% to 9.73%). In 2018, PTB rates ranged from a high of 14.13% among births to Black mothers to a low of 8.57% among Asian mothers. This means PTB rates remain 50% higher among Black women and 20% higher among American Indian/Alaska Native women compared with White women (MOD, 2018b).

The reason for the significant differences in PTB rates between racial groups is poorly understood. However, a leading hypothesis relates to underlying social and economic inequalities. Individual as well as neighborhood poverty, limited maternal education, and stress are all associated with an increased risk of PTB, yet how these factors interact with each other and modify the relationship between race and PTB is not well-established (Frey & Klebanoff, 2016). Collective research suggests that whereas social factors associated with an increased risk of PTB are more prevalent among Black individuals, maternal race is independently associated with PTB in ways we don't yet understand. Some argue that the widely used measures of socioeconomic status do not adequately capture the pervasive effect that discrimination and economic hardship have on the lives of minority women (Frey & Klebanoff, 2016).

PTB is the leading cause of neonatal mortality and the most common reason for antenatal hospitalization (AAP & ACOG, 2017). Although causes of PTB are not well-understood, the burden is clear—PTBs account for approximately 70% of neonatal deaths and 36% of infant deaths as well as 25% to 50% of cases of long-term neurologic impairment in children. An inverse relationship exists between gestational age at delivery and the risk of neonatal morbidity and mortality (Frey & Klebanoff, 2016). Average expenditures for premature or low birth weight (LBW) infants were more than 10 times as high as those for uncomplicated newborns (MOD, 2015). Preterm infants have some of the highest health-care expenditures of any patient population. In one study, infants with a diagnosis of preterm status (less than 37 weeks) incurred medical expenditures of $76,153 on average, and infants born at 24 weeks' gestation had the highest per infant average expenditures of $603,778 (Beam et al., 2020). These estimates do not consider economic challenges faced by families in long-term care of a disabled child, including out-of-pocket expenses and lost wages. However, the financial burden is only one aspect of the "cost" of PTB within families. Changes experienced by families after the birth of a preterm infant, particularly if the child was born extremely prematurely or has long-term disabilities, can be substantial.

In the 2020 Report Card, the MOD (2020) gave the United States a grade of C– on the latest key indicators of maternal and infant health. PTB and its complications are the second largest contributor to infant death in the United States, and PTB rates have been increasing for 5 years.

Identifying women who will give birth preterm is an inexact science. Researchers describe PTB as a complex cluster of problems with overlapping factors of influence. Its causes may include individual behavioral and psychosocial factors, neighborhood characteristics, environmental exposures, medical conditions, infertility treatments, biological factors, and genetics. Many of these factors occur in combination, particularly in those who are socioeconomically disadvantaged or who are members of racial and ethnic minority groups. Approximately three-quarters of all PTBs occur spontaneously, and the remainder result from medical intervention (ACOG, 2016b). Most PTBs are a result of spontaneous PTL; however, 25% of PTBs are intentional, necessary, and indicated for problems such as hypertension, preeclampsia, hemorrhage, and IUGR where early delivery would improve either maternal or fetal status. There are three main situations in which PTL and premature birth may occur (ACOG, 2012, 2021).

Spontaneous PTL and birth refers to unintentional, unplanned delivery before the 37th week of pregnancy. The pathophysiological events that trigger PTL are largely unknown but may include decidual hemorrhage (abruption), mechanical factors such as uterine overdistention or cervical incompetence, hormonal changes indicated by fetal or maternal stress, infection, and inflammation (AAP & ACOG, 2017). A history of delivering preterm is one of the strongest predictors for subsequent PTBs.

- Medically indicated PTB. In this case, the health-care provider recommends preterm delivery due to the existence of a serious medical condition such as preeclampsia. In these cases, health-care providers often take steps to keep the baby in the womb as long as possible to allow additional growth and development, while monitoring the mother and fetus for health issues. Providers also use additional interventions, such as steroids, to help improve outcomes for the baby.
- Non-medically indicated (elective) preterm delivery. Some late PTBs result from inducing labor or having a cesarean delivery in the absence of a medical reason to do so, even though this practice is not recommended. Research indicates that even babies born at 37 or 38 weeks of pregnancy are at higher risk for poor health outcomes than babies born at 39 weeks of pregnancy or later. Therefore, unless there are medical problems, health-care providers should wait until at least 39 weeks of pregnancy to induce labor or perform a cesarean delivery to prevent possible health problems.

Knowledge of the limitations of classification of spontaneous or inducted PTB has led multiple groups to propose new classification systems based on phenotype rather than

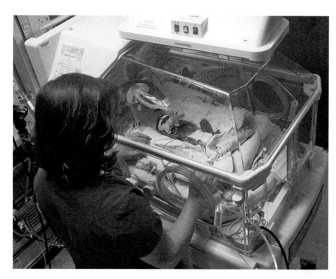

FIGURE 7–1 Premature infant in the NICU.

gestational age, risk factors, or clinical presentation, although more work is needed on this new classification (Frey & Klebanoff, 2016). The discussion in this section focuses on spontaneous PTL.

A preterm or premature infant is born before 37 weeks (36 6/7 weeks) of gestation (Fig. 7–1). More specific classifications of prematurity include (PeriStats, 2017):

- Late preterm infant: An infant born between 34 and 37 weeks of gestation (34 0/7 to 36 6/7 weeks)
- Very preterm infant: An infant born before 32 completed weeks of gestation
- Viability: The threshold for viability is at 25 and, rarely, fewer completed weeks of gestation (ACOG, 2016b)
- Periviability: Approximately 0.5% of all births occur before the third trimester of pregnancy, and these very early deliveries result in the majority of neonatal deaths and more than 40% of infant deaths. Periviable birth is delivery occurring from 20 0/7 weeks to 25 6/7 weeks of gestation (ACOG, 2017f)

Long-term sequelae for preterm infants include cerebral palsy, hearing and vision impairment, and chronic lung disease. Long-term costs include not only health-care costs but also special education costs for learning problems, costs of developmental services, and health-care costs for long-term sequelae associated with prematurity. Survival rates for extremely preterm or extremely LBW newborns born at the threshold of viability (25 or fewer completed weeks of gestation) have certainly improved in the last three decades, largely as the result of a greater use of assisted ventilation in the delivery room and surfactant therapy and increased use of antenatal and neonatal corticosteroids. However, this improvement in survival has not been associated with an equal improvement in morbidity. The incidence of chronic lung disease, sepsis, and poor growth remains high and may even have increased.

Concern exists that treatment of extremely preterm and extremely LBW newborns may result in unforeseen effects into adulthood, and that the neurodevelopmental outcome and cognitive function of extremely preterm and extremely LBW infants may be suboptimal (ACOG, 2016b; ACOG, 2017a). The goal to reduce the PTB rate to 9.4%, championed by *Healthy People 2020* and the MOD, was not achieved and remains the goal set for *Healthy People 2030* (Office of Disease Prevention and Health Promotion, Office of the Assistant Secretary for Health, Office of the Secretary, U.S. Department of Health and Human Services, 2020).

Pathophysiological Pathways of Preterm Labor

The causes of PTL and premature birth are numerous, complex, and only partly understood. Medical, psychosocial, and biological factors may all play a role in PTL and birth (Parfitt, 2021). Spontaneous PTB may be characterized by a syndrome composed of several components including uterine (PTL), chorio-amnionic-decidual (premature rupture of membranes [PROM]), and cervical (cervical insufficiency) (Owen & Harger, 2007). Yet the specific causes of spontaneous PTL and delivery are largely unknown.

PTL is characterized as a series of complex interactions of factors. No single factor acts alone, but multiple factors interact to initiate a cascade of events that result in PTL and birth (Parfitt, 2021). The pathways to PTB are thought to be multicausal and related to various contributing factors (Iams, 2007; MOD, 2018c). There are many pathways from risk factors to the terminal cascade of events resulting in labor. PTL likely occurs when local uterine factors prematurely stimulate this cascade or when suppressive factors that inhibit the cascade and maintain uterine quiescence are withdrawn prematurely. The four major factors leading to PTL are excessive uterine stretch or distention, decidual hemorrhage, intrauterine infection, and maternal or fetal stress. Uteroplacental vascular insufficiency, exaggerated inflammatory response, hormonal factors, cervical insufficiency or cervical remodeling, and genetic predisposition also play a role (Fig. 7–2), including:

- Excessive uterine stretch or distention
  - Prostaglandins can be produced, stimulating the uterus to contract when overdistended from multiple gestation, polyhydramnios, or uterine abnormalities.

- Decidual activation
  - From hemorrhage
  - From fetal-decidual paracrine system
  - From upper genital tract infection
- Premature activation of the normal physiological initiators of labor and activation of the maternal-fetal hypothalamic–pituitary adrenal (HPA) axis.
- Inflammation and infection in the decidua, fetal membranes, and amniotic fluid are associated with PTB.
- Prenatal stress has been associated with contributing to the development of PTL.

Inflammatory cytokines or bacterial endotoxins can stimulate prostaglandin release, resulting in cervical ripening, contractions, and weakening and ROM. Stress and psychosocial factors are also hypothesized to contribute to a stress response that results in uterine contractions (UCs). Studies of chronic and catastrophic stress exposures are suggestive of an association between stress and PTB. The search for a biological explanation for the pathways through which stress might affect PTB risk has led to extensive literature on the role of corticotropin-releasing hormone (CRH) as a potential mediator of this relationship. Although some studies have shown higher levels of CRH in women destined to have a PTB, these findings have not been consistent. It remains likely, however, that neuroendocrine pathways underlie the relationship between acute and chronic stressors on PTB and LBW risk (Grobman et al., 2015). Because we do not know what triggers normal labor at term, it is difficult to know what causes PTL. Extensive research has been conducted over the past three decades to predict which women are at risk to deliver preterm so that intensive interventions can be implemented to prevent prematurity.

Risk Factors for Preterm Labor and Birth

Despite its use for decades, risk factor assessment alone has a limited utility for identifying who will deliver preterm. Fifty percent of women who deliver preterm have no risk factors, and 70% of women who are at risk for preterm delivery deliver at term. Research indicates a complex interplay of multiple risk factors is responsible for preterm deliveries (PeriStats, 2017).

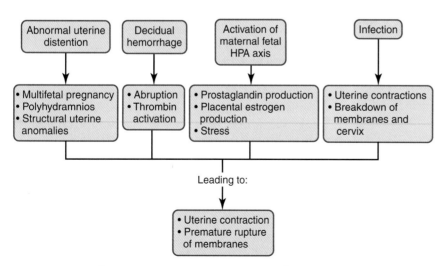

FIGURE 7–2 Pathophysiological pathways for preterm labor.

A host of behavioral, psychosocial, sociodemographic, medical, biological, and pregnancy conditions are associated with risk for PTB (MOD, 2018c). The most consistently identified risk factors include a history of PTB; for example, the additive risk associated with multiple prior PTBs is especially evident when early PTBs are considered. Women with one prior preterm delivery before 35 weeks have a 16% recurrence risk, those with two early preterm deliveries have a 41% risk, and those with three prior preterm deliveries have a 67% risk of subsequent PTB before 35 weeks (U.S. Department of Health and Human Services [DHHS], 2018). However, data are inconsistent about whether those risk factors cause PTB (AAP & ACOG, 2017).

The three most common risk factors for PTB are (Parfitt, 2021):

- Prior PTB (single most important factor, with reoccurrence rates of up to 40%)
- Multiple gestation (50% of twins delivered preterm, 90% or more higher multiples delivered preterm)
- Uterine or cervical abnormalities, shortened cervical length, history of diethylstilbestrol (DES) exposure

Other risk factors include (ACOG, 2016b):

- Fetal anomalies
- History of second-trimester loss, incompetent cervix, or cervical insufficiency
- IVF pregnancy
- Hydramnios or oligohydramnios
- Infection, especially genitourinary infections and periodontal disease
- Premature ROM
- Short pregnancy interval (less than 9 months)
- Pregnancy-associated problems such as hypertension, diabetes, and vaginal bleeding
- Chronic health problems such as hypertension, diabetes, abnormal lipid metabolism, or clotting disorders
- Inadequate nutrition, low body mass index (BMI), low pre-pregnancy weight, or poor weight gain
- Age younger than 17 or older than 35
- Late or no prenatal care
- Obesity, high BMI, or excessive weight gain
  - Working long hours, long periods of standing
  - Genetics has been an increasing focus of research and is hoped to explain up to 30% of spontaneous prematurity (Zhang et al., 2017).
  - Ancestry and ethnicity
    - PTB rates are highest for Black infants (13.3% vs. 9.6%). In the United States, the PTB rate among Black women is 48% higher than the rate among all other women (MOD, 2018a).
  - Maternal unmarried status is associated with an increased risk of PTB as well as low birth weight and small for gestational age (Shah et al., 2011).
  - PTB is more likely in the presence of intimate partner violence (IPV), mental health issues, substance abuse, and other psychosocial stressors (MOD, 2018b).
    - Maternal exposure to domestic violence is associated with significantly increased risk of LBW and PTB. Inadequate prenatal care, higher incidence of high-risk behaviors, direct physical trauma, stress, and neglect are possible mechanisms (Shah & Shah, 2010).
- Lack of social support
- Smoking, alcohol, and illicit drug use
- Lower education and socioeconomic status, poverty

Spontaneous PTB includes birth that follows PTL, preterm spontaneous ROM, and cervical insufficiency, but does not include indicated preterm delivery for maternal or fetal conditions (ACOG, 2012). Most PTBs (75%) are a result of spontaneous PTL (40%) or preterm premature rupture of membrane (PPROM) (35%) and related diagnoses (Iams, 2007; Owen & Harger, 2007). However, 25% of PTBs are clinically indicated for complications and are therefore medically indicated PTB.

SAFE AND EFFECTIVE NURSING CARE: Patient Education

Prevention of Preterm Birth

There are things you can teach your patient and her family to reduce her risk for early labor and birth. Some risk factors are things one can't change, such as having a premature birth in a previous pregnancy. However, others are things a woman can do something about, such as quitting smoking. Here are some suggestions from the MOD (2018b) for what a woman can do to reduce her risk for PTL and premature birth:

- Get to a healthy weight before pregnancy and gain the right amount of weight during pregnancy. Review the right amount of weight for her before and during pregnancy.
- Don't smoke, drink alcohol, use street drugs, or abuse prescription drugs. Ask your patient about substance and alcohol use and provide information about programs that can help.
- Go to your first prenatal care checkup as soon as you think you're pregnant. During pregnancy, encourage your patient to go to all her prenatal care checkups, even if she is feeling fine. Explain prenatal care helps make sure you and your baby are healthy.
- Get treated for chronic health conditions such as high blood pressure, diabetes, depression, and thyroid problems. Depression is a medical condition in which strong feelings of sadness last for a long time and interfere with daily life. It needs treatment to get better. All health problems need monitoring during pregnancy.
- Protect yourself from infections. Talk about vaccinations that can help protect the woman from certain infections. Remind everyone to wash their hands with soap and water after using the bathroom or blowing your nose. Remind women to not eat raw meat, fish, or eggs. Have safe sex. Don't touch cat feces or clean the litterbox.
- Reduce your stress. Encourage every woman to eat and do something active every day; ask family and friends for help around the house or in taking care of other children; and seek

Continued

help if your partner abuses you. If appropriate, suggest that your patient talk with her boss about how to lower stress at work.

- Wait at least 18 months between giving birth and getting pregnant again. Suggest to your patient the benefits of using birth control until she is ready to get pregnant again.

Prediction and Detection of Preterm Labor

Early detection of pregnant women who will give birth prematurely has been extensively researched since the 1970s with few definitive findings. No screening methods have been found consistently effective. Tests for PTB prediction include biomarkers for decidual membrane separation, such as fetal fibronectin; proteomics to identify inflammatory activity; and genomics for susceptibility for PTB. Since 1998, cervical length, bacterial vaginosis, and presence of fetal fibronectin in cervicovaginal fluid have been identified as factors most strongly linked to risk of spontaneous PTBs. Biochemical tests such as fetal fibronectin and placental alpha microglobulin-1 (PAMG-1) can reduce unnecessary hospital admissions, transfer of care, and medical interventions (Di Renzo et al., 2017).

- Transvaginal cervical ultrasonography
  - In symptomatic women, a cervical length of greater than 30 mm reliably excludes PTL.
  - A cervical length of less than 25 mm has strong positive predictive value.
- A recent systematic review and meta-analysis evaluated the accuracy of the placental alpha microglobulin-1 (PAMG-1), PartoSure, to predict PTB in women with symptoms of PTL and reported cervical PAMG-1 had a high accuracy to predict PTB within 7 and 14 days of testing in symptomatic pregnant women (Pirjani et al., 2019).
- Fetal fibronectin has a low positive predictive value but a high negative predictive value, thereby making it a useful test to predict those women who will NOT deliver preterm.

Risks for the Woman Related to Preterm Labor and Birth

- Complications related to treatment with tocolytics such as cardiac arrhythmias, pulmonary edema, and even congestive heart failure

Risks for the Fetus and Newborn Related to Preterm Labor and Birth

- Complications of prematurity and long-term sequelae associated with prematurity (see Chapter 17)

Assessment Findings

Criteria for the diagnosis of PTL have varied, and there is no universal agreement on criteria. Signs or symptoms a woman may experience include:

- Change in type of vaginal discharge (watery, mucus, or bloody)
- Increase in amount of discharge
- Pelvic or lower abdominal pressure
- Constant low, dull backache
- Mild abdominal cramps, with or without diarrhea
- Regular or frequent contractions or uterine tightening, often painless
- Possible ruptured membranes

CRITICAL COMPONENT

Diagnosis of Preterm Labor

PTB is defined as birth between 20 0/7 weeks of gestation and 36 6/7 weeks of gestation. The diagnosis of PTL generally is based on clinical criteria of regular UCs accompanied by a change in cervical dilation, effacement, or both, or initial presentation with regular contractions and cervical dilation of at least 2 cm (ACOG, 2016b). Less than 10% of women with the clinical diagnosis of PTL actually give birth within 7 days of presentation. It is important to recognize that PTL with intact membranes is not the only cause of PTB; numerous PTBs are preceded by either rupture of membranes (ROM) or other medical problems necessitating delivery.

Medical Management

Historically, nonpharmacological treatments to prevent PTBs in women with PTL have included bedrest, abstention from intercourse and orgasm, and hydration. These approaches are no longer recommended as evidence for their effectiveness is lacking and adverse effects have been reported (ACOG, 2016b). Identifying women with PTL who ultimately will give birth preterm is difficult. Approximately 30% of PTL spontaneously resolves and 50% of patients hospitalized for PTL actually give birth at term. Interventions to reduce the likelihood of delivery should be reserved for women with PTL at a gestational age at which a delay in delivery will provide benefit to the newborn. Because tocolytic therapy generally is effective for up to 48 hours, only women with fetuses that would benefit from a 48-hour delay in delivery should receive tocolytic treatment (ACOG, 2016b). Management now focuses on delaying delivery for 48 to 72 hours to administer antenatal steroids and allow time to facilitate fetal lung maturity.

Medical management includes the following measures:

- Tocolytic drugs are medications used to suppress uterine contractions (UC) in PTL. The evidence supports the use of first-line tocolytic treatment with beta-adrenergic agonist therapy, calcium channel blockers, or nonsteroidal anti-inflammatory drugs (NSAIDs) for short-term prolongation of pregnancy (up to 48 hours) to allow for the administration of antenatal steroids (ACOG, 2016b). These agents have drawbacks and potential serious adverse effects (Table 7-1). A review of evidence on tocolytic therapy revealed a small improvement in pregnancy prolongation and that extended use has little or no value (Dodd et al., 2006; Han et al., 2010). Interventions to reduce the likelihood of delivery should be reserved for women with PTL at a gestational age at which a delay in delivery will provide benefit to the newborn. Tocolytic therapy is typically administered between 24 to 34 weeks' gestation.
- Women with preterm contractions without cervical change, especially those with a cervical dilation of less than 2 cm, generally should not be treated with tocolytics.
- Maintenance therapy with tocolytics is ineffective for preventing PTB and improving neonatal outcomes and is not recommended for this purpose (ACOG, 2016b).

TABLE 7-1   Common Tocolytic Agents

AGENT OR CLASS	MATERNAL SIDE EFFECTS	FETAL OR NEWBORN ADVERSE EFFECTS	CONTRAINDICATIONS	NURSING CARE
Calcium channel blockers Ex: Nifedipine (Procardia) Relaxes myometrial muscles	Dizziness, flushing, and hypotension; tachycardia, nausea; when used with magnesium sulfate, possible suppression of heart rate, contractility, and left ventricular systolic pressure; and elevation of hepatic enzymes	No known adverse effects	Hypotension and preload-dependent cardiac lesions, such as aortic insufficiency	Assess for side effects including hypotension, dizziness, headache, nausea, palpitations, flushing, and edema. Assist woman when getting up from bed and when ambulating. Assess pulse and blood pressure before and after administration. Monitor hepatic enzymes (LFTs).
Nonsteroidal anti-inflammatory drugs Ex: Indomethacin	Nausea, esophageal reflux, gastritis, and emesis	Premature closure of fetal ductus arteriosus, interventricular hemorrhage, oligohydramnios, necrotizing enterocolitis in preterm newborns, and patent ductus arteriosus in newborn	Platelet dysfunction of bleeding disorder, hepatic dysfunction, gastrointestinal ulcerative disease, hepatitis, renal dysfunction, and asthma (in women with hypersensitivity to aspirin)	Assess for gastrointestinal upset. Assess level and characteristics of pain.
Beta-adrenergic receptor agonists (Beta-mimetics) Ex: Terbutaline, Ritodrine Works to relax smooth muscle	Tachycardia, arrhythmias, palpitations, shortness of breath, chest discomfort, pulmonary edema, hyperglycemia, hypokalemia, hypotension, tremor, nausea and vomiting Maternal death	Fetal tachycardia, alterations in fetal glucose metabolism, hyperglycemia, and hyperinsulinemia	Tachycardia-sensitive maternal cardiac disease and poorly controlled diabetes mellitus, maternal hyperthyroidism, and seizure disorders	Monitor heart rate, blood pressure, and RR. HR greater than 120 warrants continuous ECG. Strict I&O for fluid overload. Auscultate for pulmonary edema. Assess BG levels. Evaluate patient for anxiety and tremors. Use cautiously when administering to an asthma patient and monitor for respiratory distress.

Continued

TABLE 7-1 Common Tocolytic Agents—cont'd

AGENT OR CLASS	MATERNAL SIDE EFFECTS	FETAL OR NEWBORN ADVERSE EFFECTS	CONTRAINDICATIONS	NURSING CARE
Magnesium sulfate Magnesium sulfate can be used as a tocolytic, but is primarily used for fetal neuroprotection. Relaxes smooth muscle	Causes lethargy, drowsiness, flushing, diaphoresis, nausea, vomiting, headache, pulmonary edema, loss of DTRs, respiratory depression, chest pain, pulmonary edema, hypotension, and cardiac arrest; suppresses heart rate, contractility, and left ventricular systolic pressure when used with calcium channel blockers; and produces neuromuscular blockade when used with calcium-channel blockers Maternal death	Neonatal depression	Myasthenia gravis	Remain at bedside for loading dose assessing vital signs, oxygen saturation, and DTRs. Assess DTRs. Assess respiratory status, including rate, rhythm, and depth, and auscultate lungs. Monitor serum magnesium levels; therapeutic levels are 4 to 8 mg/dL. Keep calcium gluconate available for use as an antidote: 1 g (10 mL of a 10% solution). Monitor strict intake and output. If RR is lower than 12, or 4 breaths per minute below baseline or oxygen saturation lower than 95%, magnesium sulfate should be discontinued. Remember, untreated respiratory arrest will lead to cardiac arrest as the heart muscle becomes hypoxic and ischemic.

ACOG, 2016a; Parfitt, 2021.

- Antibiotics should not be used to prolong gestation or improve neonatal outcomes in women with PTL and intact membranes. This recommendation is distinct from recommendations for antibiotic use for preterm premature rupture of membranes (PPROM) and group B streptococci carrier status (ACOG, 2016d).
- Progesterone supplementation may prevent PTB for women with a history of spontaneous PTB (ACOG, 2012; Dodd et al., 2013). Data suggest that progesterone may be important in maintaining uterine quiescence in the latter half of pregnancy by limiting production of stimulatory prostaglandins and inhibiting expression of contraction-associated protein genes within the myometrium (Norwitz & Caughey, 2011). The use of progesterone is associated with benefits in infant health following administration in women at increased risk of PTB due either to a prior PTB or where a short cervix has been identified on ultrasound examination. Use of 17-alpha-hydroxyprogesterone-caproate at 250 mg/week beginning at 16 weeks to 36 weeks of gestation is considered safe. It is not recommended for prophylactic use in multiple gestation.
- Vaginal progesterone is recommended in women with a very short cervical length (less than 20 mm) before or at 24 weeks' gestation.

- Cerclage placement before 24 weeks is associated with significant decreases in PTB in women with a history of PTB, a current singleton pregnancy, and short cervical length (AAP & ACOG, 2017).
- Neonatal neuroprophylaxis with intravenous magnesium sulfate administration is recommended to reduce microcapillary brain hemorrhage in premature birth of the neonate. Accumulated available evidence suggests that magnesium sulfate reduces the severity and risk of cerebral palsy in surviving infants if administered when birth is anticipated before 32 weeks of gestation (ACOG, 2016b).
- A single course of corticosteroids is recommended for pregnant women between 24 and 34 weeks of gestation who are at risk of preterm delivery within 7 days, including those with ruptured membranes and multiple gestations.
- A single repeat course of antenatal corticosteroids should be considered in women who are less than 34 0/7 weeks of gestation, who are at risk of preterm delivery within 7 days, and whose prior course of antenatal corticosteroids was administered more than 14 days previously (ACOG, 2017a).
- Corticosteroid therapy with antenatal steroids is currently recommended to women at risk of PTB. A single course of corticosteroids is recommended for pregnant women between 24 weeks and 34 weeks of gestation who are at risk of delivery within 7 days (ACOG, 2017a). Betamethasone is an antenatal steroid given to women to accelerate fetal lung maturity, thereby decreasing the severity of respiratory distress syndrome (RDS) and other complications of prematurity in the neonate. Treatment with antenatal corticosteroids reduces the risk of neonatal respiratory distress syndrome, cerebroventricular hemorrhage, necrotizing enterocolitis, and infectious morbidity in the neonate when used between 24 and 34 weeks' gestation (Roberts et al., 2017).
- If UCs decrease to less than five per hour, women are often transferred to less acute antenatal units for further observation for several days. If they remain stable, they may be discharged to home undelivered. Discharge instructions typically include self-monitoring of uterine activity, and signs and symptoms of PTL. Maintenance tocolytic therapy has no demonstrated benefit (AAP & ACOG, 2017).

Contraindications

Contraindications to treating PTL include:

- Intrauterine fetal demise
- Lethal fetal anomaly
- Nonreassuring fetal status
- Severe preeclampsia or eclampsia
- Maternal bleeding with hemodynamic instability
- Chorioamnionitis
- PPROMs in the absence of maternal infection (tocolytics may be considered for the purposes of maternal transport, steroid administration, or both)
- Maternal contraindications to tocolysis (agent-specific)
  - Active hemorrhage
  - Severe maternal disease
  - Fetal compromise

- Chorioamnionitis
- Fetal death
- Previable gestation and PPROM

Tocolysis is generally contraindicated when the maternal and fetal risks of prolonging pregnancy or the risks associated with these drugs are greater than the risks associated with PTB (AAP & ACOG, 2017). Contraindications to tocolysis for PTL include severe preeclampsia, placental abruption, intrauterine infection, pulmonary hypertension, maternal hemodynamic instability, intrauterine fetal demise, lethal congenital or chromosomal abnormalities, fetal maturity, and fetal compromise (ACOG, 2016b).

SAFE AND EFFECTIVE NURSING CARE: Understanding Medication

Medication Antenatal Corticosteroids

The most beneficial intervention for improvement of neonatal outcomes among patients who give birth preterm is the administration of antenatal corticosteroids. A single course of corticosteroids is recommended for pregnant women between 24 and 34 weeks of gestation who are at risk of delivery within 7 days. A Cochrane meta-analysis concluded neonates whose mothers receive antenatal corticosteroids have significantly lower severity, frequency, or both of respiratory distress syndrome, intracranial hemorrhage, necrotizing enterocolitis, and death (Roberts et al., 2017).

- Indication: Given to women at 24 and 34 weeks' gestation with signs of PTL or at risk to deliver preterm in the next 7 days.
- Action: Stimulate the production of more mature surfactant in the fetal lungs to prevent respiratory distress syndrome (RDS) in premature infants. The optimal therapeutic window for delivery after corticosteroid administration is 2 to 7 days.
- Adverse reactions: Will raise blood sugar and may require temporary insulin coverage to maintain euglycemia in diabetic women.
- Route and dose: Betamethasone 12 mg IM every 24 hours × 2 doses or dexamethasone four 6-mg doses IM every 12 hours.

Because treatment with corticosteroids for less than 24 hours is still associated with significant reduction in neonatal morbidity and mortality, a first dose of antenatal corticosteroids should be administered even if the ability to give the second dose is unlikely, based on the clinical scenario (ACOG, 2017a).

A single repeat course of antenatal corticosteroids may be considered in women who are less than 34 weeks of gestation, who are at risk of preterm delivery within the next 7 days, and whose prior course of antenatal corticosteroids was administered more than 14 days previously. Rescue course corticosteroids could be provided as early as 7 days from the prior dose, if indicated by the clinical situation (AAP & ACOG, 2017; ACOG, 2017a).

Nursing Actions

Nurses can provide expertise in directing patient care, stabilizing the woman and fetus, counseling, coordinating care, and providing patient teaching. Immediate care, including assessment and stabilization, occurs in labor and delivery. If uterine activity decreases, generally to less than 5 UCs/hr with no further cervical change, women are often moved to a less intensive care setting than a labor and delivery unit. Once moved to an antenatal high-risk unit, they are often observed for several days and, if stable, discharged to home undelivered.

Immediate care:

● Review the prenatal record for risk factors and establish gestational age through history and ultrasound (ultrasound early in pregnancy is more reliable for gestational age).
● Assess the woman and fetus for signs and symptoms of:
  ● Vaginal and urinary infection
  ● ROM
  ● Sterile speculum exam to assess for ferning of amniotic fluid
  ● Vaginal bleeding or vaginal discharge
  ● Dehydration
● Assess fetal heart rate (FHR) and UCs.
  ● Report fetal tachycardia or increased UCs to the health-care provider.
● Obtain vaginal and urine cultures as per orders.
● Obtain biochemical cervical tests (fFN or PAMG-1) as per orders.
  ● This should be obtained before sterile vaginal exam. Contraindicated if ROM, bleeding, sexual intercourse, or prior collection in last 24 hours.
● Maintain strict input and output (I&O) while on tocolytics and provide oral or IV hydration.
● May restrict total intake to 3,000 mL/24 hr if on tocolytics.
● Administer tocolytic agents as per protocol.
  ● Monitor for adverse reactions (see Table 7–1).
● Administer antenatal steroids per orders.
● Position the patient on her side to increase uteroplacental perfusion and decrease pressure on the maternal inferior vena cava.
● Assess vital signs per protocol for tocolytic administered.
  ● Report to the provider blood pressure greater than 140/90 mm Hg or lower than 90/50 mm Hg; heart rate greater than 120; temperature greater than 100.4°F (38°C).
● Auscultate lungs for evidence of pulmonary edema.
● Assess cervical status with a sterile vaginal exam unless contraindicated by ROM or bleeding (may be done by the health-care provider to minimize multiple exams); cervical ultrasound may be done (cervical length of less than 30 mm may be clinically significant).
● Notify the care provider of findings.

Continuing care once the woman is stable includes the following measures.

● Provide emotional support to the woman by providing opportunities to discuss her feelings. Women often feel guilt that they caused PTL, are concerned for the infant's health, and have anxiety and sadness over loss of a "normal" newborn, pregnancy, and labor and birth.
● Facilitate a clear understanding of the treatment plan and the woman's and family's involvement in clinical decision making.
● Facilitate consultations with the neonatal staff regarding neonatal survival rates, the anticipated care of the newborn, treatments, complications, and possible long-term disabilities. The family may be taken on a tour of the NICU.
● Monitor the woman's response to treatment including FHR baseline and variability and UCs, maternal vital signs, woman's response while on tocolytics, increase in vaginal discharge, or ROM.
● Assessment of women on tocolytics is based on the tocolytic used and is detailed in Table 7-1, but generally includes monitoring of blood pressure and pulse and auscultation of lungs for pulmonary edema. Watch for:
  ● Shortness of breath, chest tightness or discomfort, cough, oxygen saturation lower than 95%, increased respiratory and heart rates
  ● Changes in behavior such as apprehension, anxiety, or restlessness
● Encourage a side-lying position to enhance placental perfusion.
● Evaluate laboratory reports such as urine and cervical cultures.
  ● White blood cell (WBC) counts are elevated in women who have received corticosteroids; therefore, elevated WBCs are not indicative of infection.
● Provide ongoing reassurance and explanations to the woman and her family.
● Explain the purpose and side effects of the medication.
● Set short-term goals such as completion of a gestational week or milestones.
● Facilitate family interactions and visiting by having flexible visiting policies.
● Assist the family in participating in a plan of care.
● Some women enjoy keeping a journal to help them deal with boredom and isolation (Parfitt, 2021).
● Provide referral information about online support groups.
● Discuss the emotional and behavioral responses they can expect from other children based on the developmental age of children.

Discharge Plan

Approximately 30% of PTL spontaneously resolves and 50% of patients hospitalized for PTL give birth at term (ACOG, 2016b). Interventions to reduce the likelihood of delivery should be reserved for women with PTL at a gestational age at which a delay in delivery would improve neonatal outcomes. All plans should be decided in consideration with the woman's and family's strengths, needs, and goals in mind and should be made with their participation (Durham, 1998; Maloni, 1998) (Fig. 7–3). Discharge instructions typically include self-monitoring of uterine activity and signs and symptoms of PTL. Maintenance tocolytic therapy has no demonstrated benefit (AAP & ACOG, 2017). Discharge teaching should include a review of warning signs and how and when to call the provider (Box 7-2).

Programs have demonstrated some improvement in outcomes with nurse phone or home care follow-up (East et al., 2019). Typically, women treated for PTL are sent home without follow-up at home except for weekly prenatal visits.

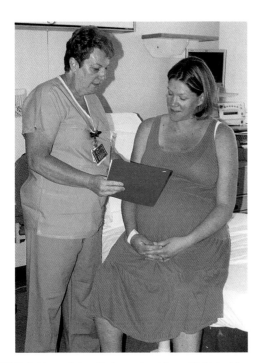

FIGURE 7–3 Nurse doing discharge teaching with high-risk pregnant woman in the hospital.

BOX 7-2 | Warning Signs of Preterm Labor

Instruct the patient to call her doctor or midwife or the hospital for any of the following:

- Bag of waters breaks
- Decreased fetal movement
- More than ____ contractions in an hour
- Low backache, menstrual-like cramps, pelvic pressure, or intestinal cramps with or without diarrhea
- Increased vaginal discharge
- Fever higher than 100.4°F (38°C)
- Feeling that something isn't right

CLINICAL JUDGMENT

When caring for a woman receiving tocolytic therapy:

- Know the potential complications of the medication your patient is receiving for tocolysis and treatment for PTL.
- Assess for symptoms of pulmonary edema such as shortness of breath, tachypnea, respiratory rate lower than 12 or greater than 24, oxygen saturation lower than 95%, apprehension, anxiety, or restlessness; and auscultate lungs.
- Remember, untreated respiratory arrest will lead to cardiac arrest as the heart muscle becomes hypoxic and ischemic (Parfitt, 2021).

- Assess I&O and maintain fluid restriction.
- Evaluate uterine activity and FHR.
- Provide psychosocial support, reinforce information and updates, and facilitate consultations.

Periviable Birth

Approximately 0.5% of all births occur before the third trimester of pregnancy, and these very early deliveries result in the majority of neonatal deaths and more than 40% of infant deaths. Periviable birth is delivery occurring from 20 0/7 weeks to 25 6/7 weeks of gestation (ACOG, 2017f; Raju et al., 2014). When delivery is anticipated near the limit of viability, families and health-care teams are faced with complex and ethically challenging decisions. Multiple factors have been found to be associated with short-term and long-term outcomes of periviable births in addition to gestational age at birth. These include, but are not limited to, nonmodifiable factors (e.g., fetal sex, weight, plurality), potentially modifiable antepartum and intrapartum factors (e.g., location of delivery, intent to intervene by cesarean delivery or induction for delivery, administration of antenatal corticosteroids and magnesium sulfate), and postnatal management (e.g., starting or withholding and continuing or withdrawing intensive care birth). Antepartum and intrapartum management options vary depending upon the specific circumstances but may include short-term tocolytic therapy for preterm labor to allow time for administration of antenatal steroids, antibiotics to prolong latency after preterm premature rupture of membranes or for intrapartum group B streptococci prophylaxis, and delivery, including cesarean delivery, for concern regarding fetal well-being or fetal malpresentation (ACOG, 2017f). Commonly, periviable births for which maternal or neonatal intervention is planned occur in centers that offer expertise in maternal and neonatal care and the capacity, including neonatal intensive care units, to support such services. Current recommendation is for treatment and resuscitation between 24 and 26 weeks' gestation; neonatal resuscitation can be considered between 22 and 24 weeks' gestation and is not recommended before 22 weeks (ACOG, 2017f).

When a decision has been made to withhold or withdraw life-sustaining treatment after birth, the newborn should receive individualized compassionate care directed toward providing warmth, minimizing discomfort, and allowing the family to spend as much time with their newborn as desired. It should be emphasized that decisions to redirect care do not mean forgoing all care but instead focusing on appropriate palliative care based on the clinical circumstances (ACOG, 2017f). Bereavement care for the family is of great importance in this situation.

Preterm Premature Rupture of Membranes and Prelabor Rupture of Membranes

Premature rupture of membranes (PROM) is rupture of membranes before the onset of labor; it is also termed prelabor rupture of membranes (ACOG, 2020e). Membrane rupture before labor and before 37 weeks of gestation is referred to as preterm PROM. Management is influenced by gestational age and presence of complications such as clinical infection, abruptio placentae, labor, or nonreassuring fetal status. Preterm premature rupture of membranes (PPROM) is rupture of membranes with a premature gestation (less than 37 weeks). It occurs in about 3% of pregnancies but causes about 30% to 40% of all PTBs. Premature rupture of membranes is rupture of the chorioamniotic membranes before the onset of labor but at term. Adding to the confusion is prolonged rupture of membranes, which is greater than 24 hours (PROM).

This section focuses on those women who have rupture of membranes preterm (PPROM) because it accounts for approximately one-third of premature births. Once the membranes rupture preterm, most women go into labor within a week. The term *latency* refers to the time from membrane rupture to delivery. Previable PROM is ROM before 23 to 24 weeks, preterm PPROM remote from term is from 24 to 32 weeks' gestation, and preterm PPROM near term is 31 to 36 weeks' gestation (Jazayeri, 2016).

Spontaneous PPROM occurs in the absence of medical intervention and is usually secondary to ascending infection. Iatrogenic PPROM occurs after medical intervention has occurred and may be secondary to invasive fetal testing such as chorionic villus sampling, amniocentesis, or fetoscopy. PPROM contributes to up to 40% of preterm (before 37 weeks) births. Spontaneous premature rupture of membranes is a multifactorial but choriodecidual infection, and inflammation appears to be an important factor, especially with preterm PROM at earlier gestations (ACOG, 2016d). Bacterial infections are thought to weaken the membranes leading to rupture, but in most cases the cause is unknown. It has also been postulated that stress and strain on the membranes from uterine activity causes the membranes to become less elastic and more prone to rupture with repeated strain. Other factors that play a role in tissue degradation and immune modulation, such as altered levels of hormones (including relaxin) and micronutrients (including vitamin C), may be important in PPROM (Crowley et al., 2016). Preterm PROM often occurs without recognized risk factors or obvious cause (ACOG, 2016d).

The optimal approach to clinical assessment and treatment of women with term and preterm PROM remains controversial. Management hinges on knowledge of gestational age and evaluation of the relative risks of delivery versus the risks of expectant management (e.g., infection, abruptio placentae, and umbilical cord accident). Current management of PPROM involves either initiating birth soon after preterm PROM or, alternatively, adopting a "wait and see" approach (expectant management). It is unclear which strategy is most beneficial for mothers and their babies. However, a recent Cochrane Review of evidence reveals no difference in the incidence of neonatal sepsis between women who delivered immediately or were managed expectantly in PPROM before 37 weeks' gestation. In pregnancies complicated by preterm premature rupture of the membranes, a policy of expectant management with careful observation is associated with better outcomes for the mother and baby (Bond et al., 2017). However, the optimal gestational age for delivery is

unclear and controversial. Regardless of obstetric management or clinical presentation, birth within 1 week of membrane rupture occurs in at least one-half of patients with preterm PROM (ACOG, 2020e). Cessation of amniotic fluid leakage with restoration of normal amniotic fluid volume may infrequently occur in the setting of spontaneous preterm PROM but can be associated with favorable outcomes (ACOG, 2020e). Women presenting with PROM before neonatal viability should be counseled regarding the risks and benefits of expectant management versus immediate delivery. Counseling should include a realistic appraisal of neonatal outcomes. Immediate delivery should be offered.

Risk Factors for Preterm PROM

- Previous preterm PROM or preterm delivery
- Bleeding during pregnancy
- Short cervical length
- Hydramnios
- Multiple gestation (up to 15% in twins, up to 20% in triplets)
- Sexually transmitted infections (STIs)
- Low body mass index (BMI)
- Low socioeconomic status
- Cigarette smoking and illicit drug use

Risks for the Woman

- Maternal infection (i.e., chorioamnionitis, endometritis). Clinically evident intraamniotic infection occurs in 15% to 35% of cases, and postpartum infection occurs in 15% to 25% of cases.
- Abruptio placenta and retained placenta in 2% to 5%
- Increased rates of cesarean birth

Risks for the Fetus and Newborn

- Fetal or neonatal sepsis
  - The earlier the fetal gestation at ROM, the greater the risk for infection.
  - The membranes serve as a protective barrier that separates the sterile fetus and fluid from the bacteria-laden vaginal canal.
- Preterm delivery and complications of prematurity including respiratory distress, sepsis, intraventricular hemorrhage, necrotizing enterocolitis, and an increased risk of neurodevelopmental impairment. However, there are no data to suggest that immediate delivery after presentation with PROM will avert these risks.
- Hypoxia or asphyxia due to umbilical cord compression or umbilical cord accidents due to decreased fluid and ROM
- Fetal deformities if preterm PROM before 26 weeks' gestation

Assessment Findings

- Confirmed premature gestational age by prenatal history and ultrasound
- Confirmed ROM with speculum exam and positive ferning test
- Oligohydramnios on ultrasound may be seen but is not diagnostic

Medical Management

The risk of perinatal complications changes drastically with gestational age at membrane rupture, so a gestational age-based approach is appropriate for medical management (ACOG, 2016d). Medical treatment is aimed at balancing the risks of prematurity and the risks of infections. Unless near-term gestation premature PROM, management is aimed at prolonging gestation for the woman who is not in labor, not infected, and not experiencing fetal compromise. Evaluation of gestational age, fetal presentation, and fetal well-being must be determined. Conservative management refers to treatment directed at continuing the pregnancy. Gestational age is a primary consideration when considering delivery versus expectant management. Nonreassuring fetal status, clinical chorioamnionitis, and significant abruptio placentae are clear indications for delivery. Otherwise, gestational age is a primary factor when considering delivery versus expectant management. According to ACOG (2020e), guidelines for management include:

Late Preterm (34 0/7 to 36 6/7 Weeks of Gestation)

- Expectant management or proceed toward delivery (induction or cesarean as appropriate or indicated)
- Single course of corticosteroids, if steroids not previously given, if proceeding with induction or delivery in no less than 24 hours and no more than 7 days, and no evidence of chorioamnionitis
- Group beta streptococcus (GBS) screening and prophylaxis as indicated
- Treat intraamniotic infection if present (and proceed toward delivery)

Preterm (24 0/7 to 33 6/7 Weeks of Gestation)

- Expectant management
- Antibiotics recommended to prolong latency if there are no contraindications. To reduce maternal and neonatal infections and gestational-age-dependent morbidity, a 7-day course of therapy of latency antibiotics with a combination of intravenous ampicillin and erythromycin followed by oral amoxicillin and erythromycin is recommended during expectant management
- Single course of corticosteroids; insufficient evidence for or against rescue course
- Treat intraamniotic infection if present (and proceed to delivery)
- A vaginal-rectal swab for GBS culture should be obtained at the time of initial presentation and GBS prophylaxis administered as indicated.
- Magnesium sulfate for neuroprotection before anticipated delivery for pregnancies at less than 32 0/7 weeks of gestation, if there are no contraindications

Periviable (Less Than 23 to 24 Weeks of Gestation)

- Patient counseling; consider neonatology and maternal-fetal medicine consultation
- Expectant management or induction of labor

- Antibiotics may be considered as early as 20 0/7 weeks of gestation.
- GBS prophylaxis is not recommended before viability.
- Corticosteroids are not recommended before viability.
- Tocolysis is not recommended before viability.
- Magnesium sulfate for neuroprotection is not recommended before viability.

Current data suggest that antenatal corticosteroids are not associated with increased risks of maternal or neonatal infection regardless of gestational age (ACOG, 2017a).

Nursing Actions

- Assess FHR and UCs.
- Assess for signs of infection including:
  - Maternal and/or fetal tachycardia
  - Maternal fever 100.4°F (38°C) or greater
  - Uterine or abdominal tenderness
  - Malodorous fluid or vaginal discharge
- Early signs and symptoms of intraamniotic infection may be subtle. In the absence of fever, other clinical criteria, such as abdominal or fundal tenderness and maternal or fetal tachycardia, have variable sensitivity and specificity for diagnosing infection.
- Serial monitoring of leukocyte counts and other markers of inflammation have not been proved to be useful and are nonspecific when there is no clinical evidence of infection, especially if antenatal corticosteroids have been administered.
- Monitor for labor and for fetal compromise. Abnormal fetal testing or evidence of intraamniotic infection are indications for delivery. Vaginal bleeding should raise concern for abruptio placentae, which should prompt consideration of delivery (ACOG, 2020f).
- Provide antenatal testing including nonstress tests (NSTs) and biophysical profiles (BPPs).
- The use of tocolytic agents in the setting of preterm PROM is controversial, and practice patterns among specialists vary widely (ACOG, 2020e).

Because either expectant management or immediate delivery in patients with PROM between 34 0/7 weeks of gestation and 36 6/7 weeks of gestation is a reasonable option, both should be carefully considered by the woman, and patients should be counseled clearly. The plan of care should be individualized through shared decision making.

Evidence-Based Practice: Cochrane Review on Social Support During At-Risk Pregnancy

East, C. E., Biro, M. A., Fredericks, S., & Lau, R. (2019). Support during pregnancy for women at increased risk of low birthweight babies. *Cochrane Database of Systematic Reviews, 4*, CD000198. https://doi.org/10.1002/14651858 .CD000198.pub3

A recent review of 25 studies, with outcome data for 11,246 mothers and babies enrolled in 21 studies, compared routine care with programs

Continued

offering additional social support for at-risk pregnant women. Results indicated a slightly reduced number of babies born with a birth weight less than 2,500 g, from 127 per 1,000 to 120 per 1,000 (risk ratio [RR] 0.94, 95% confidence interval [CI] 0.86 to 1.04; 16 studies, *n* = 11,770; moderate-quality evidence), and the number of babies born with a gestational age less than 37 weeks at birth, from 128 per 1,000 to 117 per 1,000 (RR 0.92, 95% CI 0.84 to 1.01, 14 studies, *n* = 12,282; moderate-quality evidence), though the CIs for the pooled effect for both of these outcomes just crossed the line of no effect, suggesting any effect is not large. Secondary outcomes of moderate quality suggested that there is probably a reduction in caesarean section, a reduction in the number of antenatal hospital admissions, and a reduction in the mean number of hospitalization episodes in the social support group, compared with the controls.

Cervical Insufficiency

The term *cervical insufficiency* is used to describe the inability of the uterine cervix to retain a pregnancy in the absence of the signs and symptoms of clinical contractions, or labor, or both in the middle of the second trimester or early in the third trimester (ACOG, 2014; Thakur & Mahajan, 2020) depending upon the severity of insufficiency.

Controversy exists in the medical literature pertaining to issues of pathophysiology, screening, diagnosis, and management of cervical insufficiency. The diagnosis of cervical insufficiency is challenging due to a lack of objective findings and clear diagnostic criteria. Diagnosis is based on a history of painless cervical dilation after the first trimester with subsequent expulsion of the pregnancy in the second trimester, typically before 24 weeks of gestation, without contractions or labor and in the absence of other clear pathology such as bleeding, infection, or ruptured membranes (ACOG, 2014).

Cervical incompetence may be congenital or acquired. The most common congenital cause is a defect in the embryological development or collagen deficiency that causes inadequate cervical performance, resulting in insufficiency. The most common acquired cause is cervical trauma such as lacerations during childbirth, cervical conization, LEEP (loop electrosurgical excision procedure), or forced cervical dilation during the uterine evacuation in the first or second trimester of pregnancy. In most patients, cervical changes are the result of infection or inflammation, which causes early activation of the final pathway of labor (Thakur & Mahajan, 2020). However, the pathophysiology remains poorly understood.

Various diagnostic tests in the nonpregnant woman have been suggested to confirm the presence of cervical insufficiency, but none have been validated in rigorous scientific studies and should not be used to diagnose cervical insufficiency. Based on current data, the ultrasonographic finding of a short cervical length in the second trimester is associated with an increased risk of PTB but is not sufficient for the diagnosis of cervical insufficiency (ACOG, 2014).

Risks to the Woman

- Repeated second trimester or early third trimester births
- Reported complications of cerclage include ROM, chorioamnionitis, cervical lacerations, and suture displacement

Risk to the Fetus and Newborn

- PTB and consequences of prematurity

Assessment Findings

- Patients usually are asymptomatic, but some report nonspecific symptoms such as backache, UCs, vaginal spotting, pelvic pressure, or mucoid vaginal discharge.
- Shortened cervical length or funneling of the cervix; use of ultrasound to diagnose cervical incompetence is not currently recommended (ACOG, 2014; Cunningham et al., 2018).

Medical Management

Certain nonsurgical approaches, including activity restriction, bedrest, and pelvic rest, have not been proven effective for the treatment of cervical insufficiency and their use is not recommended (ACOG, 2014; Thakur & Mahajan, 2020). Vaginal pessary has been used, but evidence is limited for potential benefit of pessary placement and has only been studied in select high-risk patients. Surgical treatment of incompetent cervix is cerclage, a type of pursestring suture placed cervically to reinforce a weak cervix (Fig. 7–4). The standard transvaginal cerclage methods currently used include modifications of the McDonald and Shirodkar techniques.

Indications for Cervical Cerclage in Women With Singleton Pregnancies

- History of one or more second-trimester pregnancy losses related to painless cervical dilation and in the absence of labor or abruptio placentae
- Prior cerclage due to painless cervical dilation in the second trimester
- Painless cervical dilation in the second trimester
- Current singleton pregnancy, prior spontaneous PTB at less than 34 weeks of gestation, and short cervical length (less than 25 mm) before 24 weeks of gestation

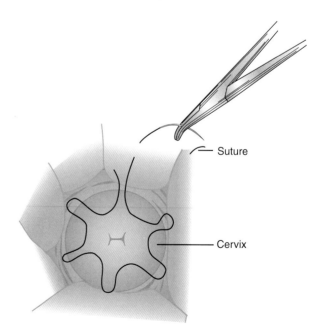

FIGURE 7–4 Cerclage.

A history-indicated cerclage (also known as prophylactic cerclage) is based on the previously noted classic historic features of cervical insufficiency. History-indicated cerclage can be considered in a patient with a history of unexplained second-trimester delivery in the absence of labor or abruptio placentae. History-indicated cerclages typically are placed at approximately 13 to 14 weeks of gestation.

Women who present with advanced cervical dilation in the absence of labor have historically been candidates for examination-indicated cerclage, also called an emergency or rescue cerclage. Women with a current singleton pregnancy, prior spontaneous PTB at less than 34 weeks of gestation, and short cervical length (less than 25 mm) before 24 weeks of gestation may benefit from cerclage placement. Evidence suggests that cerclage placement is associated with significant decreases in PTB outcomes and improved neonatal outcomes. Cerclage placement in women without a prior spontaneous PTB and a cervical length less than 25 mm detected between 16 weeks and 24 weeks of gestation has not been associated with a significant reduction in PTB. Cerclage may increase the risk of PTB in women with a twin pregnancy and an ultrasonographically detected cervical length less than 25 mm and is not recommended (ACOG, 2014).

- Most patients at risk of cervical insufficiency can be safely monitored with serial transvaginal ultrasound examinations in the second trimester, beginning at 16 weeks and ending at 24 weeks of gestation.
- Obtain transcervical ultrasound to evaluate cervix for cervical length; funneling may be done but is not diagnostic.
- Perform cervical cultures for chlamydia, gonorrhea, and other cervical infections.
  - Prophylactic cerclage may be placed in women with a history of unexplained recurrent painless dilation and second-trimester birth, generally between 12 and 16 weeks of gestation.
  - Rescue cerclage is placed after the cervix has dilated with no perceived contractions, up to about 24 weeks of gestation (Cunningham et al., 2018).
- Administer antibiotics or tocolytics; however, this has not been demonstrated to be effective and is controversial in the perioperative period (ACOG, 2014; Owen & Harger, 2007).
- A firm recommendation on whether a cerclage should be removed after premature PROM cannot be made, and either removal or retention is reasonable.
- If cervical change, painful contractions, or vaginal bleeding progress, cerclage removal is recommended. Cerclage is removed if infection occurs, or labor develops.

Postoperative Nursing Actions

- Monitor for uterine activity with palpation.
- Monitor for vaginal bleeding and leaking of fluid or ROM.
- Monitor for infection.
  - Maternal fever
  - Uterine tenderness
- Discharge teaching may include teaching the patient to:
  - Monitor for signs of uterine activity, ROM, bleeding, infection.
  - Modify activity and pelvic rest for a week.

- Transvaginal McDonald cerclage removal is recommended at 36 to 37 weeks of gestation.
- Certain nonsurgical approaches, including activity restriction, bedrest, and pelvic rest, have not been proven effective for treatment of cervical insufficiency and use is not recommended.

Multiple Gestation

Multiple gestation pregnancies are those with more than one fetus. They result from either the fertilization of one zygote that subsequently divides (monozygotic) or the fertilization of multiple ova (dizygotic, trizygotic, etc.). Twin birth rates rose about 76% from 1980 to 2012, reaching an all-time high of 33.9 per 1,000 in 2014. Since 2014, multiple gestation birth rates have been declining. In 2018, the twin birth rate was 32.6 per 1,000 births, a 2% decline from 2017. The triplet and higher-order multiple birth rate was 93.0 per 100,000 in 2018, which is an 8% decline from 2017 (Martin et al., 2019). Recent declines in triplet and higher order multiple (HOM) birth rates have been linked to changes in assisted reproductive technology (ART) procedures. The increased incidence in multifetal gestations has been attributed to two main factors: (1) a shift toward an older maternal age at conception, when multifetal gestations are more likely to occur naturally, and (2) an increased use of assisted reproductive technology (ART), which is more likely to result in a multifetal gestation. Approximately one-third of twins are monozygotic (from one egg) and two-thirds are dizygotic (from two eggs) (Fig. 7–5A,B). Multiple gestation pregnancies are associated with higher maternal and neonatal morbidity and mortality (Bowers, 2021).

- Monozygotic twins are from one zygote that divides in the first week of gestation. They are genetically identical, similar in appearance, and always have the same gender.
- Dizygotic twins result from fertilization of two eggs and may be the same or differing genders. If the fetuses are of differing gender, they are dizygotic and therefore dichorionic.
- Either of these processes can be involved in the development of HOMs.

The rate of twin-specific complications varies in relation to zygocity and chorionicity. There are two principal placental types, monochorionic (one chorion) and dichorionic (two chorions). Dizygotic twins are always dichorionic/diamniotic and may be the same or different genders. Among twin gestations, 30% are dichorionic/diamniotic, with separate placentas and amniotic sacs. About 70% are monochorionic/diamniotic with a single placenta with two amniotic sacs. Even less common are monochorionic/monoamniotic pregnancies where multiple fetuses share a single placenta and one amniotic sac, which occur in about 1% of multiple gestation pregnancies. There are increased rates of perinatal mortality and neurological injury in monochorionic, diamniotic twins compared with dichorionic pairs (see Fig. 7–5A). Monozygotic twins have morbidity and mortality rates 3 to 10 times higher than for dizygotic twins due to sharing amniotic sacs and placental resources (Bowers, 2021) (see Fig. 7–5B). Because monozygotic twins are from a single

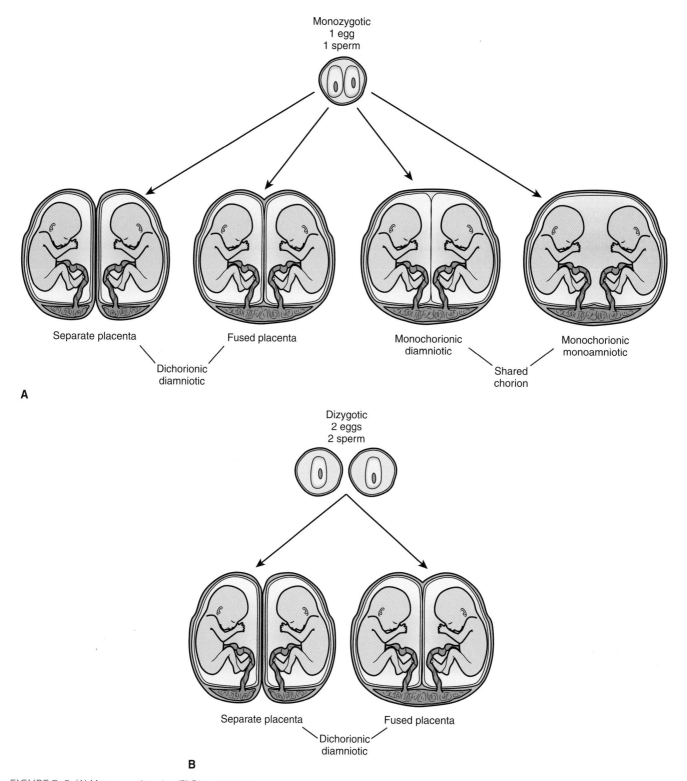

FIGURE 7–5 (A) Monozygotic twins. (B) Dizygotic twins.

fertilized ovum, they are always the same gender. Conjoined twins may result from an aberration in the twinning process ascribed to incomplete splitting of an embryo into two separate twins (Cunningham et al., 2018). Although multiple gestations are only about 3% of births in the United States, they contribute disproportionately to maternal, fetal, and neonatal morbidity and mortality. Risks for both the fetus and the woman increase with an increased number of fetuses. Compared with women with twins, women with triplets or HOMs are at even higher risk of pregnancy-related morbidities and mortality (Bowers, 2021).

Twin pregnancy is associated with higher rates of almost every potential complication of pregnancy. In multiple gestation pregnancies, there is a fivefold increased risk of stillbirth and a sevenfold increased risk of neonatal death, primarily due to complications of premature birth (ACOG, 2016c). Preterm delivery is six times more likely in multiple gestation pregnancies, which plays a major role in the increased perinatal mortality and short-term and long-term morbidity in these infants. Higher rates of fetal growth restriction and congenital anomalies also contribute to adverse outcome in twin births. In addition, monochorionic twins are at risk for complications unique to these pregnancies, such as discordant growth, or twin to twin transfusion syndrome (TTTS), which can be lethal or associated with serious morbidity (ACOG, 2016c).

Because multifetal pregnancies increase maternal and neonatal morbidity and mortality, women with multifetal pregnancies and their obstetric providers should be knowledgeable about the risks of a multifetal pregnancy and the option for multifetal pregnancy reduction. Multifetal pregnancy reduction is a procedure for reducing the number of fetuses in a multifetal pregnancy by one or more in the first trimester or early second trimester. This procedure is typically done with higher-order multiples, as they have higher risks than twin gestations (ACOG, 2017d). Risks associated with multifetal pregnancies increase with each additional fetus. Providers should offer information on risks and benefits, but only the patient can determine the best course of action for her based on her medical, ethical, religious, and socioeconomic factors. Patient autonomy must be respected and upheld (Table 7-2).

In multifetal reduction, technological, safety, and accessibility considerations influence the fetus(es) to be reduced. Selective reduction is based on health status when there is evidence of a genetic abnormality or disease risk. Decisions to reduce a multifetal pregnancy come with complex moral and ethical issues. Physicians should treat patients and these situations as professionally and as unbiased as possible whether the patient requests or declines information, intervention, or both (ACOG, 2017d).

Risks for the Woman

Twin pregnancy is associated with higher rates of almost every potential complication of pregnancy.

- Hypertensive disorders and preeclampsia, which tend to develop earlier and be more severe, are related to enlarged placenta. Hypertensive conditions associated with multifetal gestations are proportional to the total fetal number, increasing in risk with each additional fetus (ACOG, 2016c).

- Gestational diabetes due to physiological changes related to supporting multiple fetuses
- Antepartum hemorrhage, abruptio placenta, placenta previa
- Anemia related to dilutional anemia
- Peripartum cardiomyopathy, pulmonary edema, and pulmonary embolism
- Intrahepatic cholestasis
- Acute fatty liver
- Cesarean birth
- PTL

Risks for the Fetus and Newborn

- Increase in fetal morbidity and mortality due to sharing uterine space and placental circulation
  - Increased perinatal mortality is more likely (threefold higher than in singleton pregnancy).
  - Intrauterine fetal death (IUFD) of one fetus after 20 weeks' gestation increases the risks to the surviving fetus(es).
  - Twins born at less than 32 weeks of gestation are at twice the risk for developing an intraventricular hemorrhage and periventricular leukomalacia (ACOG, 2016c).
  - Delivery before term is the major reason for increased morbidity and mortality in twins. Rate of preterm delivery is 50% higher in twins and at least 90% higher in triplets and HOMs. As the number of fetuses increases, the duration of gestation decreases. Recommendations on timing of delivery may depend on the number and type of multiples, and preterm delivery may be medically indicated before 39 weeks' gestation.
- Increase of low-birth-weight (LBW) neonates (20% higher than singleton).
- Monochorionic twins have a shared fetoplacental circulation, which puts them at risk for specific serious pregnancy complications, such as TTTS and twin anemia–polycythemia sequence. These complications increase the risk for neurologic morbidity and perinatal mortality in monochorionic twins compared with dichorionic twins. In addition to the complications associated with monochorionic twinning, monoamniotic twins are also at risk for cord entanglement and conjoined twins. Morbidity and mortality rates for monozygotic twins are estimated to be 3 to 10 times higher than those for dizygotic twins (Bowers, 2021).

TABLE 7-2 Recommended Timing of Medically Indicated Preterm Delivery for Multiple Gestation

MULTIPLE GESTATION-UNCOMPLICATED		RECOMMENDED DELIVERY TIME
Dichorionic-diamniotic twins	Early term	38 0/7–38 6/7 weeks' gestation
Monochorionic-diamniotic twins	Late preterm/early term	34 0/7–37 6/7 weeks' gestation
Monochorionic-monoamniotic twins	Preterm/late preterm	32 0/7–34 0/7 weeks' gestation
Triplet and HOMs	Preterm/late preterm	Individualized

ACOG, 2021.

- Increase of intrauterine growth restriction (IUGR) and discordant growth (weight of one fetus differs significantly from the others, usually 25% or more) related to placental insufficiency and competition for nutrients (Bowers, 2021).
  - Discordant growth and twin-to-twin transfusions from sharing a placenta occur.
  - Vascular anastomosis between twins can occur with monochorionic twin placentas. Most of these vascular communications are hemodynamically balanced and do not impact fetal development and perfusion.
- In TTTS, blood is transfused from donor twin to recipient twin. Twin-to-twin transfusion is caused by an imbalance in blood flow through the vasculature of the placenta due to arteriovenous anastomosis in the placenta. This results in overperfusion of one twin and can result in circulatory overload and heart failure, underperfusion, and anemia of the co-twin.
- Increase of congenital, chromosomal, and genetic defects, in particular structural defects, may occur with monozygotic twins.
- Spontaneous loss of gestational sacs or embryos is possible and can result in preterm delivery of the other multiple (Bowers, 2021).

Assessment Findings

Ultrasound examination is the only safe and reliable method for definitive diagnosis of twin gestation. Early ultrasound assessment also provides accurate estimation of gestational age, which is important in all pregnancies, but particularly important in management of twin pregnancies due to the higher risks for preterm delivery and growth restriction. In addition, chorionicity and amnionicity can be determined by ultrasound examination.

Nearly every maternal system is affected by the physiological changes that occur in multiple gestations. These changes are greater in multiple pregnancies than in singleton pregnancies (Bowers, 2021).

- Elevation of human chorionic gonadotropin (hCG) may contribute to increased nausea and vomiting gonadotropin (hCG) and alpha-fetoprotein.
- Fundal height and size greater than dates and palpation of excessive number of fetal parts during Leopold's maneuver.
- Maternal blood volume expansion is greater than 50% to 60%, an additional 500 cc rather than 40% to 50% with singleton gestation.
- Increased cardiac output by 20% and increased stroke volume.
- Uterine growth is substantially greater, and uterine content may be up to 10 L and weigh in excess of 20 pounds. This can cause increased lower back and ligament pains and increase susceptibility to supine hypotension. Increased uterine size displaces lungs and can result in increased dyspnea and shortness of breath. Increased uterine distention increases risk of PTL and PPROM.
- Increased plasma volume 50% to 100% (results in dilutional anemia)
- Increased iron-deficiency anemia
- Increased dermatosis

Antepartal Medical Management

A woman pregnant with multiple fetuses needs ongoing, frequent surveillance of the pregnancy due to the increased rates of complications, including:

- Ultrasound for discordant fetal growth and IUGR, as well as placental sites, dividing membranes, congenital anomalies, and gender(s)
- Genetic testing for anomalies
  - Conjoined twinning has an incidence of 1 in 50,000 to 1 in 100,000 births (ACOG, 2016c).
- Monitor for PTL and prevent PTB
  - Research has associated administration of corticosteroids 1 to 7 days before birth in multiple gestation pregnancies with a decrease in newborn mortality, short-term respiratory morbidity, and severe neurological injury (see section on PTB) (ACOG, 2017a).
- Monitor for maternal anemia.
- Perform fetal surveillance including NST and biophysical profile (BPP).
- Monitor for hypertension and preeclampsia.
- Monitor for hydramnios.
- Monitor for antepartal hemorrhage.
- Monitor for intrauterine fetal demise.
  - In the first trimester, some women experience spontaneous reduction of one or more fetuses, commonly known as the "vanishing twin." The likelihood of this is about 36% for twins, 53% for triplets, and 65% for quadruplets (ACOG, 2016c).
  - When intrauterine death of one fetus occurs, immediate delivery of the second twin has not been shown to have medical benefits; thus, care should focus on the mother and surviving fetus.
- Seek a nutrition consult.
- Monitor for gestational diabetes due to increases in human placental lactogen.
- Consult with a perinatologist if complications occur.

Interventions such as prophylactic cerclage, prophylactic tocolytics, prophylactic pessary, progesterone treatment, routine hospitalization, and bedrest have not been proven to decrease neonatal morbidity or mortality and should not be used in women with multifetal gestations (ACOG, 2016c; da Silva Lopes, 2017).

Intrapartum Medical Management

Many complications of labor and birth are encountered more often in multiple gestation deliveries, including PTL, uterine contractile dysfunction, abnormal presentation, umbilical cord prolapse, abruption, and postpartum hemorrhage. The best method by which to deliver pregnancies in which only the presenting twin is cephalic remains controversial. Evidence supports a vaginal trial of labor in late preterm and term twins. Routes of delivery for preterm twins lighter than 1,500 g remains unclear, with compelling data for both planned cesarean and planned vaginal delivery. No data support planned cesarean for birth weight discordance alone. Risks of trial of labor after cesarean (TOLAC) for women with twins appear similar to risks for women with singletons, particularly for those who successfully undergo vaginal birth after cesarean (VBAC). For each of the previously noted clinical scenarios, however, two major factors remain constant: (1) Obstetricians need to be prepared for and skilled in breech extraction of the second twin; and (2) individualized patient counseling regarding mode of delivery is important when offering a vaginal trial of labor to women with a twin gestation (ACOG, 2016c; Christopher et al., 2011). See more on multiple birth in Chapter 10.

Preparation for birth of multiples includes:

- Type and cross match blood immediately available
- Ultrasound to confirm placental location and fetal positions
- Continuous electronic fetal monitoring (EFM) of all fetuses
- Cesarean birth access should be immediately available, including anesthesia, obstetricians, circulating nurse, and scrub personnel.
- Agents for hemorrhagic management are available, including medications and blood products.
- 1:1 nurse-to-patient ratio with multiple gestation labors (Bowers, 2021)
- The neonatal team available should be sufficient for all infants.
- Triplets and higher multiples are delivered by cesarean birth.

Nursing Actions

- Assess for the following possible complications:
  - UCs as PTL can be more difficult to identify in women with multiple gestations due to more discomfort, stretching, and pressure with multiple fetuses. Overdistention of the uterus results in more uterine irritability.
  - Hypertension or preeclampsia
  - Antepartal hemorrhage
- Conduct antepartal surveillance including NST, amniotic fluid index (AFI), and BPP.
- Provide information to the woman and her family regarding signs and symptoms of PTL, preeclampsia, and other possible complications related to multiple gestations.
- Facilitate nutritional consult. The woman has an increased need for iron, calcium, and magnesium to support growth of multiple fetuses.
- Parents expecting multiples have unique educational needs due to the high-risk pregnancy and unknowns of parenting multiple infants (Bowers, 2021).
- Provide emotional support to the woman and family. They often experience an increase of stress related to fear of pregnancy loss, high-risk pregnancy, and potential complications during pregnancy and delivery, as well as anxiety related to caring for more than one infant.
- Explain the plan for PNC and antenatal testing and follow-up related to multiple gestation.
- Assess the woman's and partner's response to the twin diagnosis and adaptation to multiple gestation.
  - Acknowledge feeling of distress and fear toward pregnancy.
  - Provide the family with information on multiple and support groups.
- Provide psychological support appropriate to the family's response.

- Discuss the plan of care for delivery and anticipated timing of birth (see Table 7-2). Cesarean birth is often recommended for multiples.
- Facilitate referrals such as a perinatologist, neonatologist, and social worker.

Hyperemesis Gravidarum

Hyperemesis gravidarum is vomiting during pregnancy so severe it leads to dehydration, electrolyte and acid–base imbalance, starvation ketosis, and weight loss. According to ACOG (2018g), no single accepted definition of hyperemesis gravidarum exists. It is a clinical diagnosis of exclusion based on a typical presentation in the absence of other diseases. The most commonly cited criteria include persistent vomiting not related to other causes, a measure of acute starvation (usually large ketonuria), and some discrete measure of weight loss, most often at least 5% of pre-pregnancy weight. Electrolyte, thyroid, and liver abnormalities also may be present. From an epidemiologic perspective, hyperemesis gravidarum appears to represent the extreme end of the spectrum of nausea and vomiting of pregnancy. The incidence of hyperemesis gravidarum is approximately 0.3% to 3% of pregnancies yet it is the most common indication for admission to the hospital during the first part of pregnancy and second only to PTL as the most common reason for hospitalization during pregnancy (ACOG, 2018g).

The condition is commonly defined as uncontrolled vomiting requiring hospitalization, severe dehydration, muscle wasting, electrolyte imbalance, ketonuria, and weight loss of more than 5% of body weight. Most of these patients also have hyponatremia, hypokalemia, and a low serum urea level. Ptyalism is also a typical symptom of hyperemesis. The symptoms of this disorder usually peak at 9 weeks of gestation and subside by approximately 20 weeks of gestation. Approximately 1% to 5% of patients with hyperemesis must be hospitalized. Women who experienced hyperemesis in their first pregnancy have a high risk for recurrence. Women at risk for hyperemesis also include multiple gestation, history of migraines and motion sickness, and a familial history of hyperemesis (ACOG, 2018g).

Hyperemesis appears to be related to rapidly rising serum levels of pregnancy-related hormones such as chorionic gonadotropin (hCG), progesterone, and estrogen. Other factors may include a psychological component related to ambivalence about the pregnancy, but this is controversial. A review of psychological theories proposed to explain the etiology of nausea and vomiting of pregnancy concluded that the evidence that nausea and vomiting of pregnancy is caused by a conversion disorder or an abnormal response to stress is "questionable at best" (Buckwalter & Simpson, 2002).

Regardless of the cause, a woman experiencing hyperemesis presents in the clinical situation severely dehydrated and physically and emotionally debilitated, sometimes in need of hospitalization to manage profound and prolonged nausea and vomiting (ACOG, 2018g). Hospital admission is appropriate for those with persistent vomiting after rehydration and intravenous antiemetic therapy, as well as women who present with abnormal electrolyte levels and acid–base balance (ACOG, 2018g).

The severity of nausea and vomiting dictates its effect on the embryo and fetus and research indicates a higher incidence of LBW and small-for-gestational-age infants as well as premature infants (ACOG, 2018g).

Assessment Findings

- Vomiting that may be prolonged, frequent, and severe
- Weight loss, acetonuria, and ketosis
- Signs and symptoms of dehydration including:
  - Lightheadedness, dizziness, faintness, tachycardia, or inability to keep food or fluids down for more than 12 hours
  - Dry mucous membranes
  - Poor skin turgor
  - Malaise
  - Low blood pressure

Medical Management

Most patients respond to intravenous hydration and a short period of gut rest, followed by reintroduction of oral intake and pharmacological therapy (ACOG, 2018g).

- The standard recommendation to take prenatal vitamins for 1 month before fertilization may reduce the incidence and severity of nausea and vomiting of pregnancy.
- Early treatment of nausea and vomiting of pregnancy may be beneficial to prevent progression to hyperemesis gravidarum.
- Treatment of nausea and vomiting of pregnancy with vitamin B_6 or vitamin B_6 plus doxylamine is safe and effective and should be considered first-line pharmacotherapy (ACOG, 2018g).
- Intravenous hydration should be used for the patient who cannot tolerate oral liquids for a prolonged period or if clinical signs of dehydration are present.
- In refractory cases of nausea and vomiting of pregnancy, the following medications have been shown to be safe and effective in pregnancy: antihistamine H1 receptor blockers, phenothiazines, and benzamides (ACOG, 2018g).
- Laboratory studies are performed to monitor kidney and liver function.
- Correction of ketosis and vitamin deficiency should be strongly considered. Dextrose and vitamins, especially thiamine, should be included in therapy for prolonged vomiting.
- According to ACOG (2018a), because life-threatening complications of parenteral nutrition have been described in several studies, enteral tube feeding initially should provide nutritional support to a pregnant woman with hyperemesis who cannot maintain her weight.

Nursing Actions

- Assess factors that contribute to nausea and vomiting.
- Reduce or eliminate factors that contribute to nausea and vomiting, such as triggers including stuffy rooms and odors.
- Treatment of nausea and vomiting of pregnancy with ginger has shown beneficial effects and can be considered as a non-pharmacological option.
- In refractory cases of nausea and vomiting of pregnancy, use antiemetics as ordered.

- Early treatment of nausea and vomiting of pregnancy is recommended to prevent progression to hyperemesis gravidarum.
- Provide emotional support. These patients and their families often need emotional support to help deal with stress and anxiety about the maternal illness and its effect on the fetus, and the disruption to their home- and work-related activities.
- Provide comfort measures such as good oral hygiene.
- Administer IV hydration with vitamins and electrolytes as per orders.
- Check weight daily.
- Monitor I&O and specific gravity of urine to monitor hydration. Fluids should be consumed at least 30 minutes before or after solid food to minimize the effect of a full stomach.
- Assess nausea and vomiting.
- Monitor laboratory values for fluid and electrolyte imbalances.
- Ensure that the woman remains NPO until vomiting is controlled, then slowly advance the diet as tolerated.
- Facilitate nutritional and dietary consult.
- Taking prenatal vitamins before bed with a snack, instead of in the morning or on an empty stomach, may also be helpful. Pyridoxine (vitamin B_6) can improve nausea.
- Determine and provide the woman's preferred food.
- Minimizing fluid intake with meals can decrease nausea and vomiting.
- Explore complementary therapies to manage hyperemesis, such as traditional Chinese medicine, hypnotherapy, and acupuncture (see Chapter 4). In a Cochrane Review on interventions for nausea and vomiting in pregnancy, many interventions were reviewed, including acupressure, acustimulation, acupuncture, ginger, vitamin B_6, and several antiemetic drugs (Matthews et al., 2015). Evidence regarding the effectiveness of any intervention was limited and inconsistent. There was only limited evidence from trials to support the use of pharmacological agents including vitamin B_6 and antiemetic drugs to relieve mild or moderate nausea and vomiting.

Intrahepatic Cholestasis of Pregnancy

Intrahepatic cholestasis of pregnancy (ICP), also known as obstetric cholestasis, is the most common pregnancy-specific liver disease. A reversible type of hormonally influenced cholestasis, it frequently develops in late pregnancy in individuals who are genetically predisposed. ICP is characterized by generalized itching, often with pruritus of the palms of the hands and soles of the feet with no other skin manifestations. ICP most often presents in the late second or early third trimester of pregnancy and affects approximately 1% of pregnancies in the United States.

ICP has no clear etiology and is believed to be a multifactorial disorder with environmental, hormonal, and genetic contributions. The diagnosis is based on physical examination and laboratory findings, but, in general, ICP is a diagnosis of exclusion. The incidence is 0.3% to 0.5% among the general population with up to 15% incidence in Latin American countries. Incidence also increased among those with multiple gestation (25%) and hepatitis C infection (6% to 16%) (Bowers, 2021). Affected individuals have a defect involving the excretion of bile salts, which leads to increased serum bile acids. These are deposited within the skin, causing intense pruritus.

ICP is associated with an increased risk of preterm delivery, meconium passage, intrapartum fetal heart rate (FHR) abnormalities, and fetal death as intrauterine fetal death (IUFD) incidence is most often lower than 5% in reports (Society for Maternal Fetal Medicine et al., 2017). The risk of complications for the fetus is associated with the serum level of maternal serum bile acids, and women with more severe cholestasis are at greater risk (Williamson & Geenes, 2014). The etiology of ICP is complex and appears to relate to the cholestatic effect of reproductive hormones in genetically susceptible women.

Assessment Findings

- The presenting feature of ICP is pruritus in most cases. Up to 80% of women present after 30 weeks of gestation. Pruritus is defined as an unpleasant sensation of the skin that provokes the desire to scratch. It is often the only symptom associated with ICP and may be so severe that it disturbs sleep. The pruritus typically affects the palms of the hands and the soles of the feet but may occur anywhere. It is often worse at night and gradually worsens as the pregnancy advances.
- Laboratory evidence of cholestasis includes elevated bile acids (greater than 10 umol/L). Up to 60% of patients will have elevated transaminases and 20% of patients will have increased direct bilirubin levels (Society for Maternal Fetal Medicine, 2017).
- Signs and symptoms of ICP may include systemic symptoms of cholestasis, such as dark urine and pale stools. Some women also may become clinically jaundiced, but this is rare.
- Laboratory evidence of cholestasis includes elevated bile acids (greater than 10 umol/L). Up to 60% of patients will have elevated transaminases and 20% of patients will have increased direct bilirubin levels (Society for Maternal Fetal Medicine et al., 2017).

Medical Management

- There are no preventative therapies or interventions available.
- Upon diagnosis of intrahepatic cholestasis, prenatal intervention for treatment of symptoms of cholestasis is indicated. Ursodeoxycholic acid (UDCA) has been most effective for treatment of pruritus. The starting dose of UDCA is 300 mg twice daily and can be increased to 600 mg twice daily when pruritis persists after a week of therapy. UDCA also decreases bile acids and transaminase levels though this has not been demonstrated to improve fetal outcomes. S-Adenosylmethionine can be used with UDCA for a synergistic reduction in bile acid and transaminase levels. Antihistamines, corticosteroids, or cholestyramine can be used for pruritis but are not superior to UDCA (Society for Maternal Fetal Medicine et al., 2017).
- Antihistamines are usually ineffective at relieving severe pruritus in women with ICP.
- Risk of fetal complications is increased in women whose serum bile acid level exceeds 40 micromoles/L and may be further increased if the woman has other coexistent pregnancy complications such as gestational diabetes or preeclampsia.

- In patients with ICP, the level of serum bile acids correlates with poor fetal outcomes (ACOG, 2016a).
- Antepartum fetal monitoring is recommended in antenatal management of intrahepatic cholestasis. However, type, duration, or frequency of testing has not been identified. The mechanisms of fetal death are not understood. Most demises occur late in gestation and may occur in the presence of reassuring fetal testing (Society for Maternal Fetal Medicine et al., 2017).
- Recommendation for the timing of delivery when cholestasis of pregnancy is encountered may be based on total bile acid levels (ACOG, 2021).
- ICP is associated with an increased risk of intrapartum and postpartum hemorrhage (Phillips & Boyd, 2015).
- Current consensus favors twice-weekly nonstress testing with or without Doppler testing.

Nursing Actions

- Monitor laboratory values and liver function.
- Some women find that aqueous cream with 2% menthol relieves pruritus, but it has no effect on the biochemical abnormalities associated with ICP.
- Mild itching can often be relieved with topical antipruritics and by keeping the skin well-moisturized. Emollient lotions and primrose oil may provide some relief. Increasing water intake may help keep skin hydrated and aid in excretion of toxic wastes from the body. Evaluate excoriated skin areas for possible skin infections (Phillips & Boyd, 2015).
- Resolution of pruritis usually occurs within days of delivery.
- All women with ICP should have their liver function and serum bile acids checked 6 to 8 weeks postnatally to ensure resolution.
- Explore complementary therapies to manage pruritis such as herbal remedies (e.g., milk thistle, guar gum, dandelion root, and activated charcoal); however, there is no evidence to support the use of herbal medicines or dietary supplements in the treatment of ICP.
- Medically indicated late preterm induction and birth may be based on total bile acid levels (ACOG, 2021).

DIABETES MELLITUS

In the United States, over 30 million women have diabetes mellitus, but one in four are unaware of their disease. Over the past 20 years, the number of people diagnosed with diabetes has more than tripled (Kelley & Weaver, 2019). This epidemic complicates about 7% of pregnancies per year and can significantly impact maternal and neonatal morbidity and mortality (ACOG, 2018c). There is a direct correlation between the obesity epidemic and the increased rate of diabetes and associated health risks. About 47% of gestational diabetes cases were attributed to being overweight, obese, or extremely obese (AWHONN, 2016). Though obesity predisposes women to developing diabetes, especially in pregnancy, not all women who are overweight or obese will become diabetic.

Diabetes is a complex disorder with various pathological mechanisms involved in the secretion and absorption of insulin, which results in hyperglycemia and end organ damage. It is associated with long-term harm and resulting dysfunction of the eyes, kidneys, heart, and blood vessels. Diabetes is the most common metabolic disease of pregnancy (ACOG, 2018i).

- Type 1 diabetes results from autoimmunity of beta cells of the pancreas, causing absolute insulin deficiency. It is managed with insulin. Typically, type 1 diabetics are diagnosed earlier in life and comprise about 5% to 10% of diabetic patients (Kelley & Weaver, 2019).
- Type 2 diabetes is characterized by insulin resistance and inadequate insulin production and is often diagnosed later in life. This is the most prevalent form of diabetes, making up about 90% to 95% of diabetics. Type 2 diabetes is linked to increased rates of obesity and sedentary lifestyle. Due to increasing rates of obesity, the prevalence of type 2 diabetes is rising, including in younger populations and women of childbearing age (Kelley & Weaver, 2019). It is managed primarily with diet and exercise; the addition of oral antihyperglycemic or insulin may be indicated if hyperglycemia continues. For optimum control, many women who have type 2 diabetes require insulin during pregnancy (ACOG, 2018c).

Diabetes in Pregnancy

Women with diabetes in pregnancy can be divided into two groups: pregestational diabetes and gestational diabetics (GDM). Early recognition and treatment of diabetes in pregnancy can help reduce maternal and neonatal consequences (Kelley & Weaver, 2019). For many pregnancy complications, particularly diabetes, medical management is continually under investigation and recommendations for treatment are changing. This chapter provides a general discussion of diabetes in pregnancy and then considers pregestational diabetes, followed by a discussion of gestational diabetes. Many of the same principles apply in the approach to both conditions.

- Pregestational diabetes is categorized as either type 1 or type 2 diabetes.
- Gestational diabetes mellitus (GDM) is glucose intolerance that does not present before pregnancy. Approximately 90% of diabetes cases during pregnancy are GDM (Kelley & Weaver, 2019).
- Some normal physiological changes in pregnancy present challenges for managing diabetes. These changes produce a state of insulin resistance. To spare glucose for the developing fetus, the placenta produces several hormones that antagonize insulin:
  - Human placental lactogen
  - Progesterone
  - Growth hormone
  - Corticotropin-releasing hormone

These hormones shift the primary energy sources to ketones and free fatty acids.

Most pregnant women maintain a normal glucose level in pregnancy despite increasing insulin resistance by producing increased insulin. Whether preexisting or gestational diabetes, the risk of the perinatal morbidity and mortality for the woman and neonate are significant.

For pregestational or gestational diabetes, the treatment goals are the same and management strategies are similar:

- Maintain euglycemia control.
- Minimize complications.
- Prevent prematurity.

Overall, diabetes in pregnancy is a complex health problem that requires a multidisciplinary approach to facilitate a healthy outcome for both the woman and her baby. Care for women with diabetes should begin before conception and for GDM at the time of diagnosis. The goal of preconception care is to maintain the lowest possible glycosylated hemoglobin (HbA$_1$C) without episodes of hypoglycemia (AWHONN, 2016).

- Assessment and education regarding current diabetes self-management skills
- Exploration of strategies to improve adherence to a treatment regimen
- Involvement of the woman and her family in the a treatment regimen (essential in improving adherence to treatment regimen)
- Establishment of mutual goals for glyccmic controls and self-monitoring

Pregestational Diabetes

Pregestational diabetes is used to describe blood glucose levels above the normal range but below the cutoff for overt or clinical diabetes in the nonpregnant woman (AWHONN, 2016). Although a woman may not meet the criteria for clinical diabetes, many have the components of metabolic syndrome, which include central adiposity (waste circumference greater than 35 in women), dyslipidemia, hyperglycemia, and hypertension. It is also common to see women with polycystic ovarian syndrome. It is unlikely that women diagnosed with pregestational diabetes will have improvement of their hyperglycemia once pregnant. Due to the increase of insulin resistance, women benefit from early diagnosis and management of glucose levels (ACOG, 2018i).

Pregestational diabetics have a fivefold increase in the incidence of major fetal anomalies of the heart and central nervous system (CNS). The precise mechanism for teratogenesis in diabetic women is not well-understood but is believed to be related to hyperglycemia and deficiencies in membrane lipids and prostaglandin pathways. The quality of glycemic control throughout pregnancy is key in the prevention of major complications of diabetes and the associated risks for diabetes during pregnancy (ACOG, 2018i).

Risks for the Woman

- Diabetic ketoacidosis (DKA, 1%), especially in the second trimester
- Hypertensive disorders and preeclampsia
- Metabolic disturbances related to hyperemesis, nausea, and vomiting of pregnancy
- PTL (25% risk)
- Spontaneous abortion (30% or greater risk)
- Polyhydramnios or oligohydramnios: Polyhydramnios is related to fetal anomalies and fetal hyperglycemia

(20% risk). Oligohydramnios is related to decreased placental perfusion.

- Cesarean delivery
- Labor disturbances related to increased fetal size and shoulder dystocia (ACOG, 2018i)
- Exacerbation of chronic diabetes-related conditions such as heart disease, retinopathy, nephropathy, and neuropathy
- Infection related to hyperglycemia (80% risk): urinary tract infection, chorioamnionitis, and postpartum endometritis
- Induction of labor
- Postpartum hemorrhage and subsequent anemia (ACOG, 2018i)

Risks for the Fetus and Newborn

- Congenital defects including cardiac, skeletal, neurological, genitourinary, and gastrointestinal defects related to maternal hyperglycemia during organogenesis (first 6 to 8 weeks of pregnancy)
- Growth disturbances, macrosomia related to fetal hyperinsulinemia
- Hypoglycemia related to fetal hyperinsulinemia
- Hypocalcemia and hypomagnesemia
- Polyhydramnios
- IUGR related to maternal vasculopathy and decreased maternal perfusion
- Asphyxia related to fetal hyperglycemia and hyperinsulinemia
- Respiratory distress syndrome (RDS) related to delayed fetal lung maturity
- Polycythemia (hematocrit lower than 65%) related to increased fetal erythropoietin
- Hyperbilirubinemia related to polycythemia and red blood cell (RBC) breakdown
- Prematurity due to maternal complications
- Cardiomyopathy related to maternal hyperglycemia
- Birth injury related to macrosomia
- Spontaneous abortion or stillbirth in poorly controlled maternal diabetes, especially after 36 weeks' gestation

Long-Term Risks to the Neonate

- Development of metabolic syndrome, prediabetes, and type 2 diabetes
- Impaired intellectual and psychomotor development
- Exposure to hyperglycemia in utero has been shown to affect epigenesis and is thought to change the expression of genes. As a result, it can contribute to increased risk for chronic illness later in life.

Preconception Assessment and Findings

- Classification of hyperglycemia based on abnormal blood glucose levels (HbA1c) and frequency in self-testing
- Presence of vascular or nerve dysfunction or involvement and treatment
- Evaluation of diet and proper calorie intake based on BMI
- Medication regimen evaluation and adjustment as necessary
- Evaluation of signs of metabolic syndrome or polycystic ovarian syndrome
- Evaluation of BMI

Self-Management

Comprehensive self-management of diabetes is complex yet essential for successful pregnancy outcomes. Measures include:

- Self-monitoring of blood glucose (SMBG) by checking levels four to eight times per day (before and after meals and at bedtime) in pregnancy. This is the most important parameter for determining metabolic control. Table 7-3 indicates glycemic goals for pregnancy.
- Self-monitoring of urine ketone. Women should test the first void specimen for ketones when blood glucose level is greater than 200 mg/dL, during maternal illness, or when glucose control is altered. Moderate to large amounts of ketones are an indication of inadequate food intake and should be reported to the care provider.
- Record keeping of blood glucose levels, food intake, insulin, and activity needs to be maintained for appropriate management of the treatment regimen.

TABLE 7-3   Normal Pregnancy Blood Glucose Values and Targeted Blood Glucose Values for Pregnant Women With Diabetes

NORMAL PREGNANCY BLOOD GLUCOSE VALUES		TARGET BLOOD GLUCOSE FOR PREGNANT WOMEN WITH DIABETES
Fasting	70.9 ± 7.8 mg/dL	≤ 95 mg/dL
Premeal		≤ 100 mg/dL
1 hour after meals	108.9 ± 12.9 mg/dL	≤ 140 mg/dL
2 hours after meals	99.3 ± 10 mg/dL	≤ 120 mg/dL
Mean	88 ± 10 mg/dL	100 mg/dL
A1C	4.5%–5.2%	Lower than 6%

AWHONN, 2016.

- Exercise is beneficial for glycemic control and overall well-being. Generally, exercise three times a week for at least 20 minutes is recommended, but some contraindications such as hypertension and preeclampsia do exist.
- Review signs and symptoms of maternal hypoglycemia for the prevention and management of hypoglycemic episodes. Patients should always carry a source of fast-acting carbohydrate with them, such as hard candy or fruit juice.

Medical Management

Preconception care for women with pregestational diabetes is key to decrease risks to the woman and fetus for successful pregnancy. Achieving euglycemic control for 1 to 2 months is recommended, with HbA$_1$C lower than 7%. Pregnancies complicated by preexisting diabetes are managed by a multidisciplinary team including a perinatologist, diabetes nurse educator, and dietitian. Screening at diagnosis of pregnancy may include kidney, heart, thyroid function, and ophthalmic examinations. Additional fetal diagnostic testing includes regular ultrasound examinations, intensive prenatal care schedule, and antenatal testing. The insulin needs of type 1 diabetic women increase such that by the end of pregnancy, insulin needs may be two to three times that of prepregnancy levels and may require three or four injections per day of Humulin insulin.

Medical nutritional therapy (MNT) is a cornerstone of diabetes management for pregnant women. The goal is to provide adequate nutrition, prevent diabetic ketoacidosis (DKA), and promote euglycemia. MNT needs to be individualized and continually adjusted based on blood glucose values, insulin regimen, and lifestyle. A registered dietitian should meet with the woman regularly to assess and reevaluate nutritional needs. The Institute of Medicine (IOM) recommends a calorie intake minimum of 1,800 kcals/day for pregnant women, including those who are overweight and obese. The nutritional calorie value should include intake of 40% carbohydrates, 20% protein, and 30% to 40% fat. However, all diet plans should be individualized, culturally sensitive, and set by a registered dietitian and certified diabetes educator (Roth, 2021a).

Risks of Complications During Delivery

Timing of delivery is a tremendous challenge in pregnancies complicated by diabetes. At term, the risk of stillbirth increases, as does the risk of macrosomia. However, intervention may place the woman at risk for prolonged labor and operative delivery. Thus, care providers must determine which pregnancies should be allowed to go into spontaneous labor and which are in need of labor induction. Most guidelines state that diabetes in pregnancy is not an automatic indication for scheduled cesarean delivery (ACOG, 2018i).

Complicating the issue of when and how to deliver is the fact that infants of diabetic mothers (IDM) have delayed pulmonary lung maturity and are at risk for RDS and transient tachypnea of the newborn (TTN). Excess maternal glucose levels result in excess insulin production by the fetus in utero, which is known to result in delayed surfactant production, interfering with fetal lung maturity (ACOG, 2018i).

The following are general recommendations for intrapartal care:

- Evaluate fetal lung maturity by checking if amniotic fluid is positive for phosphatidylglycerol, to try to avert RDS in the newborn who is less than 38 weeks' gestation. The lecithin/sphingomyelin (L/S) ratio is not a specific indicator for fetal lung maturity in diabetic women.
- Maintain maternal plasma glucose levels at 70 to 110 mg/dL during labor.
- Administer intravenous insulin when necessary, to achieve desired glucose levels.
- If corticosteroids are administered for risk of preterm delivery, expect insulin requirements to be increased (ACOG, 2018i).

Nursing Actions

Nurses play a key role in educating women on the importance of strict glycemic control and healthy lifestyle (Roth, 2021a). For pregnant women with type 1 diabetes, this means learning about the effects of pregnancy on diabetes management and adjustments required to the prior management regimen. The pregnancy represents new stressors and challenges for diabetic women and families. Women may feel vulnerable and anxious about their health and that of their fetus.

- Provide information on:
  - Physiological changes in pregnancy and the impact on diabetes
  - Changes in insulin requirements during pregnancy with advancing gestation
- Assist the woman in arranging for dietary counseling with a dietitian.
- Ensure dietary counseling includes the woman's preferences and pregnancy requirements along with assessment of the calorie intake and dietary pattern through 24-hour dietary recall and the importance of timing of medication if necessary.
- Review self-monitoring of blood glucose (SMBG) ketones, signs and symptoms of hyper- and hypoglycemic episode, medications including oral hypoglycemic agents or insulin, drawing up insulin and self-administering, dietary intake, and activity.
- Emphasize the importance of record keeping of dietary intake, urine ketones, glucose levels, and activity. Instruct the woman to bring records to prenatal appointments for review by the provider.
- Review signs, symptoms, and treatment of hypoglycemia (blood glucose lower than 70 mg/dL):
  - Diaphoresis; tachycardia; shakiness; cold, clammy skin; blurred vision; extreme fatigue; mental confusion and irritability; somnolence; and pallor (Roth, 2021a)
  - Ingest 15 g of carbohydrate and then wait 15 minutes for glucose level to correct before ingesting more (ACOG, 2018b)
- Review signs and symptoms of DKA, including:
  - Abdominal pain, nausea and vomiting, polyuria, polydipsia, fruity breath, leg cramps, altered mental status, and rapid respirations (Roth, 2021a)
- Care for women admitted to the hospital in DKA during pregnancy should be provided by nurses with experience in

intensive care and obstetrics. The goals of care include fluid resuscitation, restoration of electrolyte balance, reduction of hyperglycemia, and treatment of underlying cause such as infection (Roth, 2021a).

● Provide information on when and how to call the care provider:
  ● Glucose levels greater than 200 mg/dL, moderate ketones in urine, persistent nausea and vomiting, decreased fetal movement, and other indicators based on individualized plan of care (Daley, 2014)
  ● Black women are more affected by ketosis-prone type 2 diabetes (ACOG, 2018i).
● Provide information on management of nausea, vomiting, and illness:
  ● The glucose level should be checked every 1 to 2 hours during intravenous insulin infusions, urine ketones should be checked every 4 hours; insulin should still be given with vomiting (Daley, 2014).
● Provide an expected plan of prenatal care, antenatal tests, fetal surveillance, and arrange for antenatal testing.
  ● Antenatal testing generally starts at 24 to 28 weeks' gestation; includes NST and BPP.
● Provide an expected plan for labor and delivery, and plan for the possibility of an assisted birth or shoulder dystocia (Roth, 2021a).
● Assist the woman in arranging to meet with a diabetic nurse educator:
  ● Ideally, women are referred to a diabetic nurse educator to help them learn self-care management of diabetes and facilitate regulation of diabetes in pregnancy.
● Emphasize that changes in the management plan may be necessary every few weeks due to the physiological changes of pregnancy.

Gestational Diabetes Mellitus

Gestational diabetes mellitus (GDM) and pregestational diabetes have very similar predisposing factors; both are characterized by elevated blood sugar levels that do not meet criteria for clinical diabetes diagnosis. GDM is defined as glucose intolerance with onset of first recognition during pregnancy. This diagnosis applies regardless of treatment with insulin or diet modifications only and whether glucose intolerance persists after pregnancy.

GDM is divided into two clinical categories: diet controlled (GDM A1) and insulin controlled (GDM A2). Approximately 90% of pregnancies complicated by diabetes are attributed to GDM (ACOG, 2018c). When nutrition therapy is inadequate to control glucose in GDM, insulin is required. Approximately 7% of pregnancies are complicated by GDM. Increased prevalence is found in Hispanic, Black, American Indian, and Asian and Pacific Islander populations (Roth, 2021a).

Metabolic changes that occur early in pregnancy lower glucose tolerance and as a result, blood glucose levels rise and more insulin is produced. These changes promote fat storage to prepare for energy levels of a growing fetus. However, as the pregnancy develops, insulin demand increases. For most pregnant women, this is a normal physiological process. Pregnant women who

have continued hyperglycemia are diagnosed with gestational diabetes. Insulin resistance during pregnancy stems from various factors, including alterations in growth hormone and cortisol secretion (insulin antagonists), human placental lactogen secretion (produced by the placenta; affects fatty acids and glucose metabolism, promotes lipolysis, and decreases glucose uptake), and insulinase secretion (which is produced by the placenta and facilitates metabolism of insulin). In addition, estrogen and progesterone contribute to a disruption of the glucose insulin balance. Increased maternal adipose deposition, decreased exercise, and increased caloric intake also contribute to this state of relative glucose intolerance (AWHONN, 2016).

Two main contributors to insulin resistance are:

● Increased maternal adiposity
● Insulin desensitizing hormones produced by the placenta

The placenta produces human chorionic somatomammotropin (HCS), cortisol, estrogen, and progesterone. HCS stimulates pancreatic secretion of insulin in the fetus and reduces peripheral uptake of glucose. It has been proposed that as the placenta increases in size with increasing gestation, so does the production of these hormones, leading to a progressive insulin-resistant state. Women with deficient insulin secretory capacity develop GDM. Because maternal insulin does not cross the placenta, the fetus is exposed to maternal hyperglycemia and in response produces more insulin, which promotes growth and subsequent macrosomia.

The American Association of Obstetricians and Gynecologists recommends routine screening for all pregnant women at 24 to 28 weeks of gestation, with a two-step screening method for diagnosis. This two-step method was developed based on studies that showed that women with GDM have a 30% to 50% chance of developing type 2 diabetes within 20 years after pregnancy. The first step in the two-step process is a nonfasting 1-hour 50-g oral glucose tolerance test (a positive test is a result of 135 mg/dL to 140 mg/dL). Women who test positive move on to the second step, a 3-hour glucose tolerance test performed on a separate day after 8 to 12 hours of fasting. The 3-hour test is done after the woman ingests a 100-g glucose load; plasma glucose levels are drawn at 1, 2, and 3 hours post glucose load. If two or more glucose levels are above these thresholds, a diagnosis of GDM is made: fasting 95 mg/dL or higher, 1 hour of 180 mg/dL or higher, 2 hours of 155 mg/dL or higher, and 3 hours of 140 mg/dL or higher (ACOG, 2018c). Less stringent criteria have been proposed and may be used by some institutions or providers.

Risk Factors for GDM

● No known risk factors are identified in 50% of patients with GDM.
● History of fetal macrosomia
● Strong family history of diabetes
● Obesity
● Physical inactivity
● Previous history of GDM
● Polycystic ovarian syndrome
● Hypertension

Risks for the Woman

- Hypoglycemia and DKA
- Preeclampsia
- Cesarean birth
- Development of nongestational diabetes after delivery
- Hypertensive disorders
- Women with GDM who require a cesarean section may be at higher risk for delayed wound healing, infection, and postoperative mortality (Kelley & Weaver, 2019).

Risks for the Fetus and Newborn

Risks for newborns born to GDM are similar to the risks for newborns born to pregestational diabetic women, except GDM newborns are not at risk for congenital anomalies.

- Macrosomia (weight greater than the 90th percentile for gestational age and sex or a birth weight of 4,000 g to 4,500 g)
  - Macrosomia places the fetus at risk for birth injuries such as brachial plexus injury.
- IUGR
- Hypoglycemia during the first few hours post birth
- Hyperbilirubinemia
- Shoulder dystocia
- Respiratory distress syndrome
- Assisted delivery with either a vacuum or forceps
- Birth trauma
- The magnitude of fetal–neonatal complications is proportional to the severity of maternal hyperglycemia. Stillbirth related to diabetes is often due to hyperglycemia (AWHONN, 2016).

Assessment Findings

- Abnormal glucose screening results between 24 to 28 weeks of gestation
- Uncontrolled hyperglycemia may present with:
  - Polyuria
  - Polydipsia
  - Blurred vision
  - Polyphagia
  - Frequent urinary tract infections
  - Excessive fatigue and hunger
  - Recurrent vaginal candidiasis
  - Sudden weight loss
  - Episodes of hypoglycemia (see pregestational diabetes for symptoms)

Medical Management

- GDM may be managed by care providers with consultation and referral as appropriate.
- For most women with GDM, the condition is controlled with well-balanced diet and exercise.
- Up to 40% of women with GDM may need to be managed with insulin.
- Oral hypoglycemic agents may be used, but there are no currently agreed upon findings regarding their recommended use during pregnancy.

- Cesarean birth is recommended for estimated fetal weight greater than 4,500 g. Estimated fetal growth should be assessed and monitored during prenatal care appointments.
- Women with GDM need to be monitored for type 2 diabetes after the birth. Up to 70% of women with GDM will develop diabetes after pregnancy. This prevalence is highly influenced by race, as 60% of Latin American women with GDM will develop diabetes after their pregnancy (ACOG, 2018c).
- Screen women for diabetes-related comorbidities such as kidney disease, retinopathy, hypertension, neuropathy, and hyperlipidemia (Kelley & Weaver, 2019).

Nursing Actions

- The cornerstone of management of GDM is glycemic control. For women diagnosed during pregnancy with GDM, this means learning many complex skills and management strategies to maintain a healthy pregnancy.
- The goal of therapy is to maintain euglycemia throughout pregnancy.
- Teach the woman to test glucose through one fasting and three postprandial checks per day, and ask her to teach back what expected glucose levels should be (suggested glucose control is to maintain fasting glucose lower than 95 mg/dL before meals, lower than 140 mg/dL 1 hour after meals, and lower than 120 mg/dL 2 hours after meals) (Roth, 2021a) (Fig. 7–6 and Table 7-3).
- Educate the woman about the importance of glycemic control before, during, and after pregnancy, as well as the potential adverse outcomes to the mother and fetus during pregnancy from poorly controlled diabetes (Kelley & Weaver, 2019). Encourage active participation in management and decision making.
- Teach the woman to monitor fasting ketonuria levels in the morning.
- Teach proper self-administration of insulin (site selection, insulin onset, peak, duration, administration). For the gestational diabetic, it may be the first insulin administration time related to the pregnancy. Unlike for women with preexisting diabetes, this can create a tremendous change in lifestyle. Successful

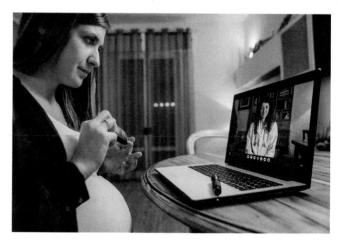

FIGURE 7–6 Blood glucose levels need to be checked regularly for any woman who has diabetes at any time during pregnancy.

self-administration of insulin requires patience, support and encouragement, and reassurance by the educator (Roth, 2021a).

- Teach the woman signs and symptoms and treatment for hypoglycemia, hyperglycemia, and DKA as previously outlined.
- Reinforce diet management. This calorie distribution will help 75% to 80% of GDM women become normoglycemic. Diet plans should be individualized and culturally sensitive. Including the person who prepares the meals in the diet planning can be helpful.
- Reinforce the plan of care related to self-management and fetal surveillance by daily fetal kick-counts and prenatal care appointments.
- Exercise has been shown to improve glycemic control by improving insulin release and sensitivity, as well as increasing caloric expenditure. Walking 10 to 15 minutes after each meal can provide benefits for glycemic control. Exercising such as brisk walking for 30 to 60 minutes per day is recommended, depending on overall physical health (Roth, 2021a). Assess the woman's mental and behavioral health. A high level of stressors, eating disorders, low self-esteem, and support systems can impact diabetes self-management by creating barriers to self-care (Kelley & Weaver, 2019).

CRITICAL COMPONENT

Key Concepts in Diabetes Management

- Pregnancy outcomes are greatly improved among women who have strict blood glucose control before and during pregnancy.
- Fetal risk and infant morbidity are relative to the level of glycemic control during pregnancy.
- Euglycemia during the preconception period reduces the risk that a woman with diabetes will spontaneously miscarry or have an infant with a congenital defect.
- Risk for gestational diabetes should be assessed early in pregnancy.
- A history of GDM increases the risk for development of overt type 2 diabetes in women (ACOG, 2018c).
- Early screening and detection may help improve outcomes for the mother and fetus (Kelley & Weaver, 2019).

HYPERTENSIVE DISORDERS IN PREGNANCY

Hypertension is identified as a systolic pressure of 140 mm Hg or greater or diastolic pressure of 90 mm Hg or greater. Hypertensive disorders of pregnancy are the most common complication of pregnancy, affecting 12% to 22% of pregnant women; they are the second leading cause of maternal death, and a significant contributor to neonatal morbidity and mortality (ACOG, 2020a). Hypertension is directly responsible for 17.6% of maternal deaths in the United States and has increased more than 50% since 1990 (Task Force on Hypertension in Pregnancy, 2013). The focus of this section is management of women with preeclampsia with severe features in the impatient setting, as that is the focus of most nursing care of women with hypertensive disorders of pregnancy.

Classifications of hypertensive disorders include:

- Chronic hypertension: Hypertension (systolic BP of 140 mm Hg or greater or diastolic pressure of 90 mm Hg or greater) before conception. Hypertension is defined as a systolic blood pressure greater than or equal to 140 mm Hg or a diastolic blood pressure greater than or equal to 90 mm Hg (ACOG, 2019b). Hypertension is diagnosed when either value is elevated; elevation of both systolic and diastolic pressures is not required for the diagnosis. Chronic hypertension is defined as hypertension present and observable before pregnancy or diagnosed before 20 weeks' gestation (ACOG, 2019b). High blood pressure is known to predate conception or detected before 20 weeks of gestation and persists beyond 12 weeks postpartum (ACOG, 2019b; Task Force on Hypertension, 2013).
- Chronic hypertension with superimposed preeclampsia includes the following scenarios:
  - Women with hypertension only in early gestation who develop proteinuria after 20 weeks of gestation
  - Women with chronic hypertension who develop new-onset or increased proteinuria and manifest other signs and symptoms such as an increase in liver enzymes or creatinine; present with thrombocytopenia; manifest with symptoms of right upper quadrant pain and headaches, blurred vision, or scotoma; and may develop pulmonary edema or congestion
- Gestational hypertension: Systolic BP of 140 mm Hg or greater or diastolic pressure of 90 mm Hg or greater for the first time after 20 weeks, without other signs and systemic finding of preeclampsia. Gestational hypertension is the onset of hypertension, generally after the 20th week of gestation, in a previously normotensive woman. If hypertension is first diagnosed during pregnancy, does not progress into preeclampsia, and is normotensive by 12 weeks postpartum. Gestational hypertension progresses to preeclampsia in 25% of cases; therefore, increased maternal-fetal surveillance is required (ACOG, 2020a).
- Preeclampsia is a multisystem hypertensive disease unique to pregnancy, with hypertension accompanied by proteinuria after the 20th week of gestation.
- Preeclampsia with severe features is preeclampsia plus at least one of the following:
  - SBP of 160 mm Hg or greater or DBP of 110 mm Hg or greater
  - Serum creatinine greater than 1.1 mg/dL or doubling of serum creatinine in the absence of renal disease
  - Platelets lower than 100,000/μL
  - Elevated serum liver enzymes to twice normal
  - New-onset cerebral or visual disturbances
  - Persistent epigastric pain
- Eclampsia is the onset of grand mal convulsions or seizures that cannot be attributed to other causes in a woman with preeclampsia. Eclampsia, the convulsive manifestation of the hypertensive disorders of pregnancy, is among the more severe manifestations of the disease.

HELLP syndrome (hemolysis, elevated liver enzymes, and low platelets) can complicate severe preeclampsia. HELLP syndrome is a clinical and laboratory diagnosis characterized by hepatic involvement as evidenced by hemolysis, elevated liver enzymes, and low platelet count. HELLP syndrome is a complication of preeclampsia or eclampsia. Due to the severity of this complication, women often require immediate treatment, urgent delivery, and transport to a tertiary care facility (ACOG, 2019b).

Preeclampsia

Preeclampsia is a hypertensive, multisystem disorder of pregnancy whose etiology remains unknown. *Williams Obstetrics* (Cunningham et al., 2018) describes preeclampsia syndrome as a pregnancy specific syndrome that can affect virtually every organ system. The rate of preeclampsia in the United States has increased 25% in the last two decades and is a leading cause of maternal and infant illness and death (ACOG, 2020a). Currently, ACOG defines preeclampsia as new-onset hypertension after 20 weeks' gestation with two blood pressure readings at least 140 mm Hg systolic and/or at least 90 mm Hg diastolic taken at least 4 hours apart. In addition, a woman will have proteinuria greater than 300 mg in 24 hours (protein/creatinine ratio of 0.3 mg/dL or higher) or new-onset systemic disease. Preeclampsia with severe features is documented when patients meet diagnostic criteria and reach severe blood pressure (systolic blood pressure of 160 mm Hg or higher and/or diastolic blood pressure of 10 mm Hg or higher) or any other diagnostic criteria aside from proteinuria.

Preeclampsia is best described as a pregnancy-specific syndrome of reduced organ perfusion secondary to vasospasm and endothelial activation (Cunningham et al., 2018). Three diagnostic considerations have emerged in recent literature. First, it is widely accepted that the disease has different presentations depending on the timing of symptom onset. Second, proteinuria is no longer an inclusion criterion for diagnosis of preeclampsia (ACOG, 2020a; Task Force on Hypertension in Pregnancy, 2013). Third, a diagnosis of mild preeclampsia is no longer appropriate based on clinical presentation, as this undermines the potential for disease progression.

Early-onset preeclampsia is defined as onset of symptoms before 34 weeks' gestation and is associated with more severe disease. Women with early-onset preeclampsia often have abnormal uterine artery Doppler waveforms and IUGR and are more likely to experience adverse perinatal outcomes, including PTB. It is proposed that poor placentation is a key factor in early-onset disease. Women with late-onset disease (onset of symptoms after 34 weeks) frequently have more favorable maternal and fetal outcomes. This disease subset is thought to be triggered by an abnormal immune response. New-onset postpartum preeclampsia appears to have yet a different clinical presentation, complicating the diagnosis.

Antepartum management as an outpatient can be considered for select women who have preeclampsia without severe features, who have access to follow-up appointments and can adhere to the treatment plan. Although management is evidence-based, preventative measures and screening tools are lacking, and treatment remains symptomatic. Delivery is no longer considered the cure.

Preeclampsia is a disease of pregnancy accompanied by underlying systemic pathology that can have severe maternal and fetal impact. It has been estimated that preeclampsia complicates 2% to 8% of pregnancies; 16% of maternal deaths can be attributed to hypertensive disorders, and, in the United States, the rate of preeclampsia increased by 25% between 1987 and 2004. In comparison with women giving birth in 1980, those giving birth in 2003 were at 6.7-fold increased risk of severe preeclampsia (ACOG, 2020a). Despite extensive research, there is no consensus as to the cause of preeclampsia.

Pathophysiology of Preeclampsia

To understand the pathophysiological mechanisms of preeclampsia, it is important to review normal physiological changes of pregnancy. Normal pregnancy is a vasodilated state in which peripheral vascular resistance decreases 25%. In the first weeks, the woman's blood pressure falls, largely due to a general relaxation of muscles within the blood vessels. Diastolic blood pressure drops 10 mm Hg at mid-pregnancy and gradually returns to prepregnant levels at term. There is a 50% rise in total blood volume by the end of the second trimester. Cardiac output increases 30% to 50%. Increased renal blood flow leads to an increased glomerular filtration rate. Because preeclampsia is a syndrome of reduced organ perfusion secondary to vasospasm and endothelial activation, the physiological changes that predispose women to preeclampsia also affect other organs and systems such as the hepatic system, renal system, coagulation system, central nervous system (CNS), eyes, fluid and electrolytes, and pulmonary system (Fig. 7–7).

Mechanisms proposed to explain the cause of preeclampsia include (Cunningham et al., 2018):

1. Placental implantation with abnormal trophoblasts invasion of uterine vessels
2. Immunological maladaptive tolerance between maternal, paternal (placental), and fetal tissues
3. Maternal maladaptation to cardiovascular changes or inflammatory changes of pregnancy
4. Genetic factors including inherited predisposing genes and epigenic influences

Disease pathways for preeclampsia are thought to involve immune system malfunction, ischemia, oxidative stress, inflammatory response, thrombosis, and endothelial dysfunction. Although signs and symptoms of preeclampsia are not evident until later in pregnancy, the pathological process most likely begins shortly after conception. It is theorized that this process involves two distinct stages: placental abnormalities and clinical manifestation of maternal disease. Fetal morbidity and mortality result from impaired or incomplete placentation. Establishment of intervillous uteroplacental circulation begins at 8 to 10 weeks' gestation and involves invasion of trophoblasts into uterine vasculature. This remodeling involves replacement of the smooth muscle layer of the spiral arteries, resulting in large-capacity dilated vessels with the low resistance necessary to increase placental circulation and oxygenation to the fetus. Incomplete transformation of the spiral arteries occurs with preeclampsia.

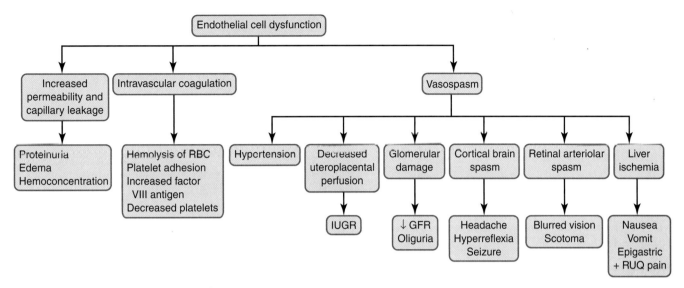

FIGURE 7-7 Pathophysiological changes of preeclampsia.

Cytotrophoblasts invade the decidua of the spiral arteries but not the myometrial portion of the artery, and this shallow invasion leads to narrow vessels with high resistance and poor placental perfusion.

An additional pathophysiologic vascular alteration occurring with preeclampsia is acute atherosis. Atherosis increases the likelihood of placental pathology, including hypoperfusion and placental infarcts. These processes may lead to placental hypoxia and ultimately fetal compromise, including IUGR, FHR decelerations, acidemia, potential developmental deficits, or fetal death (Phillips & Boyd, 2016). The placenta is evident as the root cause of preeclampsia (ACOG, 2013b).

The second stage of preeclampsia is maternal systemic disease and onset of clinical signs and symptoms. It is proposed that suboptimal placental perfusion triggers an inflammatory response, resulting in the release of pro-inflammatory cytokines, serum soluble Flt-1, and soluble endoglin into maternal circulation. Other inflammatory factors are C-reactive protein and interleukin-6. This process causes a cascading effect of endothelial damage, vasospasm, altered hemostasis, and activation of the coagulation system. Critical maternal organs affected are the brain, liver, kidneys, and vascular system. Preeclampsia is now known to have a genetic link involving inflammatory signal processing.

● Preeclampsia increases microvascular fat deposition within the liver, proposed as one cause of epigastric pain. Liver damage may be mild or progress to HELLP syndrome. Hepatic involvement can lead to periportal hemorrhagic necrosis in the liver that may cause a subcapsular hematoma, potentially resulting in right upper quadrant or epigastric pain. This may signal worsening preeclampsia.
● In 70% of preeclamptic patients, glomerular endothelial damage, fibrin deposition, and resulting ischemia reduce renal plasma flow and glomerular filtration rate (National High Blood Pressure Education Program [NHBPEP], 2000). Protein is excreted in urine. Uric acid, creatinine, and calcium clearance are decreased and oliguria develops as the condition worsens. Oliguria signifies severe preeclampsia and kidney damage.

● The coagulation system is activated in preeclampsia and thrombocytopenia occurs, possibly due to increased platelet aggregation and deposition at sites of endothelial damage, activating the clotting cascade. A platelet count lower than 100 $\times 10^9$/L is an indication of severe preeclampsia.
● Endothelial damage to the brain results in fibrin deposition, edema, and cerebral hemorrhage, which may lead to hyperreflexia and severe headaches and can progress to eclampsia.
● Retinal arterial spasms may cause blurring or double vision, photophobia, or scotoma.
● The leakage of serum protein into extracellular spaces and into urine, by way of damaged capillary walls, results in decreased serum albumin and tissue edema.
● Pulmonary edema is most commonly caused by volume overload related to left ventricular failure as the result of extremely high vascular resistance (Cunningham et al., 2018).

CRITICAL COMPONENT

Preeclampsia: Signs, Symptoms, and Severe Features

Preeclampsia is defined as new-onset hypertension after 20 weeks' gestation with two blood pressure readings of at least 140 mm Hg systolic and/or at least 90 mm Hg diastolic taken at least 4 hours apart. In addition, a woman will have proteinuria greater than 300 mg in 24 hours (protein/creatinine ratio of 0.3 mg/dL or more) or new-onset systemic disease including thrombocytopenia (platelet count lower than 100 $\times 10^9$/L), impaired liver function (hepatic transaminase levels elevated twice above normal values and/or persistent right upper quadrant or epigastric abdominal pain), creatinine level indicative of renal insufficiency (greater than 1.1 dL), new-onset cerebral or visual symptoms such as persistent headache, or visual disturbances (ACOG, 2020a; Task Force on Hypertension in Pregnancy, 2013).

Continued

CRITICAL COMPONENT—cont'd

Diagnostic Criteria for Preeclampsia
Blood pressure

- Systolic blood pressure of 140 mm Hg or more or diastolic blood pressure of 90 mm Hg or more on two occasions at least 4 hours apart after 20 weeks of gestation in a woman with a previously normal blood pressure
- Systolic blood pressure of 160 mm Hg or more or diastolic blood pressure of 110 mm Hg or more. (Severe hypertension can be confirmed within a short interval (minutes) to facilitate timely antihypertensive therapy)

and Proteinuria

- 300 mg or more per 24-hour urine collection (or this amount extrapolated from a timed collection) or
- Proteinuria during pregnancy: 300 mg/dL of protein or more in a 24-hour urine collection
- Protein/creatinine ratio of 0.3 mg/dL or more or
- Dipstick reading of 2+ (used only if other quantitative methods not available)

Or in the absence of proteinuria, new-onset hypertension with the new onset of any of the following:

- Thrombocytopenia: Platelet count lower than 100,000 × 10⁹/L
- Renal insufficiency: Serum creatinine concentrations greater than 1.1 mg/dL or a doubling of the serum creatinine concentration in the absence of other renal disease
- Impaired liver function: Elevated blood concentrations of liver transaminases to twice normal concentration
- Pulmonary edema
- New-onset headache unresponsive to medication and not accounted for by alternative diagnoses or visual symptoms

Preeclampsia With Severe Features
- Systolic blood pressure of 160 mm Hg or more, or diastolic blood pressure of 110 mm Hg or more on two occasions at least 4 hours apart (unless antihypertensive therapy is initiated before this time)
- Thrombocytopenia (platelet count lower than 100 × 10⁹/L)
- Impaired liver function that is not accounted for by alternative diagnoses and as indicated by abnormally elevated blood concentrations of liver enzymes (to more than twice the upper limit of normal concentrations), or by severe persistent right upper quadrant or epigastric pain that is unresponsive to medications
- Renal insufficiency (serum creatinine concentration more than 1.1 mg/dL or a doubling of the serum creatinine concentration in the absence of other renal disease)
- Pulmonary edema
- New-onset headache unresponsive to medication and not accounted for by alternative diagnoses
- Visual disturbances (ACOG, 2020a; Task Force on Hypertension in Pregnancy, 2013)

Risk Factors for Preeclampsia

- Nulliparity
- Maternal age older than 35 years
- Prepregnancy obesity BMI greater than 30
- Multiple gestation
- Family history of preeclampsia
- Chronic hypertension, kidney disease, systemic lupus, thrombophilia, antiphospholipid syndrome, or diabetes before pregnancy
- Previous preeclampsia or eclampsia
- Gestational diabetes
- Assisted reproduction

Although the precise role of genetic–environmental interactions is unclear, emerging data suggest the tendency to develop preeclampsia may have some genetic component. As yet no single test reliably predicts preeclampsia.

Risks for the Woman

- Cerebral edema, hemorrhage, or stroke
- Disseminated intravascular coagulation (DIC)
- Pulmonary edema
- Congestive heart failure
- Maternal sequelae resulting from organ damage include renal failure, HELLP syndrome, thrombocytopenia and disseminated intravascular coagulation, pulmonary edema, eclampsia (seizures), and hepatic failure
- Abruptio placenta
- Women with a history of preeclampsia have a 1.5 to 2 times higher risk of developing heart disease later in life. Evidence suggests that all hypertensive conditions in pregnancy are associated with later cardiovascular disease with an approximate doubling of the rate of incident cardiovascular disease and a five times higher rate of hypertension (ACOG, 2020a).

Risks for the Fetus and Newborn

- Consequences of uteroplacental ischemia include fetal growth restriction, oligohydramnios, placental abruption, and nonreassuring fetal status. Therefore, fetuses of women with preeclampsia are at increased risk of spontaneous or indicated preterm delivery.
- Fetal intolerance to labor due to decreased placental perfusion
- Stillbirth

In addition, we now know that the intrauterine environment associated with IUGR programs the fetus for adult disease later in life. Newborns with IUGR are at increased risk for metabolic and cardiovascular diseases as adults, including type 2 diabetes, obesity, metabolic syndrome, and hypertension.

Assessment Findings

Accurate assessment is essential so that early recognition of worsening disease will allow for timely intervention that may improve maternal and neonatal outcomes.

- Elevated blood pressure: Hypertension with systolic pressure of 140 mm Hg or greater and diastolic pressure of 90 mm Hg

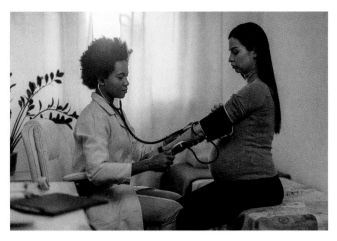

FIGURE 7–8 Take the woman's blood pressure while she is seated and with her arm at heart level.

or greater. Blood pressure should be measured with the woman at rest. The proper cuff size is one whose bladder circles at least 80% of the upper arm. A mercury sphygmomanometer is most accurate. The arm should be supported at the level of the heart (see Fig. 7–8).

- Proteinuria is no longer a diagnostic criterion. According to ACOG guidelines (2020a), the diagnosis of preeclampsia no longer requires the detection of high levels of protein in the urine (proteinuria). Evidence shows organ problems with the kidneys and liver can occur without signs of protein, and that the amount of protein in the urine does not predict how severely the disease will progress.
- Laboratory values may indicate elevations in liver function tests, diminished kidney function, and altered coagulopathies.
- Evidence tells us that preeclampsia is a dynamic process. Diagnosing a woman's condition as "mild preeclampsia" is not helpful because it is a progressive disease, progressing at different rates in different women. Appropriate care requires frequent reevaluation for severe features of the disease and appropriate actions outlined in the new guidelines.

Medical Management

Management for preeclampsia is expectant or expedient birth, depending on the severity of disease, gestational age, and fetal status. Women with early-onset preeclampsia (less than 34 weeks' gestation) will need corticosteroids to facilitate fetal lung maturity and may require magnesium sulfate. Low-dose aspirin prophylaxis is recommended for women at high risk for preeclampsia (ACOG, 2018f). Once diagnosed, the woman and fetus should be monitored weekly for indications of worsening condition, as preeclampsia is a progressive disease. However, women can also present with abrupt onset of the disease. Indications of worsening preeclampsia are treated with hospitalization and evaluation. Antihypertensive drugs are used to control elevated blood pressure. Delivery is indicated in severe preeclampsia, even before term, to protect the woman and fetus from severe sequelae. Care in labor and delivery includes use of magnesium sulfate to prevent seizures. Magnesium sulfate should be used for the prevention and treatment of seizures in women with gestational hypertension, preeclampsia with severe features, or eclampsia (ACOG, 2020a).

The primary goal in preeclampsia is to control the woman's blood pressure and prevent seizure activity and cerebral hemorrhage. Induced birth is indicated for women at less than 34 weeks' gestation with severe features of preeclampsia or for unstable maternal or fetal status at any gestation. Medical management includes the following measures:

- Magnesium sulfate, a CNS depressant, has been proven to help reduce seizure activity without documentation of long-term adverse effects to the woman and fetus.
- Antihypertensive medications are used to control blood pressure (Table 7-4).
- Outpatient management for women with mild preeclampsia is an option if the woman can adhere to activity restriction, frequent office visits, blood pressure monitoring, and antenatal testing.
- Induced birth is indicated for women at less than 34 weeks' gestation with severe features of preeclampsia or for unstable maternal or fetal status at any gestation (Cluver, 2017).
- For hypertensive disorders as a group, planned early delivery appears to be better for the mother after 34 weeks' gestation. However, it is unclear whether planned early delivery increases risks for the baby, especially at earlier gestations. More research is needed to guide practice according to a recent Cochrane Review (Cluver, 2017).
- Continued monitoring of women with gestational hypertension or preeclampsia without severe features consists of serial ultrasonography to determine fetal growth, weekly antepartum testing, close monitoring of blood pressure, and weekly laboratory tests for preeclampsia.

Nursing Actions With Hospitalized Women

- Accurate assessment is essential because early recognition of worsening disease allows timely intervention and may improve maternal and neonatal outcome.
- In women with preeclampsia without severe features, the progression to severe preeclampsia could happen within days.
- Blood pressure should be measured with the woman seated and her arm at heart level, using an appropriately sized cuff (Fig. 7–8). Placing the woman in a left lateral recumbent position is no longer recommended to evaluate blood pressure, as it gives an inaccurately low blood pressure reading (ACOG, 2020a; Cunningham et al., 2018; NHBPEP, 2000).
- Administer antihypertensive as per orders (generally for blood pressure higher than 160/110 mm Hg) (see Table 7-4).
- Administer magnesium sulfate as per orders.
- Assess for CNS changes including headache, visual changes, deep tendon reflexes (DTRs), and clonus (Box 7-3 and Fig. 7–9).

TABLE 7-4   Preeclampsia and Eclampsia Medications

DRUG NAME OR CLASS	ADMINISTRATION AND USE	CONTRAINDICATIONS
Magnesium sulfate	IV access: Load 4–6 grams 10% magnesium sulfate in 100 mL solution over 20 minutes. Maintenance dose: 1–2 grams/hour. No IV access: 10 grams of 50% solution IM (5 grams in each buttock)	Pulmonary edema, renal failure, myasthenia gravis
Antihypertensive medications	For SBP ≥160 or DBP ≥110 Labetalol: (10–20 mg for more than 2 minutes, 40 mg, 80 IV over 2 minutes, escalating doses, may repeat q 10 min). Onset of action 1 to 2 minutes. Maximum cumulative dose should not exceed 300 mg in 24 hours. Hydralazine: (5–10 mg IV over 2 minutes, may repeat q 20 min until target BP reached). Onset of action 10 to 20 minutes. Maximum cumulative IV-administered dose should not exceed 20 mg in 24 hours. Nifedipine: 10–20 mg capsules PRN may repeat in 20 minutes Use of IV labetalol, IV hydralazine, or immediate release oral nifedipine does not require cardiac monitoring.	Labetalol: Avoid in asthma or heart failure, can cause neonatal bradycardia Hydralazine: Mitral valve disease
Anticonvulsant medications	For recurrent seizures or when magnesium sulfate is contraindicated. Lorazepam (Ativan): 2–4 mg IV ×1, may repeat once after 10–15 min Diazepam (Valium): 5–10 mg IV q 5–10 min to maximum dose 30 mg *If persistent seizures, consider anticonvulsant medications and additional workup.	

ACOG, 2017a, 2019b, 2020a; Burgess, 2021.

BOX 7-3 | Assessment of Deep Tendon Reflexes

PHYSICAL ASSESSMENT	GRADE
None elicited	0
Sluggish or dull	1
Active, normal	2
Brisk	3
Brisk with transient or sustained clonus	4

See Figure 7–9.

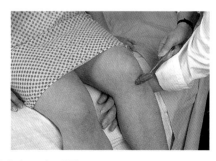

FIGURE 7–9 Assessing DTRs.

- Auscultate lung sounds for clarity and monitor the RR.
- Assess for signs and symptoms of pulmonary edema such as:
  - Shortness of breath, chest tightness or discomfort, cough, oxygen saturation lower than 95%, increased respiratory and heart rates
  - Changes in behavior, such as apprehension, anxiety, or restlessness
- Assess for epigastric pain or right upper quadrant pain indicating liver involvement.
- Assess weight daily and assess for edema to assess for fluid retention.
- Check urine for proteinuria (may include 24-hour urine collection) and specific gravity.
- Evaluate laboratory values including:
  - Elevations in serum creatinine greater than 1.1 mg/dL
  - Hematocrit levels greater than 35
  - Platelet count lower than $100 \times 10^9/L$
  - Elevated liver enzymes AST and ALT greater than 2X the upper limit of normal (Burgess, 2021)
- Perform antenatal fetal testing and FHR monitoring (NST and BPP).
- Check intake of adequate calories and protein.
- Maintain accurate I&O to evaluate kidney function. Total fluid intake may be restricted to 2,000 mL/24 hr.

- Provide a quiet environment to decrease CNS stimulation.
- Maintain bedrest in the lateral recumbent position.
- Provide information to the woman and her family. Education is key in helping with the understanding of the disease process and the plan of care.
- Report deterioration in maternal or fetal status to provider. Analysis of maternal mortality data on preeclampsia cases shows that despite triggers that clearly indicated a serious deterioration in the patient's condition, health-care providers failed to recognize and respond to these signs in a timely manner, leading to delays in diagnosis and treatment. Appendix B presents a Preeclampsia Early Recognition Tool (PERT) https://www.cmqcc.org/resource /preeclampsia-early-recognition-tool-pert as an example of tools developed by the California Maternal Quality Care Collaborative to reduce preeclampsia-related deaths with timely recognition of symptoms and a quick response to diagnosis.

SAFE AND EFFECTIVE NURSING CARE: Understanding Medication

Intravenous Administration of Magnesium Sulfate

Magnesium sulfate is indicated for women with severe features of preeclampsia. Although the exact method of action in seizure prophylaxis is not clearly understood, therapeutic levels of the drug will result in cerebral vasodilation, thereby reducing ischemia caused by vasospasm. Magnesium sulfate also slows neuromuscular conduction, depresses the vasomotor center, and decreases CNS irritability (Burgess, 2021). Magnesium sulfate is given per protocol as an IV piggyback always via a controlled infusion device.

Continuous intravenous administration:

- Loading dose: 4 to 6 g diluted in 100 mL of IV fluid administered over 15 to 20 minutes
- Continuous infusion: 1 to 2 g/hr in 100 mL of IV fluid for maintenance
- When used for seizure prophylaxis, magnesium sulfate is administered as a secondary infusion by an infusion-controlled device to achieve serum levels of approximately 4.8 to 8.4 mg/dL (4 to 7 mEq/dL).
- Laboratory evaluation: Measure serum magnesium level at 4 to 6 hours, after onset of treatment. Dosage should be adjusted to maintain a therapeutic range of 4.8 to 9.6 mg/dL (4 to 8 mEq/L).
- Duration: Intravenous infusion should continue for 24 to 48 hours postdelivery.
- The antidote for magnesium toxicity is calcium gluconate 1 g of 10% solution given IV slowly over 5 to 10 minutes.

CRITICAL COMPONENT

Care of the Woman on Magnesium Sulfate

POTENTIAL SIDE EFFECTS	NURSING ACTIONS
Maternal: Nausea Flushing Diaphoresis Blurred vision Lethargy Hypocalcemia Depressed reflexes Respiratory depression-arrest Cardiac dysrhythmias Decreased platelet aggregation Circulatory collapse	Assess baseline vital signs, DTRs, neurologic status, and urine output before beginning infusion and every 5 to 15 minutes during loading dose, then every 30 to 60 minutes until the patient stabilizes. Frequency is then determined by the patient's status and protocol.

Assess deep tendon reflexes (DTRs) every 2 hours. DTRs can be elicited by striking the tendon of a partially stretched muscle briskly using the flat or pointed surface of the reflex hammer (Burgess, 2021). Patellar, or knee-jerk, reflexes may be unreliable in women who have had regional anesthesia, and brachial reflexes should be used. Reflexes are graded on a scale of 0 to +4, with 0 being an absent reflex and +4 being a hyperactive reflex.

Educate the patient regarding side effects and provide a cool environment; offer cold packs and cool facecloth for comfort.

Clonus is associated with CNS excitability and can be elicited by dorsiflexing the foot against the nurse's hand, then releasing it suddenly. Beats of clonus occur when the foot taps against the examiner's hand instead of returning to the normal position.

Monitor strict intake and output. Some recommend intake of lower than 125 cc/hr. Consider a Foley with urimeter. Patients with oliguria or renal disease are at risk for toxic levels of magnesium.

- Monitor serum magnesium levels for a therapeutic level of 4.8 to 9.6 mg/dL (4 to 8 mEq/L). The adverse effects of magnesium sulfate (respiratory depression and cardiac arrest) come largely from its action as a smooth muscle relaxant. DTRs are lost at a serum magnesium level of 9 mg/dL (7 mEq/L), respiratory depression occurs at 12 mg/dL (10 mEq/L), and cardiac arrest occurs at 30 mg/dL (25 mEq/L). Accordingly, provided DTRs are present, more serious toxicity is avoided (ACOG, 2020a).
- Monitor for signs and symptoms of magnesium toxicity.
- Decreased reflexes could be a sign of pending respiratory depression.
- Loss of DTRs
- Respiratory depression: RR lower than 14

Continued

CRITICAL COMPONENT—cont'd

POTENTIAL SIDE EFFECTS	NURSING ACTIONS
	• breaths/min
	• Oliguria, urine output less than 30 mL/hr
	• Shortness of breath or chest pain
	• EKG changes
	• If toxicity is suspected, discontinue the infusion and notify the health-care provider. Respiration difficulty can occur with magnesium levels above 12 mEq/L.
	• Keep calcium gluconate immediately available (1 g of 10% solution).
	• Continue neurologic evaluation.
	• Maintain seizure precautions and keep resuscitation equipment nearby.
	• Patients receiving IV labetalol for blood pressure control should have cardiac monitoring.
	• Maintain continuous FHR monitoring.
	Report abnormal findings including:
	• Urine output less than 30 mL/hour
	• RR lower than 12 breaths/minute
	• SpO$_2$ lower than 95%
	• Persistent hypotension
	• Absent DTRs
	• Altered maternal levels of consciousness
	• Abnormal laboratory test values
Fetal/neonatal:	Monitor FHR. Alert the neonatal team before delivery of use of magnesium sulfate in labor.
FHR decreased variability	
Respiratory depression	
Hypotonia	
Decreased suck reflex	
Signs and symptoms of magnesium toxicity	

CLINICAL JUDGMENT

Emergent Therapy for Acute-Onset, Severe Hypertension During Pregnancy and the Postpartum Period

Acute-onset, severe systolic (greater than or equal to 160 mm Hg) hypertension; severe diastolic (greater than or equal to 110 mm Hg) hypertension; or both can occur during the prenatal, intrapartum, or postpartum periods. Pregnant women or women in the postpartum period with acute-onset, severe systolic hypertension; severe diastolic hypertension; or both require urgent antihypertensive therapy. The goal is not to normalize BP, but to achieve a range of 140–150/90–100 mm Hg to prevent repeated, prolonged exposure to severe systolic hypertension, with subsequent loss of cerebral vasculature autoregulation. In the event of a hypertensive crisis, with prolonged uncontrolled hypertension, maternal stabilization should occur before delivery, even in urgent circumstances. Treatment with first-line agents should be expeditious and occur as soon as possible within 30 to 60 minutes of confirmed severe hypertension to reduce the risk of maternal stroke.

Intravenous (IV) labetalol and hydralazine have long been considered first-line medications for the management of acute-onset, severe hypertension in pregnant women and women in the postpartum period. Immediate release oral nifedipine also may be considered as a first-line therapy, particularly when IV access is not available.

It is important to note differences in recommended dosage intervals between these options, which reflect differences in their pharmacokinetics. Protocols should be followed for maternal monitoring of blood pressure every 5 to 15 minutes. None of the recommended drugs require cardiac monitoring.

Although all three medications are appropriately used to treat hypertensive emergencies in pregnancy, each agent can be associated with adverse effects. Parenteral hydralazine may increase the risk of maternal hypotension (systolic BP, 90 mm Hg or lower). Parenteral labetalol may cause neonatal bradycardia and should be avoided in women with asthma, heart disease, or congestive heart failure. Nifedipine has been associated with an increase in maternal heart rate, and with overshoot hypotension (ACOG, 2017b, 2019b; Burgess, 2021).

Fetal Assessment

Preeclampsia exposes the fetus to an adverse intrauterine environment. Hypoperfusion of the placenta can result in chronic hypoxia, IUGR, asphyxia, and fetal death. Antenatal fetal surveillance is used to detect compromised fetal status in the hope of preventing asphyxia and stillbirth. Fetal well-being is evaluated by the following measures:

● Fetal movement is a critical component of nursing assessment; a woman's report of decreased fetal movement should always be investigated.

● Biophysical profile (BPP) can be used to screen for acute or chronic fetal hypoxia by examining five fetal parameters most affected by hypoxia: the nonstress test (NST), fetal movement, fetal breathing, fetal tone, and amniotic fluid index (AFI) (see Chapter 6). A normal score is 8 (without NST) to 10 (with reactive NST); a score of 4 or less is considered abnormal and indicative of fetal compromise.

● Oligohydramnios is associated with an increased risk of perinatal morbidity and mortality, and therefore this finding is especially concerning. Because amniotic fluid is comprised mostly of fetal urine, low fluid volume would indicate a lack of renal perfusion.

● Evaluation and decision making regarding fetal IUGR is facilitated by umbilical artery Doppler velocimetry testing. This measures hemodynamic changes in the fetal and placental circulation unit. The S/D ratio is most commonly measured, and the value should decline as a normal pregnancy progresses, reflecting increased blood flow to the fetus due to decreased placental resistance. However, when pregnancy is complicated by preeclampsia, atherosis of the placental vessels results in an increase in placental resistance. An elevated S/D ratio (greater than 3 to 4) is seen with fetal growth restriction before clinical signs of fetal distress and possibly even before an abnormal BPP. The blood flow through the umbilical arteries should be forward. If this flow, called the end diastolic flow, is an absent or reversed-end diastolic flow, this is indicative of fetal compromise and placental dysfunction and warrants increased surveillance and assessment for birth.

Eclampsia

Eclampsia is seizure activity in the presence of preeclampsia. Eclampsia is the convulsive manifestation of the hypertensive disorders of pregnancy and is among the more severe manifestations of the disease (ACOG, 2020a). Eclampsia can occur ante-, intra-, or postpartum; about 50% of cases occur antepartum. Eclampsia may be triggered by one or more of the following:

- Cerebral vasospasm
- Cerebral hemorrhage
- Cerebral ischemia
- Cerebral edema

Eclampsia often (78% to 83% of cases) is preceded by premonitory signs of cerebral irritation such as severe and persistent occipital or frontal headaches, blurred vision, photophobia, and altered mental status. However, eclampsia can occur without warning signs or symptoms.

During eclamptic seizures, prolonged FHR decelerations, even fetal bradycardia, and sometimes an increase in uterine contractility and baseline tone occur. After a seizure, due to maternal hypoxia and hypercarbia, the FHR tracing may show recurrent decelerations, tachycardia, and reduced variability. However, only after maternal hemodynamic stabilization should the team proceed with delivery (ACOG, 2020a).

Care during a seizure includes (Box 7-4):

- Remaining with the patient
- Calling for help
- Providing for patient safety by assessing airway and breathing:
  - Lower the head of the bed and turn the woman's head to one side.
  - Anticipate the need for suctioning to decrease the risk of aspiration.
  - Aspiration is the leading cause of maternal mortality (ACOG, 2020a; Burgess, 2021).
- Preventing maternal injury:
  - Keep side rails up and padded, if possible.
- Record the time, length, and type of seizure activity.
- Notify the physician.

During eclamptic seizures, there are usually prolonged FHR decelerations, even fetal bradycardia, and sometimes an increase in uterine contractility and baseline tone. After the seizure, the nurse should:

BOX 7-4 | Eclampsia Protocol

Assessment Findings

Confirm findings again within 10 minutes after calling the physician.

- SBP lower than 90 mm Hg or greater than 160 mm Hg; DBP greater than 100 mm Hg (***Not applicable for SBP lower than 90 when 30 minutes or less post-epidural and anesthesiologist present.)
- Heart rate lower than 50 bpm or greater than 120 bpm
- RR lower than 10 bpm or greater than 30 bpm
- Oxygen saturation lower than 95%
- Oliguria lower than 35 mL/hr × 2 hours
- Maternal agitation, confusion, or unresponsiveness
- Blurred vision
- Proteinuria
- Nonremitting headache or shortness of breath in a hypertensive patient

Diagnostic and Laboratory Tests to Consider

- Pulse oximeter
- CBC, CMP
- Urinalysis
- Type and screen or type and cross match if bleeding
- Magnesium level
- EKG
- CT angiogram or perfusion scan in patients with acute chest pain
- Chest x-ray if patient is short of breath, particularly if preeclamptic
- Echocardiogram

Eclampsia Nursing Interventions

- Call all emergency team members immediately and designate a team leader, checklist reader or recorder, and primary RN if needed.
- Turn the patient to the lateral recumbent position.
- Protect the airway and improve oxygenation; administer supplemental oxygen (100% nonrebreather face mask); ensure suction and bag-mask ventilation are available; maternal pulse oximetry.
- Monitor and record description, characteristics, and duration of seizure activity, if present.
- Monitor BP, RR, and pulse oximetry.
- Monitor fetal status, uterine activity, and cervical change.
- Establish and maintain IV access; draw preeclampsia laboratory results.
- Administer magnesium sulfate per protocol.
- Administer antihypertensive therapy.

Continued

BOX 7-4 | Eclampsia Protocol—cont'd

- Facilitate delivery plan, if appropriate.
- Update and communicate with patient, family, and obstetric team.

Provider Notification

- RN will notify the attending OB of the patient's status and request a bedside evaluation, and the OB physician will evaluate the patient within 10 minutes.
- The in-house OB will also be notified and will provide a bedside evaluation if the attending OB is unavailable.
- If the in-house OB is not immediately available, they will receive a verbal report and determine if further action is necessary.
- The OB will decide the planned frequency of monitoring and reevaluation, as well as criteria for immediate physician notification, and any necessary diagnostic therapeutic interventions.
- A "huddle" will take place and members, including the OB, primary RN, charge RN, and anesthesiologist, will discuss the management plan.
- If the condition persists or worsens after interventions, consider calling a rapid response.
- Seizures may lead to severe maternal hypoxia, trauma, and aspiration pneumonia. Although residual neurological damage is rare, some women may have short-term and long-term consequences such as impaired memory and cognitive function, especially after recurrent seizures or uncorrected severe hypertension leading to cytotoxic edema or infarction. Permanent white matter loss has been documented on magnetic resonance imaging (MRI) after eclampsia in up to one-fourth of women; however, this does not translate into significant neurological deficits (ACOG, 2020a).

ACOG, 2017a, 2020a; Burgess, 2021; Council on Patient Safety in Women's Health Care, 2017.

- Rapidly assess maternal and fetal status. After a seizure, due to maternal hypoxia and hypercarbia, the FHR tracing may show recurrent decelerations, tachycardia, and decreased variability.
- Assess airway; suction if needed.
- Administer supplemental oxygen: 10 L/min via mask.
- Ensure IV access:
  - Administer magnesium sulfate per orders.
  - Provide a quiet environment.
  - Seizures may lead to severe maternal hypoxia, trauma, and aspiration pneumonia. Residual neurologic damage is uncommon, although some women may have short-term and long-term consequences such as impaired memory and cognitive function; however, this does not typically result in significant neurological deficits (ACOG, 2020a).

HELLP Syndrome

The clinical presentation of hemolysis, elevated liver enzymes, and low platelet count (HELLP) syndrome is one of the more severe forms of preeclampsia because it has been associated with increased rates of maternal morbidity and mortality (ACOG, 2020a). HELLP syndrome is the acronym used to designate the variant changes in laboratory values that can occur as a complication of severe preeclampsia:

- Hemolysis results from red blood cell (RBC) destruction as the cells travel through constricted vessels.
- Elevated liver enzymes result from decreased blood flow and damage to the liver.
- Low platelets result from platelets aggregating at the site of damaged vascular endothelium, causing platelet consumption and thrombocytopenia (Cunningham et al., 2018; Sibai, 2004).

Women with severe preeclampsia have an increased risk (7% to 24%) of developing HELLP syndrome. However, HELLP may develop in women who do not present with the cardinal signs of severe preeclampsia. In fact, HELLP may appear at any time during the pregnancy in 70% of cases, and in the immediate postpartum period for 30% of cases (ACOG, 2020a). The only definitive treatment is delivery. However, some women experience worsening HELLP syndrome over the first 48-hour postpartum period. Women with only some of the laboratory changes are diagnosed with partial HELLP syndrome. HELLP is diagnosed based on the presence of:

- Hemolysis
- Abnormal peripheral smear
- LDH greater than 600 U/L
- Total bilirubin 0.2 mg/dL or greater
- Elevated liver enzymes
- Serum AST of 70 U/L or greater
- Platelet count lower than 100×10^9/L

Risks for the Woman

- Abruptio placenta
- Renal failure
- Liver hematoma and possible rupture
- Death

Risks for the Fetus and Newborn

- PTB
- Death

Assessment Findings

- In HELLP syndrome, the main presenting symptoms are right upper quadrant pain and generalized malaise in up to 90% of cases and nausea and vomiting in 50% of cases (ACOG, 2020a).
- The woman may have unexplained bruising, mucosal bleeding, petechiae, and bleeding from injection and IV sites.
- Assessment findings are related to alternations in laboratory tests associated with changes in liver function and platelets.

Medical Management

The only definitive cure for HELLP syndrome is immediate delivery of the fetus and placenta. Disease resolution generally occurs 48 hours postpartum. Medical management may include platelet replacement and is the same as for women with severe preeclampsia (Burgess, 2021).

Nursing Actions

- Perform a thorough assessment of the woman related to the diagnosis of preeclampsia.
- Evaluate laboratory tests.
- Notify the physician immediately if HELLP syndrome is suspected or laboratory values deteriorate.
- Administer platelets as per orders.
- Note that assessment and management are the same for the women diagnosed with HELLP syndrome as for the women with severe preeclampsia.
- Provide the woman and the family with information regarding HELLP and its treatment.
- Provide emotional support to the woman and her family, as the woman and family are at risk for increased levels of anxiety related to the diagnosis (Mattson & Smith, 2011).

CLINICAL JUDGMENT

Complications of Hypertensive Disorders

Complications arising from hypertensive disorders of pregnancy are among the leading causes of preventable severe maternal morbidity and mortality. Timely and appropriate treatment has the potential to significantly reduce hypertension-related complications. To assist in achieving this goal, the patient safety bundle has been developed to provide guidance to coordinate and standardize the care provided to women with severe hypertension during pregnancy and the postpartum period. Safety bundles outline critical clinical practices that should be implemented in every maternity care setting and are organized into four domains: Readiness, Recognition and Prevention, Response, and Reporting and Systems Learning. Guidelines for the response part of the Hypertension bundle include recommendations that, for every case of severe hypertension or preeclampsia, these should be standard protocols with checklists and escalation policies for management and treatment of severe hypertension, eclampsia, seizure prophylaxis, and magnesium overdosage.

Postpartum presentation of severe hypertension or preeclampsia:

Notify the physician or primary care provider if systolic BP of 160 or more or diastolic BP of 110 or more for two measurements within 15 minutes.

After the second elevated reading, treatment should be initiated ASAP (preferably within 60 minutes of verification).

Note the onset and duration of magnesium sulfate therapy.

Consider escalation measures for those unresponsive to standard treatment.

Describe the manner and verification of follow-up within 7 to 14 days postpartum.

Describe postpartum patient education for women with preeclampsia.

Develop a support plan for patients, families, and staff for ICU admissions and serious complications of severe hypertension.

Adapted from Bernstein et al., 2017.

PLACENTAL ABNORMALITIES AND HEMORRHAGIC COMPLICATIONS

Major blood loss during pregnancy is a significant contributor to both maternal and fetal morbidity and mortality. Hemorrhage predisposes a woman to hypovolemia, anemia, infection, and premature birth and maternal death. Major maternal blood loss can cause decreased perfusion and oxygen to the fetus, resulting in progressive deterioration of fetal status and even death (Salera-Vieira, 2021). Placental abnormalities and hemorrhagic complications of pregnancy are presented in this section.

The major causes of antepartum hemorrhage are placenta previa and placental abruption. The basic principles of immediate care of women with either type of antepartum hemorrhage include assessment of maternal and fetal condition, prompt maternal resuscitation if required, and consideration of early delivery if there is evidence of fetal distress and if the baby is mature enough to be potentially capable of survival. Up to 20% of maternal cardiac output, and up to 1,000 mL/min, flows through the placental bed at term; unresolved bleeding can result in maternal exsanguination in 8 to 10 minutes (Salera-Vieira, 2021).

Placental disorders such as placenta previa, placenta accreta, and vasa previa are all associated with vaginal bleeding in the second half of pregnancy. They are also important causes of serious fetal and maternal morbidity and even mortality. Moreover, the rates of previa and accreta are increasing, probably due to increasing rates of cesarean delivery, maternal age, and ART. The routine use of obstetric ultrasonography as well as improving ultrasonographic technology allows for the antenatal diagnosis of these conditions. In turn, antenatal diagnosis facilitates optimal obstetric management (ACOG, 2018h).

For the fetus, significant blood loss can result in negative alterations in maternal hemodynamic status and decreased oxygen. When bleeding decreases the blood flow to the placenta, maternal fetal gas exchange is reduced, placing the fetus at risk for progressive deterioration including hypoxemia, hypoxia, asphyxia, and death (Salera-Vieira, 2021). Risk is directly related to the amount and duration of blood loss.

CRITICAL COMPONENT

Vaginal Bleeding

A sterile vaginal exam is contraindicated in all pregnant women with extensive vaginal bleeding until the source of bleeding is identified. If a vaginal exam is performed with a placenta previa torrential, vaginal bleeding could occur related to dislodging of the placenta from maternal tissues. Maternal blood loss results in decreased oxygen-carrying capacity, which directly impacts oxygen delivery to maternal organs and placental blood flow, thus decreasing oxygen to the fetus. Therefore, the management of placenta previa and all placental abnormalities is dependent on maternal and fetal status.

Placenta Previa

The incidence of placenta previa is estimated to be 1 in 200 pregnancies at term and varies throughout the world (Cunningham et al., 2018). Placenta previa occurs when the placenta attaches to the lower uterine segment of the uterus, near or over the internal cervical os instead of in the body or fundus of the uterus (Fig. 7–10). The cause is unknown (Silver, 2015). Women with placenta previa have an approximately tenfold increased risk of antepartum vaginal bleeding. The mechanism of bleeding is uncertain but appears to be attributable to separation of the placenta from the underlying decidua, resulting from contractions, cervical effacement, cervical dilation, and/or advancing gestational age (Silver, 2015). Hemorrhage is especially likely to occur during the third trimester with development of the lower uterine segment and when UCs dilate the cervix, thereby applying shearing forces to the placental attachment to the lower segment, or when separation is provoked by vaginal examination. Placenta previa is most often diagnosed before the onset of bleeding when ultrasound is performed for other indications (Salera-Vieira, 2021).

In the past, previas were characterized as complete, partial, and marginal depending on how much of the internal endocervical os was covered by the placenta. However, the use of transvaginal ultrasonography allows for precise localization of the placental edge and the cervical os. Accordingly, the nomenclature has been modified to eliminate the terms *partial* and *marginal*. Instead, all placentas overlying the os (to any degree) are termed *previas* and those near to but not overlying the os are termed *low-lying* (Silver, 2015).

Risk Factors for Placenta Previa

- Endometrial scarring
  - Previous placenta previa
  - Prior cesarean birth
  - Abortion involving suction curettage
  - Multiparity or short pregnancy interval
- Impeded endometrial vascularization
  - Advanced maternal age (older than 35 years)
  - Diabetes or hypertension
  - Cigarette smoking
  - Uterine anomalies, fibroids, or endometritis
- Increased placental mass
  - Large placenta
  - Multiple gestation

Risks for the Woman

- Risks include hemorrhagic and hypovolemic shock related to excessive blood loss necessitating blood transfusion, hysterectomy, and maternal intensive care unit admission.
- Due to the large volume of maternal blood flow to the uteroplacental unit at term, up to 1,000 cc/min, unresolved bleeding can result in maternal exsanguinations in 8 to 10 minutes.
- Potential Rh sensitization may occur as Rh-negative women can become sensitized during any antepartum bleeding episode.
- Other risks from hemorrhage include septicemia, thrombophlebitis, and even maternal death.

Risks for the Fetus and Newborn

- IUGR
- Disruption of uteroplacental blood flow can result in progressive deterioration of fetal status, and the degree of fetal compromise is related to the volume of maternal blood loss (Salera-Vieira, 2021).

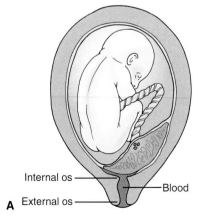
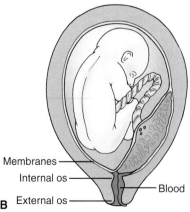
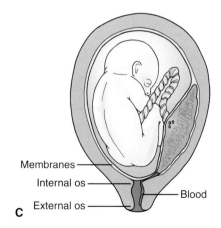

FIGURE 7–10 Placenta previa. (A) Previa. (B) Previa. (C) Low-lying placenta.

- Blood loss, hypoxia, anoxia, and death (lower than 10%) related to maternal hemorrhage may occur.
- Fetal anemia may develop due to maternal blood loss.
- Neonatal morbidity and mortality are related primarily to prematurity (Silver, 2015).

Assessment Findings

- The "classic" presentation used to be painless vaginal bleeding in the third trimester. Bleeding may be associated with abdominal pain, contractions, or both. Hemodynamic changes can be associated with blood loss.
- FHR changes are associated with maternal blood loss.
- Bleeding usually occurs near the end of the second trimester or in the third trimester of pregnancy, and initial bleeding episodes may be slight.
- The first episode of bleeding is rarely life-threatening or a cause of hypovolemic shock.
- Ultrasound confirms placental location at the cervix, and transvaginal ultrasonography also improves the accuracy of the diagnosis in the third trimester. Many placenta previas noted at mid-pregnancy during routine screening ultrasounds will no longer be present by the time of delivery. The relationship between the cervix and the placenta changes over time with the placenta typically "moving away" from the cervix. Accordingly, only approximately 10% to 20% of previas at 20 weeks of gestation will remain previas in the late third trimester.
- Maternal findings may also include fear and anxiety.
- A vaginal exam is contraindicated.

Emergency Medical Management

- Cesarean delivery is necessary when either maternal or fetal status is compromised as a result of extensive hemorrhage.
- Cesarean birth is necessary in nearly all women with placenta previa because the placenta is at the cervix, and labor and cervical dilation results in placental hemorrhage (Silver, 2015).
- Vaginal delivery may be attempted with a low-lying placenta if one can proceed with an emergency cesarean birth if needed.
- Placenta previa may be associated with placenta accreta, placenta increta, or placenta percreta.
- An increased risk of postpartum hemorrhage occurs in the setting of previa, even without accreta, and blood is transfused as needed.

Medical Management if Stable

When the maternal and fetal status is stable and bleeding is minimal (less than 250 mL), prolonging the pregnancy and delaying delivery may be possible. This expectant management or conservative management is performed when the fetus is premature to allow for fetal lungs to mature. The benefits of a planned delivery under optimal circumstances and before labor or bleeding must be weighed against the risks of prematurity. This typically includes close observation and hospitalization. If the woman and fetus remain stable and bleeding stops, discharging the woman home may be a consideration.

The mainstay of antepartum care is "expectant management." Most women with asymptomatic previa (no bleeding or contractions) are managed as outpatients. A Cochrane Review of clinical trials revealed little evidence of any clear advantage or disadvantage to a policy of home versus hospital care (Neilson, 2009). Although often prescribed, the benefits of bedrest, pelvic rest, or reduced activity remain unproven (Silver, 2015; Society for Maternal-Fetal Medicine [SMFM] & Gyamfi-Bannerman, 2018).

Nursing Actions

Nursing actions are related to maternal and fetal status and the amount of vaginal bleeding and include the following:

- Perform the initial assessment:
  - Evaluate color, character, and amount of vaginal bleeding and weight amount.
  - Arrange for ultrasound to determine placental location.
  - Determine fetal well-being, gestational age, and fetal lung maturity.
  - Continuous FHR monitoring because an indeterminant or abnormal FHR pattern may be the first sign of abnormal maternal-fetal hemodynamic compromise.
  - Assess vital signs for increased pulse and RR and falling blood pressure every 5 to 15 minutes if active bleeding. The woman can have up to a 40% maternal blood loss before exhibiting hemorrhagic hemodynamic changes in the blood pressure and pulse.
  - Assess skin color, skin temperature, and pulse oximetry mentation.
- Assess for and notify the physician of any of the following:
  - Onset of or increase in vaginal bleeding
  - Blood pressure lower than 90/60 mm Hg; pulse lower than 60 or more than 120 bpm
  - Respirations less than 14 or more than 26 breaths/min
  - Temperature greater than 100.4°F (38°C)
  - Urine output less than 30 mL/hr.
  - Saturated oxygen lower than 95%
  - Decreased level of consciousness
  - Onset or increase in uterine activity
  - Category II or III FHR pattern
- Assess abdominal pain, uterine tenderness, irritability, and contractions.
- Initiate bedrest with bathroom privileges.
- Establish and maintain IV access with large-bore IV in case blood replacement therapy is needed.
- Administer oxygen at 8 to 10 L/min per mask.
- Ensure availability of hold clot, cross match, and blood components.
- Activate massive transfusion protocols PRN; see Chapter 10.
- Assess FHR and uterine activity and facilitate antenatal testing as ordered.
- Give corticosteroids to accelerate fetal lung maturity, if indicated. Current recommendation is antenatal corticosteroids should be administered to women who are eligible and are managed expectantly if delivery is likely within 7 days, the gestational age is between 34 0/7 and 36 6/7 weeks of

gestation, and antenatal corticosteroids have not previously been administered (SMFM & Gyamfi-Bannerman, 2018).

- Monitor laboratory values including complete blood count (CBC), platelets, and clotting studies.
- Inform the patient and family of maternal and fetal status, and reassure the patient and her family. Explain interventions and the reasons they are being performed.
- Anticipate a cesarean birth if the patient or fetus is unstable.
- If undelivered and mother is RH negative, administer RhoGAM.

Placental Abruption

Placental abruption, also referred to as abruptio placentae, is bleeding at the decidual-placental interface that causes partial or complete placental detachment prior to delivery of the fetus. The diagnosis is typically reserved for pregnancies over 20 weeks of gestation. Placental abruption is initiated by hemorrhage into the decidual basalis. A hematoma forms, leading to destruction of the placenta adjacent to it. In some instances, spiral arterioles that nourish the decidua and supply blood to the placenta rupture. Bleeding into the decidua basalis results in hemorrhage and placental separation (Fig. 7–11).

Placental abruption is suspected when a woman presents with sudden onset, intense, often localized uterine pain or tenderness with or without vaginal bleeding (Salera-Vieira, 2021). She may also present with preterm contractions, uterine irritability, and back pain with or without vaginal bleeding.

Although several risk factors are known, the etiopathogenesis of placental abruption is multifactorial and not well understood. The separation may be partial or total and can be classified as grade 1 (mild), 2 (moderate), or 3 (severe). Bleeding with placental abruption is almost always maternal. This is a uniquely dangerous condition for the woman and fetus due to its potentially serious complications. Placental abruption complicates approximately 1% of pregnancies, with two-thirds classified as severe due to accompanying maternal, fetal, and neonatal morbidity.

A majority of placental abruption cases appear to have long-standing chronic etiology (Elsasser et al., 2010). The major clinical findings are vaginal bleeding and abdominal pain, often accompanied by hypertonic UCs, uterine tenderness, and a nonreassuring FHR pattern. Clinical diagnosis for abruption should include one or more of the following: retroplacental bleeding or clot, sonographic visualization of abruption, or painful vaginal bleeding accompanied by nonreassuring fetal status or uterine hypertonicity. Maternal and fetal status determine the management of the pregnancy. A concealed hemorrhage occurs in about 10% of abruptions. This results in uterine tenderness and abdominal pain. The fetal response to abruptio placenta depends on the volume of blood loss and the extent of uteroplacental insufficiency (Salera-Vieira, 2021). Management depends on maternal and fetal status and gestational age. About half of abruptions occurred before 37 weeks of gestation and 14% occurred before 32 weeks (Tikkanen, 2011).

Risk Factors

- Previous abruption increases risk up to 15%
- Hypertension, chronic, gestational hypertension, or preeclampsia
- Prior cesarean section, maternal age, multiple gestation, uterine anomalies or fibroids
- Preterm premature rupture of membranes less than 34 weeks' gestation
- Abdominal trauma, motor vehicle accident
- Cocaine, methamphetamine use, or cigarette smoking
- Thrombophilias
- Early pregnancy bleeding with subchorionic hemorrhage

Risks for the Woman

- Maternal risks include obstetric hemorrhage, need for blood transfusions, emergency hysterectomy, disseminated intravascular coagulopathy, and renal failure.
- Maternal death is rare but seven times higher than the overall maternal mortality rate.

Three Grades of Abruption Placentae

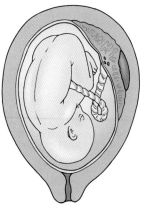

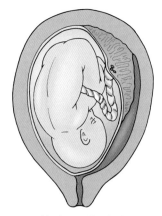

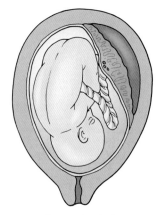

Mild Grade 1
(<15% placenta separates with concealed hemorrhage)

Moderate Grade 2
(Up to 50% placenta separates with apparent hemorrhage)

Severe Grade 3
(>50% placenta separates with concealed hemorrhage)

FIGURE 7–11 Three grades of abruptio placentae.

Risks for the Fetus and Newborn

- Perinatal consequences include low birth weight, preterm delivery, asphyxia, stillbirth, and perinatal death.
- In developed countries, approximately 10% of all PTBs and 10% to 20% of all perinatal deaths are caused by placental abruption.

Assessment Findings

- Diagnosis is made on a woman's history, clinical presentation, physical examination, and laboratory values
- Treatment depends on maternal and fetal status
- Vaginal bleeding is present in up to 80% of women with abruption. Maternal assessment findings with active bleeding include:
  - Hypovolemic shock; hypotension; oliguria; thready pulse; shallow or irregular respirations; pallor; cold, clammy skin; and anxiety
  - Vaginal bleeding (but can be concealed or occult hemorrhage)
  - Severe abdominal pain and tense abdomen or continuous, dull back pain
  - UCs, tenderness, hypertonus, increasing uterine distention
  - Nausea and vomiting
  - Decreased renal output
  - Remember, during pregnancy signs of shock are usually not present until 25% to 30% of maternal blood loss has occurred.
  - Kleihauer–Betke test in maternal blood may be positive and indicate the presence of fetal RBC.
- Ultrasound cannot accurately identify placental separation in 50% of cases (SMFM & Gyamfi-Bannerman, 2018).
- Fetal assessment findings include:
  - FHR tachycardia or bradycardia
  - Category II or III FHR patterns including loss or variability of FHR, late decelerations, decreasing baseline, sinusoidal pattern
- Maternal findings may also include fear and anxiety.

Emergency Medical Management

If abruption results in unstable or deteriorating maternal or fetal status, delivery by cesarean is indicated. Treatment includes:

- Monitoring maternal volume status and coagulation status
- Correcting coagulation defects
- Restoring blood loss
- Assessing fetal status
- Expediting delivery as indicated

Medical Management if Stable

Diagnosis is made on the woman's history, clinical presentation, physical examination, and laboratory values. If the maternal status is stable and the fetus is immature, then expectant management would include:

- Hospitalization and close monitoring of maternal and fetal status including signs and symptoms of abruption such as bleeding, uterine activity or hypertonus, and abdominal pain, as well as monitoring maternal laboratory and coagulation studies.
- Corticosteroids may be given to accelerate fetal lung maturity and tocolysis may be considered.

Current recommendation is for delivery at 36 to 37 6/7 weeks of gestation for stable women with placenta previa without bleeding or other obstetric complications (SMFM & Gyamfi-Bannerman, 2018).

Nursing Actions

- Close monitoring of maternal and fetal status including signs and symptoms of abruption such as vaginal bleeding, uterine pain, activity or hypertonus, abdominal pain, and monitoring maternal laboratory and coagulation studies.
- Palpate the uterus for contractions, tenderness, hypertonus, or increasing uterine distention.
- Monitor the maternal cardiovascular status for hypotension, tachycardia, and other signs of hypovolemic shock such as hypotension, oliguria, thready pulse, shallow or irregular respirations, low oxygen concentration with pulse oximetry, pallor, or cold, clammy skin.
  - Establish and maintain IV access with a large-bore needle.
  - Administer oxygen at 8 to 10 L/min by mask.
  - Monitor I&O.
  - Assess FHR for baseline changes, tachycardia or bradycardia, loss of variability, and periodic changes indicative of an abnormal FHR (Salera-Vieira, 2021). Continuous FHR monitoring is needed because an indeterminant or abnormal FHR pattern may be the first sign of abnormal maternal-fetal hemodynamic compromise.
  - Provide emotional support to the woman and her family, reassure the patient and her family, and provide information to the woman and her family regarding the treatment plan and status of their infant.
  - Measure and estimate blood loss.
  - Activate massive transfusion protocols PRN; see Chapter 10.
  - Anticipate a cesarean birth if the patient or fetus is unstable.
  - If undelivered and the mother is RH negative, administer RhoGAM (AAP & ACOG, 2017).
  - Give corticosteroids to accelerate fetal lung maturity, if indicated. The current recommendation is antenatal corticosteroids should be administered to women who are eligible and are managed expectantly if delivery is likely within 7 days, the gestational age is between 34 0/7 and 36 6/7 weeks of gestation, and antenatal corticosteroids have not previously been administered (SMFM & Gyamfi-Bannerman, 2018).

Placenta Accreta Spectrum

Placenta accreta spectrum (PAS), also referred to as morbidly adherent placenta, refers to the range of pathologic adherence of the placenta, including placenta increta, placenta percreta, and placenta accreta. The etiology of PAS is that a defect of the endometrial–myometrial interface leads to a failure of normal decidualization in the area of a uterine scar, which allows abnormally deep placental anchoring villi and trophoblast infiltration. Complete accreta occurs when the entire placenta is adherent, partial is when one or more cotyledons are adherent, and focal is when one is adherent (Salera-Vieira, 2020). Maternal morbidity and mortality can occur due to severe and sometimes life-threatening hemorrhage, which often requires blood transfusion.

Although ultrasound evaluation is important, the absence of ultrasound findings does not preclude a diagnosis of PAS; thus, clinical risk factors remain equally important as predictors of PAS by ultrasound findings. There are several risk factors for PAS; most common is a previous cesarean delivery. The incidence of placenta accreta increases with the number of prior cesarean deliveries. Antenatal diagnosis of PAS is highly desirable because outcomes are optimized when delivery occurs at a level III or IV maternal care facility before the onset of labor or bleeding and with avoidance of placental disruption. The most generally accepted approach to PAS is cesarean hysterectomy with the placenta left in situ after delivery of the fetus (attempts at placental removal are associated with a significant risk of hemorrhage).

Placenta accreta is a general term used to describe the clinical condition when part of the placenta, or the entire placenta, invades and is inseparable from the uterine wall. When the chorionic villi invade only the myometrium, the term *placenta increta* is appropriate, whereas *placenta percreta* describes invasion through the myometrium and serosa, and occasionally into adjacent organs, such as the bladder.

Clinically, placenta accreta becomes problematic during delivery when the placenta does not completely separate from the uterus and is followed by massive obstetric hemorrhage, leading to disseminated intravascular coagulopathy; the need for hysterectomy; surgical injury to the ureters, bladder, bowel, or neurovascular structures; adult respiratory distress syndrome; acute transfusion reaction; electrolyte imbalance; and renal failure. The average blood loss at delivery in women with placenta accreta is 3,000 to 5,000 mL (ACOG, 2018h). As many as 90% of patients with placenta accreta require blood transfusion, and 40% require more than 10 units of packed RBCs. Maternal mortality with placenta accreta has been reported to be as high as 7%. Maternal death may occur despite optimal planning, transfusion management, and surgical care (ACOG, 2018h). The incidence of placenta accreta has increased and seems to parallel the increasing cesarean delivery rate. Women at greatest risk for PAS are those with previous myometrial damage caused by previous cesarean birth with either an anterior or posterior placenta overlying the uterine scar (McMurtry Baird & Fox, 2019). Placenta accreta can be diagnosed by ultrasound prenatally but sometimes is diagnosed after delivery when the placenta is retained. If the placenta does not separate readily, rapid surgical intervention is needed (AAP &ACOG, 2017).

- Placenta accreta: Invasion of the trophoblast is beyond the normal boundary without invasion of the decidua (80% of cases).
- Placenta increta: Invasion of the trophoblast extends into the uterine myometrium (15% of cases).

- Placenta percreta: Invasion of the trophoblast extends into the uterine musculature and can adhere to other pelvic organs (5% of cases).

One of the most important modifiers of clinical outcome is prenatal diagnosis of accreta. Several studies confirm decreased hemorrhage and other maternal complications in cases diagnosed antenatally rather than intrapartum. Prenatal diagnosis allows for optimal management, typically including planned cesarean hysterectomy before the onset of labor or bleeding. Diagnosing placenta accreta before delivery allows for multidisciplinary planning to minimize potential maternal or neonatal morbidity and mortality. The diagnosis is usually established by ultrasonography and may be supplemented by MRI.

Antenatal diagnosis has significantly reduced morbidity and mortality and provides an opportunity for counseling and preparation for cesarean birth, hysterectomy and subsequent loss of fertility, and a plan to be in place for the birth (McMurtry Baird & Fox, 2019). Sometimes the woman must be hospitalized prior to birth due to repeated bleeding episodes or to optimize laboratory values. Unscheduled PTB is associated with UC, ROM, and vaginal bleeding (McMurtry Baird & Fox, 2019). In addition, established infrastructure and strong nursing leadership accustomed to managing high-level postpartum hemorrhage should be in place, and access to a blood bank capable of employing massive transfusion protocols should help guide decisions about the delivery location (ACOG, 2018h).

Risk Factors for Placenta Accreta

- Women at greatest risk of placenta accreta are those who have myometrial damage caused by a previous cesarean delivery with either anterior or posterior placenta previa overlying the uterine scar.
- The risk of placenta accreta was 3%, 11%, 40%, 61%, and 67% for the first, second, third, fourth, and fifth or greater repeat cesarean deliveries, respectively (Silver et al., 2006).
- Placenta previa without previous uterine surgery is associated with a 1% to 5% risk of placenta accreta.
- In vitro fertilization is also a risk factor.

Other risk factors include advanced maternal age, multiparity, smoking, and short interconception.

Risks for the Woman

- Hemorrhagic and hypovolemic shock related to excessive blood loss. Maternal morbidity is common and 25% to 50% of patients are admitted to an intensive care unit.
- Increased risk of infection, thromboembolism, pyelonephritis, pneumonia, adult respiratory distress syndrome, and renal failure

Risks for the Fetus and Newborn

- The average gestational age of delivery of accretas is typically 34 to 36 weeks of gestation, usually resulting from medically indicated PTB.

- At term, a placenta accreta typically does not present a risk to the fetus or neonate but presents a problem in management after delivery.

Assessment Findings

- The mainstay of antenatal diagnosis is obstetric ultrasonography.
- Another factor can be repeated bleeding episodes.

Unscheduled PTB is associated with UC, ROM, and vaginal bleeding (McMurtry Baird & Fox, 2019). Maternal assessment findings at delivery related to hypovolemic shock and hemorrhage include hypotension, oliguria, thready pulse, shallow irregular breathing, pallor, cold and clammy skin, anxiety, and confusion and agitation.

Medical Management

- The timing of delivery in cases of suspected placenta accreta must be individualized (ACOG, 2018h). This decision should be made jointly with the patient, obstetrician, and neonatologist. Patient counseling should include discussion of the potential need for hysterectomy, the risks of profuse hemorrhage, and possible maternal death.
- Generally, the recommended management of suspected placenta accreta is planned preterm cesarean hysterectomy with the placenta left in situ as removal of the placenta is associated with significant hemorrhagic morbidity.
  - Uterine preservation, referred to here as conservative management, is usually defined as removal of placenta or uteroplacental tissue without removal of the uterus.
  - Expectant management is leaving the placenta either partially or totally in situ.
  - Because PAS is potentially life threatening, hysterectomy is the typical treatment. Consideration of conservative or expectant approaches are rare and considered individually.
- Major complications of treatment of PAS are loss of future fertility, hemorrhage, and injury to other pelvic organs. To reduce complications, some advocate conservative or expectant management in patients with PAS. Therefore, surgical management of placenta accreta may be individualized (ACOG, 2018h). Current recommendation is for delivery between 34 and 37 weeks of gestation for stable women with placenta accreta (SMFM & Gyamfi-Bannerman, 2018). Corticosteroids may be given in anticipation of preterm delivery.

Nursing Actions

- Antenatal diagnosis has significantly reduced morbidity and mortality and provides an opportunity for counseling and preparation for cesarean birth, hysterectomy, and subsequent loss of fertility (McMurtry Baird & Fox, 2019).
- Provide emotional support to the woman and her family.
- Provide information to the woman and her family regarding the treatment plan and timing of birth.
- Optimal management involves a standardized approach with a comprehensive multidisciplinary care team accustomed to management of PAS. This includes an experienced team, availability of a large quantity of blood products, subspecialty providers, and an intensive care unit (McMurtry Baird & Fox, 2019).
- During hospitalization before birth, maintain large-bore IV access, cross match, type and hold 4 units of PRBC, and monitor laboratory values including CBC and clotting studies.
- Activate massive transfusion protocols PRN. Concepts related to volume resuscitation and blood component therapy are discussed in detail in Chapter 10.

CLINICAL JUDGMENT

Laboratory Values Assessed in Pregnant Women Who Are Bleeding

CBC

Fibrinogen concentration

Fibrin degradation products or fibrin split products

Platelet count

Blood type

Whole blood clotting time

Prothrombin time

Activated partial thromboplastin time

ABORTION

A little less than half of pregnancies are unplanned, and about half of unintended pregnancies end in abortion (AAP & ACOG, 2017). Abortion is the spontaneous or elective termination of pregnancy before 20 weeks' gestation. Abortions are referred to as induced, elective, therapeutic, and spontaneous. When a procedure is done or medication is taken to end a pregnancy, it is called an induced abortion. Elective abortion is termination of a pregnancy before fetal viability at the request of the woman but not for reasons of impaired health of the mother or fetal disease. Therapeutic abortion is termination of a pregnancy for serious maternal medical indications or serious fetal anomalies. An abortion is defined as legal if it was performed by a licensed clinician within the limits of state law. An abortion is defined as illegal if it was performed by any person other than a licensed clinician.

An estimated one in four women in the United States will have an abortion in her lifetime. Many factors influence or necessitate an individual's decision to have an abortion, including but not limited to contraceptive failure, barriers to contraceptive use and access, rape, incest, intimate partner violence (IPV), fetal anomalies, and exposure to teratogenic medications. Additionally, pregnancy complications such as placental abruption, bleeding from placenta previa, preeclampsia or eclampsia, chorioamnionitis, and cardiac or renal conditions may be so severe that abortion is the only measure to preserve a patient's health or save their life. According to ACOG (2020b), all terminations are considered medically indicated.

Patients who choose abortion should be counseled about all methods available as well as the risks, advantages, disadvantages, and the different features of these options. In 2017, an estimated 60% of abortions in the United States occurred at or before 10 weeks of gestation and medication abortion comprised 39% of all abortions (Jones et al., 2019). In the United States, 88% of abortions occur within the first trimester, when abortion is safest. A first-trimester abortion can be performed up to 13 weeks of pregnancy. Most induced abortions are performed during the first trimester and it is one of the safest medical procedures. It can be done safely in a health-care provider's office or clinic. Between 2006 and 2015, there was a shift in the timing of abortion, with abortions taking place at earlier gestational ages; this is likely due, in part, to the availability of medication abortion.

Medication Abortion

Most patients at 70 days of gestation or less who desire abortion are eligible for a medication abortion. Combined mifepristone-misoprostol regimens are recommended as the preferred therapy for medication abortion because they are significantly more effective than misoprostol-only regimens. Patients can safely and effectively use mifepristone at home for medication abortion. There are medical conditions for which a medication abortion may be preferable to uterine aspiration. Such examples include uterine fibroids that significantly distort the cervical canal or uterine cavity, congenital uterine anomalies, or introital scarring related to infibulation (ACOG, 2020d). Patients with asthma are candidates for medication abortion because misoprostol does not cause bronchoconstriction and actually acts as a weak bronchodilator. Multiple gestation pregnancy is not a contraindication; patients with twin gestations can be treated with the same regimens as those with singleton gestations.

Drugs used in a medical abortion cause bleeding that is much heavier than with a menstrual period. The woman may experience severe cramping. Nausea, vomiting, fever, and chills may occur and be managed with over-the-counter pain medication. The provider may prescribe stronger pain medication if needed. It can take several days or weeks for the abortion to complete.

Medication abortion is not recommended for patients with any of the following: confirmed or suspected ectopic pregnancy, intrauterine device (IUD) in place (the IUD can be removed before medication abortion), current long-term systemic corticosteroid therapy, chronic adrenal failure, known coagulopathy or anticoagulant therapy, inherited porphyria, or intolerance or allergy to mifepristone or misoprostol (ACOG, 2020d).

Surgical Abortion

A first-trimester abortion can be performed with surgery (a procedure called suction curettage) or by taking medication. Suction curettage is the most common type of abortion. After the cervix is dilated, a thin, plastic tube is inserted into the uterus. It is attached to a suction or vacuum pump that removes the pregnancy.

A second-trimester abortion takes place after 13 weeks of pregnancy. A second-trimester abortion can be performed with a surgical procedure called dilation and evacuation (D&E) or with medication (medical abortion). In the second trimester, a surgical abortion has fewer complications than a medical abortion; therefore, most women who have a second-trimester abortion have a surgical abortion. In a second-trimester abortion, general anesthesia or regional anesthesia may be used for pain relief. The fetus is removed through the vagina. Suction is used to remove any remaining tissue. Legally induced abortions have an extremely low complication rate. Serious complications from abortions are rare at all gestational ages (Upadhyay et al., 2015).

Post-abortion care should include patient counseling and a discussion of when patients should contact their clinician in the case of heavy bleeding (soaking more than two maxi pads per hour for 2 consecutive hours), fever, and when to access urgent intervention. If any of the following occur, a woman should be instructed to call her health-care provider:

● Severe abdominal or back pain
● Heavy bleeding (soaking two maxi pads per hour for 2 consecutive hours)
● Foul-smelling discharge
● A fever (above 100.4°F [38°C])

Nearly all abortions result from unintended pregnancy. Multiple factors influence the incidence of abortion, including access to health-care services, including contraception; the availability of abortion providers; state regulations, such as mandatory waiting periods or parental involvement laws, and legal restrictions on abortion providers; increasing acceptance of nonmarital childbearing; shifts in the racial or ethnic composition of the U.S. population; and changes in the economy and the resulting impact on fertility preferences and use of contraception (Jatlaoui et al., 2016). Individuals require access to safe, legal abortion. Abortion, although legal, is increasingly out of reach due to numerous restrictions imposed by the government that target patients seeking abortion and their health-care practitioners. Insurance coverage restrictions, which take many forms, constitute a substantial barrier to abortion access and increase reproductive health inequities. Adolescents, people of color, those living in rural areas, those with low incomes, and incarcerated people can face disproportionate effects of restrictions on abortion access. Stigma and fear of violence may be less tangible than legislative and financial restrictions but create powerful barriers to abortion provision nonetheless (ACOG, 2020c).

When restrictions are placed on abortion access, patients and families suffer. Abortion access is increasingly limited; research shows that restrictions dictate whether care is safely obtained as well as the quality of care. The Association of Women's Health, Obstetric and Neonatal Nurses (AWHONN, 2017) believes that any woman's reproductive health-care decisions are best made by the informed woman in consultation with her health-care provider. AWHONN believes these personal and private decisions are best made within a health-care system whose providers respect the woman's right to make her own decisions according to her personal values and preferences and to do so confidentially. However, a recent study of California nurses indicates nurses were more likely to have negative attitudes toward abortion care if they identified as Christian (_p_ lower than .001) and more positive attitudes if they identified as White (p lower than .001) independent of identifying as Christian. Additionally, nurses reported a complex range of attitudes about abortion. In some cases, these attitudes aligned or conflicted with stated religious orientation, highlighting the demographic characteristics that are associated with the attitudes and beliefs about abortion among RNs licensed in California (Swartz et al., 2020). However, because unintended pregnancy precedes nearly all abortions, efforts to reduce the incidence of abortion need to focus on helping women, men, and couples avoid unwanted pregnancies.

Early Pregnancy Loss and Miscarriage

In the first trimester, the terms *miscarriage, spontaneous abortion,* and *early pregnancy loss* are often used interchangeably. Miscarriage is generally defined as the loss of an intrauterine pregnancy before viability; spontaneous abortion is defined as a nonviable, intrauterine pregnancy with either an empty gestational sac or a gestational sac containing an embryo or fetus without fetal heart activity within the first 12 6/7 weeks of gestation; and early pregnancy loss is spontaneous pregnancy demise before 10 weeks of gestational age.

Hemorrhage in the decidua basalis followed by necrosis of the tissue usually accompanies pregnancy loss. Approximately 10% of pregnancies end in spontaneous abortion. Most (80%) occur in the first 12 weeks of gestation and are termed early abortion, and more than half of those are a result of chromosomal abnormalities (ACOG, 2018a). Early pregnancy losses typically are related to an abnormality of the zygote, embryo, fetus, or at times the placenta. Approximately 50% of all cases of early pregnancy loss are caused by fetal chromosomal abnormalities (ACOG, 2018a).

The most common risk factors identified among women who have experienced early pregnancy loss are advanced maternal age and a prior early pregnancy loss. The frequency of clinically recognized early pregnancy loss for women aged 20 to 30 years is 9% to 17%, and this rate increases sharply from 20% at age 35 years to 40% at age 40 years and 80% at age 45 years. Late pregnancy losses occur between 12 and 20 weeks' gestation. The risk of miscarriage is lowest in women with no history of miscarriage (11%), and then increases by about 10% for each additional miscarriage, reaching 42% in women with three or more previous miscarriages (Quenby et al., 2021).

A new graded model of care is being proposed for improved care for women who experience miscarriage (Lancet, 2021). This model represents a substantial move away from the current fragmented system of care, with barriers to access, and better reflects the significant mental and physical event that miscarriage is to many people. After one miscarriage, women should have their health needs evaluated and be provided with information and guidance to support future pregnancies. If a second miscarriage occurs, women should be offered an appointment at a miscarriage clinic for a full blood count and thyroid function tests and have extra support and early scans for reassurance in any subsequent pregnancies. After three miscarriages, additional tests, including genetic testing and a pelvic ultrasound, should be offered (Coomarasamy et al., 2021). Miscarriage, and especially recurrent miscarriage, is also a sentinel risk marker for obstetric complications, including PTB, fetal growth restriction, placental abruption, and stillbirth in future pregnancies, and a predictor of longer-term health problems, such as cardiovascular disease and venous thromboembolism (VTE) (Quenby et al., 2021).

Risk Factors for Early Pregnancy Loss and Miscarriage

The risk of miscarriage is lowest in women with no history of miscarriage (11%), and then increases by about 10% for each additional miscarriage, reaching 42% in women with three or more previous miscarriages (Quenby et al., 2021).

- Prior pregnancy loss
- Advanced maternal age
- Endocrine abnormalities such as diabetes or luteal phase defects
- Drug use or environmental toxins
- Immunological factors such as autoimmune diseases
- Infections
- Systemic disorders
- Genetic factors
- Uterine or cervical abnormalities
- Black women have a higher miscarriage risk.

Assessment Findings for Early Pregnancy Loss

- Uterine bleeding first, then cramping abdominal pain in a few hours to several days later
- Ultrasound confirms diagnosis. Early pregnancy loss can be diagnosed with certainty in a woman with an ultrasound-documented intrauterine pregnancy who subsequently presents with reported significant vaginal bleeding and an empty uterus on ultrasound examination.
- In other instances, the diagnosis of early pregnancy loss is not as clear. Depending on the specific clinical circumstances and how much diagnostic certainty the patient desires, a single serum β-hCG test or ultrasound examination may not be sufficient to confirm the diagnosis of early pregnancy loss.

Medical Management for Early Pregnancy Loss

Accepted treatment options for medical management include expectant management, medical treatment, or surgical evacuation depending on the classification and signs and symptoms. In patients for whom medical management of early pregnancy loss is indicated, initial treatment using 800 micrograms of vaginal misoprostol generally is recommended, with a repeat dose as needed. In women without medical complications or symptoms requiring urgent surgical evacuation, treatment plans can safely accommodate patient treatment preferences.

Women who are Rh(D) negative and unsensitized should receive 50 micrograms of Rh(D)-immune globulin immediately after surgical management of early pregnancy loss or within 72 hours of the diagnosis of early pregnancy loss with planned medical management or expectant management in the first trimester (AAP & ACOG, 2017).

Generally, no effective interventions can prevent early pregnancy loss. As with expectant management of early pregnancy loss, women opting for medical treatment should be counseled on what to expect while they pass pregnancy tissue, provided information on when to call regarding bleeding, and given prescriptions for pain medications. Counseling should emphasize that the woman is likely to have bleeding that is heavier than menses (and potentially accompanied by severe cramping). The woman should understand how much bleeding is considered too much. The patient should be advised to call her provider if she needs to change her maxi pad more than twice an hour for 2 hours. As with expectant management, it also is important to counsel patients that surgery may be needed if medical management does not achieve complete expulsion.

Patients undergoing expectant management may experience moderate-to-heavy bleeding and cramping. Educational materials instructing the patient on when and who to call for excessive bleeding and prescriptions for pain medications should be provided.

New evidence indicates vaginal micronized progesterone increases live birth rates in women with early pregnancy bleeding and a history of miscarriage. This may be a new way forward in the prevention of miscarriage (Coomarasamy et al., 2021).

A recent review of research on perinatal loss indicates that across studies, health-care professionals were an integral part of the participants' experiences regarding pregnancy loss (Berry et al., 2021). Despite the occasional positive and supportive interactions described by parents, participants primarily had negative experiences and were frustrated by the poor communication and lack of compassion shown by health-care professionals. Furthermore, communication by health-care professionals was often ambiguous and unclear. Participants reported that they were sent home without knowing when they would need to return for follow-up care. Communication and supportive, patient-centered care were especially important to families experiencing pregnancy loss.

Nursing Actions Related to Care After Early Pregnancy Loss

- Monitor vital signs per protocol and PRN.
- Monitor bleeding.
- Review laboratory results.
- Give RhoGAM if indicated.
- Follow agency guidelines and facilitate and support the family's decisions about disposition of the products of conception.
- Assess the significance of the loss to the woman and family.
  - Acknowledge feelings of sadness, distress, or relief toward pregnancy loss.
  - Give parents choices and opportunities for decision making.
  - Provide the family with information on miscarriage, pregnancy loss, and support groups.
- Provide psychological support appropriate to the family's response.

Provide resources to the patient and family to educate them about the psychological effects of pregnancy loss, because the consequences of miscarriage are both physical, such as bleeding or infection, and psychological. Psychological consequences include increases in the risk of anxiety, depression, posttraumatic stress disorder, and suicide (Quenby et al., 2021).

- Miscarriage, and especially recurrent miscarriage, is also a sentinel risk marker for obstetric complications for future pregnancies, and can be a predictor of longer-term health problems, such as cardiovascular disease and VTE (Quenby et al., 2021), so follow-up care is needed.
- Connect the patient and family with aftercare.
- Schedule a postdischarge follow-up meeting with the patient, as needed. Be sure to give written instructions for follow-up care as well.
- Provide discharge teaching related to self-care and warning signs, including:
  - Teach pericare.
  - Instruct that pelvic rest includes no tampons, douching, or sexual intercourse for several weeks.
  - Teach the patient to monitor for excessive bleeding and signs and symptoms of infection such as fever and uterine tenderness or foul-smelling discharge.
  - Teach about a diet high in iron and protein for tissue repair and RBC replacement.
  - Review the plan for follow-up with care provider and patient.
    - Follow-up typically includes confirmation of complete expulsion by ultrasound examination, but serial serum β-hCG measurement may be used instead in settings where ultrasonography is unavailable. Patient-reported symptoms also should be considered when determining whether complete expulsion has occurred.

Ectopic Pregnancy

Ectopic pregnancy is defined as a pregnancy that occurs outside of the uterine cavity. An ectopic pregnancy occurs when a fertilized egg grows outside the uterus as a result of the blastocyst implanting somewhere other than the endometrial lining of the uterus (Fig. 7–12). The embryo or fetus in an ectopic pregnancy is absent or stunted, and this is a nonviable pregnancy. Most ectopic pregnancies occur in the fallopian tube (95%), but the fertilized ovum can also implant in the ovary, cervix, or abdominal cavity (5%). Because most ectopic pregnancies are tubal, the focus of this section is on tubal ectopic pregnancy. In a tubal

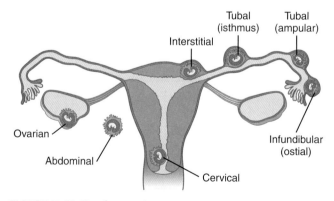

FIGURE 7–12 Sites for ectopic pregnancy.

pregnancy, the tube lacks a submucosal layer, and the fertilized ovum burrows through the epithelium of the tubal wall, tapping into the blood vessels; however, the tubal environment cannot support the rapidly proliferating trophoblast.

As the pregnancy grows, it can cause the tube to rupture (burst). If this occurs, it can cause major internal bleeding. This can be life-threatening and must be treated with surgery. The incidence of tubal pregnancy is increasing and not always reported, but is estimated at 2% (ACOG, 2018k; Panelli et al., 2015). Despite improvements in diagnosis and management, ruptured ectopic pregnancy continues to be a significant cause of pregnancy-related mortality and morbidity. In 2011 to 2013, ruptured ectopic pregnancy accounted for 2.7% of all pregnancy-related deaths and was the leading cause of hemorrhage-related mortality (Creanga et al., 2017). Women with tubal pregnancy have diverse clinical symptoms that largely depend on whether there is a rupture.

Risk Factors for Ectopic Pregnancy

Up to 50% of women diagnosed with EPs have no identifiable risk factors; however, several risk factors have been associated with EP. Prior EP is a strong risk factor for recurrent EP, with a recurrence rate of 5% to 25%, or up to 10 times the risk in the general population (Panelli et al., 2015). Women who have abnormal fallopian tubes are at higher risk of ectopic pregnancy. Abnormal tubes may be present in women who have had the following conditions:

- Pelvic inflammatory disease (PID), infection of uterus, fallopian tubes, and nearby pelvic structures
- Previous ectopic pregnancy
- Infertility
- Pelvic or abdominal surgery
- Endometriosis
- Sexually transmitted diseases (STDs)
- Prior tubal surgery (such as tubal sterilization)

Other factors that increase a woman's risk of ectopic pregnancy include the following:

- Cigarette smoking
- Exposure to the drug diethylstilbestrol (DES) during her mother's pregnancy
- Increased age

Risks for the Woman

- Hemorrhage related to rupture of fallopian tube
- Decreased fertility related to removal of fallopian tube

Assessment Findings

Most women now present prior to tubal rupture, and with advances in diagnosis and imaging, the outcomes have dramatically improved. Common findings are:

- Pelvic or abdominal pain may be present.
- Light or heavy bleeding occurs that is not at the time of your normal menstrual period (abnormal vaginal bleeding).

- Abdominal or pelvic pain occurs, which can be sudden and sharp and ache without relief or seem to come and go. It may occur on only one side.
- Blood from the ruptured tube can build up under the diaphragm, causing shoulder pain.
- Weakness, dizziness, or fainting may be caused by blood loss.
- Vital signs become unstable, indicating hypovolemia if hemorrhage is significant.

Medical Management

- Diagnosis generally is made with clinical signs, physical symptoms, serial human chorionic gonadotropin (hCG) levels, transvaginal ultrasonography, and serum progesterone levels (ACOG, 2018k).
- Early diagnosis allows for surgical or medical management of unruptured ectopic pregnancy. Treatment in stable patients is often medical, though patients meeting certain clinical criteria or with EPs outside the fallopian tube may require differing or more invasive treatment, including excision by laparoscopy or, less commonly, laparotomy.
- In clinically stable women in whom a nonruptured ectopic pregnancy has been diagnosed, laparoscopic surgery or intramuscular methotrexate administration are safe and effective treatments. Decisions for surgical management or medical management of ectopic pregnancy should be guided by the initial clinical, laboratory, and radiological data, as well as patient-informed choice based on discussion of benefits and risks of each approach (ACOG, 2018k).
- If the pregnancy is small and the tube is not ruptured, in some cases the pregnancy can be removed through a small cut made in the tube using laparoscopy. In this procedure, a slender, light-transmitting telescope is inserted through a small opening in the patient's abdomen in a hospital with general anesthesia. A larger incision in the abdomen may be needed if the pregnancy is large or the blood loss is a concern. Some or all of the tube may need to be removed.
- If the pregnancy is small and has not ruptured the tube, sometimes drugs can be used instead of surgery. Medication stops the growth of the pregnancy and permits the body to absorb it over time, allowing the woman to keep her fallopian tube. Nonsurgical medical management of ectopic pregnancy may be indicated in an unruptured and hemodynamically stable woman (ACOG, 2018k). Methotrexate, a folic acid antagonist and type of chemotherapy agent, will cause dissolution of the ectopic mass. For patients who are medically unstable or experiencing life-threatening hemorrhage, immediate surgical treatment is indicated.
- The decision to perform a salpingostomy or salpingectomy for the treatment of ectopic pregnancy should be guided by the patient's clinical status, her desire for future fertility, and the extent of fallopian tube damage (ACOG, 2018k). Surgical management of ectopic pregnancy is required when a patient is exhibiting hemodynamic instability, symptoms of an ongoing ruptured ectopic mass (such as pelvic pain), or signs of intraperitoneal bleeding.

Nursing Actions

- Ensure stabilization of cardiovascular status.
- Offer explanations and reassurance related to the plan of care.
- Assess response to the diagnosis related to anxiety, fear, and guilt.
- Provide support related to the pregnancy loss.
- Explain the plan for follow-up care, which is determined by the treatment plan, surgical or medical.
- Give RhoGAM if indicated.
- Assess the significance of the loss to the woman and family:
  - Acknowledge feelings of sadness, distress, or relief toward the pregnancy loss.
  - Give parents choices and opportunities for decision making.
  - Provide the family with information on pregnancy loss and support groups.
- Provide psychological support appropriate to the family's response.
- Offer discharge teaching related to self-care and warning signs including:
  - Teach the patient to monitor for severe abdominal pain, excessive bleeding, and signs and symptoms of infection such as fever.
  - Teach about an iron-rich diet if the woman experiences high estimated blood loss (EBL).
  - Review the plan for follow-up with the care provider.
  - Teach the patient appropriate pain management.
  - Teach the patient signs and symptoms that need to be reported, such as severe abdominal pain, fever, and bleeding.
- Special considerations for teaching women treated with methotrexate (ACOG, 2018k):
  - Because methotrexate affects rapidly dividing tissues, gastrointestinal side effects, such as nausea, vomiting, and stomatitis, are the most common. Therefore, women treated with methotrexate should be advised not to use alcohol and nonsteroidal anti-inflammatory drugs (NSAIDs).
  - It is not unusual for women treated with methotrexate to experience abdominal pain 2 to 3 days after administration, presumably from the cytotoxic effect of the drug on the trophoblast tissue, causing tubal abortion.

Gestational Trophoblastic Disease

Gestational trophoblastic disease (GTD) refers to a spectrum of placental-related tumors. GTD is a group of rare diseases in which abnormal trophoblast cells grow inside the uterus after conception (Cunningham et al., 2018). GTD is categorized into molar and nonmolar tumors. Gestational trophoblastic neoplasia (GTN) is a type of GTD that is almost always malignant. Nonmolar tumors are grouped as GTN or malignant GTD. As an example, one of the nonmalignant tumors will be described.

A hydatidiform mole (molar pregnancy) is a benign proliferating growth of the trophoblast in which the chorionic villi develop into edematous, cystic, vascular transparent vesicles that hang in grape-like clusters without a viable fetus

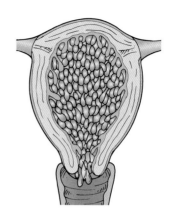

FIGURE 7–13 Hydatidiform mole.

(Fig. 7–13). A hydatidiform mole develops in 1 to 2 of 1,000 pregnancies in the United States (Cunningham et al., 2018). Most hydatidiform moles are benign, but they sometimes become cancerous. Having one or more of the following risk factors increases the risk that a hydatidiform mole will become cancer. This is a nonviable pregnancy. In a normal pregnancy, the trophoblast cells develop into the placenta and have chorionic villi that form the endometrium. With a hydatidiform mole pregnancy, there is a proliferation of the placenta and trophoblastic cells, which absorb fluid from the maternal blood. Fluid accumulates into the chorionic villi and vesicles form out of the chorionic villi (see Fig. 7–13). The erythroblastic tissue of the complete hydatidiform mole never develops into a fetus. The erythroblastic tissue of a partial hydatidiform mole may include some fetal tissue, but this is always abnormal and never matures.

Risk Factors

- Maternal age younger than 18 or older than 40 years
- Previous molar pregnancy

Risks for the Woman

- Increased risk of choriocarcinoma

Assessment Findings

In addition to vaginal bleeding and uterine enlargement, presenting signs may include:
- Pelvic pain or sensation of pressure
- Anemia
- Hyperemesis gravidarum
- Hyperthyroidism (secondary to the homology between the beta-subunits of hCG and thyroid-stimulating hormone [TSH], which causes hCG to have weak TSH-like activity)
- Gestational hypertension or preeclampsia early in pregnancy
- Amenorrhea
- Nausea and vomiting
- Abnormal uterine bleeding ranges from spotting to profuse hemorrhage
- Enlarged uterus
- Abdominal cramping and expulsion of vesicles

Diagnosis of Medical Management

- The routine use of ultrasound in early pregnancy can diagnose molar pregnancy much earlier than before.
- Other options are hCG and transvaginal ultrasound.

Medical Management

- Immediate evacuation of mole with aspiration or suction D&C is performed.
- After molar evacuation, patients should be monitored with serial hCG determinations to diagnose and treat malignant sequelae promptly. Oral contraceptives have been demonstrated to be safe and effective during posttreatment monitoring based on randomized controlled trials.
- Women with nonmetastatic GTD should be treated with single-agent chemotherapy (ACOG, 2004).
- Follow-up of hCG levels should be obtained for at least 6 months to detect trophoblastic neoplasia. After hCG levels fall to normal for 6 months, pregnancy can be considered.
- Women with metastatic GTD should be referred to specialists with experience treating this disease.

Nursing Actions for Postevacuation of Mole

- Monitor for signs and symptoms of hemorrhage such as abnormal vital signs, abdominal pain, or vaginal bleeding.
- Assess the uterus.
- Offer explanations and reassurance related to the plan of care.
- Offer emotional support related to pregnancy loss and fear of cancer risk.
- Assess response to diagnosis and treatment plan related to anxiety, fear, and guilt.
- Explain the plan for follow-up care related to serial hCG.
- Give RhoGAM if indicated.
- Assess the significance of loss to the woman and family.
  - Acknowledge feelings of sadness, distress, or relief toward pregnancy loss.
  - Give parents choices and opportunities for decision making.
  - Provide the family with information on pregnancy loss and support groups.
- Provide psychological support appropriate to the family's response.
- Offer resources to the patient and family about the psychological effects of pregnancy loss.
- Schedule a postdischarge follow-up meeting with the patient, as needed.
- Offer discharge teaching related to self-care and warning signs including (Cunningham et al., 2018; Genovese, 2016):
  - Monitor for severe abdominal pain, excessive bleeding, and signs and symptoms of infection such as fever.
  - Review the plan for follow-up with the care provider and encourage adherence to the follow-up regime.
  - Teach the patient appropriate pain management.
  - Discuss contraception options and reason to prevent pregnancy for 1 year.

- Emphasize the importance of medical follow-up with regular hCG levels due to the risk of malignant trophoblastic disease and choriocarcinoma.
- Prophylactic chemotherapy is not routinely recommended (ACOG, 2004).

CRITICAL COMPONENT

Psychosocial Consideration Related to Pregnancy Complications

A pregnant woman experiencing complications often requires increased surveillance during pregnancy and may require hospitalization. This can cause additional stress for herself, her partner, and her family (Durham, 1998). Childbearing women have a vested interest in their pregnancy and outcome; they know their bodies, preferences, concerns, and fears. Make efforts to meet their needs and desires. Provide accurate information to the woman and family in understandable terms to make sure the woman can be an informed participant in shared decision making. Communication and shared decision making improve outcomes. Hospitalization may involve not only loss of normal routine but loss of control. Establishing a plan of care includes a discussion of the risks and benefits in the context of the woman's values, preferences, obstetric history, and treatment plan so the woman can make an informed decision about her care.

Women with high-risk pregnancies may undergo unplanned cesarean birth or disruption of birth plans. High-risk pregnancies can result in financial hardship from loss of work hours and increased cost of medical care. Research has found that hospitalized antepartum women reported high levels of physical, emotional, familial, and financial hardship, and a feeling of uncertainty associated with hospitalization (Cowswell et al., 2009). Women may fear death or loss of their fetus. After a pregnancy with unplanned outcomes, a woman may experience anxiety related to future pregnancies. It is common for women with high-risk pregnancies to deliver newborns that require tertiary care in the NICU. Mothers may also experience separation from their newborns due to transport of the newborn. Some women report feeling powerless due to this separation. Maternal separation also represents a barrier for women desiring to breastfeed their newborns. These women will require lactation support. Successful breastfeeding for a duration of 6 to 12 months may decrease the risk of future health concerns for the mother and her newborn (Phillips & Boyd, 2016).

INFECTIONS

Infections are a common complication of pregnancy. Intrauterine or perinatally transmitted infections can have severe and debilitating effects on the mother, her sex partner, and the fetus. Infections can be acquired by the fetus transplacentally, such as with HIV; may ascend the birth canal; or can be acquired through contact at the time of a vaginal birth, such as herpes. The impact of infection on pregnancy depends on the infectious organism involved. A thorough history of mother and sex partner should be taken to determine the risk of STDs and counseled on perinatal testing recommendations for screening and treatment.

Some infectious agents, such as trichomoniasis and vaginosis, are easily treated and affect only the mother. Other infections, such as rubella and syphilis, can actively infect the fetus during pregnancy. The recommendations to screen pregnant women are thus based on the disease severity and sequelae of prevalence in the population, state laws requirements, and the associated costs (Centers for Disease Control and Prevention [CDC], 2015c). In the following section, infections such as HIV, gonorrhea, chlamydia, syphilis, hepatitis B, human papillomavirus (HPV), herpes simplex virus (HSV), TORCH (Toxoplasmosis, Other [hepatitis B], Rubella, and Cytomegalovirus and Herpes simplex virus) infections, urinary tract infection (UTI)/pyelonephritis, and GBS are reviewed, highlighting maternal and fetal effects, treatment, and nursing implications (CDC, 2015b).

Human Immunodeficiency Virus (HIV/AIDS)

Human immunodeficiency virus (HIV) is a chronic illness caused by the retrovirus of the lentivirus family that has an affinity for the T-lymphocytes, macrophages, and monocytes. The virus attacks the CD4 cells of the immune system (Adams, 2021). HIV/AIDS is a virus passed from one person to another through blood and sexual contact. There is an increased risk for HIV/AIDS among female adults and adolescents younger than 25 years of age (CDC, 2015c), and 19% of new HIV cases were women (CDC, 2021b). The current annual number of women with HIV infections delivering infants in the United States is about 5,000 births (Nesheim et al., 2018).

Transmission of HIV/AIDS happens through sexual contact without condoms, many partners, presence of genital sores, and presence of other STDs. It is also transmitted by exposure to blood, blood products, or by-products such as blood transfusion, needle sharing, and accidental inoculation via occupational exposure (CDC, 2015c). Transmission of HIV perinatally happens through transplacental, intrapartal, and breast milk exposure. Before use of antiviral therapy in pregnancy, risk of infection for a neonate to an HIV seropositive mother was approximately 25%, ranging from 13% to 39%. Today, most pregnant women who have HIV are on a regular antiretroviral drug regimen, decreasing their HIV viral load to undetectable. As a result, maternal-child transmission has decreased (CDC, 2015b).

Factors Associated With Increased Perinatal Transmission

- Mother who has AIDS
- Preterm delivery
- Decreased maternal CD4 count
- High maternal viral load (cesarean section recommended delivery for high viral load)
- Chorioamnionitis
- Blood exposure due to episiotomy, vaginal laceration, and forceps delivery

Risks to Fetus and Newborn

- Risk of transmission is 20% to 25% without the use of antiretroviral drugs but can be as low as 2% with appropriate antepartal drug treatment.
- Preterm delivery
- Preterm PROM
- IUGR

Assessment Findings

- Physical findings include fever, fatigue, vomiting, diarrhea, weight loss, generalized lymphadenopathy, cognitive changes, neurological disorder, PID, TORCH infections, oral gingivitis, vaginitis, and opportunistic infection.
- Psychosocial findings include anxiety, fear, lack of social support, stress, depression, denial, emotional instability, financial instability, and lack of resources.

Medical Management

- Perform routine screening starting at the first perinatal visit. CD4 counts should be tested at the first antenatal visit and every 3 months during pregnancy. HIV RNA should be tested between 36 and 38 weeks of gestation to determine the safest method of delivery (Panel on Treatment of Pregnant Women With HIV Infection and Prevention of Perinatal Transmission, 2018).
- Treatment with at least three antiretroviral drugs
- A main goal in caring for mothers with HIV is to prevent transmission to the fetus or newborn.

Nursing Actions in Antepartal Period

- Provide education and counseling on the plan of care.
- Provide education and counseling on the potential consequences of pregnancy on HIV disease progress, risk for transmission, and consequences for the neonate.
- Provide education to facilitate health promotion
  - Adequate sleep
  - Consume an adequate diet as protein deficiency can depress immunity; consume adequate zinc and vitamin A for cell growth.
  - Avoid infection.
  - Provide emotional support.
  - If the woman is diagnosed with HIV during pregnancy, she needs extensive and ongoing education and counseling on the plan of care and management.

Nursing Actions in Intrapartal Period

- Avoid using instruments during birth.
- Leave fetal membranes intact.
- Avoid fetal scalp electrode.
- Avoid episiotomy and assisted vaginal delivery.
- Provide and reinforce education.
- Provide emotional support.
- Avoid breastfeeding.

- Avoid using methergine in the immediate postpartum period for women taking antiretrovirals. The combination of these drugs can lead to exaggerated vasoconstrictive responses (ACOG, 2018e).

Hepatitis C

Hepatitis C is the most commonly reported bloodborne infection in the United States, and an estimated 2.4 million persons (1.0%) in the nation live with the disease. Percutaneous exposure is the most efficient mode of hepatitis C virus (HCV) transmission, and injection drug use (IDU) is the primary risk factor for infection. Currently, the highest rates of acute infection are among ages 20 to 39 years with new HCV infections increasing among reproductive aged adults. Rates of HCV infection nearly doubled during 2009 to 2014 among women with live births (Schillie et al., 2020). In the United States, up to 2.5% of pregnant women are infected with HCV, which carries an approximately 5% risk of transmission from mother to infant. HCV can be transmitted to the infant in utero or during the peripartum period, and infection during pregnancy is associated with increased risk of adverse fetal outcomes, including fetal growth restriction and low birth weight. Approximately 90% of HCV-infected persons can be cured of HCV infection with 8 to 12 weeks of therapy; however, direct-acting antivirals (DAAs) are not yet approved for use in pregnancy.

The postpartum period might represent a unique time to transition women who have had HCV infection diagnosed during pregnancy to treatment with DAAs. Treatment during the interconception (interpregnancy) period reduces the transmission risk for subsequent pregnancies. Identification of HCV infection during pregnancy also can inform pregnancy and delivery management issues that might reduce the likelihood of HCV transmission to the infant. In the United States, 1% to 2.5% of pregnant women are infected with HCV, which carries an approximately 5% risk of transmission from mother to infant. HCV can be transmitted to the infant in utero or during the peripartum period, and infection during pregnancy is associated with increased risk of adverse fetal outcomes, including fetal growth restriction and LBW (SMFM et al., 2017).

Current recommendations from the SMFM et al. (2017) include:

- Screen women at increased risk for hepatitis C infection by testing for anti-HCV antibodies at their first prenatal visit. If initial results are negative, hepatitis C screening should be repeated later in pregnancy in women with persistent or new risk factors for hepatitis C infection.
- Pregnant women should be counseled to abstain from alcohol.
- Antiviral treatment should be deferred to the postpartum period as DAA regimens are not currently approved for use in pregnancy.
- Cesarean delivery solely for the indication of HCV is not recommended.
- Avoid internal fetal monitoring, prolonged ROM, and episiotomy in managing labor in HCV-positive women.
- Do not discourage breastfeeding based on a positive HCV infection status.

Sexually Transmitted Infections and Diseases (STI/STD)

Sexually transmitted infections (STIs), sometimes referred to as sexually transmitted diseases (STDs), remain a major public health challenge in the United States. CDC estimates indicate that about 20% of the U.S. population, nearly 68 million people, had an STI in 2018, and STIs acquired that year will cost the American health-care system nearly $16 billion (CDC, 2021a). Of the 26 million new STIs in 2018, almost half were among youth aged 15 to 24.

As a review, prevalence is the estimated number of infections, new or existing, in a given time. Incidence is the estimated number of new infections, diagnosed or undiagnosed. In 2018, the STI prevalence and incidence in the United States for eight STIs were as follows:

- HPV prevalence was 42.5 million, incidence 13 million.
- HSV-2 prevalence was 18.6 million, incidence 572,000.
- Trichomoniasis prevalence was 2.6 million, incidence 6.9 million.
- Chlamydia prevalence was 2.4 million, incidence 4 million.
- HIV (ages 13 and older) prevalence was 984,000, incidence 32,000.
- Gonorrhea prevalence was 209,000, incidence 1.6 million.
- Syphilis (ages 14 and older) prevalence was 156,000, incidence 146,000.
- HBV (ages unavailable) prevalence was 103,000, incidence 8,300.

STIs cost the U.S. health-care system billions each year. STIs affect women of every socioeconomic and educational level, age, race, and ethnicity. The two most common reported infections in the United States are chlamydia and gonorrhea, which primarily affect women ages 15 to 24 (CDC, 2021a). Women receive routine testing for syphilis, hepatitis B, HIV, and HPV during prenatal care. Though not routinely tested, HSV screening is recommended for women with a history or new symptoms.

Table 7-5 provides a summary of fetal and maternal effects and management of STIs and STDs. Pregnant women can become infected with the same STIs as nonpregnant women. Pregnancy does not provide protection for the woman or the baby; in fact, consequences of an STI can be serious and even life-threatening for the woman and her baby. Intrauterine or perinatal transmitted STIs can have severely debilitating effects on women, their partners, and their fetuses. All women should be screened for STIs during the first prenatal visit. Women at increased risk for STIs such as those with new or multiple sex partners, sex workers, risky behaviors, or recurrent STIs during prior trimesters may be retested in the third trimester (AAP & ACOG, 2017).

Prevention and control of STIs is the best way to reduce and eliminate potential harm. Five strategies used to promote prevention are (CDC, 2015b):

- Accurate risk assessment, education, and counseling of persons at risk on ways to avoid STIs through changes in sexual behaviors and use of recommended prevention services
- Pre-exposure vaccination of persons at risk for vaccine-preventable STIs

TABLE 7-5 Summary of Fetal and Maternal Effects and Management of STIs and STDs

INFECTION	MATERNAL EFFECTS	FETAL EFFECTS	MANAGEMENT	NURSING ISSUES
Chlamydia *Chlamydia trachomatis*	Three-fourths of women have no symptoms, so it is known as a "silent" disease; may have burning on urination or abnormal vaginal discharge.	Contact at delivery may cause conjunctivitis or premature birth. The efficacy of ophthalmia neonatorum prophylaxis is unclear.	During pregnancy, treatment is with oral antibiotics such as amoxicillin, azithromycin, and erythromycin.	Can lead to PID. Treat all infected partners. Advocate for the use of expedited partner therapy as a method of preventing chlamydial reinfection when a patient's partners are unable or unwilling to seek medical care. Retest in 3 weeks.
Gonorrhea *Neisseria gonorrhoeae*	Most women have no symptoms but may have burning on urination, increased purulent yellow-green vaginal discharge, or bleeding between periods. Rectal infection can cause anal itching, discharge, and bleeding. Can lead to PID.	Contact at birth. Ophthalmia neonatorum may cause sepsis or blindness. To prevent gonococcal ophthalmia neonatorum, a prophylactic antibiotic ointment should be instilled into the eyes of all newborns.	During pregnancy, maternal treatment is with antibiotics such as cephalosporin. Neonatal treatment for women with active gonorrhea	Can lead to PID. Complete treatment. Advocate for the use of expedited partner therapy as a method of preventing gonorrhea reinfection when a patient's partners are unable or unwilling to seek medical care.
Group B *Streptococcus agalactiae* (GBS)	Women are typically asymptomatic carriers. Symptoms can include abnormal vaginal discharge, urinary tract infections, chorioamnionitis.	About 50% of women with colonized GBS will transmit it to their newborn. In about 1%–2% of infections, it can result in invasive GBS with permanent neurological sequelae.	If GBS-positive at 35–37 weeks of gestation or GBS status is unknown, treat with antibiotics in labor to prevent neonatal transmission; penicillin or ampicillin IV	Universal screening for GBS colonization. GBS-positive women receive intrapartum antibiotic prophylaxis unless a prelabor cesarean birth is performed with intact membranes.
Hepatitis B (HBV)	50% asymptomatic; may have low-grade fever, anorexia, nausea and vomiting, fatigue, and rashes. Chronic infection can lead to cirrhosis of the liver and liver cancer.	90% of infected infants have chronic infection. Cirrhosis of the liver Liver cancer	Serial testing for viral load can be completed. No specific treatment is available. Pregnant individuals who test positive for hepatitis B surface antigen (HBsAg) also should be tested for hepatitis B virus deoxyribonucleic acid (HBV DNA) to guide the use of antiviral medication to prevent perinatal transmission.	HBsAg-positive pregnant women should be reported to the state or local health department for timely and appropriate prophylaxis for their infants. Immunoprophylaxis of all newborns born to HBsAg-positive women. HBIG to neonate at delivery and hepatitis B vaccination series initiated.

TABLE 7-5   Summary of Fetal and Maternal Effects and Management of STIs and STDs—cont'd

INFECTION	MATERNAL EFFECTS	FETAL EFFECTS	MANAGEMENT	NURSING ISSUES
Hepatitis C virus (HCV)	80% of persons infected have no symptoms. Can lead to chronic liver disease, cirrhosis, and liver cancer.	Exposure transplacentally. Estimated 2%–7% transmission rate. Little research on treatment of children.	DAA treatment is contraindicated in pregnancy. Treatment postpartum	Breastfeeding is not contraindicated.
Human papillomavirus (HPV) Forty or more types infect the genital area. Most genital HPV are sexually transmitted.	The majority of HPV infections are asymptomatic but can cause genital warts. HPV infection is associated with anogenital cancer (including cervical, vaginal, vulvar, penile, and anal) and oropharyngeal cancer (back of tongue, tonsil). Genital warts are flat, papular, or pedunculated growths on the genital mucosa.	Route of transmission is unclear. Can cause respiratory papillomatosis.	Testing for HPV is done with routine Pap smear. If warts are present, they may be removed during pregnancy. HPV vaccination is not recommended during pregnancy. Treatment reduces but does not eliminate HPV infection.	The presence of genital warts is not an indication for cesarean delivery.
Syphilis *Treponema pallidum*	Ulcer or chancre, then maculopapular rash advancing to CNS and multiorgan damage.	Transplacental transmission. Congenital syphilis may cause PTB, physical deformity, neurological complications, stillbirth, or neonatal death.	Penicillin	
Trichomonas *vaginalis*	Malodorous yellow–green vaginal discharge and vulvar irritation. Can lead to premature rupture of membrane and preterm labor.	Preterm delivery and low birth weight. Respiratory and genital infection.	Metronidazole	
Candidiasis *Candida albicans**	Results from a disturbance in vaginal flora. Pruritus, vaginal soreness, dyspareunia, abnormal vaginal discharge with a yeasty odor		Topical azole therapies	
Bacterial vaginosis†	50% of women are asymptomatic. A fishy odor or vaginal discharge is present. Can result in preterm labor or premature rupture of membranes.	Premature rupture of membranes, chorioamnionitis, or PTB	Metronidazole or clindamycin	

Continued

TABLE 7-5   Summary of Fetal and Maternal Effects and Management of STIs and STDs—cont'd

INFECTION	MATERNAL EFFECTS	FETAL EFFECTS	MANAGEMENT	NURSING ISSUES
Human immunodeficiency virus (HIV/AIDS)	May be asymptomatic for years. HIV weakens the immune system. It may manifest as mononucleosis-like symptoms such as fever, fatigue, sore throat, and lymphadenopathy.	Early antiretroviral treatment has been shown to be effective in reducing maternal-fetal transmissions. Placental transmission but lower than 2% transmission with maternal treatment with antiretroviral medications. 15%–25% transmission to fetus without maternal treatment. Antibody screening is not reliable during infancy because maternally produced IgG antibodies to HIV are present for up to 18 months.	Antiviral	Cesarean birth may be considered. Breastfeeding is contraindicated. Case management follow-up is suggested for both the woman and her baby.

ACOG, 2018b; CDC, 2015a, 2015c.
*Not an STI
† A polymicrobial clinical syndrome

- Identification of asymptomatically infected persons and persons with symptoms of STIs
- Effective diagnosis, treatment, counseling, and follow-up of infected persons, and evaluation, treatment, and counseling of sex partners of persons who are infected with an STD
- Know your sexual partners. The more partners one has, the higher the risk of getting an STI.
  - Use a latex or polyurethane condom. Using a latex or polyurethane condom every time one has vaginal, oral, or anal sex reduces the risk of infection.
  - Know that some sex practices increase the risk. Sexual acts that tear or break the skin carry a higher risk of STIs. For example, anal sex poses a high risk because tissues in the rectum break easily. Body fluids also can carry STIs. Having any unprotected sexual contact with an infected person poses a high risk of getting an STI.
  - Get vaccines. Vaccines are available to help protect against hepatitis B and HPV.

Risks for the Woman

- STIs can cause PID.
- PID can lead to infertility, chronic hepatitis, and cervical and other cancers.
- STIs during pregnancy can lead to PTL, PROM, and uterine infection.

Risks for the Fetus

- STIs can pass to the fetus by crossing the placenta; some can be transmitted to the baby during delivery as the baby passes through the birth canal (see Table 7-5).
- Harmful effects to babies include PTB, low birth weight, neonatal sepsis, and neurological damage.

Assessment Findings

- Many STIs in women are "silent" without signs and symptoms, making routine screening for STIs during the first prenatal visit an important part of routine prenatal care.
- Physical findings include low-grade temperature, poor personal hygiene, genital warts, purulent urethral or cervical discharge, friable cervix, genital lesions, tender uterus, pain on motion of cervix, inguinal adenopathy, and rash on the palms and soles of the feet.
- Positive STI cultures and test results may appear.

Medical Management

- Provide routine screening of STIs and HIV at the first prenatal visit.
- Treat bacterial STIs with antibiotics.
- Prescribe antiviral medications for viral STIs to reduce symptoms.

Nursing Actions

- Provide information on STIs.
- Provide emotional support.
- Instruct the woman on the correct administration of medications and other treatments and the importance of completing treatment.
- Instruct the patient on the warning signs of complication (fever, increased pain, bleeding).
- Provide information on the importance of abstaining from intercourse until the patient and her partner are free of infection.
- Provide the partner with treatment as indicated.
- Review with the woman and partners that STIs can be transmitted through noncoital sex and infections can be transmitted through oral and anal sex (ACOG, 2013a).

TORCH Infections

TORCH is an acronym that stands for Toxoplasmosis, Other (hepatitis B), Rubella, and Cytomegalovirus and HSV. TORCH infections are unique in their pathogenesis and have potentially devastating effects on the fetus (Table 7-6). Each disease can cross the placenta and may adversely affect the developing fetus. These teratogenic effects of each disease vary depending on the developmental stage and gestational time of exposure (CDC, 2015c).

Cytomegalovirus (CMV) is the most common cause of congenital infection, and the risk of vertical transmission to the fetus in pregnancy is 30% to 40%.

CMV has been identified to cause CNS deficits such as mental retardation, cerebral palsy, seizures, chorioretinitis, and neurosensory hearing loss when transferred to the fetus. Women who develop a CMV infection in the first trimester are more likely to deliver fetuses with neurosensory birth deficits and CNS sequelae than women infected in the second or third trimester. In cases where maternal CMV infection is suspected, it is important to evaluate the risk to the fetus of being infected or symptomatically affected by CMV to provide appropriate counseling and guidance to parents (Carlson et al., 2010).

Risk Factors

Risk for these infections varies based on the route of transmission. Some, such as herpes, are STIs; others have various routes of transmission to the woman (CDC, 2015b).

Risk for the Woman

- Depends on the infectious agent (CDC, 2015b; see Table 7-6)

Risks for the Fetus

- The usual route of transmission to the fetus is transplacental (see Table 7-6).
- Infections acquired in utero can result in IUGR, prematurity, chronic postnatal infection, and even death.

Assessment Findings

- Maternal assessment findings vary with the organism (see Table 7-6).

Medical Management

- Medical management varies based on the organism, trimester of exposure, and clinical evidence of neonatal sequelae (see Table 7-6).

Nursing Actions

- Nursing considerations vary with the organism (see Table 7-6).
- Provide emotional support.
- Instruct the woman on the treatment plan.

Urinary Tract Infection and Pyelonephritis

Urinary tract infections (UTI) are the most common bacterial infections during pregnancy. They are associated with risk to both the mother and fetus and can contribute to PTL and birth, LBW, pyelonephritis, and increased risk of perinatal mortality. Pregnant women can be symptomatic or asymptomatic. Those with recurrent symptomatic UTI may receive prophylactic treatment throughout their pregnancy with oral antibiotics (Cunningham et al., 2018).

Assessment and Findings

- Infections develop from ascending colonization of preexisting vaginal, perineal, and fecal flora.
- Maternal physiological and anatomical factors can predispose women to ascending infections. Urinary retention due to an enlarging uterus and urinary stasis hormonal changes can also contribute to UTIs.
- History of previous UTI before in pregnancy or childhood.
- Increased risk related to advanced maternal age, low socioeconomic status, or underlying chronic illnesses such as preeclampsia, sickle cell trait, diabetes, and hypertension.
- Associated with poor hygiene, frequent intercourse, recent catheterization, and abdominal trauma or pelvic surgery.
- Symptoms include frequency, dysuria, hematuria, fever, chills, malaise, nocturia, malodorous urine, flank pain or tenderness, nausea, vomiting, diarrhea, and low abdominal tenderness or pain.
- Diagnostic testing of urine. A positive result is associated with more than 100,000 colonies/mL of bacteria in the urine from a clean catch midstream sample.
- *E. coli* account for 80% to 90% of UTIs.

Medical Management

- All pregnant women should have a urine culture completed at the first prenatal appointment.
- Antibiotics should be prescribed for pregnant women only for appropriate indications and for the shortest effective duration.
- During the second and third trimesters, sulfonamides and nitrofurantoins may continue to be used as first-line agents

TABLE 7-6   Torch Infections

INFECTION	MATERNAL EFFECTS	FETAL EFFECTS	PREVENTION AND MANAGEMENT	NURSING ISSUES
Toxoplasmosis *Toxoplasma gondii* Single-celled protozoan parasite Transplacental transmission	Most infections are asymptomatic but may cause fatigue, muscle pains, pneumonitis, myocarditis, and lymphadenopathy.	Severity varies with gestational age and congenital infection. Can lead to spontaneous abortion, low birth weight, hepatosplenomegaly, icterus, anemia, chorioretinitis, or neurological disease. The later in pregnancy the infection occurs, the higher the rate of transmission. The earlier in the gestation the fetus is infected, the more serious the disease.	Avoid eating raw meat and contact with cat feces. Treat with sulfadiazine or pyrimethamine after the first trimester. Treat pregnant women with acute infection; reduced risk of congenital infection, and may reduce congenital disease severity.	Teach women to avoid raw meat and cat feces. About 40% of women have an antibody to this organism.
Other Infections Hepatitis B Direct contact with blood or infected body fluid	30%–50% of infected women are asymptomatic. Symptoms include low-grade fever, nausea, anorexia, jaundice, hepatomegaly, preterm labor, and preterm delivery. Acute maternal infection in third trimester is associated with up to a 90% rate of neonatal infection.	Infants have a 90% chance of becoming chronically infected, HBV carrier, and a 25% risk of developing significant liver disease. Acute maternal infection in third trimester is associated with up to a 90% rate of neonatal infection.	Antiviral maternal treatment reduces neonatal transmission. Infant receives HBIG and hepatitis vaccine at delivery.	Universal screening recommended in pregnancy. HBV can be given in pregnancy.
Rubella (German measles) Nasopharyngeal secretions Transplacental	Erythematous maculopapular rash, lymph node enlargement, slight fever, headache, malaise	Congenital defects occur in 85% of cases of maternal infection in the first 12 weeks of gestation. Anomalies include deafness, eye defects, CNS anomalies, and severe cardiac malformation. Congenital defects are rare when infection occurs after 20 weeks of pregnancy.	Primary approach to rubella infection is immunization. If the woman is pregnant and not immune, she should not receive the vaccine until the postpartum period.	If the woman is not immune, she should not receive the vaccine until the postpartum period and be counseled to not become pregnant for 3 months.
Cytomegalovirus (CMV) Virus of herpes group Transmitted by droplet contact and transplacentally Most common congenital infection	Most infections are asymptomatic, but 15% of adults may have mononucleosis-like syndrome.	Infection to fetus is most likely with primary maternal infection and timing of infection with first- and second-trimester exposure. May result in low birth weight, IUGR, hearing impairment microcephaly, and CNS abnormalities. 30% of infected infants die and up to 80% of surviving infants have severe neurological sequalae (AAP & ACOG, 2017).	No treatment is available.	

TABLE 7-6   Torch Infections—cont'd

INFECTION	MATERNAL EFFECTS	FETAL EFFECTS	PREVENTION AND MANAGEMENT	NURSING ISSUES
Herpes simplex virus (HSV) Chronic lifelong viral infection Contact at delivery and ascending infection	Painful genital lesions. Lesions may be on external or internal genitalia.	Transmission rate of up to 60% among women who acquire genital herpes near time of delivery. Transmission rate is low (lower than 2%) among women with recurrent genital herpes. Mortality of 50%–60% if neonatal exposure to active primary lesion is related to neurological complications of massive infection sepsis and neurological complications.	No cure available. Acyclovir is used to suppress the outbreak of lesions. Antiviral treatment of primary outbreak reduces severity of symptoms and duration of viral shedding Antiviral suppressive therapy may be offered near term.	Most common viral STI. Recommendations for delivery are based on status of membrane or status of active lesions

Source: AAP & ACOG, 2017; CDC, 2015a, 2015c.

for the treatment and prevention of UTIs. Prescribing sulfonamides or nitrofurantoin in the first trimester is still considered appropriate when no other suitable alternative antibiotics are available (ACOG, 2017h).

● Obtain follow-up cultures and surveillance for recurrent UTI.

Nursing Actions

● Provide education and support of prevention and signs and symptoms of UTI.
● Instruct the patient on the use and importance of completion of antibiotic treatment with possible prophylactic treatment throughout pregnancy.
● Instruct the patient on the early labor precautions and report them immediately.
● Provide information related to proper hygiene and wiping, prompt void, and adequate daily hydration.

Group Beta Streptococcus (GBS)

Group B Streptococcus (GBS) colonizes the female genital tract and rectum. It has been known to cause UTI, pyelonephritis, chorioamnionitis, PTL, vaginal discharge, postpartum endometritis, post-cesarean section wound infection, and rarely endocarditis (AAP & ACOG, 2017). GBS is the leading cause of newborn infection. Vertical transmission of bacteria usually occurs during labor or after rupture of the membranes. Women should be screened prenatally for GBS colonization and treated appropriately with antibiotics in labor (ACOG, 2019g).

Maternal and Neonatal Risks

● Premature labor is a risk.
● Maternal intrapartum fever for prolonged ROM for more than 12 hours may occur.

● Neonatal prematurity may occur.
● Transmission rate from mother to infant at birth is 50% to 75%.
● On rare occasions, ultrasound has shown evidence of fetal hydrops and has been associated with fetal death.
● Prevalence of neonatal GBS is 0.5 per 1,000 births.
● Approximately 30% to 50% of pregnant women are carriers of GBS.

Assessment and Findings

● Common cause of sepsis, meningitis, and pneumonia
● Positive test for GBS in current pregnancy or previous pregnancy. CDC recommends routine cultures of vagina and rectum between 36 and 37 weeks' gestation (ACOG, 2019g).

Medical Management

● Collect vaginal-rectal culture for screening.
● Treat positive test results with ampicillin or penicillin during labor. For women with a penicillin allergy, cefazolin is recommended for those with a low risk for anaphylaxis and clindamycin is the alternative for women with a high anaphylactic risk (ACOG, 2019g).
● Review of previous history of GBS. If GBS status is unknown at the time the woman presents for labor, she will be treated prophylactically if she has had a prior history of GBS or risk factors.
● Women who have a cesarean before labor onset do not need treatment even with a positive test.

Nursing Actions

● Provide instruction on the importance of GBS antibiotic therapy during pregnancy.
● Assess for signs and symptoms of fever or sepsis during prenatal care through delivery.

Zika Virus

Zika virus is a flavivirus with the potential to cause adverse pregnancy and neonatal outcomes. Pregnant women should be screened for recent travel or exposure and counseled about taking trips to high-risk areas while pregnant or trying to conceive. Zika virus is spread primarily through mosquito bites and has a high potential of vertical transmission to the fetus (ACOG, 2019d).

Maternal and Neonatal Risks

- Birth defects
- PTB
- Growth restriction (IUGR)
- Miscarriage or stillbirth

Assessment Findings

- Fever
- Rash
- Arthralgia
- Conjunctivitis
- Use of ultrasonography can evaluate fetal abnormalities in women who test positive.

Medical Management

There are no current vaccines for Zika; the best method to prevent infection is to prevent exposure. The current recommendation is to counsel couples who may have been exposed to Zika to wait until a safe period has elapsed before trying to conceive. According to ACOG (2019d), if the female has tested positive, couples should use condoms or abstain from intercourse for 8 weeks. If the male or both partners have tested positive, couples should use condoms or abstain from intercourse for 3 months from symptom onset or time of exposure.

Nursing Actions

- Perform a travel assessment and screening on the woman to determine possible exposure.
- Educate patients on how to prevent Zika infection.
  - Limit travel to areas where Zika risk is high.
  - If traveling to high-risk areas, prevent mosquito bites by covering the skin at all times and use an insect repellent.

Coronavirus (COVID-19)

COVID-19 is a new viral strand of the coronavirus family that primarily affects the respiratory system. The main presenting symptoms are a cough, fever, and dyspnea. The presentation is very similar to influenza. Symptoms can range from mild to severe, and some people can be asymptomatic viral carriers. Because symptoms can be delayed or mild, it can be difficult to track the spread of infection, so coronavirus is highly contagious for a much longer period than the flu (French, 2020). The CDC suggests that pregnant patients are at increased risk for severe manifestations of COVID-19-related illnesses that could

potentially require intensive care unit admission or mechanical ventilation (Zahn, 2020). Women with additional pregnancy complications such as diabetes mellitus or obesity may be at even higher risk of developing more severe illness from COVID-19 (French, 2020).

The ACOG and the SMFM, the two leading organizations representing specialists in obstetric care, recommend that all pregnant individuals be vaccinated against COVID-19 (ACOG & SMFM, 2021). The organizations' recommendations in support of vaccination during pregnancy reflect evidence demonstrating the safe use of the COVID-19 vaccines during pregnancy from tens of thousands of reporting individuals over the last several months, as well as the current low vaccination rates and concerning increase in cases.

Data shows that COVID-19 infections disproportionately affect communities of color, especially Black, Latino, and American Indian individuals. Inequities within these populations, including limited testing, health-care resources, and other SDOH, contribute to an increased number of comorbidities. These factors predispose people of color to more severe COVID-19 manifestations and illness with fewer available resources. It is important for women's health providers to address health disparities and inequities when caring for patients and recognize the impact of racism and implicit biases on health care (French, 2020).

Maternal and Neonatal Risks

- Increased risk of severe COVID-19 manifestations and symptoms
- ICU admission
- Mechanical ventilation if respiratory status becomes severely compromised
- Preterm delivery and birth
- VTE caused by hypercoagulability of pregnancy and COVID-19

Assessment and Findings

- Symptoms may appear 2 to 14 days after exposure to the virus and can include:
  - Fever or chills
  - Cough
  - Shortness of breath or dyspnea
  - Fatigue
  - Muscle or body aches
  - Headache
  - New loss of taste or smell
  - Sore throat
  - Congestion or runny nose
  - Nausea or vomiting
  - Diarrhea

(CDC, 2020)

Medical Management

Patients with known or suspected COVID-19 should be cared for in a single-person room or isolation room and should be prioritized for testing. All providers should be educated on proper donning and doffing of personal protective equipment (PPE), and airborne and droplet precautions should be maintained. Per the CDC (2020), patients with mild to moderate illness can discontinue isolation precautions when at least 10 days have passed since symptoms first began and at least 24 hours have passed since the last fever without use of fever-reducing medications, as long as symptoms have improved. For asymptomatic patients, precautions can be discontinued when at least 10 days have passed since they first tested positive.

Infants born to mothers with a positive COVID-19 diagnosis must be tested and isolated from other healthy infants, but there is no need for maternal-infant separation solely based on a maternal positive diagnosis. For rooming-in with COVID-19 positive mothers, safety measures should be implemented to reduce the risk of transmission, including hand hygiene before contact with the neonate and maintaining 6 feet of distance between the mother and neonate as often as possible. Current research and data have determined that a COVID-19 diagnosis is not a contraindication to breastfeeding, as there is limited evidence of the COVID-19 virus in breast milk. Mothers can still transmit the virus through respiratory droplets while in close contact with their infant and should wear a face covering while breastfeeding (ACOG, 2021).

Nursing Actions

- Emphasize the importance of infection prevention methods such as hand hygiene, facial coverings, frequent disinfecting of surfaces, and social distancing (staying at least 6 feet apart and avoiding large crowds).
- Monitor fetal status by EFM.
- Help manage fear, anxiety, and stress for women and provide social support resources.
- Educate the patient about monitoring symptoms and when to get tested.
- Educate the patient about vaccinations for influenza, pneumonia, and COVID-19.
- Provide emotional support, especially if visitors are limited in the clinical setting.

Sepsis During Pregnancy

Sepsis is currently defined as a life-threatening organ dysfunction caused by a dysregulated host response to infection (Singer et al., 2016). Patients without organ dysfunction are classified as having an infection. Sepsis is a significant contributor to maternal morbidity and mortality. Sepsis screening protocols may be institution and unit specific. Whichever protocol is used, prompt recognition via positive screening or suspicion by a provider based on clinical findings warrants further investigation and prompt management. Although assessment of some parameters requires use of invasive monitoring techniques, other signs and symptoms may be detected by evaluating trends in routine clinical assessment findings such as temperature, blood pressure, heart rate, RR and effort, breath sounds, and arterial hemoglobin oxygen saturation (SaO_2). Assessment should include urine output, skin appearance, capillary refill, and mental status to further evaluate perfusion status. Fetal status should also be evaluated, depending on the estimated gestational age, as fetal compromise may be an early indicator of an adverse change in maternal status. Fetal tachycardia is often one of the first signs of maternal infection.

Compromised uteroplacental perfusion due to maternal sepsis may manifest as decreased FHR variability and late FHR decelerations (Brown & Abdel-Razeq, 2019). It cannot be emphasized enough that consistent frequency of assessment and evaluation of findings are vital for rapid detection and management of sepsis. Treatment for sepsis is predicated on timely suspicion, fluid resuscitation, and antibiotic therapy within the first hour as early antibiotic therapy for sepsis is recommended to reduce mortality (ACOG, 2019a). The goal of clinical treatment is to optimize cardiac output and oxygen transport while avoiding multiorgan system failure and death.

TRAUMA DURING PREGNANCY

Trauma is the leading cause of maternal death during pregnancy and is more likely to cause maternal death than any other complication of pregnancy. The most common cause of maternal death by trauma is abdominal injury (resulting in hemorrhagic shock) and head injury. Motor vehicle accidents and domestic violence or IPV are the predominant causes of reported trauma during pregnancy (Mendez-Figueroa et al., 2013). Injury to the pregnant woman can result from blunt or penetrating trauma. The most common cause of blunt injury is motor vehicle accidents, whereas the most common cause of penetrating trauma is from gunshot wounds. The mechanisms of maternal and fetal injury, gestational age of the fetus, and secondary complications determine the maternal-fetal response to trauma. Maternal outcome in trauma corresponds to the severity of the injury. Fetal outcome depends on injury and maternal physiological response (Salera-Vieira, 2021; Van Otterloo, 2016). The underpinning principles are that the woman's interests are paramount, and optimal fetal status is generally predicated on optimizing the maternal condition as much as possible (ACOG, 2019a). It is essential to keep in mind that at term, 15% of maternal cardiac output, 750 mL to 1,000 mL/min, flows through the placental bed; unresolved bleeding can lead to maternal exsanguination in 8 to 10 minutes (Salera-Vieira, 2021).

A wide array of complications has been associated with obstetric trauma, including maternal injury, death, shock, hemorrhage, intrauterine fetal demise, abruptio placenta, and uterine rupture; therefore, timely and efficient evaluation is critical to ensure maternal-fetal well-being. That typically includes history and physical examination, laboratory work, assessment of FHR and uterine activity, ultrasound, and radiological studies. Goals of management of the pregnant patient suffering trauma focuses on prevention of hypoxemia, acidosis, hypotension, and hyperventilation to stabilize the mother and avoid fetal hypoxia (Callahan, 2016).

A comprehensive understanding of the physiologic changes in pregnancy, complications of bleeding and PTL, and maternal fetal assessment are essential to provide safe and comprehensive care to the pregnant woman after trauma (Salera-Vieira, 2021). Pregnancy causes both anatomic and physiological changes that impact the woman's response to traumatic injury. For example, increased plasma volume by 50% and increased RBC volume of 30% can mask hemorrhage. Any condition that results in maternal hypotension, such as hemorrhage or hypovolemia, results in vasoconstriction of the uterine arteries and shunting of blood to vital organs. The shunting of blood from the uteroplacental unit maintains maternal blood pressure at the expense of perfusion to the fetus. The pregnant woman has decreased oxygen reserves and decreased blood buffering capacity, which leaves the pregnant trauma patient vulnerable to hypoxemia and less able to compensate when acidemia occurs (Baldisseri, 2016; Maharaj, 2007). Two catastrophic events can occur during pregnancy after blunt trauma to the abdomen:

- Placental abruption
- Uterine rupture

Extensive discussion of management and care during trauma in pregnancy is beyond the scope of this chapter, but key elements of stabilization of the woman and the fetus and assessments are briefly reviewed. Treatment priorities for injured pregnant women typically are directed as they would be for nonpregnant women. Some important considerations related to pregnancy are presented in the following section.

Assessment Findings

Assessment findings are based on injury. Initial maternal evaluation is the systematic evaluation performed according to standard Advanced Trauma Life Support (ATLS) protocols. Initial maternal evaluation and resuscitation take precedence over fetal evaluation. Early recognition of maternal compromise and rapid resuscitation reduce maternal mortality, which in turn reduces fetal mortality.

- Physiological changes in pregnancy might delay the usual vital sign changes of hypovolemia; blood loss of up to 1,500 mL can occur without a change in maternal vital sign changes.
- UCs more frequently than every 10 minutes and uterine irritability may be indications of placental abruption (Cunningham et al., 2018).
- Fetal well-being reflects maternal and fetal status, and conversely FHR changes may indicate maternal deterioration such as hypoxia.

Medical Management

Treatment priorities and medical management for the pregnant trauma patient are the same as for the nonpregnant woman in the initial evaluation. Admission and continuous fetal monitoring for 24 to 48 hours after stabilization, particularly for abdominal injuries due to the increased incidence of placental abruption, is common.

- Pregnant women greater than 20 weeks should be monitored for a minimum of 4 hours for uterine activity. The Kleinhauer–Betke test should be performed on all pregnant women who sustain major trauma.
- Consider obstetrical ultrasound.

Nursing Actions

- Nursing assessment and intervention for the pregnant woman who has experienced trauma are based on the clinical situation and maternal-fetal status.
- Treatment priorities for injured pregnant women typically are directed as they would be for nonpregnant women.
- Initial actions in trauma care are focused on maternal stabilization (Callahan, 2016).
- Evaluate uterine activity and fetal status and anticipate ultrasound.
- Assess for the usual signs of complications including bleeding, uterine tenderness, contractions, and possibly loss of amniotic fluid.
- All women of childbearing age should be screened for IPV.
- To improve the effectiveness of cardiopulmonary resuscitation (CPR), clinicians should perform left lateral uterine displacement by tilting the whole maternal body 25 to 30 degrees.

Pregnant women who sustain trauma present clinical challenges to the emergency, trauma, and obstetric teams. Caring for pregnant trauma patients requires understanding of physiological changes and normal anatomic changes of pregnancy. Knowledge of the mechanism of injury and the ability to assess maternal and fetal status are essential to care. A collaborative, interdisciplinary team approach is essential to optimize outcomes for the mother and fetus (Ruth & Mighty, 2019).

PREGESTATIONAL COMPLICATIONS

Women who enter pregnancy with a preexisting disease or chronic medical condition are at increased risk for complications and are considered high risk. These high-risk pregnancies require extensive surveillance and collaboration of multiple disciplines to achieve an optimal pregnancy outcome. Women often experience fear and anxiety for their health and that of the fetus regarding the impact of the chronic disease on the pregnancy outcome. Any preexisting medical disease can complicate the pregnancy or be exacerbated during pregnancy. Increasing numbers of women with chronic diseases are achieving pregnancy. Nursing care is focused on decreasing complications and providing support and education to patients and families to facilitate their participation in their health care during pregnancy.

Women and their families should participate in decision making and the plan of care to optimize outcomes for both the woman and the fetus. Maternal safety is the prime consideration in all pregnancies. The major preexisting medical complications that impact pregnancy are discussed in this chapter, although all the possible preexisting medical conditions impacting pregnancy are beyond the scope of this chapter. When caring for women who have preexisting diseases, textbooks on high-risk pregnancy management and perinatal journals are the best sources of information.

CRITICAL COMPONENT

The Importance of Patient-Centered Pregnancy Care

Women experiencing pregnancy complications are especially physiologically, psychologically, emotionally, and spiritually vulnerable. Nurses are in a unique position to explore a woman's needs and advocate for the woman's participation in management of pregnancy complications. It is essential to recognize the patient or designee as the source of control and full partner in providing compassionate and coordinated care based on respect for the patient's preferences, values, and needs.

Some suggestions to foster respect for a woman's preferences, values, and needs include:

- Elicit patient values, preferences, and expressed needs as part of the clinical interview, implementation of care plan, and evaluation of care.
- Communicate patient values, preferences, and expressed needs to other members of the health-care team.
- Value the patient's expertise with her own health and symptoms.
- Respect the patient and family preferences for degree of active engagement in the care process.

Cardiovascular Disorders

Maternal heart disease has emerged as a major threat to safe motherhood and women's long-term cardiovascular health (ACOG, 2019f). In the United States, cardiovascular disease is now the leading cause of death in pregnant women and women in the postpartum period, accounting for 4.23 deaths per 100,000 live births (Benjamin et al., 2018). The most recent data indicate that cardiovascular diseases constitute 26.5% of U.S. pregnancy-related deaths (Creanga et al., 2017). Of further concern are the disparities in cardiovascular disease outcomes, with higher rates of morbidity and mortality among nonwhite and lower-income women. Contributing factors include barriers to pre-pregnancy cardiovascular disease assessment, missed opportunities to identify cardiovascular disease risk factors during prenatal care, gaps in high-risk intrapartum care, and delays in recognition of cardiovascular disease symptoms during the puerperium (ACOG, 2019f). Pregnancy complicated by cardiovascular disease is potentially dangerous to maternal and fetal well-being and is the leading non-obstetric cause of maternal mortality. The incidence of cardiac disease among pregnant women ranges from 0.5% to 4% and varies in form and severity (Elkayam et al., 2016).

Cardiac disease during pregnancy may be categorized as congenital, acquired, or ischemic. The spectrum and severity of heart disease observed in reproductive-age women is changing. Today, congenital heart disease accounts for more than half of cardiac disease in pregnancy, and ischemic heart disease is on the rise as a result of obesity, hypertension, diabetes, and delayed childbearing (Arafeh, 2021). Some of the normal cardiac changes during pregnancy can exacerbate cardiac disease during pregnancy, including:

- Increase in total blood volume 30% to 50%
- Increase in cardiac output that peaks at 28 to 32 weeks of gestation
- Plasma volume expansion by 45%
- Increase in RBC by 20%
- Increased cardiac output by 40%
- Increased heart rate by 15%
- Decreased diastolic blood pressure by 10 to 15 mm Hg at 24 to 32 weeks (Arafeh, 2021)
- Heart slightly enlarges and displaces upward and to the left anatomically.
- The weight of the gravid uterus can lie on the inferior vena cava, causing compression and hypotension and decreasing cardiac output.
- Increased estrogen leads to vasodilatation, which lowers peripheral resistance and increases cardiac output.
- Autonomic nervous system influences are more prominent on blood pressure.

Marked hemodynamic changes in pregnancy can have a profound effect on the pregnant woman with cardiac disease and may result in exceeding the functional capacity of the diseased heart (Arafeh, 2021; Cunningham et al., 2018; Yancy, 2016), resulting in:

- Pulmonary hypertension
- Pulmonary edema
- Congestive heart failure
- Maternal or fetal death

Extensive discussion of specific cardiac disorders and their management is beyond the scope of this text. Reference to texts that deal with management of high-risk pregnancy, particularly during labor and delivery, is indicated when caring for women with underlying heart disease, but general principles are presented. The management of cardiac disease is related to the cardiac disorder present and the impact it has on cardiac function responsible for specific symptoms.

Risk Factors for Maternal Mortality

- Race/Ethnicity: Non-Hispanic Black women have a 3.4 times higher risk of dying from cardiovascular disease-related pregnancy complications compared with non-Hispanic White women. This disparity can be explained in part by exposure to structural, institutional, and systemic barriers that contribute to a higher rate of comorbidities.
- Age: Age older than 40 years increases the risk of heart disease-related maternal death to 30 times the risk for women younger than 20.
- Hypertension: Hypertensive disorders affect up to 10% of pregnancies and can lead to maternal morbidity and mortality. Severe and early-onset hypertension during pregnancy put women at an increased risk of cardiac compromise during or following delivery. In pregnancies complicated by hypertension, the incidence of myocardial infarction and heart failure

is 13-fold and 8-fold higher, respectively, than in healthy pregnancies.

● Obesity: Prepregnancy obesity increases maternal death risk due to a cardiac cause, especially if associated with moderate-to-severe obstructive sleep apnea.

The presence of one or more of these risk factors should raise the threshold for suspicion that a patient is at risk for maternal heart disease and pregnancy-related morbidity and mortality (ACOG, 2019f).

Risks for the Woman

● Maternal mortality with cardiac disorders ranges from 1% to 50% based on cardiac disorder.
● Maternal effects include severe pulmonary edema, systemic emboli, and congestive heart failure.

Risks in Labor and Birth

● Physiologic effects of labor, birth, and postpartum can post threats to women with cardiac disorders.
● Maternal cardiac output increases 50% in labor and birth, and oxygen consumption increases threefold (Krening et al., 2019).
● Generally vaginal birth is preferred due to the decreased surgical morbidity and decrease in blood loss associated with vaginal birth (Krening et al., 2019).

Risks for the Fetus and Newborn

● Fetal effects are a result of decreased systemic circulation or decreased oxygenation; the most common complications are prematurity and small for gestational age.
● If maternal circulation is compromised due to decreased cardiac function, uterine blood flow is reduced, which can result in IUGR. Fetal oxygenation is impaired when maternal oxygenation is impaired.
● Fetal hypoxia can result in permanent CNS damage depending on the length and severity of decreased oxygenation.
● If the woman has congenital heart disease, there is an increased incidence of fetal congenital cardiac anomalies (Yancy, 2016).
● Neonatal death secondary to maternal cardiac disease ranges from 3% to 50%.

Assessment Findings

● Diagnosis of cardiac disease is based on symptoms and diagnostic tests, which may include ECG, echocardiogram, and laboratory tests.
● The usual signs of deteriorating cardiac function include (Arafeh, 2021):
  ● Decreased ability to perform activities of daily living (ADLs)
  ● Breathlessness
  ● Dyspnea severe enough to limit usual activity
  ● Progressive orthopnea
  ● Paroxysmal nocturnal dyspnea
  ● Syncope during or after exertion
  ● Palpitations
  ● Chest pain with or without activity
  ● Sustained arrhythmias
  ● Loud harsh systolic murmurs
  ● Ventricular murmurs
  ● Pulmonary edema
  ● Fatigue
  ● Cyanosis
  ● Jugular venous distention less than 2 cm
  ● Thromboembolic changes
  ● Fluid retention

Medical Management

Medical management varies based on cardiac disease and should include collaboration between obstetricians, maternal fetal medicine specialists, cardiologists, anesthesiologists, and other specialists as needed. Discuss with the woman estimations of maternal and fetal mortality, potential chronic morbidity, and interventions to minimize risk during pregnancy and delivery.

● Obtain a laboratory test to evaluate renal function and profusion (electrolytes, serum creatinine, proteins, and uric acid).
● Invasive hemodynamic monitoring using pulmonary artery catheters, peripheral arterial catheters, or central venous pressure monitors may be necessary.
● Drug therapy is dependent on cardiac lesion.
● Vaginal delivery is recommended for most patients with cardiac disease.
● Preterm delivery may be indicated for deteriorating maternal or fetal status.

Nursing Actions

Risk to a woman's heart and cardiovascular system engendered by pregnancy depends upon the specific type of heart disease and clinical status of the patient. Women with known cardiovascular disease should be evaluated by a cardiologist ideally before pregnancy or as early as possible during the pregnancy for accurate diagnosis and assessment of the effect pregnancy will have on the underlying cardiovascular disease. The cardiologist will also assess the potential risks to the woman and fetus to optimize the underlying cardiac condition. A detailed history, including family history and any current cardiovascular symptoms, physical examination, and review of medical records, including prior cardiovascular testing and interventions, should be obtained (ACOG, 2019f).

● Nursing measures are directed toward prevention of complications and early identification of deteriorating cardiac status.
● Review the woman's history related to cardiovascular disorder, including previous therapies or surgery, current medications, and current functional classification of cardiac disease.
● Women with complex congenital or noncongenital heart disease should be treated by a pregnancy heart team.
● Conduct a cardiovascular assessment that includes:
  ● Auscultation of heart, lungs, and breath sounds
  ● Loss of consciousness (LOC), BP, HR, capillary refill check
  ● Evaluation of RR and rhythm
  ● Evaluation of cardiac rate and rhythm

- Body weight and weight gain
- Assessment of skin color, temperature, and turgor
- Identification of pathological edema
- Additional noninvasive assessment may include:
  - O_2 saturation via pulse oximeter
  - Arrhythmia assessment with 12-lead EKG
  - Electrocardiogram (ECG)
  - Urinary output
  - EFM
  - Review laboratory results related to renal function and perfusion.
    - Electrolytes, blood urea nitrogen (BUN), serum creatinine, proteins, uric acid
- Fetal assessment is a sensitive indicator of adequate maternal cardiac function and is a means for assessing uteroplacental perfusion (Arafeh, 2021).
- Determine patient's and family's understanding of the effect of cardiac disease on her pregnancy.
- Facilitate interdisciplinary discussion with the woman and her family, which should include the possibilities that (1) pregnancy can contribute to a decline in cardiac status that may not return to baseline after the pregnancy; (2) maternal morbidity or mortality is possible; and (3) fetal risk of congenital heart or genetic conditions, fetal growth restriction, PTB, intrauterine fetal demise, and perinatal mortality is higher (ACOG, 2019f).
- Provide information to the woman and her family regarding the status of the woman and fetus and plan of care.
  - Antepartal testing including NSTs, BPPs, and ultrasounds
  - New medications may include anticoagulation therapy; therefore, women need to learn to give self-injections.
- Provide emotional support to the woman and her family.
- Refer the patient to high-risk pregnancy support groups.
- Monitor for signs and symptoms of thromboembolism and infection.
- Review diet and activity guidelines.
- Discuss the importance of regular medical follow-up with a multidisciplinary team.
- Facilitate home health and other referrals PRN.

Pulmonary Disorders

Normal physiological changes of pregnancy can cause a woman with a history of compromised respiratory function to decompensate. As a result of cardiorespiratory changes of pregnancy, the pregnant woman has very limited cardiopulmonary reserve. It is therefore relatively easy for her to demonstrate pulmonary decompensation in the presence of any respiratory compromise. Although the etiologies of various pulmonary disorders differ, the clinical signs and symptoms of pulmonary compromise are similar. Thus, it is extremely important for the care provider to understand the basic physiology as well as predisposing factors and etiologies of these complications to facilitate accurate, timely diagnosis and treatment (Mason & Burke, 2019).

Pulmonary disease has become more prevalent in women of childbearing age. Pulmonary diseases, such as pneumonia

or tocolytic-induced pulmonary edema, can develop during pregnancy while other conditions such as asthma preexist. It is important to remember that normal respiratory changes during pregnancy can exacerbate respiratory disease. Alteration in the immune system and mechanical and anatomical changes have a cumulative effect to decrease tolerance to hypoxia and acute changes in pulmonary function (Mason & Burke, 2019; McMurtry Baird & Kennedy, 2014). These include the following:

- Increased progesterone during pregnancy results in maternal hyperventilation and increased tidal volume.
- Changes in configuration of the thorax with advancing pregnancy decrease residual capacity and volume while oxygen consumption increases.
- Increased estrogen levels result in mucosal edema, hypersecretion, and capillary congestion.
- Respiratory physiology in normal pregnancy tends toward respiratory alkalosis.
- Respiratory emergencies, such as pulmonary embolism (PE) and amniotic fluid embolism (anaphylactoid syndrome), are discussed in other sections of the chapter. Asthma is presented as an exemplar of the impact of pregnancy on a preexisting pulmonary disorder.

Asthma

Asthma, the most common form of lung disease that can impact pregnancy, complicates about 8% of pregnancies. Asthma is a chronic syndrome characterized by varying levels of airway obstruction, bronchial hyperresponsiveness, and bronchial edema. Severe and poorly controlled asthma may be associated with increased prematurity, need for cesarean delivery, preeclampsia, growth restriction, and maternal morbidity and mortality (AAP & ACOG, 2017).

Diagnosis and management goals of asthma during pregnancy are the same as for nonpregnant women. People with asthma have airways that are hyperresponsive to allergens, viruses, air pollutants, exercise, and cold air. This hyperresponsiveness is manifested by bronchospasm, mucosal edema, and mucus plugging the airways. Goals of therapy include (Yancy, 2016):

- Optimal control of asthma and maintaining adequate oxygenation of the fetus by preventing hypoxic episodes in the mother
- Maintaining normal pulmonary function
- Managing exacerbations aggressively
- Frequently assessing medication needs and response
- Identifying, avoiding, and controlling asthma triggers to protect the pulmonary system from irritants and allergen exposure
- Relief of bronchospasm
- Resolution of airway inflammation to reduce airway hyperresponsiveness
- Improvement of pulmonary function

Risks for the Woman

- Pregnancy has varying effects on asthma, with about one-third of pregnant women becoming worse, one-third improving, and one-third remaining the same (Yancy, 2016). If symptoms worsen, they tend to do so between 17 to 24 weeks' gestation.

- With aggressive management of asthma, pregnancy outcomes can be the same as for nonasthmatic pregnant women.
- Uncontrolled asthma increases the risk of preeclampsia, hypertension, and hyperemesis gravidarum.

Risks for the Fetus and Newborn

- Hypoxia to the fetus is a major complication.
- PTB
- Low birth weight
- Fetal growth restriction

Assessment Findings

- Signs and symptoms of asthma:
  - Cough (productive or nonproductive)
  - Wheezing
  - Tightness in chest
  - Shortness of breath
  - Increased RR (more than 20 breaths/min)
- Signs and symptoms of hypoxia:
  - Cyanosis
  - Lethargy
  - Agitation or confusion
  - Intercostal retractions
  - RR greater than 30 breaths/min

Medical Management

Asthma should be aggressively treated during pregnancy, as the benefits of asthma control far outweigh the risks of medication use. During pregnancy, monthly evaluation of pulmonary function and asthma history are conducted. Serial ultrasound for fetal growth and antepartal fetal testing is done for moderately or severely asthmatic women.

Medications commonly used for asthma management are considered safe during pregnancy and include bronchodilators, anti-inflammatory agents such as inhaled steroids, oral corticosteroids, allergy injections, and antihistamines. Corticosteroids should be given early to all patients with severe acute asthma (Cunningham et al., 2018).

Nursing Actions

- Take a detailed history and assessment of respiratory status, including pulmonary function tests (PFTs) and blood gases (ABGs). Pulmonary function testing should be routine in the management of chronic and acute asthma (Cunningham et al., 2018).
- Assess for signs including cough, wheezing, chest tightness, and sputum production.
- Care for women with acute asthma exacerbations includes:
  - Oxygen administration to maintain PaO_2 greater than 95%
  - Ongoing maternal pulse oximeter
  - Baseline arterial blood gases as per orders
  - Baseline PFTs performed to gather baseline data as per orders
  - Beta-agonist inhalation therapy as ordered

- Monitor maternal oxygen saturation (should be at 95% to oxygenate the fetus).
- Assess fetal well-being and for signs of fetal hypoxia.
- Evaluate PFT results and laboratory tests (i.e., arterial blood gases).
- Explain the plan of care and goals.
- Teach the woman to avoid allergens and triggers.
- Teach the woman to monitor pulmonary function daily and her normal parameters.
- Teach the woman the role of medications, correct use, and adverse effects.
- Teach the woman to recognize signs and symptoms of worsening asthma and provide a treatment plan to manage exacerbations appropriately.
- Discuss warning signs and symptoms to report to the provider, such as dyspnea, shortness of breath, chest tightness, or exacerbations of signs and symptoms beyond the woman's baseline asthma status (Yancy, 2016).

Pneumonia

Out of nonobstetric infections in the peripartum period, pneumonia is the leading cause of maternal mortality (Roth, 2021b), Pneumonia can be caused by bacteria, viruses, and aspiration of organisms. When the lower airways are infected with pathogens, the lung capillaries become more permeable and allow fluid accumulation in the alveoli. This excess fluid shows up on a chest x-ray, which can be a diagnostic feature of pneumonia (Roth, 2021b).

Risks for the Woman

- PTL
- Bacteremia or sepsis
- Pneumothorax
- Atrial fibrillation
- Pericardial tamponade
- Respiratory failure

Risks for the Fetus and Newborn

- Hypoxia to the fetus
- PTB
- Small for gestational age (SGA) or LBW infant
- Fetal death

Assessment Findings

- Vital sign abnormalities:
  - Temperature 95°F (35°C) or lower or 102.2°F (39°C) or higher
  - Respirations 30 breaths or more per minute
  - Hypotension
  - Heart rate 120 beats or more per minute
- Laboratory data abnormalities including WBC lower than 4,000 mm^3
- Anorexia
- Dry cough
- Dyspnea for several weeks

Medical Management

- Close monitoring of woman and fetus
- Antibiotics
- Oxygen supplementation (2 to 4 L/min via nasal cannula) as needed
- Antipyretics
- Adequate hydration
- Pain control
- Chest x-ray

Nursing Actions

- Obtain detailed history of symptoms.
- Perform a physical assessment including lung auscultation, PFTs, and vital signs with a continuous pulse oximeter (maternal oxygenation should be 95% or greater).
- Obtain laboratory data including WBCs, serum lactate, sputum sample, blood gases (ABGs), and blood cultures.
- Perform ongoing fetal monitoring and assessment.
- Prevent pneumonia through administration of influenza and pneumococcal vaccines.
- Assess for signs of hypoxia (irritability, restlessness, tachycardia, hypertension, cool and pale extremities, and decreased urine output).
- Position the woman in semi-Fowler's or high-Fowler's to maximize oxygenation and comfort.
- Teach the woman the role of medications, correct use, and possible side effects.

(Roth, 2021b).

Pulmonary Edema

Pulmonary edema is the accumulation of fluid in the interstitial spaces, alveoli, or lung cells that inhibits adequate diffusion of oxygen and carbon dioxide. Pulmonary edema can be divided into hydrostatic (cardiogenic) and vascular permeability (non-cardiogenic, nonhydrostatic).

Assessment Findings

- Dyspnea
- Shortness of breath
- Tachypnea
- Anxiety or agitation
- Tachycardia
- Fine or coarse crackles and wheezing; may be present with lung auscultation
- Nonproductive cough that progresses to pink, frothy sputum
- Increased work of breathing resulting in nasal flaring and retractions
- Downward trends in SpO_2

Medical Management

The woman's history is important to review when determining a diagnosis for pulmonary edema, as preexisting and pregnancy-related disease can be contributing factors. Preeclampsia, medications, fluid balance, and exposure to chemicals or anesthetics can all contribute to pulmonary edema and are therefore important to consider. Diagnostic tests to confirm pulmonary edema commonly include a chest x-ray, blood gases, trends of pulse oximetry, an ECG, and an echocardiogram. Treatment for pulmonary edema can vary dependent on the pathophysiology; however, the main goal is to maximize oxygenation to the mother and the fetus. In severe cases of pulmonary edema, the woman may require an arterial line and transfer to an intensive-care unit for closer monitoring. To optimize volume and cardiac output, antihypertensives may be ordered. Morphine sulfate can be given in small increments to assist with pain and to decrease oxygen consumption (Roth, 2021b).

Nursing Actions

- Obtain strict intake and output.
- Assess for worsening signs and symptoms of hypoxia or respiratory distress.
- Assess fetal well-being for signs of hypoxia.
- Measure serum potassium levels regularly if diuretics are administered.
- Position the woman to improve comfort and ease of breathing (high-Fowler's or on left or right side as tolerated to promote venous return).
- Monitor oxygenation levels with pulse oximeter.
- Explain to the woman the treatment plan and medications.

NEUROLOGICAL DISORDERS

Seizures

Seizure disorders include a wide range of clinical conditions associated with seizures, including epilepsy, brain infections and tumors, and traumatic brain injury. Epilepsy is a neurological syndrome characterized by recurrent convulsive seizures that usually start during childhood or adolescence (ACOG, 2020c). Epilepsy is a common disease that affects 1.5 million women of childbearing age in the United States. Approximately 24,000 women with epilepsy give birth each year (Sazgar, 2019). The following general guidelines are published by ACOG and emphasize the continuing evaluation during pregnancy of women with a history of seizure and a pregestational diagnosis of a seizure disorder (Hessler & Dolbeck, 2021).

- Measuring a baseline antiepileptic drug level before pregnancy and then monthly for the rest of pregnancy is important, particularly for lamotrigine, carbamazepine, and phenytoin due to metabolic changes during pregnancy.
- Seizure freedom for 9 months to 1 year before pregnancy is associated with a high likelihood (84% to 92%) of remaining seizure free during pregnancy.
- Risk of seizures during pregnancy includes maternal injuries and maternal sudden unexpected death in epilepsy. Potential fetal risks include hypoxia, acidosis, decreased placental blood flow, deceleration in FHR, and maternal trauma.
- The risk of poor pregnancy outcomes is primarily due to the teratogenicity of some antiepileptic drugs. Fetal antiepileptic

drug exposure is associated with a twofold to threefold increased risk of major congenital malformations, with even higher rates reported with valproate or polytherapy use (ACOG, 2021c).

- Use of valproate, phenobarbital, and topiramate during pregnancy is associated with the highest risk of major congenital malformations.
- Be sure the woman has notified her neurologist that she is pregnant.

GASTROINTESTINAL DISORDERS

A pregnant woman who presents with gastrointestinal disorders needs a workup as with any nonpregnant individual.

Cholelithiasis

Cholelithiasis is the presence of gallstones in the gallbladder. Symptomatic gallstone disease during pregnancy is common. Acute cholecystitis is the second most common nonobstetric indication for surgery during pregnancy, occurring in about 1 per 1,600 pregnancies (Cunningham et al., 2018). During pregnancy, elevated estrogen increases cholesterol secretion, whereas progesterone reduces bile acid secretion and delays gallbladder emptying, leading to the supersaturation of bile with cholesterol and predisposition to gallstone formation. Decreased muscle tone allows gallbladder distention and thickening of the bile and prolongs emptying time during pregnancy, increasing the risk of cholelithiasis. Additionally, cholesterol and biliary sludge are thought to be major factors in stone formation, and biliary sludge may increase during pregnancy (Cunningham et al., 2018; Schwulst & Son, 2020). Symptomatic cholecystitis was previously managed conservatively, but more recent data suggests high rates of recurrent symptoms (40% to 90%), increased rates of hospitalizations, PTL, and deliveries, as well as spontaneous abortions when intervention is deferred. Early surgical intervention with laparoscopic cholecystectomy after endoscopic retrograde cholangiopancreatography (ERCP) is now preferred.

Assessment Findings

- Colicky abdominal pain presents in the right upper quadrant; anorexia, nausea, and vomiting; fever.
- Gallstones are present on an ultrasound scan.

Medical Management

Cholelithiasis was typically treated with conservative management such as IV fluids, bowel rest, nasogastric suctioning, diet, and antibiotics. Increasingly, it is managed by surgical intervention with laparoscopic cholecystectomies (ACOG, 2019e; Cunningham et al., 2018). Current guidelines for nonobstetric surgeries note that pregnancy is not a reason to deny a medically necessary surgery; however, if gallbladder disease is nonacute,

surgical intervention may be delayed until postpartum. Due to the potential for preterm delivery with some nonobstetric procedures during pregnancy, corticosteroid administration for fetal benefit should be considered for viable premature gestations.

Nursing Actions

- Manage pain, administering pain medication as needed.
- Manage nausea and vomiting, minimizing environmental factors that cause nausea and vomiting such as odors.
- Administer antiemetics as needed.
- Provide comfort measures based on symptoms.
- Explain procedures and plan of care including dietary restrictions.
- Note that EFM is based on viability.
- Monitor surgical patients for signs or symptoms of PTL based on gestational age.

VENOUS THROMBOEMBOLIC DISEASE

Women who are pregnant or in the postpartum period have a fourfold to fivefold increased risk of thromboembolism compared with nonpregnant women (ACOG, 2018j). Approximately 80% of thromboembolic events in pregnancy are venous, with a prevalence of 0.5 to 2.0 per 1,000 pregnant women. VTE is one of the leading causes of maternal mortality in the United States, accounting for 9.3% of all maternal deaths (Creanga et al., 2017).

Deep vein thrombosis (DVT) and PE are collectively referred to as VTE. Approximately 75% to 80% of cases of pregnancy-associated VTE are caused by DVT, and 20% to 25% of cases are caused by PE (ACOG, 2018j). Although approximately one-half of these events occur during pregnancy and one-half occur during the postpartum period, the risk per day is greatest in the weeks immediately after delivery. VTE is a blood clot that starts in a vein. It is the third leading vascular diagnosis after heart attack and stroke, affecting about 300,000 to 600,000 Americans each year. There are two types of VTE: DVT is a clot in a deep vein, usually in the leg, but sometimes in the arm or other veins. PE occurs when a DVT clot breaks free from a vein wall, travels to the lungs, and blocks some or all of the blood supply. Blood clots in the thigh are more likely to break off and travel to the lungs than blood clots in the lower leg or other parts of the body.

Thromboembolism is a blood clot that can potentially block blood flow and damage the organs, a leading cause of maternal morbidity and mortality in the United States. The risk of venous thrombosis and PE in otherwise healthy women is considered highest during pregnancy and postpartum (Cunningham et al., 2018). Pregnancy is a hypercoagulable state with increased fibrin generation and coagulation factors and decreased fibrinolytic activity. Venous stasis in the lower extremities, increased blood volume, and compression of the inferior vena cava and pelvic veins with advancing gestation combine to increase risk fivefold over risk for nonpregnant women.

Physiological and anatomic changes during pregnancy increase the risk for thromboembolism. Hypercoagulability, increased venous stasis, decreased venous outflow, uterine compression of the inferior vena cava and pelvic veins, reduced mobility, and changes in levels of coagulation factors normally regulating hemostasis all result in an increased thrombogenic state. Risk for DVT during pregnancy is greatest in the left lower extremity. About half of the cases of VTE during pregnancy are associated with a common risk factor for thrombophilia. Acquired or inherited thrombophilia are associated with severe preeclampsia, abruption, IUGR, intrauterine fetal demise (IUFD), PTB, and recurrent miscarriage.

Thrombophilia can be an inheritable hypercoagulable condition caused by mutations in clotting mechanisms. The most common acquired thrombophilia during pregnancy is antiphospholipid antibody syndrome (APLA). These antibodies are a result of antigenic changes in endothelial and platelet membranes, which promote thrombosis. Besides a personal history of thrombosis, or the presence of a thrombophilia, or both, the primary risk factors for the development of pregnancy-associated VTE are the physiological changes that accompany pregnancy and childbirth. Cesarean delivery, particularly when complicated by postpartum hemorrhage or infection, as well as medical factors or pregnancy complications such as obesity, hypertension, autoimmune disease, heart disease, sickle cell disease, multiple gestation, and preeclampsia also increase the risk of VTE (ACOG, 2018j). Medical conditions such as diabetes, heart disease, hypertension, renal disease, sickle cell disease, smoking, or serious infections increase the risk of complications in pregnancy (AAP & ACOG, 2017).

Assessment Findings

- The two most common initial symptoms of DVT, present in more than 80% of women with pregnancy-associated DVT, are pain and swelling in an extremity. Difference in calf circumference of 2 cm or more is particularly suggestive of DVT in a lower extremity (ACOG, 2018j).
- Classic signs of DVT are dependent edema, abrupt unilateral leg pain, erythema, low-grade fever, and positive Homan's sign (i.e., pain with dorsiflexion of foot).
- A PE may present with shortness of breath, tachypnea, tachycardia, dyspnea, pleural chest pain, fever, and anxiety.

Medical Management

Objective tests for DVT include Doppler ultrasound, magnetic resonance venography, and pulsed Doppler study. Chest x-ray, CT, and electrocardiography are used to diagnose PE. ACOG (2018j) recommends preventive treatment with anticoagulant medication for women who have a history of acute VTE during pregnancy, a history of thrombosis, or significant risk for VTE during pregnancy and postpartum, such as women with high-risk acquired or inherited thrombophilias. Women with a history of thrombosis should be evaluated for underlying causes to determine if anticoagulation

medication is appropriate during pregnancy. Most women who take anticoagulation medications before pregnancy must continue during pregnancy and postpartum. Common anticoagulation medications include low-molecular-weight heparin (LMWH), unfractionated heparin, and warfarin. In general, preferred anticoagulants in pregnancy are heparin compounds.

Treatment goals include prevention of further clot propagation, prevention of PE, and prevention of further venous thromboembolism.

- Anticoagulation therapy is required for women experiencing a DVT during pregnancy with heparin compounds titrated to achieve an activated partial thromboplastin time (aPTT) of 1.5 to 2.5 times control values. Intravenous anticoagulation should be maintained for at least 5 to 7 days, after which treatment is converted to subcutaneous heparin (Cunningham et al., 2018).
- Early reviews concluded that LMWH is safe and effective for use throughout pregnancy. The ACOG (2018j) concluded that risks associated with LMWH use were rare and that no cause-and-effect relationship has been established between LMWH and congenital anomalies or maternal hemorrhage (Cunningham et al., 2018).
- Treatment of PE is to stabilize a woman with a life-threatening PE and transfer her to the ICU. Thromboembolic therapy and catheter or surgical embolectomy may be done.

Nursing Actions

- Begin ambulation after symptoms dissipate (Cunningham et al., 2018).
- Administer elastic stockings.
- Manage pain, administering pain medication as needed.
- Teach the woman how to administer heparin SQ to her abdomen.
- Instruct the woman to report side effects such as bleeding gums, nosebleeds, easy bruising, or excessive trauma at injection sites.

Evidence-Based Practice: Venous Thromboembolism Bundle

D'Alton, M., Friedman, A., Smiley, R., Montgomery, D., Paidas, M., D'Oria, . . . Clark, S. (2016). National Partnership for Maternal Safety: Consensus bundle on venous thromboembolism. *Journal of Obstetric, Gynecologic & Neonatal Nursing, 45*(5), 706–717.

Obstetric VTE is a leading cause of severe maternal morbidity and mortality. Maternal death from thromboembolism is amenable to prevention, and thromboprophylaxis is the most readily implementable means of systematically reducing the maternal death rate. Observational data support the benefit of risk-factor-based prophylaxis in reducing obstetric thromboembolism. This bundle, developed by a multidisciplinary working group and published by the National Partnership for Maternal Safety under the

Continued

guidance of the Council on Patient Safety in Women's Health Care, supports routine thromboembolism risk assessment for obstetric patients, with appropriate use of pharmacological and mechanical thromboprophylaxis. Safety bundles outline critical clinical practices that should be implemented in every maternity unit. The bundle is divided into four domains: The *Readiness* domain supports establishment of risk-assessment strategies throughout pregnancy. Risk assessment should occur at four time points in pregnancy: (1) during the first prenatal visit, (2) during all antepartum admissions, (3) immediately postpartum during a hospitalization for childbirth, and (4) on discharge home after a birth. The *Recognition* domain reviews clinical recommendations from major existing guidelines for patients recognized to be at increased risk for thromboembolism. The *Response* domain outlines specific recommendations for prophylaxis for at-risk patients from the NPMS working group, and the *Reporting and Systems Learning* domain includes recommendations for quality assurance and surveillance.

MATERNAL OBESITY

Maternal obesity, defined as a BMI of 30 or greater, has long been recognized as a risk factor in pregnancy. Severe obesity is a BMI greater than 40. The prevalence of obesity was 42.4% in 2017–2018; the prevalence of obesity increased from 30.5% to 42.4%, and the prevalence of severe obesity increased from 4.7% to 9.2% (Hales et al., 2020). The overall prevalence of obesity was similar among men and women, but the prevalence of severe obesity was higher among women. Additionally, the prevalence of obesity was highest among non-Hispanic Black adults compared with other races and Hispanic-origin groups, overall and among women. Non-Hispanic Asian adults had the lowest (Hales et al., 2020).

Obesity is associated with higher rates of diabetes, hypertension, high cholesterol, stroke, heart disease, certain types of cancer, and surgical complications such as wound infections and VTE (ACOG, 2019c; ACOG 2021b). Approximately one-third of all women of childbearing age are overweight or obese. Obesity in pregnancy is associated with an increased risk of early pregnancy loss, prematurity, stillbirth, fetal anomalies, fetal macrosomia and LBW, gestational diabetes, hypertension, preeclampsia, and cesarean delivery (ACOG, 2019c; ACOG, 2021b; Opray et al., 2015). Obesity during pregnancy increases the risk of morbidity and mortality for both the mother and baby and is a well-established risk factor for the development of comorbid conditions such as preeclampsia, gestational and type 2 diabetes, and thrombosis (ACOG, 2015b). Many of the systemic physiological alterations that occur during pregnancy may be altered when the pregnant woman is obese. For example:

- The typical increase in cardiac output associated with pregnancy is compounded when a woman is obese and is influenced by the degree and duration of obesity. Cardiac output increases by 30 to 50 mL/min for every 100 g of fat deposited. Blood volume is increased as well. A degree of cardiac hypertrophy is normal during pregnancy, but obesity exaggerates the hypertrophy and contributes to myocardial dilation.

- Although obese women can experience more frequent episodes of obstructive sleep apnea (OSA) than women with normal BMI, pregnancy may exert a protective effect on OSA occurrence.

- Pregnant women are more prone to gastric reflux, given associated hormonal and anatomic changes. The incidence of hiatus hernia is greater in obese patients, and abdominal pressure and intragastric volume are increased.

- Pregnancy is a hypercoagulable state, and obesity further increases the risk of thrombosis by promoting venous stasis, increasing blood viscosity, and promoting activation of the coagulation cascade.

- A large panniculus, a thick layer of adipose tissue in the abdominal area sometimes called a fatty apron, may contribute to uterine compression and exaggerate vena cava syndrome that may affect pregnant women.

Risks for the Woman

- Preeclampsia
- Deep vein thrombosis
- Urinary tract infections
- Gestational diabetes
- PTB
- Cesarean delivery
- Operative and postoperative complications
  - Prolonged operating times
  - Excessive blood loss
  - Wound infection and wound dehiscence
  - Thromboembolism
  - Endometritis

Risks for the Fetus and Newborn

- Congenital anomalies, including neural tube defects, cardiovascular anomalies, diaphragmatic hernia, cleft lip and palate, anorectal atresia, hydrocephaly, and limb reduction
- IUGR
- Prematurity related to medically indicated PTB due to maternal complications and comorbidities and conditions associated with prematurity
- Neonatal macrosomia
- Fetal death
- Low Apgar scores
- Birth trauma
- Neonatal acidemia
- Neonatal intensive care unit admission
- Neonatal respiratory complications
- Childhood, adolescent, and adult obesity

Assessment Findings

- BMI of 30 kg/m^2 or higher. BMI calculated at the first prenatal visit should be used to provide diet and exercise counseling guided by IOM recommendations for gestational weight gain during pregnancy (AAP & ACOG, 2017; ACOG, 2015b).

Medical Management

- Provide specific information on maternal risks of obesity in pregnancy.
- Early pregnancy screening for glucose intolerance (gestational diabetes or overt diabetes) should be based on risk factors, including maternal BMI of 30 or greater, known impaired glucose metabolism, or previous gestational diabetes (ACOG, 2015b).
- Provide specific information on the increased risk for an infant with a neural tube defect and for a stillborn infant.
- These risks require heightened and ongoing evaluation of the pregnant woman and fetus.
- Given the limited data on pregnancy weight gain by obesity class, the IOM recommendation for weight gain is 5.0 to 9.1 kg (11 to 20 lb.) for all obese women (ACOG, 2015b).
- The woman contemplating pregnancy after bariatric surgery has special nutritional needs and should be evaluated to offer appropriate supplementation.

Nursing Actions

- Measure and record the height and weight of the woman and calculate BMI.
- Generally, women can be expected to gain 3 to 6 lb. during the first trimester and 0.5 to 1 lb. each week thereafter until birth; however, for women with obesity, it is important to try to avoid gaining more than the recommended weight. Proper maternal nutrition can have a positive influence on improving the woman's overall health and birth of a healthy baby of an appropriate weight (AAP & ACOG, 2017).
- Reinforce information on maternal and fetal risks associated with obesity.
- Provide teaching on signs and symptoms of preeclampsia, diabetes, sleep apnea, and vena cava syndrome.
- Ensure the woman understands the plan of care for increased and ongoing evaluation of pregnancy.
- Because pregnancy presents an ideal time during which to initiate simple healthy behaviors, such as walking and proper diet, that can be maintained after birth, offer suggestions and encouragement for lifestyle changes.
- Appropriately defining obesity as a medical condition helps focus the approach to obesity on helping patients address the disease and its implications for health.
- Obese women who have even small weight reductions before pregnancy may have improved pregnancy outcomes. Interpregnancy weight loss in obese women may decrease the risk of a large-for-gestational-age neonate in a subsequent pregnancy (ACOG, 2015b).
- Provide referrals to a dietitian for nutritional counseling and reinforce guidelines for diet and weight gain. Recommended weight gain in obese women is 11 to 20 pounds (Cunningham et al., 2018).
- Use caution when shifting the panniculus to assess for fetal heart sounds or when providing personal hygiene, as the redistributed weight may alter maternal hemodynamics and increase the risk of vena cava compression.

- Encouraging the woman to sleep in a sitting position may help, as effects of obesity on the respiratory system are decreased in this position.
- Make appropriate environmental changes to accommodate the larger patient, such as assuring that patient beds, examining tables, and chairs can support at least 400 pounds.
- Body weight is the result of genes, metabolism, behavior, environment, culture, and socioeconomic status. Interventions should be focused on health (Maher, 2021). In many cases, people with obesity are blamed for irresponsible overeating or inactivity, or both. Women with obesity also face barriers to optimal care that arise from obesity bias in our society and in our medical institutions. Such negative attitudes and biases place the patient–physician relationship at risk by reducing patient satisfaction and the quality of the patient encounter, which can lead to negative patient outcomes (ACOG, 2019c). Remember that patients with obesity may have had negative experiences with other health-care professionals regarding their weight, and they should approach the topic with sensitivity, empathy, and an understanding of the emotional consequences of obesity stigma.
- Nurses, and all care providers, should be mindful of the tendency to harbor implicit bias toward patients with obesity, engage in self-reflection to identify any personal implicit bias, and take steps to address any identified bias to help ensure that it does not interfere with the delivery of respectful care for patients with obesity.
- Care of the woman with obesity during childbirth and postpartum can be challenging and will be addressed in other chapters.

THYROID DISORDERS

The production, circulation, and disposal of thyroid hormones are altered in pregnancy to support maternal metabolic changes and fetal growth and development. Increased vascularity and hyperplasia of the thyroid gland result in increased hormone production and an increase in thyroid size (Blackburn, 2021). Thyroid disorders are common in young women and thus managed frequently in pregnancy. There is an intimate relationship between maternal and fetal thyroid function, which makes identifying thyroid disorders an important aspect of antenatal assessment and care. Care of thyroid disorders during pregnancy is essential to both the mother and baby because maternal TSH-receptor-blocking antibodies can cross the placenta and cause fetal thyroid dysfunction. However, identifying thyroid disorders in pregnancy can be difficult because many symptoms can mirror those of pregnancy itself (Cunningham et al., 2018).

Inadequate management of hyperthyroidism or hypothyroidism is associated with adverse pregnancy outcomes such as miscarriage and PTB (AAP & ACOG, 2017). Screening for symptoms of hypothyroidism and hyperthyroidism during pregnancy is challenging because pregnancy is commonly associated with heat intolerance, tachycardia, wide pulse pressure, and vomiting (all signs seen with hyperthyroidism). Fatigue, constipation, weight gain, and muscle cramps are also seen with hypothyroidism). Poor control during pregnancy can result in PTL, fetal loss, or thyroid crisis in these women. Diagnosis of abnormal thyroid function in the pregnant woman requires an understanding of the normal changes in thyroid function during pregnancy in order to appropriately interpret results of laboratory tests.

Hyperthyroidism

Hyperthyroidism or symptomatic thyrotoxicosis is caused by hyperfunctioning of the thyroid gland, resulting in excessive amounts of thyroid hormone. Graves' disease is responsible for 90% to 95% of hyperthyroidism cases in pregnant women (ACOG, 2020g; Van Otterloo, 2016).

Distinctive features of Graves' disease are ophthalmopathy (signs include lid lag and lid retraction) and dermopathy (signs include localized or pretibial myxedema) (ACOG, 2020g). Compared with controlled maternal hyperthyroidism, inadequately treated maternal hyperthyroidism is associated with a greater risk of preterm delivery, severe preeclampsia, and heart failure with an increase in medically indicated preterm deliveries, LBW infants, and possible fetal loss (ACOG, 2020g).

Assessment Findings

- Screening for symptoms of hyperthyroidism during pregnancy is challenging because the heat intolerance, tachycardia, wide pulse pressure, and vomiting common in pregnancy are also signs of hyperthyroidism.
- Overt hyperthyroidism is characterized by decreased TSH level and increased free T4 level.

Medical Management

- Pregnant women with overt hyperthyroidism should be treated with antithyroid drugs (thioamides). Either propylthiouracil or methimazole, both thioamides, can be used to treat pregnant women with overt hyperthyroidism. The choice of medication is dependent on the trimester of pregnancy, response to prior therapy, and whether the thyrotoxicosis is predominantly T4 or T3. Women should be counseled about the risks and benefits of the two thioamides described in the text that follows, using shared decision making to develop an appropriate treatment plan (ACOG, 2020g).
- Medication must be used cautiously, as many antithyroid drugs can cause birth defects and fetal thyroid problems (Van Otterloo, 2016).
- Use of iodine 131 for treatment of Graves' disease after the first trimester can destroy the fetal thyroid gland, so it is contraindicated during pregnancy (AAP & ACOG, 2017).
- Monitor fetal growth and development through ultrasound testing and fundal height measurement.
- Assess thyroid hormone levels (TSH and thyroxine) periodically throughout pregnancy and adjust medication dosage accordingly.

- Monitor hepatic enzymes.
- Monitor WBC for leukopenia.

Nursing Actions

- Provide teaching on signs and symptoms of hyperthyroidism and the treatment plan, including daily medication and side effects.
- Educate the woman and family on the plan of care for increased and ongoing evaluation of pregnancy, including frequent monitoring of thyroid levels to ensure that the lowest possible amount of antithyroid medication is administered for control of the patient's symptoms while minimizing fetal exposure to antithyroid medications (Van Otterloo, 2016).
- Provide nutritional counseling to meet additional calorie requirements.
- Discuss information regarding fetal status and potential maternal and fetal complications associated with hyperthyroidism in pregnancy.

Hypothyroidism

Hypothyroidism is caused by inadequate thyroid hormone production and is associated with elevated TSH levels and decreased FT4 levels. Maternal thyroid hormone is critical for fetal CNS development, especially in early pregnancy, when the CNS undergoes critical development until the fetus is able to produce T4. Adverse perinatal outcomes such as spontaneous abortion, preeclampsia, PTB, abruptio placentae, and stillbirth are associated with untreated overt hypothyroidism (ACOG, 2020g). Untreated maternal hypothyroidism increases the risk of altered fetal brain development and later neurocognitive impairment and neurodevelopmental problems (Blackburn, 2021).

Assessment Findings

- Screening for symptoms of hypothyroidism during pregnancy is challenging because pregnancy is commonly associated with fatigue, constipation, weight gain, and muscle cramps, which are also seen with hypothyroidism.
- Other clinical findings include edema, dry skin, hair loss, and a prolonged relaxation phase of DTRs.
- Hypothyroidism is diagnosed based on laboratory values with a TSH above the upper limit of normal and a free T4 below the lower limit of normal (ACOG, 2020f).
- Subclinical hypothyroidism is defined by an elevated serum TSH level and normal serum thyroxine.

Medical Management

- Pregnant women with overt hypothyroidism should be treated with adequate thyroid hormone replacement to minimize the risk of adverse outcomes. Recommended treatment of overt hypothyroidism in pregnancy is T4 replacement therapy, beginning with levothyroxine in dosages of 1 to 2 micrograms/kg daily or approximately 100 micrograms daily (ACOG, 2020g).

- Surveillance of TSH and thyroxine levels is measured at 4- to 6-week intervals.
- If replacement therapy is inadequate or not instituted during pregnancy, there is a high risk of fetal mortality and morbidity.

Nursing Actions

- Reinforce information on maternal and fetal risks associated with hypothyroidism.
- Provide teaching on signs and symptoms of hypothyroidism and the treatment plan, including daily medication.
- Ensure the woman and family understand the plan of care for increased and ongoing evaluation of pregnancy.

Systemic Lupus Erythematosus

Systemic lupus erythematosus (SLE) is one of the most common systemic autoimmune diseases in young women. SLE is a heterogeneous autoimmune disease characterized by immune system abnormalities, including overactive B lymphocytes. These overactive lymphocytes result in tissue and cellular damage and immunosuppression. SLE involves the skin, joints, kidneys, serous membranes, nervous system, and blood. Usually, the onset occurs during puberty or early adulthood, and SLE affects women more than men. Pregnancy in patients with SLE is considered high risk (ACOG, 2020f). Almost 90% of lupus cases are in women, and the disease is encountered relatively frequently in pregnancy (Cunningham et al., 2018). With modern management, the survival of SLE patients has greatly improved; however, SLE remains the fifth or sixth leading cause of death in Black and Hispanic women younger than 35 (ACOG, 2020f).

Pregnancy in patients with SLE is associated with increased maternal mortality and morbidity, particularly preeclampsia and GDM. SLE increases the risk of spontaneous abortion, intrauterine fetal death, preeclampsia, IUGR, and PTB. Prognosis for both mother and child is best when SLE is quiescent for at least 6 months before the pregnancy and when the mother's underlying renal function is stable and normal or near normal (Khurana, 2017). Lupus nephritis can get worse during pregnancy. In general, pregnancy does not cause flares of SLE.

Assessment Findings

- Malaise
- Fever
- Weight loss
- Arthritis
- Rash
- Pleuro-pericarditis
- Photosensitivity
- Anemia
- Cognitive dysfunction

Medical Management

- There is no cure for SLE; thus, lupus management consists primarily of monitoring maternal clinical and laboratory conditions as well as fetal well-being (Cunningham et al., 2018).
- Low-dose aspirin may be used throughout pregnancy.
- Monitor for complications of pregnancy such as spontaneous abortion, intrauterine fetal death, preeclampsia, IUGR, and PTB.
- The provider needs to balance control of disease activity against the fetal toxicity of some of the commonly used lupus medications (ACOG, 2020f).
- Corticosteroids may be used during acute flare-up.
- Methylprednisolone is also an option.

Nursing Actions

- Monitor and identify flare-ups.
- Provide teaching on the signs and symptoms of SLE and the disease process, as well as the treatment plan throughout pregnancy.
- Ensure the woman and family understand the plan of care for increased and ongoing evaluation during pregnancy.
- Reinforce a low-salt diet is recommended in pregnancy to prevent weight increase and hypertension. Calcium and vitamin D supplementation may be advised to prevent osteoporosis.
- More than 22% to 45% of patients with SLE also have fibromyalgia. Fibromyalgia also causes chronic muscle pain, which is not a manifestation of SLE. Daily stretching and aerobic exercise are recommended and should be reinforced for symptom management (ACOG, 2020f).
- Reinforce adherence to an exercise program may help prevent bone loss and depression. Strenuous activity is best avoided when women have flare-ups.

SUBSTANCE USE

Alcohol abuse and other substance use disorders are major, often underdiagnosed health problems for women, regardless of age, race, ethnicity, and socioeconomic status, and have resulting high costs for individuals and society (ACOG, 2015a). Substance use disorder is commonly defined as a pathological pattern of behaviors related to the use of any of 10 separate classes of substances, including alcohol and licit and illicit substances.

Alcohol, cigarette, and illicit drug use during pregnancy can cause poor pregnancy and birth outcomes including LBW, developmental disabilities, PTB, and infant mortality. The first 8 weeks of pregnancy are the most critical in terms of embryonic development, and substances ingested in that period can have a teratogenic effect (Sullivan, 2016). In 2018, 5.4% of women reported using illicit drugs during pregnancy. The drug most commonly used by pregnant women was marijuana (Substance Abuse and Mental Health Services Administration [SAMHSA], 2019). The findings in this report suggest that many U.S. women, particularly those in the third trimester, are getting the message and abstaining from substance use. Still, a sizable proportion of women in the first trimester of pregnancy were past-month users of alcohol,

BOX 7-5 | Substances That Are Commonly Misused or Abused

Alcohol (ethanol)

Cannabinoids (marijuana and hashish)

Club drugs (methylenedioxymethamphetamine [MDMA], flunitrazepam, and gamma-hydroxybutyrate [GHB])

Dissociative drugs (ketamine, phencyclidine [PCP] and analogs, Salvia divinorum, and dextromethorphan)

Hallucinogens (lysergic acid diethylamide [LSD], mescaline, and psilocybin)

Opioids (heroin and opium)

Other compounds (anabolic steroids and inhalants)

Prescription medications (central nervous system depressants, stimulants, and opioid pain relievers)

Stimulants (cocaine, amphetamine, and methamphetamine)

Tobacco

National Institute on Drug Abuse, 2013.

BOX 7-6 | Nursing Interventions With Substance-Using Patients

The nurse caring for a pregnant woman who abuses substances should take the following measures.

- Advocate for intervention and treatment referral for those patients with positive screening results (Box 7-8).
- Provide health education about the risks to the fetus of substance use during pregnancy and facilitate early diagnosis and appropriate intervention and referral.
- Maintain a nonjudgmental and nonpunitive attitude; remember, addiction is a disease.
- It has been proposed that government policies can be viewed as either "facilitative" or "adversarial." Facilitative policies improve women's access to prenatal care, food, shelter, and treatment. Adversarial policies propose that women who fail to seek treatment are liable to criminal prosecution and may diminish utilization of prenatal care and support services, such as housing, education and job training, financial support services, parenting education, legal services, and aftercare.
- Nurses have a responsibility to treat their patients with substance use disorder with dignity and respect and to try to establish a therapeutic alliance with these patients.
- Encourage prenatal visits and ongoing assessment for pregnancy complications and provide information on fetal growth and development.
- Provide specific suggestions to decrease smoking, alcohol intake, and substance use.
- Provide written information of resources at the appropriate educational level.
- Nurses should familiarize themselves with resources available through their local hospital and community to appropriately and effectively discuss treatment options for patients.
- Nurses should be aware of strategies for safe and effective pain management in women with long-term opioid exposure, which results in tolerance and hyperalgesia.
- Nurses should communicate the unique needs of pregnant women and position themselves as advocates for the benefit of timely and ongoing treatment that will improve perinatal and neonatal outcomes rather than focus on their criminalization.

cigarettes, or cannabis, and one in seven women used cigarettes in the second or third trimester (Box 7-5). In addition, many women resume use of these substances after childbirth, and that resumption appears to be rapid given the higher rates for mothers of infants younger than 3 months old compared with pregnant women in the second or third trimesters. Effective interventions for women to further reduce substance use during pregnancy and to prevent postpartum resumption of use could improve the overall health and well-being of mothers and infants (Box 7-6).

Polydrug abuse among pregnant women with substances such as alcohol and tobacco with marijuana or cocaine has become very common. In these cases, it can be difficult to determine which complications are associated with which substance. For example, recent research shows that smoking tobacco or marijuana, taking prescription pain relievers, or using illegal drugs during pregnancy is associated with double or even triple the risk of stillbirth. Specifically, for tobacco use there is a 1.8 to 2.8 times greater risk of stillbirth, with the highest risk found among the heaviest smokers. Marijuana use carries a 2.3 times greater risk of stillbirth; evidence of any stimulant, marijuana, or prescription pain reliever use has a 2.2 times greater risk of stillbirth; and passive exposure to tobacco carries a 2.1 times greater risk of stillbirth (SAMHSA, 2014).

Risks of specific complications vary based on the substance used; however, general risks resulting from substance abuse for both the woman and fetus or newborn are presented. Pregnant women using illicit substances often fear legal consequences and may avoid seeking prenatal care. A nonjudgmental and factual approach with attention toward reducing risks offers the best approach for these complex pregnancies. Chemically

dependent pregnant women may also engage in other risky behaviors. A holistic, comprehensive approach to care that deals not only with the prenatal aspects of care, but also with the complex social and psychological contributing factors, is needed. The AWHONN opposes laws and other reporting requirements that result in incarceration or other punitive legal actions against women due to a substance abuse disorder in pregnancy (AWHONN, 2015). Box 7-6 reviews nursing interventions with substance-using patients.

Smoking and Tobacco Use

Smoking is one of the most important modifiable causes of poor pregnancy outcomes in the United States, and is associated with maternal, fetal, and infant morbidity and mortality (ACOG, 2020h). Smoking has been linked to doubling a woman's risk of having an LBW baby, slowing fetal growth, and increasing the risk of preterm delivery, spontaneous abortion, and stillbirth. Compared with babies of nonsmokers, babies whose mothers smoked during pregnancy are up to three times more likely to die from sudden infant death syndrome (SIDS). Furthermore, smoking during pregnancy doubles a woman's risk of experiencing placenta previa and placenta abruption, both of which can cause heavy bleeding that adversely affects mother and baby. An estimated 5% to 8% of preterm deliveries, 13% to 19% of term deliveries of infants with LBW, 23% to 34% of cases of sudden unexplained infant death (SUID), and 5% to 7% of preterm-related infant deaths can be attributed to prenatal maternal smoking (ACOG, 2020h). The risks of smoking during pregnancy extend beyond pregnancy-related complications. Children born to mothers who smoke during pregnancy are at an increased risk of asthma, infantile colic, and childhood obesity (ACOG, 2020h).

In 2016, 7.2% of women who gave birth smoked cigarettes during pregnancy (Drake et al., 2018). Statistics show that 910 infant deaths occur due to smoking during pregnancy and an estimated $350 million is spent each year in health care due to the effects of smoking while pregnant (National Institute on Drug Abuse [NIDA], 2013). Although quitting smoking before 15 weeks of gestation yields the greatest benefits for the pregnant woman and fetus, quitting at any point can be beneficial. Pregnancy influences many women to stop smoking, and approximately 50% of women who smoke before pregnancy quit smoking directly before or during pregnancy (ACOG, 2020h). Conflicting evidence exists as to whether nicotine replacement therapy increases abstinence rates in pregnant smokers.

The physiological effects of smoking are a result of transient intrauterine hypoxemia and are dose-dependent. The more the woman smokes, the greater the risk. Cigarette smoke contains many chemicals, particularly nicotine and carbon monoxide, that cause adverse pregnancy outcomes such as LBW and prematurity (NIDA, 2020b). Nicotine reduces uterine blood flow and carbon monoxide binds to hemoglobin, reducing the oxygen-carrying capacity of the blood, which increases the risk of fetal morbidity and mortality.

Assessment and Findings

- Gather a history of prior tobacco use, current use, quantity of use daily, and exposure to other family members that smoke.
- Inquire about all types of tobacco or nicotine use, including cigarette smoking, use of e-cigarettes or vaping products, hookahs, snus (a pulverized, moist tobacco product that is placed under the lip), lozenges, patches, and gum, during the prepregnancy, pregnancy, and postpartum periods.
- Physical findings include a cough, congestion, and smell of tobacco in the air or on clothing.
- Psychosocial findings include denial, anxiety, depression, anger, and guilt.
- An ultrasound can be performed as a diagnostic test to detect intrauterine fetal growth (IUGR).

Medical Management

- Provide education with smoking cessation education and information around smoking and its health hazards to the woman and fetus (American Cancer Society, 2015).

Nursing Management

Health-care professionals have a responsibility to routinely screen patients for tobacco use, to implement or support evidence-based smoking cessation strategies, and to refer patients to smoking cessation programs and resources. Nurses have the expertise in health promotion, disease prevention, women's health issues, and holistic care to provide the continuity of care necessary during and after pregnancy to support and monitor a woman's efforts to quit smoking. Additionally, AWHONN supports educational programs at the federal, state, and local levels that increase public awareness of the health risks for women and their babies related to smoking during pregnancy, increasing smoking bans, and taxation of cigarettes. Although quitting smoking before 15 weeks of gestation yields the greatest benefits for the pregnant woman and fetus, quitting at any point can be beneficial (ACOG, 2017h). Nurses should:

- Assess patients' smoking habits and timing. Inquire about all types of tobacco or nicotine use, including cigarette smoking, use of e-cigarettes or vaping products, hookahs, snus, lozenges, patches, and gum.
- Support the patient in decreasing smoking intake.
- Provide and help the patient identify alternative coping mechanisms instead of smoking. Examples are having a nutritious snack, walking to relieve stress, and relaxation as a substitute.
- Women should be advised of the significant perinatal risks associated with tobacco use, including orofacial clefts, fetal growth restriction, placenta previa, abruptio placentae, preterm prelabor ROM, LBW, increased perinatal mortality, ectopic pregnancy, and decreased maternal thyroid function (ACOG, 2020h).
- Because smoking continuation during pregnancy is associated with the likelihood of other substance use, screening for alcohol and other substance use is an important component of care (ACOG, 2020h).
- Refer the patient to appropriate programs for stress reduction and smoking cessation support (Sullivan, 2016) (Box 7-7).
- Current evidence suggests addiction to and dependence on cigarettes is physiological and psychological, and cessation techniques should include psychosocial interventions and pharmacological therapy. Two counseling techniques with positive effects on smoking and nicotine cessation in pregnant women are motivational interviewing and cognitive behavioral therapy. Specific aspects of cognitive behavioral therapy shown to benefit pregnant women include developing a sense of self-monitoring and control, learning to manage

BOX 7-7 | Patient Referrals for Information and Support on Quitting Substance Use During Pregnancy

Alcoholics Anonymous

    www.aa.org

Narcotics Anonymous

    www.na.org

Smoking Cessation

    www.ahrq.gov/consumer/tobacco/quits.htm

    www.helppregnantsmokersquit.org/quit/toll_free.asp

    1-800-QUIT-NOW

    www.cancer.org

    www.marchofdimes.org

    CDC.gov/quit

    Smokefree.gov

    TEXT PROGRAM: SmokefreeTXT at smokefree.gov/smokefreetxt

    MOBILE APP: QuitSTART at smokefree.gov/apps-quitstart

cravings, managing situations of stress and anxiety, promoting self-efficacy, and goal setting and action planning. Counseling, financial incentives, and feedback-based interventions such as cognitive behavioral therapy are associated with a reduction in smoking during pregnancy and decreased risk for infants with LBW (ACOG, 2020h).

● Intervention context and strategies should be individualized.

Marijuana

Marijuana, or cannabis, is the most commonly used illicit drug during pregnancy, and its use is rising (NIDA, 2018a, 2018b). Aggregate data from 2002 to 2012 indicated almost 15% of pregnant women were current marijuana users; however, the authors state that this likely underestimates actual use due to underreporting and social desirability bias (Young-Wolff et al., 2017). Current national estimates show that between 3% and 7% of pregnant women report using marijuana while pregnant. In 2018, there was a significant decline in illicit drug use by pregnant women. The decrease in marijuana uses among pregnant women between 2017 and 2018 (7.1% to 4.7%) contributed to this overall decline (SAMHSA, 2019). Marijuana is the drug most commonly used by pregnant women. Notably, 34% to 60% of women who use marijuana continue use during pregnancy, with many believing that it is relatively safe to use during pregnancy and less expensive than tobacco (SAMHSA, 2019).

Marijuana use causes tachycardia and low blood pressure, which can result in orthostatic hypotension. Research has shown that neonates born to mothers who used marijuana during pregnancy can have an altered response to visual stimuli, increased tremulousness, and even a high-pitched cry that may indicate a problem with neurological development and developmental problems (ACOG, 2017c; Mark et al., 2016; Sullivan, 2016).

With increasing legalization of cannabis, pregnant women may think the drug is safe to treat pregnancy-related ailments, such as morning sickness. The results research indicates this assumption is unwarranted (NIDA, 2020a). Cannabis use during pregnancy can affect the developing fetus, because THC can enter the fetal brain from the mother's bloodstream. It may disrupt the endocannabinoid system, which is important for a healthy pregnancy and fetal brain development (U.S. Surgeon General's Advisory, 2019). Fetal effects include CNS abnormalities and IUGR, small for gestational age, LBW, prematurity, and stillbirth.

Alcohol

Alcohol consumption during pregnancy is a major health problem, and prenatal exposure to alcohol remains the leading known preventable cause of birth defects in the United States. One report indicates 11.5% of pregnant women reported current drinking in the past 30 days and 3.9% of pregnant women reported binge drinking; in other words, among pregnant women, one in nine reported alcohol use (Denny et al., 2019). In another study, pregnant respondents in the first trimester reported higher current alcohol use than respondents in the second or third trimester. Among first-trimester respondents, 19.6% reported current alcohol use and 10.5% reported binge drinking; among second- or third-trimester respondents, current drinking and binge drinking were reported by 4.7% and 1.4%, respectively. Importantly, 40% of pregnant females reporting current drinking also reported current use of other substances (England et al., 2020).

Because a safe level of alcohol intake during pregnancy cannot be determined, both the U.S. Surgeon General and the March of Dimes Foundation recommend that pregnant women not consume any alcohol. The National Institute on Alcohol Abuse and Alcoholism defines at-risk alcohol use for healthy women as more than three drinks per occasion or more than seven drinks per week and any amount of drinking for women who are pregnant or at risk of pregnancy. Binge drinking is defined as more than four drinks per occasion. Almost 50% of binge drinking occurs among otherwise moderate drinkers. Heavy alcohol use is binge drinking on 5 or more days in the past month, whereas moderate drinking is defined as one drink per day. Alcohol use disorder (AUD) is a medical condition that doctors diagnose when a patient's drinking causes distress or harm. When evaluating a patient's drinking habits, it is important to verify the description of "a drink" to determine the actual amount of alcohol consumed.

Pregnant women age 15 to 17 years may need alcohol prevention services tailored for their age group, as nearly 16% of them used alcohol in the past month. Pregnant women in this age group consumed an average of 24 drinks in the past month (i.e., they drank on an average of 6 days during the past month and an average of about four drinks on the days that they drank).

Alcohol is a teratogen. Fetal alcohol spectrum disorder (FASD) is the most severe result of prenatal drinking, affecting

40,000 newborns in the United States annually. Recent reports from specific U.S. sites report the prevalence of FAS to be two to seven cases per 1,000, and the prevalence of FASD to be as high as 5% (MOD, 2016). Evidence shows that the brain was the most severely impacted organ of the body systems discussed. However, prenatal alcohol exposure causes several abnormalities within the heart, kidney, liver, gastrointestinal tract, and endocrine system (Caputo et al., 2016).

Alcohol use during pregnancy is associated with a range of complications and poor reproductive outcomes and can cause FASDs, characterized by lifelong physical, behavioral, and intellectual disabilities (Green et al., 2016). The estimated prevalence of FASDs, based on a community study of first grade students in the United States, ranges from 2% to 5%, but FASDs are completely preventable if a woman does not drink alcohol at any time while she is pregnant.

When a pregnant woman drinks, alcohol passes swiftly to the fetus through the placenta. Because alcohol is processed more slowly in the fetus's liver, the alcohol level can be even higher and remain elevated longer. Drinking alcohol during pregnancy can result in a wide range of physical and mental birth defects. For example, FASD is associated with abnormalities, growth defects, and facial dysmorphia. However, for every child born with FASD, many more are born with neurobehavioral defects caused by prenatal alcohol exposure. Other alcohol-related birth defects include growth deformities, facial abnormalities, CNS impairment, behavioral disorders, and impaired intellectual development.

Alcohol can affect a fetus at any stage of pregnancy, and the cognitive defects and behavioral problems that result from prenatal alcohol exposure are lifelong. In early pregnancy during organogenesis and perhaps before the patient's recognition of pregnancy, the fetus may be particularly vulnerable to maternal binge or heavy alcohol use. Even moderate alcohol consumption during pregnancy may alter psychomotor development, contribute to cognitive defects, and produce emotional and behavioral problems in children, although patient denial and underreporting make it difficult to quantify these effects. Evidence supports varying susceptibility to alcohol's effect on the developing fetus. Although alcohol consumption may have negative consequences for any pregnant woman, these effects may be more potent in mothers who are older, in poor health, or who also smoke or use drugs. Chapter 17 provides additional information on FASDs.

Assessment Findings

- Providers should advise women not to drink at all if they are pregnant or there is any chance they might be pregnant.
- Five criteria for determining risk for FAS are drinking during pregnancy, cluster of birth defects, facial abnormalities, brain damage, and fetal growth restriction.
- History of prenatal care should be taken from a nonjudgmental perspective.
- Screening with the Four P's of pregnancy (Chasnoff et al., 2007) includes the following questions:
  - Have you ever used drugs or alcohol during pregnancy?
  - Have you had a problem with drugs or alcohol in the past?
  - Does your partner have a problem with drugs or alcohol?
  - Do you consider one of your parents to be an addict or alcoholic? (Chasnoff et al., 2007)
- Risk factors include history of substance abuse, current or recent drug use, previous child with FAS, smoking, multiple sex partners, recent abuse, and mental health problems.
- Physical findings: Poor nutrition or hygiene, tremors, edema, agitated, memory loss, and hepatomegaly
- Psychological findings: Depression, fear, anxiety, lack of family support, denial, hostility, anger, unplanned pregnancy, and low self-esteem
- Diagnostic studies: Blood alcohol level, STI testing, and serial sonogram

Medical Management

- Offer inpatient or outpatient treatment for alcohol or other drugs.
- Provide written information of resources at appropriate educational level.
- Offer case management and increasing prenatal visits.

Nursing Management

- Health education should be provided on the effects of alcohol and potential dangers.
- Women wanting a pregnancy should be advised to stop drinking at the same time contraception is discontinued.
- One study found that approximately 3.3 million women aged 15 to 44 years reported drinking alcohol in the past month even though they had sex and did not use contraception, and thus were at risk for an alcohol-exposed pregnancy. Raising awareness about the dangers of alcohol use among reproductive-aged women is important, especially if contraception is not being used (Green et al., 2016).
- Refer to community support and resources (see Box 7-7).
- Assess risk factors and physical or psychological effects.

Illicit Drugs

An average of 5.4% of pregnant women use illicit drugs such as cocaine, amphetamines, and heroin (SAMHSA, 2019). The effect of the drug on placental function and fetal development depends on its nature. For example, cocaine causes vasoconstriction that can impact the placenta and uterus, resulting in placental abruption or PTB (Sullivan, 2016). Women who use illicit drugs are counseled to stop, except for heroin users, for whom methadone treatment is recommended to prevent stillbirth.

Methamphetamine

The abuse of methamphetamine has been increasing in the United States since the late 1980s. After alcohol and marijuana, methamphetamine is the drug most frequently abused in many western and midwestern states. Methamphetamine is a more potent stimulant drug than its parent compound, amphetamine.

Both cocaine and methamphetamine block reuptake of dopamine at nerve endings, but methamphetamine also increases the release of dopamine, leading to higher concentrations of dopamine in the synapse, which may be toxic to nerve terminals. The half-life of methamphetamine is approximately 12 hours compared with approximately 1 hour for cocaine. Cardiovascular and neurological complications such as hypertension, tachycardia, UCs, myocardial infarction, dysrhythmias, subarachnoid hemorrhage, thrombocytopenia, seizures, and even sudden death have been described among patients who abuse methamphetamine or cocaine. Stimulants such as cocaine, crank, and crystal meth are correlated to the abnormal neurobehavioral affects in the neonate as a result of direct exposure instead of association of withdrawal symptoms (Hudak et al., 2014). Acute use of cocaine during the third trimester can result in PTL, a greater incidence of PROM, abruptio placentae, precipitous delivery, increased risk for meconium staining, and premature and LBW infants (Forray, 2016). Methamphetamine use may be associated with an increase in defects of the fetal CNS, cardiovascular system, and gastrointestinal system, as well as oral cleft and limb defects, prematurity, and small for gestational age issues (ACOG, 2011).

Opioid Use

The prevalence of opioid use disorder in the United States continues to rise and is a public health crisis. Opioid use in pregnancy has escalated dramatically in recent years, paralleling the epidemic observed in the general population. Nationally, rates of opioid use disorder at delivery hospitalization more than quadrupled during 1999 to 2014 (Haight et al., 2018). Over time, the repeated administration of any opioid may result in tolerance and dependence. Tolerance refers to an individual's response to a drug so that the person needs more of a substance to get the desired effect. Drug dependence occurs after repeated use when adaptations in the brain trigger physical withdrawal symptoms if the substance is not used. The time from the beginning of opioid use to drug dependence is highly variable, and many factors influence this complex phenomenon, such as type of opioid, dose, and exposure frequency.

Opioid use disorder is a pattern of opioid use characterized by tolerance, craving, inability to control use, and continued use despite adverse consequences. Opioid use disorder is a chronic, treatable disease that can be managed successfully by combining medications with behavioral therapy and recovery support (NIDA, 2014). It is thus increasingly important for providers to be educated on opioid prescribing and patients to have access to accurate information and appropriate treatment (ACOG, 2017e).

Opioid abuse in pregnancy includes use of heroin and misuse of prescription opioid analgesic medications. Opioid exposure during pregnancy is linked to adverse health effects for both mothers and their babies. Long-term opioid use has been linked to poor fetal growth, PTB, stillbirth, specific birth defects, and neonatal abstinence syndrome. The effects of prenatal opioid exposure on children over time are largely unknown. During pregnancy, addiction to heroin is associated with lack of prenatal care, increased risk of fetal growth restriction, abruptio placentae, fetal death, PTL, and intrauterine passage of meconium (ACOG, 2017e).

In addition to the use of screening tools, certain signs and symptoms may suggest a substance use disorder in a pregnant woman. Pregnant women with opioid addiction often seek prenatal care late in pregnancy; exhibit poor adherence to their appointments; experience poor weight gain; or exhibit sedation, intoxication, withdrawal, or erratic behavior. Opioid-assisted therapy during pregnancy can prevent complications of illicit opioid use and narcotic withdrawal, encourage prenatal care and drug treatment, reduce criminal activity, and avoid risks of associating with a drug culture. Comprehensive opioid-assisted therapy that includes prenatal care reduces the risk of obstetric complications. For pregnant women with an opioid use disorder, opioid agonist pharmacotherapy is the recommended therapy and is preferable to medically supervised withdrawal because withdrawal is associated with high relapse rates, which lead to worse outcomes (ACOG, 2017e).

Methadone maintenance, as prescribed and dispensed daily by a registered substance abuse treatment program, is part of a comprehensive package of prenatal care, chemical dependency counseling, family therapy, nutritional education, and other medical and psychosocial services as indicated for pregnant women with opioid dependence (ACOG, 2017e).

Heroin abuse during pregnancy is linked to adverse consequences for both mother and fetus. Hazards of heroin to the fetus are believed to be directly related to the physiological dependence effect on the fetus and the maternal lifestyle associated with heroin use. Opioids such as heroin, morphine, and methadone are CNS depressants that can cross the placenta and blood-brain barrier, potentially causing withdrawal signs in the neonate (Hudak et al., 2014). The primary effects of heroin include analgesia, sedation, feeling of well-being, and euphoria.

Women who use heroin during pregnancy typically do not seek early prenatal care for fear of detection of heroin use and are at an increased risk to exposure to serious infections such as STDs, hepatitis, and HIV. The neonatal effects of prenatal heroin exposure include withdrawal symptoms, increased incidence of meconium aspiration at birth, increased incidence of sepsis, IUGR, and neurodevelopmental behavioral problems (Sullivan, 2016).

Assessment Findings in Women With Substance Use Disorder During Pregnancy

Screening for smoking, alcohol use, and illicit drugs is recommended to start at the first prenatal visit and may use various screening tools. Universal screening should take a supportive and nonjudgmental manner. One simple screening tool includes asking the following four questions for a yes or no response, described as Ewing's 4 P's (Taylor et al., 2002).

- Have you ever used alcohol or drugs during this pregnancy?
- Have you had a problem with drugs or alcohol in the past?
- Does your partner have a problem with drugs or alcohol?
- Do you consider one of your parents to have a problem with drugs or alcohol?

A yes answer to any of these questions should trigger further evaluation of habits. Additionally, a toxicology screen of a urine sample can be attained to evaluate for certain drug use.

Medical Management

- Screen for substance use in pregnancy with all pregnant women (ACOG, 2017e).
- Refer to multispecialty clinics.
- Refer to drug treatment programs.
- Screen for domestic violence.
- Conduct frequent urine toxicology tests.
- Use targeted ultrasound to rule out congenital anomalies.
- Provide patient education.
- Conduct antepartal testing.

Risks for the Woman With Substance Use Disorder During Pregnancy

- PTL
- PPROM
- Poor weight gain and nutritional status
- Placental abnormalities (placenta previa, abruptio placentae)

Nursing Actions for the Woman With Substance Use Disorder During Pregnancy

Women are more receptive to treatment and lifestyle changes during pregnancy; therefore, pregnancy may be a window of opportunity for chemically dependent women to enter treatment. To facilitate this, nurses must be armed with the knowledge and information necessary to screen and identify women who abuse substances during pregnancy. Due to the substantial costs and repercussions of drug use during pregnancy for newborns, women, and society, it is essential to devise methods of intervention that decrease this risky behavior. Many women who need substance abuse treatment may not receive it due to lack of money or child care, fear of losing custody of their children, or other barriers.

For successful recovery, women often need a continuum of care for an extended period, including comprehensive inpatient or outpatient treatment for alcohol and other drugs, case management for coordination of prenatal care, counseling, and other mental health treatment (see Box 7-7). The AWHONN (2019) opposes laws and other reporting requirements that result in incarceration or other punitive legal actions against women due to a substance use disorder (SUD) in pregnancy and the postpartum period. AWHONN supports universal verbal screening for substance use during pregnancy using a validated tool that should begin at entry into prenatal care and continue periodically throughout pregnancy. Early identification and treatment of women with SUD or dependence is a critical component of preconception and prenatal care and is important to support healthy birth outcomes. Exposure to STIs and victimization; lack of or inconsistent use of contraception and knowledge of safe sex practices; and inadequate mental health, dental, and well-woman care place women with SUD at greater risk for significant, long-term health concerns.

Treatment for SUD should be family focused and nonstigmatizing. It is important to remember that abstinence will not be immediately possible for some women and substitution treatment or harm reduction approaches may be the most appropriate. Substance use disorders are characterized by periods of remission and relapse; thus, treatment must be tailored to address this variable course. Given substance dependence is a chronic relapsing disorder, and a high proportion of pregnancies are reported to be unplanned, the focus of treatment should be one of long-term follow-up to support the woman. Appropriate treatment will also depend on factors including other mental and physical health problems, access to services including transport, and severity of the problem.

In addition to psychosocial treatments, if the woman is substance dependent, it may be necessary to provide a supervised detoxification. Depending on the substance and severity of the dependence, this may be as an inpatient. Proper addiction treatment differs from most medical conditions in that it requires access to focused behavioral health treatment and support for standard social services, such as housing, transportation, and communication. Nurses and other health-care professionals should be familiar with laws on mandatory reporting and referral in their states and comply as applicable.

Nursing actions include the following:

- Pregnancy provides an important opportunity to identify and treat women with substance use disorders. Substance use disorders affect women across all racial and ethnic groups and all socioeconomic groups, and affect women in rural, urban, and suburban populations. Therefore, it is essential that screening be universal (ACOG, 2017e).
- Screening for substance use should be a part of comprehensive obstetric care and should be done at the first prenatal visit in partnership with the pregnant woman.
- Provide health education about the risks to the fetus of substance use during pregnancy and facilitate early diagnosis and appropriate intervention and referral.
- Pregnant women with substance use disorders are often judged harshly and stigmatized by family, friends, society, and even health-care providers, who may see the abuse as a weakness that needs to be punished rather than a health condition that needs to be treated (Keough & Fantasia, 2017).
- Some states criminalize opioid abuse during pregnancy, further adding to stigma, suspicion of health-care providers, removal of children from the home, and reluctance to enter care.
- Laws governing drug screening during pregnancy vary from state to state. Nurses must be aware of laws and local guidelines for toxicology screening of pregnant women, treatment options, and availability of programs, as many programs do not accept pregnant women.
- Urine drug testing has been used to detect or confirm suspected substance use, but should be performed only with the patient's consent and in compliance with state laws.
- Counsel women who test positive for drug or alcohol use and those who smoke during pregnancy to stop and supply referrals to assist with cessation and refer to local treatment centers for pregnant women (see Box 7-7).
- Maintain a nonjudgmental and nonpunitive attitude; remember that addiction is a disease.

- Nurses should remain up to date with current treatment approaches and strategies regarding addiction management in pregnancy (Box 7-8).
- Women with addiction often suffer from poor nutrition, and many have disrupted support systems leading to social service needs. Identifying these problems during pregnancy with referral for specialized multidisciplinary care is important to achieve optimal care.
- The nurse should provide evidence-based information and emphasize health promotion, disease prevention, and holistic care. Consistent screening, education, testing, and retesting of pregnant women is imperative and reduces the potential for discriminatory testing.
- Remember addiction is a chronic, relapsing biological and behavioral disorder with genetic components, and substance use is addictive in some individuals. Drug enforcement policies that deter women from seeking prenatal care are contrary to the welfare of the mother and fetus (ACOG, 2017e).
- Advocate for culturally specific public health campaigns that help women and their families better understand potential effects of marijuana and other drug use on the woman, fetus, and newborn (AWHONN, 2018).
- Advocate for increased access to interventions for use of all substances that are high-quality, affordable, and logistically feasible, including in the home or integrated into the maternity care setting.

It has been proposed that government policies can be viewed as either "facilitative" or "adversarial." Facilitative policies improve women's access to prenatal care, food, shelter, and treatment. Adversarial policies, in contrast, propose that women who fail to seek treatment are liable to criminal prosecution and may diminish utilization of prenatal care and support services, such as housing, education and job training, financial support services, parenting education, legal services, and aftercare. Research shows that residential substance abuse treatment designed specifically for pregnant women and women with children can have substantial benefits in terms of recovery, pregnancy outcomes, parenting skills, and women's ability to maintain or regain custody of their children.

BOX 7-8 | Resources for Further Information on Substance Abuse Treatment for Health Professionals

Alcoholics Anonymous (AA)
Check your local phone book for listings in your area
Internet address: http://www.aa.org

National Council on Alcoholism and Drug Dependence, Inc. (NCADD)
217 Broadway, Suite 712
New York, NY 10007
Phone: (212) 269–7797; Fax: (212) 269–7510
HOPE LINE: (800) NCA–CALL (24-hour Affiliate referral)
Email: national@ncadd.org
Internet address: http://www.ncadd.org

National Institute on Alcohol Abuse and Alcoholism
5635 Fishers Lane
Bethesda, MD 20892–9304
(301) 443–3860; Fax: (301) 480–1726
Internet address: http://www.niaaa.nih.gov

National Organization on Fetal Alcohol Syndrome
900 17th Street, NW, Suite 910
Washington, DC 20006
(800) 66–NOFAS; Fax: (202) 466–6456
Internet address: http://www.nofas.org

March of Dimes
Internet address: https://www.marchofdimes.org/

Substance Abuse and Mental Health Services Administration (SAMHSA)
Treatment Facility Locator
(800) 662–HELP
Internet address: http://www.findtreatment.samhsa.gov

CONCEPT MAP |

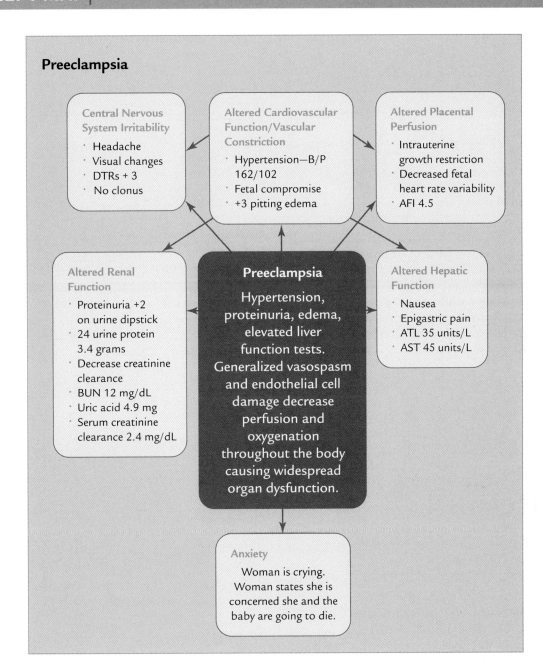

Preeclampsia

Central Nervous System Irritability
- Headache
- Visual changes
- DTRs + 3
- No clonus

Altered Cardiovascular Function/Vascular Constriction
- Hypertension—B/P 162/102
- Fetal compromise
- +3 pitting edema

Altered Placental Perfusion
- Intrauterine growth restriction
- Decreased fetal heart rate variability
- AFI 4.5

Altered Renal Function
- Proteinuria +2 on urine dipstick
- 24 urine protein 3.4 grams
- Decrease creatinine clearance
- BUN 12 mg/dL
- Uric acid 4.9 mg
- Serum creatinine clearance 2.4 mg/dL

Preeclampsia
Hypertension, proteinuria, edema, elevated liver function tests. Generalized vasospasm and endothelial cell damage decrease perfusion and oxygenation throughout the body causing widespread organ dysfunction.

Altered Hepatic Function
- Nausea
- Epigastric pain
- ATL 35 units/L
- AST 45 units/L

Anxiety
Woman is crying. Woman states she is concerned she and the baby are going to die.

CARE PLANS

Problem 1: Central nervous system irritability

Goal: Prevent seizures and cerebral edema.

Outcome: Patient will remain seizure free and not develop neurological sequelae.

Nursing Actions

1. Monitor CNS changes including headache, dizziness, blurred vision, and scotoma.
2. Maintain seizure precautions.
3. If treated with magnesium sulfate, see Critical Component: Care of the Woman on Magnesium Sulfate.
4. Restrict fluids to total of 125 mL/hr or as ordered.
5. Monitor I&O.
6. Assess DTRs.
7. Maintain bedrest in the lateral position.
8. Provide an environment that is conducive to decreased stimulation, such as low lights, decreased noise, and uninterrupted rest periods.
9. Teach the patient relaxation techniques.

Continued

Problem 2: Altered cardiovascular function and vasoconstriction
Goal: Normal blood pressure
Outcome: Blood pressure within acceptable limits, below 140/90 mm Hg

Nursing Actions

1. Monitor BP every hour or more frequently if elevated.
2. Administer antihypertensive medication as ordered related to hypertensive parameters.
3. Assess edema.
4. Assess lungs for pulmonary edema.
5. Maintain bedrest in the left lateral position.

Problem 3: Anxiety related to harm for self and fetus
Goal: Decreased anxiety.
Outcome: Patient verbalizes that she feels less anxious.

Nursing Actions

1. Be calm and reassuring in interactions with the patient and her family.
2. Explain all procedures.
3. Explain results of test and procedures.
4. Teach patient relaxation and breathing techniques.
5. Encourage the patient and family to verbalize their feelings regarding recent hemorrhage by asking open-ended questions.

Problem 4: Altered renal function
Goal: Maintain adequate renal function.
Outcome: The patient will maintain adequate renal function.

Nursing Actions

1. Monitor and maintain strict I&O.
2. Report urine output less than 30 mL/hr.

3. Check urine protein and specific gravity.
4. Evaluate kidney function tests.
5. Report changes in urine output or worsening kidney function laboratory values to the care provider.
6. Assess edema.

Problem 5: Altered hepatic function
Goal: Maintain adequate hepatic function.
Outcome: The patient will maintain adequate hepatic function.

Nursing Actions

1. Assess epigastric pain, right upper quadrant pain, nausea, and vomiting.
2. Interpret laboratory tests related to liver function (AST, LDH).
3. Report changes in liver function tests to the care provider.

Problem 6: Altered placental perfusion
Goal: Maintain fetal oxygenation.
Outcome: Assessments of fetal status remain within normal limits.

Nursing Actions

1. Assess FHR baseline, variability, and for Category II or III FHR patterns.
2. Provide interventions for intrauterine resuscitation of fetus (IV fluid, O_2, lateral position).
3. Report any abnormal FHR patterns to the care provider.
4. Facilitate antenatal testing.
5. Instruct the woman in daily kick counts.

Case Study

As the nurse, you evaluate Mallory Polk in triage in the labor and delivery unit. She presented in the triage unit at 8 p.m. at 32 weeks' gestation with complaints of a persistent low, dull backache; increased vaginal discharge; and pelvic pressure in her vagina for 2 days with some vaginal spotting this evening when she went to the bathroom. She attributed the discomforts of backache and pulling to working long hours for the past week in arbitration on a "big case," as she is a partner in a large law firm. Mallory is a 42-year-old single Black woman. She is accompanied by her sister Alison, who is visiting for the week from out of state. When placed on the monitor, Mallory is having contractions every 5 to 7 minutes that she reports as "menstrual cramping." The FHR is in the 150s baseline with accelerations to 170s with moderate variability. A review of her prenatal record reveals she is a G2 P0 and the pregnancy is a result of in vitro fertilization. She has received regular prenatal

visits. She does not smoke or drink alcohol. Her prenatal laboratory results are as follows:

- Blood type A+
- RPR NR
- GBS negative
- Hgb 12.4
- Hct 32.1
- Hepatitis negative

Prenatal Care Summary

Mallory began prenatal care at 10 weeks' gestation and receives regular prenatal care. She conceives after three attempts at in vitro fertilization. She has no prior medical complications and has experienced a normal pregnancy. Her first pregnancy was terminated at 6 weeks of gestation. She is allergic to shellfish and is allergic to sulfa drugs. An ultrasound at 12 weeks confirms a gestational age of 32 weeks.

Detail the aspects of your initial assessment and what you would report to her physician.

Within 40 minutes of arrival, you phone her physician, who is completing a delivery, and report your assessment findings. The physician comes to the unit in 10 minutes to evaluate Mallory. Based on her assessment, she orders an IV lactated Ringer's 300-mL bolus, a CBC, and urinalysis clean catch; does a fetal fibronectin; and does a sterile vaginal exam that reveals her cervix is 2 cm dilated/75% effaced/0 station. Her physician orders a 4 g magnesium sulfate bolus over 30 minutes, then 2 g per hour. Betamethasone is to be given 12 mg now and to be repeated in 24 hours. An ultrasound is ordered for fetal size and position. Her physician discusses the plan of care for treatment of PTL with Mallory and answers her questions, and Mallory agrees to the plan to attempt to stop the contractions and delay delivery.

What are your immediate priorities in nursing care for Mallory?

Discuss the rationale for the priorities.

State the nursing diagnosis, expected outcome, and interventions related to this problem.

List Mallory's risk factors for PTL.

What teaching would you include?

Within 10 minutes of starting the magnesium sulfate bolus, Mallory reports feeling hot and flushed and feels burning at the IV site. After the magnesium sulfate bolus is complete, you start the magnesium sulfate infusion at 2 g per hour. At midnight, her contractions slow down to every 15 minutes or 4 to 5 contractions/hour. The FHR baseline is in the 140s with minimal variability and periodic accelerations. An ultrasound reveals the fetus is vertex, estimated fetal weight (EFW) is 1,560 g, and fetal fibronectin is positive.

What are the assessments for a woman treated for PTL on magnesium sulfate?

Discuss the rationale for the assessments.

What teaching would you include in the nursing action plan?

At 7 a.m. when you sign off, Mallory is sleeping intermittently. Her contractions are 23 per hour and the FHR is normal. Mallory is very concerned about giving birth to a premature baby. She is concerned that a baby will not survive at this gestation and states, "I have always wanted to be a mother and was so happy when I was finally ready to have a baby and conceived with IVF." She is worried about not being able to return to work over the next few days and weeks, as she has many active cases pending over the next few weeks. She states that she is not ready for the baby to come and has not set up the crib or finished the nursery. She feels guilty that she did not come to the hospital sooner and considered the backache as just part of pregnancy discomforts. Before you leave, you have requested Mallory be seen that day by the neonatal clinical specialist to review status and care for neonates born prematurely and to have Mallory's sister tour the NICU.

Detail the aspects of your psychosocial assessment for a woman with a high-risk pregnancy.

Discuss the rationale for the assessment.

Discuss nursing diagnosis, nursing actions, and expected outcomes related to this psychosocial assessment.

The next night, you come onto your shift at 7 p.m. and care for Mallory again. She remains on the magnesium sulfate and appears to be tolerating the medication. Her magnesium level is 5.6 mEq/L. She still feels warm and somewhat lethargic with sore muscles from being in bed all day. She is due for her second dose of betamethasone. Her I&O for the past 24 hours are: I: 2,500 mL; O: 2,300 mL. The plan is to stop the magnesium sulfate, transfer her to the antenatal unit in the morning, and observe her for a day or so.

Detail the aspects of your ongoing assessment for a woman treated with magnesium sulfate and diagnosed with PTL.

Discuss the rationale for the assessment.

At 3:20 p.m. Mallory reports feeling a gush of fluid from her vagina after a strong contraction. Between her legs is a large amount of clear fluid. The FHR is baseline 140s with minimal variability and accelerations. Mallory appears frightened and anxious. She is crying and her sister is at her side holding her hand and reassuring her.

What are your immediate priorities in nursing care for Mallory?

Discuss the rationale for the priorities.

Within 45 minutes, the physician comes in to see Mallory and does a sterile vaginal examination (SVE). She is 5 cm, 90% effaced, and +1 station, and an ultrasound reveals the fetus is vertex. The physician recommends they turn off the magnesium sulfate and anticipate a vaginal birth due to the advanced PTL. Mallory agrees with the plan.

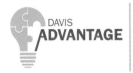
DAVIS ADVANTAGE

Go to Davis Advantage to complete your learning: strengthen understanding, apply your knowledge, and prepare for the Next Gen NCLEX®.

REFERENCES

Adams, E. (2021). Antenatal care. In K. Simpson, P. Creehan, N. Obrien-Abel, C. Roth, & A. Rohan (Eds.), *Perinatal nursing* (5th ed., pp. 65–97). Wolters Kluwer.

American Academy of Pediatrics and the American College of Obstetricians and Gynecologists. (2017). *Guidelines for perinatal care* (8th ed.). Authors.

American Cancer Society. (2015). *Smoking while you are pregnant or breastfeeding.* https://www.cancer.org/cancer/cancer-causes/tobacco-and-cancer/smoking-while-you-are-pregnant-or-breastfeeding.html

American College of Obstetricians and Gynecologists. (2004). Diagnosis and treatment of gestational trophoblastic disease. ACOG Practice Bulletin No. 53. *Obstetrics & Gynecology, 93*(3), 575–585. https://doi.org/10.1016/j.ygyno.2004.05.013

American College of Obstetricians and Gynecologists. (2011). Methamphetamine abuse in women of reproductive age. Committee Opinion No. 479. *Obstetrics & Gynecology, 117,* 751–755.

American College of Obstetricians and Gynecologists. (2012). Prediction and prevention of preterm birth. Practice Bulletin No. 130. American College of Obstetricians and Gynecologists. *Obstetrics & Gynecology, 120*, 964–973.

American College of Obstetricians and Gynecologists. (2013a). Addressing health risks of noncoital sexual activity. Committee Opinion No. 582. *Obstetrics & Gynecology, 122*, 1378–1383.

American College of Obstetricians and Gynecologists. (2013b, November). *Hypertension in pregnancy. Practice Guideline. Obstetrics & Gynecology, 122*(5). 1122–1131. https://doi.org/10.1097/01.AOG.0000437382.03963.88

American College of Obstetricians and Gynecologists. (2014). Cerclage for the management of cervical insufficiency. ACOG Practice Bulletin No. 142. *Obstetrics & Gynecology, 123*, 372–379.

American College of Obstetricians and Gynecologists. (2015a). Alcohol abuse and other substance use disorders: Ethical issues in obstetric and gynecologic practice. Committee Opinion No. 633. *Obstetrics & Gynecology, 125*(6), 1529–1537.

American College of Obstetricians and Gynecologist. (2015b). Obesity in pregnancy. ACOG Practice Bulletin No. 150. *Obstetrics & Gynecology, 126*(6), e112–e126.

American College of Obstetricians and Gynecologists. (2016a). Clinical updates in women's health care: Liver disease. *General Pathophysiology, Diagnosis, and Management, XV*(6).

American College of Obstetricians and Gynecologists. (2016b). Management of preterm labor. ACOG Practice Bulletin No. 171. *Obstetrics & Gynecology, 128*, e155–164.

American College of Obstetricians and Gynecologists. (2016c). Multifetal gestations: Twin, triplet, and higher-order multifetal pregnancies. ACOG Practice Bulletin No. 169. *Obstetrics & Gynecology, 127*, e1–e16.

American College of Obstetricians and Gynecologists. (2016d). Premature rupture of membranes. Practice Bulletin No. 172. *Obstetrics & Gynecology, 128*, e165–e177.

American College of Obstetricians and Gynecologists. (2017a). Antenatal corticosteroid therapy for fetal maturation. Committee Opinion No. 713. *Obstetrics & Gynecology, 130*, e102–e109.

American College of Obstetricians and Gynecologists. (2017b). Emergent therapy for acute-onset, severe hypertension during pregnancy and the postpartum period. Committee Opinion No. 692. Obstetrics Period. *Obstetrics & Gynecology, 129*, e90–e95.

American College of Obstetricians and Gynecologists. (2017c). Marijuana use during pregnancy and lactation. Committee Opinion No. 722. *Obstetrics & Gynecology, 130*, e205–e209.

American College of Obstetricians and Gynecologists. (2017d). Multifetal pregnancy reduction. Committee Opinion No. 719. *Obstetrics & Gynecology, 130*(3), e158–e163. https://doi.org/10.1097/AOG.0000000000002302

American College of Obstetricians and Gynecologists. (2017e). Opioid use and opioid use disorder in pregnancy. Committee Opinion No. 711. *Obstetrics & Gynecology, 130*, e81–e94.

American College of Obstetricians and Gynecologists. (2017f). Periviable birth. Obstetric Care Consensus No. 6. American College of Obstetricians and Gynecologists. *Obstetrics & Gynecology, 130*, e187–e199.

American College of Obstetricians and Gynecologists. (2017h). Sulfonamides, nitrofurantoin, and risk of birth defects. Committee Opinion No. 717. *Obstetrics & Gynecology, 130*, e150–e152.

American College of Obstetricians and Gynecologists. (2018a). Early pregnancy loss. ACOG Practice Bulletin No. 200. *Obstetrics & Gynecology, 132*, e197–e207.

American College of Obstetricians and Gynecologists. (2018b). Expedited partner therapy. ACOG Committee Opinion No. 737. *Obstetrics & Gynecology, 131*, e190–193.

American College of Obstetricians and Gynecologists. (2018c). Gestational diabetes mellitus. ACOG Practice Bulletin No. 190. *Obstetrics & Gynecology, 131*, e49–e64.

American College of Obstetricians and Gynecologists. (2018d). Importance of social determinants of health and cultural awareness in the delivery of reproductive health care. Committee Opinion No. 729. *Obstetrics & Gynecology, 131*(1), e43–e48. https://doi.org/10.1097/AOG.0000000000002459

American College of Obstetricians and Gynecologists. (2018e). Labor and delivery management of women with human immunodeficiency virus infection. ACOG Committee Opinion No. 751. *Obstetrics & Gynecology, 132*, e131–e137.

American College of Obstetricians and Gynecologists. (2018f). Low-dose aspirin use during pregnancy. ACOG Committee Opinion No. 743. *Obstetrics & Gynecology, 132*, e44–e52.

American College of Obstetricians and Gynecologists. (2018g). Nausea and vomiting of pregnancy. ACOG Practice Bulletin No. 189. *Obstetrics & Gynecology, 131*, e15–e30.

American College of Obstetricians and Gynecologists. (2018h). Placenta accreta spectrum. Obstetric Care Consensus No. 7. *Obstetrics & Gynecology, 132*, e259–e275.

American College of Obstetricians and Gynecologists. (2018i). Pregestational diabetes mellitus. ACOG Practice Bulletin No. 201. *Obstetrics & Gynecology, 132*, e229–e248.

American College of Obstetricians and Gynecologists. (2018j). Thromboembolism in pregnancy. ACOG Practice Bulletin No. 196. *Obstetrics & Gynecology, 132*, e1–e17.

American College of Obstetricians and Gynecologists. (2018k). Tubal ectopic pregnancy. ACOG Practice Bulletin No. 193. *Obstetrics & Gynecology, 131*, e91–e103.

American College of Obstetricians and Gynecologists. (2019a). Critical care in pregnancy. ACOG Practice Bulletin No. 211. *Obstetrics & Gynecology, 133*, e303–e319.

American College of Obstetricians and Gynecologists. (2019b). Emergent therapy for acute-onset, severe hypertension during pregnancy and the postpartum period. ACOG Committee Opinion No. 767. *Obstetrics & Gynecology, 133*, e174–e180.

American College of Obstetricians and Gynecologists. (2019c). Ethical considerations for the care of patients with obesity. ACOG Committee Opinion No. 763. *Obstetrics & Gynecology, 133*, e90–e96.

American College of Obstetricians and Gynecologists. (2019d). Management of patients in the context of Zika virus. ACOG Committee Opinion No. 784. *Obstetrics & Gynecology, 134*, e64–e70.

American College of Obstetricians and Gynecologists. (2019e). Nonobstetric surgery during pregnancy. ACOG Committee Opinion No. 775. *Obstetrics & Gynecology, 133*, e285–e286.

American College of Obstetricians and Gynecologists. (2019f). Pregnancy and heart disease. ACOG Practice Bulletin No. 212. *Obstetrics & Gynecology, 133*, e320–e356.

American College of Obstetricians and Gynecologists. (2019g). Prevention of group B streptococcal early-onset disease in newborns. ACOG Committee Opinion No. 782. *Obstetrics & Gynecology, 135*, e51–e72.

American College of Obstetricians and Gynecologists. (2020a). Gestational hypertension and preeclampsia. ACOG Practice Bulletin No. 222. *Obstetrics & Gynecology, 135*, e237–e260.

American College of Obstetricians and Gynecologists. (2020b). Gynecologic management of adolescents and young women with seizure disorders. ACOG Committee Opinion No. 806. *Obstetrics & Gynecology, 135*, e213–e220.

American College of Obstetricians and Gynecologists. (2020c). Increasing access to abortion. ACOG Committee Opinion No. 815. *Obstetrics & Gynecology, 136*, e107–e115.

American College of Obstetricians and Gynecologists. (2020d). Medication abortion up to 70 days of gestation. ACOG Practice Bulletin No. 225. *Obstetrics & Gynecology, 136*, e31–e47.

American College of Obstetricians and Gynecologists. (2020e). Prelabor rupture of membranes. ACOG Practice Bulletin No. 217. American College of Obstetricians and Gynecologists. *Obstetrics & Gynecology, 135*, e80–e97.

American College of Obstetricians and Gynecologists. (2020f). Systemic lupus erythematosus. *Clinical Updates in Women's Health Care, XIX*(4), 136(1), 226. https://doi.org/10.1097/AOG.0000000000003942

American College of Obstetricians and Gynecologists. (2020g). Thyroid disease in pregnancy. ACOG Practice Bulletin No. 223. *Obstetrics & Gynecology, 135*, e261–e274.

American College of Obstetricians and Gynecologists. (2020h). Tobacco and nicotine cessation during pregnancy. ACOG Committee Opinion No. 807. *Obstetrics & Gynecology, 135*, e221–e229.

American College of Obstetricians and Gynecologists. (2021a). Medically indicated late-preterm and early-term deliveries. ACOG Committee Opinion No. 818. *Obstetrics & Gynecology, 137*, e29–e33.

American College of Obstetricians and Gynecologists. (2021b, June). Obesity in Pregnancy. *Obstetrics & Gynecology, 137*(6), e128–e144.

American College of Obstetricians and Gynecologists. (2021c, January). *Seizures.* Clinical Updates in Womens Health.

American College of Obstetricians and Gynecologists and Society for Maternal Fetal Medicine. (2021). *ACOG and SMFM recommend COVID-19 vaccination for pregnant individuals.* News Release, July 30.

Arafeh, J. (2021). Cardiac disease in pregnancy. In K. Simpson, P. Creehan, N. Obrien-Abel, C. Roth, & A. Rohan (Eds.), *Perinatal nursing* (5th ed., pp. 199–219). Wolters Kluwer.

Association of Women's Health, Obstetric and Neonatal Nurses. (2015). Criminalization of pregnant women with substance use disorders position statement 2015. *Journal of Obstetric, Gynecologic, & Neonatal Nursing, 44,* 155–157. https://doi.org/10.1111/1552-6909.1253

Association of Women's Health, Obstetric and Neonatal Nurses. (2016). The nursing care of the woman with diabetes in pregnancy: Evidence-based clinical practice guideline. Evidence-Based Clinical Practice Guideline Development Team. Association of Women's Health, Obstetric and Neonatal Nurses, Washington, DC.

Association of Women's Health, Obstetric and Neonatal Nurses. (2017). Access to health care position statement. *Journal of Obstetric, Gynecologic, & Neonatal Nursing, 46*(1), 44, 155–157. https://doi.org/10.1111/1552-6909.1253

Association of Women's Health, Obstetric and Neonatal Nurses. (2018). Marijuana use during pregnancy. AWHONN position statement. *Journal of Obstetric, Gynecologic, & Neonatal Nursing, 47*(5), 719–721.

Association of Women's Health, Obstetric and Neonatal Nurses. (2019). *Standards for professional nursing practice in the care of women and newborns* (8th ed.). Author.

Baldisseri, M. (2016). *Shock and pregnancy.* https://www.uptodate.com/contents/shock in pregnancy

Beam, A. L., Fried, I., Palmer, N., Agniel, D., Brat, G., Fox, K., . . . Armstrong, J. (2020). Estimates of healthcare spending for preterm and low-birthweight infants in a commercially insured population: 2008–2016. *Journal of Perinatology, 40,* 1091–1099. https://doi.org/10.1038/s41372-020-0635-z

Benjamin, E. J., Virani, S. S., Callaway, C. W., Chamberlain, A. M., Chang, A. R., Cheng, S., . . . Muntner, P.; American Heart Association Council on Epidemiology and Prevention Statistics Committee and Stroke Statistics Subcommittee. (2018). Heart disease and stroke statistics—(2018) update: A report from the American Heart Association. *Circulation, 137*(12), e67–e492. https://doi.org/10.1161/CIR.0000000000000558.

Bernstein, P. S., Martin, J. N., Barton, J. R., Shields, L. E., Druzin, M. L., Scavone, B. M., . . . Menard, M. K. (2017). National partnership for maternal safety. *Obstetrics & Gynecology, 130*(2), 347–357. https://doi.org/10.1097/AOG.0000000000002115

Berry, S., Marko, T., & Oneal, G. (2021). Qualitative interpretive metasynthesis of parents' experiences of perinatal loss. *Journal of Obstetric, Gynecologic & Neonatal Nursing, 50*(1), 20–29.

Blackburn, S. (2021). Physiologic changes of pregnancy. In K. Simpson, P. Creehan, N. Obrien-Abel, C. Roth, & A. Rohan (Eds.), *Perinatal nursing* (5th ed., pp. 47–64). Wolters Kluwer.

Bond, D., Middleton, P., Levett, K., van der Ham, D., Crowther, C., Buchanan, S., & Morris, J. (2017). Planned early birth versus expectant management for women with preterm prelabour rupture of membranes prior to 37 weeks' gestation for improving pregnancy outcome. *Cochrane Database of Systematic Reviews, 3,* CD004735. https://doi.org/10.1002/14651858.CD004735.pub4

Bowers, N. (2021). Multiple gestation. In K. Simpson, P. Creehan, N. Obrien-Abel, C. Roth, & A. Rohan (Eds.), *Perinatal nursing* (5th ed., pp. 248–294). Wolters Kluwer.

Bryant, A., Worjoloh, A., Caughey, A., & Washington. A. (2010). Racial/ethnic disparities in obstetric outcomes and care: Prevalence and determinants. *American Journal of Obstetrics & Gynecology, 202*(4), 335–343.

Brown, K. E., & Abdel-Razeq, S. S. (2019). Sepsis in pregnancy. In N. Troiano, P. Witcher, & S. McMurtry Baird (Eds.), *High risk & critical care obstetrics* (4th ed., pp. 296–319). Wolters Kluwer.

Buckwalter, J. G., & Simpson, S. W. (2002). Psychological factors in the etiology and treatment of severe nausea and vomiting in pregnancy. *American Journal of Obstetrics & Gynecology, 186,* S210–S214.

Burgess, A. (2021). Hypertensive disorders of pregnancy. In K. Simpson, P. Creehan, N. Obrien-Abel, C. Roth, & A. Rohan (Eds.), *Perinatal nursing* (5th ed., pp. 98–122). Wolters Kluwer.

Callahan, L. (2016). Management of non-obstetrical surgery and trauma in pregnancy. In S. Mattson & J. E. Smith (Eds.), *Core curriculum for maternal-newborn nursing* (5th ed.). Elsevier.

Caputo, C., Wood, E., & Jabbour, L. (2016). Impact of fetal alcohol exposure on body systems: A systematic review. Birth defects research. Part C. *Embryo Today: Reviews, 108*(2), 174–180. https://doi.org/10.1002/bdrc.21129

Carlson, A., Norwitz, E. R., & Stiller, R. J. (2010). Cytomegalovirus infection in pregnancy: Should all women be screened? *Reviews in Obstetrics & Gynecology, 3*(4), 172–179.

Centers for Disease Control and Prevention. (2015a). *Fact sheet. Reported STDs in the United States. 2015 National Data for chlamydia, gonorrhea and syphilis.* https://www.cdc.gov/nchhstp/newsroom/docs/factsheets/std-trends-508.pdf

Centers for Disease Control. (2015b). Sexually transmitted disease treatment guidelines. *Morbidity and Mortality Weekly Report. Recommendations and Reports, 64*(3), 1–135.

Centers for Disease Control and Prevention. (2015c). *Sexually transmitted disease surveillance.*

Centers for Disease Control and Prevention. (2020). *Discontinuation of transmission-based precautions and disposition of patients with SARS-CoV-2 infection in healthcare settings.* https://www.cdc.gov/coronavirus/2019-ncov/hcp/disposition-hospitalized-patients.html

Centers for Disease Control and Prevention. (2021a). *Sexually transmitted infections prevalence, incidence, and cost estimates in the United States.* https://www.cdc.gov/std/statistics/prevalence-incidence-cost-2020.htm

Centers for Disease Control and Prevention. (2021b). *Women and HIV, March 2021.* https://www.cdc.gov/hiv/pdf/group/gender/women/cdc-hiv-women.pdf

Chasnoff, I. J., Wells, A., McGourty, R. F., & Bailey, L. K. (2007). Validation of the 4P's Plus© screen for substance use in pregnancy. *Journal of Perinatology, 27,* 744–748.

Christopher, D., Robinson, B., & Peaceman, A. (2011). An evidence-based approach to determining route of delivery for twin gestations. *Reviews in Obstetrics & Gynecology, 4*(3–4), 109–116.

Cluver, C. (2017). Planned early delivery versus expectant management for hypertensive disorders from 34 weeks gestation to term. *Cochrane Database of Systematic Reviews, 1.* https://doi.org/10.1002/14651858.CD009273.pub2

Coomarasamy, A., Dhillon-Smith, R. K., Papadopoulou, A., Al Memar, M., Brewin, J., Abrahams, V. M., . . . Quenby, S. (2021). Recurrent miscarriage: Evidence to accelerate action. *Lancet, 397*(10285), 1675–1682. https://doi.org/10.1016/S0140-6736(21)00681-4

Council on Patient Safety in Women's Health Care. (2016). *Reduction in peripartum racial/ethnic disparities.* http://safehealthcareforeverywoman.org

Council on Patient Safety in Women's Health Care. (2017). *Hypertension safety bundle: Severe hypertension in pregnancy.* http://safehealthcareforeverywoman.org/patient-safety-bundles/severe-hypertension-in-pregnancy/

Cowswell, T., Middleton, P., & Weeks, A. (2009). Antenatal day care units versus hospital admission for women with complicated pregnancy. *Cochrane Database of Systematic Reviews, 4,* CD001803. https://doi.org/10.1002/14651858.CD001803.pub2

Creanga, A. A., Syverson, C., Seed, K., & Callaghan, W. M. (2017). Pregnancy-related mortality in the United States, 2011–2013. *Obstetrics & Gynecology, 130,* 366–373.

Crowley, A., Grivell, R., & Dodd, J. (2016). Sealing procedures for preterm prelabour rupture of membranes. *Cochrane Database of Systematic Reviews, 7,* CD010218. https://doi.org/10.1002/14651858.CD010218.pub2

Cunningham, F., Leveno, K., Bloom, S., Dashe, J., Hoffman, B., Casey, B., & Spong, C. (2018). *Williams obstetrics* (25th ed.). McGraw-Hill.

Daley, J. (2014). Diabetes in pregnancy. In K. Simpson & P. Creehan, *Perinatal nursing* (4th ed., pp. 181–198). Lippincott, Williams & Wilkins.

D'Alton, M., Friedman, A., Smiley, R., Montgomery, D., Paidas, M., D'Oria, R., . . . Clark, S. (2016). National Partnership for Maternal Safety: Consensus bundle on venous thromboembolism. *Journal of Obstetric, Gynecologic & Neonatal Nursing, 45*(5), 706–717.

da Silva Lopes, K. (2017). Bed rest with and without hospitalization in multiple pregnancy for improving perinatal outcomes. *Cochrane Database of Systematic Reviews, 4.* https://doi.org/10.1002/14651858.CD012031.pub2

Denny, C. H., Acero, C. S., Naimi, T. S., & Kim, S. Y. (2019). Consumption of alcohol beverages and binge drinking among pregnant women aged 18–44 years—United States, 2015–2017. *Morbidity and Mortality Weekly Report, 68,* 365–368. https://doi.org/10.15585/mmwr.mm6816a1

Di Renzo, G. C., Pacella, E., Di Fabrizio, L., & Giardina, I. (2017). Preterm birth: Risk factors, identification and management. In A. Malvasi, A. Tinelli, & G. Di Renzo (Eds.), *Management and therapy of late pregnancy complications.* Springer. https://doi.org/10.1007/978-3-319-48732-8_6

Dodd, J., Crowther, C., Dare, M., & Middleton, P. (2006). Oral betamimetics for maintenance therapy after threatened preterm labour. *Cochrane Database of Systematic Reviews, 1,* CD003927. https://doi.org/10.1002/14651858.CD003927.pub2

Dodd, J., Jones, L., Flenady, V., Cincotta, R., & Crowther, C. (2013). Prenatal administration of progesterone for preventing preterm birth in women considered to be at risk of preterm birth. *Cochrane Database of Systematic Reviews, 7,* CD004947. https://doi.org/10.1002/14651858.CD004947.pub3

Drake, P., Driscoll, A. K., & Mathews, T. J. (2018). *Cigarette smoking during pregnancy: United States, 2016. NCHS Data Brief No. 305.* National Center for Health Statistics. https://www.cdc.gov/nchs/data/databriefs/db305.pdf

Durham, R. (1998). Strategies women engage in when managing preterm labor at home. *Journal of Perinatology, 18,* 61–64.

East, C. E., Biro, M. A., Fredericks, S., & Lau, R. (2019). Support during pregnancy for women at increased risk of low birthweight babies. *Cochrane Database of Systematic Reviews, 4,* CD000198. https://doi.org/10.1002/14651858.CD000198.pub3

Elkayam, U., Goland, S., Pieper, P. G., & Silverside, C. K. (2016). High-risk cardiac disease in pregnancy: Part I. *Journal of American College of Cardiology, 68,* 396–410.

Elsasser, D., Ananth, C., Prasad, V., Vintzileos, A., & New Jersey-Placental Abruption Study Investigators. (2010). Diagnosis of placental abruption: Relationship between clinical and histopathological findings. *European Journal of Obstetrics, Gynecology, and Reproductive Biology, 148*(2), 125. http://doi.org/10.1016/j.ejogrb.2009.10.005

England, L. J., Bennett, C., Denny, C. H., Honein, M. A., Gilboa, S. M., Kim, S. Y., . . . Boyle, C. (2020). Alcohol use and co-use of other substances among pregnant females aged 12–44 years—United States, 2015–2018. *Morbidity and Mortality Weekly Report, 69,* 1009–1014. https://doi.org/10.15585/mmwr.mm6931a1

Forray, A. (2016). *Substance use during pregnancy. F1000Research, 5, F1000 Faculty Rev–887.* http://doi.org/10.12688/f1000research.7645.1

French, V. (2020). *Coronavirus (COVID-19) and women's health care: A message for patients.* American College of Obstetrics and Gynecology. https://www.acog.org/womens-health/faqs/coronavirus-covid-19-and-womens-health-care?utm_source=redirect&utm_medium=web&utm_campaign=int

Frey, H. A., & Klebanoff, M. A. (2016). The epidemiology, etiology, and costs of preterm birth. *Seminars in Fetal and Neonatal Medicine, 21*(2), 68–73. https://doi.org/10.1016/j.siny.2015.12.011

Genovese, S. K. (2016). Hemorrhagic disorders. In S. Mattson & J. E. Smith (Eds.), *Core curriculum for maternal-newborn nursing* (5th ed.). Elsevier.

Geronimus, A. T. (1992). The weathering hypothesis and the health of African-American women and infants: Evidence and speculations. *Ethnicity & Disease, 2,* 207–221.

Green, P. P., McKnight-Eily, L. R., Tan, C. H., Mejia, R., & Denny, C. H. (2016). Vital signs: Alcohol-exposed pregnancies—United States, 2011–2013. *Morbidity and Mortality Weekly Report, 65,* 91–97. https://doi.org/10.15585/mmwr.mm6504a6external.icon

Grey, B. (2006). A ticking uterus. *Lifelines, 10,* 380–389.

Grobman, W. A., Bailit, J. L., Rice, M. M., Wapner, R. J., Reddy, U. M., Varner, M. W., . . . VanDorsten, J. P. for the Eunice Kennedy Shriver National Institute of Child Health and Human Development (NICHD) Maternal-Fetal Medicine Units (MFMU) Network. (2015). Racial and ethnic disparities in maternal morbidity and obstetric care. *Obstetrics & Gynecology, 125*(6), 1460–1467. https://doi.org/10.1097/AOG.0000000000000735

Haight, S. C., Ko, J. Y., Tong, V. T., Bohm, M. K., & Callaghan, W. M. (2018). Opioid use disorder documented at delivery hospitalization—United States, 1999–2014. *Morbidity and Mortality Weekly Report, 67,* 845–849.

Hales, C. M., Carroll, M. D., Fryar, C. D., & Ogden, C. L. (2020). *Prevalence of obesity and severe obesity among adults: United States, 2017–2018. NCHS Data Brief, no 360.* National Center for Health Statistics.

Han, S., Crowther, C., & Moore, V. (2010). Magnesium maintenance therapy for preventing preterm birth after threatened preterm labour. *Cochrane Database of Systematic Reviews, 7,* CD000940. https://doi.org/10.1002/14651858.CD000940

Hessler, A., & Dolbeck, K. (2021). Clinical updates in women's health care. Seizures. *Obstetrics & Gynecology, 137*(1), 207. https://doi.org/10.1097/AOG.0000000000004211

Howell, E. A., Brown, H., Brumley, J., Bryant, A. S., Caughey, A. B., Cornell, A. M., . . . Grobman, W. A. (2018). Reduction of peripartum racial and ethnic disparities: A conceptual framework and maternal safety consensus bundle. *Obstetrics & Gynecology, 131*(5), 770–782. https://doi.org/10.1097/AOG.0000000000002475

Hudak, M. L., Tan, R. C., & Committee on Drugs and Committee on Fetus and Newborn. (2014). Neonatal drug withdrawal. *Pediatrics, 133*(5), 937–938.

Iams, J. (2007). Predication and early detection of preterm labor. In J. Queenan (Ed.), *High risk pregnancy.* American College of Obstetricians and Gynecologists.

Jackson, F., Rashied-Henry, K., Braveman, P., Dominguez, T., Ramos, D., Maseru, N., . . . James, A. (2020). A prematurity collaborative birth equity consensus statement for mothers and babies. *Maternal and Child Health Journal, 24,* 1231–1237. https://doi.org/10.1007/s10995-020-02960-0

Jatlaoui, T., Ewing, A., Mandel, M., Simmons, K., Suchdev, D., Jamieson, D., & Pazol, K. (2016). Abortion surveillance—United States, 2013. *MMWR Surveillance Summary, 65*(12), 1–44. https://www.cdc.gov/mmwr/volumes/65/ss/ss6512a1.htm

Jazayeri, A. (2016). *Premature rupture of membranes.* https://emedicine.medscape.com/article/261137-overview

Jones, R. K., Witwer, E., & Jerman, J. (2019). *Abortion incidence and service availability in the United States, 2017.* Guttmacher Institute. https://www.guttmacher.org/report/abortion-incidence-service-availability-us-2017

Kelley, C., & Weaver, A. (2019). *Diabetes mellitus. Clinical updates in women's health care.* American College of Obstetricians and Gynecologists.

Keough, L., & Fantasia, H. (2017). Pharmacologic treatment of opioid addiction during pregnancy. *Nursing for Women's Health, 21*(1), 34–44.

Khurana, R. (2017). *Systemic lupus erythematosus and pregnancy.* https://emedicine.medscape.com/article/335055-overview

Krening, C., Troiano, N., & Shah, S. (2019). Maternal cardiac disorders. In N. Troiano, P. Witcher, & S. McMurtry Baird (Eds.), *High risk & critical care obstetrics* (4th ed., pp. 134–154). Wolters Kluwer.

Lancet. (2021). Miscarriage: Worldwide reform of care is needed. *Lancet, 397*(10285), 1597. https://doi.org/10.1016/S0140-6736(21)00954-5

Maharaj, D. (2007). Intrapartum fetal resuscitation: A review. *Internet Journal of Gynecology and Obstetrics, 9*(2), 1–11.

Maher, M. (2021). Obesity in pregnancy. In K. Simpson, P. Creehan, N. Obrien-Abel, C. Roth, & A. Rohan (Eds.), *Perinatal nursing* (5th ed., pp. 295–313). Wolters Kluwer.

Maloni, J. A. (1998). *Antepartum bedrest: Case studies, research & nursing care.* Association of Women's Health, Obstetric and Neonatal Nurses.

March of Dimes. (2015). *Perinatal data snapshots: United States: Maternal and infant health overview.* http://www.marchofdimes.com

March of Dimes. (2016). *Fetal alcohol syndrome disorders.* http://www.marchofdimes.com

March of Dimes. (2018a). *Guiding principles to achieving equity in preterm birth.* https://www.marchofdimes.org/materials/PC18-02%20PrematurityCollaborative2018SummitReport_F.pdf

March of Dimes. (2018b). *Preterm labor and preterm birth: Are you at risk?* https://www.marchofdimes.org/complications/preterm-labor-and-preterm-birth-are-you-at-risk.aspx

March of Dimes. (2018c). *2018 Premature birth report card.* https://www.marchofdimes.org/mission/prematurity-reportcard.aspx

March of Dimes. (2020). *March of Dimes report card 2020 United States.* https://www.marchofdimes.org/mission/prematurity-reportcard.aspx

Mark, K., Desai, A., & Terplan, M. (2016). Marijuana use and pregnancy: Prevalence, associated characteristics, and birth outcomes. *Archives Women's Mental Health, 19*(1), 105–111.

Martin, J. A., Hamilton, B. E., Osterman, M. J. K., & Driscoll, A. K. (2019). Births: Final data for 2018. *National Vital Statistics Reports, 68*(13), 1–44. National Center for Health Statistics.

Mason, B. A., & Burke, C. (2019). Pulmonary disorders in pregnancy. In N. Troiano, P. Witcher, & S. McMurtry Baird (Eds.), *High risk & critical care obstetrics* (4th ed., pp. 155–175). Wolters Kluwer.

Matthews, A., Haas, D. M., O'Mathúna, D. P., & Dowswell, T. (2015). Interventions for nausea and vomiting in early pregnancy. *Cochrane Database of Systematic Reviews, 9,* CD007575. https://doi.org/10.1002/14651858.CD007575.pub4

Mattson, S., & Smith, J. E. (Eds.). (2011). *Core curriculum for maternal-newborn nursing* (4th ed.). Elsevier Saunders.

McMurtry Baird, S., & Fox, K. (2019). Morbidly adherent placenta. In N. Troiano, P. Witcher, & S. McMurtry Baird (Eds.), *High risk & critical care obstetrics* (4th ed., pp. 244–257). Wolters Kluwer.

McMurtry Baird, S., & Kennedy, B. (2021). Pulmonary complications in pregnancy. In K. Simpson, P. Creehan, N. Obrien-Abel, C. Roth, & A. Rohan (Eds.), *Perinatal nursing* (5th ed., pp. 220–247). Wolters Kluwer.

Mendez-Figueroa, H., Dahlke, J. D., Vrees, R. A., & Rouse, D. J. (2013). Trauma in pregnancy: An updated systematic review. *American Journal of Obstetrics & Gynecology, 209,* 1.

National Academies of Sciences, Engineering, and Medicine. (2019). *Vibrant and healthy kids: Aligning science, practice, and policy to advance health equity.* The National Academies Press.

National High Blood Pressure Education Program. (2000). *Working group report on high blood pressure in pregnancy* (NHBPEP Publication No. 00-3029). National Heart Lung and Blood Institute.

National Institute on Drug Abuse. (2013). *Commonly abused drugs.* https://www.drugabuse.gov/

National Institute on Drug Abuse. (2014). *America's addiction to opioids: Heroin and prescription drug abuse.* National Institute on Drug Abuse. https://www.drugabuse.gov/about-nida/legislative-activities/testimony-to-congress/2016/americas-addiction-to-opioids-heroin-prescription-drug-abuse

National Institute on Drug Abuse. (2018a). *Marijuana drug use increasing during pregnancy.* https://www.drugabuse.gov/news-events/science-highlight/marijuana-drug-use-increasing-during-pregnancy

National Institute on Drug Abuse. (2018b). *What science says about tobacco + marijuana + pregnancy.* https://www.drugabuse.gov/news-events/science-highlight/what-science-says-about-tobacco-marijuana-pregnancy

National Institute on Drug Abuse. (2020a). *Prenatal cannabis exposure alters brain reward circuitry in male rats.* https://www.drugabuse.gov/news-events/nida-notes/2020/08/prenatal-cannabis-exposure-alters-brain-reward-circuitry-in-male-rats

National Institute on Drug Abuse. (2020b). *What are the risks of smoking during pregnancy?* https://www.drugabuse.gov/publications/research-reports/tobacco-nicotine-e-cigarettes/what-are-risks-smoking-during-pregnancy

Neilson, J. (2009). Interventions for suspected placenta previa. *Cochrane Database of Systematic Reviews, 1.* https://doi.org/10.1002/14651858.CD001998

Nesheim, S. R., FitzHarris, L. F., Lampe, M. A., & Gray, K. M. (2018). Reconsidering the number of women with HIV infection who give birth annually in the United States. *Public Health Reports, 133*(6), 637–643. https://doi.org/10.1177/0033354918800466

Norwitz, E., & Caughey, A. (2011). Progesterone supplementation and the prevention of preterm birth. *Reviews in Obstetrics & Gynecology, 4*(2), 60–72.

Office of Disease Prevention and Health Promotion, Office of the Assistant Secretary for Health, Office of the Secretary, U.S. Department of Health and Human Services. (2020). *Preterm births.* https://www.healthypeople.gov/2020/healthy-people-in-action/story/the-ohio-perinatal-quality-collaborative-an-evidence-based-data-driven-approach-to-reducing-preterm

Opray, N., Grivell, R., Deussen, A., & Dodd, J. (2015). Directed preconception health programs and interventions for improving pregnancy outcomes for women who are overweight or obese. *Cochrane Database of Systematic Reviews, 7,* CD010932. https://doi.org/10.1002/14651858.CD010932.pub2

Owen, J., & Harger, J. (2007). Cerclage and cervical incompetency. In J. Queenan (Ed.), *High risk pregnancy.* American College of Obstetrics and Gynecologists.

Panel on Treatment of Pregnant Women With HIV Infection and Prevention of Perinatal Transmission. (2018). *Recommendations for use of antiretroviral drugs in transmission in the United States.* https://health.gov/healthypeople/tools-action/browse-evidence-based-resources/recommendations-use-antiretroviral-drugs-pregnant-women-hiv-infection-and-interventions-reduce-perinatal-hiv-transmission-united-states

Panelli, D., Phillips, C., & Brady. P. (2015). Incidence, diagnosis and management of tubal and nontubal ectopic pregnancies: A review. *Fertility Research and Practice, 1,* 15.

Parfitt, S. (2021). Preterm labor and birth. In K. Simpson, P. Creehan, N. Obrien-Abel, C. Roth, & A. Rohan (Eds.), *Perinatal nursing* (5th ed.). Wolters Kluwer.

PeriStats. (2017). *National Center for Health Statistics, final natality data.* http://www.marchofdimes.com/peristats

Phillips, C., & Boyd, M. (2015). Intrahepatic cholestasis of pregnancy. *Nursing for Women's Health, 19*(1), 46–57.

Phillips, C., & Boyd, M. (2016). Assessment, management, and health implications of early-onset preeclampsia. *Nursing for Women's Health, 20*(4), 402–414.

Pirjani, R., Moini, A., Almasi-Hashiani, A., Farid Mojtahedi, M., Vesali, S., Hosseini, L., & Sepidarkish, M. (2021). Placental alpha microglobulin-1 (PartoSure) test for the prediction of preterm birth: a systematic review and meta-analysis. *The Journal of Maternal-Fetal & Neonatal Medicine, 34*(20), 3445–3457. https://doi.org/10.1080/14767058.2019.1685962

Prather, C., Fuller, T. R., Jeffries, W. L., Marshall, K. J., Howell, A. V., Belyue-Umole, A., & King, W. (2018). Racism and African American women, and their sexual and reproductive health: A review of historical and contemporary evidence and implications for health equity. *Health Equity, 2*(1), 249–259.

Quenby, S., Gallos, I. D., Dhillon-Smith, R. K., Podesek, M., Stephenson, M. D., Fisher, J., . . . Coomarasamy, A. (2021). Miscarriage matters: The epidemiological, physical, psychological, and economic costs of early pregnancy loss. *Lancet, 397*(10285), 1658–1667. https://doi.org/10.1016/S0140-6736(21)00682-6

Raju, T. N., Mercer, B. M., Burchfield, D. J., & Joseph, G. F., Jr. (2014). Periviable birth: Executive summary of a joint workshop by the Eunice Kennedy Shriver National Institute of Child Health and Human Development, Society for Maternal-Fetal Medicine, American Academy of Pediatrics, and American College of Obstetricians and Gynecologists. *Obstetrics & Gynecology, 123,* 1083–1096.

Roberts, D., Brown, J., Medley, N., & Dalziel, S. R. (2017). Antenatal corticosteroids for accelerating fetal lung maturation for women at risk of preterm birth. *Cochrane Database of Systematic Reviews, 3,* CD004454. https://doi.org/10.1002/14651858.CD004454.pub3

Roth, C. (2021a). Diabetes in pregnancy. In K. Simpson, P. Creehan, N. Obrien-Abel, C. Roth, & A. Rohan (Eds.), *Perinatal nursing* (5th ed., pp. 181–198). Wolters Kluwer.

Roth, C. (2021b). Pulmonary complications in pregnancy. In K. Simpson, P. Creehan, N. Obrien-Abel, C. Roth, & A. Rohan (Eds.), *Perinatal nursing* (5th ed., pp. 220–247). Wolters Kluwer.

Ruth, D., & Mighty, H. (2019). Trauma in pregnancy. In N. Troiano, P. Witcher, & S. McMurtry Baird (Eds.), *High risk & critical care obstetrics* (4th ed.). Wolters Kluwer.

Salera-Vieira, J. (2021). Bleeding in pregnancy. In K. Simpson, P. Creehan, N. Obrien-Abel, C. Roth, & A. Rohan (Eds.), *Perinatal nursing* (5th ed., pp. 123–140). Wolters Kluwer.

Sazgar, M. (2019). Treatment of women with epilepsy. *Continuum, 25,* 408–430.

Schillie, S., Wester, C., Osborne, M., Wesolowski, L., & Ryerson, A. B. (2020). CDC recommendations for hepatitis C screening among adults—United States, 2020. *Morbidity and Mortality Weekly Report, 69*(RR-2), 1–17. https://doi.org/10.15585/mmwr.rr6902a1

Schwulst, S. J., & Son, M. (2020). Management of gallstone disease during pregnancy. *Journal of the American Medical Association Surgery, 155*(12), 1162–1163. https://doi.org/10.1001/jamasurg.2020.3683

Shah, P., & Shah, J. (2010). Maternal exposure to domestic violence and pregnancy and birth outcomes: A systematic review and meta-analyses. *Journal of Women's Health, 19*(11), 2017–2031. https://doi.org/10.1089/jwh.2010.2051

Shah, P., Zao, J., & Ali, S. (2011). Maternal marital status and birth outcomes: A systematic review and meta-analyses. *Maternal & Child Health Journal, 15*(7), 1097–1109. https://doi.org/10.1007/s10995-010-0654-z

Sibai, B. (2004). Diagnosis, controversies, and management of the syndrome of hemolysis, elevated liver enzymes, and low platelet count [High Risk Pregnancy Series: An expert's view]. *Obstetrics & Gynecology, 103,* 981–991.

Silver, R. (2015). Abnormal placentation: Placenta previa, vasa previa, and placenta accreta. *Obstetrics & Gynecology, 26*(3), 654–668.

Silver, R. M., Landon, M. B., Rouse, D. J., Leveno, K. J., Spong, C. Y., Thom, E. A., . . . Mercer, B. M. (2006). Maternal morbidity associated with multiple repeat cesarean deliveries. National Institute of Child Health and Human Development Maternal-Fetal Medicine Units Network. *Obstetrics & Gynecology, 107,* 1226–1232.

Singer, M., Deutschman, C. S., Seymour, C. W., Shankar-Hari, M., Annane, D., Bauer, M., . . . Angus, D. C. (2016). The Third International Consensus Definitions for Sepsis and Septic Shock (Sepsis-3). *Journal of the American Medical Association, 315,* 801–810.

Society for Maternal-Fetal Medicine & Gyamfi-Bannerman, C. (2018). Society for Maternal-Fetal Medicine consult series #44: Management of bleeding in the late preterm period. *American Journal of Obstetrics and Gynecology, 218*(1), B2–B8. https://doi.org/10.1016/j.ajog.2017.10.019

Society for Maternal-Fetal Medicine, Hughes, B. L., Page, C. M., & Kuller, J. A. (2017). Hepatitis C in pregnancy: Screening, treatment, and management. *American Journal of Obstetrics and Gynecology, 217*(5), B2–B12. https://doi.org/10.1016/j.ajog.2017.07.039

Substance Abuse and Mental Health Services Administration, (2014). *Substance Abuse and Mental Health Services Administration, Results from the 2013 National Survey on Drug Use and Health: Summary of National Findings,* NSDUH Series H-48, HHS Publication No. (SMA) 14-4863. Rockville, MD:

Substance Abuse and Mental Health Services Administration. (2019). *Key substance use and mental health indicators in the United States: Results from the 2018 National Survey on Drug Use and Health.* Center for Behavioral Health Statistics and Quality, SAMHSA.

Sullivan, C. (2016). Substance abuse in pregnancy. In S. Mattson & J. E. Smith (Eds.), *Core curriculum for maternal-newborn nursing* (5th ed.). Elsevier.

Swartz, A., Hoffmann, T. J., Cretti, E., Burton, C. W., Eagen-Torkko, M., Levi, A. J., . . . McLemore, M. R. (2020). Attitudes of California registered nurses about abortion. *Journal of Obstetric, Gynecologic & Neonatal Nursing, 49*(5), 475–486. https://www.jognn.org/article/S0884-2175%2820%2930106-4/fulltext

Sweetland, J. (2018). *Evidence based messaging on birth equity.* FrameWorks Institute

Task Force on Hypertension in Pregnancy and American College of Obstetricians and Gynecologists. (2013). *Hypertension in pregnancy.* https://journals.lww.com/greenjournal/Fulltext/2013/11000/Hypertension_in_Pregnancy__Executive_Summary.36.aspx. https://www.acog.org/Clinical-Guidance-and-Publications/Task-Force-and-Work-Group-Reports/Hypertension-in-Pregnancy

Taylor, P., Zaichkin, J., & Bailey, D. (2002). *Substance abuse during pregnancy: Guidelines for screening.* http://contentmanager.med.uvm.edu/docs/default-source/vchip-documents/vchip_screening_for_preg_subabuse.pdf?sfvrsn=2

Thakur, M., & Mahajan, K. (2020). Cervical incompetence. *StatPearls.* https://www.ncbi.nlm.nih.gov/books/NBK525954/

Tikkanen, M. (2011). Placental abruption: Epidemiology, risk factors and consequences. *Acta Obstetricia et Gynecologica Scandinavica, 90,* 140.

Upadhyay, U. D., Desai, S., Zlidar, V., Weitz, T. A., Grossman, D., Anderson, P., & Taylor, D. (2015). Incidence of emergency department visits and complications after abortion. *Obstetrics & Gynecology, 125,* 175–183. https://doi.org/10.1097/AOG.0000000000000603

U.S. Department of Health and Human Services. (2018). *Recommendations for the use of antiretroviral drugs in pregnant women with HIV infection and interventions to reduce perinatal HIV transmission in the United States.* Author. https://aidsinfo.nih.gov/guidelines

U.S. Surgeon General. (2019). U.S. Surgeon General warning on marijuana use in adolescence and during pregnancy. https://nida.nih.gov/news-events/emerging-trend/us-surgeon-general-warning-marijuana-use-in-adolescence-during-pregnancy on 2022

Van Otterloo, L. (2016). Trauma in pregnancy. In S. Mattson & J. E. Smith (Eds.), *Core curriculum for maternal-newborn nursing* (5th ed.). Elsevier.

Williamson, C., & Geenes, V. (2014). Intrahepatic cholestasis of pregnancy. *Obstetrics & Gynecology, 124,* 120–133. https://doi.org/10.1097/AOG.0000000000000346

Yancy, M. (2016). Other medical complications. In S. Mattson & J. E. Smith (Eds.), *Core curriculum for maternal-newborn nursing* (5th ed.). Elsevier.

Young-Wolff, K. C., Tucker, L. Y., Alexeeff, S., Armstrong, M. A., Conway, A., Weisner, C., & Goler, N. (2017). Trends in self-reported and biochemically tested marijuana use among pregnant females in California from 2009–2016. *Journal of the American Medical Association, 318*(24), 2490–2491. https://doi.org/10.1001/jama.2017.17225

Zahn, C. (2020). *ACOG statement on COVID-19 and pregnancy.* American College of Obstetricians and Gynecologists. https://www.acog.org/news/news-releases/2020/06/acog-statement-on-covid-19-and-pregnancy

Zhang, G., Feenstra, B., Bacelis, J., Liu, X., Muglia, L. M., Juodakis, J., . . . Muglia, L. J. (2017). Genetic associations with gestational duration and spontaneous preterm birth. *New England Journal of Medicine, 377*(12), 1156–1164.

The Intrapartal Period

8

Labor and Birth

Susan Forsyth, PhD, RN

LEARNING OUTCOMES

Upon completion of this chapter, the student will be able to:
1. Describe the four stages of labor and the related nursing and medical care.
2. Demonstrate understanding of supportive care of laboring women.
3. Identify the five Ps of labor.
4. Describe the mechanism of spontaneous vaginal delivery and related nursing care.
5. Describe both pharmacological and nonpharmacological pain relief interventions.

CONCEPTS

Caring
Clinical Judgment
Collaboration
Comfort
Communication
Elimination
Evidence-Based Practice
Family
Fluid and Electrolytes
Grief and Loss
Infection
Mobility
Mood and Affect
Oxygenation
Perfusion
Safety
Self
Stress and Coping
Tissue Integrity

Nursing Diagnosis

- Deficient knowledge related to the birthing process
- Risk for acute pain related to uterine contractions (UCs), and stretching of the cervix, birth canal, and introitus
- Risk for anxiety related to fear of the unknown, such as fear of the birthing process
- Risk for fatigue related to the child birthing process

Nursing Outcomes

- The woman and support people will understand the processes and interventions related to labor.
- The woman will be educated on and offered appropriate pain interventions.
- The woman will verbalize satisfaction with pain control interventions.

Continued

Nursing Diagnosis—cont'd

- Risk of infection related to tissue trauma, multiple vaginal exams, episiotomy/laceration, and prolonged rupture of membranes (ROM)
- Risk of impaired tissue integrity related to passage of the fetus through the birth canal
- Risk of ineffective fetal oxygen perfusion related to interference with maternal-fetal gas exchange
- Risk for impaired urinary elimination related to the birthing process, tissue trauma, or epidural administration
- Risk of fluid volume deficit related to the excessive loss of blood
- Risk of impaired family coping related to situational crises

Nursing Outcomes—cont'd

- The woman will be continually physically and emotionally supported during the laboring process by the RN and the woman's chosen support people.
- The woman and fetus will remain physiologically stable throughout the laboring process.
- The woman and fetus or newborn will be free of signs and symptoms of infection.

INTRODUCTION

The intrapartum period begins with the onset of regular uterine contractions (UCs) and lasts until the expulsion of the placenta. This process is called labor and consists of three distinct stages: dilation and effacement, expulsion of the fetus, and expulsion of the placenta. More recently, a fourth recovery stage has been added to highlight the importance of the immediate postpartum period. This chapter discusses the intrapartum or childbirth process, including the factors affecting labor and delivery, progression of labor and delivery, the immediate postpartum period, and the nursing care involved.

LABOR TRIGGERS

Labor is a multifactorial physiological process involving sequential and coordinated changes of the cervix, myometrium, and decidua resulting in delivery of the fetus and the placenta from the uterus. How labor is initiated is still an area of active research. We do know that initiation of labor is a complex process involving stretching of uterine muscles and the inhibition of progesterone (the "pro pregnancy" hormone) and other hormones that quiet the uterus (uterine quiescent hormones). With the suppression of hormones that have kept the uterus quiet, hormones that promote uterine contractility are activated, primarily estradiol, oxytocin, and prostaglandins (Ravanos et al., 2015). These hormones work together to inhibit calcium binding in muscle cells, raising intracellular calcium levels and activating contractions. The fetus appears to also help control the timing of labor through the activation of the fetal hypothalamic-pituitary-adrenal axis. This results in a sharp rise in fetal cortisol production, which stimulates the placenta to produce corticotropin-releasing hormone. This results in an inflammatory process and the release of prostaglandins, promoting the start of labor (Norwitz et al., 2021) (Fig. 8–1).

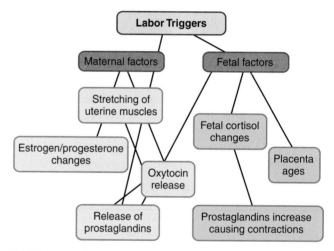

FIGURE 8–1 Labor triggers.

Maternal Factors

- Uterine muscles are stretched to the threshold point, leading to the release of prostaglandins and oxytocin that stimulate contractions.
- Increased pressure on the cervix stimulates the nerve plexus, causing the release of oxytocin by the maternal pituitary gland, which then stimulates contractions.
- Estrogen levels increase, enhancing the ability of uterine myometrium to produce contractions.
- Progesterone is functionally withdrawn.
- Oxytocin and prostaglandins, which have been previously inhibited by progesterone, together soften the cervix and stimulate myometrial contractions.

Fetal Factors

- Prostaglandin synthesis by the fetal membranes and the decidua stimulates contractions.
- Produced by the fetal hypothalamic-pituitary-adrenal axis, fetal cortisol levels increase, and, acting on the placenta, cause an inflammatory response and an increased level of prostaglandins, stimulating the uterus to contract.

SIGNS OF IMPENDING LABOR

A few weeks before labor begins, the body begins to exhibit signs and symptoms in preparation. These changes are also referred to as premonitory signs of labor.

- Lightening: In primiparas, approximately 2 weeks before labor begins, the fetus descends into the true pelvis. Women may feel they can breathe more easily as the pressure of the diaphragm decreases, but they often experience urinary frequency at this stage from increased bladder pressure. In subsequent pregnancies, this may not occur until labor begins.
- Braxton-Hicks: All women will experience Braxton-Hicks contractions. These irregular, uncoordinated contractions do not result in cervical change and are associated with "false labor." They are commonly felt in the second and third trimester and may feel similar to mild menstrual cramps over a specific section of the abdomen. They do not increase in frequency, duration, or intensity and will disappear entirely only to reappear at a later time. They are thought to prepare the uterus for true labor by toning it, and are sometimes called "practice labor" (Raines & Cooper, 2021).
- Cervical changes: The cervix ripens, becomes soft, moves from a posterior position to an anterior position, and may become partially effaced or thinned out and begin to dilate.
- Losing the mucus plug: The mucus plug is a viscous collection of mucus that seals the cervix shut. Many women lose it before the beginning of labor.
- An increase in vaginal discharge: As the cervix begins to soften and open, small blood vessels are broken, resulting in pink or red streaked discharge; along with the mucus plug, this is known as "bloody show."
- Nesting: Some women experience a burst of energy or feel the need to put everything in order, which is sometimes referred to as nesting.
- Less commonly, some women experience a 1- to 3-pound weight loss and others experience diarrhea, nausea, or indigestion preceding labor.
- Women may experience low backache and sacroiliac discomfort due in part to the relaxation of the pelvic joints.

FACTORS AFFECTING LABOR

The onset of labor is defined as progressive cervical dilation and effacement with regular uterine contractions (UC) (AAP Committee on Fetus and Newborn and ACOG Committee on Obstetric Practice, 2017). For vaginal delivery, labor must first occur, resulting in complete dilation and effacement of the cervix, culminating in the descent of the fetus through the cervix, vagina, and introitus. Factors identified as essential to successful vaginal birth include the 5 "Ps."

- Powers (the contractions and pushing efforts)
- Passage (the pelvis and birth canal)
- Passenger (the fetus)
- Psyche (the response of the woman)
- Position (positions that facilitate labor and birth)

Powers

The powers of labor are divided into two categories: (1) involuntary UCs resulting in dilation and effacement of the cervix, known as primary powers; and (2) the voluntary expulsive efforts of the birthing woman during the second stage of labor, known as secondary powers. As the pregnant body begins the laboring process, the uterine muscle, the myometrium, becomes highly sensitive to oxytocin. Oxytocin, synthesized by the hypothalamus and released by the posterior pituitary, is the most potent uterotonic (contraction promoting) hormone produced (Norwitz et al., 2021). Although still being studied, research suggests that contractions are controlled by pacemaker-type myocytes that send electrical pulses initiating coordinated myometrial contractile responses (Garfield et al., 2021). Contractions begin in the fundus (apex) of the uterus and proceed in a peristaltic manner down the uterine walls toward the cervix, both propelling the fetus downward and dilating and effacing the cervix.

Primary Powers: Uterine Contractions

- The myometrium contracts and shortens during the first stage of labor. The myometrium has two segments:
  - The muscular upper uterine segment, composed of the upper two-thirds of the uterus, which contracts to push the fetus down.
  - The less muscular and more elastic lower uterine segment, composed of the lower third of the uterus and the cervix, which allows the cervix to become thinner and pulled upward.
- UCs are responsible for the dilation (opening) and effacement (thinning) of the cervix in the first stage of labor.
- UCs are rhythmic and intermittent.
- Each contraction has a resting phase or uterine relaxation period that allows the uterine muscle a pause for rest. At term, the uteroplacental blood flow is estimated to be 500 to 750 mL/min. During a contraction, the blood flow is decreased in proportion to the strength of the contraction, decreasing the oxygen transfer from parent to fetus. Fetuses have multiple compensatory mechanisms to cope and usually are able to tolerate this stress (Turner et al., 2020). The period between contractions allows uteroplacental blood flow to be restored, the fetus to be reoxygenated, and waste to be removed.
- UCs are described in the following ways (Fig. 8–2):
  - Frequency: Time from beginning of one contraction to the beginning of another. It is recorded in minutes (e.g., occurring every 3 to 4 minutes).
  - Duration: Time from the beginning of a contraction to the end of the contraction. It is recorded in seconds (e.g., each contraction lasts 45 to 50 seconds).
  - Intensity: Strength of the contraction. The intensity may be evaluated by palpation or with an intrauterine pressure

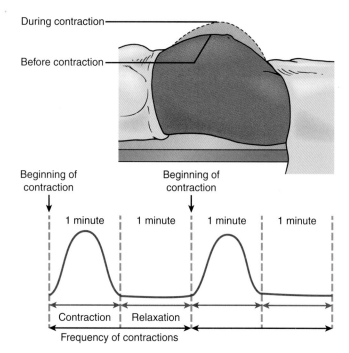

FIGURE 8-2 Frequency and duration of a contraction.

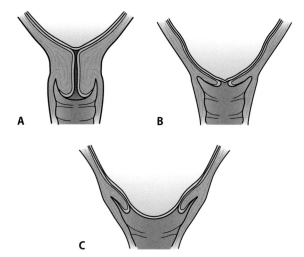

FIGURE 8-3 Cervical effacement and dilation. (A) Cervix before labor is closed and not effaced. (B) Cervix in latent phase of labor is effaced and starting to dilate. (C) Cervix in labor is effaced and dilating.

catheter (IUPC). An IUPC is an internal monitor placed in the uterus to allow accurate measurement of the strength, duration, and frequency of contractions. If using palpation, contractions are categorized as:

- Mild: The uterine wall is easily indented during contraction. It feels similar to the tip of a nose.
- Moderate: The uterine wall is resistant to indentation during a contraction. It feels similar to a chin.
- Strong: The uterine wall cannot be indented during a contraction. It feels similar to a forehead.
- If an IUPC is used, the intensity is measured in mm Hg.
- Uterine resting tone between contractions: assessed between contractions and described as either hard or soft, or in mm Hg if using an IUPC.
- A contraction has three phases (see Fig. 8–2):
  - Increment phase: The buildup of the contraction that begins in the fundus and spreads throughout the uterus; the longest part of the contraction.
  - Acme phase: Peak of intensity but the shortest part of the contraction.
  - Decrement phase: The relaxation of the uterine muscle.
- Contractions facilitate cervical changes (Fig. 8–3A, B, C).
  - Dilation and effacement occur during the first stage of labor when UCs push the presenting part of the fetus toward the cervix, causing it to open and thin out as the musculofibrous tissue of the cervix is drawn upward (see Fig. 8–3B).
  - Dilation is the enlargement or opening of the cervical os.
    - The cervix dilates from closed (or less than 1 cm diameter) to 10 cm diameter (see Fig. 8–3C).
    - When the cervix reaches 10 cm dilation, it is considered completely dilated and can no longer be palpated on vaginal examination.

- Effacement is the softening, shortening, and thinning of the cervix (Fig. 8–3).
  - Before the onset of labor, the cervix is 2 to 3 cm long (Fig. 8–3A).
  - When completely effaced, the cervix is just a few sheets of paper thick.
  - The degree of effacement is measured in percentage and goes from 0% (not effaced) to 100% (completely effaced).
  - Effacement often precedes dilation in a first-time pregnancy.

Secondary Powers: Voluntary Expulsive Efforts

Once the cervix is fully dilated (10 cm) and the woman feels the urge to push, she will often involuntarily bear down. Epidurals may blunt this urge. Women should not attempt to push before the cervix is fully dilated as this may damage and/or swell the cervix. As the fetus descends through the cervix and the presenting part reaches the pelvic floor, the Ferguson reflex is triggered, activating stretch receptors that send impulses to the hypothalamus, resulting in an acceleration of oxytocin release stimulating stronger contractions (Uvnäs-Moberg et al., 2019).

The most effective method of pushing for maintaining fetal homeostasis and maternal well-being has been continually debated. The active pushing phase of labor is the most stressful phase for the fetus and has the highest likelihood of negatively affecting fetal acid–base balance. Current research has not found a clear difference in outcomes for the fetus or parent when nurse-directed pushing is used (the nurse directs the patient to Valsalva and keep a closed glottis during the pushing efforts) versus spontaneous pushing, where the patient is directed to push the way her body tells her, including keeping an open glottis (Barasinski et al., 2020; Lemos et al., 2017)

Current guidelines suggest that the woman be encouraged to push for 6 to 8 seconds, followed by a slight exhale, repeating the effort three to four times per contraction as tolerated by the parent and the fetus. Some birthing women may choose open-glottis pushing with expiratory noises, whereas others sustained hold their breath. Sustained, strong pushing coupled with prolonged breath-holding should be discouraged and the nurse should not use directed counting techniques (for example, counting to 10 while the woman pushes) (Association of Women's Health, Obstetric and Neonatal Nurses [AWHONN], 2019).

Passage

The passage includes the bony pelvis and the soft tissues of the cervix, pelvic floor, vagina, and introitus (external opening to the vagina). Although all these anatomical structures play a role in the birth, the size and shape of the maternal pelvis are the most important determinants in whether the fetus will deliver vaginally. Assessment of the pelvis is performed manually through palpation with a vaginal exam by the care provider during pregnancy.

Pelvis

- Types of bony pelvis (Fig. 8–4):
  - Gynecoid: Most common type occurring in 41% to 42% of women and considered optimal for childbearing due to its rounded shape (King et al., 2019).
  - Android: Inlet is heart-shaped with limited space in the posterior pelvis for accommodating the fetal head. This shape may make vaginal birth more difficult (King et al., 2019).
  - Anthropoid: Inlet is oval shaped, with a narrower pubic arch, which is usually adequate for childbirth (King et al., 2019).
  - Platypelloid: Least common type found in about 3% of women. Has a flat inlet and a short anterior-posterior diameter, making childbirth more difficult (King et al., 2019).

- The anatomical structures of the pelvis include the ileum, the ischium, the pubis, the sacrum, and the coccyx (Fig. 8–5).
- The bony pelvis is divided into:
  - False pelvis, which is the shallow upper section of the pelvis.
  - True pelvis, which is the lower part of the pelvis and consists of three planes, the inlet, the midpelvis, and the outlet. The measurement of these three planes defines the obstetric capacity of the pelvis.
- The pelvic joints include the symphysis pubis, the right and the left sacroiliac joints, and the sacrococcygeal joints.
- During pregnancy, the hormones estrogen and relaxin soften cartilage and increase elasticity of the ligaments, allowing the joints to stretch, making room for the fetal head.
- Station refers to the relationship of the ischial spines to the presenting part of the fetus and assists in assessing fetal descent during labor (Fig. 8–6). At 0 station, the fetal head is even with the ischial spines. Station 0 is also the narrowest diameter the fetus must pass through during a vaginal birth.

Soft Tissue

- The cervix is made up of fibrous connective tissues that efface and dilate during labor, allowing the fetus to descend into the vagina.
- Ideally, when the fetal head encounters resistance from the pelvic floor muscles, the mentum (fetal chin) is flexed toward the fetal thorax, and the occiput is directed toward the maternal symphysis, resulting in an optimal position for moving through the pelvis.
- The soft tissue of the vagina expands to allow passage of the fetus.
- A full bladder may impede the progress of the fetus through the pelvis.

	Shape	Inlet	Midpelvis	Outlet
Gynecoid				
Android				
Anthropoid				
Platypelloid				

FIGURE 8–4 Pelvic types: gynecoid, android, anthropoid, and platypelloid.

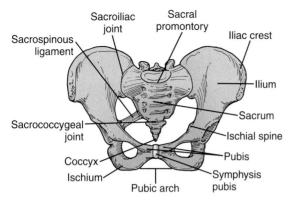

FIGURE 8–5 Anatomical structures of the pelvis.

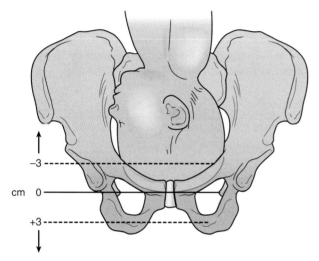

FIGURE 8–6 Station of presenting part: Fetal head in relation to ischial spines.

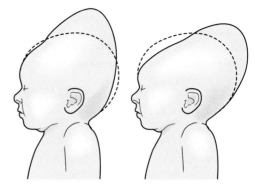

FIGURE 8–7 Molding of the fetal head.

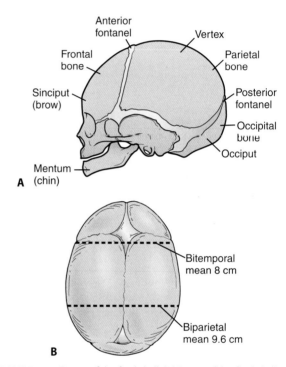

FIGURE 8–8 Bones of the fetal skull. (A) Bones of the fetal skull (side view). (B) Diameter of the fetal skull.

Passenger

The fetus is the passenger. The fetus must successfully transit through the passageway for a vaginal birth to occur. The relationship between the fetus and the passageway is affected by the fetal skull shape and size, fetal attitude, fetal lie, fetal presentation, fetal position, and fetal size. Each of these factors plays an important role in determining the route of delivery.

Fetal Skull

- The fetal head usually accounts for the largest portion of the fetus to come through the birth canal.
- The fetal head is able to mold. Molding is the ability of the fetal head to change shape to accommodate or fit through the maternal pelvis (Fig. 8–7).
- The fetal skull comprises two parietal bones, two temporal bones, the frontal bone, and the occipital bone (Fig. 8–8A).
  - The biparietal diameter (BPD) (mean of 9.6 cm at 40 weeks) (Kiserud et al., 2017) is the largest transverse measurement and an important indicator of head size (see Fig. 8–8B).
  - The membranous spaces between the bones are called the cranial sutures. Fontanels, also called soft spots, are the

intersections of these sutures. There are two fontanels in the fetal skull, the anterior and posterior. Together, sutures and fontanels allow the skull bones to overlap and mold to fit through the birth canal (see Fig. 8–8).
- Fontanels are used to identify the positioning of the fetal head during a vaginal exam. By identifying the anterior fontanel in relationship to the pelvis, the examiner can determine the position of the head and the degree of rotation that has occurred. Identification of the posterior fontanel may be obscured by molding or caput that can occur in labor.

Fetal Attitude or Posture

Fetal attitude or posture is the relationship of fetal parts to one another, noted by the flexion or extension of the fetal joints (Fig. 8–9).

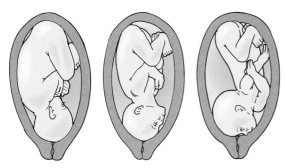

FIGURE 8–9 Fetal attitude or posture (flexed, deflexed, extended).

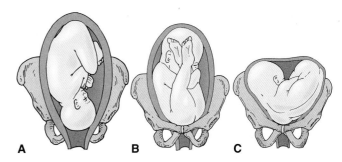

FIGURE 8–11 Fetal presentation. (A) Cephalic. (B) Breech. (C) Shoulder.

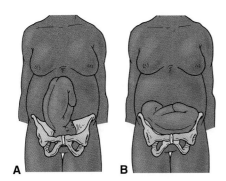

FIGURE 8–10 Fetal lie. (A) Longitudinal lie. (B) Transverse lie.

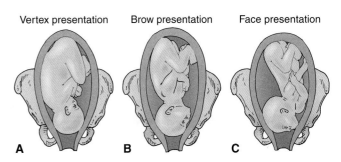

FIGURE 8–12 Cephalic presentation. (A) Vertex. (B) Brow. (C) Face.

Fetal Presentation

Fetal presentation is determined by the part of the fetus that enters the pelvic inlet first. There are three main presentations (Fig. 8–11):

- Cephalic (head first) (Fig. 8–11A)
- Breech (pelvis first) (Fig. 8–11B)
- Shoulder (shoulder first) (Fig. 8–11C)

Presenting Part

The presenting part is the specific fetal structure lying nearest to the cervix. It is determined by the attitude or posture of the fetus. Each presenting part has an identified reference point used to describe the fetal position in the pelvis.

- Cephalic presentations: The presenting part is the head (Fig. 8–12).
  - Cephalic presentations account for nearly 97% of all births (Cunningham et al., 2018).
  - The degree of flexion or extension of the head and neck further classifies cephalic presentations.
    - Vertex or occiput presentation indicates that the head is sharply flexed and the chin is touching the thorax. The reference point is the occiput.
    - Frontum or brow presentation indicates partial extension of the neck with the brow as the presenting part. The reference point is the frontum.
    - Face presentation indicates that the neck is sharply extended and the back of the head (occiput) is arching to the fetal back. The reference point is the mentum-chin.
- Breech presentations: The presenting part is the buttock or feet (Fig. 8–13).

Toward the end of pregnancy, the fetus usually assumes a rounded shape that corresponds to the shape of the uterine cavity. The fetal back becomes convex and the head is flexed so that the chin is almost in contact with the chest, the thighs are flexed over the abdomen, and the legs are bent at the knee.

- Abnormal exceptions to this attitude occur if the fetal head becomes progressively more extended instead of flexed. This results in a progressive change in fetal attitude from a convex (flexed) to a concave (extended) contour of the vertebral column (Cunningham et al., 2018). This position presents a larger diameter head to move through the birth canal, making vaginal birth more difficult.
- The most conducive attitude to vaginal childbirth occurs when the head is in complete flexion (fetal chin to chest), allowing an easier passage through the true pelvis.

Fetal Lie

Fetal lie refers to the long axis (spine) of the fetus in relationship to the long axis of the woman.

- The two primary lies are longitudinal and transverse (Fig. 8–10A & B).
  - In a longitudinal lie, the long axes of the fetus and the woman are parallel, occurring in 99% of labors (Cunningham et al., 2018).
  - In a transverse lie, the long axis of the fetus is perpendicular to the long axis of the woman. The fetal head is positioned in one iliac fossa and the buttocks and feet are in the other.
    - A fetus cannot be delivered vaginally in the transverse lie.

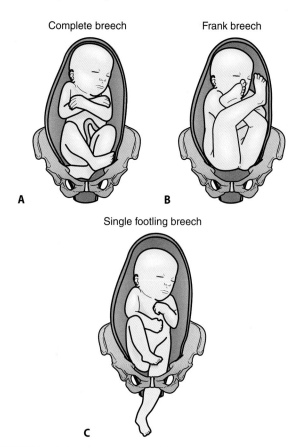

Complete breech   Frank breech

A   B

Single footling breech

C

FIGURE 8–13 Breech presentation. (A) Complete. (B) Frank. (C) Incomplete (Footling).

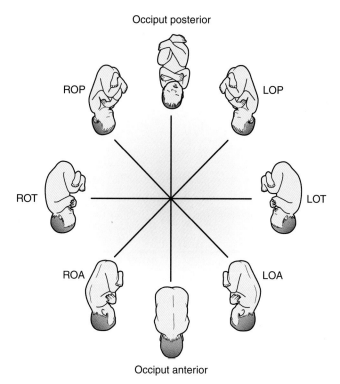

Occiput posterior

ROP   LOP

ROT   LOT

ROA   LOA

Occiput anterior

FIGURE 8–14 Variety of fetal positions with vertex presentation.

Fetal Position

The fetal position refers to the relation of the reference point to the maternal pelvis (Fig. 8–14).

- There are six positions for each presentation: right anterior, right transverse, right posterior, left anterior, left transverse, and left posterior.
- The occiput is the specific fetal structure for a cephalic presentation (see Fig. 8–11A).
- The sacrum is the specific fetal structure for a breech presentation (see Fig. 8–11B).
- The acromion is the specific fetal structure for a shoulder presentation (see Fig. 8–11C).
- The mentum is the specific fetal structure for a face presentation (see Fig. 8–12C).
- Position is designated by a three-letter abbreviation (Fig. 8–14):
  - First letter: Designates location of presenting part to the left (L) or right (R) of the woman's pelvis
  - Second letter: Designates the specific fetal part presenting: occiput (O), sacrum (S), mentum (M), and shoulder (A)
  - Third letter: Designates the relationship of the presenting fetal part to the woman's pelvis such as anterior (A), posterior (P), or transverse (T)

Psyche

Nursing care of the laboring woman should also focus on providing emotional support and information to empower the woman's decision making, with the goal of making the woman and family feel cared-for and safe (AAP Committee on Fetus and Newborn and ACOG Committee on Obstetric Practice, 2017). Coming

- Breech presentations account for 3% of all births. The reference point for breech presentations is the sacrum (Hofmeyr, 2021).
- Breech presentations are further classified as follows:
  - Complete breech: The knees are bent and the buttocks and feet are close to the cervix, with the fetus sitting cross-legged over the cervix. At term, 5% to 10% of breech fetuses are in this position (Hofmeyr, 2021) (Fig. 8–13A).
  - Frank breech: Complete flexion of thighs and legs, with the feet adjacent to the fetal head. At term, 50% to 70% of breech fetuses are in this position (Hofmeyr, 2021) (Fig. 8–13B).
  - Incomplete breech: Extension of one or both thighs and legs so that one or both feet are presenting, often called footling breech. At term, 10% to 40% of breech fetuses are in this position (Fig. 8–13C).
- Transverse presentation: The presenting part is usually the shoulder. The reference point for transverse presentations is the acromion (see Fig. 8–10B).
  - This usually is associated with a transverse lie.
- Compound presentation: An extremity prolapses along with the presenting part and both present together in the pelvis. This occurs in about 0.1% of labors. If the prolapse is an arm next to the fetal head, it will often not interfere with labor (Cunningham et al., 2018).

into a hospital environment is stressful and anxiety provoking for many. Although incomplete, research suggests that increased anxiety and stress result in slower labors with a greater number of interventions, including greater use of uterotonic medications, instrumented deliveries, and cesarean sections. Biochemical research has shown that self-reported anxiety and epinephrine level were significantly correlated. Higher epinephrine levels were significantly associated with decreased uterine activity resulting in longer labors (Hishikawa et al., 2019).

Nurses can have a significant impact on the patient's experience of labor. Providing warmth, care, education, and guidance, and asking about and honoring patient preferences and desires, may help decrease stress and anxiety, resulting in better labor experiences and outcomes. Many factors influence the woman's coping mechanisms including culture and expectations, overall support system, type of support during labor, and the nurse's understanding of historic and current inequities in maternity care.

Culturally Sensitive Patient-Centered Care

Culture influences the woman's reaction to labor expectations and interactions with others. Culture is also highly individualized and nurses should not make assumptions about someone based on outward appearance. Instead, nurses should practice patient-centered care by being aware and sensitive to the needs and practices of the individual. Ways to do this include asking about and then integrating individual cultural and religious values, beliefs, and practices into a mutually acceptable plan of care. Sensitive communication also includes effective verbal and nonverbal interactions in a context of creating a mutual understanding and respect for the patient's values, beliefs, preferences, and culture (Brooks et al., 2019). Questions that the nurse should consider asking include:

- Who does the patient want in the room during the labor and birth?
- What has been the patient's previous experience with the health-care system and how can their needs and preferences be met during this hospitalization?
- What are the patient's preferences for use of pharmacological and nonpharmacological pain management in labor?
- What needs to be known in order to give the patient the best care possible?
- What are the patient's expectations and concerns about the birthing process?

Culture and Equity

Every patient brings their unique histories, beliefs, concerns, and experiences, which all influence their experience of care, desires, and preferences. To provide equitable and inclusive care to all laboring people, nurses should examine their existing biases. One method of doing this is to adopt an anti-racist stance. Anti-racism is structured around conscious efforts and deliberate actions to provide equitable opportunities for all people, not privileging one set of cultural ideas or beliefs over another, and the understanding that racial groups are equal in all of their apparent differences (Kendi, 2019). It is important to understand that in the United States, health inequities have been racialized, meaning that birthing women of color often are not afforded the

same resources and experiences given to White birthing women (Roberts, 2011). When caring for patients in labor, the nurse should always keep the ANA Code of Ethics in mind (American Nurses Association, 2015). Particularly relevant provisions for maternity are the inherent dignity and uniqueness of all individuals regardless of race, class, or religion and the requirement to practice with compassion and respect for human needs without prejudice as well as the patient's right to complete and accurate information for autonomous decision making. For more about culturally competent nursing care, please see Chapter 5.

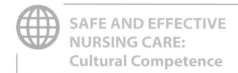

SAFE AND EFFECTIVE NURSING CARE: Cultural Competence

Creating an Equitable Birthing Environment for All Patients

To successfully provide respectful and culturally appropriate care while supporting a woman through the laboring process, nurses must acknowledge and respect the variety of cultural experiences and contexts in which people live, including structural issues that have affected their lives (Crear-Perry et al., 2021). The White experience in the United States has been too often seen as normal, and therefore invisible, with cultural experiences of non-White individuals seen as different or "not the norm." To provide appropriate support to all laboring people and to strive toward equity in birthing experiences and outcomes, nurses need to shift our view from a majority group's perspective to those who have been marginalized, accounting for implicit bias, structural determinants of health, and historical and current racism (Hardeman et al., 2016).

Laboring in a hospital can be particularly stressful for people of color. The maternal death rate for Black birthing women is 2.5 times higher than it is for White birthing women (Hoyert & Miniño, 2020). In 2018, infant mortality for Black infants was 10.8 per 1,000 live births, whereas White infant mortality was 4.6 (Ely & Driscoll, 2020). A recent study indicated that Black and Latina birthing women had a significantly higher rate of severe morbidity within the same large urban hospital, regardless of insurance type or other socioeconomic factors (Howell et al., 2020). Another study demonstrated that when Latina women were subjected to the stress and fear of deportation and discrimination, the rate of preterm birth increased by 24% (Novak et al., 2017).

Science has repeatedly demonstrated that there are no biological differences between racial groupings and that race categories are socially constructed (Kendi, 2016; Roberts, 2011), meaning these differences in outcomes must be due to other factors such as racism and other structural determinants of health. Racism is a system of oppression that operates on many levels, including internalized, interpersonal, institutional, and structural levels causing race-associated differences in health outcomes (Jones, 2000). Structural racism involves systematic laws and processes used to differentiate access to services, goods, and opportunities in society by racial groups. Exposure to structural racism has been linked to higher incidences of preterm birth and infant mortality, even after controlling for other factors (Chambers et al., 2019). These issues, as well as other historical and current abuses of people of color in the health-care system, need to be considered when caring for patients in labor (Washington, 2006).

Considerable evidence supports women of color reporting that their concerns were dismissed and they were not listened to. Strategies for providing safe, equitable, and respectful care for birthing women of color should include, but are not limited to:

- Ask patients what their preferred name is; if you're having trouble pronouncing it, ask the patient how to correctly say her name. Respect starts with addressing a patient with her name, without claims of her name being too difficult to pronounce or understand.
- When caring for women of color or non-English-speaking patients, use eye contact and nonverbal language. Body language can tell the patient a lot about how we feel and affects the nurse–patient relationship. For example, a teen mom may already feel a sense of embarrassment. Cold blank stares could intimidate the patient and increase her stress and anxiety about her birthing experience and the process.
- When developing the plan of care, be sure to include the patient in a process of shared decision making. For example, rather than saying: "We are going to induce you and start Pitocin," you could say "Our thoughts on your suggested plan of care involve an induction with Pitocin. How do you feel about that? Do you have any questions?" Including the patient and asking open-ended questions along the way can foster open dialogue and increase satisfaction in the birthing family.
- Do not gossip about or exoticize patients (discussing personal opinions about employment status, type of insurance coverage or lack thereof, non-English-speaking patients, obesity-shaming, and details about the patient's personal information on social media). Remember, we are in a professional environment; our personal opinions of patients' social situations should not be the focus or determine the level of care anyone receives.
- Do not use negative stereotypes to describe patients, such as lazy, difficult, and aggressive. These attitudes and terms have been grossly overgeneralized to describe large groups of people of color. Treat each patient as an individual and avoid lumping groups of patients into categories that lead to false assumptions, such as "Black women do not want to breast-feed." Generalizations such as these are damaging, untrue, and historically have been created from bias and discrimination. It also gives an easy way out or an excuse to dismiss the patient or provide the best care because she is "difficult," "drug-seeking," or any other biased assumption.
- Remember, care for all laboring patients should be respectful, kind, and equitable. Nurses must consider each patient individually and practice culture humility and patient-centered care.

A recent qualitative study on pregnancy and birth care experiences of birthing people of color found that when providers spent quality time with patients, worked on relationship building, and provided individualized person-centered care, it improved the person's experience of care (Altman et al., 2020).

CRITICAL COMPONENT

Nursing Support of Laboring Patients

The AWHONN asserts that continuous labor support from a registered nurse is critically important to achieve improved birth outcomes. Together with the laboring woman, the RN assesses, implements, and evaluates an individually constructed care plan based on physical, psychological, and sociocultural needs, incorporating the laboring patient's desires for and expectations of the process of labor. The RN also coordinates the laboring patient's support team, which may include a partner, family, friends, or a doula, to assist the patient to achieve the desired childbirth goals (AWHONN, 2018). Evidence also suggests that in addition to regular nursing care, continuous one-to-one emotional support provided by support personnel such as a doula is associated with improved outcomes for women in labor (Committee on Obstetric Practice, 2017). A Cochrane Review found that continual labor support resulted in:

- Increased rates of spontaneous vaginal birth
- Decreased reports of negative ratings of or feelings about their childbirth experience
- Decreased use of any intrapartum analgesia
- Shorter labors
- Having a cesarean birth
- Less likelihood of having an instrumental vaginal birth
- Less likelihood of having regional analgesia
- Less likelihood of having a baby with a low 5-minute Apgar score (Bohren et al., 2017).

Caring for Laboring Patients Who Identify as Transgender

Not all patients who present to labor and delivery identify as women; however, all patients deserve supportive, gender-affirming care during labor. Gender identity is separate from physiological sex assigned at birth and describes whether individuals identify themselves as a man, a woman, or somewhere else on the spectrum of gender. People who identify as transgender (people whose identified gender is different from their assigned birth sex) have reported high levels of mistreatment when seeking health care. In a large survey completed in 2015, 33% of those who saw a health-care provider had at least one negative experience related to being transgender, such as being verbally harassed or refused treatment because of their gender identity. Additionally 23% of respondents reported that they did not seek the health care they needed in the year prior due to fear of being mistreated as a transgender person, and 33% did not go to a health-care provider when needed because they could not afford it (James et al., 2016).

People who have a uterus but do not necessarily identify as female have the right to choose to become pregnant as a method of family building. Labor and delivery units historically have been highly gendered spaces, and when people who do not identify as women enter, they have often been faced with discrimination, barriers to care, and stigma (Richardson et al., 2019). Labor units should be safe, supportive places for all pregnant people, and it is important that nursing staff receive education to make it so. Although limited research has been done on this topic, one study indicates that nurses may feel uncomfortable around transgender patients, have difficulty using the correct pronouns, use dehumanizing language, or gossip about or exoticize these patients (Carabez et al., 2016). Strategies for creating safe spaces for patients on the gender spectrum include, but are not limited to, the following:

● Ask patients what their preferred gender pronouns are and use them consistently.
● Ask patients what their preferred name is and use it consistently.
● Understand that patients on the gender spectrum desire the same things that patients who identified as cisgender (people whose identified gender is the same as their assigned birth sex) desire: a safe, supportive, affirming delivery resulting in a positive outcome for the delivering parent and the infant.
● Ask patients which terms they wish the nurse to use to refer to body parts. For example, some patients prefer the term *chest feeding* to breastfeeding. Use the preferred terms.
● Do not gossip about or exoticize transgender patients. As with all laboring patients, care should be respectful, kind, and equitable.
● Learn about caring for transgender patients. A few resources include *The Center of Excellence for Transgender Health* and *The National Center for Transgender Equality*.

Birthing Women Who Have Made an Adoption Plan

For pregnant women who have made an adoption plan for their infants, the nursing care plan should consider issues surrounding labor support, who will be with the birth mother, and the extent of the adoptive parents' involvement in the labor and after birth. When preparing the care plan, birth mothers should be asked if they want the prospective adoptive parents to be present for the birth, whether in the waiting room or labor room itself, or whether they prefer the adoptive parents remain at home during labor and birth. The birth mother is always the decision maker.

Commonly, birth mothers decide to have some time alone at the hospital with the infant. This gives them a chance to feel settled in the decision and make peace before placement. Supporting the wishes of the birth mother is the priority and duty of the nurse caring for the laboring woman. The experience of birth and the moments after belong to the birth mother, and nurses must allow the birth family to have time with the infant if desired. Although adoption laws vary by state in the United States, in general, birthing parents are the decision makers for their infants until they consent to and sign legal forms terminating their parental rights. The birth mother decides when the adoptive parents will have contact with the newborn in most situations.

Although adoption is common, society still views adoption as nonnormative and less preferable to biologically based families, leading to stigmatization of those involved with the adoption triad, particularly of the relinquishing parent (Coleman & Garratt, 2016). Because the child is still alive and the birth

parent(s) has made the decision to relinquish, there is often no societal expectation of grief expression by the birthing parent. One researcher called this phenomenon "disenfranchised grief," indicating that society does not expect birthing parents to grieve, but instead to "move on" with their lives (Aloi, 2009). However, the relinquishing parent values and needs someone who will support them and their interests at this vulnerable point in their lives. The attitudes of the health-care provider can affect how much control the relinquishing mother has over the adoption process (Clutter, 2014). Nurses involved with women at the time of relinquishment can be of significant help in the resolution of grief. In addition to providing supportive and compassionate nursing care, it is important to assess whether the patient desires post-hospital follow-up. The nurse should assess and provide resources regarding support groups and make referrals to social work or counseling.

Gestational surrogacy involves a woman known as a gestational carrier who agrees to bear a genetically unrelated child with the help of assisted reproductive technologies for an individual or couple who intend to be the legal and rearing parents, referred to as the intended parents (American College of Obstetricians and Gynecologists [ACOG], 2016). In gestational surrogacy, legal contracts are signed before embryo transfer. Everyone involved in surrogacy may need early and ongoing support, education, care options, and counseling. Remember the gestational surrogate is the patient and is always the nurses' primary concern. Again, the birth mother decides when legal parents have contact with the newborn in most situations.

Caring for Adolescents in Labor

Nurses are responsible for providing safe, high-quality confidential care to adolescent laboring patients. When caring for adolescents, as with all patients, communication is critical. Nursing communication with adolescents should be nonjudgmental and nonpatronizing. Nurses should respect adolescents' ability to make decisions, accept responsibility, and problem-solve regarding their own health care (Edwards et al., 2016). The position of the AWHONN is that "Adolescents are entitled the same legal rights to confidentiality as adults, and nurses should ensure that these rights are guaranteed. Nurses should provide confidential services as appropriate and promote policies in health care settings that protect these services" (AWHONN, 2017, p. 889). However, not all states in the United States currently protect adolescent confidentiality. As of 2021, only 33 states and Washington, DC, explicitly allow adolescents under the age of 18 to consent to prenatal care. Of those, 14 states allow, but do not require, the physician to inform parents that their child is seeking prenatal care. One state allows the adolescent to consent to care during the first trimester but requires parental consent for care in the second and third trimester. Four states allow young people who are considered "mature" to consent to care, and 13 states have no explicit policy or relevant case law (The Guttmacher Institute, 2021). It is important for nurses to know the relevant federal and state laws and regulations as well as the individual hospital policy so that accurate information can be provided to adolescent pregnant patients.

Position

The position of the woman during labor and birth is the fifth "P." Laboring in the hospital has historically included spending most of the labor in bed. However, when allowed and encouraged to do so, most laboring women will move frequently and assume many different positions (Fig. 8–15) Frequent position changes during labor enhance maternal comfort and promote optimal fetal positioning, and should be supported if the positions allow appropriate maternal and fetal monitoring (ACOG, 2019a). (Remember, not all patients will need to be continuously monitored.) Laboring patients should have unlimited access and assistance to assume positions that are safe for the mother and fetus, restful, and comfortable.

- A Cochrane Review found that laboring patients who walked, stood, sat, or kneeled during the first stage of labor shortened the first stage by more than 80 minutes compared with patients who maintained a recumbent, supine, or lateral position. Birthing women in upright positions were also less likely to have a C-section (Lawrence et al., 2013) (Fig. 8–16A).
- During the second stage of labor, upright or lateral positions were associated with a decrease of the length of the second stage, a decrease in oxytocin use, fewer medical interventions, and greater satisfaction. Upright positioning was also associated with greater oxygenation of the fetus (AWHONN, 2019) (Fig. 8–16B).
- Maintaining an upright position during the second state of labor may increase the pelvic diameter by up to 30%, making it easier for the fetus to move through the pelvis. (AWHONN, 2019) (Fig. 8–16B).
- Supine positions should be avoided. The pressure of the uterus against the spine causes compression of the inferior vena cava, aorta, and iliac arteries, causing supine hypotension for the birthing parent and impairing oxygen flow to the fetus (Simpson & James, 2005).

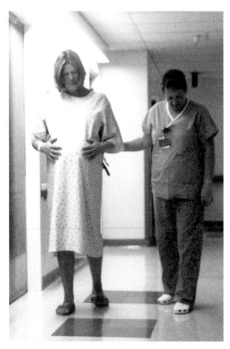

FIGURE 8–15 Woman walking in labor with her nurse.

- Nurses are integral to helping laboring patients move and choose positions that are conducive to labor progress and patient comfort and needs. RNs provide advice, support, and encouragement to empower patients to take advantage of their options during labor.
- Resting places other than beds, such as rocking chairs and birthing balls, may be suggested. If appropriate, laboring in the shower or the tub during the first stage of labor may provide comfort and pain relief.
- Registered nurses should also be knowledgeable about positioning techniques for patients with epidural analgesia, and they play a key role in supporting position changes that facilitate the birth process, promote comfort, and maintain patient safety.

ONSET OF LABOR

As the woman comes closer to term, the uterus becomes more sensitive to oxytocin; progesterone is functionally withdrawn, resulting in increased contraction frequency and intensity. This can be an anxious time for the woman and her support people as they decide when to come to the birthing center for evaluation. Teaching people about the signs of labor can help to alleviate some of these fears.

True Labor Versus False Labor

True labor contractions occur at regular intervals and increase in frequency, duration, and intensity (Fig. 8–17). True labor contractions cause changes in cervical effacement and dilation. False labor is characterized by irregular contractions with little or no cervical change.

Assessment of Rupture of the Membranes (ROM)

Spontaneous rupture of the membranes (SROM) may occur before the onset of labor but typically occurs during labor. When the amniotic sac ruptures at term, but before the onset of labor, approximately 77% to 79% of women will go into labor spontaneously within 12 hours, and 95% will start labor spontaneously within 24 to 28 hours (ACOG, 2019a). Once the amniotic sac ruptures, the risk of infection begins to increase for the fetus and the pregnant woman, rising over time (Middleton et al., 2017). If there are no medical reasons to expedite the delivery, and the woman and fetus are stable, it is reasonable to wait 12 to 24 hours to see if labor starts spontaneously before inducing labor (ACOG, 2019a). When the provider ruptures the membranes using an amnihook, it is called artificial rupture of membranes (AROM).

Assessing the Status of Membranes

Different techniques may be used to confirm rupture of membranes (ROM):

- Speculum, fern, and nitrazine exams
  - A speculum exam may be done to assess for amniotic fluid in the vaginal vault (pooling). The patient may be asked to cough during the exam to enhance the flow of amniotic fluid.

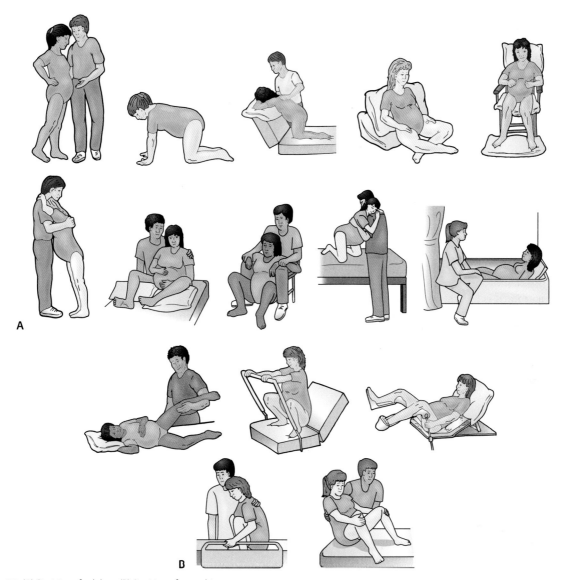

FIGURE 8–16 (A) Positions for labor. (B) Positions for pushing.

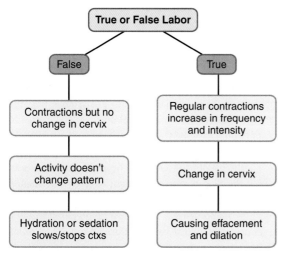

FIGURE 8–17 True versus false labor.

- Ferning: During a sterile speculum exam, a sample of fluid in the upper vaginal area is obtained, placed on a slide, and assessed for a "ferning pattern" under a microscope (Fig. 8–18A). Amniotic fluid dries in a fern pattern. If a ferning pattern is seen, it suggests ROM. However, the results of this test can be equivocal, and should be interpreted with other clinical findings.
- Nitrazine paper: This special paper turns blue when in contact with amniotic fluid. The paper may be dipped in the vaginal fluid or a fluid-soaked Q-tip can be used to transfer the fluid to the paper (Fig. 8–18B). This method is no longer common due to its high rate of false negatives and positives.
- Laboratory tests:
  - AmniSure: The AmniSure ROM Test is a rapid, non-invasive monoclonal immunoassay that detects placental alpha microglobulin-1 (PAMG-1), an amniotic protein that appears in vaginal secretions if ROM has occurred. In large-scale testing, AmniSure has a sensitivity rate (the test states the

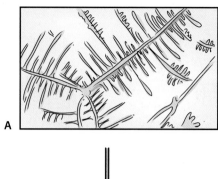

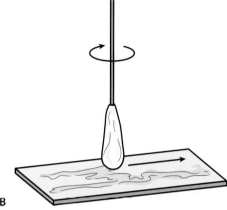

FIGURE 8–18 Assessment of rupture of membranes. (A) Ferning pattern of dried amniotic fluid seen under microscope. (B) Placing fluid on nitrizine paper with a Q-tip.

patient is ruptured and the patient is actually ruptured—true positive) of 94.9% to 98.9%, and a specificity rate (the test states the patient is not ruptured and the patient is actually not ruptured—true negative) of 87.5% to 100% (Duff, 2021). Although highly accurate, it should be used in conjunction with other clinical findings to confirm rupture.

- Actim PROM: The Actim PROM Test tests for growth factor binding protein-1 (GFBP-1), which is secreted by decidual and placental cells and has a very high concentration in amniotic fluid compared with other bodily fluids. Sensitivity ranges from 95% to 100% and specificity ranges from 93% to 98% (Duff, 2021).
- ROM Plus: The ROM Plus test detects two protein markers found in amniotic fluid. The test's sensitivity is 99% and its specificity is 91%.

Nursing Actions After Rupture of Membranes

- Assess the fetal heart rate (FHR).
  - The fetal environment has dramatically changed, and the priority after rupture is to assess fetal well-being by assessing the fetal response.
    - There is an increased risk of umbilical cord prolapse with ROM.
      - The risk is higher when the presenting part is not engaged in the true pelvis.
- Assess the amniotic fluid for color, amount, and odor.
  - Normal amniotic fluid is clear or cloudy with a normal odor that is similar to that of ocean water or the loam of a forest floor.

- Foul-smelling amniotic fluid suggests infection.
- Fluid can be meconium-stained; this must be reported to the care provider as it may indicate fetal compromise in utero, which requires intervention at birth.
- Document the date and time of ROM, characteristics of the fluid, and FHR.

Guidelines for Going to the Birthing Facility

By law, all pregnant women in labor or experiencing complications must have access to medical care regardless of their ability to pay (Box 8-1). By discussing when to go to the birthing facility with the pregnancy care provider before labor happens, women will have less anxiety and be more prepared when labor begins. This decision depends on each person's past pregnancy history, location of the birth center, and risk status of the pregnancy. Often, the advice for first-time pregnancy without risk factors is to wait until contractions are 5 minutes apart, last 60 seconds, and are regular for at least an hour. However, the woman should go to the birthing center immediately when:

- The membrane ruptures, or water breaks.
- The woman is experiencing intense pain.
- Bloody show markedly increases or there is frank bleeding.
- There is a marked decrease in fetal movement.
- The patient experiences a severe headache, blurred vision, or epigastric pain, or other marked changes in maternal well-being.

BOX 8-1 | Emergency Medical Treatment and Active Labor Act

The Emergency Medical Treatment and Active Labor Act (EMTALA) is a federal act passed in 1986 as part of the Consolidated Omnibus Reconciliation Act (COBRA) in response to "patient dumping"—the policy of hospitals refusing to treat patients based on insurance and ability to pay. The act states that any person who presents either to a hospital emergency department or to a labor and delivery unit must receive a medical screening examination by a qualified professional. If a patient is assessed to be stable (for OB, this means not in labor and without other high-risk signs and symptoms), the patient may be discharged. If a medical emergency exists, including obstetric emergencies or if a person is in labor, the hospital must treat the patient until they are stabilized or the condition is resolved, regardless of their ability to pay. The hospital may transfer the patient, if the patient consents, to a hospital with a higher level of care, if the type of care the patient needs is unavailable at the current hospital. Because of this important act, RNs staffing triage in labor and delivery units must be prepared to see and treat all pregnant people, even if they have not had prenatal care within the hospital system.

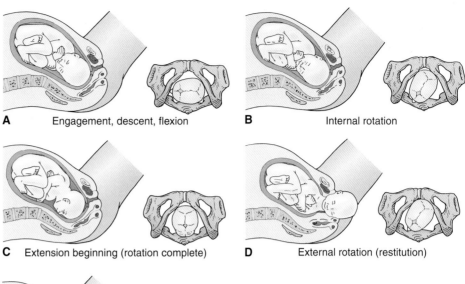

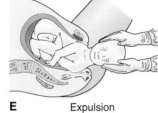

FIGURE 8-19 Cardinal movements of labor. (A) Engagement, descent, and flexion. (B) Internal rotation. (C) Extension. (D) External rotation. (E) Expulsion.

MECHANISMS OF LABOR

The positional changes of the fetal presenting part (most often the occiput) required to navigate the birth canal constitute the mechanisms of labor. These mechanisms are also called the cardinal movements of labor (Fig. 8–19).

- Engagement: When the greatest diameter of the fetal head passes through the pelvic inlet; can occur late in pregnancy or early in labor (see Fig. 8–19A).
- Descent: Movement of the fetus through the birth canal during the first and second stages of labor (see Fig. 8–19A).
- Flexion: When the chin of the fetus moves toward the fetal chest; occurs when the descending head meets resistance from maternal tissues; results in the smallest fetal diameter to the maternal pelvic dimensions; normally occurs early in labor (see Fig. 8–19A).
- Internal rotation: When the rotation of the fetal head aligns the long axis of the fetal head with the long axis of the maternal pelvis; occurs mainly during the second stage of labor (see Fig. 8–19B).
- Extension: Facilitated by resistance of the pelvic floor that causes the presenting part to pivot beneath the pubic symphysis and the head to be delivered; occurs during the second stage of labor (see Fig. 8–19C).
- External rotation and restitution: The sagittal suture moves to a transverse diameter and the shoulders align in the antero-posterior diameter. The sagittal suture maintains alignment with the fetal trunk as the trunk navigates through the pelvis

(see Fig. 8–19D). Head and shoulders rotate to move under the symphysis pubis.
- Expulsion: The anterior shoulder usually comes first followed by the remainder of the body (see Fig. 8–19E).

CRITICAL COMPONENT

Reduction of Peripartum Racial and Ethnic Disparities: A Conceptual Framework and Maternal Safety Consensus Bundle

A joint statement from key professional organizations acknowledged that racial and health inequities exist both in maternal and perinatal outcomes and in health-care quality, and that health-care quality cannot fully be realized until health-care equity has gained. Consistent with a large body of previous work, the review of evidence found that racial and ethnic minority women experience more maternal deaths, comorbid illnesses, and adverse perinatal outcomes than White women (Howell et al., 2018). They identify unequal delivery of care to racial and ethnic minorities as one cause of these disparities. As part of the bundle, signees of the joint statement recommend that every clinical encounter:

- Engage in best practices for shared decision making.
- Ensure a timely and tailored response to each report of inequity or disrespect.
- Address reproductive life plan and contraceptive options not only during or immediately after pregnancy, but at regular intervals throughout a woman's reproductive life.

- Establish discharge navigation and coordination systems post childbirth to ensure that women have appropriate follow-up care and understand when it is necessary to return to their health-care provider.
- Provide discharge instructions that include information about what danger or warning signs to look out for, whom to call, and where to go if they have a question or concern.
- Design discharge materials that meet the patients' health literacy, language, and cultural needs.

   Every clinical unit must:

- Build a culture of equity, including systems for reporting, response, and learning similar to ongoing efforts in safety culture.
- Develop a disparities dashboard that monitors process and outcome metrics stratified by race and ethnicity, with regular dissemination of the stratified performance data to staff and leadership.
- Implement quality improvement projects that target disparities in health-care access, treatment, and outcomes.
- Consider the role of race, ethnicity, language, poverty, literacy, and other social determinants of health, including racism at the interpersonal and system level when conducting multidisciplinary reviews of severe maternal morbidity, mortality, and other clinically important metrics.
- Add as a checkbox on the review sheet: Did race or ethnicity (i.e., implicit bias), language barrier, or specific social determinants of health contribute to the morbidity (yes/no/maybe)? And if so, are there system changes that could be implemented that could alter the outcome?

(Howell et al., 2018)

STAGES OF LABOR AND CHILDBIRTH

Labor is the process in which the fetus, placenta, and membranes are expelled through the uterus and out the introitus of the vagina. The care of pregnant women and families during labor and delivery requires astute and ongoing assessments of the biopsychosocial adaptation of the woman and fetus. Because childbirth is a natural process, care should move forward on a continuum from least invasive interventions to more invasive, and from nonpharmacological to pharmacological interventions according to the desires of the woman and assessment of health-care providers. Teamwork and collaboration among physicians, midwives, nurses, patients, and those who support them in labor can facilitate women achieving their goals for labor and birth by using techniques that require minimal interventions and avoiding many common obstetric practices that are of limited or uncertain benefit for low-risk women in spontaneous labor (ACOG, 2019a).

In 2017, in the United States, 98.4% of all infants were delivered in hospitals. Out-of-hospital deliveries represented only 1.6% of births. Physicians delivered 90.6% of hospital-based births and certified nurse-midwives (CNMs) delivered 8.7% (MacDorman & Declercq, 2019). Nurses in intrapartal settings have key roles in providing comprehensive and individualized care for women and their families. To do so, nurses must have a clear understanding of the processes of labor and birth and the immediate postpartum period. By understanding the stages and phases of labor, nurses can facilitate, assist, and provide care for laboring patients, the fetus, and the patient's support systems (see Concept Map).

CRITICAL COMPONENT

Care Practices That Support and Promote Normal Physiological Birth

A normal physiologic labor and birth is powered by the innate human capacity of the woman and fetus. This birth is more likely to be safe and healthy because no unnecessary intervention disrupts normal physiologic processes. Supporting the normal physiologic processes of labor and birth can enhance best outcomes for the mother and infant.

The World Health Organization (WHO) and Lamaze International identified six birth practices that support and promote normal physiologic birth:

1. Labor begins on its own: Support the normal physiological process.
2. Freedom of movement throughout labor: Allow women to move around and adapt positions of their choosing.
3. Continuous labor support from family, friends, doulas, or nursing staff.
4. Minimize interventions to allow healthy labor progress.
5. Allow spontaneous pushing in nonsupine positions.
6. Allow NO separation of mother and baby.

American College of Nurse-Midwives (ACNM), 2016; American College of Obstetrics and Gynecologists, 2019a; Romano & Lothian, 2008.

Labor and birth are divided into four stages (Table 8-1, Fig. 8–20):

- The first stage begins with onset of labor and ends with complete cervical dilation.
- The second stage begins with complete dilation of the cervix and ends with delivery of the baby.
- The third stage begins after delivery of the baby and ends with delivery of the placenta.
- The fourth stage begins after delivery of the placenta and is completed after the stabilization of the birth parent and infant; it is the immediate postpartum period (see Fig. 8–20).

First Stage

The first stage of labor begins when the cervix starts to thin and open. The completion of this process marks the end of the first stage. The first stage is divided into two phases: latent phase and

TABLE 8-1   Stages and Phases of Labor

STAGES	FIRST		SECOND		THIRD	FOURTH
Phases	Latent	Active	Latent	Active		
Length	Mean length: 11.8 hours for primiparas, 9.3 hours for multiparas	Mean rate of dilation: 1.2–1.5 cm/hr. More rapid for multiparas	0–2 hours, depending on patient status, urge to push, and risk factors	Most primiparas will deliver within 3 hours of active pushing; multiparas will deliver within 2 hours	Mean length: 5 mins, 90% will deliver the placenta within 13–15 minutes	2–4 hours
Cervix	Effacing, dilation from 0–5 cm	Effacement 80% or more, dilation from 6–10 cm	Completely dilated and effaced	Completely dilated and effaced	Closing	Closing
Uterine contractions	Becoming stronger, more regular, and increasing in frequency	Moderate, regular, frequency: every 2–3 minutes, no more than 5 in a 10-minute period	Moderate, frequency: every 2–3 minutes, no more than 5 in a 10-minute period	Moderate/strong with an urge to bear down. Frequency: every 2–3 minutes	Mild contractions to deliver the placenta	Mild contractions to assist with uterine involution
Vaginal discharge	Blood-tinged mucus	Increased blood-tinged mucus	Bloody mucus	Bloody mucus	Gush of blood before placenta delivery	Lochia rubra
Membranes	Intact or ruptured	Intact or ruptured	Usually ruptured	Usually ruptured	Check placenta for completeness after delivery	
Biological response	Cramps, backache, may request pain medication, may be excited to begin labor, talkative. Good time to do patient education. May stay home if stable.	May turn more inward, focused on contractions, may become worried, or panicked May request pain medications. Benefits from continuous labor support.	Assess for urge to push when fetus reaches the pelvic floor. If the patient has an epidural, client may use this time to rest and prepare for pushing.	Urge to bear down, focused on pushing fetus out. Perineum flattens and bulges.	Cord lengthens, gush of blood, then delivery of the placenta. Relieved, skin-to-skin time with infant	Uterus is involuting. Resting, recovering, and bonding with new infant
Maternal assessment	Upon admission, full systems assessment, review prenatal and medical history Assess maternal well-being at least every 30 minutes. P, R, and BP every hour; T every 2 hours unless ROM, then every hour. SVE only as needed; limit SVE to prevent infection.	Assess maternal well-being at least every 30 minutes. P, R, and BP every hour; T every 2 hours unless ROM, then every hour. SVE only as needed; limit SVE to prevent infection. Assess labor status every 30 minutes.	Assess maternal well-being at least every 5–15 minutes. P, R, and BP every hour; T every 2 hours unless ROM, then every hour. SVE only as needed; limit SVE to prevent infection.	Assess maternal well-being at least every 5–15 minutes. P, R, and BP every hour; T every 2 hours unless ROM, then every hour. SVE only as needed; limit SVE to prevent infection.	Assess maternal well-being. BP and pulse every 15 minutes Assess for signs of impending placental delivery.	Assess maternal well-being. Assess uterus and lochia every 15 minutes, BP and pulse every 15 minutes for 2 hours. Assess pain.

Continued

TABLE 8-1   Stages and Phases of Labor—cont'd

STAGES	FIRST		SECOND		THIRD	FOURTH
Phases	Latent	Active	Latent	Active		
	Assess labor status every 30 minutes. Assess bladder status, and encourage voiding every 2 hours. Assess pain every 30 minutes; work with the laboring woman to devise ongoing pain control strategies.	Assess bladder status, encourage voiding every 2 hours, catheterize if necessary. Assess pain every 30 minutes; work with the laboring woman to devise ongoing pain control strategies.	Assess bladder status, encourage voiding every 2 hours, catheterize if necessary. Assess readiness to push. Prepare for delivery.	Assist with pushing efforts. Prepare for delivery.		
Maternal interventions	Assist with positioning; encourage movement. Avoid supine position. Monitor fetal response to position changes. Implement pain control strategies. Respond to changes in maternal status.	Assist with positioning; encourage movement. Avoid supine position. Monitor fetal response to position changes. Implement pain control strategies. Respond to changes in maternal status.	Many women will want to rest; assist the patient into a comfortable resting position, changing positions as needed. Monitor fetal response to position changes. Avoid supine position. Implement pain control strategies. Respond to changes in maternal status.	Assist patient into comfortable and effective pushing positions; change positions as needed to assist the fetus's descent. Monitor fetal response to position changes. Avoid supine position. Implement pain control strategies. Respond to changes in maternal status.	Administer uterotonic medication per order. Respond to changes in maternal status.	Assist patient into comfortable positions, which facilitates bonding with the infant. Implement pain control strategies. Respond to changes in maternal status.
Fetal assessments	Assess FHR and response to labor every 30 minutes. Leopold's maneuvers for fetal position	Assess FHR and response to labor every 30 minutes.	Assess FHR and response to labor every 5–15 minutes.	Assess FHR and response to labor every 5–15 minutes. Observe for crowning.	Ask: Term infant? Crying or breathing? Good tone? Apgar scores at 1 and 5 minutes	Ongoing newborn assessments
Fetal interventions	Institute uterine resuscitation interventions for category II and III fetal heart tracings.	Institute uterine resuscitation interventions for category II and III fetal heart tracings.	Institute uterine resuscitation interventions for category II and III fetal heart tracings.	Institute uterine resuscitation interventions for category II and III fetal heart tracings.	Skin-to-skin if stable, immediately begin newborn resuscitation measures if needed. Maintain warmth.	Ongoing assessments Maintain warmth. Assist with breastfeeding. Administer newborn medications.

TABLE 8-1   Stages and Phases of Labor—cont'd

STAGES	FIRST		SECOND		THIRD	FOURTH
Phases	Latent	Active	Latent	Active		
Social systems	Welcome the laboring woman and her support system. Work with the woman and support system to assess needs, expectations, and desires for this labor. Provide patient education regarding the laboring process and on all interventions. Be kind and empathetic.	Assist the support system to help the laboring patient cope with labor. Provide patient education regarding the laboring process and on all interventions. Be kind and empathetic.	Prepare the support people for delivery. Assist the support system to help the laboring patient cope with labor. Provide patient education regarding the laboring process and on all interventions. Be kind and empathetic.	Assist support person in supporting the patient during pushing. Prepare the support people for delivery. Be kind and empathetic.	Assist support people in welcoming the new infant. Be kind and empathetic.	Support people to remain with the patient and infant. Assist with bonding. Provide patient education on the recovery process and newborn care. Be kind and empathetic.

BP, blood pressure; FHR, fetal heart rate; P, pulse; R, respirations; ROM, rupture of membranes; SVE, sterile vaginal examination.

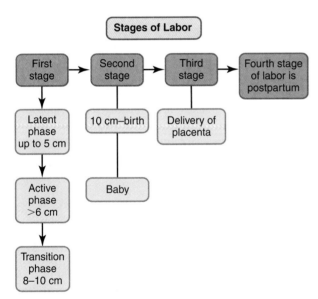

FIGURE 8-20 Stages of labor.

active phase. Characteristics of the first stage of labor are as follows (see Table 8-1):

- It begins with the onset of true labor and ends with complete cervical dilation (10 cm) and complete effacement (100%).
- Stage 1 is the longest stage, with the latent phase typically moving much more slowly than the active phase. For example, the median rate for a primigravida to dilate from 2 to 3 cm is 5.3 hours and the median rate to dilate from 9 to 10 cm is 0.5 hours (Abalos et al., 2020).

- The first stage of labor may tremendously vary in length (Oladapo et al., 2018).
- The bag of waters usually ruptures during this stage.
- The laboring patient's cardiac output increases. Cardiac output increases by 15% to 25% during the first stage above pre-labor levels. During contractions, blood from the uterine sinuses is pushed out to the systemic vasculature, increasing preload (Oladapo et al., 2018). This may also increase the laboring patient's pulse.
- Gastrointestinal motility decreases, which leads to delayed gastric emptying time (Simpson & O'Brien-Abel, 2021).
- As the patient moves through stage 1 of labor, she usually feels increased pain. The patient and the care team should devise a flexible plan to help the patient cope, including both pharmacological (if desired) and nonpharmacological pain control interventions.
- Cervical changes are used in assessing progression through each phase of the first stage of labor: latent phase, 0 to 5 cm; active phase, 6 to 10 cm (Simpson & O'Brien-Abel, 2021).

Assessment

Assessment during all phases of the first stage of labor includes:

- Vital signs
- The patient's response to labor and pain
- FHR and UCs
- Cervical changes
- Fetal position and descent in the pelvis

Nursing Actions

Nursing actions during all phases of the first stage of labor are related to:

- Diet and hydration
  - There is active debate about oral intake of fluids and food during labor.
    - ACOG endorses a moderate amount of clear liquids during labor for uncomplicated patients (AAP Committee on Fetus and Newborn and ACOG Committee on Obstetric Practice, 2017).
    - The ACNM recommendations include facilitating self-determination of appropriate oral intake in healthy women experiencing normal labors. and that midwives and physicians should discuss the potential benefits of oral intake during labor with women (ACNM, 2016).
    - A 2013 Cochrane meta-analysis identified no benefits or harms of restricting foods and fluids during labor in women who were at low risk of needing anesthesia (Singata et al., 2013).
    - A 2017 meta-analysis found that low-risk patients who were allowed to eat more freely during labor had a shorter duration of labor. A policy of less-restrictive food intake during labor did not influence other obstetric or neonatal outcomes nor did it increase the incidence of vomiting. Operative delivery rates were similar (Ciardulli et al., 2017).
  - Nurses should follow hospital policy and individual patient orders while staying current on research on oral intake during labor. They should advocate for evidence-based practice changes as appropriate.
- Activity and rest
  - Encouraging frequent position changes and upright positions assists labor progression, facilitates fetal descent, and decreases pain perception.
- Elimination
  - Frequent emptying of the bowel and bladder assists in comfort of the laboring woman, provides more pelvic room as the baby descends, and decreases pressure and injury to the urethra and bowel.
- Comfort
  - Providing comfort measures facilitates labor progress, decreases pain perception, and supports maternal coping to manage the labor process.
- Support and family involvement
  - Encouraging the patient's identified family to provide emotional and physical support to the patient results in decreased stress and facilitates labor progress.
- Education
  - Providing education and information about labor, procedures, and hospital policies will decrease anxiety and fear. It also empowers laboring women and their support people to make informed decisions.
- Safety
  - Providing a safe, friendly, and affirming environment will enhance the birthing experience.
- Documentation of labor admission and progression (Fig. 8–21 and Fig. 8–22)

Stage One: Latent Phase (0 to 5 cm Cervical Dilation)

The latent phase is the early phase of labor when cervical dilation is typically slow. For patients having their first baby, the mean duration of the latent phase is 11.8 hours, with 95% of patients completing latent phase by 30 hours. For multiparous patients, the mean duration of the latent phase is 9.3 hours, with 95% of patients completing latent phase by 24.5 hours (Tilden et al., 2019). During the latent phase, women experience contractions that become stronger, more regular, and more frequent over time and are associated with cervical change.

In the beginning of the latent phase, laboring patients are often both excited and apprehensive about the start of labor. They may be talkative and able to relax with the contractions. Many laboring women choose to stay home during this phase, although some are admitted to the birth center. Indications for admittance include but are not limited to cervical change and ROM, fetal intolerance of labor, maternal complications, or pain uncontrolled by at-home comfort measures. Most can go home at this stage and return to the birth center when labor progresses. However, because of the length of this phase, laboring patients may also begin to feel distressed and lose confidence in themselves. A 2017 Cochrane Review found that providing assessment and support in the form of telephone calls and home visits during this phase may increase satisfaction and reduce epidural and oxytocin use, although more research needs to be done to confirm these findings (Kobayashi et al., 2017)

Medical Interventions

- Laboratory tests, which may include complete blood count (CBC); a hold clot or a type-and-screen, depending on risk profile; urinalysis, including protein and glucose; and possible drug screening. Additional screening may include laboratory tests to assess for preeclampsia or other pregnancy complications.
- Order IV or saline lock.
- Order intermittent fetal monitoring or continuous fetal and uterine monitoring, depending on patient condition.
- Provide pain control management as decided by the patient and the care team.

Nursing Actions (see Clinical Pathway and Concept Map)

- Admit to the labor unit and orient the laboring woman and support people to the labor room.
- Review the prenatal record, which should include the following:
  - All laboratory tests and ultrasounds (for estimated date of delivery [EDD] and placental location) as well as any prior obstetrical history (pregnancy, births, abortions, and living children)
  - Review of allergies and medications
  - Trends in vital signs and weight gain
  - Chronic conditions
  - Pregnancy-related complications
  - All prenatal laboratory tests, including CBC, blood type, Rh status, HBsAg, rapid plasma reagin (RPR), rubella, results of the glucose tolerance test, HIV, group B streptococci (GBS), and other tests that may have been done to check for complications, such as preeclampsia.

Labor and Delivery Admission Record

PT. NAME: _____   AGE: _____   CARE PROVIDER: _____

ADMIT DATE/TIME: _____

EDC	LMP	Weeks of Gestation	Gravida	Para	Term	Preterm	Spontaneous Abortion	Elective Abortion	Living	Stillborn	C-Section	VBAC

T	P	R	BP	Height	Weight	Pre-Pregnant Weight	Weight Gain	How Admitted		Accompanied By	

Date/Time Care Provider Notified	Date/Time Seen by Care Provider	Reason for Admission

Onset of Labor	Contraction Frequency (Min)

Dilatation (cm)	Effacement (%)	Station

Contraction Duration (Sec)   Contraction Quality
None   Mild   Moderate   Strong

Pelvic Exam By:

Pain Level Assessment: *Pain scale 0–10*

Admission Membranes: Intact   Ruptured   Bulging   Unknown

Fern: N/A   Negative   Positive   Equivocal

AROM/SROM (Date/Time):

Amniotic Fluid:
Amount: None   N/A   Copious   Large   Moderate   Small   Scant
Color: N/A   Clear   Bloody   Meconium   Heavy   Light   Particulate
Odor: None   N/A   Normal   Foul
Amniotic Fluid Comments:

Vaginal Bleeding: None   Normal   Frank bleeding
Describe Vaginal Bleeding:

Mental Status: Alert   Anxious   Confused

Feeding Preference: Breast   Bottle   Breast/Bottle   Undecided

Support Person: None   Husband   Partner   Other
Support Person(s) Name:

Anesthesia Plans: None Local Epidural Spinal General Pudendal
Paracervical
Anesthesia Plans Other:

Anesthesia Class: Yes   No   Yes, Previous Pregnancy

Attended Prenatal Class: Yes   No   Yes, Previous Pregnancy

Labor Teaching Initiated: Yes   No   N/A
   Fetal Well-being   Yes   No   N/A
   Labor Progress   Yes   No   N/A
   Pain Relief Measures   Yes   No   N/A
   Other

Nutritional screen:
[ ] N/A
[ ] History of Diabetes/Gestational Diabetes
[ ] History of Eating Disorder
[ ] Multiple Pregnancy
[ ] Special Diet/Vegetarian Diet
[ ] Pt. is 18 Years Old or Younger
[ ] Failure to Gain at Least 1/2 lb. per Wks. of Gestation
[ ] Food Allergies
[ ] Other _____

Describe Last Solid Intake (Include Date/Time):

Describe Last Fluid Intake (Include Date/Time):

In-Pt. Dietary Referral Entered in Computer: Yes No N/A	In-Pt. Dietary Referral Entered in Computer: Yes No N/A

Medication Allergy: Yes   No
Medication Allergy Detail:

Food Allergies: Yes   No
Food Allergy Detail:

Latex Allergy: Yes   No
Describe Latex Reaction:

Allergy Sticker on Chart: Yes N/A	Allergy Band on Patient: Yes N/A

Prenatal Vitamins This Pregnancy: Yes No	Anticoagulants Describe: This Pregnancy: Yes No

For current prescription/over-the-counter medications taken during pregnancy see Home Medication Order Sheet.

Prescription/over-the-counter medications previously taken during pregnancy:

Addressograph

(continued on next page)

FIGURE 8–21 Labor and delivery admission sheet.

Labor and Delivery Admission Record *(continued)*

PT. NAME:

GBS Tested: Yes No **Results:** Negative Positive Unknown **Results Date:**

Blood Type/Rh: Rhogam **This Pregnancy:** N/A Yes No No Record

Rubella: Immune Non-immune Unknown **HBsAg:** Negative Positive Unknown **RPR:** Non-reactive Reactive Unknown

Hemoglobin = ______ g/dL **Initials:** ______
Reference Range: 11–14 g/dL (pregnancy) **HIV:** Non-reactive Reactive

Heart Disease: Yes No **Hypertension:** Yes No

MVP: Yes No **Diabetes:** Yes No

Asthma: Yes No **DVT:** Yes No

Blood Transfusion: Yes No
Blood Transfusion Reason/Yr:

Sexually Transmitted Diseases: Denies Chlamydia Syphilis Gonorrhea HIV HPV/Genital Warts Herpes Other ______

Exposure to Infectious Disease This Pregnancy: Denies Measles Mumps HIV/AIDS Chicken Pox TB Hepatitis Other ______

Cervical Procedures: Denies D&C LEEP Cervical Biopsy Laser Cryo/Cautery Other ______

History of Major Illness or Surgery:

Patient History Detail:

Past Pregnancy Complications: None PIH Cystitis Pyelitis Preterm Labor Preterm Birth Anemia Rh Sensitization Positive GBS Other ______
Comments:

Complications Current Pregnancy: None PIH Cystitis Preterm Labor Anemia Rh Sensitization Placental Abnormalities ______ Other ______
Comments:

Fetal Assessments Done This Pregnancy: None Non-Stress Test OCT CVS BPP US Amnio

Previous Labor Durations:

Sibling History:

Family History: N/A Adopted Heart Disease HTN Diabetes Cancer Bleeding Disorder Other ______
Family History Comments:

Drug Use: Denies Yes *If Yes, Describe:*
Drug Use Comments:

Contact Lenses: Yes No Soft Lenses Hard Lenses Lenses In Lenses Out

Glasses: Yes No **Dentures:** Yes No

Body Piercing: Yes No **Body Piercing Location/Removed:**

Support System After Birth: Family Friends Community None
If None, Social Service Referral Entered In Computer: Yes No N/A

History of Abuse: Denies Emotional Physical Sexual Other ______ *If Other, Describe*
Social Service Referral Entered in Computer: Yes No N/A

Special Needs: None Spiritual Cultural Emotional Other ______ Hearing/Vision Impaired: Yes No *If Other, Describe*

Social Service Referral Entered in Computer: Yes No N/A **Pastoral Service Referral Entered in Computer:** Yes No N/A

Interpreter needed? Yes No Primary Language: ______

Psychosocial Comments:

Room Orientation: EFM Bed Phone Call Light Visitors Computer

Does the Patient Have an Advance Directive?

Yes — **If Yes, is Copy in Chart?** Yes No — **If No Copy on Chart, Remind Pt. to Have Family Member Bring Copy AND Send Advance Directive Referral to Pastoral Services** — **Referral Entered in Computer:** Yes No

No — **If No, Does Pt. Want Additional Information or Assistance?** Yes No — **If Yes, Was Referral Sent to Pastoral Care?** Yes No — **Referral Entered in Computer:** Yes No

Disposition of Valuables: Sent Home Kept with Pt. Valuables in Security Office Pt. Encouraged to Take Valuables Home Other ______
Valuables Comments:

Pt. Wants Other Physician or Family Notified: Yes No

Other Physician/Family Notified:

Smoke Use/Frequency: Denies <5 per day 5–10 per day >10 per day >20 per day

Alcohol Use: Denies Occasional 3–5 Drinks/Week 6 or More Drinks/Week

Morse Fall Scale Score:
[ ] <45, low fall risk; initiate appropriate interventions
[ ] >50, high fall risk; initiate appropriate interventions
[ ] ≥4 medications associated with increased fall risk; high fall risk; initiate appropriate interventions

Initiate Care Plan if:
[ ] Anticipated physiological fall risk
[ ] Unanticipated physiological fall risk
[ ] Accidental fall risk

Immunization History
Vaccines: Influenza Yes No Date ______
Pneumonia Yes No Date ______
Tetanus Yes No Date ______
PPD Yes No Date ______

Nursing Assessment Summary: ______

Requests Cord Blood Banking: Y N
Cord Blood Banking Type: ☐ NA
☐ St. Louis Cord Blood Bank
☐ Private Cord Blood Bank

Addressograph

FIGURE 8–21 cont'd

Patient Name:		Physician/CNM:			KEY
	DATE:				**Variability**
	TIME:				Ab = Absent (undetectable)
Cervix — Dilation					Min = Minimal (>0 out ≤5 bpm)
Cervix — Effacement					Mod = Moderate (6–25 bpm)
Cervix — Station					Mar = Marked (>25 bpm)
Fetal Heart — Baseline Rate					**Accelerations**
Fetal Heart — Variability					+ = Present and appropriate for gestational age
Fetal Heart — Accelerations					∅ = Absent
Fetal Heart — Decelerations					**Decelerations**
Fetal Heart — STIM/pH					E = Early
Fetal Heart — Monitor Mode					L = Late
					V = Variable
					P = Prolonged
Uterine Activity — Frequency					**Stim/pH**
Uterine Activity — Duration					+ = Acceleration in response to stimulation
Uterine Activity — Intensity					∅ = No response to stimulation
Uterine Activity — Resting Tone					Record number for scalp pH
Uterine Activity — Monitor Mode					**Monitor mode**
Uterine Activity — Oxytocin milliunits/min					A = Auscultation/Palpation
					E = External u/s or toco
					FSE = Fetal spiral electrode
					IUPC = Intrauterine pressure catheter
Pain					**Frequency of uterine activity**
Coping					∅ = None
Maternal Position					Irreg = Irregular
O2/LPM/Mask					**Intensity of uterine activity**
IV					M = Mild
					Mod = Moderate
Nurse Initials					Str = Strong
					By IUPC = mm Hg
					Resting tone
					R = Relaxed
					By IUCP = mm Hg
Narrative notes:					**Coping**
					W = Well
					S = Support provided
					For pain use 0–10 scale
					Maternal position
					A – Ambulatory
					U = Upright
					SF = Semi-Fowler's
					RL = Right Lateral
					LL = Left Lateral
					MS = Modified Sims'

FIGURE 8-22 Key labor documentation example.

- Complete labor and delivery admission record (see Fig. 8–21).
- Review childbirth plan and discuss the laboring woman's expectations.
  - Pregnant patients may present with a birth plan. A birth plan is a document where the pregnant woman has listed her desires and preferences for labor and delivery. Spend time with the patient reading the plan and supporting the desired choices. Have a clear discussion with the patient about what is available and clarify what is not and why. Communicate with the provider about the birth plan. Using clear, open, and compassionate communication techniques will show respect and understanding of the patient's desires.
- Teach and reinforce relaxation and breathing techniques.
  - Support what they have been practicing or teach techniques as needed to decrease pain and anxiety.
- Obtain laboratory tests as per orders.
  - Provides information on patient status and health.
- Start IV or insert saline lock, if ordered.
  - Provides access for fluids or medications if needed.
- Review the patient's report of onset of labor.
- Assess and record (see Fig. 8–21 and Clinical Pathway and Concept Map):
  - Maternal vital signs
  - FHR
  - UCs
  - Cervical dilation and effacement; as well as fetal presentation, position, and station by performing a sterile vaginal examination (SVE) (Fig. 8–23, Box 8-2).
    - This may be delayed if the patient is ruptured, to decrease the possibility of infection.
  - Status of membranes

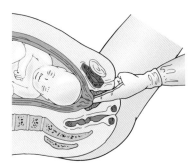

FIGURE 8–23 Sterile vaginal exam.

BOX 8-2 | Sterile Vaginal Exam

Intrapartal Sterile Vaginal Exam

To perform a vaginal exam, the labia are separated with a sterile gloved hand. Fingers are lubricated with a water-soluble lubricant. The first and second fingers are inserted into the introitus; the cervix is then located and the following parameters are assessed (see Fig. 8–23):

- Cervical dilation: This measurement estimates the dilation of the cervical opening by sweeping the examining finger from the margin of the cervical opening on one side to that on the other.

- Cervical effacement: This measurement estimates the shortening of the cervix from 2 cm to paper-thin measured by palpation of the cervical length with the fingertips. The degree of cervical effacement is expressed in terms of the length of the cervical canal compared with that of an unaffected cervix. When it is reduced by one-half (1 cm), it is 50% effaced. When the cervix is thinned out completely, it is 100% effaced.

- Position of cervix: Relationship of the cervical os to the fetal head, which is characterized as posterior, midposition, or anterior.

- Station: Level of the presenting part in the birth canal in relationship to the ischial spines. Station is 0 when the presenting part is at the ischial spines or engaged in the pelvis.

- Presentation: Cephalic (head first), breech (pelvis first), or shoulder (shoulder first).

- Fetal position: Locate the presenting part and specific fetal structure to determine the fetal position in relation to the maternal pelvis.

- Amniotic fluid for color, amount, consistency, and odor
- Vaginal bleeding or bloody show for amount and characteristics of vaginal discharge
- Fetal position with Leopold's maneuvers (Fig. 8–24, Box 8-3)
- Deep tendon reflexes
- Signs of edema
- Heart and lung sounds
- Emotional status
- Pain and discomfort

BOX 8-3 | Leopold's Maneuvers

The purpose of Leopold's maneuvers is to inspect and palpate the maternal abdomen to determine fetal position, station, and size (see Fig. 8–24).

- The first maneuver is to determine what part of the fetus is located in the fundus of the uterus.

- The second maneuver is to determine the location of the fetal back.

- The third maneuver is to determine the presenting part.

- The fourth maneuver is to determine the location of the cephalic prominence.

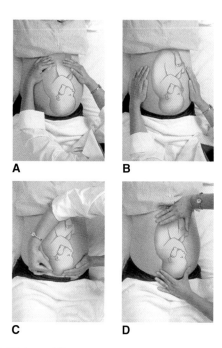

FIGURE 8–24 Leopold's maneuver.

- Review current laboratory results, noting blood Rh status, hematocrit and hemoglobin, and urine dipstick or urinalysis for glucose and protein.
- Review GBS status. If the woman is GBS positive, intrapartum IV antibiotic prophylaxis should be started. The GBS culture should have been completed within the previous 5 weeks (ACOG, 2020)
  - GBS, also known as *Streptococcus agalactiae,* is the leading cause of newborn infection. The primary risk factor for the newborn is birth parent GBS colonization of the GI and GU tracts. Between 10% and 30% of pregnant women are colonized with GBS.
  - Approximately 50% of pregnant women who are colonized will transmit GBS to their newborn via vertical transmission, occurring after the ROM. Without prophylaxis, 1% to 2% of those newborns will go on to develop GBS early-onset disease (EOD).
  - EOD commonly manifests as pneumonia, sepsis, or meningitis, with significant morbidly and mortality rates.

- Implementation of national guidelines for intrapartum antibiotic prophylaxis since the 1990s has resulted in an approximate 80% reduction in the incidence of early-onset neonatal sepsis due to GBS. Penicillin remains the drug of choice, with ampicillin as an alternative. If a patient is allergic to penicillin, cefazolin, clindamycin, or vancomycin may be used (ACOG, 2020).
- Intrapartum GBS prophylaxis is indicated in women who have had (ACOG, 2020):
  - A previous infant with invasive GBS disease
  - GBS bacteriuria (GBS cultured from the urine) during any trimester of current pregnancy
  - Positive GBS vaginal-rectal screening culture at 36 0/7 weeks' gestation or more during the current pregnancy, unless a cesarean birth is performed before the onset of labor, with unruptured membranes.
  - Intrapartum nucleic acid amplification testing (NAAT) positive.
    - NAAT may also be used intrapartum, with a 1- to 2-hour turnaround time, but is less sensitive, with a 7% to 10% failure rate.
  - Intrapartum NAAT negative, but risk factors develop (less than 37 weeks' gestation, or ROM greater than 18 hours, or temperature greater than 100.4°F [38.0°C]).
  - Unknown GBS status at onset of labor with any of the following:
    - Less than 37 weeks' gestation, or ROM greater than 18 hours, or temperature greater than 100.4°F (38.0°C), or known positive GBS status in a previous pregnancy
- Document allergies, history of illness, and last food intake.
- If provider orders allow, encourage fluid intake; food may or may not be restricted.
- Provide comfort measures such as pillows, warm showers, warm blankets, and linen changes as needed.
- Encourage the laboring woman to move as much as possible by:
  - Explaining the importance of walking or maintaining an upright position in facilitating labor progression, fetal descent, rotation, and efficient UCs
  - Being present with the patient may provide comfort, reassurance, distraction, and encouragement.
- Be kind, supportive, and actively listen to the patient's concerns and individual needs, incorporating these into the care plan and establishing a therapeutic relationship. Use translation services if the RN does not speak the patient's preferred language.
- Incorporate understanding of the couple's maturity level, educational level, and previous experience into nursing care.
- Review the labor plan with the laboring woman and her support system.
- Provide clear explanations and updates on progress.
- These nursing actions will provide information to the nurse to facilitate teaching moments, decrease patient anxiety, and support the plan of care.
- Recent recommendations have targeted modifiable obstetric practices that are thought to influence this high C-section rate, such as admitting uncomplicated laboring women to the labor unit with a cervical dilation of less than 3 to 4 cm. A growing body of research suggests that waiting for admission until active labor, if there are no other risk factors and the birthing parent is in agreement, may decrease the need for C-sections and other interventions. Nurses should continue to examine new evidence.

Stage One: Active Phase (6 to 10 cm)

The active phase of labor is the inflection point where labor begins to move more rapidly. It is characterized by regular contractions that require the focus and attention of the birthing woman, significant effacement (80% or more), and greater than 5 cm dilation with ongoing cervical change (Lagrew et al., 2018). During the active phase, the cervix typically dilates at a rate of 1.2 to 1.5 centimeters per hour, much more quickly than the latent phase. Multiparas tend to demonstrate even more rapid cervical dilation (Hutchison et al., 2021) (see Table 8-1). Laboring patients in this phase may have decreased energy and experience fatigue. They become more serious and turn attention to internal sensations. Characteristics of this phase include the following:

- Fetal descent continues.
- Contractions increase in intensity, occurring every 2 to 5 minutes with duration of 45 to 60 seconds.
- Discomfort increases; this is typically when patients come to the birth center or hospital if they have not done so already.
- As the patient moves closer to 10 cm dilation, the patient may experience:
  - Exhaustion and increased difficulty concentrating
  - Increase of bloody show
  - Nausea and vomiting
  - Backache: complaints of back pressure, hand goes over hip, pressing on area
  - Trembling
  - Diaphoresis, especially along the upper lip and facial area
  - May have a strong urge to bear down or push and become more vocal with primal noises and facial expressions.

Medical Interventions

- Evaluate fetal status by fetal monitoring as indicated, either intermittent or continuous.
- Perform internal monitoring with application of internal fetal scalp electrode (FSE) or an IUPC, if necessary.
- These are both invasive interventions and should be used only if external monitoring is not feasible or does not provide enough information to make safe clinical decisions.
  - Pain assessment: Order pain medication or epidural anesthesia.
  - Evaluate progression in labor.
    - If there is slow progress in the active phase of labor, the provider may order an oxytocin drip or an oxytocin drip combined with an amniotomy. An amniotomy alone has not been shown to increase labor progress (Alhafez & Berghella, 2020).

Nursing Actions (see Clinical Pathway and Concept Map)

- If using intermittent monitoring, assess the fetus every 15 to 30 minutes for low-risk patients and every 15 minutes for high-risk patients or consider using continuous monitoring

(Lyndon & Usher Ali, 2015). Intervene for abnormal fetal heart patterns (see Chapter 9).

- Low-risk patients usually include (Simpson & O'Brien-Abel, 2021):
  - No meconium staining, intrapartum bleeding, or abnormal or undetermined fetal test results before birth or at initial admission
  - No increased risk of developing fetal acidemia during labor (e.g., congenital anomalies, intrauterine growth restriction)
  - No maternal condition that may affect fetal well-being (e.g., prior cesarean scar, diabetes, hypertensive disease)
  - No requirement for oxytocin induction or augmentation of labor
- Monitor maternal pulse, blood pressure (BP), and respiratory rate (RR) every hour; temperature every 2 hours, unless ruptured, then every 1 hour.
- Perform intrapartal vaginal exams as needed to assess cervical changes and fetal descent (see Box 8-2).
  - Care should be taken to limit the number of vaginal exams to only those that are necessary. Researchers found that performing five or more vaginal exams during labor was independently associated with increases of febrile morbidity, both intrapartum and postpartum. Compared with patients who received four or less vaginal examinations, patients who received five to six vaginal exams were 1.5 times as likely to become febrile, and patients who received nine or more vaginal exams were 2.6 times as likely to become febrile (Gluck et al., 2020).
- Assess pain (location and degree).
- Administer analgesia as per orders and desire of the laboring patient.
- Monitor and evaluate the effectiveness of epidural or other pain medication.
- Monitor intake and output (I&O), hydration status, and for nausea and vomiting.
- Offer oral fluids as per orders (ice chips, ice pops, carbohydrate liquids, and water). Encourage the patient to listen to her body regarding hydration and nausea and allow her to decide when she has had enough intake.
- Offer clear explanations and updates of progress.
- Promote comfort measures.
- Assist with elimination (bladder distention can hinder fetal descent).
- Encourage breathing and relaxation methods (Box 8-4).
  - Review and reinforce relaxation techniques.
  - Maintain eye contact and physical proximity to the laboring patient.
  - Develop a rhythm and breathing style to deal with each contraction.
  - Use a direct and gentle voice and have a calm and confident manner, speaking slowly in a low, soothing tone, giving short and clear directs such as: "You are in control"; "It is normal to feel so much pressure as the baby moves down"; "You are doing a great job working with your contractions."
  - Use touch or massage if acceptable to the patient.
- Communicate clearly and promptly with other members of the health-care team regarding updates on the patient's

---

BOX 8-4 | Standard of Practice. AWHONN Position Statement: Continuous Labor Support for Every Woman

The AWHONN asserts that continuous labor support from an RN is critical to achieve improved birth outcomes. In partnership with the woman, the RN conducts an assessment, then implements and evaluates an individualized plan of care based on the woman's physical, psychological, and sociocultural needs. This plan incorporates the woman's desires for and expectations of the process of labor. The RN coordinates the woman's support team, which may include a partner, family, friends, or a doula, to assist the woman to achieve her childbirth goals. Care and support during labor are powerful nursing functions, and it is incumbent on health-care facilities to provide a level of staffing that facilitates the unique patient–RN relationship during childbirth. AWHONN recognizes that childbirth education and doula services contribute to the woman's preparation for and support during childbirth and supports consideration of these services as a covered benefit in public and private health insurance plans.

The support provided by the RN should include the following:

- Assessment of the physiological and psychological processes of labor;
- Facilitation of normal physiological processes (e.g., allow movement in labor);
- Provision of physical comfort measures, emotional support, information, and advocacy;
- Evaluation of maternal and fetal status, including uterine activity and fetal oxygenation;
- Instruction regarding the labor process and comfort and coping measures;
- Role modeling to facilitate the participation of the family and companions during labor and birth; and
- Direct collaboration with other members of the health-care team to coordinate patient care.

AWHONN, 2018.

---

progress and changes in status. Use the SBAR technique (Situation, Background, Assessment, Recommendation) to facilitate clear communication.

- Incorporate the support person in care of the patient by:
  - Role modeling and teaching supportive behaviors
  - Carefully listening to and addressing the support person's desires and concerns
  - Assisting the partner with food and rest
  - Providing breaks if desired or needed
- Explain procedures before initiating, asking permission from the patient.
- Adjust the environment as necessary, including dimming the lights, decreasing noise, and limiting interruptions.
- Provide reassurance, updates on progress, and positive reinforcement.

- Attend to the patient's hygiene needs, such as providing cool cloths to wipe her face, providing pericare, and changing chux.
- Check all the supplies necessary for a safe delivery, including all infant resuscitation equipment, delivery equipment, and emergency equipment.

Second Stage

The second stage of labor begins when cervical dilation is complete (10 cm) and ends with the birth of the baby (see Table 8-1) (Fig. 8–25). The second stage is divided into two phases: the latent phase, where the woman is fully dilated but has not begun to push, and the active pushing phase, where the woman is actively bearing down and using expulsive efforts (Simpson & O'Brien-Abel, 2021). Whether a woman feels the immediate need to push when fully dilated depends on whether she has an epidural, the density of the epidural, the station of the fetus, and the individual. Laboring patients often describe the urge to push as intense rectal pressure, similar to the strong need to have a bowel movement. When a patient begins to push, care should be individualized based on maternal and fetal condition (Simpson & O'Brien-Abel, 2021). Some patients, especially those who have neuraxial anesthesia, may elect to have a longer latent phase, also called passive descent, or "laboring down," allowing the fetus to descend farther into the vaginal tract, without active effort by the woman. Others may begin to push immediately.

Research on immediate pushing versus delayed pushing is mixed. In a 2020 meta-analysis, there was no difference found between immediate and delayed pushing in relation to spontaneous vaginal delivery rates, operative vaginal delivery, cesarean section, intrapartum fever, endometritis, postpartum hemorrhage (PPH), episiotomy, or severe perineal lacerations. Women who were in the delayed pushing group had shorter periods of active pushing, but longer overall second stages of labor. Women in the delayed pushing groups also had greater risk of chorioamnionitis (9.1% vs. 6.6%) and low umbilical cord pH (2.7% vs. 1.3%) (DiMascio et al., 2020). However, practice may shift on delayed pushing as current recommendations from ACOG (2019a) indicate data support pushing at the start of the second stage of labor for nulliparous women receiving neuraxial analgesia. Delayed pushing has not been shown to significantly improve the likelihood of vaginal birth. Risks of delayed pushing, including infection, hemorrhage, and neonatal acidemia, should be shared with nulliparous women receiving neuraxial analgesia who consider such an approach. According to AWHONN (2019), each woman and baby represent an individual clinical situation. Therefore, the entire clinical scenario should be reviewed when considering how long to continue the second stage of labor. Fetal status, progress of fetal descent, maternal wishes, maternal fatigue, and duration of active pushing are clinical assessment factors that may help inform this decision.

Characteristics of the second stage include the following:

- Women may feel an intense urge to push or bear down when the baby reaches the pelvic floor, which is known as the Ferguson reflex.

- Women, especially women who do not have an epidural, may feel a burning sensation as the fetus crowns. This is due to tissue stretching.
- It is uncommon for primiparas to actively push more than 3 hours and for multiparas to actively push more than 2 hours.
  - However, even after 4 hours of pushing, approximately 78% of primiparas who continued with active pushing had a vaginal delivery and more than 97% did not have adverse neonatal outcomes.
  - Similarly, after more than 2 hours of pushing, approximately 82% of multiparas who continued active pushing delivered vaginally and more than 97% did not have adverse neonatal outcomes (Grobman et al., 2016).
- Contractions are intense and may occur with greater frequency.
- Bloody show increases.
- The second stage may last longer for women with epidurals.
- The perineum flattens and the rectum and vagina bulge.

Pushing

Preferred pushing techniques, which vary in practice, are an area of active research. Pushing techniques should be individualized for each patient, based on patient preference, patient progress, and fetal status. Pushing techniques include the following (AWHONN, 2019):

- Closed glottis, also referred to as the Valsalva technique, involves a voluntary or directed strenuous bearing-down effort against a closed glottis for at least 10 seconds. The woman is instructed to take a deep breath and hold it for as long as she can (during each count of 10) throughout the entire contraction. This method usually involves two to three pushes of 10 seconds each with each contraction. It is no longer recommended.
- Directed pushing refers to instructions from care providers to the woman concerning how to push and often includes directions to hold your breath (closed glottis or Valsalva technique) for a count of 10 or more seconds. Instructions also may be given concerning positioning during pushing—often a supine or semi-Fowler's position—rather than encouraging the woman to choose her own position of comfort.
- Mother-initiated spontaneous pushing refers to the laboring woman's response to the natural urge to push or a bearing-down effort that comes and goes several times during each contraction. It does not involve timed breath holding or counting to 10.
- Nondirected pushing refers to care providers encouraging the woman to choose whatever method she feels is effective to push her baby out, including choosing the position during pushing, deciding whether to hold her breath during pushing, and determining the duration of each pushing effort. This type of pushing effort may also include maternal vocalizations.
- Open glottis refers to spontaneous, involuntary bearing down accompanying the forces of the UC and is usually characterized by expiratory grunting or vocalizations.

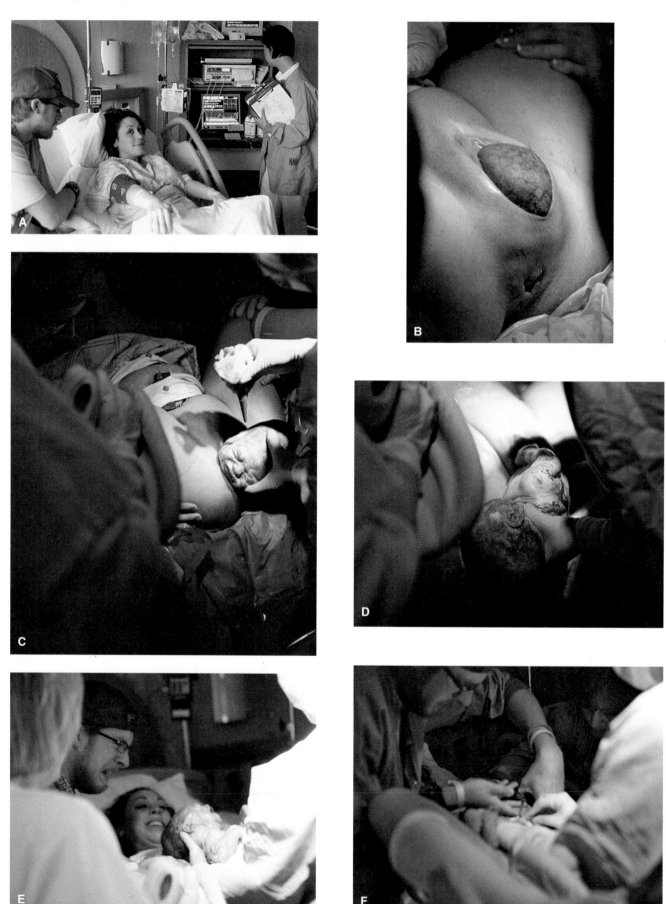

FIGURE 8–25 Vaginal birth sequence. (A) Pushing in an upright position allows the use of gravity to promote fetal descent. (B) Crowning. (C) Birth of the head. (D) Birth of the shoulders. (E) The infant is shown to the new parents. (F) The baby's father cuts the umbilical cord.

To maximize pushing efforts, the nurse should assess the woman's knowledge of pushing techniques, expectations for pushing, presence of Ferguson's reflex, intensity of UCs, readiness to push, and the fetal presentation, position, and station. With adequate information, the woman can actively participate in the decision to start pushing. AWHONN recommends encouraging women to push for 6 to 8 seconds followed by a slight exhale and repeat of this pattern for three to four pushes per contraction or as tolerated by the woman and fetus.

Perineal Stretching

The perineum is at risk for lacerations during the birthing process as the head stretches the perineal tissue. Various measures have been used to enhance perineal stretching and decrease perineal trauma, including application of warm compresses, gentle perineal massage and stretching, and perineal massage with warm oil during the second stage of labor. Moderate quality evidence indicates that warm compresses and massage on the perineum may effectively reduce the incidence of third- and fourth-degree lacerations compared with no warm compresses and no massage (Aasheim et al., 2017).

Evidence-Based Practice

AWHONN's Recommendations for the Management of the Second Stage of Labor

AWHONN recommends the following for the management of the second stage of labor, the latent (passive descent) phase (AWHONN, 2019):

- Maternal assessment
  - Assess the knowledge of the laboring woman regarding her position during the second stage.
  - Assess factors that may affect the ability to change position or push effectively.
  - Assess fetal presentation, position, station, and descent and progress toward birth.
  - Assess maternal vital signs every 4 hours or more frequently when indicated and as per institution protocol.
  - Assess the woman's comfort level to ensure adequate pain relief if she desires.
    - If the patient has chosen an epidural form of pain relief, continue epidural analgesia and anesthesia.
  - Assess the woman's urinary bladder status periodically.
    - Avoid use of continuous indwelling urinary (e.g., Foley) catheters during labor.
    - Encourage the mother to void on the bedpan; if she is unable, consider use of an intermittent catheter (in-and-out) if the bladder needs to be emptied.
- Maternal positioning:
  - Avoid the supine position during the second stage of labor.
  - Encourage repositioning at least every 30 minutes whenever possible.
  - Assist the woman in changing her position if she has not done so herself.

- Incorporate the use of upright positioning aids as tolerated and with assistance from the nurse or the woman's support person.
  - Positioning aids may include but are not limited to a birthing ball, a peanut ball, cushions, towel pull, squat bar, and birthing stool. The peanut ball offers nurses and women a low-tech, high-touch intervention to possibly improve chances for a vaginal birth (Hickey & Savage, 2019).
- Passive fetal descent
  - When a patient is fully dilated, assess the following parameters to determine when the woman should begin pushing:
    - Assess the woman's urge to push and feelings of perineal pressure.
    - Assess fetal presentation, station, and position.
- Provide information to the woman about options for immediate or delayed pushing, including risks and benefits.
- If delayed pushing until urge to push is chosen as an option, these time frames are considered: up to 2 hours for nulliparous women and up to 1 hour for multiparous women with regional anesthesia.
- However, there may be a shift in practice on delayed pushing as current recommendations from the ACOG (2019a) indicate data support pushing at the start of the second stage of labor for nulliparous women receiving neuraxial analgesia. Delayed pushing has not been shown to significantly improve the likelihood of vaginal birth, and risks of delayed pushing, including infection, hemorrhage, and neonatal acidemia, should be shared with nulliparous women receiving neuraxial analgesia who consider such an approach.
- Fetal evaluation during the passive phase
  - Promote fetal well-being by assessing the FHR.
  - During the second stage passive fetal descent phase, assess and document the FHR every 30 minutes.

AWHONN recommends the following for the management of the second stage of labor, the active (pushing) phase:

- Maternal assessment
  - Assess the knowledge of the laboring woman and her support persons about positioning during the active phase.
    - Maintaining upright, hands-and-knees, or lateral positions during active pushing
    - Ability to push effectively
    - Avoiding supine position
  - Assess maternal vital signs every 4 hours or more frequently when indicated and as per institution protocol.
  - Assess the woman's comfort level to ensure she has adequate pain relief, including continuing analgesia or anesthesia if the woman has chosen this method of pain relief. Data indicate discontinuation of epidural analgesia or anesthesia has not been shown to be beneficial for maternal pushing efforts, shortening the second stage of labor, or decreasing the risk of operative vaginal birth.
  - Continue to assess the woman's bladder status periodically.
    - Encourage the mother to void on the bedpan; if she is unable, consider use of an in-and-out catheter if the bladder needs to be emptied.
    - If an indwelling urinary catheter was used during labor, it is typically discontinued during pushing.

- Positioning:
  - Engage in shared decision making by offering choices of birthing positions. More upright positions have been associated with a shorter second stage of labor.
  - Encourage and assist with frequent material position changes at least every 30 minutes whenever possible and assist as needed.
    - Evaluate the effectiveness of position changes on fetal well-being, fetal descent, and maternal comfort.
    - Incorporate the use of positioning aids.
- Active pushing:
  - When conditions are physiologically appropriate for active pushing, women can be encouraged to bear down and "do whatever comes naturally."
    - Help the woman with open-glottis pushing for 6 to 8 seconds with a slight exhale for approximately three to four pushes per contraction or as tolerated by the woman and fetus.
  - Discourage holding the breath for more than 8 seconds; do not count to 10 during pushing.
  - Assess progress during active pushing, including pushing effort and descent and rotation of the fetal presenting part.
  - If appropriate for fetal and maternal conditions, allow at least 2 hours of pushing for multiparas and 3 hours for primiparas. Longer periods of pushing may be appropriate on an individualized basis, based on assessment of progress and maternal or fetal tolerance.
- Fetal assessment during active phase
  - Assess and promote fetal well-being during active pushing.
  - Use fetal assessment data to guide pushing efforts.
    - Assess and document FHR every 5 to 15 minutes depending on fetal status.
  - Most fetuses tolerate decelerations during pushing, although some fetuses enter the second stage of labor with less physiologic reserve than others. The same intrauterine resuscitation measures appropriate in first-stage labor can be applied to second-stage labor.
  - If FHR is category II or III, provide intrauterine resuscitation measures and notify the provider. These interventions are detailed in Chapter 9.
  - Modify pushing efforts, based on fetal status. For example, push every other or every third contraction.
    - Stop pushing temporarily if fetal condition warrants.
  - Assess uterine activity to avoid uterine tachysystole (more than five contractions in a 10-minute period), and treat tachysystole if it occurs.
  - Differentiate between maternal and FHR periodically.

Medical Interventions

- Prepare for delivery.
- Provide reassurance to the woman while she pushes and brings the baby through the birth canal.
- Support the fetal head and the maternal perineum to minimize lacerations.
- Episiotomies should not be routinely done (Box 8-5).
- Assist the woman in birthing her child.

BOX 8-5 | Episiotomy Types and Lacerations

An episiotomy is an incision made in the perineum by the delivering provider to provide more space for the presenting part at delivery (see Fig. 8–28). Routine use of episiotomy at delivery is no longer typical. However, it may be used when clinical circumstances warrant; for example, if there is a need to deliver the fetus quickly due to fetal heart tracing concerns or shoulder dystocias.

- The most common types of episiotomies are midline (cut at a 90-degree angle toward the rectum) and mediolateral (cut at a 45-degree angle) (see Fig. 8–29).
  - Midline episiotomies are associated with higher risks of severe perineal trauma, including third- and fourth-degree lacerations (Pergialiotis et al., 2020).
  - Mediolateral episiotomies were thought to be protective against severe perineal trauma, but recent research indicates that they are neither helpful or harmful, and should not be used for that reason (Pergialiotis et al., 2020)
- Lacerations can occur in the cervix, vagina, or the perineum, either on their own or in addition to episiotomies. Perineal lacerations are most common (see Fig. 8–29A).
- A first-degree laceration of the perineum involves injury to the skin and subcutaneous tissue of the perineum and vaginal epithelium only. The perineal muscles remain intact (see Fig. 8–29B).
- A second-degree laceration of the perineum involves skin, mucous membranes, and fascia of the perineal body. The anal sphincter muscles remain intact (see Fig. 8–29C).
- A third-degree laceration involves skin, mucous membranes, and muscles of the perineal body and extend into, but not through, the rectal sphincter (see Fig. 8–29D).
- A fourth-degree laceration extends into the rectal mucosa and exposes the lumen of the rectum (see Fig. 8–29E).

Nursing Actions (see Clinical Pathway)

- Instruct the woman to bear down with the urge to push.
- Assess fetal response to pushing; check FHR every 5 to 15 minutes or after each contraction.
- Explain the need for vaginal examinations and the pressure or pain sensations anticipated. Negotiate when exams will be performed whenever possible. Perform vaginal exams only as needed, share findings with the woman and her partner, and acknowledge and apologize for the discomfort caused during these procedures.
- Provide comfort measures and assist with position changes.
- Provide reassurance, empathy, and encouragement to the woman by methods such as acknowledging the stress and work of labor, acknowledging unpleasant sensations, and encouraging the woman's spontaneous pushing efforts.
- Attend to perineal hygiene as needed. Passing stool is common during pushing efforts. Reassure the woman that passing stool is a normal and expected part of pushing.

- Encourage rest between contractions by breathing with the patient and through therapeutic touch.
  - Decreases fatigue and hypoxia in the fetus by providing increased oxygenation.
- Review and reinforce pushing technique by:
  - Maintaining eye contact
  - Developing a rhythm and pushing style to deal with each contraction that maximizes the woman's urge to push
  - Using direct, simple, and focused communication, while avoiding unnecessary conversation
- Advocate on the woman's behalf for her desires of the delivery plan. Facilitate collaboration or negotiation among other caregivers on behalf of the woman to support care decisions and preferences whenever possible.
- Check that all infant resuscitation equipment is ready and set for immediate use.
- Assure that the staff that should be present at the birth (additional RN, provider, NICU staff if required, etc.) have been notified and are available to immediately come when called.
- Evaluate the birth partner's knowledge of physical, emotional, and psychosocial support needed during labor and augment as needed to meet the individual woman's needs.
- Assist the support people and birth partner.
  - Role model supportive behaviors.
  - Offer support, praise, and encouragement.
  - Assist with food and rest and provide breaks.

Third Stage

The third stage of labor begins immediately after the delivery of the fetus and involves separation of the placenta from the wall of the uterus and expulsion of the placenta and membranes from the uterus and vagina (see Table 8-1). As the infant is born, the uterine myometrium spontaneously contracts, reducing its surface area and resulting in shearing forces at the placental attachment site and subsequent placental separation. Once the placenta separates from the wall of the uterus, the uterus continues to contract until the placenta is expelled (Fig. 8–26). In term pregnancies, the mean length of the third stage is 5 minutes, with 90% of all placentas delivered by 15 minutes (AAP & ACOG, 2019). Signs that signify the impending delivery of the placenta include:

- Rising of the uterus into a ball shape
- Lengthening of the umbilical cord at the introitus
- Sudden gush of blood from the vagina

Once the infant is delivered, many providers start active management of the third stage, rather than expectant management (waiting without intervention for the placenta to deliver). Although the evidence is of low quality, and more research needs to be done, active management appears to reduce the incidence of maternal hemorrhage and the need for blood transfusion (Begley et al., 2019). Active management includes the delivery of prophylactic uterotonic drugs (drugs that cause UCs, such as oxytocin) either after the delivery of the anterior shoulder or the delivery of the entire infant, often combined with controlled traction on the umbilical cord. Some protocols also add uterine massage (Berghella, 2021). Evidence shows that administration of uterotonic medication has been the most effective component of the triad (King et al., 2019).

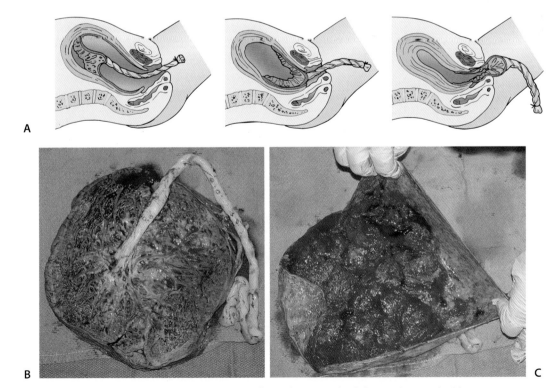

FIGURE 8–26 (A) Delivery of the placenta. (B) Delivered placenta (fetal side). (C) Inside of placenta (maternal side).

CLINICAL JUDGMENT

Quantification of Blood Loss After Birth

Average blood loss for a vaginal birth is approximately 500 mL within 24 hours (King et al., 2019). Historically, providers would visually scan the bloody items after birth and assign an estimated blood loss amount to their assessment. This method, sometimes called "a glance and a guess," is subjective, imprecise, and frequently resulted in underestimations of blood loss by 33% to 50%, particularly when large volumes are lost (Main et al., 2015). Inaccuracies around the amount of blood lost after a delivery may delay the identification of a postpartum hemorrhage (PPH), defined as blood loss over 1,000 mL. Obstetric hemorrhage is the most common serious complication of childbirth and the most preventable cause of maternal mortality (see Chapter 14), making it critical that RNs are able to accurately quantify blood loss after delivery. Both AWHONN (AWHONN, 2015c) and ACOG (ACOG, 2019b) recommend that cumulative blood loss be formally measured or quantified after every birth.

Tips to do a quantified blood loss include:

- Create a list of dry weights of all items that might absorb blood during a delivery.
- Begin quantification of blood loss immediately after the infant's birth, but before the delivery of the placenta, using a calibrated under-buttocks drape.
  - Before delivery of the placenta, fluid collected is likely amniotic fluid, urine and stool, and should not be considered in the count.
- Record the total fluid amount in the calibrated-under buttocks drape after the delivery of the placenta, subtracting pre-placenta fluid volume from the post-placenta volume.
  - The fluid collected after the delivery of the placenta is likely to be blood.
- Weigh all blood-soaked materials (chux, laps, etc.). Subtract the dry weight of each item. This will give an estimate of the amount of blood absorbed by each item.
  - Formula: Wet item gram weight – Dry item gram weight = Amount of blood.
- Add the totals from the calibrated drape and the blood-soaked materials. If irrigation was used, subtract the amount of irrigation.
- This will produce a quantified blood loss.
- Remember: 1 gram of blood = 1 mL of blood.

Adapted from Association of Women's Health, Obstetric and Neonatal Nurses (AWHONN). (2015b). Practice brief. Quantification of blood loss: AWHONN practice brief number 1. Journal of Obstetric, Gynecologic, and Neonatal Nursing, 44, 158–160.

Some hospitals are beginning to use computer-assisted devices to help quantify blood loss. These devices are still under study, but research is promising. To use these devices, the nurse holds up each blood-soaked item to the screen, and the device, using sensitive algorithms, is able to estimate the amount of blood on the item versus other types of fluid, and keeps a running tally of blood loss (Saoud et al., 2019). If shown to be accurate, this method of quantifying blood loss may become more common.

SAFE AND EFFECTIVE NURSING CARE: Understanding Medication

Uterotonics

Uterotonics are pharmacological agents used to induce contractions and to increase tonicity of the uterus. The use of uterotonics during the third stage of labor and in the immediate postpartum period for the prevention of PPH is recommended for all births by both ACOG and AWHONN (Main et al., 2015). Oxytocin is the recommended first-line uterotonic drug for the prevention of PPH. Other medications may be used to augment oxytocin, if oxytocin does not control the bleeding adequately.

Oxytocin (Pitocin)

- Classification: hormone or oxytocic.
- Route or dosage:
  - Intravenous (IV) infusion: Commonly used dosages include 10 to 40 international units of oxytocin in 500 to 1,000 mL normal saline (NS), with the rate adjusted to uterine tone, up to 500 mL/hr.
  - Intramuscularly (IM): 10 international units for women without IV access. Oxytocin should not be administered by IV push.
- As a high-alert medication, IV oxytocin premixed bags should be:
  - Infused via an IV infusion pump to control oxytocin administration.
  - Prominently and clearly labeled with bright-colored labeling.
  - Stored separately to prevent a 1,000 mL IV bag with oxytocin from being mistaken for a plain 1,000 mL bag used for IV fluid resuscitation bolus.
- Administer IV oxytocin by providing a bolus dose followed by a total minimum infusion time of 4 hours after birth, or per hospital policy. For women at high risk for a PPH, continuation beyond 4 hours is recommended. Rate and duration should be titrated according to uterine tone and bleeding (AWHONN, 2015a).
- Actions: Stimulates uterine smooth muscle that produces intermittent contractions. Has vasopressor and antidiuretic properties.
- Side effects: Hypotension, tachycardia, water retention.
- Indications: Control of postpartum bleeding after placental expulsion

Methylergonovine (Methergine)

- Classification: Oxytocic or ergot alkaloids.
- Route or dosage:
  - PO 0.2 mg three to four times daily in the puerperium for 7 days (maximum 1 week).
  - IM 0.2 mg after delivery of anterior shoulder, after delivery of placenta, or during puerperium; may be repeated every 2 to 4 hours.
  - IV administration should only be considered during life-threatening situations.

- Actions: Increases the tone, rate, and amplitude of contractions on the smooth muscles of the uterus, producing sustained contractions and reducing blood loss.
- Indications: Prevent or treat PPH, uterine atony, or subinvolution. This is used as a second-line medication.
- Monitor: BP, central nervous system (CNS) status, and vaginal bleeding on a regular basis. May cause nausea. Patient may require antiemetic.
- Contraindicated in hypertensive and preeclamptic patients. May cause severe vasoconstriction (Lexi-Comp, 2021a).

Carboprost Tromethamine (Hemabate)

- Classification: Prostaglandin F2a analog.
- Route or dosage: IM 0.25 mg injected into a large muscle or the uterus. Total doses are not to exceed 2 mg.
- Actions: Increases contractions of the uterine smooth muscles.
- Indications: Uterine atony. Second-line medication. Carboprost is a treatment alternative to methylergonovine for patients with hypertensive disorders. It also may be used in hemorrhage situations refractory to methylergonovine and oxytocin.
- Common side effects: nausea, vomiting, and diarrhea.
- Use cautiously in patients with asthma, as Carboprost can stimulate vasospasm (Vallera et al., 2017).

Misoprostol (Cytotec)

- Classification: synthetic analog of prostaglandin E.
- Originally developed to treat peptic ulcers, it is now used widely in obstetrics, including off-label use (non-FDA-approved use) to manage postpartum bleeding. Second-line medication.
- Route or dosage:
  - Oral (only FDA-approved route), sublingual, buccal, 200 to 400 mcg
  - Rectal 800 to 1,000 mcg
- Action: Acts as a prostaglandin analogue causing UCs.
- Common side effects: abdominal pain, diarrhea, fever, and chills.
- Indications: To control PP hemorrhage. Misoprostol may be used as a first-line medication in low-resource areas where oxytocin is not available (Vallera et al., 2017).

Tranexamic Acid

- Classification: antifibrinolytic.
- Although relatively new in obstetrics, use has become standard of care as a second-line medication in treatment of women with PPH and as a prevention strategy for women at high risk for PPH.
- Route or dosage: 1 gram IV over 10 to 20 minutes.
- Action: inhibits fibrinolysis (stops the breakdown of clots).
- Common side effects: abdominal pain, headache (Lexi-Comp, 2021b), nausea, vomiting, and diarrhea.

Medical Interventions

- At delivery, the neonate is often placed skin-to-skin on the mother's chest and dried. Assessment of respiratory status is immediately performed; if the neonate does not display adequate respiratory effort, the neonate is taken to the warmer for further evaluation and treatment.
- Await delivery of placenta and begin active management of the third stage of labor (Begley et al., 2019).
- If the third stage of labor is longer than 30 minutes, it is known as "prolonged third stage" or "retained placenta." Retained placenta is associated with increased risk of hemorrhage and infection, which may be partially due to complications arising from the need for the provider to manually remove the placenta (King et al., 2019).
- Order pain medications and uterotonics if necessary.

Nursing Actions (see Clinical Pathway and Concept Map)

- Administer uterotonics per provider order after the delivery of the neonate.
- Assess maternal vital signs every 15 minutes.
- Encourage the woman to breathe with contractions and relax between contractions.
- Encourage mother–baby interactions by providing immediate skin-to-skin contact if the newborn is stable.
- Administer pain medications as per order.
- Complete documentation of the delivery (Fig. 8–27).
  - Documentation includes labor summary, delivery summary for mother and baby, infant information, Apgar, infant resuscitation, and documentation of personnel in attendance.
- Explain all forthcoming procedures.
- Stay with the woman and her family.

Fourth Stage

The fourth stage begins after delivery of the placenta and typically ends with the stabilization of the mother. After the placenta delivers, the primary mechanism by which hemostasis is achieved at the placental site is vasoconstriction produced by a well-contracted myometrium. During the fourth stage, usually lasting at least 2 hours, the nurse is caring for both the woman and her newborn child and should have no other nursing responsibilities (Simpson & O'Brien-Abel, 2021) (see Table 8-1). The nurse must focus both on the transition of the newborn from intrauterine to extrauterine life and the mother's safe recovery from childbirth. This stage also begins the postpartum period (see Chapter 12 for a discussion of the postpartum period).

Medical Interventions

- Repair the episiotomy or laceration (see Box 8-5) (Figs. 8–28 and 8–29).
- Complete all sponge, needle, and instrument counts with the RN.
- Inspect the placenta after delivery: Intact, three-vessel cord, cord attachment to placenta. If any part of the placenta is left in the uterus, including membranes, it becomes a risk factor for a PPH.
- Assess the fundus for firmness. Uterine atony is the most common cause of PPH.
- Order uterotonics, as needed.
- Order pain medications, if necessary.

Delivery/Newborn Record

LABOR SUMMARY   Time   Date

Regular contractions began: _____
Time of Oxytocin start: _____
BOW ruptured: _____
(best estimate) 4 cm: _____
10 cm: _____

Amniotic fluid rupture:
- [ ] Spontaneous
- [ ] Artificial

Color:
- [ ] Clear
- [ ] Light mec. (stain)
- [ ] Medium mec.
- [ ] Thick mec.
- [ ] Cloudy
- [ ] Bloody

Labor description:
- [ ] Spontaneous
- [ ] AROM for induction
- [ ] Augmented, oxytocin
- [ ] No labor
- [ ] Induced, oxytocin

Fetal monitoring in labor:
- [ ] Auscultation only
- [ ] External monitor
- [ ] Internal monitor
- [ ] Both
- [ ] IFM site

- [ ] Cervical ripening agent _____
- [ ] IUPC
- [ ] Amino infusion
   Previous C/S: [ ] No   VBAC   [ ] No
                  [ ] Yes attempted: [ ] Yes

Analgesics: before delivery

Drug	Dose	Time
_____	_____	_____

Labor analgesia:
- [ ] None
- [ ] Epidural
- [ ] Narcotic
- [ ] Both
- [ ] Cervical dil @ epid _____

Steroids for lung maturity: Date ___ Time ___ Date ___ Time ___
Antibiotic started: (prior to birth): [ ] <4 hrs [ ] ≥4 hrs [ ] >24 hrs
   Why: [ ] GBS ⊕ Pending / Preterm   # Doses before birth _____
         [ ] Cardiac prophylaxis
         [ ] Fever/Chorioamnionitis
         [ ] Other: _____
Peak maternal temp   [ ] <99.5   [ ] 99.5–101.9   [ ] ≥102

GROUP B STREP SCREEN

Universal Risk Factors
- [ ] Previous GBS infected infant
- [ ] ⊕ Urine cx for GBS in current pregnancy

Culture Based
- [ ] Negative
- [ ] Positive
- [ ] Not available

Risk Based (Intrapartum)
- [ ] No risk factors
- [ ] < 37 weeks
- [ ] ROM ≥ 18 hours
- [ ] Maternal temp ≥ 100.4

APGAR SCORE

	1 min	5 min
Heart Rate		
Respiratory Effort		
Muscle Tone		
Reflex Irritability		
Color		
TOTAL		

Cord around neck X ☐

Umbilical Vessel Number: ☐

- [ ] Voided in DR
- [ ] Stool in DR

DELIVERY–MOTHER

Method of Delivery:
- [ ] Vertex, Vaginal
- [ ] Breech, Vaginal
- [ ] Cesarean Section
- [ ] Vacuum
- [ ] Forceps

Episiotomy/Laceration:
- [ ] None
- [ ] Median
- [ ] Mediolateral
- [ ] Laceration
- [ ] Repaired

PLACENTA:
- [ ] Spontaneous
- [ ] Assist
- [ ] Manual
Abnormalities:

Medications at Delivery:

Drug	Dose	Time
Pitocin IV IM	_____ units	_____
_____	_____	_____
_____	_____	_____

PEDIATRICIAN: _____

DELIVERY SUMMARY

Baby [____] of a [____] gestation
   Birth Order   Plurality

	Time	Date
DELIVERY:		
PLACENTA:		
C/S start time:		
Uterine incis. time:		
C/S finish time:		

INFANT   (circle)   Boy   Girl

Weight _____ lb _____ gm
Length _____ in _____ cm
Head circ _____ in _____ cm

Delivery Outcomes:
- [ ] Live birth admitted for regular care
- [ ] Live birth admitted to trans. nursery
- [ ] Live birth admitted to NICU
- [ ] Neonatal death in delivery room
- [ ] Fetal death before admission
- [ ] Fetal death after admission

Feeding:
- [ ] Breast
- [ ] Bottle

Gest. Age @ Delivery _____

I.D. BAND #: [_____]
Bands Checked by:
_____ RN   _____ RN

Cord Blood to Lab: [ ] Yes   [ ] No
Cord Gases Sent: [ ] Yes   [ ] No
Specimen to Lab: [ ] Type _____
Culture to Lab: [ ] Type _____

RESUSCITATION

Respirations: [ ] Spontaneous   [ ] Delayed _____ min

Check ALL that apply:
- [ ] Suction
- [ ] Oxygen
- [ ] Mask vent
- [ ] Intubation for resuscitation
- [ ] Chest compression
- [ ] Medications
- [ ] Volume

- [ ] Narcan Given
   Time: _____
   Dose: _____
   Route: _____
   By whom: _____

For Meconium Babies:
- [ ] Not intubated
- [ ] Intubated—∅ Below cords
- [ ] Intubated—Meconium noted

Note: _____
_____
_____
_____

Newborn attended by _____ RN/MD
- [ ] Newborn admitted time: _____ am/pm
MR # _____   Pat # _____
Pediatrician notified of delivery: K # _____
   Name _____ MD
   Date _____ Time _____ am/pm
   Via _____ by _____

DELIVERING PHYSICIAN/CNM:	APN/NICU STAFF AT DELIVERY:	ANESTHESIOLOGIST:
ASSIST MD/CNM:	OB/RN AT DELIVERY:	RN SIGNATURE DATE/TIME:

Patient's Data/Addressograph

FIGURE 8-27 Documentation of delivery.

CRITICAL COMPONENT

Newborn–Family Attachment: The Golden Hour

The "golden hour" is defined as the first 60 minutes after childbirth. This critical period is a time of transition for the neonate and the new family. If it is physiologically safe to do so, the infant should remain on the birthing parent's chest the entire time. The three key components of the golden hour are delayed cord clamping until the umbilical cord has stopped pulsating (usually between 1 and 5 minutes); maternal-neonatal skin-to-skin contact, including performing all assessments while the infant is on the maternal abdomen; and early breastfeeding. Skin-to-skin contact is described as holding the unclothed, diapered newborn on the mother's or caretaker's bare chest, usually in an upright position. Routine interventions that are not time-sensitive should be delayed.

These three components of the golden hour reduce the risk for neonatal hypoglycemia, help regulate newborn temperature, and decrease newborn and maternal stress levels. Because skin-to-skin promotes oxytocin letdown, which is critical for uterine involution, it helps stabilize the mother. Implementing the golden hour is also associated with increased rates and duration of breastfeeding. If the maternal condition excludes a golden hour, the infant may also be placed skin-to-skin with the birth partner (Neczypor & Holley, 2017). AWHONN recommends all stable infants greater than 37 weeks and 0 days' gestation born by vaginal or cesarean birth should be placed in immediate skin-to-skin contact for at least the first hour of life or until the first breastfeeding is completed (AWHONN, 2016).

Nursing Actions (see Clinical Pathway and Concept Map)

- Explain all procedures.
- Assess the uterus at least every 15 minutes for position, tone, and location, intervening with fundal massage as necessary.
  - The majority of hemorrhages occur during the fourth stage labor from uterine atony, making ongoing and careful assessment crucial (King et al., 2019).
- Assess lochia for color, amount, and clots at least every 15 minutes.

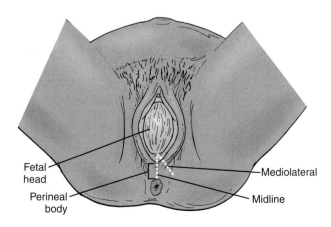

FIGURE 8–28 Episiotomy lacerations.

- Assess maternal vital signs at least every 15 minutes.
- Complete quantified blood loss measurements.
- Administer medications as per orders.
- Assist the care provider with repair of lacerations or episiotomy.

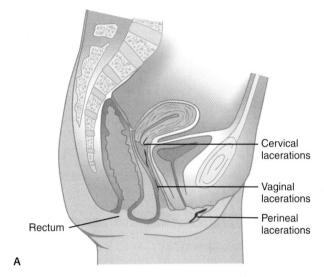

A

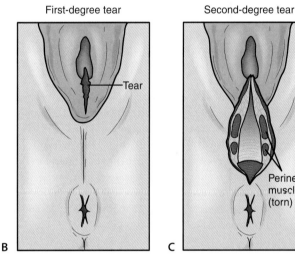

B   C

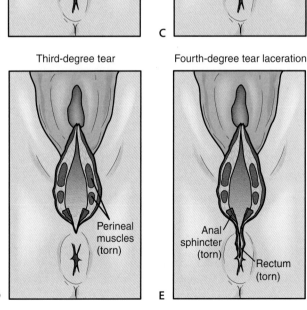

D   E

FIGURE 8–29 (A) Potential locations of lacerations. (B) First-degree tear. (C) Second-degree tear. (D) Third-degree tear. (E) Fourth-degree tear.

- Complete all sponge, needle, and instrument counts with the provider.
- Monitor perineum for unusual swelling or hematoma formation.
- Apply ice packs to the perineum.
- Assess for return of full motor-sensory function if epidural or spinal anesthesia is used.
- Monitor for bladder distention
  - If the woman has full motor-sensory function, assist her to the bathroom and measure the void. Stay to aid with peri-care and monitor for orthostatic hypotension.
  - If the woman does not have full motor-sensory function and the bladder is distended, resulting in a change in uterine position and increased lochia amount, offer the patient a bedpan. If unable to void, consider inserting a straight catheter to drain the bladder.
- Assess pain levels and intervene per patient desire.
- Stay with the mother and family.
- Offer congratulations and reassurance on a job well done to the woman and family.
- Explore with the family any requests they have for keeping the placenta. The placenta was the active interface between the fetus and the mother, and many people have rituals attached to its disposition (Burns, 2014). Efforts should be made to accommodate those requests.
  - There has been a recent trend for parents to take the placenta home and consume it, either raw, cooked, or via encapsulation for alleged health benefits and ability to aid in recovery from childbirth. However, researchers have not found scientific evidence of any clinical benefit of placentophagy (eating the placenta) among humans and evidence of actual risk of harm. In 2017, the Centers for Disease Control and Prevention (CDC) found evidence of late-onset GBS transmission from mother to infant due to maternal ingestion of encapsulated placenta (Farr et al., 2018).
- Provide an opportunity for the support person to interact with the newborn (Fig. 8–30).

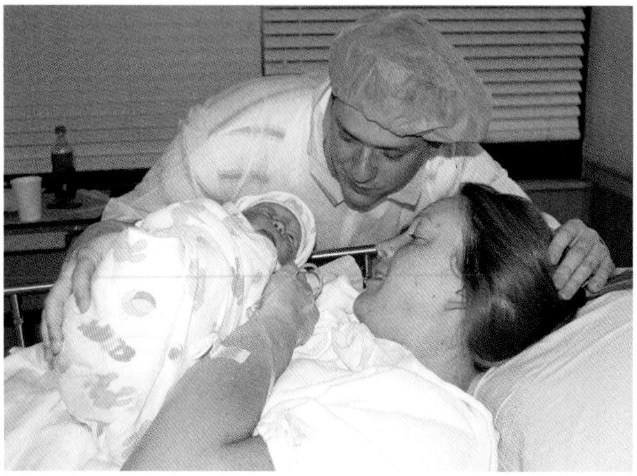

Courtesy of Fisher family

FIGURE 8–30 Newly delivered baby in the delivery room with family.

THE NEWBORN

Newborn transition and initial care typically occur in the labor and delivery room. Initial assessments can be safely done with the infant skin-to-skin on the mother's abdomen after delivery if the infant is stable. It is critical that the nurse monitor the newborn's respiratory transition. The newborn must begin to breathe; if the newborn does not breathe or is gasping, immediate intervention is needed. Remember, "bonding is beautiful, breathing is better." Temperature, heart and respiratory rates, skin color, adequacy of peripheral circulation, type of respiration, level of consciousness, tone, and activity should be monitored and recorded at least every 30 minutes until the newborn's condition has remained stable for at least 2 hours.

Apgar Scores

Apgar scores should be obtained at 1 minute and 5 minutes after birth. If the 5-minute Apgar score is less than 7, additional scores should be assigned every 5 minutes up to 20 minutes. The Apgar score is a rapid assessment of five physiological signs that indicate the physiological status of the newborn and includes (Table 8-2):

- Heart rate based on auscultation
- Respiratory rate based on observed movement of chest
- Muscle tone based on degree of flexion and movement of extremities
- Reflex irritability based on response to tactile stimulation
- Color based on observation

  Each component is given a score of 0, 1, or 2. An Apgar score of:

- 0 to 3 indicates severe distress.
- 4 to 6 indicates moderate difficulty with transition to extrauterine life.
- 7 to 10 indicates stable status.

TABLE 8-2   Neonatal Apgar Score

SIGN	SCORE 0	1	2
Respiratory effort	Absent	Slow, irregular	Good cry
Heart rate	Absent	Slow, below 100 bpm	Above 100 bpm
Muscle tone	Flaccid	Some flexion of extremities	Active motion
Reflex activity	None	Grimace	Vigorous cry
Color	Pale, blue	Body pink, blue extremities	Completely pink

The Apgar score is not used to determine the need for resuscitation, nor is it predictive of the long-term neurological outcome of the neonate. Rather, it is a rapid, objective, convenient shorthand for reporting the status of the newborn and the response to resuscitation immediately after birth (AAP Committee on Fetus and Newborn and ACOG Committee on Obstetric Practice, 2015).

Overview of Neonatal Resuscitation

It is estimated that 10% of all infants need help to begin breathing and 1% need extensive resuscitation at birth. At every delivery, one person should be solely responsible for assessing the neonate response to the birth and initiating resuscitation of the neonate if needed (Aziz et al., 2021). It is beyond the scope of this chapter to fully describe the steps of neonatal resuscitation. However, briefly, upon birth, the newborn should be assessed for the following:

- Was the infant a term gestation?
- Is the newborn crying or breathing?
- Is there good muscle tone?

If the answer to all three questions is "yes," the neonate does not need resuscitation and should not be separated from the mother. The infant should be dried, placed skin-to-skin with the mother, and covered with dry linen to maintain temperature. Observation of breathing, activity, and color should be ongoing (Aziz et al., 2021).

If the infant does not meet these criteria, however, the infant should be placed under a warmer, positioned with the head in a "sniffing" position to open the airway. If at initial assessment visible fluid obstructs the airway or a concern exists about obstructed breathing, the mouth and nose may be suctioned. Avoiding unnecessary suctioning helps prevent the risk of induced bradycardia because of suctioning of the airway. Do not use routine suctioning for vigorous and nonvigorous infants born with meconium-stained amniotic fluid (Aziz et al., 2021).

Resuscitation should proceed in this order:

- **Airway:** Perform initial steps to open the airway (reposition, open mouth, clear secretions if necessary).
- **Breathing:** Newborns with apnea or bradycardia may need positive-pressure ventilation (PPV). PPV is the most important intervention for infants who are apneic or gasping. Most infants will successfully respond to this intervention.
- **Circulation:** If the newborn has severe and persistent bradycardia despite assisted ventilation, perform chest compressions coordinated with PPV.
- **Drugs:** If assisted ventilation and coordinated compressions are unsuccessful and severe bradycardia persists, administer epinephrine and continue with PPV and chest compressions.

Initial Newborn Procedures

One of the first procedures after birth is newborn identification. Perinatal nurses must be meticulous when recording the identification band number, birth, and newborn information. ID bands should be secured as soon as possible to mothers, birth partner, and newborns. Many hospitals use electronic infant security bands. These bands will set an alarm off if the infant is taken out of a specified area. Electronic security bands should also be applied as soon as possible after birth. It is important to be familiar with individual institutional policies for newborn identification and newborn safety as they may vary.

Three medications are routinely administered to newborns:

- Erythromycin ointment is administered to the eyes shortly after birth as prophylaxis to prevent gonococcal and chlamydia infections.
- Vitamin K is administered shortly after birth via intramuscular injection to prevent hemorrhagic disease caused by vitamin K deficiency.
- Hepatitis B virus vaccine is recommended before discharge for all newborns (AAP Committee on Fetus and Newborn and ACOG Committee on Obstetric Practice, 2017)
- Newborn care is discussed in Chapter 15.

MANAGEMENT OF PAIN AND DISCOMFORT DURING LABOR AND DELIVERY

A woman's experience of pain during childbirth is a complex, individual, and multidimensional response to sensory stimuli generated by parturition (Lowe, 2002). The experience of pain may lead to emotional distress, anxiety, and fear, all impacting the woman's experience of the labor process and its progression (Burke, 2021). When women evaluate their experience of labor, four factors predominate: the amount of support received from caregivers, the quality of relationships with caregivers, the level of involvement with decision making, and high expectations or experiences that exceed expectations (Bohren et al., 2017).

Multiple modalities exist to help a laboring woman effectively and safely manage her pain. Labor nurses should be comfortable assisting women with a variety of pain control techniques, adapting them to meet the individual needs of the patient. The nurse educates women about their options for pain relief during labor and provides information about the benefits and risks associated with various types of analgesia and anesthesia (AWHONN, 2020).

Many physiologic reasons exist for pain during labor, resulting in a pain experience that can be multifaceted for the laboring patient. During the first stage of labor, pain may be caused by:

- UCs leading to uterine muscle hypoxia
- Lactic acid accumulation
- Cervical and lower uterine segment stretching
- Traction on the fallopian tubes, ovaries, and ligaments
- Pressure on the bony pelvis
- Perineal stretching on the urethra, bladder and rectum (Burke, 2021)

In addition, during the second stage of labor, pain may be caused by:

● Continued perineal stretching on the urethra, bladder, and rectum
● Mechanical stretching of the lower uterine segment, cervix, and vagina
● Descent of the fetal head causing pressure on the roots of the lumbosacral plexus and other structures, resulting in pain in the thighs, legs, vagina, perineum, and rectum
● Back pain may be present during both stages of labor, if the fetal occiput is resting on the maternal sacrum (Burke, 2021).

Other factors that may influence a laboring woman's perception of pain include:

● Rate of cervical dilation and strength of contractions
● Size and position of fetus
● Sleep deprivation and exhaustion from a long labor
● The support the woman receives from the people around her, including the RN
● Previous birth experiences
● Extent of childbirth preparation and knowledge about the process
● Expectations of the birth experience.

The Experience of Pain

Pain is experienced universally, although the way pain is outwardly expressed may depend on individual and community upbringing. Research demonstrates no difference in self-reported labor pain intensity ratings among ethnic groups (Lowe, 2002). Research also demonstrates no biological differences between how groups of people experience pain (D. E. Roberts, 2011). Multiple myths exist about the experience of pain related to race. For example, in a 2016 study on racial bias, half of White medical trainees believed myths such as that Black people have thicker skin or have less sensitive nerve endings than White people

(Hoffman et al., 2016). Although not specific to labor pain, a 2012 meta-analysis found that Black patients were 22% less likely to receive medication for pain as compared with White patients with similarly painful conditions (Meghani et al., 2012). It is critically important that nurses work with patients sensitively and individually to understand their goals for pain control and develop plans to meet those goals. Treating patients based on assumptions and stereotypes is unethical, does not support the goal of patient autonomy, and is poor nursing practice.

Gate Control Theory of Pain

Understanding the gate control theory of pain can assist in choosing interventions to manage the pain of labor (Fig. 8–31). This theory postulates that there are two different nerve fibers, large diameter and small diameter, which transmit sensations to the brain. These fibers encounter various "gates" along the neural pathway, which filter the signals that reach the brain. Small diameter fibers transmit painful sensations, and large diameter fibers transmit sensations such as touch, pressure, and vibration. The theory proposes that the gates that control the level of noxious input to the brain via the small-fiber neurons can be modulated by activating the large-fiber neurons, thus "closing the gate" to the painful stimuli. This allows an alternate, less painful sensation to replace or decrease the sensation of the more noxious one (Moayedi & Davis, 2013). The gate control theory of pain helps explain how the application of pressure to certain areas of the body, effleurage (gentle stroking of the abdomen), and the use of heat or cold may have a direct effect on decreasing pain sensations.

Childbirth Preparation

Although more research needs to be done, studies show that women who attended childbirth education classes reported greater satisfaction with the birthing experience than those who did not (Mueller et al., 2020; Taheri et al., 2018). A recent Cochrane Review found that women who attended a variety of

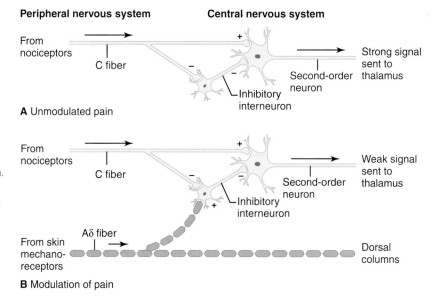

FIGURE 8–31 Gate control theory of pain modulation. (A) Normally C-fibers carrying slow pain signals block inhibitory interneurons and transmit their signals across the synapse unimpeded. (B) A-delta fibers carrying pleasurable signals from touch excite inhibitory interneurons, which then block the transmission of slow pain signals (+ equals transmission, – equals no transmission).

types of childbirth education also had lower cesarean section rates than those who did not attend (Chen et al., 2018).

Childbirth classes, by providing education about the birth process and teaching coping strategies, help decease the stress and anxiety of the unknown and promote informed decision making during labor. Most classes provide the information on signs and stages of labor, positioning for labor and birth, ways to control pain, and strategies to work through labor pains to help stay relaxed and in control. Classes usually include practice of the techniques taught. Most classes also include information on postpartum care for the birthing mother and infant. Classes generally include the birth partner and many classes also provide a tour of the birthing facility.

Popular types of childbirth education classes include:

- Lamaze: Lamaze offers childbirth education classes grounded in the idea that women have an innate ability to give birth.
  - Letting labor begin on its own, freedom of movement in labor, labor support, no routine interventions, spontaneous pushing in nonsupine positions, and keeping mother and baby together (Lothian, 2014).
- The Bradley method: This method emphasizes natural childbirth with the birth partner as coach. This method encourages concentrated awareness that works through pain rather than blocking it. Parents are taught deep abdominal breathing, massage, and an understanding of the labor and delivery process.
- The International Childbirth Education Association (ICEA): Classes sponsored by the ICEA do not emphasize any particular approach to childbirth but offer general information about the process of labor and birth. They discuss natural childbirth, teach various methods of dealing with the pain of labor and birth, and present the options available for pain relief. All instructors are certified by the ICEA.
- Hypnobirthing: These childbirth classes focus on teaching pregnant women to use self-hypnosis techniques, breathing, relaxation, nutrition, meditation, and visualization to control pain and remain in control during labor.
- *Birthing From Within*: A holistic approach to childbirth, *Birthing From Within* offers parents a general informative teaching experience. Activities and processes teach parents specific skills to holistically inform and prepare them for birth.
- Hospital-based birthing classes: Many hospitals offer birthing classes for parents planning to give birth at their facility. These classes may follow a specific method or a combination of methods, with the goal of preparing the mother and birth partner for labor and postpartum.

Nonpharmacological Management of Labor Discomfort

Nonpharmacological management of labor pain includes a wide array of interventions. The advantages of nonpharmacological methods are that they are often simple to use, allow the birth partner to become actively involved, promote a sense of control for the laboring woman, and lack serious side effects (Burke,

2021). In the *Listening to Mothers III* survey, 73% of women reported using at least one nonpharmacological method of pain control during labor, led by breathing techniques (48%), position changes (40%), hands-on (e.g., massage) techniques (22%), and mental strategies (e.g., relaxation) (21%) (Declercq et al., 2014). Nurses should be comfortable assisting women with a range of nonpharmacological pain management techniques. Some of those techniques include:

- Relaxation and breathing techniques: Teaching focused breathing patterns may promote relaxation and feeling of control during labor. Most childbirth preparation methods teach some form of relaxation and breathing techniques (Fig. 8–32). Women are often taught to take a deep breath at the beginning of the contraction to signal its onset and then to breathe slowly during the contraction. As labor pain increases, the woman may need to breathe in a more rapid and shallow manner. On occasion, a woman will experience hyperventilation from this type of breathing. Symptoms are related to respiratory alkalosis and include tingling of the fingers or circumoral numbness, lightheadedness, or dizziness. This undesirable side effect can be eliminated by having the woman breathe into a bag or cupped hands. This causes her to rebreathe carbon dioxide and reverses the respiratory alkalosis.
- Massage and effleurage: Some women may find effleurage on the abdomen during a contraction useful. Effleurage is lightly stroking a body part in a circular motion with the palm of the hand. Massage is also often used, employing firmer longer strokes on the legs and back, per the woman's request. Although the evidence was of low quality, a Cochrane Review found that the use of massage during labor reduced pain and provided a greater sense of control and satisfaction (Smith, Levett, et al., 2018).

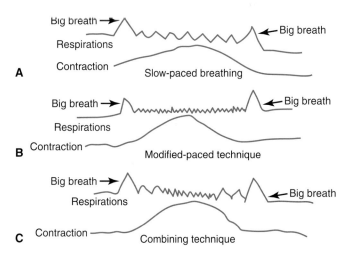

FIGURE 8–32 Space breathing technique graph. (A) Slow-paced breathing is with a big breath at the beginning and end of the contraction; the typical rate is fewer than 10 breaths per minute. (B) Modified-paced breathing is with a big breath at the beginning and end of the contraction and rapid shallow breaths that are comfortable for the woman at a rate of about twice normal respirations. (C) Combining technique. Big breath at the beginning and end of the contraction with more rapid and shallow breathing at the peak of the contraction.

- Counterpressure: Sacral counterpressure involves using an open hand, fist, or object to press downward on the woman's sacrum during a contraction, using as much force as is comfortable for the woman. Some women also find relief with bilateral hip pressure, where the support person provides a "hip squeeze" during contractions. These techniques are especially helpful for women experiencing back pain in labor.
- Hydrotherapy: Hydrotherapy, in the form of warm baths or showers, is an effective method of pain management during labor. Warm water provides soothing stimulation of nerves in the skin and promotes vasodilation, reversal of sympathetic nervous system response, and reduction in catecholamine production. Hydrotherapy also provides pain relief through the perception of warmth by nerve receptors in the skin, initiating the gate mechanism (Burke, 2021). Using hydrotherapy is associated with a reduction in epidural use (Cluett et al., 2018). The water temperature should be maintained between 96.8°F and 99.5°F (36°C and 37.5°C) to promote relaxation and maintain warmth. Warmer water may raise both maternal and fetal temperature and lead to fetal tachycardia and elevated neonatal temperature, so both should be monitored and cool drinks provided to the woman.
- Warm and cold packs: These may provide pain relief when applied. Warm packs may increase blood flow and relax muscles, and cold packs may provide a numbing effect. These should not be used with epidurals, however, as epidurals cause decreased sensation and the laboring woman may not be aware of the temperature of the packs.
- Guided imagery, relaxation, distraction, and focal points: These techniques are easy to use and require no special equipment. During early labor, providing alternative activities such as games, watching TV, listening to music, or talking with friends may help women cope. Nurses can also provide positive guided imagery, such as, "Imagine the baby moving down the birth canal" or "Imagine your cervix gently opening up." Having a woman focus on a certain object, usually one of meaning to her, as a focal point during contractions may help her maintain control. Encouraging and reminding women to use the relaxation techniques that they learned in childbirth class may also help them cope with contractions.
- Acupuncture and acupressure: Acupuncture has a long history of use in Asia for pain control and requires a trained practitioner to place the needles. To apply acupressure, however, the provider uses their hand and fingers to apply pressure to the same points as used in acupuncture. Nurses may learn how to apply acupressure in their practice. A recent Cochrane Review found that acupuncture when compared with a placebo increased satisfaction with pain management and reduced the use of pharmacological analgesia. Acupressure, when compared with a combined control and usual care, reduced labor pain intensity. However, the evidence was of low quality and more research should be done (Smith et al., 2020).
- Positioning: Although changing position is important to the progress of labor, it may also help with pain control. Assisting the laboring woman with using a birth ball, ambulating, sitting up in a comfortable chair, or any other position that the woman finds comfortable may help the woman to feel in more control and better able to cope with pain (Ondeck, 2014).
- Aromatherapy: Aromatherapy with lavender may be effective in reducing pain and anxiety during the first stage of labor (Liao et al., 2021). The mechanism of action is unclear, and it may be that aromatherapy works by distracting the patient from the pain. However, no negative side effects are associated with the use of lavender in labor. Always check with the patient before use, as some women are sensitive to smell.
- Continuous labor support: This is perhaps the most important nonpharmacological intervention. Women who received continuous labor support from an RN, a doula, or a family member used less pain medication, reported being more satisfied with the experience, and had shorter labors. Continuous labor support may include emotional support (continuous presence, reassurance, and praise) and information about labor progress. It may also include advice about coping techniques, comfort measures (comforting touch, massage, warm baths or showers, encouraging mobility, promoting adequate fluid intake and output), and speaking up when needed on behalf of the woman (Bohren et al., 2017).

Assessing Labor Pain

Unlike other experiences with pain, which often signal pathology, labor pain is nonpathological and is associated with bringing new life into the world. Asking a laboring patient to simply rate her pain on a 1 to 10 scale does not adequately assess whether the woman is coping with the pain, nor does it account for the complexity of the sensations experienced. Many birth centers are moving from a numeric pain scale to a tool that assesses the laboring patient's ability to cope. Asking the open-ended question, "How are you coping with labor?" and assessing for signs that the woman is coping makes room for the laboring woman to say that while she is in pain, she is coping with the current interventions in place. If the woman states or exhibits signs that she is not coping, this signals the RN that new interventions should be implemented. Once new interventions have been implemented, the RN should reassess the patient's coping status.

Cues that indicate the woman is coping include:

- She states that she is coping.
- She exhibits rhythmic activity such as rocking or swaying during contractions.
- She uses rhythmic breathing during contractions.
- She vocalizes during contractions by chanting, counting, or moaning.
- She is focused inward.
- She is able to relax during contractions.
- Some cues that may indicate the woman is not coping:
- She states she is not coping.
- She is crying, tearful, and tense.
- She speaks with a tremulous voice.
- She cannot focus or concentrate.
- She is panicked during contractions.
- She is thrashing, clawing, or biting.
- She is sweaty or jittery (Roberts et al., 2010, Simpson & O'Brien-Abel, 2021).

Pharmacological Management of Labor Discomfort

In addition to nonpharmacological interventions, many patients elect to have pharmacological interventions. It is important for nurses to be nondirectional in their counseling to patients about pain control choices. Some women may feel as if they have "given in" or failed if they decide to use medication. Other patients may feel pressured by the nurse to use a certain intervention. Nurses have a responsibility to present accurate, nonjudgmental, accessible information, then support the woman in the choices she has made, in collaboration with the provider. Women should be reassured about their pain choices. Existing data suggest that administering pain medication during labor has no effect on an infant's later mental or neurological development. Maternal request for pain medication during labor is a sufficient indication for its administration (AAP Committee on Fetus and Newborn and ACOG Committee on Obstetric Practice, 2017).

The use of medication in the relief of pain during labor falls into two major categories: Analgesia (Table 8-3) and anesthesia (Table 8-4).

TABLE 8-3　Common Analgesic Medications in Labor

DRUG NAME AND CLASSIFICATION	DOSAGE	ONSET OF ACTION	DURATION OF ACTION	COMMENTS
Fentanyl or opioid	50–100 mcg IV 10–25 mcg every 10–12 min in a PCA	2–4 min IV	30–60 min	Short acting, potent respiratory depressant, often used in PCAs
Morphine or opioid	2–5 mg IV 5–10 mg IM	5–10 min IV 20–30 min IM	1–3 or 2–4 hours	Not frequently used in active labor due to long half-life. Monitor neonate for respiratory depression.
Butorphanol or mixed opioid agonist or antagonist	1–2 mg IV or IM	5–10 min IV 30–60 min IM	4–6 hours	Less respiratory depression than other narcotics due to the mixed opioid effects
Nalbuphine or mixed opioid agonist or antagonist	10–20 mg IV, SQ, or/IM	2–3 min IV 10–15 min SQ or IM	2–4 hours	Less respiratory depression than other narcotics due to the mixed opioid effects
Remifentanil or opioid	0.15–0.5 mcg/kg every 2 mins in a PCA	20–90 seconds	2–4 min	PCA only. Ultra-short acting, potent respiratory depressant, continuously monitor oxygen and respiratory rate. 1:1 nursing highly recommended.

IM, intramuscular; IV, intravenous; PCA, patient-controlled analgesia; SQ, subcutaneously.
AAP Committee on Fetus and Newborn and ACOG Committee on Obstetric Practice, 2017; Burke, C. (2021). Pain labor: Nonpharmacologic and pharmacologic management.
In K. Simpson, P. Creehan, N. Obrien-Abel, C. Roth, & A. Rohan (Eds.), Perinatal nursing (5th ed., pp. 325-411). Wolters Kluwer.

TABLE 8-4　Common Types of Anesthesia in Labor

TYPE OF ANESTHESIA	TIME GIVEN AND EFFECTS	ADVERSE EFFECTS	NURSING IMPLICATIONS
LOCAL: Anesthetic injected into perineum at episiotomy site	Second stage of labor, immediately before delivery Anesthetizes local tissue for episiotomy and repair	Risk of a hematoma Risk of infection	Monitor for: Return of sensation to area Increased swelling at site of injection
REGIONAL: Pudendal Block: Anesthetic injected in the pudendal nerve (close to the ischial spines) via needle guide known as "trumpet"	Second stage of labor, before time of delivery Anesthetizes vulva, lower vagina, and part of perineum for episiotomy and use of low forceps	Risk of local anesthetic toxicity Risk of a hematoma Risk of infection	Monitor for: Return of sensation to area Increased swelling Signs and symptoms of infection Urinary retention

Continued

TABLE 8-4   Common Types of Anesthesia in Labor—cont'd

TYPE OF ANESTHESIA	TIME GIVEN AND EFFECTS	ADVERSE EFFECTS	NURSING IMPLICATIONS
Epidural Block: Anesthetic injected in the epidural space: Located outside the dura mater between the dura and spinal canal via an epidural catheter	First stage or second stage of labor Can be used for both vaginal and cesarean births Can be used with opioids such as Sublimaze to allow walking during the first stage of labor and effective pushing in the second stage of labor	Most common complication is hypotension. Other side effects include nausea, vomiting, pruritis, respiratory depression, and alterations in FHR.	Pre-anesthesia care: Obtain consent. Check laboratory values—especially for bleeding or clotting abnormalities, or platelet count. IV fluid bolus with normal saline or lactated Ringer's Ensure emergency equipment is available. Do time-out procedure verification.
			Post-procedure care: Monitor maternal vital signs and FHR every 5 minutes initially and after every re-bolus, then every 15 minutes and manage hypotension or alterations in FHR. Urinary retention is common and catheterization may be needed. Assess pain and level of sensation and motor loss. Position woman as needed (on side to prevent inferior vena cava syndrome). Assess for itching, nausea and vomiting, and headache and administer meds PRN. When catheter discontinued, note intact tip when removed.
Spinal Block: Anesthetic injected in the subarachnoid space	Second stage of labor or in use for cesarean section Rapid acting with 100% blockage of sensation and motor functioning. Can last up to 3 hours.	Adverse effects are similar to the epidural with the addition of a spinal headache. A blood patch often provides relief.	Interventions are same as for epidural. Monitor site for leakage of spinal fluid or formation of hematoma. Observe for headache.
GENERAL ANESTHESIA: Use of IV injection or inhalation of anesthetic agents that render the woman unconscious.	Used mainly in emergency cesarean birth	Risk for fetal depression Risk for uterine relaxation Risk for maternal vomiting and aspiration	Obtain consent. Ensure woman is NPO. IV with large-bore needle. Place indwelling urinary catheter. Administer medications to decrease gastric acidity as ordered such as antacids: Bicitra or proton pump inhibitor: Protonix. Place wedge to hip to prevent vena cava syndrome. Assist with supportive care of newborn.

- Basic principles when using analgesia include:
- Select medication that provides relief to the woman with minimal risk to the baby.
- Neonatal respiratory depression may occur if opioids are given close to delivery. The nurse should have Narcan (naloxone) available if needed.
- Women with opioid use disorder may need higher doses of medication to achieve a therapeutic effect.
- Basic principles for anesthesia include:
  - Local anesthesia is used at the time of delivery for episiotomy and for the episiotomy and laceration repair.
  - Regional anesthesia is used during labor and at delivery.
    - Regional anesthesia includes pudendal block, epidural block, and spinal block (Fig. 8–33 and Fig. 8–34).
    - Regional or general anesthesia is used for cesarean deliveries. Chapter 11 addresses the care of cesarean birth women (Fig. 8–35).

Parenteral Opioids

Use of various parenteral opioid agonists and opioid agonist-antagonists is common during labor. Opioids provide pain relief by binding to opioid receptor sites and blocking transmission of pain signals to the brain. Opioids also work by causing an emotional detachment from the pain. The pain is still there, but the laboring woman is less concerned about it (Burke, 2021). Using parenteral opioids does not provide long-term or complete pain relief. A recent Cochrane Review found that parenteral opioid use during labor provided some pain relief, although many women still reported moderate or severe pain. Opioids were also associated with increased nausea, vomiting, and drowsiness (Smith, et al., 2018). Opioids may cause maternal respiratory depression. The RN must assess maternal respiratory status after opioid administration. All opioids cross the placental barrier and may cause a transient decrease in fetal

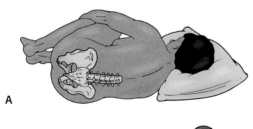

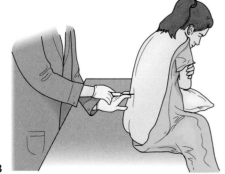

FIGURE 8–33 Lateral (A) and sitting (B) positions for placement of spinal and epidural block.

heart variability and contribute to neonatal respiratory depression after birth. The RN must be prepared and ready to intervene. Advantages of parenteral opioids include availability, ease of administration, cost, and continued mobility. Laboring patients may select this method of pain relief while waiting for an epidural or to provide a pain respite to allow for a period of rest and relaxation during labor.

Nitrous Oxide Analgesia

Nitrous oxide may increasingly be a vital component in high-quality maternity care, and intrapartum nurses are in an ideal situation to offer and initiate nitrous oxide use (AWHONN, 2020). Intermittent inhalation of nitrous oxide provides analgesia for labor but does not eliminate the pain of UCs. Inhaled nitrous oxide allows freedom of movement during labor and does not require additional monitoring. Inhaled nitrous oxide may be combined with nonpharmacological pain management techniques and be used during the placement of regional anesthesia and afterward if the relief provided by anesthesia is suboptimal (AWHONN, 2020).

Inhaled nitrous oxide (laughing gas) has been used effectively for decades for labor pain, although it has been used more widely in Europe than in the United States. In one study, even though women reported that inhaled nitrous oxide did not provide pain control equal to an epidural, women who used nitrous oxide reported higher satisfaction rates than those who used an epidural (Richardson et al., 2017).

Nitrous oxide has been found to be safe for the laboring woman and the fetus. It is transmitted to the fetus via the placenta, but it is quickly eliminated once the infant begins to breathe. Other advantages include:

- It does not limit mobility.
- Patient can control the amount of medication received.
- Administration does not require IV access.
- It does not interfere with the labor process.
- Quick termination of effects occurs when the mask is removed.

Reported side effects include nausea, vomiting, dizziness, and drowsiness. Nitrous oxide is self-administered via a handheld mask or mouthpiece with a mix of 50% nitrous oxide and 50% oxygen. The delivering apparatus must use a demand valve so that medication is only administered when a breath is taken from the mask to limit environmental exposure to others.

Regional Anesthesia

Regional (neuraxial) anesthesia refers to the epidural or spinal administration of opioids combined with a local anesthetic. This results in the partial or total loss of sensation below the T8 to T10 level, with or without motor blockade (Richardson et al., 2017). Approximately 75% of women in the United States use regional anesthesia for pain control during labor (Burke, 2021). The administration of regional anesthesia requires specialized knowledge, experience, and training, and only qualified anesthesia personnel, such as anesthesiologists and certified registered nurse anesthetists (CRNA), should administer and manage this type of anesthesia during labor and birth (AWHONN, 2020).

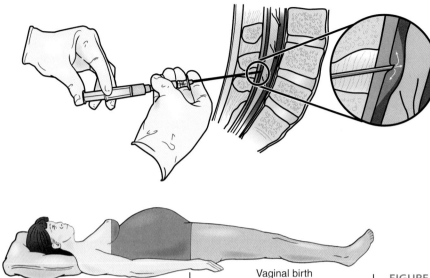

FIGURE 8–34 Technique for epidural block.

Vaginal birth

Cesarean birth

FIGURE 8–35 Levels of anesthesia necessary for vaginal and cesarean births.

The scope of registered nursing practice may vary from state to state. Registered nurses caring for women receiving regional anesthesia should refer to their state's board of nursing. Nurses should also be familiar with their facility's guidelines, policies, and procedures. There are several common types of regional anesthesia used in obstetrics:

- Spinal anesthesia: Spinal administration is a single injection of medication into the subarachnoid space in the spinal column via a fine needle. It causes rapid and complete loss of sensation in the lower half of the body. It is most often used in planned cesarean sections.
- Epidural anesthesia: Epidural administration is the administration of medication into the epidural space around the spinal cord. Epidural anesthesia is generally delivered via a small catheter placed into the epidural space between the lumbar vertebrae and below the termination of the spinal column. A needle is introduced into the location by a skilled provider, and the catheter is threaded through the needle. The needle is removed and the catheter taped in place. Medication may be delivered by continuous infusion or patient control epidural administration (PCEA), where the laboring woman can dose herself as needed. It is most often used to manage labor pain but can be used for a cesarean section with proper dosage.
- Combined spinal-epidural anesthesia (CSE): This method combines the rapid onset of pain relief from the spinal with the long-term pain relief benefits of an epidural. The provider inserts an epidural needle into the epidural space, then inserts a smaller spinal needle through the epidural needle and into the subarachnoid space, administering the spinal. The spinal needle is removed, and an epidural catheter is inserted via the epidural needle. The needle is then removed, and the catheter is taped into place.

Research demonstrates that the administration of regional anesthesia, even early in labor, does not increase cesarean rates nor affect fetal outcomes when compared with women who did not receive epidurals (Anim-Somuah et al., 2018; Sng et al., 2014). Regional anesthesia may be associated with increased numbers of instrumented deliveries when high concentrations of local anesthetic are in the admixture. However, newer anesthesia protocols use lower concentrations of local anesthetic and more recent studies detect a difference in instrumented deliveries between women who received epidurals and women who did not (Anim-Somuah et al., 2018).

Common side effects and risks associated with regional anesthesia include (Burke, 2021):

- Maternal hypotension: Epidurals result in sympathetic nerve blockade and vasodilation, resulting in maternal hypotension. Maternal hypotension may decrease blood flow to the uterus, decreasing fetal oxygenation. Pre-epidural hydration of 500 to 1,000 mL of crystalloid is usually ordered to blunt this effect. Careful monitoring of post-procedure BP and FHR are required.
- Headache: If the dura is punctured inadvertently during the epidural placement, it may result in a "wet tap," causing a severe headache. The incidence of a wet tap is about 1:100, with 70% of those affected complaining of a headache. To treat this type of headache, blood is withdrawn aseptically from the affected woman, and injected into the site of the leak, forming a blood patch over the leak.
- Hyperthermia: There appears to be an association between epidural use and an increase in maternal temperature, although the etiology is incompletely understood.
- Urinary retention: Regional anesthesia may make it difficult to detect a full bladder and void. The woman may need assistance voiding, and a catheter should be placed as needed.
- Pruritus: Itching is a common side effect of regional anesthesia. Medication may be used to relieve the itching.
- Systemic toxicity: If the epidural catheter is inadvertently placed into the intrathecal space and the infusion is started, an immediate high spinal block occurs, resulting in loss of thoracic sensation and a severe lower extremity motor blockade. If the medication travels to the brainstem, respiratory

paralysis, loss of consciousness, and autonomic blockage can occur. To prevent this from happening, a test dose of a local anesthetic and epinephrine are injected into the epidural before any medication administration.

CLINICAL JUDGMENT

The Role of the Registered Nurse in Regional Anesthesia Administration

The AWHONN maintains that RNs who are not licensed anesthesia providers should *monitor* but not *manage* the delivery of analgesia and anesthesia by catheter techniques to pregnant women (2020). Following stabilization of vital signs after initial insertion, initial injection, bolus injection, re-bolus injection, or initiation of continuous infusion by a qualified anesthesia provider, RNs in communication with the maternity care team and anesthesia provider may:

- Monitor the woman's vital signs, level of mobility, level of consciousness, and perception of pain and level of pain relief.
- Monitor the status of the fetus, pause, or stop the infusion to replace empty infusion syringes or infusion bags with new, pre-prepared solutions that contain the same medication and concentration according to orders from the anesthesia provider; restart the infusion.
- Stop the continuous infusion if there is a safety concern or the woman has given birth.
- Remove the catheter if the RN has the appropriate educational training, criteria have been met, and institutional policy and state law allow. Removal of the catheter by an RN is contingent upon receipt of a specific order from a qualified anesthesia provider or physician.
- Initiate emergency therapeutic measures if complications arise according to institutional policy, protocol, and RN scope of practice.
- Communicate clinical assessments and changes in patient status to the maternity and anesthesia care providers as indicated by institutional policy.

RNs who are not qualified anesthesia providers should not (AWHONN, 2020):

- Administer medications (via bolus or re-bolus) for the purpose of providing neuraxial analgesia or anesthesia by injecting doses into the catheter.
- Manipulate doses of neuraxial analgesia or anesthesia medications delivered by continuous infusion.
- Manipulate doses of neuraxial analgesia or anesthesia medications or dosing intervals for PCEA.
- Increase or decrease the rate of a continuous infusion.
- Reinitiate an infusion once it has been stopped for any reason other than to introduce a new bag.
- Be responsible for obtaining informed consent for analgesia and anesthesia procedures; however, the nurse may witness the patient signature for informed consent before analgesia and anesthesia administration (AWHONN, 2020).

Nursing Responsibilities for Patients Receiving Regional Anesthesia

As adapted from the AWHONN Guidelines on Anesthesia and Analgesia during the intrapartum period (Hale et al., 2020), follow these guidelines before placement of regional anesthesia:

- Verify informed consent has been obtained by the anesthesia provider.
- Assess fetal status and maternal baseline, including pain level, BP, pulse, respiratory rate, temperature, oxygen status, and labor progress.
- Obtain and review labs as requested by the anesthesia care provider. These include but are not limited to a CBC and platelet count.
- Obtain a fetal heart tracing before an epidural.
- Administer an IV bolus as ordered by the provider. If preload is ordered, initiate an IV fluid bolus 10 to 15 minutes before the procedure. If co-load is ordered, administer a rapid infusion of IV fluid bolus in conjunction with (during and throughout) the regional analgesia or anesthesia procedure.
- Conduct a time-out before regional anesthesia administration.
- Provide patient education on the selected pain control method.

During regional anesthesia placement:

- Assist the woman to an appropriate position, either sitting, lateral, or pendant position.
- Assist with maintaining the position and with breathing and relaxation.
- Monitor for adverse maternal reactions during and immediately after the test dose.
- Monitor for adverse fetal reactions during initiation medication.

After regional anesthesia placement:

- Assess fetal response frequently to regional anesthesia, and intervene as necessary.
- Assist with maternal positioning, and avoid the supine position.
- Assess maternal BP after initiation or re-bolus of a regional block, including PCEA.
  - BP should be assessed at least every 5 minutes for the first 15 minutes, and then repeated at 30 minutes and 1 hour after the procedure.
  - More frequent BP monitoring may be warranted.
  - Initiate interventions to resolve maternal hypotension according to provider orders and facility protocol, such as lateral positioning, and administer additional crystalloid fluid boluses or vasopressors.
- Assess uterine activity every 5 minutes for the first 15 minutes.
- Monitor the woman for signs of sedation and respiratory depression (Fig. 8–35).
- Assess the level of motor blockade hourly throughout the period of analgesia or anesthesia.
  - Monitor maternal temperature every 2 to 4 hours after anesthesia.

● Assess for urinary retention and bladder distention at a minimum of every 4 hours and assist with bladder emptying as needed.
  ● Assist the woman to void using a bedpan.
  ● Perform intermittent urinary catheterization using a straight catheter if she is unable to void spontaneously.
  ● If frequent bladder catheterizations are indicated, consider the use of an indwelling urinary catheter.
● Assess for sedation level, nausea, vomiting, and pruritis.

Evidence-Based Practice: Expectant Fathers and Labor Epidurals

Chapman, L. (2000). Expectant fathers and labor epidurals. *Maternal Child Nursing, 25,* 133–138.

A qualitative research study using grounded theory methodology was conducted to describe and explain the expectant father's experience during labor and birth when epidural anesthesia or analgesia was used for labor pain management. Based on the research data, a theory, "cruising through labor," was developed. The epidural labor process is different from non-epidural labor and is comprised of six phases:

• Holding out

• Surrendering

• Waiting

• Getting

• Cruising

• Pushing

Expectant fathers explained that before the epidural they felt as if they were "losing" their partner as the increasing pain caused the woman to focus inward and away from interaction with those in the labor room. The expectant fathers explained that they felt a loss of connection with their partner and a loss of control. They felt that the pain of labor overtook their partner and was all-encompassing. The men further explained that they felt helpless, frustrated, and a sense of losing her to the pain of labor.

The men explained that the labor nurse played a significant role in supporting them during this time. The major supportive behaviors by the nurse were:

• Remaining in the labor room

• Explaining what was happening to their partner

• Including the men in the care of their partner

Expectant fathers reported that once the epidural was administered and the woman experienced relief from labor pain, they saw a dramatic change in their partner's behavior. They often stated, "She's back," that she was comfortable and able to interact with those around her. One man stated, "She wasn't in pain. Her color was back. Her pain was gone. She wasn't throwing up. She was back. She was comfortable."

Men further explained that the effects of the epidural in decreasing the degree of labor pain allowed the men to shift their focus from labor pain management to enjoying the labor and birthing experience (Fig. 8–36 and Fig. 8–37).

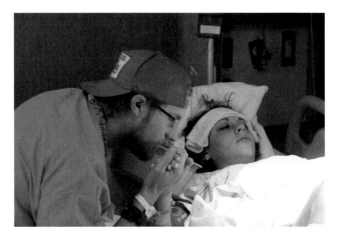

FIGURE 8–36 Partners experiencing labor together.

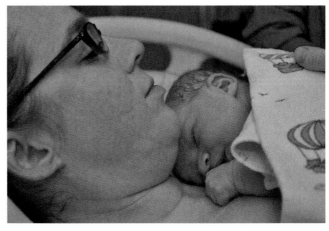

Courtesy of Chapman family

FIGURE 8–37 A new family.

Clinical Pathway for Intrapartal Maternal and Fetal Assessment

	Active Labor	Second Stage Labor (Active Pushing)	Third Stage of Labor (Delivery of Placenta)	Fourth Stage of Labor (Immediate Postpartum)
Maternal vital signs	P, R, and BP every hour; temp every 2 hours unless ROM, then every hour	P, R, and BP every hour; temp every 2 hours unless ROM, then every hour	P, R, and BP every 15 minutes	P, R, and BP every 15 minutes
FHR	Every 15–30 minutes*	Assessment every 5–15 minutes*	NA	Initiate neonatal transition care
Uterine activity	Every 15–30 minutes**	Assessment every 5–15 minutes**	NA	NA Fundal and lochia checks every 15 minutes
Pain status	Every 30 minutes and PRN	Assessment every 15 minutes	Assessment every 15 minutes	Assessment every 15 minutes
Response to labor	Every 30 minutes and PRN	Assessment every 15 minutes	Assessment every 15 minutes	
Comfort measures	Every 30 minutes and PRN	Assessment every 15 minutes and PRN	Assessment every 15 minutes and PRN	Assessment every 15 minutes and PRN
Maternal position	Every 30 minutes and PRN	Change every 30 minutes and PRN		
Vaginal examination, fetal station, and progress in descent	As needed	As needed	NA	NA
Intake and output	Every 8 hours	Assess bladder distention		Assess bladder distention

BP, blood pressure; FHR, fetal heart rate; P, pulse; R, respirations; ROM, rupture of membranes.
*FHR characteristics include baseline rate, variability, and presence or absence of accelerations and periodic or episodic decelerations.
**Uterine activity included contraction frequency, duration, intensity, and uterine resting tone.
AWHONN, 2018; O'Brien-Abel, & Simpson, 2021; Simpson & O'Brien-Abel, 2021.

CONCEPT MAP

Latent phase send home

Labor management

Admit

First stage

Review prenatal records

Vital signs Pain

Comfort measures

Assess for risk factors

Labs

Maternal assessment Cervical exam UC monitoring

Fetal monitoring

Facilitate ambulation intake and output

Natural childbirth

Complementary therapies

Medical management IV

Epidural/ medication assessment

Second stage

More frequent maternal and fetal assessment

Comfort measures for pushing efforts

Assess for pain and epidural assessment

Support and encourage

Communicate with interdisciplinary team Prepare for delivery

BABY IS HERE

If stable to mother's chest

Apgar

Stabilize baby

Initiate breastfeeding

Baby assessment

Third stage

Facilitate family bonding

Assess maternal stability and comfort

Manage newborn Resuscitation and stability

Prepare for delivery of placenta Uterotonics if needed

Fourth stage

Maternal assessment every 15 minutes

Assess bladder, fundus lochia, and vital signs

Hydrate and feed the new family

Initiate breastfeeding

CARE PLANS

For Labor and Birth

First Stage of Labor

Goal: Safe delivery for mother and baby

Outcome: Safe delivery for mother and baby

Nursing Actions

1. Perform admission procedures and orient patient to setting.
2. Review prenatal records.
3. Assess FHR and uterine activity.
4. Assess maternal vital signs and pain.
5. Assist with ambulation and maternal position changes.
6. Provide comfort measures.
7. Discuss pain management options.
8. Administer pain meds PRN.
9. Monitor I&O and provide oral or IV hydration as indicated.
10. Provide ongoing assessment of labor progress.
11. Request an immediate bedside evaluation by a physician or CNM.

Second Stage of Labor

Goal: Safe delivery for mother and baby

Outcome: Safe delivery for mother and baby

Nursing Actions

1. Perform more frequent maternal and fetal assessment.
2. Review prenatal records.
3. Assess FHR and uterine activity.
4. Assess maternal vital signs and pain.
5. Encourage open glottis pushing efforts.
6. Provide comfort measures for pushing efforts.
7. Provide ongoing assessment and encouragement of labor progress.
8. Communicate with interdisciplinary team.
9. Prepare for delivery.

Third Stage of Labor

Goal: Safe delivery of placenta and transition for baby

Outcome: Safe delivery of placenta and transition for baby

Nursing Actions

1. Facilitate family bonding.
2. Assess maternal vital signs and pain.
3. Assess maternal stability.
4. Prepare for delivery of placenta and need for uterotonics.

Fourth Stage of Labor

Goal: Safe recovery of mom and baby

Outcome: Safe recovery of mom and baby

Nursing Actions

1. Facilitate family bonding.
2. Assess maternal vital signs and pain.
3. Assess maternal stability, fundus, lochia, bladder, and perineum.
4. Provide comfort measures and pain meds.
5. Initiate breastfeeding.
6. Provide food and fluids for patient when stable.

Case Study

As the nurse, you admit Margarite Sanchez to the labor and delivery unit. She arrived in the triage unit at midnight in early labor with UCs that were 5 minutes apart for 3 hours. Patient is a 28-year-old G3 P1 Hispanic woman. She is 39 weeks' gestation. José, her husband, has accompanied her to the unit. Two years ago, she had a normal spontaneous vaginal delivery NSVD after an 18-hour labor for a baby girl, Sonya, who was 7 lbs., 3 oz.

Margarite's cervix is now 4 cm/80%/0 station and fetal position is left occiput anterior (LOA).

Prenatal Laboratory Test Results

Blood type O+

RPR NR

GBS negative

Hepatitis B negative

Hgb

Hct

Vital signs: BP 110/60; pulse 84 bpm; respiratory rate 18; temperature 98.6°F (37°C).

Began prenatal care at 10 weeks of gestation and received regular prenatal care. Margarite gained 22 pounds during pregnancy, and her current weight is 164 lbs. She is 5 feet, 4 inches tall. She has no prior medical complications and has experienced a normal pregnancy. Her first pregnancy ended in miscarriage at 8 weeks' gestation. She has no allergies to food or medication. She does not have a birth plan and states, "I just hope for a normal delivery and a healthy baby."

Detail the aspects of your initial assessment.

Electronic fetal monitor (EFM) reveals an FHR pattern that is normal, category I, with an FHR baseline of 140s moderate variability with accelerations to 160s for 20 seconds. She is uncomfortable with contractions and rates her pain at 5. She requests ambulation, as she feels more comfortable with walking.

At 0120 she has SROM for a large amount of clear amniotic fluid. FHR is baseline 130s with moderate variability, and accelerations and contractions are every 3 minutes and feel moderate to palpation. Her SVE reveals her cervix is 6 cm/90/0 station. She is very uncomfortable with contractions but does not want pain medication at this time. José appears anxious and at a loss for how to help his wife.

What are your immediate priorities in nursing care for Margarite and José Sanchez?

Discuss the rationale for the priorities.

What teaching would you include?

State nursing diagnosis, expected outcome, and interventions related to managing labor pain.

What are appropriate interventions to manage her labor pain nonpharmacologically?

At 0200 Margarite is increasingly uncomfortable with contractions and cries out that she can no longer take the pain. Her cervical examination is 6/100/0. She requests pain medication and is given a dose of Nubain (nalbuphine hydrochloride) at 0215 for pain relief in active labor. José asks how much longer the labor will be and when the baby will be born.

Detail the aspects of your ongoing assessment.

What are your current priorities in nursing care for Margarite Sanchez?

Discuss the rationale for the priorities.

State nursing diagnosis, expected outcome, and interventions related to this problem.

At 0410 Margarite is very uncomfortable with contractions and cries out that she feels more pressure. She vomits a small amount of bile-colored fluid and is perspiring and breathing hard with contractions. Her cervical exam is 8/100%/0. She requests pain medication and is given a dose of Nubian at 0440 for pain relief in transition.

What are appropriate interventions?

At 0630 Margarite reports an urge to bear down and push with contractions; she is very uncomfortable with contractions, and cries out that she feels more pressure. Her SVE reveals she is 10 cm/100% and +1 station. She has a strong urge to push with contractions that are every 2 minutes and strong to palpation. The FHR is 130 with moderate variability, and the FHR drops to 90 bpm for 40 seconds with pushing efforts.

What are your immediate priorities in nursing care for Margarite Sanchez?

Discuss the rationale for the priorities.

What does the FHR indicate?

State nursing diagnosis, expected outcome, and interventions related to managing labor pain.

Margarite continues to bear down, using open glottis pushing with contractions, and the fetal head is descending with contractions. The FHR is 130 with moderate variability and the FHR drops to 90 bpm for 40 seconds with pushing efforts. At 0730. Margarite is increasingly unfocused with contractions and states, "I can't push . . . call my doctor to get the baby out!" José is at her side, holding her hand and encouraging her pushing efforts.

What are your immediate priorities in nursing care for Margarite Sanchez?

Discuss the rationale for the priorities.

At 0815 Margarite continues to bear down with contractions and the fetal head is descending with contractions. The FHR is 130 with moderate variability and the FHR drops to 90 bpm for 40 seconds with pushing efforts. Margarite is focused with contractions. The fetal head is starting to crown with pushing efforts.

What are your immediate priorities in nursing care for Margarite Sanchez?

Discuss the rationale for the priorities.

Her doctor comes into the labor and delivery room and she delivers a baby boy at 0839, with a second-degree perineal laceration. Her son weighs 3,800 g and 1- and 5-minute Apgar scores are 8 and 9.

Both Margarite and José begin to cry when their son is born, and José holds his son and hugs his wife. The placenta is delivered apparently intact at 0845. Both Margarite and her son are stable, and you initiate immediate postpartum and transition care for the mother and baby.

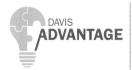

Go to Davis Advantage to complete your learning: strengthen understanding, apply your knowledge, and prepare for the Next Gen NCLEX®.

REFERENCES

AAP Committee on Fetus and Newborn and ACOG Committee on Obstetric Practice. (2015). The Apgar score. *Pediatrics, 136*(4), 819. https://doi.org/10.1542/peds.2015-2651

AAP Committee on Fetus and Newborn and ACOG Committee on Obstetric Practice. (2017). *Guidelines for perinatal care* (8th ed.). The American College of Obstetricians and Gynecologists. http://ebooks.aappublications.org/content/9781610020886/9781610020886

Aasheim, V., Nilsen, A. B. V., Reinar, L. M., & Lukasse, M. (2017). Perineal techniques during the second stage of labour for reducing perineal trauma. *Cochrane Database of Systematic Reviews* (6). https://doi.org/10.1002/14651858.CD006672.pub3

Abalos, E., Chamillard, M., Díaz, V., Pasquale, J., & Souza, J. P. (2020). Progression of the first stage of spontaneous labour. *Best Practice & Research Clinical Obstetrics & Gynaecology, 67*, 19–32. https://doi.org/10.1016/j.bpobgyn.2020.03.001

Alhafez, L., & Berghella, V. (2020). Evidence-based labor management: First stage of labor (part 3). *American Journal of Obstetrics & Gynecology MFM, 2*(4), 100185. https://doi.org/10.1016/j.ajogmf.2020.100185

Aloi, J. A. (2009). Nursing the disenfranchised: Women who have relinquished an infant for adoption. *Journal of Psychiatric and Mental Health Nursing, 16*(1), 27–31. https://doi.org/10.1111/j.1365-2850.2008.01324.x

Altman, M. R., McLemore, M. R., Oseguera, T., Lyndon, A., & Franck, L. S. (2020). Listening to women: Recommendations from women of color to improve experiences in pregnancy and birth care. *Journal of Midwifery & Women's Health, 65*(4), 466–473. https://doi.org/10.1111/jmwh.13102

American College of Nurse-Midwives. (2016). Providing oral nutrition to women in labor. *Journal of Midwifery & Women's Health, 61*(4), 528–534. https://doi.org/10.1111/jmwh.12515

American College of Obstetricians and Gynecologists. (2016). Committee Opinion No. 660: Family building through gestational surrogacy. *Obstetrics & Gynecology, 127*(3), e97–e103. https://doi.org/10.1097/AOG.0000000000001352

American College of Obstetricians and Gynecologists. (2019a). ACOG Committee Opinion No. 766: Approaches to limit intervention during labor and birth. *Obstetrics & Gynecology, 133*(2), e164–e173. https://doi.org/10.1097/AOG.0000000000003074

American College of Obstetricians and Gynecologists. (2019b). ACOG Committee Opinion No. 794: Quantitative blood loss in obstetric hemorrhage. *Obstetrics & Gynecology, 134*(6), e150–e156. https://doi.org/10.1097/aog.0000000000003564

American College of Obstetricians and Gynecologists. (2020). ACOG Committee Opinion Summary, Number 797: Prevention of group B streptococcal early-onset disease in newborns: *Obstetrics & Gynecology, 135*(2), 489–492. https://doi.org/10.1097/aog.0000000000003669

American Nurses Association. (2015). *Code of ethics*. American Nurses Association. https://www.nursingworld.org/practice-policy/nursing-excellence/ethics/code-of-ethics-for-nurses/coe-view-only

Anim-Somuah, M., Smyth, R. M. D., Cyna, A. M., & Cuthbert, A. (2018). Epidural versus non-epidural or no analgesia for pain management in labour. *Cochrane Database of Systematic Reviews* (5). https://doi.org/10.1002/14651858.CD000331.pub4

Association of Women's Health, Obstetric and Neonatal Nurses. (2015a). AWHONN Practice Brief Number 2: Guidelines for oxytocin administration after birth. *Nursing and Women's Health, 19*(1), 99–101. https://doi.org/10.1111/1751-486x.12199

Association of Women's Health, Obstetric and Neonatal Nurses. (2015b). AWHONN Practice Brief Number 1: Quantification of blood loss. *Journal of Obstetric, Gynecologic, and Neonatal Nursing, 44,* 158–160. https://www.nwhjournal.org/article/S1751-4851%2821%2900085-4/pdf

Association of Women's Health, Obstetric and Neonatal Nurses. (2015c). AWHONN Practice Brief Number 1: Quantification of blood loss. *Nursing and Women's Health, 19*(1), 96–98. https://doi.org/10.1111/1751-486x.12198

Association of Women's Health, Obstetric and Neonatal Nurses. (2016). AWHONN Practice Brief Number 5: Immediate and sustained skin-to-skin contact for the healthy term newborn after birth. *Journal of Obstetric, Gynecologic & Neonatal Nursing, 45*(6), 842–844. https://doi.org/10.1016/j.jogn.2016.09.001

Association of Women's Health, Obstetric and Neonatal Nurses. (2017). Confidentiality in adolescent health care. *Journal of Obstetric, Gynecologic & Neonatal Nursing, 46*(6), 889–890. https://doi.org/10.1016/j.jogn.2017.09.003

Association of Women's Health, Obstetric and Neonatal Nurses. (2018). Continuous labor support for every woman. *Journal of Obstetric, Gynecologic & Neonatal Nursing, 47*(1), 73–74. https://doi.org/10.1016/j.jogn.2017.11.010

Association of Women's Health, Obstetric and Neonatal Nurses. (2019). Nursing care and management of the 2nd stage of labor (Evidence-Based Clinical Practice Guideline, 3rd ed.). Washington, DC: Author.

Association of Women's Health, Obstetric and Neonatal Nurses. (2020). Position statement: Role of the registered nurse in the care of the pregnant woman receiving analgesia and anesthesia by catheter techniques. *Journal of Obstetric, Gynecologic & Neonatal Nursing. 41*(3), 327–329

Aziz, K., Lee, C. H. C., Escobedo, M. B., Hoover, A. V., Kamath-Rayne, B. D., Kapadia, V.S., . . . Zaichkin, J. (2021, Jan). Part 5: Neonatal resuscitation 2020 American Heart Association guidelines for cardiopulmonary resuscitation and emergency cardiovascular care. *Pediatrics, 147*(Suppl 1); S524–S550. https://doi.org/10.1542/peds.2020-038505E

Barasinski, C., Debost-Legrand, A., & Vendittelli, F. (2020). Is directed open-glottis pushing more effective than directed closed-glottis pushing during the second stage of labor? A pragmatic randomized trial—the EOLE study. *Midwifery, 91,* 102843. https://doi.org/10.1016/j.midw.2020.102843

Begley, C. M., Gyte, G. M., Devane, D., McGuire, W., Weeks, A., & Biesty, L. M. (2019, Feb 13). Active versus expectant management for women in the third stage of labour. *Cochrane Database of Systematic Reviews, 2*(2), Cd007412. https://doi.org/10.1002/14651858.CD007412.pub5

Berghella, V. (2021). Management of the third stage of labor after vaginal delivery: Prophylactic drug therapy to minimize hemorrhage. In T. Post (Ed.), *UpToDate.* https://www.uptodate-com.ucsf.idm.oclc.org/contents/management-of-the-third-stage-of-labor-after-vaginal-delivery-prophylactic-drug-therapy-to-minimize-hemorrhage?sectionName=GENERAL%20APPROACH&search=3rd%20stage%20of%20labor&topicRef=4445&anchor=H7&source=see_link#H7

Bohren, M. A., Hofmeyr, G. J., Sakala, C., Fukuzawa, R. K., & Cuthbert, A. (2017, Jul 6). Continuous support for women during childbirth. *Cochrane Database of Systematic Reviews, 7*(7), Cd003766. https://doi.org/10.1002/14651858.CD003766.pub6

Brooks, L. A., Manias, E., & Bloomer, M. J. (2019). Culturally sensitive communication in healthcare: A concept analysis. *Collegian, 26*(3), 383–391. https://doi.org/10.1016/j.colegn.2018.09.007

Burke, C. (2021). Pain labor: Nonpharmacologic and pharmacologic management. In K. Simpson, P. Creehan, N. Obrien-Abel, C. Roth, & A. Rohan (Eds.), *Perinatal nursing* (5th ed., pp. 325-411). Wolters Kluwer

Burns, E. (2014, Winter). More than clinical waste? Placenta rituals among Australian home-birthing women. *Journal of Perinatal Education, 23*(1), 41–49. https://doi.org/10.1891/1058-1243.23.1.41

Carabez, R. M., Eliason, M. J., & Martinson, M. (2016). Nurses' knowledge about transgender patient care: A qualitative study. *Advances in Nursing Science, 39*(3), 257–271. https://doi.org/10.1097/ans.0000000000000128

Chambers, B. D., Baer, R. J., McLemore, M. R., & Jelliffe-Pawlowski, L. L. (2019). Using index of concentration at the extremes as indicators of structural racism to evaluate the association with preterm birth and infant mortality-California, 2011–2012. *Journal of Urban Health, 96*(2), 159–170. https://doi.org/10.1007/s11524-018-0272-4

Chapman, L. (2000). Expectant fathers and labor epidurals. *Maternal Child Nursing, 25,* 133–138.

Chen, I., Opiyo, N., Tavender, E., Mortazhejri, S., Rader, T., Petkovic, J., . . . Betran, A. P. (2018, Sep 28). Non-clinical interventions for reducing unnecessary caesarean section. *Cochrane Database of Systematic Reviews,* (9), Cd005528. https://doi.org/10.1002/14651858.CD005528.pub3

Ciardulli, A., Saccone, G., Anastasio, H., & Berghella, V. (2017). Less-restrictive food intake during labor in low-risk singleton pregnancies: A systematic review and meta-analysis. *Obstetrics & Gynecology, 129*(3), 473–480. https://doi.org/10.1097/aog.0000000000001898

Cluett, E. R., Burns, E., & Cuthbert, A. (2018). Immersion in water during labour and birth. *Cochrane Database of Systematic Reviews* (5). https://doi.org/10.1002/14651858.CD000111.pub4

Clutter, L. B. (2014). Adult birth mothers who made open infant adoption placements after adolescent unplanned pregnancy. *Journal of Obstetric, Gynecologic, and Neonatal Nursing 43*(2), 190.

Coleman, P. K., & Garratt, D. (2016). From birth mothers to first mothers: Toward a compassionate understanding of the life-long act of adoption placement. *Issues in Law & Medicine, 31*(2), 139–163.

Committee on Obstetric Practice. (2017). Committee Opinion No. 687: Approaches to limit intervention during labor and birth. *Obstetrics & Gynecology, 129*(2), e20-e28. https://journals.lww.com/greenjournal/Fulltext/2017/02000/Committee_Opinion_No__687__Approaches_to_Limit.43.aspx

Crear-Perry, J., Correa-de-Araujo, R., Lewis Johnson, T., McLemore, M. R., Neilson, E., & Wallace, M. (2021). Social and structural determinants of health inequities in maternal health. *Journal of Women's Health (Larchmt), 30*(2), 230–235. https://doi.org/10.1089/jwh.2020.8882

Cunningham, F. G., Leveno, K. J., Bloom, S. L., Dashe, J. S., Hoffman, B. L., Casey, B. M., & Spong, C. Y. (2018). Abnormal labor. In *Williams obstetrics* (25th ed.). McGraw-Hill Education. http://accessmedicine.mhmedical.com/content.aspx?aid=1160775319

Declercq, E. R., Sakala, C., Corry, M. P., Applebaum, S., & Herrlich, A. (2014). Major survey findings of listening to mothers (SM) III: Pregnancy and birth: Report of the Third National U.S. Survey of Women's Childbearing Experiences. *The Journal of Perinatal Education, 23*(1), 9–16. https://doi.org/10.1891/1058-1243.23.1.9

DiMascio, D., Saccone, G., Bellussi, F., Al-Kouatly, H. B., Brunelli, R., Benedetti Panici, P., . . . Berghella, V. (2020). Delayed versus immediate pushing in the second stage of labor in women with neuraxial analgesia: A systematic review and meta-analysis of randomized controlled trials. *American Journal of Obstetrics and Gynecology, 223*(2), 189–203. https://doi.org/10.1016/j.ajog.2020.02.002

Duff, P. (2021). Preterm prelabor rupture of membranes: Clinical manifestations and diagnosis. In T. Post (Ed.), *UpToDate.* UpToDate. 1-24. https://www.uptodate-com.ucsf.idm.oclc.org/contents/preterm-prelabor-rupture-of-membranes-clinical-manifestations-and-diagnosis?search=amnisure&source=search_result&selectedTitle=1~1&usage_type=default&display_rank=1

Edwards, M., Lawson, C., Rahman, S., Conley, K., Phillips, H., & Uings, R. (2016). What does quality healthcare look like to adolescents and young adults? Ask the experts! *Clinical Medicine, 16*(2), 146. https://doi.org/10.7861/clinmedicine.16-2-146

Ely, D., & Driscoll, A. (2020). Infant mortality in the United States, 2018: Data from the period linked birth/infant death file. *National Vital Statistics Reports, 69*(7), 1–18. https://www.cdc.gov/nchs/data/nvsr/nvsr69/NVSR-69-7-508.pdf

Farr, A., Chervenak, F. A., McCullough, L. B., Baergen, R. N., & Grünebaum, A. (2018, Apr). Human placentophagy: A review. *American Journal of Obstetrics & Gynecology, 218*(4), 401.e401–401.e411. https://doi.org/10.1016/j.ajog.2017.08.016

Garfield, R. E., Murphy, L., Gray, K., & Towe, B. (2021, Mar). Review and study of uterine bioelectrical waveforms and vector analysis to identify electrical and mechanosensitive transduction control mechanisms during labor in pregnant patients. *Reproductive Science, 28*(3), 838–856. https://doi.org/10.1007/s43032-020-00358-5

Gluck, O., Mizrachi, Y., Ganer Herman, H., Bar, J., Kovo, M., & Weiner, E. (2020, Apr 25). The correlation between the number of vaginal examinations during active labor and febrile morbidity, a retrospective cohort study. *BMC Pregnancy Childbirth, 20*(1), 246. https://doi.org/10.1186/s12884-020-02925-9

Grobman, W. A., Bailit, J., Lai, Y., Reddy, U. M., Wapner, R. J., Varner, M.W., . . . Tolosa, J. E. (2016, Apr). Association of the duration of active pushing with obstetric outcomes. *Obstetrics & Gynecology, 127*(4), 667–673. https://doi.org/10.1097/aog.0000000000001354

Hale, S., Hill, C. M., Hermann, M., Kinzig, A., Lawrence, C., McCaughin, N., & Parker, C. (2020). Analgesia and anesthesia in the intrapartum period. *Nursing for Women's Health, 24*(1), e1–e60. https://doi.org/10.1016/j.nwh.2019.12.002

Hardeman, R. R., Medina, E. M., & Kozhimannil, K. B. (2016, Dec 1). Structural racism and supporting Black lives—The role of health professionals. *New England Journal of Medicine, 375*(22), 2113–2115. https://doi.org/10.1056/NEJMp1609535

Hickey, L., & Savage, J. (2019). Effect of peanut ball and position changes in women laboring with an epidural. *Nursing for Women's Health, 23*(3), 245–252. https://doi.org/10.1016/j.nwh.2019.04.004

Hishikawa, K., Kusaka, T., Fukuda, T., Kohata, Y., & Inoue, H. (2019). Anxiety or nervousness disturbs the progress of birth based on human behavioral evolutionary biology. *Journal of Perinatal Education, 28*(4), 218–223. https://doi.org/10.1891/1058-1243.28.4.218

Hoffman, K. M., Trawalter, S., Axt, J. R., & Oliver, M. N. (2016). Racial bias in pain assessment and treatment recommendations, and false beliefs about biological differences between Blacks and Whites. *Proceedings of the National Academy of Sciences, 113*(16), 4296. https://doi.org/10.1073/pnas.1516047113

Hofmeyr, G. (2021). Overview of breech presentation. In V. Barss (Ed.), *UpToDate*. UpToDate. https://www-uptodate-com.ucsf.idm.oclc.org/contents/overview-of-breech-presentation?search=breech%20presentation&source=search_result&selectedTitle=1~54&usage_type=default&display_rank=1

Hoyert, D. L., & Miniño, A. M. (2020). Maternal mortality in the United States: Changes in coding, publication, and data release, 2018. *National Vital Statistics Reports: From the Centers for Disease Control and Prevention, National Center for Health Statistics, National Vital Statistics System, 69*(2), 1–18.

Howell, E. A., Brown, H., Brumley, J., Bryant, A., Caughey, A., Cornell, A., . . . Grobman, W. (2018). Reduction of peripartum racial and ethnic disparities: A conceptual framework and maternal safety consensus bundle. *Journal of Obstetric, Gynecologic & Neonatal Nursing, 47*(3), 275–289. https://doi.org/10.1016/j.jogn.2018.03.004

Howell, E. A., Egorova, N. N., Janevic, T., Brodman, M., Balbierz, A., Zeitlin, J., & Hebert, P. L. (2020, Feb). Race and ethnicity, medical insurance, and within-hospital severe maternal morbidity disparities. *Obstetrics & Gynecology, 135*(2), 285–293. https://doi.org/10.1097/aog.0000000000003667

Hutchison, J., Mahdy, H., & Hutchison, J. (2021). Stages of labor. In *StatPearls*. StatPearls Publishing.

James, S., Herman, J., Rankin, S., Keisling, M., Mottet, L., & Anafi, M. A. (2016). *The report of the 2015 US transgender survey*. National Center for Transgender Equality. https://transequality.org/sites/default/files/docs/usts/USTS-Full-Report-Dec17.pdf

Jones, C. P. (2000, Aug). Levels of racism: A theoretic framework and a gardener's tale. *American Journal of Public Health, 90*(8), 1212–1215. https://doi.org/10.2105/ajph.90.8.1212

Kendi, I. X. (2016). *Stamped from the beginning: The definitive history of racist ideas in America.* Hachette UK.

Kendi, I. X. (2019). *How to be an antiracist*. One World.

King, T. L., Brucker, M. C., Osborne, K., & Jevitt, C. (2019). *Varney's midwifery* (6th ed.). Jones & Bartlett Learning.

Kiserud, T., Piaggio, G., Carroli, G., Widmer, M., Carvalho, J., Neerup Jensen, L., . . . Platt, L. D. (2017, Jan). The World Health Organization fetal growth charts: A multinational longitudinal study of ultrasound biometric measurements and estimated fetal weight. *PLOS Med, 14*(1), e1002220. https://doi.org/10.1371/journal.pmed.1002220

Kobayashi, S., Hanada, N., Matsuzaki, M., Takehara, K., Ota, E., Sasaki, H., . . . Mori, R. (2017). Assessment and support during early labour for improving birth outcomes. *Cochrane Database of Systematic Reviews* (4). https://doi.org/10.1002/14651858.CD011516.pub2

Lagrew, D. C., Low, L. K., Brennan, R., Corry, M. P., Edmonds, J. K., Gilpin, B.G., . . . Jaffer, S. (2018). National partnership for maternal safety: Consensus bundle on safe reduction of primary cesarean births—Supporting intended vaginal births. *Obstetrics & Gynecology, 131*(3), 503–513. https://doi.org/10.1097/aog.0000000000002471

Lawrence, A., Lewis, L., Hofmeyr, G. J., & Styles, C. (2013). Maternal positions and mobility during first stage labour. *Cochrane Database of Systematic Reviews* (10). https://doi.org/10.1002/14651858.CD003934.pub4

Lemos, A., Amorim, M. M., Dornelas de Andrade, A., de Souza, A. I., Cabral Filho, J. E., & Correia, J. B. (2017, Mar 26). Pushing/bearing down methods for the second stage of labour. *Cochrane Database of Systematic Reviews, 3*(3), Cd009124. https://doi.org/10.1002/14651858.CD009124.pub3

Lexi-Comp. (2021a). *Methylergonovine*. http://www.crlonline.com.ucsf.idm.oclc.org/lco/action/doc/retrieve/docid/patch_f/7280?cesid=85ZSiQMQ7Rn&searchUrl=%2Flco%2Faction%2Fsearch%3Fq%3Dmethergine%26t%3Dname%26va%3Dmethergine

Lexi-Comp. (2021b). *Tranexamic acid.* http://www.crlonline.com.ucsf.idm.oclc.org/lco/action/doc/retrieve/docid/patch_f/7798?cesid=4CBLEHnxe08&searchUrl=%2Flco%2Faction%2Fsearch%3Fq%3Dtranexamic%252520acid%26t%3Dname%26va%3Dtranexamic%252520acid#pha

Liao, C. C., Lan, S. H., Yen, Y. Y., Hsieh, Y. P., & Lan, S. J. (2021). Aromatherapy intervention on anxiety and pain during first stage labour in nulliparous women: A systematic review and meta-analysis. *Journal of Obstetrics & Gynaecology, 41*(1), 21–31. https://doi.org/10.1080/01443615.2019.1673707

Lothian, J. A. (2014, Fall). Promoting optimal care in childbirth. *Journal of Perinatal Education, 23*(4), 174–177. https://doi.org/10.1891/1058-1243.23.4.174

Lowe, N. K. (2002). The nature of labor pain. *American Journal of Obstetrics & Gynecology, 186*(5 Suppl Nature), S16–S24.

Lyndon, A., & Usher Ali, L. (2015). *Fetal heart monitoring principles and practices* (5th ed.). Kendall-Hunt.

MacDorman, M. F., & Declercq, E. (2019). Trends and state variations in out-of-hospital births in the United States, 2004–2017. *Birth, 46*(2), 279–288. https://doi.org/10.1111/birt.12411

Main, E. K., Goffman, D., Scavone, B. M., Low, L. K., Bingham, D., Fontaine, P. L., . . . Levy, B. S. (2015). National partnership for maternal safety: Consensus bundle on obstetric hemorrhage. *Obstetrics & Gynecology, 126*(1), 155–162. https://doi.org/10.1097/aog.0000000000000869

Meghani, S. H., Byun, E., & Gallagher, R. M. (2012). Time to take stock: A meta-analysis and systematic review of analgesic treatment disparities for pain in the United States. *Pain Medicine, 13*(2), 150–174. https://doi.org/10.1111/j.1526-4637.2011.01310.x

Middleton, P., Shepherd, E., Flenady, V., McBain, R. D., & Crowther, C. A. (2017). Planned early birth versus expectant management (waiting) for prelabour rupture of membranes at term (37 weeks or more). *Cochrane Database of Systematic Reviews* (1). https://doi.org/10.1002/14651858.CD005302.pub3

Moayedi, M., & Davis, K. D. (2013). Theories of pain: From specificity to gate control. *Journal of Neurophysiology, 109*(1), 5–12. https://doi.org/10.1152/jn.00457.2012

Mueller, C. G., Webb, P. J., & Morgan, S. (2020). The effects of childbirth education on maternity outcomes and maternal satisfaction. *The Journal of Perinatal Education, 29*(1), 16–22. https://doi: 10.1891/1058-1243.29.1.16.

Neczypor, J. L., & Holley, S. L. (2017). Providing evidence-based care during the golden hour. *Nursing for Women's Health, 21*(6), 462–472. https://doi.org/10.1016/j.nwh.2017.10.011

Norwitz, E., Lockwood, C., & Barss, V. (2021). Physiology of parturition at term. In T. Post (Ed.), *UpToDate*. UpToDate. https://www-uptodate-com.ucsf.idm.oclc.org/contents/physiology-of-parturition-at-term?search=labor&source=search_result&selectedTitle=4~150&usage_type=default&display_rank=4#H24

Novak, N. L., Geronimus, A. T., & Martinez-Cardoso, A. M. (2017). Change in birth outcomes among infants born to Latina mothers after a major immigration raid. *International Journal of Epidemiology, 46*(3), 839–849. https://doi.org/10.1093/ije/dyw346

O'Brien-Abel, N., & Simpson, K. (2021). Fetal assessment during labor. In K. Simpson, P. Creehan, N. Obrien-Abel, C. Roth, & A. Rohan (Eds.), *Perinatal nursing* (5th ed., pp. 412-464). Wolters Kluwer.

Oladapo, O. T., Diaz, V., Bonet, M., Abalos, E., Thwin, S. S., Souza, H., . . . Gülmezoglu, A. M. (2018). Cervical dilatation patterns of "low-risk" women with spontaneous labour and normal perinatal outcomes: A systematic review. *BJOG: An International Journal of Obstetrics & Gynaecology, 125*(8), 944–954. https://doi.org/10.1111/1471-0528.14930

Ondeck, M. (2014, Fall). Healthy birth practice #2: Walk, move around, and change positions throughout labor. *Journal of Perinatal Education, 23*(4), 188–193. https://doi.org/10.1891/1058-1243.23.4.188

Pergialiotis, V., Bellos, I., Fanaki, M., Vrachnis, N., & Doumouchtsis, S. K. (2020, Apr). Risk factors for severe perineal trauma during childbirth: An updated meta-analysis. *European Journal of Obstetrics & Gynecology and Reproductive Biology, 247*, 94–100. https://doi.org/10.1016/j.ejogrb.2020.02.025

Raines, D. A., & Cooper, D. B. (2021). Braxton Hicks contractions. In *StatPearls*. StatPearls Publishing.

Ravanos, K., Dagklis, T., Petousis, S., Margioula-Siarkou, C., Prapas, Y., & Prapas, N. (2015). Factors implicated in the initiation of human parturition in term and preterm labor: A review. *Gynecological Endocrinology, 31*(9), 679–683. https://doi.org/10.3109/09513590.2015.1076783

Richardson, B., Price, S., & Campbell-Yeo, M. (2019). Redefining perinatal experience: A philosophical exploration of a hypothetical case of gender diversity in labour and birth. *Journal of Clinical Nursing, 28*(3-4), 703–710. https://doi.org/10.1111/jocn.14521

Richardson, M. G., Lopez, B. M., Baysinger, C. L., Shotwell, M. S., & Chestnut, D. H. (2017). Nitrous oxide during labor: Maternal satisfaction does not depend exclusively on analgesic effectiveness. *Anesthesia and Analgesia, 124*(2), 548–553. https://doi.org/10.1213/ane.0000000000001680

Roberts, D. E. (2011). *Fatal invention: How science, politics, and big business re-create race in the twenty-first century*. New Press.

Roberts, L., Gulliver, B., Fisher, J., & Cloyes, K. G. (2010). The coping with labor algorithm: An alternate pain assessment tool for the laboring woman. *Journal of Midwifery & Women's Health, 55*(2), 107–116. https://doi.org/10.1016/j.jmwh.2009.11.002

Saoud, F., Stone, A., Nutter, A., Hankins, G. D., Saade, G. R., & Saad, A. F. (2019, Sep). Validation of a new method to assess estimated blood loss in the obstetric population undergoing cesarean delivery. *American Journal of Obstetrics & Gynecology, 221*(3), 267.e261–267.e266. https://doi.org/10.1016/j.ajog.2019.06.022

Simpson, K. R., & James, D. C. (2005). Efficacy of intrauterine resuscitation techniques in improving fetal oxygen status during labor. *Obstetrics & Gynecology, 105*(6), 1362–1368. https://doi.org/10.1097/01.AOG.0000164474.03350.7c

Simpson, K., & O'Brien-Abel, N (2021). Labor and birth. In K. Simpson, P. Creehan, N. Obrien-Abel, C. Roth, & A. Rohan (Eds.), *Perinatal nursing* (5th ed., pp. 325-411). Wolters Kluwer.

Singata, M., Tranmer, J., & Gyte, G. M. L. (2013). Restricting oral fluid and food intake during labour. *Cochrane Database of Systematic Reviews* (8). https://doi.org/10.1002/14651858.CD003930.pub3

Smith, C. A., Collins, C. T., Levett, K. M., Armour, M., Dahlen, H. G., Tan, A. L., & Mesgarpour, B. (2020). Acupuncture or acupressure for pain management during labour. *Cochrane Database of Systematic Reviews* (2). https://doi.org/10.1002/14651858.CD009232.pub2

Smith, C. A., Levett, K. M., Collins, C. T., Dahlen, H. G., Ee, C. C., & Suganuma, M. (2018). Massage, reflexology and other manual methods for pain management in labour. *Cochrane Database of Systematic Reviews* (3). https://doi.org/10.1002/14651858.CD009290.pub3

Smith, L. A., Burns, E., & Cuthbert, A. (2018). Parenteral opioids for maternal pain management in labour. *Cochrane Database of Systematic Reviews* (6). https://doi.org/10.1002/14651858.CD007396.pub3

Sng, B. L., Leong, W. L., Zeng, Y., Siddiqui, F. J., Assam, P. N., Lim, Y., . . . Sia, A. T. (2014). Early versus late initiation of epidural analgesia for labour. *Cochrane Database of Systematic Reviews* (10). https://doi.org/10.1002/14651858.CD007238.pub2

Taheri, M., Takian, A., Taghizadeh, Z., Jafari, N., & Sarafraz, N. (2018). Creating a positive perception of childbirth experience: Systematic review and meta-analysis of prenatal and intrapartum interventions. *Reproductive Health, 15*(1), 73. https://doi.org/10.1186/s12978-018-0511-x

The Guttmacher Institute. (2021). *An overview of consent to reproductive health services by young people*. https://www.guttmacher.org/state-policy/explore/overview-minors-consent-law

Tilden, E. L., Phillippi, J. C., Ahlberg, M., King, T. L., Dissanayake, M., Lee, T. S., . . . Caughey, A. B. (2019). Describing latent phase duration and associated characteristics among 1281 low-risk women in spontaneous labor. *Birth, 46*(4), 592–601. https://doi.org/10.1111/birt.12428

Turner, J. M., Mitchell, M. D., & Kumar, S. S. (2020). The physiology of intrapartum fetal compromise at term. *Ameican Journal of Obstetrics & Gynecology, 222*(1), 17–26. https://doi.org/10.1016/j.ajog.2019.07.032

Uvnäs-Moberg, K., Ekström-Bergström, A., Berg, M., Buckley, S., Pajalic, Z., Hadjigeorgiou, E., . . . Dencker, A. (2019). Maternal plasma levels of oxytocin during physiological childbirth—a systematic review with implications for uterine contractions and central actions of oxytocin. *BMC Pregnancy and Childbirth, 19*(1), 285. https://doi.org/10.1186/s12884-019-2365-9

Vallera, C., Choi, L. O., Cha, C. M., & Hong, R. W. (2017). Uterotonic medications: Oxytocin, methylergonovine, carboprost, misoprostol. *Anesthesiology Clinics, 35*(2), 207–219. https://doi.org/10.1016/j.anclin.2017.01.007

Washington, H. A. (2006). *Medical apartheid. The dark history of medical experimentation on Black Americans from colonial times to the present*. Doubleday Books.

Williams, J. W., Cunningham, F. G., Leveno, K. J., Bloom, S. L., Spong, C. Y., & Dashe, J. S. (2018). *Williams obstetrics* (25th ed.). McGraw-Hill Education Medical.

Fetal Heart Rate Assessment

9

Janice Stinson, RNC, PhD

LEARNING OUTCOMES

Upon completion of this chapter, the student will be able to:

1. Define terms used in electronic fetal monitoring (EFM).
2. Identify the modes of fetal heart rate (FHR) assessment: auscultation, palpation, EFM.
3. Describe the components of FHR and uterine contraction (UC) patterns essential to interpretation of monitor strips.
4. Articulate the physiology of FHR patterns.
5. Distinguish between Category I, II, and III FHR patterns and appropriate nursing actions based on these interpretations.

CONCEPTS

Acid Base
Clinical Judgment
Collaboration
Comfort
Communication
Evidence-Based Practice
Family
Mobility
Oxygenation
Perfusion
Stress and Coping

Nursing Diagnosis

- Risk for disturbed maternal fetal dyad
- Deficient knowledge of EFM assessment and interventions
- Impaired fetal oxygenation and perfusion related to impaired uteroplacental perfusion
- Risk of fetal injury related to respiratory or metabolic acidemia

Nursing Outcomes

- The pregnant woman and family will verbalize basic understanding of fetal monitoring.
- Intrauterine resuscitation strategies will be initiated for Category II or III EFM patterns.

INTRODUCTION

This chapter introduces basic fetal monitoring concepts which include both intermittent auscultation (IA) and electronic fetal monitoring (EFM). Fetal heart rate (FHR) assessment began almost 200 years ago when Swiss surgeon Francois-Isaac Mayor (1818) and nobleman Vicomte de Kergaradec (1821) reported the presence of fetal heart sounds via auscultation (hearing sounds via ear-to-abdomen, Picard horn, or stethoscope) (Freeman et al., 2003, Simpson & Creehan, 2014). Electronic monitors that could continually record indirect abdominal phono and fetal electrocardiography (ECG) were developed in the 1950s (Edward H. Hon in the United States, Roberto Caldeyro Barcia in Uruguay, and Konrad Hammacher in Germany). Hon compared heart rate and patterns of FHR changes with labor variables and neonatal outcomes (Freeman, 2002; Tucker et al., 2009).

A 1968 study (Benson et al.) of 24,000 births called the Collaborative Perinatal Project showed that auscultation during labor was unreliable in determining abnormal fetal outcomes except in extreme cases of terminal bradycardia. Hence, in the 1970s, FHR assessment transitioned from an auditory skill to visual assessment of data and continues to be the primary method for intrapartum fetal surveillance despite subsequent clinical trials regarding its efficacy and ability in failing to improve neonatal outcomes (Freeman, 2002; Tucker et al., 2009). This included failure to decrease perinatal mortality and cerebral palsy.

Additionally, a four-fold increase in operative delivery due to a high sensitivity of EFM resulted in many false-positive interpretations of abnormality but low specificity (Simpson & Creehan, 2014). However, many clinicians (Cibils, 1996) feel that it is better to make a clinical decision using a continuous, more precise recording of the FHR and uterine contractions (UCs), especially for high-risk conditions during labor; this process is recommended by the American College of Obstetrics and Gynecologists (ACOG; 2009b).

Current practice indicates that EFM is used for virtually all women during labor in the United States. While it is essential in the assessment of maternal and fetal well-being in antepartal and intrapartal settings, keep in mind that other evidence-based options such as IA are also appropriate for laboring women (True & Bailey, 2016; Wisner & Holschuh, 2018). Both IA and EFM will be covered in this chapter.

The goal of fetal monitoring is to interpret and continually assess fetal oxygenation (Lyndon & Ali, 2015) and prevent significant fetal acidemia while minimizing unnecessary interventions and promoting a satisfying family-centered birth experience (O'Brien-Abel & Simpson, 2021). IA and EFM are techniques for fetal assessment based on the fact that the FHR reflects fetal oxygenation (Lyndon & Ali, 2015) (Box 9-1).

Nurses are expected to independently assess, interpret, and intervene based on interpretations of EFM patterns. Assessments and interactions with monitored women and families are individualized to provide information and explanation, as well as reduce anxiety (Box 9-2). Clear and accurate communication with care providers and the perinatal team is essential for optimizing perinatal outcomes.

TEAMWORK AND COLLABORATION

Teamwork and collaboration imply effective function within nursing and interprofessional teams, open communication, mutual respect, and shared decision making to achieve quality patient care. Communication and collaboration are particularly essential in EFM and the care of women in labor. In 2004, The Joint Commission published *Sentinel Event Alert* Issue #30, Preventing Infant Death and Injury During Delivery. The Joint Commission analyzed 47 cases of perinatal death or permanent disability and found that 72% of root causes identified were related to communication issues among health-care providers. It is not uncommon for disagreements in the interpretation of FHR patterns to exist between team members.

BOX 9-1 | Principles of Fetal Monitoring

Overall Goals
- Support maternal coping and labor progress.
- Maximize uterine blood flow.
- Maximize umbilical blood flow.
- Maximize oxygenation.
- Maintain appropriate uterine activity.

Nursing Actions
- Review plans and expectations with the woman and her family
- Maintain a calm environment
- Stay at the bedside as much as possible
- Monitor only at the level needed for this patient
- Frequent position changes; upright positioning
- Judicious use of technology
- Avoid:
  - Unnecessary interventions
  - Tachysystole
  - Supine position
  - Coached pushing
  - Valsalva pushing

BOX 9-2 | AWHONN Fetal Heart Monitoring Clinical Position Statement

The AWHONN asserts that care by registered nurses (RNs) skilled in fetal heart monitoring (FHM) techniques, including auscultation and EFM, is essential to maternal and fetal well-being during antepartum care, labor, and birth. EFM requires advanced assessment and clinical judgment. It is within the nurse's scope of practice to implement customary interventions in response to FHM data and clinical assessment. Interprofessional policies should support the RN in making decisions regarding fetal monitoring practice, intervening independently when appropriate to maternal or fetal condition.

A woman's preferences and clinical presentation should guide selection of FHM techniques with consideration given to use of the least invasive methods. In general, the least invasive method of monitoring is preferred to promote physiological labor and birth. Labor is dynamic; therefore, consideration of maternal preferences and identification of risk factors should occur upon admission to the birth setting and be ongoing throughout labor.

AWHONN, 2018.

Some suggestions to foster your development in this area include:

● Remembering effective communication is timely, direct, respectful, and identifies the level of concern and urgency. For example, if the situation is acute, "I need you to come now" is a clear and concise request for immediate action (O'Brien-Abel & Simpson, 2021).
● Appreciating the importance of intra- and interprofessional collaboration to improve patient outcomes.
● Integrating the contributions of others who play a role in helping the patient and her family achieve a healthy birth.
● Respecting the centrality of the patient and family as core members of any health-care team.
● Acknowledging your own potential to contribute to effective team functioning in this critical setting.
● Practicing the use of consistent fetal heart monitoring terminology among perinatal-care providers as one strategy to improve communication (Box 9-3)

TERMINOLOGY RELATED TO FETAL ASSESSMENT

Definitions used in this chapter are from the National Institute of Child Health and Human Development (NICHD) Research Planning Workshop (1997a, 1997b) and the 2008 NICHD Workshop Report on Electronic Fetal Monitoring: Update on Definitions, Interpretations and Research Guidelines publications (ACOG, 2010; Macones et al., 2008). There is a current movement to standardize language for FHR interpretations.

BOX 9-3 | Common Abbreviations for Electronic Fetal Monitoring

BPM	Beats per minute
ED	Early deceleration
EFM	Electronic fetal monitoring
FHR	Fetal heart rate
FSE	Fetal scalp electrode
IA	Intermittent auscultation
IUPC	Intrauterine pressure catheter
LD	Late deceleration
MVU	Montevideo units
PD	Prolonged deceleration
TOCO	Tocodynamometer
UC	Uterine contractions
US	Ultrasound
VD	Variable deceleration
VAS	Vibroacoustic stimulation
VE	Vaginal examination

It is critical for labor units to select one set of definitions for FHR patterns for all types of professional communications (Association of Women's Health, Obstetric and Neonatal Nurses [AWHONN], 2018; Simpson, 2004b) (Table 9-1; Box 9-3). Clinicians should be familiar with these definitions and use them consistently in clinical practice.

TABLE 9-1 Terminology Related to Fetal Heart Rate Assessment

TERMINOLOGY	DEFINITION
Baseline FHR	FHR rounded to increments of 5 bpm during a 10-minute window. There must be at least 2 minutes of identifiable baseline segments (not necessarily contiguous). Does not include accelerations or decelerations or periods of marked variability (amplitude greater than 25 bpm). • Periodic: Changes in baseline of FHR occur in relation to UCs. • Episodic: Changes in baseline of FHR occur independent of UCs. • Recurrent: Changes in baseline of FHR occur in greater than or equal to 50% of the contractions in a 20-minute period. • Intermittent: Changes in baseline of FHR in less than 50% of the contractions in a 20-minute period.
Baseline variability	Fluctuations in the baseline FHR that are irregular in amplitude and frequency. The fluctuations are visually quantified as the amplitude of the peak to trough in bpm. It is determined in a 10-minute window, excluding accelerations and decelerations. It reflects the interaction between the fetal sympathetic SNS and parasympathetic nervous system. • Absent: Amplitude range is undetectable. • Minimal: Amplitude range is visually detectable at 5 bpm or less. • Moderate: Amplitude from peak to trough is 6 bpm to 25 bpm. • Marked: Amplitude range greater than 25 bpm.
Indeterminant FHR	FHR that does not meet the criteria of baseline FHR.

Continued

TABLE 9-1   Terminology Related to Fetal Heart Rate Assessment—cont'd

TERMINOLOGY	DEFINITION
Accelerations	Visually apparent, abrupt increase in FHR above the baseline. The peak of the acceleration is 15 bpm or greater over the baseline FHR for 15 or more seconds and less than 2 minutes. • Before 32 weeks' gestation, acceleration is 10 beats or greater over the baseline FHR for 10 or more seconds. • Prolonged accelerations are 2 minutes or more but 10 minutes or less.
Deceleration	Transitory decrease in the FHR from the baseline. • Early deceleration is a visually apparent gradual decrease in FHR from baseline to nadir (lowest point of the deceleration) taking more than 30 seconds. The nadir occurs at the same time as the peak of the UC. Onset, nadir, and recovery match the onset, peak, and end of the UC. It's always periodic. • Variable deceleration is a visually apparent abrupt decrease in the FHR from baseline to nadir taking less than 30 seconds. The decrease in FHR is greater or equal to 15 bpm and less than 2 minutes in duration. It can be periodic or intermittent. • Late deceleration is a visually apparent gradual decrease of FHR from baseline to nadir taking more than 30 seconds. Nadir occurs at the peak of the UC. Onset, nadir, and recovery occur after the respective onset, peak, and end of the UC. It is always periodic. • Prolonged deceleration is a visually apparent abrupt or gradual decrease in FHR below baseline that is 15 bpm or greater lasting 2 minutes or more but 10 minutes or less. It can be periodic or intermittent.
Variation in baseline	Sinusoidal pattern: Visually apparent smooth sine wave similar to undulating pattern in FHR baseline with a cycle frequency of 3 to 5 minutes that persists for 20 minutes or greater. Benign sinusoidal patterns contain accelerations that last less than 20 minutes. A sinusoidal-appearing FHR pattern can occur following maternal administration of some opioids (butorphanol and fentanyl). This undulating FHR pattern is of short duration and is also referred to as pseudosinusoidal or medication-induced sinusoidal (O'Brien-Abel & Simpson, 2021).
Tachycardia	• Baseline FHR of greater than 160 bpm lasting 10 minutes or longer.
Bradycardia	• Baseline FHR of less than 110 bpm lasting for 10 minutes or longer.
Normal FHR	• Category I (see Critical Component: Three-Tier FHR Interpretation System) reflects absence of metabolic acidemia at the time the EFM pattern is observed (O'Brien-Abel & Simpson, 2021), and reflects favorable physiological response to maternal-fetal environment.
Abnormal FHR	• Category II and III (see Critical Component: Three-Tier FHR Interpretation System) reflects unfavorable physiological response to maternal fetal environment.

EFM, electronic fetal monitor; FHR, fetal heart rate; PSNS, parasympathetic nervous system; SNS, sympathetic nervous system; UC, uterine contraction.
ACOG, 2010; Lyndon & Ali, 2015; Macones et al., 2008.

MODES OR TYPES OF FETAL AND UTERINE MONITORING

Preparation for fetal monitoring includes a discussion of the risks and benefits of methods of fetal assessment in the context of the woman's values, preferences, obstetric history, and treatment plan so the woman can make an informed decision about monitoring (O'Brien-Abel & Simpson, 2021). Types of fetal and uterine monitoring include auscultation and palpation for IA; ultrasound and tocodynamometer (shortened to TOCO) for external EFM; and internal fetal spiral electrode (FSE) and intrauterine pressure catheter (IUPC) for internal EFM.

Auscultation

Auscultation refers to the use of the fetoscope or Doppler to listen to the FHR without use of a paper recorder (Feinstein et al., 2008) (Fig. 9–1A&B). Auscultation with a fetoscope allows the practitioner to hear sounds associated with opening and closing of ventricular valves via bone conduction. A Doppler, by contrast, uses sound waves that are deflected from fetal heart movements similar to that used on an EFM external ultrasound transducer. This ultrasound device then converts information into a sound that represents cardiac events.

A paper recorder provides additional information on a tracing for clinician assessment, such as determining the difference

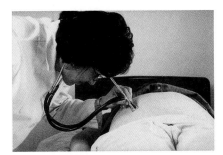

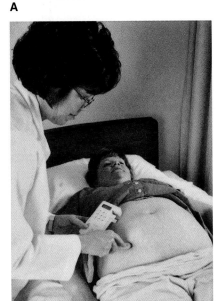

FIGURE 9–1 Auscultation of fetal heart rate. (A) Fetoscope. (B) Doppler ultrasound stethoscope.

> ## BOX 9-4 | Guidelines and Procedure for Auscultation
>
> 1. Explain the procedure to the woman and her family.
> 2. Palpate the maternal abdomen to determine fetal position (Leopold's maneuvers).
> 3. Place the Doppler over the area of maximum intensity of fetal heart tones, generally over the fetal back.
> 4. Palpate the maternal radial artery to differentiate MHR from FHR.
> 5. Determine the relationship between UCs and FHR by palpating for UCs during the period of FHR auscultation.
> 6. Count FHR between contractions for at least 30 to 60 seconds to determine the baseline rate.
> 7. Determine differences between baseline FHR and fetal response to contractions by counting FHR after a UC using multiple consecutive 6- to 10-second intervals for 30 to 60 seconds (protocols may differ based on location).
>
> ———
> Killion, 2015.

between categories in the three-tiered FHR interpretation system. Auscultation limits assessment data to FHR baseline, rhythm, and changes from baseline and cannot detect certain types of decelerations and variability that can be detected by a combination of a paper recorder and ultrasound technology (part of electric monitoring).

A Cochrane Review found that use of a handheld Doppler and intermittent EFM in labor were associated with an increase in caesarean sections due to fetal distress. There was no clear difference in neonatal outcomes, but long-term outcomes for the infants were not reported. The authors reported a range in quality of the evidence and noted that uncertainty remains regarding the use of IA and intermittent FHR in labor (Martis et al., 2017). Research evidence supports the use of structured intermittent auscultation (SIA) as a method of fetal surveillance during labor for low-risk pregnancies (Feinstein et al., 2008; Lyndon & Ali, 2015; True & Bailey, 2016). An updated position statement from the ACOG supports IA in low-risk pregnancy in labor (ACOG, 2017, 2019).

Normal findings of SIA include normal baseline between 110 and 160 beats per minute (bpm) and regular rhythm; presence of FHR increases from baseline, and the absence of FHR decreases from baseline. To identify the baseline rate, the FHR should be auscultated and counted between contractions when the fetus is not moving for at least 30 to 60 seconds. Once the baseline is established, the FHR is then auscultated and counted while palpating maternal pulse for 15 to 60 seconds between contractions (Killion, 2015) (see Box 9-4). Successful implementation of SIA can be achieved by considering the following guidelines:

- Presence of nurses and providers experienced in auscultation and recognition of auditory changes in FHR
- Institutional policy developed to address the technique and frequency of assessment
- Clinical interventions (e.g., change to EFM) when concerning findings are present
- Nurse to laboring women ratio of 1:1
- User-friendly documentation tools for recording SIA findings
- Ready availability of auscultation devices
- Culture embracing the normalcy of childbirth and minimization of unnecessary interventions (True & Bailey, 2016)

In summary, fetoscope and Doppler obtain information differently but are both appropriate in certain auscultation clinical situations.

Palpation of Contractions

When the uterus contracts, the musculature becomes firm and tense and can be palpated with the fingertips by the nurse. The frequency, duration, tone, and intensity of contractions can be assessed by palpation (Lyndon & Ali, 2015). This is a subjective assessment and can be biased by the fat distribution around the pregnant woman's uterus.

● Palpation of UCs is done by the nurse placing her fingertips on the fundus of the uterus and assessing the degree of tension as the contractions occur.
● The intensity of contractions is measured at the peak of the contraction and is rated as:
  ○ Mild or 1+ feels similar to the tip of the nose (easily indented uterus).
  ○ Moderate or 2+ feels similar to the chin (can slightly indent uterus).
  ○ Strong or 3+ feels similar to the forehead (cannot indent uterus).
● Resting tone is measured between contractions and listed as either soft or firm uterine tone.
● Palpation is a subjective assessment and can be biased by the fat distribution on the pregnant woman's abdomen.

External Electronic Fetal and Uterine Monitoring

External electronic fetal and uterine monitoring uses an ultrasound device to detect FHR and a pressure device attached to a paper recorder to assess uterine activity (Fig. 9–2 and Box 9-5).

● The FHR is measured via an ultrasound transducer, an external monitor.
  ○ External EFM detects FHR baseline, variability, accelerations, and decelerations.
  ○ External heart rate monitors receive waveforms from the fetal heart interpreted by the computer in the fetal monitor to produce sound and visual tracing to reflect FHR.
  ○ Fetal monitors average three consecutive beat-to-beat intervals and then assign the FHR (Killion, 2015). Although autocorrelation now minimizes doubling and halving of the FHR (erroneous readings), this can still occur. Therefore, providers are instructed to take precautions against misinterpretations by verification of FHR through monitoring of

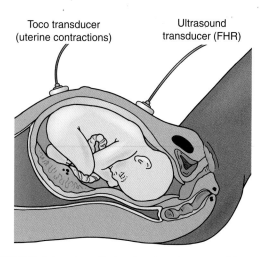

Toco transducer (uterine contractions)   Ultrasound transducer (FHR)

FIGURE 9–2 External monitoring showing placement of the ultrasound and tocodynamometer.

---

maternal heart rate via palpating the maternal radial pulse and maternal pulse oximetry (Killion, 2015).
● Today, many EFMs allow the monitoring of both the FHR and the maternal heart rate via sensors within the TOC, with both appearing on the printout paper. Maternal heart rate usually is significantly lower than the FHR and tends to increase as labor progresses and during contractions and pushing efforts.
● Location of the FHR via EFM changes in maternal position and as the fetus descends during labor, especially in the second stage (Lyndon & Ali, 2015).
● Erratic FHR recordings or gaps on a paper recorder may be caused by inadequate conduction of ultrasound signal, displacement of the transducer (may be picking up maternal heart rate), fetal or maternal movement, inadequate ultrasound gel, or fetal arrhythmia (may need to auscultate to verify).
● Contractions are measured via TOCO, as well as an external uterine monitor.
  ○ The relative frequency and duration of UCs and relative resting tone, the tone of the uterus between contractions, can be measured by this method.
  ○ An external contraction monitor, TOCO, is a strain gauge that detects skin tightness or contour changes resulting from UCs. It should be placed via palpation at the uterine fundus, during maximum UC intensity, ideally at a smooth part of the uterus where no fetal small parts are felt. Appropriate placement of the TOCO may change during labor. Also, it may be more difficult to monitor tightening of the skin with increased fat distribution around the maternal abdomen.
  ○ External uterine monitors cannot measure the pressure or intensity of contractions.
  ○ Pressure or intensity of the contraction must be estimated by the palpation of contractions.

- Contractions not recording on a paper recorder may occur when the transducer is placed away from the strongest area of contraction or when the resting tone is not dialed to 10 to 20 mm Hg when the uterus is relaxed.
- Abdominal surface electrodes measuring electrohysterogram (EHG) is a more reliable and reasonable alternative to TOCO with the advantage of being noninvasive and more sensitive in detecting contractions than TOCO (Parameshwari & Shenbaga, 2020).

Internal Electronic Fetal and Uterine Monitoring

Internal EFM uses a fetal scalp electrode (FSE) or internal scalp electrode applied to the presenting part of the fetus to directly detect FHR. Internal electronic uterine monitoring involves an IUPC placed in the uterine cavity to directly measure UCs (Fig. 9–3 and Box 9-6). Membranes must be ruptured for both methods.

The decisions to insert an FSE are based on the need for continuous FHR tracing when troubleshooting methods do not alter the quality of tracing. A nurse or care provider certified to attach this should be aware of relative contraindications to direct methods of monitoring. These include chorioamnionitis, active maternal genital herpes, HIV, positive group B streptococcus testing and conditions that preclude vaginal exams (e.g., placenta previa and undiagnosed vaginal bleeding).

The contraction and resting tone intensity is a combination of pressure from myometrial muscle contraction and intrauterine hydrostatic pressure (pressure exerted from amniotic fluid above the catheter). Positioning of patient-measuring IUPC pressures in left, right, supine, and lateral prevents possible erroneous conclusions about induction or augmentation management.

- FHR is measured via FSE.
- Internal EFM detects FHR baseline, variability, accelerations, decelerations, and limited information on some types of arrhythmias.
- It is attached to the presenting part of the fetus by the nurse or care provider.

IUPC monitoring is initiated based on clinical need for additional uterine activity information. It may be used when external

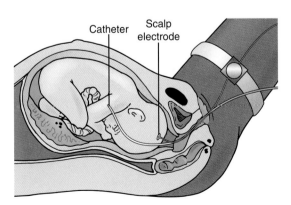

FIGURE 9–3 Internal monitoring, showing placement of the fetal scalp electrode and intrauterine pressure catheter.

BOX 9-6 | Guidelines for Placement of an Internal Electronic Fetal Monitor

Explain the procedure to the woman and her family. For example: "The internal fetal scalp electrode allows us to directly monitor your baby's heart rate. It is clipped on the baby's scalp during a vaginal exam and the monitor is attached to your leg. You can still move around and go to the bathroom.

"The intrauterine pressure catheter tells us exactly how strong your contractions are. It is a direct measurement of the pressure of your contractions. It is placed in your uterus during a vaginal examination."

FETAL HEART RATE	UTERINE CONTRACTIONS
Placement of the FSE requires skills and techniques of vaginal examination and EFM. There are risks, limitations, and contraindications, such as abnormal presentation, placenta previa, or preexisting infections such as herpes, HIV, or group B streptococcus.	Placement of an IUPC is an invasive procedure where the nurse should have knowledge and understanding of indications and contraindications, as well as risks of internal monitoring. For placement of the IUPC, the manufacturer directions are reviewed as there are several types of IUPC with different set-up guidelines. The IUPC and the guide tube are inserted in the vagina with a vaginal examination, and the catheter is advanced through the cervix into the amniotic cavity. The membranes must be ruptured for placement and cervix dilated to 2 cm.
For placement of the FSE, a vaginal examination is performed and the guide tube with the electrode is advanced and attached to the presenting part of the fetus. The membranes must be ruptured for placement and cervix dilated to 2 cm.	

Killion, 2015.

---

monitoring is inadequate due to maternal obesity or lack of progress in labor when quantitative analysis of uterine activity is needed for clinical decision making. An IUPC may be inserted to treat a worsening Category II tracing (e.g., recurrent variable decelerations with nadir greater than 60 mm Hg from baseline) via amnioinfusion. IUPCs provide an objective measure of frequency, duration, and intensity of contractions (as opposed to palpation, which is subjective) and resting tone, both expressed in mm Hg.

- Contractions are measured via IUPC.
  - IUPC provides an objective measure of the pressure of contractions, expressed as mm Hg.
  - IUPC monitoring can detect actual frequency, duration, and strength of UCs and resting tone in mm Hg.
  - UC intensity is measured using an IUPC = Peak pressure minus the baseline pressure in mm Hg.
  - Contraction intensity varies during labor, from 30 mm Hg in early spontaneous labor to 70 mm Hg in transition to 70 to 90 mm Hg in the second stage.
  - Peak pressure is the maximum uterine pressure during a contraction measured with an IUPC.
  - Resting tone or baseline pressure is the uterine pressure between contractions and should be about 5 to 20 mm Hg.

- The contraction and resting tone intensity is a combination of pressure from myometrial muscle contraction as well as intrauterine hydrostatic pressure (pressure exerted from amniotic fluid above the catheter). Therefore, positioning of the patient—measuring IUPC pressures in left, right, supine, and lateral—will prevent possible erroneous conclusions about induction or augmentation management.
- UC may also be quantified via Montevideo units (MVUs) measured by the peak pressure for each contraction in a 10-minute period. ACOG has recommended at least 200 MVUs every 10 minutes for 2 hours as adequate UC intensity for normal progress of labor (Cunningham et al., 2018).
- An IUPC can be used to perform an amnioinfusion.
- The IUPC is inserted by the care provider. Some institutions may have protocols for nurses to insert IUPCs; nurses need to check hospital policy on IUPC insertion.

Telemetry

Telemetry is a type of continuous EFM that involves connecting the patient to a radio frequency transmitter that allows her to walk and take a bath without having to be connected to the monitor via cables. Nurses can oversee the fetal and uterine information as if the patient were connected directly to the monitor (Tucker et al., 2009). It can be used in all phases of labor.

Monitor Paper Used for the Electronic Fetal Monitor

Monitor paper is used for the EFM (Fig. 9–4). At a paper speed of 3 cm per minute (standard for the United States), each dark

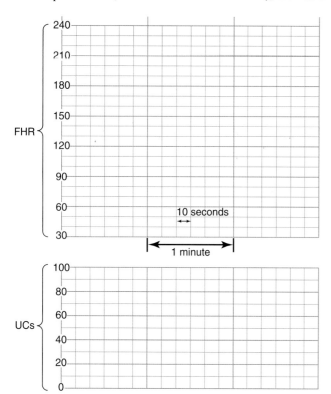

FIGURE 9–4 Monitor paper indicating timing on a grid.

vertical line represents 1 minute and each lighter vertical line represents 10 seconds.

FHR is recorded on the top grid of the paper in bpm while UCs are recorded on the lower grid in mm Hg with IUPC and relative height for TOCO. Some EFM systems allow for maternal pulse to be recorded on the top grid of the paper. Maternal pulse can be obtained via a blood pressure cuff or pulse oximetry; some TOCOs now have sensors that can detect maternal pulse. Clinicians may need this additional information to distinguish between maternal and FHR. Both external and internal fetal monitors may inadvertently pick up maternal rate, which is especially critical if the fetus is not tolerating labor or has died (Lyndon & Ali, 2015).

AWHONN STANDARDS FOR FREQUENCY OF FETAL HEART RATE ASSESSMENT

Frequency of FHR assessment is based on assessment of risk status, stage of labor, and ongoing clinical assessment (Lyndon & Ali, 2015).

- IA (Table 9-2): Absent risk factors:
  - Every 1 hour in latent phase
  - Every 5 to 30 minutes in active and transition phases
- Intermittent EFM
  - Latent and active phase of first stage for low-risk labors (Category I) need EFM for 10 to 30 minutes every 1 to 2.5 hours, with particular attention to baseline, variability, and accelerations and decelerations for 30 seconds before, during, and after a UC.
  - Need continuous EFM during the second stage.
- Continuous EFM
  - Continuous fetal monitoring requiring external or internal monitoring became a part of routine maternal care during the 1970s.
  - By 2002, 85% of live births (3.4 million out of 4 million) were monitored by continuous monitoring.
  - This method of monitoring led to an increase in cesarean and instrumental (vacuum, forceps) vaginal births.
  - A decrease in neonatal seizures is the sole benefit of this method of perinatal management (Alfirevic et al., 2017).
  - It is considered necessary if risk factors are present (Table 9-3).
- With risk factors, women should be monitored every 30 minutes during the latent phase, every 15 minutes during the active phase, and every 5 minutes during the second stage.
  - Thick meconium upon rupture of membranes (ROM)
  - ROM (greater than 24 hours at term)
  - Maternal fever
  - Vaginal bleeding in labor
  - Intrauterine infection or chorioamnionitis
  - Previous cesarean section
  - Abnormal vital signs
  - Fetal conditions (anomalies, anemia, intrauterine growth restriction (IUGR), multiple gestation, breech presentation, prematurity, isoimmunization)

TABLE 9-2   Assessment and Documentation Recommendations of Fetal Status During Labor With Intermittent Auscultation

	LATENT PHASE (LESS THAN 4 CM)	LATENT PHASE (4 TO 5 CM)	ACTIVE PHASE (6 CM OR GREATER)	SECOND STAGE (PASSIVE FETAL DESCENT)	SECOND STAGE (ACTIVE PUSHING)
Low-risk without oxytocin	Insufficient evidence to make a recommendation Frequency at the discretion of the midwife or physician	Every 15–30 minutes	Every 15–30 minutes	Every 15 minutes	Every 5–15 minutes

Assessment frequency should also be determined by maternal-fetal condition and may need to be done more frequently depending on the clinical situation. AWHONN, 2018; O'Brien-Abel & Simpson, 2021.

TABLE 9-3   Electronic Fetal Heart Monitoring Assessment Recommendations for Fetal Status During Labor

	LATENT PHASE (LESS THAN 4 CM)	LATENT PHASE (4 TO 5 CM)	ACTIVE PHASE (6 CM OR GREATER)	SECOND STAGE (PASSIVE FETAL DESCENT)	SECOND STAGE (ACTIVE PUSHING)
Low-risk without oxytocin	Insufficient evidence to make a recommendation Frequency at the discretion of the midwife or physician	Every 30 minutes	Every 30 minutes	Every 30 minutes	Every 15 minutes
With oxytocin or risk factors	Every 15 minutes with oxytocin, every 30 minutes without	Every 15 minutes	Every 15 minutes	Every 15 minutes	Every 5 minutes

Assessment frequency should also be determined by maternal-fetal condition and may need to be done more frequently depending on the clinical situation. AWHONN, 2018; O'Brien-Abel & Simpson, 2021.

- Fetal intolerance of labor (as evidenced by late decelerations, variable decelerations, nadir below 60 bpm)
- Decreased fetal activity
- Maternal conditions (e.g., hypertensive disorders, diabetes, cholestasis, preexisting diseases, morbid obesity, labor dystocia)
- Augmentation or induction of labor with use of uterine stimulants (misoprostol, dinoprostone, oxytocin)
- Epidural, other maternal analgesic interventions
- Preterm labor (less than 37 weeks)
- Post-term pregnancy (greater than 42 weeks)
- Category II or III upon admission to labor and delivery unit
- The frequency of assessment increases:
  - When indeterminate Category II or abnormal Category III FHR characteristics are heard
  - Before and after ROM or administration of medication
- When indeterminate or abnormal characteristics are heard, electronic FHR monitoring is used to:
  - Clarify pattern interpretation.
  - Assess baseline variability.
  - Further assess fetal status.

It is common practice for all women to have a baseline EFM tracing of at least 20 minutes at the time they are first evaluated in labor. Routine continuous FHR monitoring remains controversial.

Continuous EFM was introduced to reduce the incidence of perinatal death and cerebral palsy and as an alternative to the practice of IA. However, the widespread use of continuous EFM has not been shown to significantly affect such outcomes as perinatal death and cerebral palsy when used for women with low-risk pregnancies (ACOG, 2019). Even a recent statement from the ACOG (2019) suggests adopting protocols and training staff to use a handheld Doppler device for low-risk women for intermittent monitoring. Nurses should be a part of policy development for EFM on their units to advocate for EBP related to fetal and maternal assessment in labor. Some experts advocate for use of a decision tree to help guide fetal assessment (ACOG, 2010; Lyndon & Ali, 2015) and standardized algorithms may play an important part in management of FHR patterns in the future (O'Brien-Abel & Simpson, 2021).

Evidence-Based Practice

Electronic Fetal Heart Rate Monitoring for Fetal Assessment During Labor

Alfirevic, Z., Devane, D., Gyte, G. M. L., & Cuthbert, A. (2017). Continuous cardiotocography (CTG) as a form of electronic fetal monitoring (EFM) for fetal assessment during labour. *Cochrane Database of Systematic Reviews, 2.* Art. No., CD006066. https://doi.org/10.1002/14651858.CD006066.pub3

EFM, also referred to as *cardiotocography*, records changes in the FHR and their temporal relationship to UCs. The aim of EFM is to identify babies who may be short of oxygen (hypoxic) to guide additional assessments of fetal well-being and determine if the baby needs to be delivered by caesarean section or instrumental vaginal birth.

A systematic review of randomized and quasi-randomized controlled trials was conducted to evaluate the effectiveness and safety of continuous cardiotocography (CTG) when used as a method to monitor fetal well-being during labor.

This review included 13 trials involving over 37,000 women. One trial (4,044 women) compared continuous CTG with intermittent CTG; all other trials compared continuous CTG with IA. Compared with IA, continuous CTG showed no significant improvement in overall perinatal death rate (risk ratio [RR] 0.86, 95% confidence interval [CI] 0.59 to 1.23) but was associated with halving neonatal seizure rates (RR 0.50, 95% CI 0.31 to 0.80). There was no difference in cerebral palsy rates (RR 1.75, 95% CI 0.84 to 3.63). However, there was an increase in caesarean sections associated with continuous CTG (RR 1.63, 95% CI 1.29 to 2.07). Women were also more likely to have instrumental vaginal births (RR 1.15, 95% CI 1.01 to 1.33). There was no difference in the incidence of cord blood acidosis (RR 0.92, 95% CI 0.27 to 3.11) or use of any pharmacological analgesia (RR 0.98, 95% CI 0.88 to 1.09).

Compared with intermittent CTG, continuous CTG made no difference to caesarean section rates (RR 1.29, 95% CI 0.84 to 1.97) or instrumental births (RR 1.16, 95% CI 0.92 to 1.46). Less cord blood acidosis was observed in women who had intermittent CTG; however, this result could have been due to chance (RR 1.43, 95% CI 0.95 to 2.14).

Overall, methodological quality of the studies reviewed was mixed. Authors concluded that EFM during labor is associated with reduced rates of neonatal seizures, but no clear differences in cerebral palsy, infant mortality, or other standard measures of neonatal well-being. However, continuous CTG was associated with an increase in cesarean sections and operative vaginal births. The authors believe the real challenge is how best to convey this uncertainty to women to enable them to make an informed choice without compromising the normality of labor.

INFLUENCES ON FETAL HEART RATE

An understanding of FHR physiology aids in the interpretation of FHR patterns, because FHR responds to multiple physiological factors. The following sections review the influences of these factors on the FHR.

Uteroplacental Unit

At term, about 10% to 15% of maternal cardiac output (600 cc to 750 cc) perfuses the uterus per minute. Oxygenated blood from the mother is delivered to the intervillous space in the placenta via uterine arteries. Maternal-fetal exchange of oxygen, carbon dioxide, nutrients, waste products, and water occurs in the intervillous space across the membranes that separate fetal and maternal circulations. Oxygen and carbon dioxide diffuse across membranes rapidly and efficiently.

- Effective transfer of oxygen and carbon dioxide between fetal and maternal bloodstreams is dependent on:
  - Adequate uterine blood flow
  - Sufficient placental area
  - Unconstricted umbilical cord
- Appropriate oxygenation to the fetus depends on:
  - Adequate oxygenation of the mother
  - Adequate blood flow to the placenta
  - Adequate uteroplacental circulation
  - Adequate umbilical circulation
  - The fetus's own innate ability to initiate compensatory mechanisms to regulate FHR
- Additional factors in the fetal environment that influence fetal oxygenation include:
  - Uteroplacental function
  - Uterine activity
  - Umbilical cord issues
  - Maternal physiological function

A basic understanding of the extrinsic influence on FHR, such as normal physiological changes in pregnancy, uterine and placental blood flow, and umbilical blood flow, improves the nurse's ability to assess FHR patterns (Lyndon & Ali, 2015). The influences related to labor are discussed in Chapter 10.

Autonomic Nervous System

The autonomic nervous system is divided into the parasympathetic and sympathetic nervous systems.

Parasympathetic Nervous System

- Parasympathetic stimulation decreases the FHR.
- The parasympathetic nervous system (PSNS) is primarily mediated by the vagus nerve innervating the sinoatrial and atrioventricular nodes in the heart.
- Vagus nerve stimulation slows FHR and helps maintain variability.
  - Variability in FHR develops at 28 to 30 weeks' gestation.

Sympathetic Nervous System

- Sympathetic nervous system (SNS) stimulation increases the FHR.
- Nerves are distributed widely in the fetal heart, and stimulation increases the strength of the fetal heart contraction.

- SNS is responsible for FHR variability.
- Action occurs through release of norepinephrine.
- Stimulation of SNS increases FHR.
- SNS may be stimulated during hypoxemia.

Baroreceptors

- Baroreceptors are stretch receptors in the aortic arch and carotid arch that detect pressure changes.
- They provide a protective homeostatic mechanism for regulating heart rate by stimulating a vagal response and decreasing FHR, fetal blood pressure, and cardiac output.

Central Nervous System (CNS)

- The CNS is the integrative center responsible for variations in FHR and baseline variability related to fetal activity.
- The CNS regulates and coordinates autonomic activities, mediates cardiac and vasomotor reflexes, and responds to fetal movement.

Chemoreceptors

- Chemoreceptors are located in the aortic arch and the CNS.
- They respond to changes in fetal O_2 and CO_2 and pH levels. Decreased O_2 and increased CO_2 cause peripheral chemoreceptors to stimulate the vagal nerve and slow the heart rate, and central chemoreceptors respond to an increased heart rate and increased blood pressure.

Hormonal Regulation

- The fetus responds to a decrease in O_2 or uteroplacental blood flow by releasing hormones that maximize blood flow to vital organs, such as the heart, brain, and adrenals.
- Epinephrine, norepinephrine, catecholamines, and vasopressin facilitate hemodynamic changes in response to changes in fetal oxygenation. Fetal hypoxia causes a release of epinephrine and norepinephrine that increases FHR and blood pressure. Vasopressin increases blood pressure in response to hypoxia.
- Renin-angiotensin secreted by the kidneys produces vasoconstriction in response to hypovolemia.

FETAL RESERVES

Placental reserve describes the reserve oxygen available to the fetus to withstand the transient changes in blood flow and oxygen during labor (Lyndon & Ali, 2015). In a healthy maternal-fetal unit, the placenta provides oxygen and nutrients beyond the baseline needs of the fetus.

- When oxygen is decreased, blood flow is deferred to vital fetal organs to compensate.

- When placental reserves of oxygen are depleted, the fetus may not be able to adapt to or tolerate decreased oxygen that occurs during a labor contraction.
- Fetal adaptation to the stresses of labor occurs through homeostatic mechanisms.
  - Prolonged or repeated hypoxemia may deplete reserves, resulting in decompensation.
  - Interpretation of FHR data requires the ability to differentiate three types of fetal responses:
    - Nonhypoxic reflex responses such as FHR accelerations
    - Compensatory responses to hypoxemia, such as variable decelerations
    - Impending decompensation responses such as late decelerations (Lyndon & Ali, 2015)

Umbilical Cord Blood Acid–Base Analysis After Delivery

Umbilical cord blood acid–base acidosis analysis can be a useful, objective way to quantify fetal acid–base balance at birth and may be critical in evaluating whether a poor neonatal outcome is due to a hypoxic event before or during labor. An understanding of respiratory and metabolic acidosis and acidemia and associated clinical applications is required to interpret the findings (O'Brien-Abel & Simpson, 2021).

Although maternal and fetal components of oxygen transport are similar, some features of oxygen transport are unique to the fetus. Fetal oxygen transport is directly dependent on the maternal transport system. The fetus has lower oxygen tension (30%) than the adult (100%). Fetuses have higher oxygen affinity (due to different fetal hemoglobin) than adults. The amount of oxygen transported to the fetus may be affected by the sufficiency of blood flow to the uterus and placenta, the integrity of the placenta, and the blood flow through the umbilical cord.

Normally, the fetus can maintain normal aerobic metabolism even though there are transient decreases in blood flow to the uterus. However, when available oxygen in the intervillous space falls below 50% of normal levels, a sequential process occurs:

1. Redistribution of blood to vital organs (heart, brain, and adrenal glands). In scenarios where oxygen is altered chronically, fetal growth will decelerate and lead to intrauterine growth restriction (IUGR).
2. Fetal myocardium will change in oxygen consumption, leading to changes in FHR, such as FHR variability.
3. Fetus will convert from aerobic to anaerobic metabolism.

In fetal heart muscle cells, normal cellular metabolism utilizes glucose and oxygen for aerobic metabolism. Carbon dioxide and water are the waste products that need to be taken away from the muscle cell by the fetal blood flow and increase of hydrogen ions in tissue (acidosis).

When the fetus experiences hypoxia, it may switch to anaerobic metabolism, which is non-oxygen dependent. The waste product produced during this process is lactic acid. Accumulation of this acid leads to cell death and eventually to acidemia (increase of hydrogen ions in the blood). Should blood flow decrease, resulting in significant hypoxia, the peripheral tissues shift into anaerobic metabolism, utilizing glucose as well as any stored glycogen while creating lactic acid. When the amount of lactic acid exceeds fetal buffering capacity, metabolic acidosis is the result. Should the hypoxia become severe enough (or prolonged enough), metabolic acidosis may occur not only in the peripheral tissues, but also in the vital organs (brain, heart, adrenals) where blood flow was initially redistributed as a protective mechanism. Once metabolic acidosis reaches these vital organs, the fetus is at risk for organ damage. Because clinicians cannot directly measure metabolic *acidosis* (tissues), cord gases are evaluated for *acidemia* (blood) as the blood levels represent what is happening in the tissues. Most clinicians use the terms *acidosis* and *acidemia* interchangeably in clinical practice, but it is important to note that when reviewing the fetal response to ongoing hypoxemia, the progression is always hypoxemia → hypoxia → metabolic acidosis → metabolic acidemia.

Shortly after birth, blood may be drawn from the umbilical vein and one of the umbilical arteries. The umbilical vein represents oxygen supply available to the fetus, and the arterial blood best represents fetal usage of oxygen because it is the end point of fetal metabolism as blood returns to the placenta.

Respiratory acidosis occurs when an elevated Pco_2 level is present. An elevated Pco_2 indicates that the fetus is still processing oxygen via aerobic metabolism. It can develop rapidly in the fetus during acute hypoxia but can also be corrected rapidly when carbon dioxide is allowed to diffuse. Base excess with acidemia, during anaerobic metabolism, can become elevated. A normal Pco_2 may reflect a prolonged hypoxic insult (Tucker et al., 2009).

Table 9-4 contains normal values for umbilical cord blood. Note that greater absolute values for base deficit or excess (bicarbonate concentration, which increases to compensate for greater hydrogen ion concentration) are associated with acidemia. Also, acidemia is determined by the pH level. Our goal for a vigorous infant at birth is a pH of 7.1 or higher and a base excess of more than −12 (base deficit of 12 or less) (Lyndon & Ali, 2015).

TABLE 9-4 Normal Umbilical Cord Blood Gas Values

ARTERIAL CORD BLOOD MEASURES	NORMAL VALUES	TARGET VALUES
pH	7.20–7.29	≥7.10
Pco_2 (mm Hg)	49.2–56.3	<60
HCO^3 (mEq/L) bicarbonate	22–24	>22
Base excess (mEq/L)	2.7–8.3	>−12
Po_2 (mm Hg)	15–24	>20

Cypher, 2015.

NICHD Criteria for Interpretation of Fetal Heart Rate Patterns

A variety of systems and terminology have been used in the interpretation of FHR patterns. The FHR should be interpreted within the context of the overall clinical circumstances. Clinical conditions that impact FHR patterns include gestational age, prior results of fetal assessment, medications, maternal medical conditions, and fetal conditions. FHR patterns are dynamic, transient, and require frequent assessment. A careful review of current evidence has resulted in a new recommendation for FHR interpretation in the intrapartum period from NICHD based on a three-tier category system (see Critical Component: Three-Tier FHR Interpretation System) for use in the interpretation of EFM during the intrapartum period.

- Category I FHR tracings are normal. They are strongly predictive of a well-oxygenated, nonacidotic fetus with a normal fetal acid–base balance. They may be followed in a routine manner and no action is required.
- Category II FHR tracings are indeterminate. They do not predict abnormal fetal acid–base status, yet there is not adequate evidence to classify them as Category I or III. They require evaluation, continued surveillance, and reevaluation in the context of the clinical circumstances.
- Category III FHR tracings are abnormal. They are predictive of abnormal fetal acid–base status and require prompt evaluation. Depending on the clinical situation, efforts to resolve the underlying cause of the abnormal FHR pattern should be made expeditiously and should include intrauterine resuscitation or potentially expediting birth.

A more complex five-tier system has also been proposed to standardize management of FHR but has not been widely adopted (Parer & Ikeda, 2007; Parer et al., 2018).

CRITICAL COMPONENT

Three-Tier FHR Interpretation System
Category I Normal
FHR tracings include *all* of the following:

- Baseline rate 110 to 160 bpm
- Baseline variability moderate
- Late or variable deceleration absent
- Early decelerations absent or present
- Accelerations absent or present

Category II Indeterminate
FHR tracings include all FHR tracings not categorized as Category I or III. They include *any* of the following:

- Bradycardia not accompanied by absent variability
- Tachycardia
- Minimal baseline variability
- Absent baseline variability not accompanied by recurrent decelerations
- Marked baseline variability
- Absence of induced accelerations after fetal stimulation

- Recurrent variable decelerations with minimal or moderate baseline variability
- Prolonged decelerations greater than 2 minutes but less than 10 minutes
- Recurrent late decelerations with moderate baseline variability
- Variable decelerations with other characteristics, such as slow return to baseline "overshoots" or "shoulders"

Category III Abnormal

FHR tracings that are *either*:

- Absent variability with any of the following:
  - Recurrent late decelerations
  - Recurrent variable decelerations
  - Bradycardia
- Sinusoidal pattern

FETAL HEART RATE AND CONTRACTION PATTERN INTERPRETATION

Three major areas are assessed when interpreting an FHR pattern: FHR baseline, periodic and episodic changes, and uterine activity.

- Interpretation of an FHR baseline includes:
  - Baseline rate
  - Baseline variability
- Interpretation of periodic and episodic changes includes:
  - Accelerations
  - Decelerations (early, variable, late, and prolonged)

- Interpretation of uterine activity includes:
  - Frequency
  - Duration
  - Intensity
  - Resting tone
  - Relaxation time between UCs

Baseline Fetal Heart Rate

Baseline FHR is the mean FHR rounded to increments of 5 bpm during a 10-minute window, excluding accelerations, decelerations, or marked variability (Fig. 9–5). There must be at least 2 minutes of identifiable baseline segments (not necessarily contiguous) in a 10-minute period or the baseline for that period is indeterminate.

Characteristics

- The normal range is 110 to 160 bpm.
- FHR baseline above 160 bpm for at least 10 minutes is tachycardia.
- FHR baseline below 110 bpm for at least 10 minutes is bradycardia.

Medical Management

- Assess the baseline over a 10-minute period.

Nursing Actions

- Assess the baseline over a 10-minute period.

TABLE 9-5   Intrauterine Resuscitation

GOAL	TECHNIQUES AND METHODS
Promote fetal oxygenation	• Lateral positioning (left or right side) • IV fluid bolus of ≥500 mL lactated Ringer's solution • Discontinue oxytocin, remove dinoprostone insert, or withhold next dose of misoprostol • Alter pushing to every other contraction or every third contraction, or temporarily stop pushing (during second stage of labor) • Administer oxygen at 10 L/min via nonrebreather face mask (discontinue as soon as possible based on fetal response)
Reduce uterine activity	• Discontinue oxytocin, remove dinoprostone insert, or withhold next dose of misoprostol • IV fluid bolus of ≥500 mL lactated Ringer's solution • Lateral positioning (left or right side) • If no response, consider administration of 0.25 mg subcutaneous terbutaline
Alleviate umbilical cord compression	• Repositioning • Amnioinfusion (during first-stage labor) • Alter pushing to every other contraction or every third contraction, or temporarily stop pushing (during second stage of labor) • If umbilical cord prolapse is noted, elevate the presenting fetal part while preparations are made for an expedited birth
Correct maternal hypotension	• Lateral positioning (left or right side) • IV fluid bolus of ≥500 mL lactated Ringer's solution • If no response, consider ephedrine 5–10 mg IV push

Lyndon & Ali, 2015.

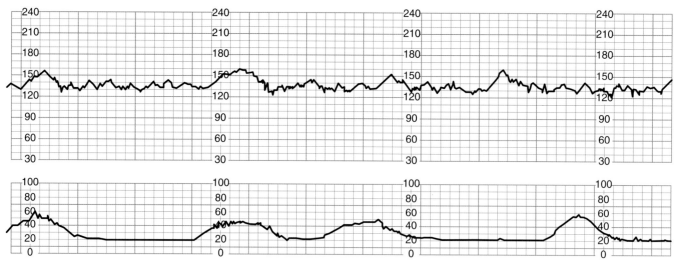

FIGURE 9–5 Normal fetal heart rate with moderate variability. (Top) Fetal heart rate. (Bottom) Contractions.

Fetal Tachycardia

Tachycardia is an FHR above 160 bpm that lasts for at least 10 minutes (Fig. 9–6A).

- Tachycardia may be a sign of early fetal hypoxemia, especially with decreased variability and decelerations. Deceleration area is the most predictive EFM pattern for acidemia, and combines with tachycardia for a significant risk of morbidity (Cahill et al., 2018).
- If tachycardia persists above 200 to 220 bpm, fetal demise may occur.
- Fetal tachycardia greater than 200 bpm may be an arrhythmia.
- Some causes of fetal tachycardia, such as maternal fever or exposure to medications such as terbutaline, do not reflect a risk of abnormal acid–base balance.

Characteristics

- Baseline FHR above 160 bpm that lasts for at least 10 minutes.
- It is often accompanied by a decreased or absent baseline variability due to the relationship to the increased parasympathetic and sympathetic tone.

Causes

Maternal-related causes include:

- Fever
- Infection
- Chorioamnionitis
- Dehydration
- Anxiety
- Anemia
- Medications such as beta-sympathomimetic, sympathomimetic, ketamine, atropine, phenothiazines, epinephrine, terbutaline, and ephedrine
- Illicit drugs such as cocaine

  Fetal-related causes include:

- Compensatory effort following acute hypoxemia
- Infection or sepsis
- Activity or stimulation
  - Chronic hypoxemia
- Fetal tachyarrhythmia
- Cardiac abnormalities
- Anemia

Medical Management

- Treat the underlying cause of tachycardia, such as antibiotics for infection, antipyretics for fever, or fluids for dehydration.
- Consider delivery.

Nursing Actions

- Assess FHR variability and consider the need for position change or oxygen to promote fetal oxygenation (see Table 9-5).
- Assess maternal vital signs (particularly temperature and pulse), as maternal fever and tachycardia increase FHR.
- Initiate interventions to decrease maternal temperature, if elevated.
  - Give medications as ordered (e.g., antibiotics, antipyretics).
  - Use ice packs to decrease maternal fever.
- Assess hydration by checking skin turgor, mucous membranes, urine-specific gravity, and intake and output.
  - Hydrate the woman by oral intake or IV fluids.
- Reduce anxiety by explaining, reassuring, and encouraging.
- Decrease or discontinue oxytocin.
- Notify the physician or midwife.

Fetal Bradycardia

Fetal bradycardia is a baseline FHR of less than 110 bpm (Fig. 9–6B).

- A decreased FHR can lead to decreased cardiac output, which causes a decrease in umbilical blood flow that leads to decreased oxygen to the fetus, causing fetal hypoxia.
- Unresolved bradycardia may result in fetal hypoxia and needs immediate intervention.

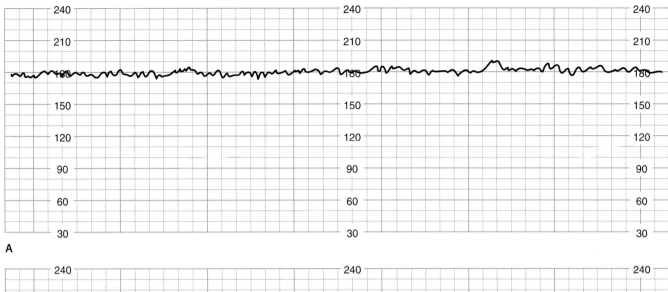

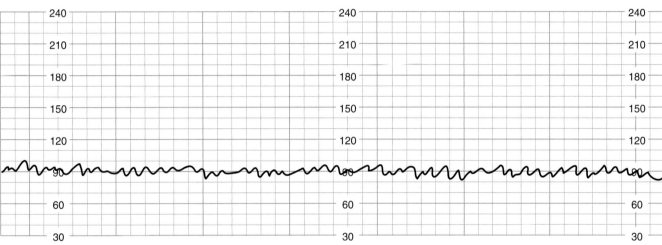

FIGURE 9-6 (A) Fetal tachycardia. (B) Fetal bradycardia.

● Sudden profound bradycardia (less than 80 bpm) is an obstetrical emergency.
● Bradycardia may be tolerated by the fetus if the FHR remains above 80 bpm with variability.
● Bradycardia with normal variability may be benign.
● Bradycardia with loss of variability or late decelerations is associated with current or impending fetal hypoxia (NICHD, 1997a).

Characteristics

● FHR less than 110 bpm for more than 10 minutes

Causes

Maternal-related causes include:

● Supine position
● Dehydration
● Hypotension
● Acute maternal cardiopulmonary compromise (cardiac arrest, seizures)
● Rupture of uterus or vasa previa

● Placental abruption
● Medications such as anesthetics and adrenergic receptors

  Fetal-related causes include:

● Fetal response to hypoxia
● Umbilical cord occlusion
● Acute hypoxemia
● Late or profound hypoxemia
● Hypothermia
● Hypokalemia
● Chronic fetal head compression
● Fetal bradyarrhythmias

Medical Management

● Intervene related to the cause of bradycardia.
● Consider delivery.

Nursing Actions

● Confirm if EFM is monitoring FHR versus MHR.
● Assess fetal movement.

- Assess the fetal response to fetal scalp stimulation. This is done when FHR is between contractions and when it is determined that the baseline has changed.
- Perform a vaginal exam and assess for a prolapsed cord.
- Assess maternal vital signs (especially blood pressure).
- Assess hydration and hydrate as needed to reduce UCs and promote fetal oxygenation.
- Depending on FHR variability and other FHR characteristics (see Table 9-5), consider:
  - Changing maternal position (left or right lateral) to promote fetal oxygenation
  - Discontinuing oxytocin to reduce UCs
  - Giving oxygen 10 L/min via nonbreather face mask to promote fetal oxygenation
  - Modifying pushing to every other contraction or stop pushing until the FHR recovers to promote fetal oxygenation
  - Encouraging open glottis pushing efforts
  - Discouraging prolonged or sustained breath holding with pushing
  - Supporting the woman and her family
  - Notifying the physician or midwife

Misidentification of Heart Rate: Maternal Versus Fetal

Fetal monitors may record maternal heart rate patterns that mimic FHR patterns, which may result in the provider's failure to diagnose fetal demise on a patient's admissions or a delay in diagnosis of fetal compromise or death during labor. The phenomenon of MHR being recorded through an FSE has been extensively recorded. Maternal heart rate has unique features such as doubling when the ultrasound feature is used and accelerations with painful contractions during second labor. Once the maternal signal source has been confirmed, actions must be taken to confirm fetal life and to obtain an accurate fetal signal (Murray, 2004).

Baseline Variability

Baseline variability refers to the fluctuations in the baseline FHR that are irregular in amplitude and frequency. Cycles portray the peak to trough (rise and fall) of the heart rate within its baseline range over a minute. It is the most important predictor of adequate fetal oxygenation and fetal reserve during labor (O'Brien-Abel & Simpson, 2021). Baseline variability reflects an intact pathway from the cerebral cortex to the midbrain (medulla oblongata) to the vagus nerve and finally to the heart, as well as an interaction between the fetal sympathetic and parasympathetic nervous system. Accelerations and decelerations are excluded from the evaluation of baseline variability.

Characteristics

- Variability is described as follows:
  - Absent: Amplitude range is undetectable (Fig. 9–7A).
  - Minimal: Amplitude range is undetectable below 5 bpm range (Fig. 9–7B).
  - Moderate: Amplitude from peak to trough, 6 bpm to 25 bpm (Fig. 9–7C). Moderate variability reliably predicts a well-oxygenated fetus with normal acid–base balance at the time.
  - Marked: Amplitude range is greater than 25 bpm (Fig. 9–7D).

Minimal or absent variability can occur when the fetus is in a sleep cycle, sedated by certain CNS depressants such as opiates or magnesium sulfate, or has a previous CNS injury. Minimal or absent variability can also be significant for the presence of fetal hypoxia or acidosis, especially if persisting 40 minutes despite interventions as listed in the text that follows (Lyndon & Ali, 2015).

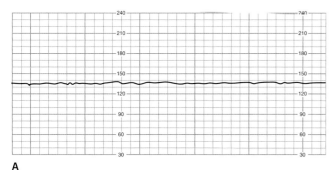

A

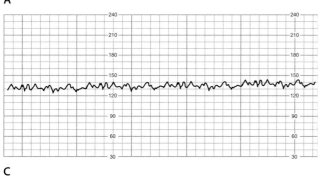

C

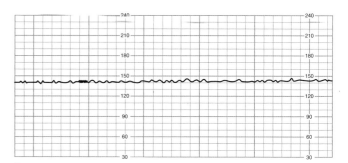

B

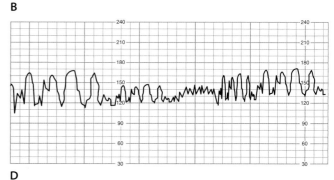

D

FIGURE 9–7 Types of variability. (A) Absent variability (abnormal). (B) Minimal variability. (C) Moderate variability (normal). (D) Marked variability.

Causes of Minimal or Absent Variability

- Maternal-related:
  - Supine hypotension
  - Cord compression
  - Uterine tachysystole
  - Drugs (prescription, illicit drugs, alcohol)
- Fetal-related:
  - Fetal sleep
  - Prematurity
  - Hypoxia
  - Acidosis

Medical Management

- Consider artificial rupture of membranes (AROM) and more invasive internal monitoring with FSE.
- Manage cause of decreased variability.
- Consider expedited delivery.

Nursing Actions

- Change the maternal position to promote fetal oxygenation.
- Assess fetal response to fetal scalp stimulation or vibroacoustic stimulation (VAS).
- Assess hydration. Give IV bolus to reduce uterine activity and promote uterine perfusion.
- Discontinue oxytocin to reduce uterine activity.
- Deliver oxygen to the woman at 10 L/min via nonbreather face mask to promote fetal oxygenation.
- Consider invasive monitoring, such as internal FSE.
- Support the woman and her family.
- Notify the physician or midwife and if variability is absent request a bedside evaluation.

Periodic and Episodic Changes

Periodic changes are accelerations or decelerations in the FHR that are related to UCs and persist over time. They include accelerations and four types of decelerations: early, variable, late, and prolonged. Episodic changes are acceleration and deceleration patterns not associated with contractions. Accelerations are the most common episodic change.

Fetal Heart Rate Accelerations

The presence of FHR accelerations is predictive of adequate central fetal oxygenation and reflects the absence of fetal acidemia. They identify a well-oxygenated fetus and require no intervention. The absence of FHR accelerations, especially in the intrapartum period, however, does not reliably predict fetal acidemia.

Characteristics

FHR accelerations are the visually abrupt, transient increases (onset to peak less than 30 seconds) in the FHR above the baseline (Fig. 9–8).

- In a fetus more than 32 weeks' gestation, they are 15 beats above the baseline and last from 15 seconds to less than 2 minutes.
- Before 32 weeks' gestation, accelerations are defined as acceleration of 10 bpm or greater over the baseline FHR for 10 or more seconds.
- Prolonged accelerations are 2 or more minutes but less than 10 minutes.

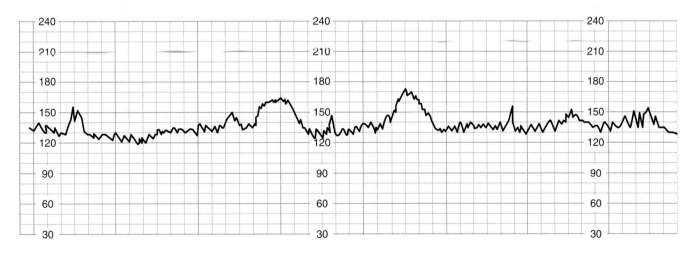

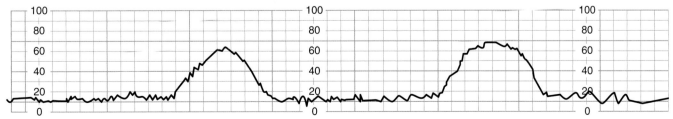

FIGURE 9–8 Fetal heart rate accelerations.

Causes

● Sympathetic response to fetal movement
● Transient umbilical vein compression

Medical Management

● None

Nursing Actions

● Record accelerations in the woman's labor documentation.

Fetal Heart Rate Decelerations

FHR decelerations are transitory decreases in the FHR baseline. They are classified as early, variable, late, and prolonged decelerations according to their shape, timing, and duration in relationship to the contraction.

● Decelerations are defined as recurrent when they occur with at least 50% of UCs over a 20-minute period.
● Decelerations are defined as intermittent when they occur with fewer than 50% of UCs over a 20-minute period.

Early Decelerations

Early decelerations are visually apparent, usually symmetrical, and have a gradual decrease and return of FHR associated with a UC (Fig. 9–9). They do not occur early or before the contraction starts; thus, this term is something of a misnomer.

Characteristics

● The nadir (the lowest point of the deceleration) occurs at the peak of the contraction.
● Generally, the onset, nadir, and recovery mirror the contraction.

Causes

● When a UC occurs, the fetal head is subjected to pressure that stimulates the vagal nerve.
● Fetal head compression results in increased intracranial pressure, decreased transient cerebral blood flow, and corresponding decrease in Po_2 with stimulation of a cerebral chemoreceptor (Fig. 9–10).

Medical Management

● None

Nursing Actions

● Early decelerations are benign and no intervention is needed.

Variable Decelerations

A variable deceleration is a visually apparent abrupt decrease in the FHR of less than 30 seconds from baseline to nadir.

● They are the most common decelerations seen in labor.
● When variable decelerations persist over time, fetal tolerance is confirmed by the presence of variability or accelerations in the FHR (Lyndon & Ali, 2015).
● Recurrent variable decelerations that become deeper and last longer are more likely to be associated with fetal acidemia (ACOG, 2010).

Characteristics

● They can be periodic or episodic and may vary in duration, depth or nadir, and timing in relation to UCs (Fig. 9–11).
● Decrease in FHR is at least 15 bpm lasting at least 15 seconds but less than 2 minutes in duration.

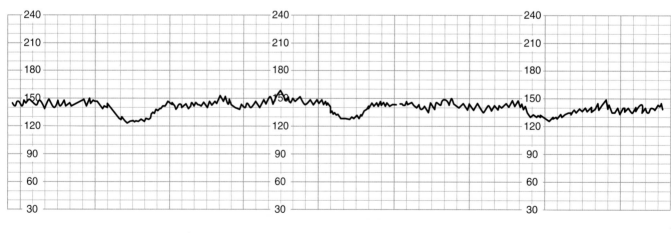

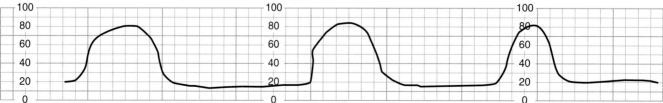

FIGURE 9–9 Early decelerations.

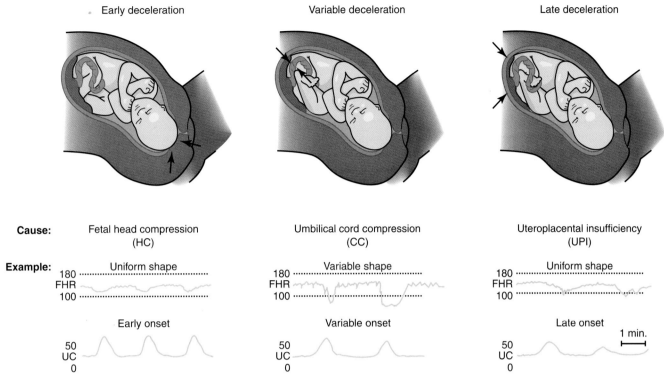

FIGURE 9-10 Causes and examples of periodic decelerations.

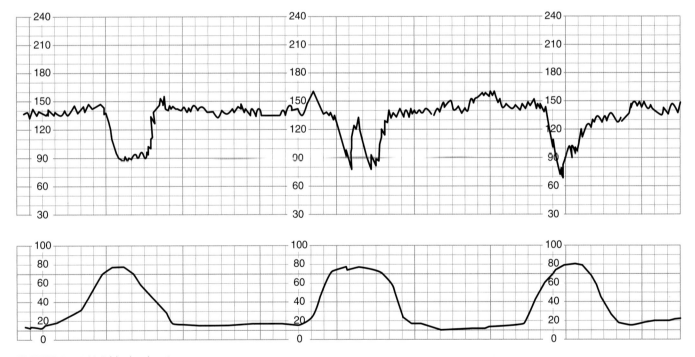

FIGURE 9-11 Variable decelerations.

● Depth (nadir) of variable deceleration of less than 60 would lead to an amnioinfusion intervention in the first stage.
● Alter frequency in the second stage.
● Accelerations at the beginning and end of decelerations ("overshoots") are not associated with acidemia.
● Characteristics of normal variable decelerations include:
  ● Duration of less than 60 seconds
  ● Rapid return to baseline
  ● Normal baseline and variability

● Characteristics of indeterminate or abnormal variable decelerations include:
  ● Prolonged return to baseline
  ● Persistence to less than 60 bpm and greater than 60 seconds
  ● Presence of overshoots tachycardia
  ● Repetitive overshoots and absent variability

Causes

● Umbilical cord occlusion (see Fig. 9–10).

● Umbilical cord compression triggers a vagal response that slows the FHR, usually related to decreased cord perfusion.
● This results in initial compression of the umbilical vein (decreased Po_2 and chemoreceptor stimulation) and then compression of the more muscular umbilical arteries (fetal hypertension with resultant baroreceptors stimulation; remember that hypertension is often accompanied with a corresponding drop in heart rate) (see Fig. 9–11).
● Prolonged cord compression produces a decrease in Po_2 with direct myocardial depression, adrenal activation, and sometimes rebound tachycardia.
● Variable decelerations can also occur with sudden descent of the vertex late in the active phase of labor (i.e., head compression).
● These appear different from early decelerations in that they are usually not repetitive or smooth or regular in shape.

Medical Management

● Consider amnioinfusion (see description later in chapter under interventions)
● Consider tocolytics.
● Consider delivery.

Nursing Actions

● Change the maternal position to promote fetal oxygenation (Fig. 9–12, Table 9-5).
● Perform a sterile vaginal examination (SVE) to evaluate cord and labor progress and perform fetal scalp stimulation.
● Perform amnioinfusion if ordered to alleviate umbilical cord compression by increasing the volume of fluid in the uterus and thereby correcting umbilical cord compression (see Critical Component: Amnioinfusion).
● Administer O_2 at 10 L/min via nonrebreather face mask to improve fetal oxygen status.
● Decrease or discontinue oxytocin.
● Consider the need for tocolytic to reduce UCs.
● Consider more invasive monitoring with fetal spiral electrode.
● Modify pushing.
● Support the woman and her family to decrease anxiety or pain.
● Notify the physician or midwife.
● Plan for delivery and care of the neonate.

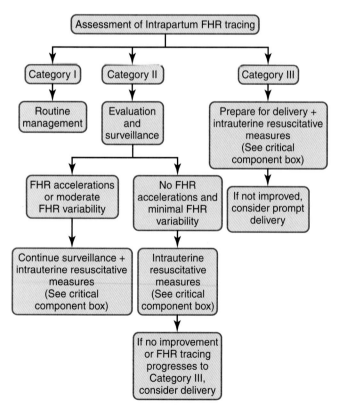

FIGURE 9–12 Management of EFM tracings.

CLINICAL JUDGMENT

Intrauterine Resuscitation Interventions
Interventions for Category II and III indeterminate or abnormal FHR patterns are referred to as intrauterine resuscitation. These interventions maximize uterine blood flow, umbilical circulation, and maternal fetal oxygenation (Lyndon & Ali, 2015; Simpson, 2004a, 2015; Simpson & James, 2005). Interventions to promote fetal oxygenation include:

• Promote maternal positioning to minimize or correct cord compression, decrease frequency of UCs, and improve uterine blood flow (either left or right).
• Administer an IV bolus of at least 500 mL of lactated Ringer's to maximize maternal intravascular volume and improve utero-placental perfusion.
• Correct maternal hypotension with positioning, hydration, and ephedrine as needed.
• Category II and Category III tracings require evaluation of the possible etiology.
• Administer O^2 at 10 L/min via nonrebreather face mask to improve fetal oxygen status. There is some controversy about the values of oxygen administration during labor to improve FHR patterns; however, it remains a common practice (Garite et al., 2015).
• Reduce uterine activity if UCs are too frequent, as there may be insufficient time for blood to perfuse the placenta.
• Decrease or discontinue oxytocin.
• Remove cervical ripening agent, if possible.
• Terbutaline may be used to relax the uterus.
• Amnioinfusion has been used to resolve variable FHR deceleration by alleviating umbilical cord compression as a result of oligohydramnios in the first stage of labor.
• Amnioinfusion is a procedure in which a saline solution at room temperature is introduced transcervically via an IUPC to correct the FHR decelerations associated with cord compression or decreased amniotic fluid.
• Encourage physiological pushing techniques, alter pushing efforts, or stop pushing, or encourage pushing with every other or every third UC to provide time for the fetus to recover when FHR is indeterminate or abnormal during the second stage.
• Support the woman and her family to decrease anxiety or pain, improve uterine blood flow, and maximize oxygenation to the fetus.

- Obtain fetal acid–base status if possible, with scalp or VAS (the safety and efficacy of VAS in the intrapartal period is debated) or fetal scalp sampling if available. See Chapter 6 for more on VAS.
- Correct maternal hypotension.
- Abnormal FHR patterns are associated with fetal acidemia. When this occurs:
  - Notify the primary provider; the presence of one of the abnormal patterns warrants immediate bedside evaluation by a physician who can initiate a cesarean birth.
  - Notify or activate OR, anesthesia, and pediatric teams as indicated.
  - Move the patient to OR as indicated.
- When a Category II or III FHR pattern is identified, initial assessment may also include:
  - Assessment of maternal vital signs, especially:
    - Maternal temperature for maternal fever and maternal blood pressure for hypotension
    - Assessment of uterine activity for uterine tachysystole
  - Cervical examination to assess for:
    - Umbilical cord prolapse
    - Rapid cervical dilation
    - Rapid descent of fetal head

CRITICAL COMPONENT

Amnioinfusion

Amnioinfusion is a therapeutic option for recurrent variable decelerations because of decreased amniotic fluid. Amnioinfusion is a reasonable and effective measure used to treat recurrent variable FHR decelerations during the first stage of labor that have not been resolved with maternal repositioning. Amnioinfusion has been found to significantly resolve patterns of "moderate" or "severe" variable decelerations but does not affect late decelerations or patterns with absent variability (Simpson & O'Brien-Abel, 2021). During amnioinfusion, room temperature normal saline or lactated Ringer's is infused into the uterus transcervically via an IUPC to increase intraamniotic fluid to cushion the umbilical cord and reduce cord compression. Usually a bolus of 250 to 500 mL is given over a 20- to 30-minute period; however, sometimes a continuous infusion of 120 to 180 mL/hour may be given up to 1,000 mL.

Indications: Variable decelerations in the first stage of labor

Contraindications: Vaginal bleeding, uterine anomalies, and active infection such as HIV or herpes. Because recurrent variable decelerations may be a sign of impending uterine rupture during a trial of labor after a cesarean (TOLAC), careful consideration should be made before amnioinfusion (Simpson, 2015; Simpson & O'Brien-Abel, 2021).

Careful monitoring of maternal and fetal response is needed; documentation of fluid infused and fluid returned is also important to avoid iatrogenic polyhydramnios.

Lyndon & Ali, 2015; Simpson, 2015.

Late Decelerations

Late deceleration is a visually apparent symmetrical gradual decrease of FHR associated with UCs.

- Late decelerations can be a sign of fetal intolerance to labor.
- Fetal tolerance of late decelerations is assessed by evaluating the baseline, the presence of variability, and the presence of accelerations.

Characteristics

- Onset is gradual with onset to nadir at least 30 seconds (Fig. 9–13).
- Nadir (lowest point) of the deceleration occurs after the peak of the contraction.
- In most cases, the onset, nadir, and recovery of the deceleration occur after the respective onset, peak, and end of the UC.
- Nadir decreases 10 to 20 bpm and rarely 30 to 40 bpm (Freeman et al., 2003).

Causes

- Fetal response to transient or chronic uteroplacental insufficiency (see Fig. 9–10)
- Decreased availability of O_2 because of uteroplacental insufficiency
- Suppression of the fetal myocardium
- Late decelerations are not completely understood:
  - Usually related to placental insufficiency (in which case they are often accompanied by decreased or absent FHR variability).
  - Late decelerations with moderate variability reflect a compensatory response and are not associated with significant fetal acidemia.
  - Late decelerations with minimal or absent variability reflect hypoxia and represent a risk of significant fetal acidemia.
  - Fetal hypoxia stimulates chemoreceptors when it is acute (i.e., recently occurring) and, if prolonged, results from direct myocardial depression.
  - Maternal-related factors associated with decreased uteroplacental circulation include:
    - Hypotension from regional anesthesia, supine positioning, or maternal hemorrhage
    - Maternal hypertension, gestational or chronic
    - Placental changes affecting gas exchange such as postmaturity or placental abnormalities
    - Decreased maternal hemoglobin or oxygen saturation from severe anemia or cardiopulmonary disease
    - Uterine tachysystole

Medical Management

- Interventions are directed at causes of late decelerations.
- Consider tocolytics.
- Consider delivery.

Nursing Actions

- The degree to which the deceleration is abnormal depends on the status and response of the fetus after the deceleration.
- Change the maternal position to promote fetal oxygenation (see Fig. 9–12; Table 9-5).

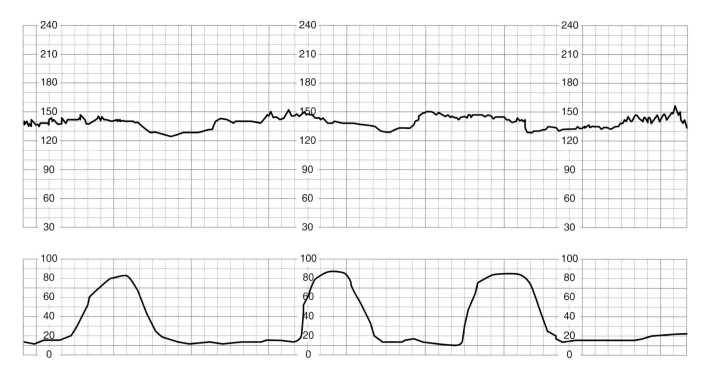

FIGURE 9–13 Late decelerations.

- Discontinue oxytocin (consider terbutaline) to reduce uterine activity.
- Assess hydration. Give an IV bolus to promote fetal oxygenation.
- Consider fetal scalp stimulation or VAS to assess fetal status (the safety and efficacy of VAS in the intrapartal period is debated; see Chapter 6 for more information on VAS).
- Administer O_2 at 10 L/min via nonrebreather face mask to improve fetal oxygen status.
- Consider more invasive monitoring with fetal spiral electrode.
- Support the woman and her family.
- Notify the physician or midwife.
- Plan for delivery and care of the neonate.

Prolonged Decelerations

Prolonged deceleration is a visually apparent abrupt decrease in FHR below baseline that is greater than 15 bpm, lasting longer than 2 minutes but less than 10 minutes (Fig. 9–14). Prolonged decelerations that are not recurrent and are preceded and followed by normal baseline and moderate variability are not associated with fetal hypoxemia.

Characteristics

- Episodic decelerations that last longer than 2 minutes but less than 10 minutes
- May be abrupt or gradual

Causes

- May be any mechanism that causes a profound change in the fetal O_2
- Interruption of uteroplacental perfusion
  - Tachysystole

- Maternal hypotension
- Abruptio placenta
- Interruption of umbilical blood flow
  - Cord compression
  - Cord prolapse
- Vagal stimulation
  - Profound head compression
  - Rapid fetal descent

Medical Management

- Treat the cause of prolonged deceleration.
- Consider amnioinfusion.
- Consider tocolytics.
- Consider delivery.

Nursing Actions

- Assess baseline variability preceding and following deceleration.
- Change the maternal position to improve fetal oxygenation (see Table 9-5).
- Discontinue oxytocin (consider terbutaline) to decrease the UCs.
- Administer O_2 at 10 L/min via nonrebreather face mask to improve fetal oxygen status.
- Assess hydration. Give an IV bolus to promote fetal oxygenation.
- Perform SVE to assess labor and cord.
- Perform amnioinfusion, if ordered, to alleviate umbilical cord compression.
- Consider more invasive monitoring with fetal spiral electrode.
- Support the woman and her family.
- Notify the physician or midwife.
- Plan for delivery and care of the neonate.

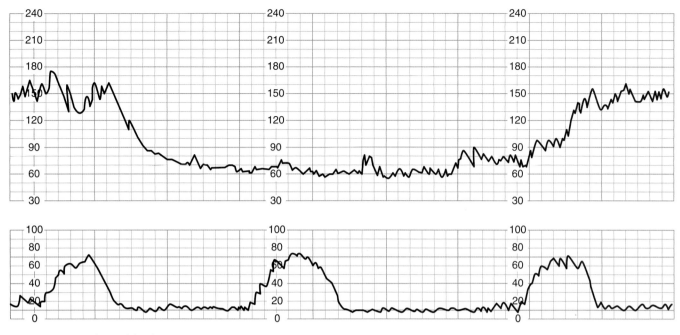

FIGURE 9–14 Prolonged deceleration.

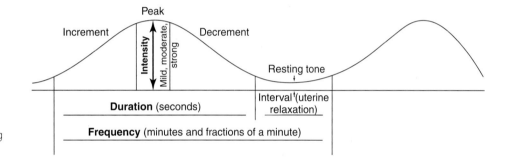

FIGURE 9–15 Example of contraction frequency, duration, intensity, and resting tone.

Uterine Activity and Contraction Patterns

Interpretation of the FHR pattern is done in concurrence with uterine activity. Interpretation of uterine activity includes assessment of the contractions' frequency, duration, and intensity, and the uterine resting tone (Fig. 9–15). Uterine activity can be monitored by palpation or via IUPC.

- Frequency of contractions is expressed in minutes or seconds and is determined by counting the number of contractions in a 10-minute period, counting from the start of one contraction to the start of the next contraction in minutes. It is recorded in minutes (i.e., frequency of contractions is every 3 minutes). Frequency of contractions can be expressed in a range: for example, UCs every 2 to 3 minutes.
- Duration of contractions is measured in seconds by counting from the beginning to the end of one contraction. Because contractions often vary in their duration, this is typically calculated for several contractions and expressed as a range.
- Intensity is the strength of the contraction and measured by palpation, or internally by an IUPC in mm Hg.

- Resting tone is the pressure in the uterus between contractions. It is measured by an IUPC when internal fetal monitoring is used or by palpation when an external monitor is used. When an IUPC is being used, it is described as the number of mm Hg when the uterus is not contracting and as "soft" if the uterus feels relaxed by palpation.
- Normal: Five or fewer contractions in 10 minutes averaged over a 30-minute window (Fig. 9–16A).
- Tachysystole: More than five contractions in 10 minutes over a 30-minute window.

Tachysystole

Tachysystole, formerly called hyperstimulation, is excessive uterine activity and is the most concerning side effect of oxytocin because it can result in a progressive adverse effect on fetal status (Simpson & O'Brien-Abel, 2021). Similar to duration, frequency of contractions is expressed in minutes and often given in seconds. UCs cause an intermittent decrease in blood flow in the intervillous space where oxygen exchange occurs. The decreased intervillous blood flow associated with tachysystole leads to decreased oxygen to the fetus. Tachysystole can result in progressive deterioration in fetal status and hypoxemia that result in an abnormal FHR. Tachysystole may result in abruptio placenta or uterine rupture, which are rare complications (ACOG, 2009a).

- These contraction patterns may contribute to fetal hypoxia.
- Tachysystole should be treated regardless of fetal response.
- Tachysystole can result in decreased uteroplacental blood flow and result in indeterminate or abnormal FHR patterns.

Characteristics

- More than five contractions in 10 minutes (Fig. 9–16B)
- Contractions lasting 2 minutes or longer (Fig. 9–16C)
- Contractions occurring within 1 minute of each other (Fig. 9–16D)

- Increasing resting tone greater than 20 to 25 mm Hg, peak pressure greater than 80 mm Hg, or MVUs greater than 400

Causes

- Tachysystole can be spontaneous or stimulated labor.
- The most common cause is medications used for cervical ripening, induction, and augmentation of labor.
- Abruption may also lead to tachysystole accompanied with increased vaginal bleeding.
- Women with a history of motor vehicle accidents, domestic violence, dehydration, preeclampsia, or methamphetamine use may be at higher risk.

Medical Management

- Manage cause of tachysystole (e.g., discontinuing oxytocin, removing cervical ripening medication). See Chapter 10.

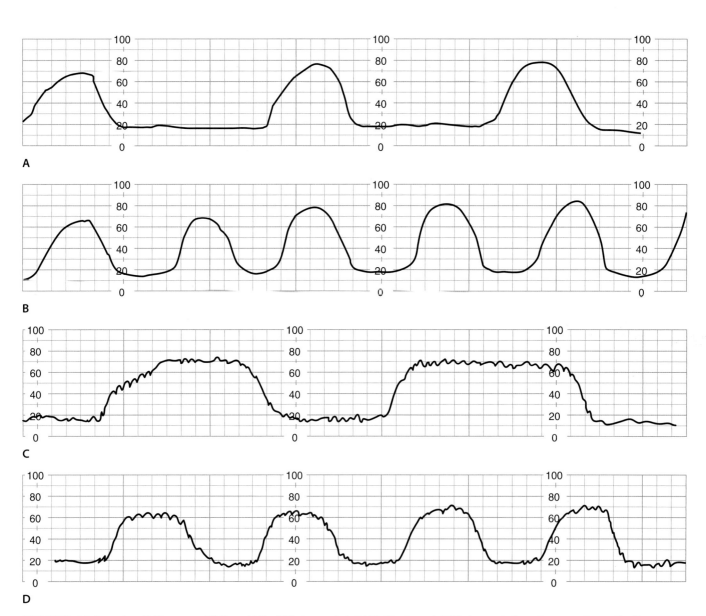

FIGURE 9–16 Examples of UC patterns. (A) Normal UCs. (B) Tachysystole (<5 UCs 10 minutes). (C) Tachysystole (tetanic contraction verified by palpation). (D) Tachysystole (inadequate interval of resting tone between UCs).

Nursing Actions

- A variety of interventions can effectively reduce uterine activity, such as the following (these practices are known as intrauterine resuscitation):
  - Changing maternal position
  - Providing hydration
  - Using IV fluid bolus
  - Reducing maternal anxiety or pain
  - Administering a tocolytic (terbutaline)
  - Supporting woman and family

SPECIAL MONITORING CIRCUMSTANCES

In some cases, women require special monitoring to ensure her health and that of the fetus.

Monitoring the Preterm Fetus

As noted in Chapter 7, preterm labor can be defined as the onset of labor at less than 37 weeks' gestation. The U.S. preterm birth rate rose to 10.02% in 2018, a 1% rise from 2017, and the fourth straight year in which this rate increased (Martin et al., 2019). With the preterm birth rate continuing to rise, most obstetric units monitor a preterm fetus during the antepartum and intrapartum. Two important points to remember when caring for the mother with a preterm fetus:

- Physiological responses of the preterm fetus depend on the stage of fetal development.
- Physiological responses and tolerance to stress (maternal tachycardia and sepsis) in the preterm fetus can be different (more rapid deterioration) from those in the term fetus.

Some preterm FHR characteristics:

- Baseline is higher but still within the normal FHR range.
- Accelerations may be of lower amplitude—accelerations of at least 10 bpm of baseline lasting 10 seconds are considered acceptable for a fetus less than 32 weeks' gestation. However, once the preterm fetus (sometimes as early as 24 to 26 weeks) demonstrates accelerations of 15 bpm above baseline that last for 15 seconds, the fetus is generally held to that criteria in subsequent evaluations.
- Variability may be decreased, although specific parameters have not been quantified.
- Variable decelerations may occur more frequently in the preterm fetus even in the absence of contractions (ACOG, 2009b). During labor, variable decelerations occur in approximately 70% to 75% of preterm fetuses compared with 30% to 50% in term fetuses.
- Late and prolonged decelerations occur at the same frequency in preterm labor as in term labor. Conditions associated with late decelerations, such as IUGR, preeclampsia, and abruption, are more commonly present during preterm labor (Simpson, 2004b).

- Magnesium sulfate (now used for neuroprotection of the preterm fetus rather than tocolytics) decreases FHR variability and acceleration amplitude in preterm infants.
- Beta-sympathomimetics (e.g., terbutaline) are associated with tachycardia in both mother and fetus.
- Indomethacin, other antiprostaglandin medications, and calcium channel blockers (e.g., nifedipine) have minimal effect on the preterm fetus.

The preterm fetus is more likely to be subjected to hypoxia, including conditions such as preeclampsia, abruption, and intrauterine infection that frequently are either the indication for or cause of preterm delivery. The loss of variability in a preterm fetus is more predictive of acidosis and depressed Apgar scores at birth than for a term infant (Macones et al., 2008). It is therefore important to continually evaluate trends and assess the maternal and fetal condition when making clinical decisions regarding the antepartum and intrapartum management of the preterm fetus.

Monitoring the Woman With Multiple Gestation

Current monitors have the capability of monitoring twins and higher multiples at the same time with two ultrasound transducers on the same monitor. The dual tracings distinguish each fetus by a thicker or darker tracing for one fetus and a thinner or lighter tracing for the other. To more clearly distinguish between the fetuses, their positions on the mother's abdomen can be documented and transducers appropriately labeled. In identifying twins or higher multiples, the more advanced (lower in uterus) fetus is labeled as A, the next one B, and so on. Once the membranes are ruptured, it is recommended that the more advanced fetus is monitored by a scalp electrode to distinguish it from the other fetus. Two monitors are required for higher multiples, with the third fetus on the second monitor, which has an identical clock setting to the first one (Tucker et al., 2009). At the time of birth, the first twin that is delivered may not necessarily be twin A, especially with cesarean sections. In that case, the medical chart should be written as first twin (B) and second twin (A) or vice versa.

Other Topics

Monitoring of fetal arrhythmias and sinusoidal pattern (a Category III or impending decompensation fetal response) is beyond the scope of this chapter. Resources are cited for more in-depth exploration and advanced concepts in fetal monitoring. Antenatal fetal surveillance and testing are discussed in Chapter 6.

DOCUMENTATION OF ELECTRONIC MONITORING INTERPRETATION—UTERINE ASSESSMENT

Documentation of fetal monitoring consists of the elements described in Table 9-6 and Fig. 9–17.

TABLE 9-6   Assessment and Documentation of Electronic Fetal Monitoring

FETAL HEART RATE External/Ultrasound	UTERINE CONTRACTION External/Tocodynamometry
• FHR baseline • Baseline variability • Presence of accelerations • Periodic or episodic decelerations	• Frequency • Duration • Palpate strength of UCs and resting tone
Internal/Fetal Scalp Electrode	**Internal/Intrauterine Pressure Catheter**
• FHR baseline • Baseline variability • Presence of accelerations • Periodic or episodic decelerations • FHR dysrhythmias	• Frequency • Duration • Strength of uterine contractions and resting tone (in mm Hg)

Patient Name:		Physician/CNM:			KEY
	DATE:				**Variability**
	TIME:				Ab = Absent (undetectable) Min = Minimal (>0 out ≤5 bpm)
Cervix	Dilation				Mod = Moderate (6–25 bpm)
	Effacement				Mar = Marked (>25 bpm)
	Station				**Accelerations**
Fetal Heart	Baseline Rate				+ = Present and appropriate for gestational age
	Variability				∅ = Absent
	Accelerations				**Decelerations**
	Decelerations				E = Early L = Late
	STIM/pH				V = Variable
	Monitor Mode				P = Prolonged
Uterine Activity	Frequency				**Stim/pH** + = Acceleration in response to stimulation
	Duration				∅ = No response to stimulation Record number for scalp pH
	Intensity				**Monitor mode**
	Resting Tone				A = Auscultation/Palpation E = External u/s or toco
	Monitor Mode				FSE - Fetal spiral electrode
	Oxytocin milliunits/min				IUPC = Intrauterine pressure catheter
	Pain				P = Palpation
	Coping				T = Telemetry
	Maternal Position				**Frequency of uterine activity** ∅ = None
	O2/LPM/Mask				Irreg = Irregular
	IV				**Intensity of uterine activity** M = Mild
	Nurse Initials				Mod = Moderate Str = Strong
Narrative notes:					By IUPC = mm Hg
					Resting tone R = Relaxed By IUCP = mm Hg
					Coping W = Well S = Support provided For pain use 0–10 scale
					Maternal position A = Ambulatory U = Upright SF = Semi-Fowler's RL = Right Lateral LL = Left Lateral MS = Modified Sims'

FIGURE 9–17 Example of FHR documentation.

CONCEPT MAP |

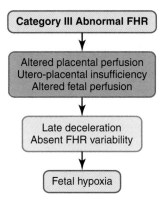

CARE PLANS

Problem 1: Category III FHR
Altered Placental Perfusion—Uteroplacental Insufficiency
Recurrent late decelerations
Absent FHR variability
Category III FHR pattern
Late decelerations and absent FHR variability
Goal: Improve placental perfusion. Fetus will become well perfused and oxygenated; cord gases indicate no respiratory or metabolic acidosis.
Outcome: Fetus will become well perfused and oxygenated; cord gases indicate no respiratory or metabolic acidosis.

Nursing Actions
1. Change maternal position (left, right, lateral, or hands and knees).
2. Administer 500 mL IV bolus of fluid.
3. Perform cervical exam to assess cord prolapse, rapid cervical dilation, or rapid descent of the fetal head.
4. Assess uterine activity for uterine tachysystole.
5. Assess maternal vital signs, especially temperature for maternal fever and blood pressure for hypotension.
6. Administer O_2 at 10 L/min via nonrebreather face mask to improve fetal oxygen status.
7. Consider discontinuing oxytocin if in use.
8. Consider use of terbutaline to stop UCs, unless mother is a drug user, has previous preeclampsia, or has a heart rate greater than 120 bpm.
9. Alter pushing efforts, or stop pushing, or push with every other or every third UC to provide time for fetus to recover when FHR is Category III during second stage.
10. Request an immediate bedside evaluation by a physician or midwife.

Problem 2: Maternal fear and anxiety
Woman is crying.
Woman states that she is concerned that her baby is going to die.
Patient is G2 P1 at term, 10 cm and pushing.
Goal: Decreased anxiety
Outcome: Patient verbalizes that she feels less anxious.

Nursing Actions
1. Be calm and attentive in interactions with the patient and her family.
2. Explain all procedures and interventions.
3. Explain current fetal status.
4. Assist patient with breathing and relaxation techniques.
5. Encourage the patient and family to verbalize their feelings regarding concern for the fetus.
6. Remain with the patient and her family.
7. Provide accurate information to the woman and her family in understandable terms to make sure the woman is able to be an informed participant in shared decision making.

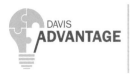

Go to Davis Advantage to complete your learning: strengthen understanding, apply your knowledge, and prepare for the Next Gen NCLEX®.

REFERENCES

Alfirevic, Z., Devane, D., Gyte, G. M. L., & Cuthbert, A. (2017). Continuous cardiotocography (CTG) as a form of electronic fetal monitoring (EFM) for fetal assessment during labour. *Cochrane Database of Systematic Reviews, 2.* https://doi.org/10.1002/14651858.CD006066.pub3

American College of Obstetricians and Gynecologists. (2009a, reaffirmed, 2019). Induction of labor. Practice Bulletin #107. *Obstetrics & Gynecology, 114*(2 Pt 1), 386–397. https://doi.org/10.1097/AOG.0b013 e3181b48ef5

American College of Obstetrics and Gynecologists. (2009b). Intrapartum fetal heart rate monitoring: Nomenclature, interpretation, and general management principles. Practice Bulletin #70. *Obstetrics & Gynecology, 114*(1), 192–202. https://doi.org/10.1097/AOG.0b013e3181aef106

American College of Obstetrics and Gynecologists. (2010). Management of intrapartum fetal heart rate tracing. Practice Bulletin #116. *Obstetrics & Gynecology, 116*(5), 1232–1240. https://doi.org/10.1097/AOG.0b013e3182004fa9

American College of Obstetrics and Gynecologists. (2017). Approaches to limit intervention during labor and birth. Committee Opinion Number 687. *Obstetrics & Gynecology, 129*(5), 20–28.

American College of Obstetricians and Gynecologists. (2019). Approaches to limit intervention during labor and birth. ACOG Committee Opinion No. 766. *Obstetrics & Gynecology, 133*, e164–e173.

Association of Women's Health, Obstetric and Neonatal Nurses. (2018). *Fetal heart monitoring* (Position Statement). Author. https://doi.org/10.1016/j.jogn.2018.09.007

Benson, R. C., Shubeck, E., Deutschberge, J., Weiss, W., & Berenes, H. (1968). Fetal heart rate as a predictor of fetal distress. A report from the collaborative project. *Obstetrics & Gynecology, 32*(2), 259–266.

Cahill, A. G., Tuuli, M. G., Stout, M. J., Lopez, J. D., & Macones, G. A. (2018). A prospective cohort study of fetal heart rate monitoring: Deceleration area is predictive of fetal acidemia. *American Journal Obstetrics & Gynecology, 218*, 523.e1.

Cibils, L. A. (1996). On intrapartum fetal monitoring. *American Journal of Obstetrics and Gynecology, 174*(4), 1382–1389.

Cunningham, F., Leveno, K., Bloom, S., Dashe, J., Hoffman, B., Casey, B., & Spong, C. (2018). *Williams obstetrics* (25th ed.). McGraw-Hill.

Cypher, R. (2015). Assessment of fetal oxygenation and acid–base balance. In A. Lyndon & L. U. Ali (Eds.), *Fetal heart monitoring: Principles and practices* (5th ed.). Kendall Hunt Publishing.

Feinstein, N., Sprague, A., & Trepanier, M. (2008). *Fetal heart rate auscultation* (2nd ed.). Association of Women's Health, Obstetric and Neonatal Nurses.

Freeman, R. (2002). Problems with intrapartum fetal heart rate monitoring interpretation and patient management. *American College of Obstetricians and Gynecologists, 100*(4), 813–826. https://doi: 10.1016/s0029-7844(02)02211-1

Freeman, R., Garite, T., & Nageotte, M. (2003). *Fetal heart rate monitoring* (3rd ed.). Lippincott Williams & Wilkins.

Garite, T. J., Nageotte, M. P., & Parer, J. T. (2015). Should we really avoid giving oxygen to mothers with concerning fetal heart rate patterns? *American Journal of Obstetrics and Gynecology, 212*(4), 459–460, 459.e1. Epub 2015

Killion, M. M. (2015). Techniques for fetal heart and uterine activity assessment. In A. Lyndon & L. U. Ali (Eds.), *Fetal heart monitoring: Principles and practices* (5th ed.). Kendall Hunt Publishing.

Lyndon, A., & Ali, L. U. (2015). *Fetal heart monitoring: Principles and practices* (5th ed.). Kendall Hunt Publishing.

Macones, G., Hankins, G., Spong, C., Hauth, J., & Moore, T. (2008). The 2008 National Institute of Child Health and Human Development Workshop Report on Electronic Fetal Monitoring: Update on definition, interpretation, and research guidelines. *Journal of Obstetric, Gynecologic, & Neonatal Nursing, 37*(5), 510–515.

Martin, J. A., Hamilton, B. E., Osterman, M. J. K., & Driscoll, A. K. (2019). Births: Final data for 2018. *National Vital Statistics Reports, 68*(13). National Center for Health Statistics.

Martis, R., Emilia, O., Nurdiati, D. S., & Brown, J. (2017). Intermittent auscultation (IA) of fetal heart rate in labour for fetal well-being. *Cochrane Database of Systematic Reviews, 2.* https://doi.org/10.1002/14651858.CD008680.pub2

Murray, M. L. (2004). Maternal or fetal heart rate? Avoiding intrapartum misidentification. *Journal of Obstetrical & Gynecological Neonatal Nursing, 33*(1), 93–102.

National Institute of Child Health and Human Development. (1997a). Electronic fetal heart rate monitoring: Research guidelines for interpretation. *American Journal of Obstetrics and Gynecology, 177*(6), 1385–1390.

National Institute of Child Health and Human Development. (1997b). Electronic fetal heart rate monitoring: Research guidelines for interpretation. *Journal of Obstetric Gynecology and Neonatal Nursing, 26*(6), 635–640.

O'Brien-Abel, N., & Simpson, K. (2021). Fetal assessment during labor. In K. Simpson, P. Creehan, N. O'Brien-Abel, C. Roth, & A. Rohan (Eds.), *Perinatal nursing* (5th ed., pp. 412–464). Wolters Kluwer.

Parameshwari R., & Shenbaga D. (2020). Acquisition and analysis of electrohysterogram signal. *Journal of Medical Systems, 44*(3), 66. https://doi.org/10.1007/s10916-020-1523-y

Parer, J. T., & Ikeda, T. (2007). A framework for standardized management of intrapartum fetal heart rate patterns. *American Journal of Obstetrics and Gynecology, 197*, 26.e1–26.e6.

Parer, J. T., King, T. L., & Ikeda, T. (2018). Electronic fetal heart rate monitoring: The 5-tier system (3rd ed.). Jones & Bartlett Learning.

Simpson, K. (2004a). Fetal assessment in the adult intensive care unit. *Critical Care Nursing Clinics of North America, 16*, 233–242. https://doi: 10.1016/j.ccell.2004.02.003

Simpson, K. (2004b). Standardized language for electronic fetal heart rate monitoring. *American Journal of Maternal/Child Nursing, 29*(5), 336.

Simpson, K. (2015). Physiologic interventions for fetal heart rate patterns. In A. Lyndon & L. U. Ali (Eds.), *Fetal heart monitoring: Principles and practices* (5th ed.). Kendall Hunt Publishing.

Simpson, K., & Creehan, P. A. (2014). *Perinatal nursing.* Wolters Kluwer.

Simpson, K., & James, D. (2005). Efficacy of intrauterine resuscitation techniques in improving fetal oxygen status during labor. *American College of Obstetricians and Gynecologists, 105*(6), 1362–1368. https://doi.10.1097/01.AOG.0000164474.03350.7c

Simpson, K. R., & O'Brien-Abel, N. (2021). Labor and birth. In K. Simpson, P. Creehan, N. O'Brien-Abel, C. Roth, & A. Rohan (Eds.), *Perinatal nursing* (5th ed., pp. 325–411.). Wolters Kluwer.

The Joint Commission. (2004). Preventing infant death and injury during delivery. *Sentinel Event Alert, 30.* https://www.jointcommission.org/Sentinel Events/SentinelEventAlert/sea_30.

True, B. A., & Bailey, R. E. (2016). Intrapartum fetal surveillance. In *Advanced life support in obstetrics, provider syllabus* (pp. 125–145). American Academy of Family Physicians Pediatrics and American College of Obstetricians and Gynecologists.

Tucker, S., Miller, S., & Miller, D. (2009). *Fetal monitoring, A multidisciplinary approach* (6th ed.). Mosby.

Wisner, K., & Holschuh, C. (2018). Fetal heart rate auscultation, 3rd edition. *Nursing for Women's Health, 22*(6), e1–e32.

Complications of Labor and Birth

10

Roberta F. Durham, RN, PhD

LEARNING OUTCOMES

Upon completion of this chapter, the student will be able to:

1. Describe the primary causes of dystocia and the related nursing and medical care.
2. Identify potential complications of dystocia in labor and related nursing and medical care.
3. Demonstrate understanding of knowledge and care related to induction of labor and augmentation of labor.
4. Identify and manage complications of labor and birth to promote healthy outcomes for the mother and infant.
5. Describe the key obstetrical emergencies and the related nursing and medical care.

CONCEPTS

Caring
Collaboration
Comfort
Communication
Family
Grief and Loss
Infection
Oxygenation
Perfusion
Safety

Nursing Diagnosis

- Risk of maternal injury related to interventions implemented for dystocia
- Risk of maternal injury related to obstetrical emergencies
- Risk of fetal injury related to complications of labor and birth
- Anxiety related to labor and birth complications

Nursing Outcomes

- The woman will understand causes of dystocia and interventions to achieve a safe birth.
- The woman will give birth without maternal or fetal injury.
- The woman will give birth to a healthy infant without complications.
- The woman verbalizes understanding of the situation and plan of care and uses effective coping strategies.

INTRODUCTION

Most pregnant women go into labor spontaneously and have a normal labor and spontaneous vaginal birth. However, interventions to initiate or accelerate labor and birth are increasingly common. This chapter presents problems encountered during labor and birth and interventions related to those complications. Nurses have a key role in identifying complications and implementing nursing actions to achieve a safe birth and improve maternal and neonatal outcomes. Nurses are also in an ideal position to take a leadership role in improving maternity care in the United States, especially with complications in labor and birth, and reduce the risk of preventable adverse outcomes (Simpson, 2021). Outdated ways of providing care to childbearing women should be replaced with collaborative decision-making approaches. The old patriarchal culture that involves telling women what to do, expecting them to follow without questions, and treating them disrespectfully when they are unable or unwilling to "comply" is being slowly transformed to include women and their families as true partners in care.

DYSTOCIA

Labor dystocia (i.e., slow abnormal progression of labor) is the leading indication for primary cesarean birth in the United States (American Academy of Pediatrics [AAP] & American College of Obstetricians and Gynecologists [ACOG], 2017). Abnormal labor results from abnormalities of the power, the passenger, or the passage. The terms *dystocia* and *failure to progress* are both used to characterize an abnormally long labor. However, this diagnosis is often mistakenly made before the woman has entered the active phase of labor and, therefore, before adequate trial of labor (Simpson & O'Brien-Abel, 2021). Unrealistic expectations of faster labor based on outdated evidence contributes to excessive unnecessary interventions such as labor augmentation techniques as well as primary and repeat cesarean birth in the United States (ACOG, 2019d). Additionally, a prolonged latent phase (e.g., greater than 20 hours in nulliparous women and greater than 14 hours in multiparous women) should not be an indication for cesarean delivery (ACOG, 2019a, 2019d). When the first stage of labor is protracted or arrested, oxytocin is commonly recommended.

Dystocia is related to the same factors that influence normal labor; these "Ps" are discussed in detail in Chapter 8. It can be helpful to look at the factors that influence labor within the 5 Ps to understand complications in labor and birth as well. Dystocia is related to 3 of the 5 Ps; powers, passenger and pelvis.

- Powers of labor (uterine contractions [UCs] and maternal expulsive effort)
- Passenger (fetal presentation, position, or development)
- Passage (maternal bony pelvis or soft tissue)

The primary issues impacting nursing care with regard to dystocia are related to uterine factors, which are described in this chapter. Other factors are presented in Chapter 8 and are briefly discussed in the following section. Risk factors for dystocia include:

- Congenital uterine abnormalities such as bicornate uterus
- Malpresentation of the fetus such as occiput posterior, or face presentation
- Cephalopelvic disproportion
- Tachysystole of the uterus with oxytocin
- Maternal fatigue and dehydration
- Administration of analgesia or anesthesia early in labor
- Extreme maternal fear or exhaustion, which can result in catecholamine release interfering with uterine contractility

Uterine Dystocia

Dystocia, or slow, abnormal labor, includes lack of progressive cervical dilation, lack of descent of the fetal head, or both. Uterine dystocia indicates weak or uncoordinated UCs in labor, characterized as either hypertonic or hypotonic uterine dysfunction.

Hypertonic Uterine Dysfunction

Hypertonic uterine dysfunction is uncoordinated uterine activity. Contractions are frequent and painful but ineffective in promoting dilation and effacement. When this occurs in early labor, it may be referred to as prodromal labor. Women who experience hypertonic uterine dysfunction are at risk for exhaustion related to prolonged labor, and the fetus is at risk for fetal intolerance of labor and asphyxia related to decreased placental profusion.

Risk Factors

- Nulliparous women are more subject to abnormal early labor.

Assessment Findings

- Painful, frequent UCs with inadequate uterine relaxation between UCs with little cervical changes (Fig. 10–1B)
- May be Category II (indeterminate) or Category III (abnormal) fetal heart rate (FHR) related to prolonged labor and inadequate uterine relaxation

Medical Management

- Evaluate labor progress.
- Evaluate the cause of labor dysfunction.
- Hydrate to improve uterine perfusion and coordination of UCs.
- Provide pain management to allow the woman to sleep and prevent exhaustion.

Nursing Actions

- Promote rest to try to break the pattern of frequent but ineffective UCs. The pattern typically becomes effective when the woman sleeps for a period of several hours and awakens in a normal pattern of active labor. Methods used to promote uterine rest are:
  - Administration of pain medication such as morphine as per order to decrease labor contractions and allow the uterus to rest.
  - Promotion of relaxation.
    - Warm shower or tub bath
    - Quiet environment
    - Minimal interruptions to allow for long period of sleep
- Hydrate the woman with IV or PO fluids if tolerated. Dehydration can result in dysfunctional labor.
- Assess FHR and UCs.
- Evaluate labor progress with a sterile vaginal examination (SVE).
- Inform the woman and family of the progress of labor and explain interventions.
- Inform the care provider of the woman's response and progress in labor.

Hypotonic Uterine Dysfunction

Hypotonic uterine dysfunction occurs when the pressure of the UC is insufficient (intrauterine pressure catheter [IUPC] measurement less than 25 mm Hg) to promote cervical dilation and effacement. Typically, in this situation, the woman makes normal progress during the latent phase of labor, but during active labor the UCs become weaker and less effective for cervical changes and labor progress (Fig. 10–1A). The woman is at risk

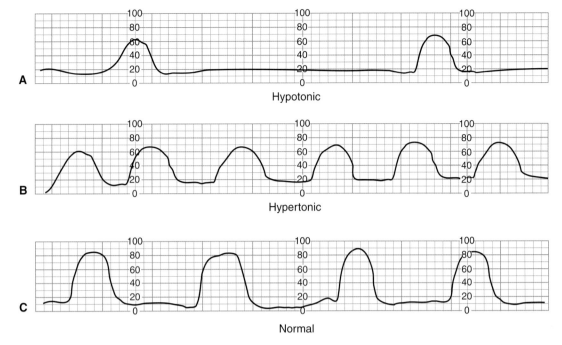

FIGURE 10–1 Hypertonic versus hypotonic versus normal uterine contractions. (A) Hypotonic UC pattern. (B) Hypertonic UC pattern. (C) Normal UC pattern.

for exhaustion and infection related to the prolonged labor, and the fetus is at risk for fetal intolerance of labor and asphyxia. Figure 10–1C shows a normal UC pattern.

Risk Factors

- Multiparous women often have more problems in the active phase.
- Extreme fear may result in catecholamine release, interfering with uterine contractility.

Assessment Findings

- Decreased frequency, strength, and duration of UCs
- Little or no cervical change in active labor
- Less than 0.5 cm/hr progress in cervical dilation for a primiparous woman in active labor; primiparous women likely have cervical dilation less than 0.5 cm/hr in earlier active labor and faster in later active labor (Simpson & O'Brien, 2021)
- Less than 1 cm/hr progress in cervical dilation for a multiparous woman in active labor less than or equal to 6 cm
- Increased fear and anxiety levels

Medical Management

- Evaluate labor progression.
- Determine the cause of the dysfunction.
- Consider obstetrical interventions:
  - Augment labor with oxytocin.
  - Perform amniotomy.
  - Perform cesarean birth when other interventions have failed or when there are signs of fetal intolerance of labor.

Nursing Actions

- Assess uterine activity.
- Assess maternal and fetal status.

- Stimulate uterine activity to achieve a normal labor pattern using the following methods:
  - Ambulate and change the woman's position to promote comfort and labor progress.
  - Hydrate with IV or PO as per orders, as dehydration can result in dysfunctional labor.
  - Administer IV fluids to maximize maternal fluid volume, correct maternal hypotension, and improve placental perfusion.
  - Augment labor with oxytocin as per protocol.
- Evaluate labor progress with SVE.
- Inform the woman and the family of labor progress and explain interventions.
- Provide emotional support and labor support. Anxiety levels can increase due to prolonged labor; increased anxiety and fear can interfere with effective UCs.
- Maintain good aseptic technique to minimize the risk of infection if there is rupture of membranes (ROM).
  - Minimize vaginal exams.
  - Maintain perineal cleanliness.
- Inform the care provider of the woman's response and progress in labor.

Active Phase Disorders

In both spontaneous and induced labor, diagnosis of an arrest disorder should not be made before the patient has entered the active phase of labor at greater than or equal to 6 cm. Definitions of arrest disorders vary somewhat in published criteria. Current guidelines regarding labor progress challenge our long-held practices based on the Friedman curve. For example, the active phase of labor is now classified at 6 cm dilation (rather than the previously recognized 4 cm), and multiparous women appear to have a steeper acceleration phase than previously thought (Simpson, 2020; Spong et al., 2012).

The current working definition of arrest of labor in the first stage in spontaneous labor (ACOG, 2014c) uses a dilation of more than or equal to 6 cm with membrane rupture and one of the following:

- 4 hours or more of adequate contractions (e.g., more than 200 Montevideo units)
- 6 hours or more of inadequate contractions and no cervical change

As long as fetal and maternal status are reassuring, cervical dilation of 6 cm should be considered the threshold for the active phase of most women in labor. Before 6 cm of dilation is achieved, standards of active phase progress should not be applied. Further, cesarean delivery for active phase arrest in the first stage of labor should be reserved for women at or beyond 6 cm of dilation with ruptured membranes who fail to progress despite 4 hours of adequate uterine activity, or at least 6 hours of oxytocin administration with inadequate uterine activity and no cervical change (ACOG, 2014c).

Second-Stage Disorders

The second stage of labor begins when the cervix becomes fully dilated, 10 cm, and ends with delivery of the neonate. Parity, delayed pushing, use of epidural analgesia, maternal body mass index (BMI), birth weight, occiput posterior position, and fetal station at complete dilation all have been shown to affect the length of the second stage of labor (ACOG, 2014c). Additionally, the duration of the second stage was approximately 1 hour longer in women who received epidural analgesia than in those who did not.

Prolonged second-stage labor for nulliparous women, as defined by ACOG and AAP (2017), is lack of continuing progress toward birth for 3 hours with regional anesthesia or 2 hours without regional analgesia or anesthesia and for multiparous women as a lack of continuing progress for 2 hours with regional anesthesia or 1 hour without regional anesthesia. Multiparous women experiencing a second stage of 3 hours or longer are at increased risk for operative birth, peripartum morbidity, and adverse neonatal outcomes.

The literature supports that for women, longer time in the second stage of labor is associated with increased risks of morbidity and a decreasing probability of spontaneous vaginal delivery. However, this may be due to provider actions and interventions. Given the available literature, before diagnosing arrest of labor in the second stage and if the maternal and fetal conditions permit, at least 2 hours of pushing in multiparous women and at least 3 hours of pushing in nulliparous women should be allowed according to current ACOG guidelines (2019a). Inadequate expulsive forces occur in the second stage of labor when the woman is not able to push or bear down. It was previously thought that limiting the second stage to

---

BOX 10-1 | Definitions of Arrest Disorders

First-Stage Arrest

Spontaneous labor: Greater than 6 cm dilation with membrane rupture and more than 4 hours of adequate contractions (e.g., more than 200 Montevideo units) or more than 6 hours if contractions are inadequate with no cervical change

Induced labor: Greater than 6 cm dilation with membrane rupture or greater than 5 cm without membrane rupture and more than 4 hours of adequate contractions (e.g., more than 200 Montevideo units), or more than 6 hours if contractions are inadequate with no cervical change

Second-Stage Arrest

Prolonged second-stage labor for nulliparous women, as defined by the ACOG and AAP (2017), is a lack of continuing progress for 3 hours with regional anesthesia or 2 hours without regional analgesia or anesthesia, and for multiparous women as a lack of continuing progress for 2 hours with regional anesthesia or 1 hour without regional anesthesia. Multiparous women experiencing a second stage of 3 hours or longer are at increased risk for operative birth, peripartum morbidity, and adverse neonatal outcomes. No progress (descent or rotation) for 4 hours or more in nulliparous women with an epidural, 3 hours or more in nulliparous women without an epidural, 3 hours or more in multiparous women with an epidural, or 2 hours or more in multiparous women without an epidural is an indication.

American Academy of Pediatrics & American College of Obstetricians and Gynecologists (AAP and ACOG), 2017; Spong et al., 2012.

---

2 hours was essential to decrease fetal morbidity and mortality. However, it is now known that waiting beyond 2 hours is safe for the fetus and the 2-hour time frame is no longer clinically valid (see Box 10-1).

- The fetus is at higher risk for asphyxia related to a prolonged second stage of labor.
- The woman with a prolonged second stage, beyond 4 hours, is at risk for operative vaginal birth and perineal trauma.

Risk Factors

- Maternal exhaustion
- Epidural anesthesia because woman may not feel the urge to push

Assessment Findings

- Inadequate or ineffective pushing with little or no descent of the fetal head with expulsive pushing efforts
- Potential for Category II (indeterminate) or Category III (abnormal) FHR

Medical Management

- Evaluate the woman's progress, maternal-fetal status, and likelihood of vaginal birth.
- Augment with oxytocin.
- Assist birth with vacuum or forceps.
- Perform cesarean birth when other interventions are ineffective or signs of fetal intolerance to labor.

Nursing Actions

- Assess fetal descent and station with SVE.
- Evaluate fetal response to expulsive pushing.
- Facilitate the second stage of labor by doing the following:
  - Coaching the woman in bearing-down efforts
  - Minimizing the Valsalva maneuver by using open glottis push strategies detailed in Chapter 8
  - Maintaining adequate pain relief for the woman with labor epidurals
  - Helping the woman shift to a more upright position to facilitate fetal descent
  - Supporting the woman's involuntary pushing efforts

Precipitous Labor And Birth

Precipitous labor is an extremely rapid labor and birth lasting fewer than 3 hours from onset. The estimated rate of precipitous labor for women is less than 3% (Cunningham et al., 2018). Women who experience a precipitous labor often have higher anxiety and pain levels related to the rapid and intense labor experience. Precipitous labor or birth places the woman at risk for postpartum hemorrhage related to uterine atony or lacerations. It places the fetus or neonate at risk for hypoxia and at risk for central nervous system (CNS) depression related to hypoxia from rapid birth.

Risk Factors

- Grand multiparity
- History of precipitous labor

Assessment Findings

- Hypertonic UCs (tetanic UCs) occurring every 2 minutes or more frequently, lasting greater than 60 seconds and strong (Fig. 10–2)

- Potential for Category II (indeterminate) or Category III (abnormal) FHR and nursing actions are based on FHR pattern (see Chapter 9)
- Rapid cervical dilation such that labor is less than 3 hours

Medical Management

- Prepare for and stand by for precipitous birth.

Nursing Actions

- Remain in the room with the woman since birth is often very rapid with precipitous labor.
- Monitor FHR and UCs at least every 15 minutes.
- Assess labor progress and cervical change closely with SVEs.
  - Assess the cervix if the woman states she feels pressure or feels as if the baby is coming. This may be a sign of impending birth.
- Support the woman and the family. This type of labor can be frightening, overwhelming, and painful.
- Anticipate potential maternal postpartum complications such as hemorrhage from uterine atony and lacerations.
- Anticipate potential neonatal complications such as hypoxia and CNS depression related to rapid birth.
- Prepare for delivery.

Fetal Dystocia

Fetal dystocia may be caused by excessive fetal size, malpresentation, multifetal pregnancy, or fetal anomalies. The fetus can move through the birth canal most effectively when the head is flexed and is presenting anterior to the woman's pelvis (occiput anterior position). This allows the smallest diameter of the fetal head to enter the maternal pelvis and the most flexible part of the fetal body, the back of the neck, to adapt to the curve of the birth canal. When the fetal position is other than flexed and vertex of the fetus is large in comparison with the maternal pelvis, labor may be difficult and vaginal birth a challenge. Complications of fetal dystocia are:

- Neonatal asphyxia related to prolonged labor
- Fetal injuries, such as bruising
- Maternal lacerations
- Cephalopelvic disproportion (CPD)

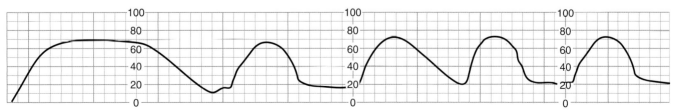
Tachysystole (tetanic contractions)

FIGURE 10–2 Tetanic UCs.

CRITICAL COMPONENT

Fetopelvic or Cephalopelvic Disproportion

Fetopelvic disproportion arises from diminished pelvic capacity, excessive fetal size, or both (Cunningham et al., 2018). CPD is a condition in which the size, shape, or position of the fetal head prevents it from passing through the lateral aspect of the maternal pelvis or when the maternal pelvis is of a size or shape that prevents the descent of the fetus through the pelvis. A diagnosis of CPD often necessitates a cesarean birth. CPD can rarely be diagnosed until labor has progressed for some time.

The success of any labor depends on the complex interrelationship of several factors:

• Fetal size, presentation, and position
• Size and shape of the maternal pelvis
• Quality of the UCs

Risk Factors

● Contraction or narrowing of the pelvic inlet, the midpelvis, or the pelvic outlet
● Abnormal fetal presentation or position such as asynclitism, face, brow presentation, or breech or transverse lie (Table 10-1)
● Fetal anomalies, such as hydrocephalus, or any other fetal anomaly that interferes with fetal descent through the birth canal
● Fetal macrosomia; birth weight greater than 4,500 g. However, prediction of birth weight is imprecise by ultrasonography or clinical measurement (ACOG, 2020b).

Assessment Findings

● FHR may be heard above the umbilicus versus in the lower uterine segment; this is a sign that the fetus may be in a position other than vertex.
● The SVE reveals the buttocks or face when malpresentation is the cause of dystocia.
● The presenting part is not engaged in the maternal pelvis.
● There is no fetal descent through the pelvis.

Medical Management

● Confirm the fetal position with SVE and ultrasound.
● Determine the type of obstetrical interventions, such as use of vacuum extractor, forceps, or need for cesarean birth.

Nursing Actions

● Perform Leopold's maneuver as described in Chapter 8 to determine the fetal position.
● Assess the location of the FHR.
● Assess the fetal position with SVE.
● Alert the care provider if there is any question regarding fetal presentation, position, or absence of fetal descent.

Pelvic Dystocia

Pelvic dystocia is related to the contraction of one or more of the three planes of the pelvis. During the prenatal period, the care provider determines the general pelvic size and configuration by vaginal examination. Pelvic measurements are not typically done. Descent and engagement of the fetal head in labor indicate adequate pelvic inlet. The outcome of labor is dependent on the interrelationship of the size and shape of the pelvis, fetal size, presentation and position, and quality of the UCs. The three contractions of the pelvic planes are:

● Inlet contraction, which occurs when the widest part of the pelvis is small.
● Midpelvis contraction, which is related to prominent ischial spines, convergent pelvic side walls, and a narrow sacrosciatic notch; this may arrest the descent of the vertex.
● Outlet contraction, which can be estimated by measuring the transverse diameter of the pelvis. Normally, the anteroposterior diameter is 14 cm.

Risk Factors

● Small pelvis
● Abnormal pelvic shape

Assessment Findings

● Delayed descent of the fetal head

Medical Management

● Evaluate the pelvis for contraction of one or more of the planes of the pelvis.
● Evaluate the descent and engagement of the fetal head.

Nursing Actions

● Perform SVE to evaluate the progress of labor and fetal descent into the pelvis (i.e., check station).

LABOR INTERVENTIONS

Most pregnant women go into labor spontaneously at term (37 to 42 weeks' gestation) and progress through the labor and birth experience without complications. Increasingly, the approach to labor has shifted from a natural process to one that should be "managed" by the woman, nurse, and care provider. Management of labor has resulted in an increase in labor interventions, including induction of labor (which may also include cervical ripening) and augmentation to speed up labor. This section reviews interventions to induce (initiate) and augment (strengthen) labor.

Induction of labor is the stimulation of UCs to initiate labor. Examples of methods include, but are not limited to, artificial

TABLE 10-1   Malpresentation of the Fetus

MALPRESENTATION	DESCRIPTION	IMPLICATIONS
Occiput posterior	The occiput of the fetus is in the posterior portion of the pelvis rather than the anterior. As the fetus moves through the birth canal, the occiput bone presses on the woman's sacrum. Rotation of the fetal head may occur during fetal descent.	Prolonged labor and prolonged second stage Severe back pain
Face presentation	Fetal head is in extension rather than flexion as it enters the pelvis.	Labor and pushing may be prolonged. Cesarean delivery may be indicated. The neonate's face may have extensive bruising.
Brow presentation	Fetal head presents in a position midway between full flexion and extreme extension. This causes the largest diameter of the head to engage in the pelvis.	Prolonged second stage of labor
Shoulder presentation or compound presentation	Shoulder presentation: The fetal spine is vertical to the maternal pelvis. Compound presentation: One or more fetal extremities accompany the presenting part.	Higher risk of prolapsed cord. Cesarean delivery is typically indicated.

Continued

TABLE 10-1   Malpresentation of the Fetus—cont'd

MALPRESENTATION	DESCRIPTION	IMPLICATIONS
Breech presentations: Frank breech Complete breech Footling breech (single) Footling breech (double)	Frank breech: Thighs flexed alongside body; feet are close to the head. Complete breech: One or both knees are flexed. Footling breech: Either one (single footling) or both (double footling) feet present before the buttocks.	Dysfunctional labor. Fetal injury. Increased risk of prolapsed cord. Typically, cesarean birth is indicated.

rupture of membranes (AROM), balloons, oxytocin, prostaglandin, laminaria, or other cervical ripening agents (ACOG, 2014b). Augmentation of labor is the stimulation of UCs using pharmacological methods or AROM to increase their frequency or strength following the onset of spontaneous labor or contractions following spontaneous rupture of membranes (SROM). Cervical ripening is the process of effecting physical softening and distensibility of the cervix in preparation for labor and birth. Cervical ripening can occur naturally or by use of mechanical or pharmacological methods (ACOG, 2014b).

Labor interventions are medically indicated when either the condition or safety of the woman or fetus would be improved with birth. Because spontaneous labor is associated with fewer complications than induced labor, induction of labor without a medical indication is discouraged. Despite risks to the woman and fetus (such as increased rates of cesarean birth), labor interventions such as elective induction are at an all-time high. Because of the potential risks associated with induction of labor, elective induction should be undertaken only after fully informing the woman of risks and benefits and establishing a gestational age of 39 weeks or greater. The primary role of the labor nurse during cervical ripening, labor induction, or labor augmentation is ongoing maternal and fetal assessment to support safe care and birth. The goal is labor progression without excessive uterine activity or fetal compromise. The nurse providing care for the woman during cervical ripening, induction, or augmentation of labor should be aware of the indications, actions, expected results, and potential risks of each agent. Before any agent is used, maternal status and fetal well-being should be established and cervical status should be assessed and documented (Simpson & Knox, 2009).

Labor Induction

Induction of labor is the deliberate stimulation of UCs before the onset of spontaneous labor to facilitate a vaginal delivery. Induction of labor refers to techniques for stimulating UCs to accomplish delivery before the onset of spontaneous labor. According to the National Center for Health Statistics (Martin et al., 2019), in 2018 (the most recent year for which detailed natality data is available), rates of induction and augmentation of labor in the United States were 27.1% and 21.5%, respectively, for all births. The 2018 induction rate (27.1%) was 184% higher than the 1990 rate (9.5%) and the highest since these data have been recorded from birth certificates. The induction rate increased by 5% from 2017 (25.7%) to 2018 (27.1%). Induction rates in 2018 differed by race: White women were at 30.3%, Black women at 25.2%, and Hispanic women at 22.8%. The augmentation rate increased slightly (1.26%) from 2017 (21.28%) to 2018 (21.55%). Augmentation rates are similar among the three categories of race reported, and all are between 21% and 22%.

Data show that outcomes for newborns are greatly improved when gestation is longer than 39 weeks. Yet studies indicate that almost a third of babies delivered in the United States are electively delivered—most for convenience. This impacts short-term neonatal morbidity. New guidelines are being set by The Joint Commission to decrease elective inductions of labor before 39 weeks' gestation. Labor induction should be performed only for medical indication; if done for nonmedical indications, the gestational age should be 39 weeks or more to avoid the risk of iatrogenic prematurity, and the cervix should be favorable (Bishop score of 8 or higher), especially in the nulliparous patient (AAP & ACOG, 2017) (Box 10-2).

Women who are undergoing induction of labor should have adequate, objective information with which to make informed decisions about the potential risks and benefits of induction. This information should include indications for induction, agents and methods of cervical ripening and labor stimulation, and their risks (AAP & ACOG, 2017; AWHONN, 2019). The nurse may face a dilemma when women are admitted for induction or cervical ripening without documented indications for it. It is the nurse's responsibility to ensure that the woman is fully informed by her provider before beginning a procedure (Simpson, 2020). If it is apparent during admission that the woman is not fully informed about the intended method of labor induction, the health-care provider who ordered the induction or their physician designee should be notified and should speak to the woman either on the telephone or in person about the potential risks and benefits of the process and ensure that her questions and concerns have been addressed before proceeding (Simpson, 2020).

As part of the informed consent process, women considering labor induction should be aware that it typically is not an isolated intervention. Labor induction often results in a cascade of other interventions and activities that have the potential to negatively

SAFE AND EFFECTIVE NURSING CARE:
Patient Education

Go the Full 40

One source of information women can use when considering childbearing options is the Association for Women's Health Obstetric and Neonatal Nurses' (AWHONN's) "Don't Rush Me . . . Go the Full 40" consumer-awareness campaign, launched in 2012. It seeks to empower women to make labor and delivery decisions that are in their best interests and is designed to help women understand 40 key reasons for carrying her baby to term, challenging the common myth that it's okay for babies to be born just a little early. In fact, babies need the benefit of a full-term pregnancy. Inducing labor before 40 weeks is associated with prematurity, cesarean surgery, hemorrhage, and infection. Babies born before 37 completed weeks of gestation are at risk for breathing problems, feeding issues, jaundice, low blood sugar, and problems stabilizing their own body temperature (www.health4mom.org).

Gestational age at birth is classified (ACOG, 2014b) as the following:

Preterm: less than 37 weeks and 0 days,

Late preterm: 34 weeks and 0 days through 36 weeks and 6 days, and

Term: greater than or equal to 37 weeks and 0 days using best estimated due date and is divided into the following categories:

Early term: 37 weeks and 0 days through 38 weeks and 6 days, +

Full term: 39 weeks and 0 days through 40 weeks and 6 days, +

Late term: 41 weeks and 0 days through 41 weeks and 6 days, and +

Post term: Greater than or equal to 42 weeks and 0 days.

Healthy Mom & Baby, the consumer magazine from AWHONN, can also be helpful for women considering induction.

BOX 10-2 | Criteria, Indications, and Contraindications for Labor Induction and Cervical Ripening

Criteria

Generally, induction of labor has merit as a therapeutic option when the benefits of expeditious delivery outweigh the risks of continuing the pregnancy. The benefits of labor induction need to be weighed against the potential maternal and fetal risks associated with this procedure. Before 41 0/7 weeks of gestation, induction of labor generally should be performed based on maternal and fetal medical indications. Inductions at 41 0/7 weeks of gestation and beyond should be performed to reduce the risk of cesarean birth and the risk of perinatal morbidity and mortality.

- Gestational age, cervical status, pelvic adequacy, fetal size, and fetal presentation should be assessed.
- Any potential risks to the mother and fetus should be considered.
- The medical record should document that a discussion was held between the pregnant woman and her health-care provider about the indications; the agents and methods of labor induction, including the risks, benefits, and alternative approaches; and the possible need for a repeat induction or cesarean birth.
- A nulliparous woman undergoing elective induction of labor with an unfavorable cervix should be counseled about a twofold increased risk of cesarean birth.
- Cervical ripening and induction agents should be administered by trained personnel familiar with their effects on mother and fetus.
- Prostaglandin preparations should be administered where uterine activity and FHR can be monitored continuously for an initial observation period. FHR monitoring should be continued if regular UCs persist.
- FHR and UCs should be monitored closely during induction and augmentation as for any high-risk patient in active labor.
- A physician capable of performing a cesarean birth should be readily available.
- For women undergoing trial of labor after cesarean (TOLAC), induction of labor for maternal or fetal indications remains an option.
- Misoprostol should not be used for third-trimester cervical ripening, or for labor induction in women who have had a cesarean birth or major uterine surgery.

Indications

Indications for induction of labor are not absolute but should take into account maternal and fetal conditions; gestational age; and assessment of the cervix, pelvis, and fetal size and presentation.

These are examples of maternal or fetal conditions that may be indications for induction of labor:

- Abruptio placentae
- Chorioamnionitis (intraamniotic infection)
- Fetal demise
- Gestational hypertension
- Preeclampsia, eclampsia
- PROM
- Post-term pregnancy for women at greater than or equal to 41 0/7 weeks' gestation; induction should be performed to reduce risks of cesarean birth and perinatal morbidity and mortality
- Maternal medical conditions (e.g., diabetes mellitus, renal disease, chronic pulmonary disease, chronic hypertension, or antiphospholipid syndrome)
- Fetal compromise (e.g., severe fetal growth restriction, isoimmunization, oligohydramnios)

Labor may also be induced for logistical reasons (e.g., risk of rapid labor, distance from the hospital, or psychosocial indications). In such circumstances, at least one of the following criteria should be met, or fetal lung maturity should be established:

- Ultrasound measurement at less than 20 weeks' gestation supports gestational age of 39 weeks or greater.
- Fetal heart tones have been documented as present for 30 weeks by Doppler ultrasonography.
- It has been 36 weeks since a positive serum or urine human chorionic gonadotropin pregnancy test result.
- Testing for fetal lung maturity should not be performed and is contraindicated when delivery is mandated for fetal or maternal indications. Conversely, a mature fetal lung maturity test result before 39 weeks' gestation, in the absence of appropriate clinical circumstances, is not an indication for elective labor induction.

Examples of medical indications in late preterm or early term births include the following:

- Preeclampsia, eclampsia, gestational hypertension, or complicated chronic hypertension
- Oligohydramnios
- Previous classical cesarean birth or prior myomectomy
- Placenta previa or placenta accreta
- Multiple gestation
- Fetal growth restriction
- Pregestational diabetes with vascular disease
- Poorly controlled pregestational or gestational diabetes
- PROM
- Cholestasis of pregnancy
- Alloimmunization of pregnancy with known or suspected fetal growth effect

---

BOX 10-2 | Criteria, Indications, and Contraindications for Labor Induction and Cervical Ripening—cont'd

Contraindications

Generally, the contraindications for labor induction are the same as those for spontaneous labor and vaginal birth. They include, but are not limited to, the following:

- Vasa previa or complete placenta previa
- Transverse fetal lie
- Umbilical cord prolapse

- Previous classical cesarean birth
- Active genital herpes infection
- Previous myomectomy entering the endometrial cavity

American Academy of Pediatrics & American College of Obstetricians and Gynecologists, 2017; American College of Obstetrics and Gynecologists, 2009a; American College of Obstetricians and Gynecologists & Society for Maternal-Fetal Medicine, 2014; Simpson, 2020.

---

affect the childbirth process. Labor induction in the United States requires the establishment of IV access, bedrest, and continuous electronic fetal monitoring (EFM). Amniotomy, significant discomfort, the use of epidural analgesia or anesthesia, and a prolonged stay on the labor unit are also frequently involved. Use of oxytocin and prostaglandin agents increases the risk of fetal compromise during labor and neonatal depression at birth, primarily as a result of uterine tachysystole (Simpson, 2020; Simpson & Atterbury, 2003; Simpson & O'Brien-Abel, 2021).

AWHONN published clinical practices based on the best available evidence that promote the safest care possible for mothers and babies during labor induction (Simpson & O'Brien-Abel, 2021). These include, but are not limited to, the following:

- Awaiting spontaneous labor until 41 weeks' gestation
- Informed consent with the woman and her family as true partners in care. (Information should be at the appropriate literacy level, in understandable language, evidence based, unbiased, and individualized and include potential benefits and risks.)
- If elective, not performing labor induction before 39 completed weeks of gestation
- Cervical readiness before labor induction achieved without pharmacological agents (if induction is elective)
- Standard physiological oxytocin protocol including a standard concentration and standard dosing regime with agreed upon definition of tachysystole, appropriate and timely interventions for tachysystole, standardizing one nurse for each woman undergoing induction of labor and assessment of fetal well-being based on national guidelines for interpretation and frequency of assessment, and also a common understanding among members of the perinatal team regarding how labor induction will be conducted and an agreement that all team members will participate

---

CRITICAL COMPONENT

Elective Induction of Labor

It is estimated that 25% to 50% of inductions are elective or nonmedical. Before elective induction, fetal maturity must be confirmed to be 39 weeks or greater by the following:

1. Ultrasound before 20 weeks' gestation confirms gestational age of 39 weeks or greater.

---

2. Fetal heart tones have been documented as present by Doppler for 30 weeks.
3. It has been 36 weeks since a positive serum or urine pregnancy test was confirmed.

According to the American College of Obstetricians and Gynecologists (ACOG, 2011), for certain medical conditions, available data and expert opinion support optimal timing of delivery in the late-preterm or early-term period for improved neonatal and infant outcomes. However, for nonmedically indicated early-term deliveries, such an improvement has not been demonstrated. Morbidity and mortality rates are greater among neonates and infants delivered during the early-term period compared with those delivered between 39 and 40 weeks' gestation. Nevertheless, the rate of nonmedically indicated early-term deliveries continues to increase in the United States. ACOG recommends implementing a policy to decrease the rate of nonmedically indicated deliveries before 39 weeks' gestation. In addition, AWHONN (2014) advises that until we better understand the complex physiology of the hormones involved in labor and birth and the implications of interrupting this powerful hormonal process, we should limit induction and augmentation of labor to situations for which there are medical indications. (ACOG, 2011; AWHONN, 2014). A recent large randomized controlled trial (RCT) (Grobman et al., 2018), found that elective labor induction at 39 weeks of gestation did not result in a greater frequency of perinatal adverse outcomes than expectant management and resulted in fewer instances of cesarean delivery.

The increase in the elective induction rate over the past two decades has profoundly changed the practice of perinatal nursing. Instead of predominantly caring for women who present in spontaneous active labor, many labor nurses now spend significant time titrating oxytocin infusions and managing the side effects of oxytocin. Given the results of the ARRIVE trial (Grobman et al., 2018), there is potential for an increase in the rate of elective induction and a concomitant escalation of the medicalization of childbirth.

Numerous methods of labor induction have been proposed as being effective in initiating labor. When the decision has been made to induce labor, the next important question raised is how to induce labor. When deciding on the method of induction, certain clinical factors are considered, including parity, status of membranes (ruptured or intact), status of the cervix (favorable or unfavorable), and history of previous cesarean births.

All these factors or clinical situations are considered important to the provider's decision about which method of labor induction should be used. Labor induction is thought to be less successful when the cervix is unfavorable (not ripe). It is more successful in parous women than in nulliparous women. Little attention has been given to the combination of these factors, which may be important to women and clinicians when attempting to make informed decisions about the induction of labor (Kelly et al., 2009).

The nurse providing care for the woman during cervical ripening, as well as induction and augmentation of labor, must be aware of appropriate indications for the use of each mechanical method and pharmacological agent, as well as their actions, expected results, and potential risks. Additionally, before any cervical ripening or labor induction agent is used, maternal status and fetal well-being should be established and findings from an assessment of the cervix, pelvis, fetal size, and presentation documented in the medical record by the provider and an estimation of fetal weight and size and assessment of the maternal pelvis should be determined and documented by the provider (AAP & ACOG, 2017).

Oxytocin Induction

A pharmacological method for labor induction is administration of oxytocin, the most common induction agent used worldwide. It has been used alone, in combination with amniotomy, or after cervical ripening with other pharmacological or nonpharmacological methods. Before the introduction of prostaglandin agents, oxytocin was used as a cervical ripening agent as well.

- Endogenous oxytocin is a peptide synthesized by the hypothalamus that is transported to the posterior lobe of the pituitary gland, where it is released in the maternal circulation in response to vaginal and cervical stretching. The release of oxytocin stimulates UCs.
- Synthetic oxytocin is identical to endogenous oxytocin.
- Uterine response to oxytocin usually occurs within 3 to 5 minutes after IV administration begins, with a half-life of 10 minutes (Simpson, 2020).
- Considerable controversy exists related to dose and rate increase intervals when oxytocin is used for induction of labor.

There appears to be no advantage to continuing oxytocin once active labor is established (Simpson & O'Brien-Abel, 2021). Some data indicated reducing or discontinuing oxytocin may result in an equal or shorter length of labor compared with labor for women for whom oxytocin is continued or incrementally increased after active labor is achieved. Continued increases in oxytocin rates over a prolonged period can result in oxytocin receptor desensitization or down-regulation, making oxytocin less effective in producing normal UCs and having the opposite result than intended. Prolonged oxytocin infusion at higher-than-appropriate doses can result in side effects such as dysfunctional uterine activity patterns and uterine tachysystole.

A trend to use higher doses of oxytocin, termed "active management of labor" (see Box 10-1), was based on research conducted in the 1970s in Dublin, Ireland. However, current evidence supports lower-dose infusions (Simpson, 2020), with research reporting more successful vaginal births, fewer operative vaginal deliveries, and less tachysystole and lower cesarean birth rates. See Box 10-2 for indications and contraindications.

Risks Associated With Induction

- Tachysystole leading to Category II (indeterminate) or Category III (abnormal) FHR pattern is the primary complication of oxytocin in labor.
- Failed induction of labor: Failure to generate regular (e.g., every 3 minutes) contractions and cervical change after at least 24 hours of oxytocin administration, with artificial membrane rupture if feasible.
- Side effects of oxytocin use are primarily dose related; tachysystole and subsequent FHR decelerations are common side effects (ACOG, 2011).
- Water intoxication can occur with high concentrations of oxytocin with large quantities of hypotonic solutions, but usually only with prolonged administration with at least 40 mU/min.

Assessment Findings

- The woman understands the indication for induction.
- Assessment findings and prenatal records reflect an indication for induction.
- If elective induction, confirm gestational age of at least 39 weeks.

Medical Management

- Advise of indication for induction of labor and order induction of labor as per institutional protocol.
- Be available to respond to complications.

CRITICAL COMPONENT

Administering Oxytocin in Labor

Nursing responsibility during oxytocin infusion involves careful titration of the drug to the maternal-fetal response. The titration process includes decreasing the dosage rate or discontinuing the medication when contractions are too frequent, discontinuing the medication when fetal status is indeterminate or abnormal, and increasing the dosage rate when uterine activity and labor progress are inadequate. Often during oxytocin infusion, physicians and nurses are focused on the rate-increase section of the protocol while ignoring the clinical criteria for dosage increases. For example, if cervical effacement is occurring or if the woman is progressing in labor as expected, based on parity and other individual clinical factors, there is no need to increase the oxytocin rate, even if contractions appear to be mild and infrequent. Labor progress and maternal-fetal response to the medication should be the primary considerations (Simpson, 2020). The goal of oxytocin use in labor is to establish UC patterns that promote cervical dilation of about 1 cm/hr once in active labor.

Generally, the UC pattern consists of:

- Three UCs in 10 minutes, lasting 40 to 60 seconds, intensity of 25 to 75 mm Hg with IUCP with resting tone less than 20 mm Hg with 1 minute between each UC.
- Oxytocin is administered intravenously and is piggybacked to a mainline IV solution at the port most proximal to the venous site.
- Oxytocin is always infused via a pump.
- There is variation in the concentrations of oxytocin, and it should be prepared by the pharmacy, as it is a high-alert medication.
  - Typical concentrations are:
    - 10 units of oxytocin in 1,000 mL of lactated Ringer's result in an infusion rate of 1 mU/min = 6 mL/hr.
    - 20 units of oxytocin in 1,000 mL of lactated Ringer's result in an infusion rate of 1 mU/min = 3 mL/hr.
    - The key issue is consistency in practice within each institution.
- Bedrest is not required during infusion. EFM telemetry can be used during ambulation or while sitting on a chair or birthing ball.
- Administer in labor and birth suite, where uterine activity and FHR can be recorded continuously via EFM and evaluated at a minimum of every 15 minutes during the first stage of labor and every 5 minutes during the second stage of labor.
- Current dose recommendations are for low-dose oxytocin starting at 0.5 mU/min and increasing the dose by 1 to 2 mU/min every 30 to 60 minutes until adequate labor progress is achieved (i.e., cervical effacement or cervical dilation of 0.5 to 1 cm/hr) and regular UCs every 2 to 3 minutes lasting 45 to 60 seconds.
  - Generally, starting doses of 1 to 2 mU/min with increases in 1 to 2 mU/min increments every 30 to 60 minutes are most appropriate and commonly used.
  - Nursing responsibilities during oxytocin infusion involve careful titration of the drug to the maternal and fetal response.
  - The titration process includes decreasing dosage rates or discontinuing infusion when UCs are too frequent.
  - Discontinue oxytocin when FHR is abnormal (Simpson, 2020; Simpson & O'Brien-Abel, 2021).
  - Increase doses when UCs are inadequate; however, the lowest possible dose should be used to achieve labor progress (Simpson & Atterbury, 2003).
- Once active labor is established, oxytocin should be discontinued to avoid downregulation. Contemporary labor patterns suggest that the active phase of first-stage spontaneous labor likely does not start until 6 cm for nulliparous women and 5 cm for multiparous women (Simpson & O'Brien-Abel, 2021).
- Careful close monitoring for women with a history of prior cesarean birth or uterine scar; use lowest dose possible to achieve labor progress.
- Titrate dose to maternal-fetal response to labor.
- Use the lowest dose possible to achieve adequate progress of labor (progressive cervical effacement and cervical dilation of approximately 0.5 to 1.0 cm/hr once active labor has been achieved; expectation for labor progress is based on maternal parity).

- Reevaluate clinical situation if oxytocin dosage rate reaches 20 mU/min.
- Contractions should not be more frequent than every 2 minutes.
- Maternal-fetal response to oxytocin is the primary consideration. If the frequency, intensity, duration, or resting tone of the contraction is increased by oxytocin, this can impede uterine blood flow and can cause fetal compromise, resulting in a Category II or Category III FHR pattern. Thus, oxytocin must be administered with careful monitoring and prompt recognition and interventions for tachysystole to prevent fetal acidosis.
  - Avoid tachysystole because it frequently results in a Category II (indeterminate) or Category III (abnormal) FHR pattern.
  - Continuous EFM is typically used with oxytocin administration. During oxytocin induction or augmentation, FHR monitoring should be as per high-risk patients (AAP & ACOG, 2017) and therefore via continuous EFM.
  - In the absence of risk factors, intermittent auscultation is permitted with evaluation of FHR and UCs at least every 30 minutes in active labor and every 15 minutes in the second stage.
- The absence of fetal well-being necessitates direct bedside evaluation by a physician or certified nurse-midwife (CNM), interdisciplinary discussion, and written documentation of further clinical management plans (Simpson, 2021). For Category II (indeterminate) or Category III (abnormal) FHR patterns, interventions include the following actions:
  - Discontinue oxytocin.
  - Change maternal position to left lateral position.
  - Initiate IV hydration of at least 500 mL lactated Ringer's.
  - Administer O_2 by nonrebreather mask at 10 L/min.
  - Consider terbutaline if no response.
  - Notify provider, observe, and reevaluate.
  - Notify provider and request bedside evaluations for Category III abnormal FHR.
  - Assess emotional response of patient and support person to induction of labor. Provide information and reassurance as needed to alleviate feelings of failure.
  - Assess patient's level of fear and provide information and reassurance.
- If oxytocin has been discontinued for 20 to 30 minutes, the FHR is reassuring, and no uterine tachysystole is present, oxytocin may be restarted at half the rate that caused tachysystole and gradually increased every 30 minutes based on maternal-fetal response. If oxytocin has been discontinued for more than 30 to 40 minutes, exogenous oxytocin is metabolized; therefore, oxytocin must be restarted at the initial dose (2 mU per minute) (ACOG, 2011).
- Terminate the oxytocin infusion if there is tachysystole of the uterus, as previous defined; precipitous labor; nonreassuring FHR pattern; if the provider is unexpectedly unavailable; there is an inability to monitor the patient's FHR or UC at recommended intervals; or the desired labor pattern is achieved. If unable to continuously monitor FHR during an epidural administration, stop oxytocin infusion and restart infusion at half strength and increase per protocol once FHR continuous monitoring can be reestablished (ACOG, 2011).

Nursing Actions

- Ensure informed consent has been obtained by providing information about induction and discussing the agents, methods, options, and risks (Gilbert, 2011; Simpson, 2020). Nurses can play an important role in advocating for women who want to wait for labor to progress naturally but face pressure from their families or obstetric providers to undergo nonmedically indicated induction. Nurses can also play an important role in ensuring women have the information needed to make informed decisions regarding labor augmentation (AWHONN, 2014; Simpson, 2020).
- Review prenatal record with woman for indication for labor induction.
- Intermittent auscultation done appropriately is an acceptable method for labor management when heart rate remains within normal limits (Category I of the FHR categories).
- In the presence of risk factors, continuous EFM is recommended and FHR should be evaluated and documented every 15 minutes in active labor and every 5 minutes in the second stage.
- Monitor strength, frequency, and duration of UCs as an indicator of oxytocin efficacy every 30 minutes.
- Evaluate uterine resting tone by palpation or IUPC pressure below 20 mm Hg to ensure uterine relaxation between contractions.
- Decrease or discontinue oxytocin in the event of uterine tachysystole or indeterminate or abnormal fetal status. The current recommendation when decreasing oxytocin is to lower the dose by half.
- Assess FHR in response to UCs (see Chapter 9).
- Monitor labor progress with SVE for cervical dilation and fetal descent. Cervical change of 1 cm/hr indicates sufficient progress.
- Assess the character and amount of amniotic fluid.
- Assess the character and amount of bloody show.
- Assess the maternal response, including level of discomfort and pain and effectiveness of pain management and labor support PRN every 30 minutes.
- Assess vital signs (VS) per policy, generally every 2 hours.
- Assess input and output (I&O) for fluid overload; output should mirror intake. Signs and symptoms of fluid overload include decreased urine output, edema, increased blood pressure (BP), and pulmonary edema.
- Ensure adequate hydration, assess I&O every 8 hours.
- Greater than 50% of all legal settlements involved perinatal cases, with 40% to 50% of these cases related to management of oxytocin (Jonsson et al., 2007). Nurses must minimize the risk of patient harm by being well-educated regarding oxytocin risks as well as being proactive with interventions when there is evidence of tachysystole or abnormal FHR patterns.
- Follow the constitutions of chain of command if nursing disagrees with the plan of care (Gilbert, 2011).
- During the infusion of the oxytocin, the attending or another licensed provider who has assumed responsibility for the patient's care will be available within 30 minutes to manage any complications that may arise. A physician with privileges to perform a cesarean section should also be readily available (ACOG, 2011).

SAFE AND EFFECTIVE NURSING CARE: Understanding Medication

Oxytocin: High-Alert Medication

In 2007, IV oxytocin was designated as a high-alert medication. Drugs in this category carry a heightened risk of causing significant patient harm when they are used in error. Errors with high-alert medications may or may not be more common than with other drugs; however, patient injury and consequences of associated errors may be more devastating.

Patient injury from drug therapy is the single most common type of adverse event that occurs in the inpatient setting (Agency for Healthcare Research & Quality, 2001; Institute for Healthcare Improvement, 2007). When medication errors result in patient injury, there are significant costs to the patient, the health-care providers, and the institution. Special considerations and precautions are required before and during administration of high-alert medications (Institute for Safe Medication Practices, 2007). This is significant for perinatal care providers because oxytocin is a drug that they use quite frequently. Errors that involve IV oxytocin administration for labor induction or augmentation are most commonly dose-related and often involve lack of timely recognition and appropriate treatment of excessive uterine activity (i.e., tachysystole) (Clark et al., 2009).

Other types of oxytocin errors involve mistaken administration of IV fluids with oxytocin for IV fluid resuscitation during Category II or III FHR patterns or maternal hypotension and inappropriate elective administration of oxytocin to women who are less than 39 completed weeks' gestation. Oxytocin medication errors and subsequent patient harm are generally preventable (Simpson & Knox, 2009). The perinatal team can develop strategies to minimize risk of maternal-fetal injuries related to oxytocin administration consistent with safe care practices used with other high-alert medications. As with other high-alert medications, the lowest possible dose to achieve the desired therapeutic effect should be used (Simpson, 2020).

1. Requirement that women having elective labor induction be at least 39 completed weeks' gestation
2. Standard order sets and protocols that reflect a standardized clinical approach to labor induction and augmentation based on current pharmacological and physiological evidence
3. Standard concentration of oxytocin prepared by the pharmacy
4. Standard definition of uterine tachysystole that does not include a Category III or II (abnormal or indeterminate) FHR pattern (a contraction frequency of more than five in 10 minutes, a series of single contractions lasting 2 minutes or more, contractions of normal duration occurring within 1 minute of each other)
5. Standard treatment of oxytocin-induced uterine tachysystole guided by fetal status

Agency for Healthcare Research and Quality, 2001; Clark et al., 2009; Institute for Healthcare Improvement, 2007; Institute for Safe Medication Practices, 2007; Simpson, 2020; Simpson & Knox, 2009.

CLINICAL JUDGMENT

Tachysystole

Tachysystole is excessive uterine activity and can be either spontaneous or induced. It is defined as more than five contractions in 10 minutes, averaged over 30 minutes (ACOG, 2009a, 2011; Macones et al., 2008). Additional features of excessive uterine activity include contractions lasting 2 minutes or longer, contractions of normal duration occurring within 1 minute of each other, or insufficient return of uterine resting tone between contractions via palpation or intraamniotic pressure above 25 mm Hg between contractions via IUPC (ACOG, 2009a).

The placenta serves as the fetal lungs in utero. Uteroplacental circulation allows oxygen to be exchanged for the carbon dioxide and waste products from the fetus. During a contraction, the myometrial pressure exceeds the arterial pressure and the uterine blood flow is interrupted, causing a cessation in oxygen delivery to the placenta and the fetus. The fetus can withstand the stresses of labor during recurring periods of transient hypoxemia through a physiological compensatory mechanism known as the fetal oxygen reserve. However, if contractions are either too long or too strong, hypoxemia may result. Complications of uterine tachysystole for the fetus include hypoxia that can lead to acidemia, worsening to acidosis, ultimately leading to brain damage and even fetal death (Kunz et al., 2013).

Tachysystole, previously referred to as hyperstimulation, is excessive uterine activity and is the most concerning side effect of oxytocin because it can result in a progressive adverse effect on fetal status (Simpson, 2020; Simpson & O'Brien-Abel, 2021) (Fig. 10–3). UCs cause an intermittent decrease in blood flow in the intervillous space where oxygen exchange occurs. The decreased intervillous blood flow associated with tachysystole leads to decreased oxygen to the fetus. Tachysystole can result in progressive deterioration in fetal status and hypoxemia that result in an abnormal FHR. Tachysystole may result in abruptio placenta or uterine rupture, which are rare complications (ACOG, 2009a).

Tachysystole is defined as:

- Five or more UCs in 10 minutes over a 30-minute window
- A series of single UCs lasting 2 minutes or longer
- UCs occurring within 1 minute of each other
- Insufficient return of uterine resting tone between contractions via palpation or intraamniotic pressure above 25 mm Hg between contractions via IUPC

Nursing actions for tachysystole with Category I (normal) FHR pattern:

- Assist mother to a lateral position.
- Provide IV fluid bolus of at least 500 mL lactated Ringer's (unless contraindicated).
- If uterine activity has not returned to normal after 10 to 15 minutes, decrease oxytocin rate by at least half; if uterine activity has not returned to normal after 10 to 15 more minutes, discontinue oxytocin until uterine activity is normal.

Resume oxytocin after resolution of tachysystole. If oxytocin has been discontinued for less than 20 to 30 minutes, the FHR is normal, and the contraction frequency, intensity, and duration are normal, resume oxytocin at no more than half the rate that caused the tachysystole, and gradually increase the rate as appropriate based on unit protocol and maternal-fetal status. If the oxytocin is discontinued for more than 30 to 40 minutes, resume oxytocin at the initial dose ordered (Simpson & O'Brien-Abel, 2021).

Nursing actions for tachysystole with a Category II (indeterminate) or Category III (abnormal) FHR pattern would also include (Lyndon & Ali, 2008):

- Discontinue oxytocin and notify the provider.
- Assist with maternal repositioning (left or right lateral).
- Administer an IV fluid bolus of at least 500 mL lactated Ringer's (unless contraindicated).
- Give O_2 at 10 L/min by nonrebreather mask (discontinue as soon as possible based on the FHR pattern).
- Notify the provider of actions taken and maternal-fetal response.
- With category III FHR pattern, request an immediate bedside evaluation.
- Consider terbutaline if no response to above measures.

Resume oxytocin after resolution of tachysystole. If oxytocin has been discontinued for less than 20 to 30 minutes, the FHR is normal, and the contraction frequency, intensity, and duration are normal, resume oxytocin at no more than half the rate that caused the tachysystole, and gradually increase the rate as appropriate based on unit protocol and maternal-fetal status. If the oxytocin is discontinued for more than 30 to 40 minutes, resume oxytocin at the initial dose ordered (Simpson, 2020).

Normal UCs produce intermittent diminution of blood flow to the intervillous space where oxygen exchange occurs. The decreased intervillous blood flow associated with tachysystole ultimately leads to decreased oxygen transfer to the fetus (Simpson & James, 2008). When fetal oxygenation is sufficiently impaired to produce fetal metabolic acidosis from anaerobic glycolysis, direct myocardial depression occurs. If the intermittent interruption in blood flow caused by excessive uterine activity exceeds a critical level, the fetus responds with evolving hypoxia, acidosis, and ultimately asphyxia. Therefore, every effort should be made to avoid tachysystole and treat it appropriately when identified (Simpson & Knox, 2009). Waiting until the FHR is indeterminate or abnormal to treat tachysystole is not consistent with fetal safety (Simpson, 2020).

When tachysystole occurs during induced or augmented labor and the FHR pattern is normal, ACOG (2010) recommends decreasing oxytocin. If there are changes in the FHR pattern, further interventions such as discontinuation of oxytocin, maternal repositioning, and an IV fluid bolus should be considered (ACOG, 2010; Simpson, 2020). Simultaneous initiation of maternal repositioning, an IV fluid bolus, and discontinuation of oxytocin will usually resolve oxytocin-induced tachysystole within 6 to 10 minutes (Simpson & James, 2008).

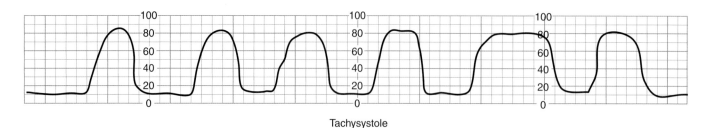

Tachysystole

FIGURE 10-3 Uterine tachysystole (hyperstimulation).

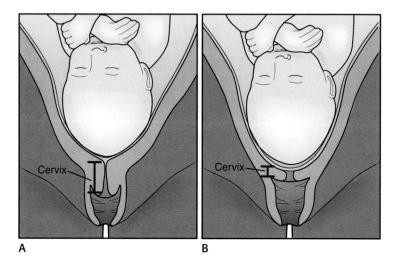

FIGURE 10-4 (A) Unripe cervix, cervix is not effaced or dilated. (B) Ripe cervix, cervix is 100% effaced and 1 cm dilated.

A   B

Cervical Ripening

Cervical ripening is the process of physical softening, thinning, and dilating of the cervix in preparation for labor and birth (Simpson, 2020). The cervix, composed of connective tissue, is typically closed until labor begins. At the onset of labor, it undergoes rapid changes, including ripening, effacement, and dilation (Fig. 10–4A and B).

Cervical ripening typically begins before the onset of labor contractions and is necessary for cervical dilation and the passage of the fetus. A series of complex biochemical processes, ending with rearrangement and realignment of the collagen molecules, allows the cervix to ripen. The cervix thins, softens, relaxes, and dilates in response to UCs, allowing the cervix to easily pass over the presenting fetal part during labor.

Because cervical status is the most important predictor of successful labor induction, it is crucial for cervical status to be assessed before beginning this process. Typically, cervical status is assessed via the Bishop score (Table 10-2). A Bishop score greater than 8 generally confers the same likelihood of vaginal delivery with induction of labor as that following spontaneous labor, and thus has been considered to indicate a favorable cervix (see Fig. 10–4A). Conversely, a Bishop score of 6 or less has been used to denote an unfavorable cervix in many studies and has been associated with a higher risk of cesarean delivery when labor is induced compared with spontaneous labor (Fig. 10–4B). A score of 6 or more is considered favorable for successful induction of labor. However, when the score is unfavorable (a Bishop score of less than 6), cervical ripening is usually considered.

A modified Bishop score is sometimes used to evaluate cervical status and includes three factors: fetal station, dilation of

TABLE 10-2 Bishop Score to Assess Cervical Ripeness

	0	1	2	3
Dilation cm	Closed	1–2	3–4	5–6
Effacement %	0–30	40–50	60–70	80
Station	–3	–2	–1,0	+1/+2
Consistency of cervix	Firm	Medium	Soft	___
Cervical position	Posterior	Midposition	Anterior	___

Bishop, 1964.

cervix, and length of cervix or cervical effacement (Grobman et al., 2018). Scores range from 1 to 12; less than 5 is considered an unripe cervix. A mechanical or pharmacological cervical ripening agent may be used and sometimes stimulates labor.

Mechanical Cervical Ripening

Mechanical cervical ripening methods are devices that are inserted through the vagina and into the cervix to promote cervical dilation. They are among the oldest methods to initiate labor. Pharmacological prostaglandins have partially replaced mechanical methods (Jozwiak et al., 2012). These methods have a lower risk of tachysystole compared with pharmacological methods. Examples of mechanical methods are:

- Hygroscopic dilators (laminaria, Lamicel, or Dilapan): Several products are available that are placed in the cervix to promote dilation by water absorption. Laminaria is made from dried seaweed. Commercial products, such as Dilapan and Lamicel, are produced from synthetic hygroscopic material. Several dilators are inserted into the cervix—as many as will fit—and they expand over 12 to 24 hours as they absorb water. Absorption of water from the cervical tissue leads to expansion of the dilators and opening of the cervix, which releases local prostaglandin. They function similarly as the balloon catheter. Women do not need prophylactic antibiotics for the balloon catheter or hygroscopic dilators, unless specific indications exist such as the need for subacute bacterial endocarditis prophylaxis. Today, they are used primarily during pregnancy termination rather than for cervical ripening in term pregnancies (Simpson, 2020).

- Transcervical balloon catheters: A Cook balloon or deflated Foley catheter (#16–#18, french, with a 30-mL balloon) is inserted into the extra-amniotic space and inflated above the internal os with 30 to 60 mL of sterile water. The inflated balloon is then retracted to rest against the internal os. This appears effective for preinduction, cervical ripening by causing direct pressure, overstretching of the lower uterine segment and cervix, and stimulating the release of local prostaglandin. The balloon catheter usually falls out when cervical dilation occurs. A double-balloon device designed for cervical ripening can be used (Simpson, 2020).

Indications

- When the woman has little or no cervical effacement
- When pharmacological methods are contraindicated, such as with prior uterine incision

Contraindications

- Active herpes
- Fetal malpresentation
- Nonreassuring fetal surveillance
- History of prior traumatic delivery
- Regular contractions
- Unexplained vaginal bleeding
- Placenta previa
- Vasa previa
- Prior uterine myomectomy involving the endometrial cavity or classical cesarean delivery

A history of a prior low transverse cesarean delivery was considered a contraindication to induction of labor. According to the ACOG Practice Bulletin on vaginal birth after previous cesarean delivery, induction of labor is not contraindicated in women with a prior low transverse cesarean delivery; however, use of prostaglandins should be avoided in these patients due to a significantly increased risk of uterine rupture. A relative contraindication to cervical ripening is ruptured membranes. No current evidence shows that cervical ripening followed by delayed induction of labor reduces the rate of cesarean delivery.

Risks Associated With Mechanical Cervical Ripening

- Higher infection rate
- Premature rupture of membranes (PROM)

Assessment Findings

- The cervix is unripe based on SVE and Bishop score.
- Prenatal record reflects indications for induction.

Medical Management

- The physician or midwife places the mechanical dilators, which usually stay in place for 6 to 12 hours before being removed by the care provider.

Nursing Actions

- Obtain informed consent following an informative discussion as to the procedure, and so on.
- Prepare the patient and assist with the insertion procedure.
- Instruct the patient that she might experience discomfort or cramping during insertion.
- Provide ongoing emotional and informational support and encourage relaxation.
- Record the type of dilator and number of dilators or the size of the balloon placed.
- Assess onset of UCs.
- Assess FHR.
- Assess maternal temperature, as the woman is at higher risk for infection.
- Assess for ROM and vaginal bleeding.
- Assess maternal and fetal status as per institutional policy.

Pharmacological Methods of Cervical Ripening

Pharmacological methods of cervical ripening in preparation for labor induction include a variety of hormonal preparations (Table 10-3). Agents available to induce cervical ripening include prostaglandin E2 (PGE2) preparations (dinoprostone, e.g., Prepidil gel or Cervidil insert) and prostaglandin E1 (PGE1) preparations (misoprostol, e.g., Cytotec). These preparations, which are placed in or near the cervix, produce cervical ripening by causing softening and thinning of the cervix. Occasionally these agents can stimulate labor contractions.

Indications

- See indications for induction in Table 10-2.

Risks Associated With Pharmacological Methods of Cervical Ripening

- Tachysystole of the uterus

Assessment Findings

- Unripe cervix based on SVE and Bishop score of 6 or less
- Prenatal record reflecting indication for induction

Medical Management

- Determine the need for cervical ripening.
  - The ACOG Committee on Obstetrics Practice recommends that misoprostol not be used to induce labor after previous cesarean section or major uterine surgery, due to a significant risk of uterine rupture.

TABLE 10-3   Pharmacological Cervical Ripening Agents

MEDICATION	CERVIDIL (DINOPROSTONE INSERT)	MISOPROSTOL PGE1 (CYTOTEC)
Dose	The Cervidil vaginal insert is a thin, flat, rectangular-shaped, cross-linked, polymer hydrogel that releases dinoprostone from a 10-mg reservoir.	25 micrograms (mcg) inserted in the posterior vaginal fornix Q3–6 hrs Not to exceed 50 mcg When used for cervical ripening or induction of labor, 25 mcg placed in the posterior vaginal fornix should be considered for the initial dose. Tachysystole and indeterminate or abnormal FHR changes have been associated with this medication. A recent review reports the possibility of rare but serious adverse events, particularly uterine rupture, with misoprostol use. Oral administration is not as effective. Oral administration is associated with fewer indeterminate or abnormal FHR patterns and episodes of tachysystole (ACOG, 2009a).
Nursing actions	Cervidil may be inserted by the perinatal nurse when the nurse has demonstrated competence in insertion, and the activity is within the scope of practice as defined by the state. The woman should remain in the supine or lateral position for 2 hours after insert. Continuous FHR and UC monitoring while medication is in place and for 15 minutes after removal. One major advantage of Cervidil is that the system can be easily and quickly removed in the event of uterine tachysystole or other complications. Oxytocin should be delayed for 30–60 minutes after removal.	Continuous FHR and UC monitoring. Oxytocin should be delayed until at least 4 hours after the last dose.
Contraindications	Not recommended for women with previous cesarean section or uterine scar.	Not recommended for women with previous cesarean section or uterine scar.
Actions	UCs after 5–7 hours, tachysystole can occur within 1 hour in up to 5% of patients. Remove if tachysystole or Category II or III FHR.	Wide variations in onset of UCs. Peak action 1–2 hours. Tachysystole more common with misoprostol than with prostaglandins or oxytocin.

Simpson, 2020; Simpson & O'Brien-Abel, 2021.

- Insert the pharmacological agent.
- Administration of the agent should be done at or near the labor and birthing unit.

Nursing Actions

- Obtain informed consent.
- Evaluate prenatal record for indications and contraindications for induction (see Box 10-2).
- Prostaglandin preparations for cervical ripening (e.g., misoprostol or vaginal insert) should be administered where FHR and uterine activity can be monitored continuously for an initial observation period (4 hours after intravaginal misoprostol and 2 hours after oral misoprostol). With the dinoprostone (Cervidil, PGE) vaginal insert, FHR and uterine activity should be monitored continuously while in place and for at least 15 minutes after removal.
- The major risk of the previously noted prostaglandin preparations is uterine hyperstimulation. The woman and fetus must be monitored for contractions, fetal well-being, and changes in the cervical Bishop score.

● Document baseline cervical exam and Bishop score with SVE.
● Obtain baseline FHR.
● Monitor FHR and uterine activity as indicated based on medication and institutional policies.

Sweeping or Stripping the Membranes

Sweeping or stripping the membranes involves digital separation of the chorionic membrane from the wall of the cervix and lower uterine segment during a vaginal exam done by a primary care provider to stimulate labor. The exact mechanism of action is unclear, but it is commonly believed it releases prostaglandins and may cause maternal oxytocin release. It is most effective in first-time pregnancies with an unripe cervix. Sweeping involves digital separation of the chorioamniotic membrane from the wall of the cervix and lower uterine segment by inserting a gloved finger beyond the internal cervical os and rotating the finger 360 degrees along the lower uterine segment. This can be performed during an office visit for a pregnant woman at 39 weeks' gestation or greater with a partially dilated cervix to hasten the onset of spontaneous labor.

Routine membrane stripping is not recommended given there is no evidence of improved maternal or neonatal outcomes. Manual separation of the amniotic membranes from the cervix is thought to induce cervical ripening and the onset of labor. The mechanism is unknown, but mechanical disruption of this tissue has been postulated to increase local prostaglandins by the induction of phospholipase A2 in the cervical and membrane tissues. Such a postulation is certainly consistent with the known stimulation of cervical ripening by prostaglandins. Membrane sweeping is associated with a decreased risk of late-term and post-term pregnancies. Although some studies of membrane sweeping have yielded conflicting results, the most recent Cochrane Review (Finucane et al., 2020) reports membrane sweeping is probably effective in increasing the likelihood of achieving a spontaneous onset of labor. When compared with expectant management, it potentially reduces the risk of formal induction of labor. Women report positive experiences as a method of preventing a formal induction of labor. Two small studies report that membrane sweeping potentially offers significant savings in health-care costs.

Women with late-term or post-term pregnancies who are considering membrane sweeping should be counseled that the procedure can be associated with vaginal bleeding and maternal discomfort. Contraindications to membrane sweeping include placenta previa and other contraindications to labor and vaginal delivery. There is insufficient data on the risks of membrane sweeping in women who are colonized with group B streptococci (GBS). Therefore, the decision to perform membrane sweeping in these women should be based on clinical judgment (ACOG, 2014b).

● The procedure is usually done in the care provider's office.
● The care provider is responsible for explaining the procedure and its risks.
● The FHR should be assessed before and after the procedure.
● The woman might experience some spotting after the procedure.
● The woman might experience mild cramping immediately after the procedure.

Indications

● See indications for oxytocin induction.

Risks Associated With Membrane Sweeping

● Infection
● Bleeding from undiagnosed placental problem
● The woman should call her maternity care provider or come to the hospital if the membranes rupture, bleeding occurs, fetal activity decreases, fever develops, regular contractions begin, or discomfort persists between UCs (Simpson, 2020).
● Unplanned ROM

Assessment Findings

● Intact membranes
● Presenting part engaged
● Term gestation

Amniotomy

Amniotomy, the artificial rupture of membranes (AROM), is used to induce or augment labor with an amnihook during an SVE (Fig. 10–5A and B). Amniotic fluid release increases the conversion of prostaglandins following the amniotomy. For women with normally progressing labor and no evidence of fetal compromise, routine amniotomy need not be undertaken unless required to facilitate monitoring (ACOG, 2019a).

Amniotomy is a common intervention in labor and may be used to facilitate fetal or intrauterine pressure monitoring. Amniotomy also may be used alone or in combination with oxytocin to treat slow labor progress. However, whether elective amniotomy is beneficial for women without a specific indication is now in question.

Amniotomy is most typically used to augment or shorten labor but may also be used to induce labor. There is insufficient

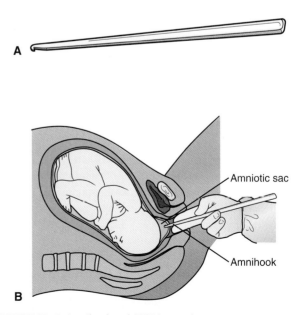

FIGURE 10–5 Amnihook and AROM procedure.

Amniotic sac

Amnihook

evidence to support the value of this as a sole intervention for induction (Bricker & Luckas, 2000). This procedure is done by the primary care provider and only if an emergency delivery can be performed nearby (Gilbert, 2011). It is most effective in multiparous women who are dilated to 2 cm or more. Amniotomy in early labor increases the risk of cesarean birth for abnormal FHR.

Indications

● To stimulate labor

Contraindications

● Fetal head not engaged in the maternal pelvis
● Maternal infection such as HIV, viral hepatitis, or active genital herpes

Risks Associated With Amniotomy

● Severe variable decelerations.
● Bleeding from undiagnosed vasa previa or other placental abnormality.
● Umbilical cord prolapse when presenting part is not engaged.
● Intraamniotic infection increases with duration of the rupture.
● A Cochrane Review of trials noted early intervention with amniotomy and oxytocin appears to be associated with a modest reduction in cesarean births (Wei et al., 2013).

Assessment Findings

● The woman leaks amniotic fluid vaginally.

Medical Management

● The procedure is done by the primary care provider with an SVE when the head is engaged in the pelvis.

Nursing Actions

● Assess the FHR before, during, and immediately following ROM because of the risk of umbilical cord prolapse.
● Offer comfort and support to the woman, as the procedure may be uncomfortable.
● Assess the color, amount, and odor of amniotic fluid.
● Monitor FHR and UC pattern.
● Document the time of the AROM as well as the indication for amniotomy; amount, color, and odor of amniotic fluid; FHR characteristics before amniotomy; fetal response after the procedure; cervical status; and fetal station.
● Assess maternal temperature every 4 hours or more frequently if signs and symptoms of infection occur.
● Administer pericare as the woman continues to leak fluid after AROM.
● Typically, nurses do not perform an amniotomy. However, there may be individual institutional policies allowing nurses to perform AROM under specific criteria.

External Cephalic Version

External cephalic version (ECV) refers to a procedure in which the fetus is rotated from the breech to the cephalic presentation by manipulation through the mother's abdomen (Fig. 10–6). The goal of ECV is to increase the proportion of vertex presentations among fetuses that were formerly in the breech position near term. Breech presentation occurs in approximately 3% to 4% of term pregnancies, and there is a high cesarean birth rate for breech presentation. Once a vertex presentation is achieved, the chances for a vaginal delivery increase. ECV provides a means of reducing cesarean births, but implementation of ECV varies, with an estimated 20% to 30% of eligible women not being offered ECV.

It is typically performed as an elective procedure in nonlaboring women at or near term to improve their chances of having a vaginal cephalic birth. Women most likely to opt for ECV are those who are well informed, encouraged to undergo the procedure, believe in its safety, and desire a vaginal birth. Women may choose not to undergo ECV because of fear of the procedure, incomplete information, and preference for scheduled cesarean delivery (ACOG, 2020a).

The effectiveness of ECV, estimated at about 65%, is based on its ability to increase the proportion of fetuses in cephalic presentation at birth and decrease the frequency of cesarean delivery (ACOG, 2020a). The procedure is done by the primary care provider only if an emergency delivery can be performed nearby (ACOG, 2020a).

Indications

● Breech presentation to reposition a fetus to vertex

Contraindications

● Placental abnormalities

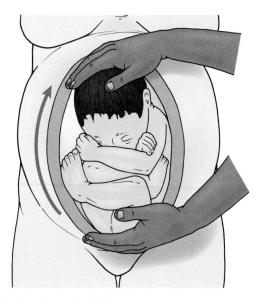

FIGURE 10–6 External cephalic version.

Risks Associated With ECV

- Adverse events after ECV have been reported and include abruptio placentae, umbilical cord prolapse, ROM, stillbirth, and fetomaternal hemorrhage; all occurred at rates of less than 1%.
- Severe variable decelerations are related to umbilical cord compression.

Assessment Findings

- Leopold's maneuver indicates nonvertex presentation and FHR may be located in the upper maternal abdomen.

Medical Management

- Before attempting ECV, an ultrasound is necessary to confirm the malpresentation of the fetus and rule out the presence of any anomalies that would complicate a vaginal delivery. Informed consent is needed and may include risks and benefits of the procedure as well as use of tocolysis and neuraxial analgesia if they are to be used for an ECV. Fetal well-being and contraction pattern should be assessed by a nonstress test or biophysical profile before and after the procedure. ECV should be attempted only in settings in which cesarean delivery services are readily available (ACOG, 2020a).
- The current recommendation for ECVs at term could reduce the need for cesarean delivery and prevent unnecessary prematurity at the expense of a potentially small increase in cesarean delivery risk.

Nursing Actions

- Fetal well-being and contraction pattern should be assessed by a nonstress test or biophysical profile before and after the procedure (ACOG, 2020a). Testing should continue for at least 30 minutes after the procedure. Anti-D immune globulin should be given to Rh-negative mothers who have no plans for delivery within 72 hours after ECV.
- Offer comfort and support to the woman, as the procedure may be uncomfortable.
- Evidence supports the use of parenteral tocolysis to improve the success of ECV.
- Neuraxial analgesia in combination with tocolytic therapy is now considered a reasonable intervention to increase the ECV success rate (ACOG, 2020a).
- ECV should be attempted only in settings in which cesarean delivery is readily available.

Labor Augmentation

Augmentation of labor is the stimulation of UCs when spontaneous contractions have failed to result in progressive cervical dilation or descent of the fetus (Simpson, 2020). Wide variations in labor progress and duration occur among women in labor, and there is no consensus among experts as to the appropriate length of labor. The terms *dystocia* and *failure to progress* are sometimes used to characterize an abnormally long labor. However, this diagnosis is often mistakenly made before the woman has entered the active phase of labor and, therefore, before an adequate trial of labor has been achieved. Some women have a cesarean birth because of "failure to progress in labor" for the diagnosis of lack of labor progress; yet, active labor has not begun or labor has not been abnormally long (ACOG, 2014c).

Many providers believe decreasing the length of labor through augmentation with oxytocin has benefits (Simpson, 2020). Data on augmentation are usually similar to the induction rate at about 20%, but other reports estimate about half the women laboring in the United States have artificial labor stimulation (AWHONN, 2014). Generally, maternal-fetal status and individual clinical situations are the basis for labor management decisions. According to the ACOG, contraindications to augmentation are similar as for labor induction and may include placenta or vasa previa, umbilical cord presentation, prior classical uterine incision, active genital herpes infection, pelvic structural deformities, or invasive cervical cancer. Labor augmentation is the stimulation of ineffective UCs after onset of spontaneous labor to manage labor dystocia. Principles of oxytocin induction apply to use of oxytocin for augmentation of labor.

Lower doses of oxytocin are required for augmentation of labor because cervical resistance is lower in women in labor who have some cervical effacement and dilation. This may not be indicated in induction protocols, as some protocols have been influenced by research on active management of labor (Box 10-3).

Indications

- To strengthen and regulate UCs
- To shorten the length of labor

Contraindications

- Any contraindications for vaginal birth
- Previous vertical (classical) uterine scar or prior transfundal uterine scar
- Placental abnormalities such as complete placenta previa or vasa previa
- Abnormal fetal position
- Umbilical cord prolapse
- Active genital herpes
- Pelvic abnormalities

Risks Associated With Augmentation

- Tachysystole leading to a Category II or Category III FHR pattern is a primary complication of oxytocin in labor.

Assessment Findings

- Prolonged labor
- Inadequate UCs and inadequate labor progress

Medical Management

- Determine the need for labor augmentation.
- Be available to respond to complications of using oxytocin to augment labor.

BOX 10-3 | Indications and Contraindications for Labor Augmentation

Indications

Augmentation refers to stimulation of UCs when spontaneous contractions have not resulted in progressive cervical dilation, or descent of the fetus. Expectations for labor progress should be based on the most recent data regarding what constitutes normal progress of labor, based on parity and other maternal factors.

- Before augmentation, assessment of maternal pelvis and cervix and fetal position, station, and well-being should be performed.
- Augmentation should be considered if the frequency of the contractions is less than 3 contractions per 10 minutes, or if the intensity of contractions is less than 25 mm Hg above baseline, or both.

Contraindications

Contraindications to augmentation of labor are the same or very similar to those for induction of labor and may include, but are not limited to, the following:

- Placenta or vasa previa
- Umbilical cord presentation
- Prior classical uterine incision
- Active genital herpes infection
- Pelvic structural deformities
- Invasive cervical cancer

Simpson, 2020.

Nursing Actions

- Administer low-dose oxytocin starting at 0.5 mU/min and increasing the dose by 1 to 2 mU/min every 30 to 60 minutes as recommended.
- Monitor FHR and UCs. FHR and UCs are typically continuously monitored, but intermittent monitoring is within the standard of care (see Chapter 9).
- Follow the same principles of nursing care for induction of labor.
- Decrease or discontinue oxytocin in the event of uterine tachysystole or Category II (indeterminate) or Category III (abnormal) FHR.

Complementary Therapies to Stimulate Labor

The use of complementary therapies is increasing as more and more women look to these methods during pregnancy and childbirth to be used instead of, or more commonly alongside, conventional medical practice. Acupuncture involves the insertion of very fine needles into specific points of the body.

Acupressure is using the thumbs or fingers to apply pressure to specific points. The limited observational studies to date suggest acupuncture for induction of labor has no known adverse effects to the fetus, and may be effective. However, the evidence regarding the clinical effectiveness of this technique is limited. A Cochrane Review concluded acupuncture does not appear to reduce the need for caesarean section but may improve the cervical readiness for labor (Smith et al., 2017). No evidence indicated benefit from acupressure in nonlaboring women. The main limitation of research reviewed was limited reporting of health outcomes. Acupuncture and acupressure appear safe and the review suggests some potential benefit, but the specific timing and how many treatments remain unclear.

Over decades, many strategies have been proposed to initiate or augment labor. Other practices include bowel stimulation with castor oil or an enema to increase prostaglandin production. Cochrane Reviews of complementary therapies indicate further research is needed to determine the effectiveness of most therapies to stimulate or induce labor (Kelly et al., 2013). Complementary therapies may include castor oil, herbal preparations such as black cohosh and evening primrose oil, or sexual intercourse.

OPERATIVE VAGINAL DELIVERY

Operative vaginal delivery is birth that is assisted by vacuum extraction or forceps. In the United States, about 3.1% of all deliveries are accomplished via an operative vaginal approach (Martin et al., 2017). Forceps deliveries accounted for 0.56% of vaginal births, and vacuum deliveries accounted for 2.58% of vaginal births. However, there is a wide range in the prevalence of operative vaginal delivery both across and within geographic regions in the United States (1% to 23%), which suggests that evidence-based guidelines for operative vaginal delivery are either inadequate or randomly applied, or familiarity and expertise with the technique is declining (Wegner & Bernstein, 2021).

Use of forceps and vacuum extraction continues to decline. Use of either method of instrumental delivery is decreasing to about 3% of births (down from 9.01% in 1990). Use of forceps remained steady in 2015 at less than 1%, compared with vacuum extraction at less than 3% (Martin et al., 2017). Since 1996, the rate of cesarean birth has increased and the percentage of operative vaginal deliveries with either forceps or vacuum extraction has decreased.

Indications for operative vaginal delivery are to improve maternal or fetal status by shortening the second stage of labor. Examples include maternal exhaustion and an inability to push effectively; medical indications such as maternal cardiac disease and a need to avoid pushing in the second stage of labor; prolonged second stage of labor, arrest of descent, or rotation of the fetal head; and nonreassuring FHR patterns in the second stage of labor. Operative vaginal birth is beneficial for women because it avoids cesarean birth and its associated morbidities (ACOG, 2020d).

For the fetus showing signs of possible compromise, successful operative vaginal birth can shorten the exposure to additional labor and reduce or prevent the effect of intrapartum insults. Often, operative vaginal birth can be safely accomplished more quickly than cesarean birth. Facilitating birth and shortening the second stage of labor can be performed only by care providers with hospital privileges for these procedures. Although sometimes indicated, operative vaginal birth is not without risk of complications to the woman and the fetus. Specific guidelines for the use of forceps and vacuum extraction are provided, and use of only one method, either forceps or vacuum, for an individual patient is recommended. If attempts are unsuccessful, the physician proceeds with a cesarean birth.

Although operative vaginal delivery is acceptable in appropriate circumstances, it requires an operator who understands the indications and prerequisites and is skilled in the technique. Operative vaginal birth should be performed only by experienced obstetricians and obstetric care providers with privileges for such procedures after the patient has agreed and been informed of the risks and benefits of the procedure. The provider must be able to perform emergency cesarean birth if operative vaginal birth is unsuccessful (ACOG, 2020d). The rate of failed operative vaginal birth is about 2.9% to 6.5% (ACOG, 2020d). Diminishing training and experience in operative vaginal delivery nationally is of concern (ACOG, 2020d; Spong et al., 2012).

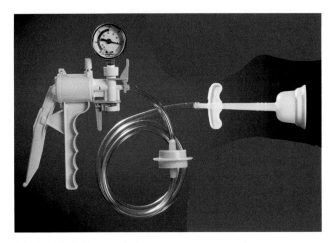

FIGURE 10–7 Vacuum device. *Source: © CooperSurgical.*

Vacuum-Assisted Delivery

Vacuum-assisted delivery or vacuum extraction is a birth involving the use of a vacuum cup on the fetal head to assist with delivery of the head (Fig. 10–7). The cup is placed on the fetal head and suction is increased gradually until a seal is formed. Gentle traction is then applied to deliver the fetal head (Fig. 10–8). Only gentle augmentation of the natural rotation that occurs with maternal pushing and fetal descent is recommended (ACOG, 2020d).

The rate of vacuum-assisted delivery, which increased by 77% between 1989 (3.5%) and 1997 (6.2%), has since decreased to below 3% (Martin et al., 2017). Some advantages to use of vacuum over forceps include:

● Easier application
● Less anesthesia required
● Less maternal soft tissue damage
● Fewer fetal injuries

Current guidelines for vacuum application are as follows:

● The fetal head needs to be engaged and the cervix completely dilated.
● Guidelines from the manufacturer should be followed regarding the specific suction cup device and policies should be in place for the use of vacuum to decrease clinical disagreements.
● Commonly the provider should make no more than three attempts for a period of 15 minutes: the "three-pull rule."
● Cup detachment from the fetal head (pops off the vacuum) is a warning sign that too much pressure or ineffective force is being exerted on the fetal head.

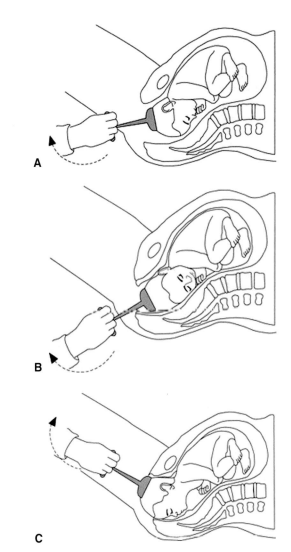

FIGURE 10–8 Vacuum delivery. *Source: © CooperSurgical.*

● The physician should proceed with cesarean birth when vacuum attempts are not successful.
● Vacuum birth is contraindicated if the fetal head is not engaged in the maternal pelvis, if the position of the vertex cannot be determined, or it is less than 34 weeks' gestation.

Indications

- Suspicion of immediate or potential fetal compromise
- Need to shorten the second stage for maternal benefit
- Prolonged second stage
  - Nulliparous woman with lack of continuing progress for 3 hours with regional anesthesia, or for 2 hours without anesthesia
  - Multiparous woman with lack of continuous progress for 2 hours with regional anesthesia, or for 1 hour without regional anesthesia (ACOG, 2015)

Risks for the Woman

- Vaginal and cervical lacerations; vacuum extractor use has been associated with a twofold increased risk of third- and fourth-degree perineal tears compared with patients who had a spontaneous delivery (ACOG, 2020d)
- Extension of episiotomy
- Hemorrhage related to uterine atony or uterine rupture
- Bladder trauma
- Perineal wound infection

Risks for the Newborn

- Traction applied to the fetal scalp with the vacuum can result in laceration, cephalohematoma formation (15%), and subgaleal or intracranial hemorrhage or retinal hemorrhages; increased rates of hyperbilirubinemia also have been reported.
- Cephalohematoma (Fig. 10–9) is more likely as the duration of vacuum application increases.

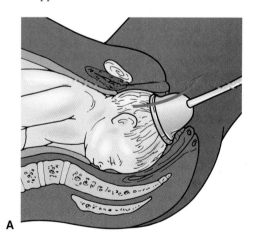

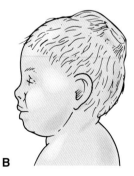

FIGURE 10–9 Cephalohematoma.

Assessment Findings

- Cervix fully dilated and retracted
- Membranes ruptured
- Engagement of the fetal head
- Position of the fetal head has been determined
- Fetal weight estimation performed
- Pelvis thought to be adequate for vaginal birth
- Adequate anesthesia
- Maternal bladder has been emptied
- Patient has agreed after being informed of the risks and benefits of the procedure
- Fetus at greater than 34 weeks' gestation and the fetal head is engaged, at least 0 station in the maternal pelvis (Cunningham et al., 2018)

Medical Management

- Explain the procedure and obtain the woman's consent.
- Place the vacuum appropriately.
- Routine use of episiotomy is no longer recommended because of prolonged healing, increased pain, and potential for third- and fourth-degree tears (ACOG, 2020d).
- After three unsuccessful attempts, proceed with a cesarean birth.
- The recommendations of the manufacturer of the vacuum device should be followed.
- Documentation of fetal station, duration of application, pressure, and number of pulls and pop-offs should be included in the medical record by the provider performing the procedure.

Nursing Actions

- Assess the woman's anesthesia level and comfort level.
- Urinary bladder may be emptied by provider or nurse to decrease risk of trauma.
- Educate and reassure the woman and her family.
- Anticipate potential complications for the woman and the newborn. Nurses should also be aware of potential complications related to the use of vacuums and observe both the mother and baby for associated signs and symptoms.
- Pump up the vacuum manually per the manufacturer guidelines to the pressure indicated on the pump, not to exceed 500 to 600 mm Hg.
  - Cup detachment (pop-off) is a warning sign that too much ineffective force is being exerted on the fetal head.
- Pressure should be released between contractions.
- The nurse may indicate in the medical record that vacuum-assisted birth was performed as well as any related nursing interventions. Responsibility for the documentation of station, the position before application of the vacuum and the complete procedure, rests with the provider who performs the operative birth (Simpson & O'Brien-Abel, 2021).
- The vacuum procedure should be timed from insertion of the cup into the vagina until the birth, and the cup should not be on the fetal head for longer than 15 to 20 minutes.
  - Adherence to the guidelines for the vacuum device related to pressure and maximum time will minimize nurse liability in vacuum-assisted vaginal births.

Forceps-Assisted Delivery

Forceps-assisted birth is one in which an instrument is used to assist with delivery of the fetal head, typically done to improve the health of the woman or the fetus. The rate of forceps delivery has decreased over the last 20 years from 5.55% to only 1% (Martin et al., 2011). Outlet forceps are used when the head is visible on the perineum and the skull has reached the pelvic floor, and rotation is less than 45 degrees (Fig. 10–10). Low forceps are used when the skull is at +2 station or lower in the maternal pelvis and not on the pelvic floor, and rotation is greater than 45 degrees (Fig. 10–11). Without rotation: Rotation is 45 degrees or less (right or left occiput anterior to occiput anterior, or right or left occiput posterior to occiput posterior). With rotation: Rotation is greater than 45 degrees. Midforceps is when the station is above +2 cm but the head is engaged. Typically, only outlet and low forceps are currently recommended for use in assisting delivery. Midforceps and rotational forceps deliveries may be appropriate in select clinical circumstances (ACOG, 2020d).

Indications

- The fetal head is engaged and the cervix completely dilated. Operative vaginal birth is contraindicated if the fetal head is not engaged in the maternal pelvis or the position of the vertex cannot be determined.

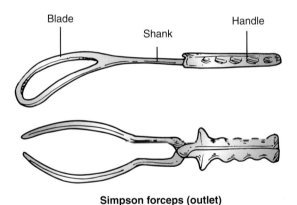

Simpson forceps (outlet)

FIGURE 10–10 Outlet forceps.

- There is suspicion of immediate or potential fetal compromise.
- This is used to shorten the second stage for maternal benefit (maternal exhaustion or fetal compromise).
- Prolonged second stage:
  - Nulliparous woman with lack of continuing progress for 3 hours with regional anesthesia, or for 2 hours without anesthesia
  - Multiparous woman with lack of continuous progress for 2 hours with regional anesthesia, or for 1 hour without regional anesthesia
- High level of regional anesthesia inhibits pushing.
- Maternal cardiac or pulmonary disease contraindicates pushing efforts.

Risks for the Woman

- Vaginal and cervical lacerations; forceps use is associated with a sixfold increase in the risk of third- and fourth-degree perineal tears compared with patients who had a spontaneous delivery.
- Extension of episiotomy
- Hemorrhage related to uterine atony and uterine rupture
- Perineal hematoma
- Bladder trauma
- Perineal wound infection

Risks for the Newborn

- Reported injuries have included facial lacerations and facial nerve palsy, corneal abrasions and external ocular trauma, skull fracture, and intracranial hemorrhage.

Assessment Findings

- Cervix fully dilated and retracted
- Membranes ruptured
- Engagement of the fetal head
- Position of the fetal head has been determined
- Fetal weight estimation performed
- Pelvis thought to be adequate for vaginal birth
- Adequate anesthesia
- Maternal bladder has been emptied

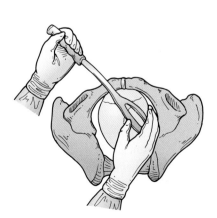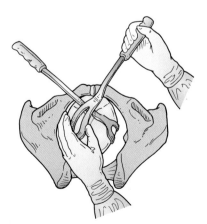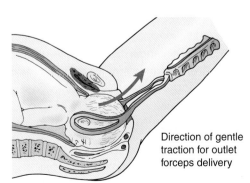

Direction of gentle traction for outlet forceps delivery

FIGURE 10–11 Forceps delivery.

Medical Management

- Use only on a fetus that is at least 34 weeks' gestation (ACOG, 2015).
- Explain the procedure and obtain the woman's consent.
- Routine use of episiotomy is no longer recommended because of prolonged healing, increased pain, and potential for third- and fourth-degree tears (ACOG, 2020d).
- Place forceps appropriately.
- Complete documentation of the operative birth procedure rests with the provider who performed the procedure.

Nursing Actions

- Assess the woman's anesthesia level and comfort level.
- Insert a straight catheter to empty the bladder to decrease the risk of bladder trauma and increase room for the fetal head and forceps.
- Provide emotional support for the woman and her partner, since use of forceps can increase anxiety level.
- Document the type of forceps, number of applications, and time of application.
- Anticipate potential complications for the woman and the neonate. Nurses should be aware of potential complications related to the use of forceps and vacuums and observe both the mother and baby for associated signs and symptoms.

OPERATIVE BIRTH

In 2019, the U.S. cesarean delivery rate remained stable at 31.7% (Martin et al., 2021). Between 1970 and 2016, the cesarean rate increased from 5% to 31.9%, peaking in 2009 at 32.9% after increasing every year since 1996. That means one in three women who give birth in the United States do so by cesarean delivery. Cesarean birth can be lifesaving for the fetus, the mother, or both in certain cases. However, the rapid increase in cesarean birth rates in the past decades without clear evidence of decreases in maternal or neonatal morbidity or mortality raises significant concern that cesarean delivery is overused. Current guidance from the American College of Obstetricians and Gynecologists and the Society for Maternal-Fetal Medicine recommends that if the maternal and fetal status allow, cesarean births for failed induction of labor in the latent phase can be avoided by allowing longer durations of the latent phase (up to 24 hours or longer) and requiring that oxytocin be administered for at least 12 to 18 hours after membrane rupture before deeming the induction a failure (ACOG, 2014c). Because the needs and experiences of cesarean birth couples are distinctly different from those of couples who experience a vaginal birth, Chapter 11 is devoted to care of women who have cesarean births and their families (Figure 10–12).

Vaginal Birth After a Cesarean

The vaginal birth after a cesarean (VBAC) rate measures vaginal births among women who had a previous cesarean delivery. In 2018, 13.3% of women with a previous cesarean delivered vaginally, up 4% from 12.8% in 2017 (Martin et al., 2019). A trial

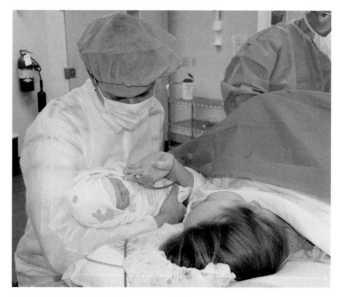

FIGURE 10–12 Family in cesarean birth.

of labor after cesarean (TOLAC) offers women the opportunity to achieve a VBAC. Evidence suggests that benefits of VBAC outweigh risks in women with lower uterine transverse cesarean birth who have no contraindications for a vaginal birth.

In addition to providing an option for those who want to experience a vaginal birth, VBAC is associated with several potential health advantages for women. For example, women who achieve VBAC avoid major abdominal surgery; have lower rates of hemorrhage, thromboembolism, and infection; and have shorter recovery than women who have an elective repeat cesarean delivery). For those considering future pregnancies, VBAC may decrease the risk of maternal consequences related to multiple cesarean deliveries (e.g., hysterectomy, bowel or bladder injury, transfusion, infection, and abnormal placentation such as placenta previa and placenta accreta [ACOG,2019d]).

According to the ACOG, most women with one previous cesarean birth with a low transverse incision are candidates for vaginal birth after cesarean birth and should be counseled about VBAC and offered a trial of labor (ACOG, 2019d). This is reportedly related to more conservative ACOG practice guidelines, legal pressure, and the continuing debate over the harms and benefits of vaginal birth compared with cesarean birth and an increase in repeat cesarean births. VBAC is associated with a small but important risk of uterine rupture (less than 1%), which increases with each additional cesarean birth. Nurses should know these important definitions regarding VBAC delivery:

- A TOLAC is a planned attempt to labor by a woman who has previously undergone a cesarean delivery and desires a subsequent vaginal delivery.
- A VBAC is a "successful" trial of labor resulting in a vaginal birth.
- A TOLAC may result in either a "successful" VBAC or a "failed" trial of labor, resulting in a repeat cesarean delivery.
- A repeat cesarean delivery may be planned and scheduled beforehand and thus is an elective repeat cesarean delivery. If the woman who plans an elective repeat cesarean delivery enters

spontaneous labor before the scheduled date, this is still considered an elective repeat cesarean delivery even if delivery is unscheduled. The woman with a failed TOLAC undergoes a repeat cesarean delivery that is unplanned and unscheduled.

Benefits of VBAC

The benefits of a TOLAC resulting in a VBAC include the following:

- Shorter hospital stays and postpartum recovery in most cases
- Fewer complications, such as postpartum fever, wound or uterine infection, thromboembolism (blood clots in the leg or lung), and need for blood transfusion
- Fewer neonatal breathing problems

Risks of VBAC

The risks of an attempted VBAC or TOLAC include:

- Risk of failed TOLAC; however, 60% to 80% of TOLAC are successful VBACs.
- Risk of rupture of the uterus, resulting in an emergency cesarean delivery. Common sequelae associated with uterine rupture includes excessive hemorrhage requiring surgical exploration; the need for hysterectomy; the need for blood product transfusion; hypovolemia; hypovolemic shock; injury to the bladder or ureters; bowel laceration; extrusion of any part of the fetus, cord, or placenta through the disruption; emergent cesarean birth for suspected rupture; emergent cesarean birth for indeterminate or abnormal fetal status; and general anesthesia. Many women with uterine rupture experience more than one of these complications (Simpson & O'Brien-Abel, 2021).
- Risks to the baby associated with uterine rupture are significant and can be catastrophic: Hypoxemia, neurologic depression, pathologic fetal acidosis, seizures, asphyxia, hypoxic ischemic encephalopathy, cerebral palsy, and death (Simpson & O'Brien-Abel, 2021).
- The risk of uterine rupture may be related in part to the type of uterine incision made during the first cesarean delivery. A previous transverse uterine incision has the lowest risk of rupture (less than 1%). Vertical or T-shaped uterine incisions have a higher risk of uterine rupture (4% to 9%). Remember that the direction of the skin incision does not indicate the type or direction of the uterine incision; a woman with a transversal (bikini) skin incision may have a vertical uterine incision.
- Although women who attempt TOLAC and VBAC have a low risk of uterine rupture, the risk of uterine rupture is higher with VBAC than with RCD.
- The risk of fetal death is very low with both VBAC and ERCD, but the likelihood of fetal death is higher with VBAC than ERCD. Maternal death is very rare with either delivery.

Candidates for TOLAC and VBAC

- Both ACOG (2019d) and the National Institutes of Health (NIH; 2010) suggest that a TOLAC to attempt a VBAC is an acceptable option for a woman who has undergone one prior cesarean delivery with a low transverse uterine incision, assuming there are no other conditions that would normally require a cesarean delivery such as placenta previa.
- ACOG further suggests that a woman with two prior low transverse uterine incisions, or a woman with a twin pregnancy, or a woman who requires induction of labor may also be considered candidates for VBAC with appropriate counseling.
- TOLAC with anticipated VBAC should be attempted only in those facilities capable of performing emergency cesarean deliveries and those with an appropriate nursing staff, anesthesia team, operating room, and obstetrician or other surgeon immediately available in case an emergency cesarean delivery becomes necessary.
- A woman considering VBAC should discuss with her health-care provider the risks and benefits of VBAC versus elective repeat cesarean delivery, and the discussion should include plans for intervention in case of uterine rupture or another indication for an emergency cesarean delivery.
- Unlike most medical decisions in which patients are comparing risks and benefits for themselves, the pregnant patient must compare risks and benefits for both herself and her fetus, and the risks and benefits for these two individuals sometimes do not align. A decision that increases maternal risk may be associated with fetal benefit.
- Good, consistent evidence exists indicating that a woman who has had only one previous cesarean delivery using a transverse lower segment hysterotomy incision has the lowest risk of uterine scar separation during a subsequent trial of labor; thus, TOLAC is a reasonably safe option for delivery for these women. In this setting, the body of evidence suggests a TOLAC success rate of 60% to 80%, with an estimated uterine rupture rate of less than 1%. Success rates are higher in patients with additional characteristics, such as a prior vaginal delivery (Cunningham & Wells, 2017).

Management During Labor

In many ways, a woman who attempts VBAC is managed similarly to other women anticipating vaginal delivery. A fetal monitor may be used to observe the baby's heart rate and detect early signs of fetal distress. Medications to induce labor or improve contractions (e.g., oxytocin) are used cautiously since they can increase risk of uterine rupture. If problems occur during labor, a cesarean delivery will likely be recommended. Waiting for spontaneous labor, thus avoiding cervical ripening agents and oxytocin, appears to significantly decrease the risk of uterine rupture for women attempting VBAC. ACOG supports the use of oxytocin for induction and augmentation of labor in women with a previous cesarean delivery. Misoprostol (PGE1) should not be used for cervical ripening or labor induction in the third trimester in women with prior uterine incisions, and use of other prostaglandins is also strongly discouraged.

Consistent with the principle of respect for patient autonomy, patients should be allowed to accept increased levels of risk; however, women should be clearly informed of the potential increases in risk and management alternatives (ACOG, 2019d, Simpson & O'Brien-Abel, 2021). Evaluation of a patient's individual likelihood of VBAC and risk of uterine rupture are central to these considerations. Because of the risks associated with TOLAC, and because uterine rupture and other complications may be unpredictable, ACOG recommends that TOLAC be attempted in facilities that can provide cesarean delivery for situations that are immediate threats to the life of the woman or fetus. When resources for emergency cesarean delivery are not available, ACOG recommends that care providers and women considering TOLAC discuss the hospital's resources and availability of obstetric, pediatric, anesthesiology, and operating room staffs.

VBAC Success Rates

In general, 60% to 80% of women considered candidates for a TOLAC who attempt a VBAC will have a successful vaginal birth (Cunningham & Wells, 2017). Factors that increase the chances for a successful VBAC include:

- A previous vaginal delivery, especially a previous VBAC
- Spontaneous onset of labor (labor is not induced)
- Normal progress of labor, including dilation and effacement (thinning) of the cervix
- Prior cesarean delivery performed because the baby's position was abnormal (e.g., breech)
- Only one prior cesarean delivery
- The prior cesarean delivery was performed early in labor, and not after full cervical dilation.
- Factors that negatively influence the likelihood of VBAC include the first cesarean delivery was performed because of an arrest of labor disorder, use of labor induction or augmentation, increasing maternal age, high BMI, high birth weight, and more than 40 weeks' gestation.

Indications

- Experts suggest a TOLAC to attempt a VBAC is an acceptable option for a woman who has undergone one prior cesarean delivery with a low transverse uterine incision.
- Guidelines also suggest that a woman with two prior low transverse uterine incisions, a woman with a twin pregnancy, or a woman who requires induction of labor may also be considered candidates for VBAC with appropriate counseling.
- One or two TOLAC with anticipated VBAC should be attempted only in those facilities capable of performing emergency cesarean.
- Clinically adequate pelvis is desired.
- Physician and OR team are immediately available to perform emergent cesarean birth.

Contraindications

- Those at high risk of uterine rupture (e.g., those with a previous classical or T-incision, prior uterine rupture, or extensive transfundal uterine surgery) (Fig. 10–13)
- Pelvic abnormalities

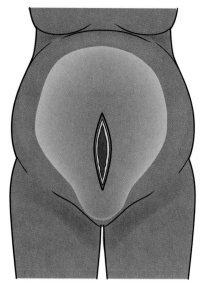

FIGURE 10–13 Vertical uterine incision.

- Medical or obstetric complications that preclude a vaginal birth
- Inability to perform an emergent cesarean birth if necessary, because of insufficient personnel such as surgeons, anesthesia, or facility
- Those in whom vaginal delivery is otherwise contraindicated (e.g., those with placenta previa) are not generally candidates for planned TOLAC.
- Because of the unpredictability of complications requiring emergency medical care, home birth is contraindicated for women undergoing TOLAC (ACOG, 2019d).

Risks Associated With VBAC

- Uterine rupture and complications associated with uterine rupture (1%)
  - Waiting for spontaneous labor and avoiding use of prostaglandins and oxytocin reduces the risk of uterine rupture.
- A failed TOLAC is associated with more complications than elective repeat cesarean delivery.
- Uterine rupture or dehiscence is the outcome associated with TOLAC that most significantly increases the chance of additional maternal and neonatal morbidity.
- Neonatal morbidity is higher in the setting of a failed TOLAC than in a VBAC.

Assessment Findings

- Records confirm prior transverse uterine scar.

Medical Management

- Explain the risks and benefits of VBAC.
- Induction of labor for maternal or fetal indications remains an option in women undergoing TOLAC.
- Use of misoprostol for cervical ripening is contraindicated.
- The physician and surgical team must be available to perform a cesarean birth if necessary.

Nursing Actions

- Review the prenatal record for documentation of prior uterine scar because VBAC is contraindicated in vertical uterine incisions.
- Closely and continuously monitor uterine activity and FHR.
- Assess the progress of labor.
- Provide information, reassurance, and support to the woman.
- Report any complaints of severe pain and be alert to signs of uterine rupture such as vaginal bleeding and ascending station of fetal presenting part.

OBSTETRIC COMPLICATIONS

Complications during birth can emerge abruptly without warning or risk factors. More often, they result from pregnancy-associated or preexisting risks. Regardless, women experiencing complications in labor and birth need special attention and support provided by nurses in the perinatal setting.

Pregnancy-Related Complications in Labor

Most pregnancy-related complications have the potential to impact labor. For example, diabetic women in labor need continuous glucose monitoring because hyperglycemia impacts placental perfusion. Another example is preeclampsia, where vasospasm related to the pathophysiology of preeclampsia also diminishes perfusion and impacts both maternal and fetal outcomes. Refer to Chapter 7 for management and care of patients with these disorders. Several pregnancy-related complications are presented here as examples.

CRITICAL COMPONENT

Nursing Care and Support for Birth Complications

Perinatal nurses can have a profound influence on the labor and birth care provided in the hospital setting, thereby influencing birth outcomes (Adams et al., 2016). Ideally, a hospital perinatal nurse is present with a family for the entire labor and birth process. In a high-risk pregnancy, the woman and her family may be known to the nurses, and the same nurse may care for the woman over several days. In this situation, the nurse can form a stronger bond with the patient and enhance trust and therapeutic communication through continuity of care.

Nurses are responsible for assessing maternal and fetal well-being; administering procedures and monitoring their effectiveness; providing nursing interventions to assist with a laboring woman's physical, emotional, and spiritual needs; rendering care related to the birth process, whether vaginal or cesarean; initiating newborn care; and providing care during the early postpartum period. Perinatal nurses also advocate and teach women during the birth process, communicate with health-care providers, and document care (Adams et al., 2016).

When a woman develops complications in labor or during birth, she experiences increased fear and anxiety for herself and her baby. Effective therapeutic communication with the woman and her family is essential and may help the woman remain an active decision maker. Women experiencing complications or emergencies need ongoing information they can understand, reassurance, and physical, emotional, and spiritual support to help them navigate the sometimes treacherous path of labor and birth.

The complexity of communication between mothers and health-care team members during labor and birth increases the potential for error and safety issues. The combination of physiological, emotional, relational, and contextual factors that influence labor contribute to the challenge of communication, and nuanced and quickly evolving situations make it more difficult to maintain the shared understanding necessary for successful teamwork. Unrecognized differences in clinical goals and divergent understandings of risks and benefits may increase safety threats (Jacobson et al., 2013).

Post-Term Pregnancy and Birth

Post-term pregnancy refers to a pregnancy that has reached or gone beyond 42 weeks' gestation, dated from the last menstrual period; a late-term pregnancy reaches between 41 0/7 weeks and 41 6/7 weeks of gestation. In 2018, the incidence of post-term pregnancy in the United States was less than 1% and has decreased steadily over the prior 5 years. The late-term birth rate is less than 6% and decreasing (Martin et al., 2019).

The incidence of post-term pregnancies may vary by population, in part as a result of differences in regional management practices for pregnancies that go beyond the estimated date of delivery. Accurate determination of gestational age is essential for accurate diagnosis and appropriate management of late-term and post-term pregnancies. Antepartum fetal surveillance and induction of labor have been evaluated as strategies to decrease the risks of perinatal morbidity and mortality associated with late-term and post-term pregnancies (ACOG, 2014b). The etiology of most pregnancies that are late-term or post-term is unknown. However, several risk factors for post-term pregnancy have been identified, including nulliparity, prior post-term pregnancy, carrying a male fetus, and maternal obesity (ACOG, 2014b).

Postmaturity refers to the abnormal condition of the newborn resulting from prolonged pregnancy. Both the woman and infant are at increased risk of adverse events when the pregnancy continues beyond term. After 41 weeks, risk of neonatal and postneonatal death increases significantly (ACOG, 2014b; Gülmezoglu et al., 2006). ACOG (2014b) concludes that induction of labor between 41 0/7 and 42 0/7 weeks can be considered and induction of labor after 42 0/7 weeks and by 42 6/7 weeks of gestation is recommended based on evidence of an increase in perinatal morbidity and mortality.

The risk of stillbirth increases beyond 41 weeks. Additional fetal risks of post-term pregnancies include macrosomia, which increases the likelihood of operative vaginal deliveries, cesarean deliveries, and shoulder dystocia, as well as neonatal seizures, meconium aspiration syndrome (MAS), and low 5-minute Apgar scores. Oligohydramnios is more common in post-term pregnancies and has been associated with cord compression, FHR abnormalities, meconium-stained amniotic fluid, and fetal acidosis. Maternal risks are generally those associated with macrosomia and related dysfunctional labors, including severe perineal lacerations, infection, and postpartum hemorrhage:

- Induction of labor with an unfavorable cervix
- Cesarean birth
- Prolonged labor
- Postpartum hemorrhage
- Traumatic birth

Some of these unwanted outcomes likely result from intervening when the uterus and cervix are not ready for labor. First-trimester pregnancy ultrasound is associated with a reduced incidence of post-term pregnancy, possibly by avoiding incorrect dating and misclassification of postdates. Induction of labor is widely practiced to try to prevent the previously mentioned problems and to improve the health outcome for women and their infants.

- Labor induction may itself cause problems, especially when the cervix is not ripe.
- The ideal timing for induction of labor is not clear. In the past, there was a tendency to await spontaneous labor until 42 completed weeks.
- Current practice is to offer induction of labor between 41 and 42 weeks. Data indicating an increased risk of stillbirth at or beyond 41 weeks' gestation and initiation of antepartum fetal surveillance at or beyond 41 weeks' gestation is common (ACOG, 2014b).
- The gestational age and the cervix being unfavorable (unripe) may affect the success of the induction of labor and result in an increase in cesarean birth rates.
- When the cervix is favorable (usually a Bishop score of 6 or more), induction is often carried out via oxytocin and AROM.
- If the cervix is not favorable, usually a prostaglandin gel or tablet is placed in the vagina or cervix to ripen the cervix and to initiate the UCs and labor. Many protocols are used with varying repeat intervals and transition to oxytocin and amniotomy depending on the onset of UCs and progress of cervical dilation.

Risks to the Mother

Risks to the mother are related to the larger size of post-term fetuses and include difficulties during labor, an increase in injury to the perineum (including the vagina, labia, and rectum), and an increased rate of cesarean birth with its associated risks of bleeding, infection, and injury to surrounding organs (Norwitz, 2017). Obstetric complications are more likely with increased gestational age, and risks of severe perineal laceration, infection, postpartum hemorrhage, and cesarean delivery increase in women with late-term and post-term pregnancies. In addition, some studies suggest that maternal anxiety increases as post-term approaches (ACOG, 2014b).

Because late-term and post-term pregnancies are associated with an increased risk of perinatal morbidity and mortality, induction of labor between 41 and 42 weeks' gestation may be considered. Induction of labor after 42 0/7 weeks and by 42 6/7 weeks of gestation is recommended given evidence of an increase in perinatal morbidity and mortality (ACOG, 2014b). Initiation of antepartum fetal surveillance at or beyond 41 weeks' gestation may be indicated, and a trial of labor after cesarean delivery is an option for uncomplicated post-term pregnancies (ACOG, 2014b).

Risks to the Fetus

- Stillbirth or neonatal death: The incidence of stillbirth or infant death is increased in pregnancies that continue beyond 42 weeks. However, the risk is relatively small, with only four to seven deaths per 1,000 deliveries. By comparison, the risk of stillbirth or infant death in pregnancies between 37 and 42 weeks is two to three per 1,000 deliveries.
- Macrosomia: Post-term fetuses have a greater chance of developing complications related to larger body size (macrosomia), which is defined as weighing more than 4,500 grams, or about 10 pounds. There is a twofold increase in macrosomia believed to contribute to the increased risks of operative vaginal delivery, cesarean delivery, and shoulder dystocia observed in post-term pregnancies.
- Fetal dysmaturity: Also called post-maturity syndrome, this refers to a fetus whose growth in the uterus after the due date has been restricted, usually due to a problem with delivery of placental blood flow to the fetus. Post-maturity syndrome complicates 10% to 20% of post-term pregnancies. Post-mature fetuses have decreased subcutaneous fat and lack vernix and lanugo. Meconium staining of the amniotic fluid, skin, membranes, and umbilical cord often is seen in association with a post-mature newborn.
- Oligohydramnios: This occurs more frequently in post-term pregnancies than in pregnancies at less than 42 weeks' gestation. Oligohydramnios increases the risk of FHR abnormalities, umbilical cord compression, meconium-stained fluid, umbilical cord artery blood pH of less than 7, and lower Apgar scores (ACOG, 2014b). Oligohydramnios has been commonly defined as a single deep vertical pocket of amniotic fluid of 2 cm or less (not containing umbilical cord or fetal extremities) or an amniotic fluid index of 5 cm or less.
- Meconium aspiration: Beyond term, the fetus is more likely to have a bowel movement, called meconium, into the amniotic fluid. A stressed fetus may inhale some of this meconium-stained amniotic fluid; this can cause breathing problems when the baby is born.
- Prolonged pregnancy: This results in a decrease in amniotic fluid volume and may impact fetal status because amniotic fluid cushions the fetus and cord from pressure and injury and amniotic fluid volume is an indicator of placental function.
- Decreased placental reserve: This occurs as the placenta begins to age, as there are increased areas of infarction and deposition of calcium and fibrin within its tissue (Fig. 10–14).

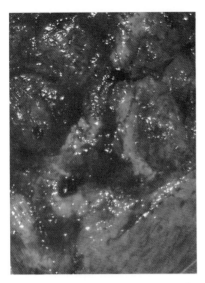

FIGURE 10–14 Calcified placenta are white areas in the placenta.

- Meconium-stained fluid: This occurs in 25% to 30% of post-term pregnancies and creates an increased risk for meconium aspiration of the neonate at birth.
- Fetal macrosomia: There is an increased risk for this as the fetus increases in size, approximately 1 ounce per day after term.

Assessment Findings

- Category II or III FHR related to decreased amniotic fluid and uteroplacental insufficiency
- Pregnancy with aging placenta
- Meconium-stained fluid
- Women report increased anxiety and frustration with prolonged pregnancy
- Fetal macrosomia

Medical Management

- Antenatal surveillance
- Induction of labor offered at 41 weeks' gestation

Nursing Actions

- Review the plan of care with the woman.
- Confirm prolonged pregnancy on the prenatal record.
- Anticipate management with induction of labor and possible cervical ripening agents.
- Monitor FHR because of increased incidence of uteroplacental insufficiency.
- Assess amniotic fluid for amount and meconium staining with ROM (see Concept Map for post-term pregnancy and labor induction).

Meconium-Stained Fluid and Birth

In 10% to 20% of deliveries, meconium enters the amniotic fluid. In utero, meconium passage results from neural stimulation of a maturing gastrointestinal (GI) tract, usually due to fetal hypoxic stress. As the fetus approaches term, the GI tract matures, and vagal stimulation from head or spinal cord compression may cause peristalsis and relaxation of the rectal sphincter, leading to meconium passage. Meconium-stained amniotic fluid may be aspirated by the fetus before or during labor and delivery. Aspiration of meconium results in respiratory distress that in severe cases can be life-threatening. There is strong suggestive evidence that prevention of meconium aspiration, by its removal from the respiratory tract, can ameliorate or prevent most cases of severe MAS. This aspiration induces hypoxia via four major pulmonary effects: airway obstruction, surfactant dysfunction, chemical pneumonitis, and pulmonary hypertension (Geis, 2017).

Risks Associated With Meconium-Stained Fluid

- MAS in the neonate

Assessment Findings

- Meconium-stained amniotic fluid

Medical Management

- Infants with meconium-stained amniotic fluid, regardless of whether they are vigorous or not, should no longer routinely receive intrapartum suctioning (ACOG, 2017a).
- Resuscitation should follow the same principles for infants with meconium-stained fluid as for those with clear fluid.

Nursing Actions

- Alert the neonatal team, as meconium-stained amniotic fluid is a condition that requires notification and availability of an appropriately credentialed team with full resuscitation skills, including endotracheal intubation.
- Gentle clearing of meconium from the mouth and nose with a bulb syringe may be done if necessary.
- Infants with meconium-stained amniotic fluid, regardless of whether they are vigorous or not, should no longer routinely receive intubation.
- Meconium-stained amniotic fluid is a condition that requires the notification and availability of an appropriately credentialed team with full resuscitation skills, including endotracheal intubation. Resuscitation should follow the same principles for infants with meconium-stained fluid as for those with clear fluid (ACOG, 2017a).

Multiple Gestation Birth

The patient with a multiple gestation pregnancy is at higher risk for many complications during the intrapartum period, including preterm birth, preeclampsia, and hemorrhage. Women with multifetal gestations are 6 times more likely to give birth preterm and 13 times more likely to give birth before 32 weeks of gestation than women with singleton gestations (ACOG, 2016).

Preparing for delivery of multiples is both high-risk and complex. Decisions on the method of delivery are dependent on numerous factors, including the number of fetuses; position of presentation of fetuses, particularly the presenting fetus (twin A); and fetal weight. If the first twin is in a vertex presentation, vaginal delivery may be attempted. It is common for women to be delivered by cesarean birth with twins, though in some cases both twins can be born vaginally or twin A vaginally and twin B by cesarean. There are three routes for twin births: both vaginal, both by cesarean, or twin A vaginally and twin B by cesarean. The optimal route of delivery in women with twin gestations depends on the type of twins, fetal presentations, gestational age, and experience of the clinician performing the delivery. A twin gestation in and of itself is not an indication for cesarean delivery. Women with monoamniotic twin gestations should undergo cesarean delivery to avoid an umbilical cord complication of the nonpresenting twin at the time of the initial twin's delivery (ACOG, 2016). Women with diamniotic twin gestations whose presenting fetus is in a vertex position are candidates for a vaginal birth. Nearly all triplets (94.14%) and other higher-order multiples (HOMs) are delivered by cesarean (Centers for Disease Control and Prevention [CDC], 2019).

Labor in multiple gestations appears to progress differently from singleton labor. Most data are from twin labors, with limited information from triplets (Bowers, 2021). Factors affecting labor progress may include fetal weights, presentations, and use of epidural anesthesia. After birth of the first infant, ultrasound should be used to assess presentation of the second twin and to exclude a funic presentation (cord between the fetal vertex and the internal cervical os) (Malone & D'Alton, 2014). Membrane rupture of the second twin should be delayed until contractions are reestablished and the presenting part is engaged in the pelvis to minimize risk of cord prolapse. Once the presenting part of the next fetus is accessible and membranes are ruptured, a scalp electrode may be applied for continuous fetal monitoring of the remaining fetus(es). In all vaginal delivery scenarios, clinicians should be alert for changes in fetal presentation and maternal and fetal well-being and be ready for emergent cesarean delivery (Bowers, 2021). The use and choice of anesthesia depends on the potential need for uterine manipulation, operative birth, version of the second twin, emergent cesarean birth, and the increased risks for uterine atony and postpartum hemorrhage (ACOG, 2016). See Chapter 7 for more on multiple gestation pregnancy and Chapter 9 for fetal monitoring with multiples.

The 2018 twin birth rate was 32.6 twins per 1,000 births, a 2% decline from the 2017 rate. The twinning rate rose 76% from 1980 to 2009, and was generally stable from 2009 through 2012. The 2014 rate of 33.9 was the highest ever reported. The triplet and HOM birth rate (triplet/+) was 93.0 per 100,000 births for 2018 (an 8% decline from 2017) and down 52% from the 1998 peak (Martin et al., 2019). The increased incidence in multifetal gestations over several decades has been attributed to two main factors: (1) a shift toward an older maternal age at conception, when multifetal gestations are more likely to occur naturally, and (2) an increased use of assisted reproductive technology (ART), which is more likely to result in a multifetal gestation (ACOG, 2016).

Risks Associated With Multiple-Gestation Labor and Delivery

- Preterm labor
- Labor dystocia
- Antepartum hemorrhage (i.e., abruptio placentae)
- Stillbirth

Assessment Findings

- On admission, ultrasound should be used to confirm viability, placental location, and fetal presentation.
- Multiple fetuses may be assessed by Leopold's maneuver, but ultrasound is the most definitive assessment for fetal position with more than one fetus.

Medical Management

- On admission, ultrasound should be used to confirm viability, placental location, and fetal presentation (Bowers, 2021).
- Method of delivery is determined based on fetal presentation, subsequent fetal position, and medical considerations (AAP & ACOG, 2017; ACOG, 2016; Malone & D'Alton, 2014).
- Hospital birth is performed with a Level II or Level III nursery.
- Two experienced obstetricians or one OB and one CNM are available.
- Delivery is done in a surgical suite as a double setup.

Nursing Actions

- Expectant parents' birth plans and desires should be respected as much as possible, acknowledging the unique aspects of the birth for these families.
- The mother and support persons should be given anticipatory guidance for all labor and birth procedures.
- Discuss the number of persons and personnel present at the multiple birth (Bowers, 2021).
- Ensure placement of large-bore IV for fluid replacement in case of hemorrhage or need for emergency fluid replacement and anesthesia administration (Parfitt, 2016).
- Continuous FHR monitoring for each fetus and, once membranes are ruptured, internal monitoring for twin A.
- Have a hemorrhage cart or medications available.
- Anesthesia provider, circulating nurse, and scrub nurse should be present.
- Ensure ultrasound access to confirm position of twin B after birth of twin A.
- Neonatal team should be present for each twin.
- Have type and cross-match blood available.

Stillbirth or Intrauterine Fetal Demise

Stillbirth, or intrauterine fetal demise (IUFD), is defined as a fetal death after 20 weeks' gestation. Stillbirth is one of the most common adverse pregnancy outcomes, occurring in 1 in 160 deliveries in the United States. Approximately

23,600 stillbirths at 20 weeks or greater of gestation are reported annually. Perinatal mortality (late fetal death at 28 weeks or more and early neonatal death under age 7 days) can indicate the quality of health care before, during, and after delivery (Gregory et al., 2018). The method and timing of delivery after a stillbirth depend on the gestational age when death occurred, obstetric history, and maternal preference. Although most patients desire prompt delivery, the timing may not be critical as coagulopathies associated with prolonged fetal retention are uncommon (ACOG, 2020c).

Before 28 weeks of gestation, vaginal misoprostol is reported to be the most efficient method of induction regardless of cervical Bishop score, although high-dose oxytocin infusion also is an acceptable choice (ACOG, 2020c). After 28 weeks of gestation, induction of labor should be managed according to usual obstetric protocols. In general, cesarean delivery for fetal demise would be reserved for unusual circumstances because it is associated with potential maternal morbidity without any fetal benefit. Further discussion of the care of families experiencing a stillbirth can be found related to postpartum nursing care in Chapter 17.

Risk Factors

- The most prevalent risk factors associated with stillbirth are Black race, nulliparity, advanced maternal age, obesity, preexisting diabetes, chronic hypertension, smoking, alcohol use, having a pregnancy using ART, multiple gestation, male fetal sex, unmarried status, and past obstetric history (ACOG, 2020c)
- Five selected causes of fetal death accounted for 89.5% of fetal deaths (Hoyert & Gregory, 2020). By order of frequency, these were:
  - Fetal death of unspecified cause (unspecified cause);
  - Fetus affected by complications of placenta, cord, and membranes (placental, cord, and membrane complications);
  - Fetus affected by maternal complications of pregnancy (maternal complications);
  - Congenital malformations, deformations, and chromosomal abnormalities (congenital malformations); and
  - Fetus affected by maternal conditions that may be unrelated to present pregnancy (maternal conditions unrelated to pregnancy).
- Although maternal and gestational factors play a role in determining risk factors for stillbirth and IUFD, nearly half of cases have an unknown etiology.
- Disparities in fetal mortality among women of different races demonstrate an association between stillbirth and both low-income and minimal access to quality health care; however, the disparity remains unexplained. Health-care access and socioeconomic and education levels also play a vital role.
- Severe medical maternal complications with diabetes, renal disease, cardiovascular disease, thyroid disease, connective tissue disease, autoimmune disease, malnutrition, maternal trauma, placental abruption, or obesity.
- The stillbirth rate among twin pregnancies is approximately 2.5 times higher than that of singletons (ACOG, 2020c).

Risks Associated With Stillbirth

- Prolonged retention of the dead fetus may lead to the development of disseminated intravascular coagulation (DIC) in the mother and puts the mother at higher risk for infection, which can result in sepsis or endometritis.

Assessment Findings

- Decreased or absent fetal movement for several hours or more
- Symptoms related to underlying cause of stillbirth
- Stillbirth is confirmed by visualization of the fetal heart with absence of heart activity on an ultrasound (ACOG, 2009c).

Medical Management

- The method and timing of delivery after a stillbirth depend on the gestational age, maternal obstetric history, and maternal preference.
- Induction of labor within 24 to 48 hours of confirmed diagnosis is typical.
- Vaginal misoprostol may be used if less than 28 weeks.
- Cervical ripening and induction of labor are assessed.

Nursing Actions

- The emotional worry from the time of suspecting a problem to an actual diagnosis can be devastating for a woman, her family, and the health-care team. Women bond with their babies and feel deep sadness from this loss.
- Provide anticipatory guidance in slow, small increments. When communicating with family and staff, the term *stillbirth* is preferred over *fetal demise* or *death* (Parfitt, 2016). Talk to the patient and family directly and give simple explanations.
- Allow the patient to make decisions related to the plan of care.
- During the admission process, it is crucial that a woman have the support of people who will be there both mentally and physically.
- To maintain a woman's comfort and sense of control, nurses can find out how she wants to birth and what pain management options, either epidural or intravenous narcotic, she wants to consider before starting any medications (Sousou & Smart, 2015). Provide comforting touch to the patient.
- Maintain continuity of care; prevent unnecessary moves from the labor room to delivery to recovery.
- To maintain privacy and comfort, a card of an appropriate image should be hung on the door to notify staff and personnel of the woman's status and minimize unnecessary interruptions.
- Offer the opportunity for mother and family to hold and touch the infant and allow unlimited time with the infant after delivery (Parfitt, 2016).
- Provide the patient and family with mementos such as baby clothing, photos of the baby with family and patient, measuring tape, baby comb, blanket, footprints, and handprints.
- In caring for a family with stillbirth, nurses are part of an interdisciplinary team that also includes physicians, midwives, social workers, chaplains, geneticists, genetic counselors, lactation specialists, funeral directors, volunteers, and psychologists (Sousou & Smart, 2015).

- The interdisciplinary team must be mindful of the approach taken when caring for grieving families and should be available both physically and emotionally while anticipating and meeting the needs of the family.
- Nurses can build trust with the women and families they care for while keeping in mind that decisions made are based on their unique cultural and individual identity.
- Suggestions for helping grieving families include listening more than talking, allowing for silence, being genuine and caring, allowing them to express their feelings, and listening to their story without passing judgment (Sousou & Smart, 2015).
- Recognize that feelings of guilt or anger in parents who have experienced a stillbirth are common and may be magnified when there is an abnormal child or a genetic defect.
- It is important for health-care professionals to not use any clichés that belittle the situation; they should not avoid discussing the experience or the baby but should not provide advice or make commentary about the situation.
- Rituals related to the perinatal bereavement process may include naming the infant, having a spiritual blessing or baptism, and arranging a memorial or burial service.
- Mementos are an important part of grieving. Memory boxes can be created on behalf of the family by nursing staff. Items often included are photographs of the infant, locks of hair, name bracelets, footprints, measuring tape, name certificates, quilts, clothing, poems, and sympathy cards.
- Bereavement care should recognize parents' individual personal, cultural, or religious needs.
- Components of bereavement care after a stillbirth include good communication; shared decision making; recognition of parenthood; acknowledgment of a partner's and families' grief; acknowledgment that grief is individual; awareness of burials, cremation, and funerals; ongoing emotional and practical support; and health professionals trained in bereavement care (ACOG, 2020c).
- Referral to a bereavement counselor, peer support group, or mental health professional may help with grief and depression.
- Parents who have had a stillborn baby are more likely to have another stillbirth than parents who do not have this history. In their next pregnancy, parents often experience anxiety, depression, and worry about whether their baby will survive. It is important to implement evidence-based interventions in planning subsequent pregnancies and, if relevant, manage a mother's health before conception to address issues and assist with high-risk behaviors or risk factors such as being overweight or using substances (Wojcieszek et al., 2018).

Intraamniotic Infection, Chorioamnionitis, and Triple 1

Intraamniotic infection, also referred to as chorioamnionitis, is an infection with inflammation of any combination of the amniotic fluid, placenta, fetus, fetal membranes, or decidua (ACOG, 2017b). Chorioamnionitis refers to a heterogeneous group of conditions that includes inflammation as well as infections of varying degrees of severity and duration. Inflammation includes a reaction that results in tissue edema, swelling, and irritation. Infection includes inflammation with concurrent invasion of bacteria, virus, fungus, or another infectious agent. Often a diagnosis of chorioamnionitis is made when any combination (or even one) of the following elements is noted: maternal fever, maternal or fetal tachycardia or both, elevated maternal white blood cell (WBC) count, uterine tenderness, and purulent fluid or purulent discharge from the cervical os. However, the presence of one (or even more than one) of these signs and symptoms does not necessarily indicate intrauterine infection or chorioamnionitis is present (Higgins et al., 2016).

The term *intraamniotic infection* is common since infection often involves the amniotic fluid, fetus, umbilical cord or placenta, and the fetal membranes. To clarify this issue, an expert panel recommended terminology to differentiate the presence of fever from infection, inflammation, or both, and clarify that inflammation can occur without infection. Therefore, given the historical inconsistency in use, experts proposed to discontinue the intrapartum use of the term *chorioamnionitis* and instead use *intrauterine inflammation or infection or both* or *Triple I*.

Isolated maternal fever is defined as a maternal oral temperature of 102.2°F (39°C) or greater on any one occasion, and it is a documented fever that should be reported to the health-care team. If the oral temperature is between 100.4°F (38°C) and 102.2°F (39°C), repeat the measurement in 30 minutes; if the repeat value remains at least 100.4°F (38°C), it is a documented fever and should be reported (Higgins et al., 2016).

Suspected Triple I is fever without a clear source plus any of the following:

- Baseline fetal tachycardia (greater than 160 beats per minute [bpm] for 10 minutes or longer, excluding accelerations, decelerations, and periods of marked variability)
- Maternal WBC counts greater than 15,000 per mm^3 in the absence of corticosteroids
- Definite purulent fluid from the cervical os

Confirmed Triple I includes all of the previously noted items as well as at least one of the following:

- Amniocentesis-proven infection through a positive Gram stain
- Low glucose or positive amniotic fluid culture
- Placental pathology revealing diagnostic features of infection

Fever in the absence of any of these criteria should be categorized as "isolated maternal fever." Isolated maternal fever can include but is not limited to fever secondary to epidural anesthesia, prostaglandin use, dehydration, hyperthyroidism, and excess ambient heat. In the clinical situation of labor with fever and unknown GBS status at 37 weeks' gestation or greater, intrapartum prophylaxis should be initiated as per CDC guidelines. Clinical use of the term *chorioamnionitis* is outdated and overused and implies the presence of infection. Use of the phrase *maternal chorioamnionitis* has significant implications for both mother and neonate. The expert panel recommended the use of new terminology, specifically Triple I, with the term *chorioamnionitis* restricted to pathological diagnosis.

Risk Factors

- Migration of cervicovaginal flora through the cervical canal is the most common path for this infection. Intraamniotic infection is often polymicrobial, commonly involves aerobic and anaerobic bacteria, and frequently originates from the vaginal flora (ACOG, 2017b).
- Prolonged ROM lasts greater than 24 hours.
- Obstetric risk factors for intraamniotic infection at term have been delineated, including low parity, multiple digital examinations, use of internal uterine and fetal monitors, meconium-stained amniotic fluid, and the presence of certain genital tract pathogens (e.g., GBS infection and sexually transmitted infections) (ACOG, 2017b).
- Intraamniotic infection can be associated with acute neonatal morbidity, including neonatal pneumonia, meningitis, sepsis, and death, as well as long-term infant complications such as bronchopulmonary dysplasia and cerebral palsy.

Risks Associated With Triple I

- For the mother, intrauterine infection may lead to serious complications such as sepsis, prolonged labor, wound infection, need for hysterectomy, postpartum endometritis, postpartum hemorrhage, adult respiratory distress syndrome, intensive care unit admission, and, in rare instances, maternal mortality (ACOG, 2017b; Higgins et al., 2016).
- Intraamniotic infection can be associated with acute neonatal morbidity, including neonatal pneumonia, meningitis, sepsis, and death, as well as long-term infant complications such as bronchopulmonary dysplasia and cerebral palsy. Risk of neonatal infection increases as the duration of ruptured membranes lengthens.

Assessment Findings

- Fetal tachycardia (greater than 160 bpm for 10 minutes or longer)
- Maternal WBC count greater than 15,000 in the absence of corticosteroids
- Purulent fluid from the cervical os (cloudy or yellowish thick discharge confirmed visually on speculum examination to be coming from the cervical canal)
- Biochemical or microbiologic amniotic fluid results consistent with microbial invasion of the amniotic cavity
- Be alert for and report characteristic clinical signs of chorioamnionitis, including:
  - Maternal fever (intrapartum temperature higher than 100.4°F [37.8°C])
  - Significant maternal tachycardia (greater than 120 bpm)
  - Fetal tachycardia (greater than 160 to 180 bpm)
  - Purulent or foul-smelling amniotic fluid or vaginal discharge
  - Uterine tenderness
  - Maternal leukocytosis (total blood leukocyte count greater than 15,000 to 18,000 cells/μL)
  - Hypotension
  - Diaphoresis
  - Cool or clammy skin

Medical Management

- Administration of intrapartum antibiotics is recommended whenever an intraamniotic infection is suspected or confirmed. Antibiotics should be considered in the setting of isolated maternal fever unless a source other than intraamniotic infection is identified and documented (ACOG, 2017b).
- The choice of antimicrobial agents in the case of suspected Triple I should be guided by the prevalent microorganisms causing intrauterine infection. In general, a combination of ampicillin and gentamicin should cover most relevant pathogens. The use of intrapartum antibiotic treatment given either in response to maternal GBS colonization or in response to evolving signs of intraamniotic infection during labor has been associated with a nearly 10-fold decrease in GBS-specific neonatal sepsis (ACOG, 2017b).
- Controlling maternal temperature with antipyretics and judicious hydration may be required.

Nursing Actions

- Communicate findings of maternal tachycardia, fetal tachycardia, maternal WBC count above 15,000, maternal GBS status, duration of ROM, duration of labor, purulent fluid, amniotic fluid evaluation, highest maternal temperature, epidural use of anesthesia, prostaglandin use, antimicrobial agent(s) or antipyretic used, spontaneous preterm birth, and prior spontaneous preterm birth to all obstetrical and neonatal team members.
- Administer antipyretics and antibiotics as ordered.

Pregestational Complications Impacting Intrapartal Period

Maternal morbidity includes physical and psychological conditions that result from or are aggravated by pregnancy and have an adverse effect on a woman's health (Behling & Renaud, 2015). The most severe complications of pregnancy, generally referred to as severe maternal morbidity (SMM), affect more than 50,000 women in the United States every year. Based on recent trends, this burden has been steadily increasing. Consequences of increasing SMM rate are wide-ranging and include higher health service use, higher direct medical costs, extended hospitalization stays, and long-term rehabilitation. For example, labor complicated by cardiovascular disease is potentially dangerous to maternal and fetal outcomes. Marked hemodynamic changes in labor profoundly affect labor, placental perfusion, and fetal status.

Extensive discussion of specific pregestational complications and their management in labor is beyond the scope of this text, but the impact of obesity in labor is presented as an exemplar. Refer to Chapter 7 for additional information on management of pregestational complications.

Maternal Obesity

The World Health Organization (WHO) and the NIH define *obesity* as a BMI of 30 or greater. Maternal obesity was first recognized as a risk factor in pregnancy more than 50 years ago. A global epidemic of obesity is unfolding, including an even greater prevalence in Black and Latina women, resulting in new challenges for the management of obesity in up to 40% of women aged 20 to 39 years old (ACOG, 2021). The obstetric complications for women with obesity are generally related to issues of maternal pre-pregnancy obesity rather than excessive weight gain during pregnancy. Maternal obesity is a well-established risk factor for the development of preeclampsia, gestational diabetes, and thrombosis. However, the impact on pregnancy also translates to complications in labor, including spontaneous abortion, labor induction, cesarean births, endometritis, and failed vaginal birth after cesarean. Obesity in labor also puts the laboring woman at increased risk of emergent complications of wound rupture or dehiscence, with a twofold increase in maternal morbidity and fivefold increase in neonatal injury associated in TOLAC (ACOG, 2021).

Female obesity is so prevalent that its implications for pregnancy are often unrecognized or overlooked. Therefore, understanding of obesity management during labor is essential to maternal and neonatal health. It is currently recommended that every perinatal department have policies and practices specific to this patient population (ACOG, 2021; Maher, 2021). Obesity is a medical condition associated with bias among health-care professionals, which may result in disrespectful or inadequate care of patients who have obesity (ACOG, 2019c). Remember, the term *obese patient,* which suggests that obesity defines the patient, should be avoided in favor of people-first terminology, such as *patient with obesity,* which identifies a patient as having the condition of obesity All care providers need to work within their units and advocate for the best possible resources to provide optimal care for patients with obesity.

Risks at Delivery

- Abnormal progress of labor
- Fetal macrosomia
- Shoulder dystocia
- Higher rates of operative vaginal birth and cesarean birth
- Performing epidural or spinal anesthesia on women with morbid obesity can be extremely problematic. The use of epidural or spinal anesthesia for intrapartum pain relief is recommended but may be technically difficult because of body habitus and loss of landmarks. The risk of epidural analgesic failure is greater in obese women.
- Pregnant women with obesity undergoing a trial of labor after a previous cesarean delivery have an almost twofold increase in composite maternal morbidity and a fivefold increased risk of neonatal injury. Not only do women with obesity experience higher rates of failed VBAC, but they also have higher rates of infection with VBAC.
- Increased risk of hemorrhage
- Intraoperative challenges and complications can include difficulty with IV access, difficulty monitoring BP, prolonged cesarean surgical and recovery time, poor operative exposure, difficulty with transfers, increased aspiration, and thromboembolic risk. Increased postoperative complications include wound infection, delayed wound healing, excessive blood loss, deep vein thrombosis, and endometritis (ACOG, 2021).

- Consultation with anesthesia service should be considered for obese pregnant women with obstructive sleep apnea (OSA) because they are at an increased risk of hypoxemia, hypercapnia, and sudden death (ACOG, 2021).

Assessment Findings

- Delayed descent of fetal head, abnormal labor progress, or labor dystocia (Parfitt, 2016)

Nursing Actions

- Anticipate the impact of the previously listed pregnancy complications on labor and birth.
- Challenges caring for obese women in labor can include difficulty gaining IV access; difficulty with monitoring BP, fetal heart tones (FHTs), and UCs; and transferring or moving patients.
- Anticipate the need for additional staff for position changes, monitoring and assistance at birth, and transfer and transport (Maher, 2021).
- Assess progress of labor; internal monitoring may be necessary.
- Ensure that all equipment is available for labor, delivery, possible cesarean, and recovery, and check that equipment weight limits are adequate to support the patient's weight.
- Birthing beds capable of supporting an obese gravida for a vaginal delivery with appropriate monitoring equipment should be available. Other common requirements include large chairs, BP cuffs, and wheelchairs.
- Facilitate an anesthesia consultation in early labor to allow adequate time to develop an anesthetic plan that addresses the availability of proper equipment for BP monitoring, venous access, and the influence of comorbid conditions such as sleep apnea.
- Facilitate patient positioning for administering epidural analgesia to obese women. Use of epidural or spinal anesthesia for intrapartum pain relief is recommended but may be technically difficult because of body habitus and loss of landmarks.
- A sensitive and empathic approach to the woman and her family is essential to meet the specialized needs of an obese woman in labor, birth, and recovery.
- When there are challenges in care due to the patient's weight status, such as IV access, epidural catheter placement, external fetal monitoring, or extra steps or equipment for patient transfer and anesthesia management, it is important to avoid reminding the woman that these clinical issues are related to her obesity (Maher, 2021).
- Promote a caring environment that does not cause embarrassment, guilt, or self-esteem problems. The focus of care should be centered on her safety and clinical needs as it is with women with other chronic diseases (ACOG, 2021).

OBSTETRICAL EMERGENCIES

Obstetrical emergencies are urgent clinical situations that place either the mother or fetus at risk for increased morbidity and mortality. Intrapartum emergencies may be related to one or more maternal, fetal, uterine, cord, or placental factors. The physiological effects of intrapartum emergencies on the woman and fetus may cause rapid deterioration in oxygenation and perfusion.

Intrapartum emergencies may place the woman and fetus at risk of exceeding oxygen and perfusion reserves. Interventions are directed at stabilizing maternal status, which in turn stabilizes fetal status.

Perinatal nurses practice in an environment where emergencies will occur. Preparation for these situations requires allocation of resources and supplies, planning, and collaboration. Inpatient emergencies can be mitigated by a rapid response team that has designated roles, streamlined communication, prompt access to emergency supplies, and ongoing education and training. Specific criteria or triggers used to activate a rapid response team should be defined to reflect the populations cared for by the institution and disseminated among interprofessional staff. Protocols with standardized interventions and on-site drills will improve the care given in an emergency. Prompt recognition of and response to critical clinical scenarios, teamwork, and training enhance patient safety and mitigate the severity of adverse outcomes (ACOG, 2014a). We can improve management of hospitalized patients with the use of a rapid response team that has designated roles, streamlined communication, prompt access to emergency supplies, and ongoing education and training (ACOG, 2014a). Tools include:

- Availability of appropriate emergency supplies in a resuscitation cart (crash cart) or kit
- Development and implementation of a rapid response team
- Development and implementation of protocols that include clinical triggers
- Use of standardized communication tools for huddles and briefs such as SBAR (situation, background, assessment, recommendation)
- Implementation of emergency drills and simulations

SMM includes unexpected outcomes of labor and delivery that result in significant short- or long-term consequences to a woman's health. It is not entirely clear why SMM is increasing, but changes in the overall health of the women giving birth may be contributing to increases in complications. For example, increases in maternal age, pre-pregnancy obesity, four preexisting chronic medical conditions, and cesarean delivery have been documented (CDC, 2017b). In the United States, the pregnancy-related mortality ratio rose from 10 deaths per 100,000 live births in 1990 to 17.4 in 2018 per 100,000 births, which is more than double the 1978 rate of 7.2 deaths per 100,000 live births (CDC, 2017a; CDC, 2021). Significant racial disparity exists in the pregnancy-related mortality ratio; for example, Black women have a pregnancy-related mortality risk three times greater than that of White women (CDC, 2017a; CDC, 2021). Additionally, complications associated with delivery and specifically for postpartum hemorrhage have increased 75%. Identifying potential problems early, developing written protocols that outline a clear plan of response for common emergencies, and using mock drills to train staff in protocol responses can help ensure that no tasks are redundant or omitted and ultimately create a more controlled environment that promotes positive health outcomes (Roth et al., 2015). Communication and teamwork are essential parts of safety and improving patient outcomes. Effective, patient-centered communication facilitates interception and correction of potentially harmful conditions and errors. All team members, including women, their families, physicians, midwives, and nurses, have roles in identifying the potential for harm during labor and birth (Lyndon et al., 2015).

CLINICAL JUDGMENT

Examples of Trigger Threshold Parameters

Some events, referred to as "triggers," mandate further actions by the health-care team according to protocol, such as bringing the attending physician to the patient's bedside immediately. Some emergencies are preceded by a period of instability during which timely intervention may help avoid disaster. OB emergency teams, sometimes referred to as OB stat team for obstetrical emergencies, are rapid response teams in labor and delivery. Nurses need to recognize that certain changes in a patient's condition can indicate an emergency that requires immediate intervention. A "red" trigger typically mandates an immediate bedside evaluation and a "yellow" trigger indicates further clinical evaluation (ACOG, 2014a).

	RED TRIGGER	YELLOW TRIGGER
Temperature; °C	<35 or >38	35–36
Systolic BP; mm Hg	<90 or >160	150–160 or 90–100
Diastolic BP; mm Hg	>100	90–100
Heart rate; beats/min	<40 or >120	100–120 or 40–50
Respiratory rate; breaths/min	<10 or >30	21–30
Oxygen saturation; %	<95	

BP, blood pressure.

CRITICAL COMPONENT

Intrapartum Care Communication

Intrapartum care is inherently dynamic and nuanced, and crucial communication gaps can occur. Road signs may be unclear or change quickly, leading care providers to have completely different interpretations of clinical situations and divergent ideas of the right thing to do. Conflicting approaches are easily exacerbated by the dynamic nature of labor; differences of opinion and prioritization occur with some regularity (Lyndon et al., 2014). Key steps toward improving communication include assuming the best motives of others, recognizing that we all make assumptions that reflect our own worldviews, seeking first to understand others' views and then to be understood, and avoiding stereotyping. Differences of opinion and judgment occur naturally in complex situations such as labor and birth. Ensuring that patients' interests are the focus of action at all times serves as a powerful resource for proactive problem-solving (Lyndon et al., 2015). Communication issues, most notably between providers, were identified in 41% of cases and included the lack of timely acknowledgment and effective communication. Other factors were the lack of appreciation for clinical significance or decline, variation in willingness to escalate concerns about care, and poor communication due to lack of team structure and function that often led to delays in care management and effective response.

Shoulder Dystocia

Shoulder dystocia is a birth complication that requires additional maneuvers to relieve impaction of the fetal shoulder. This unpredictable and unpreventable obstetric emergency places the laboring mother and neonate at risk of injury and complications (ACOG, 2017c). Shoulder dystocia refers to difficulty encountered during delivery of the shoulders after the birth of the head, which often occurs when the passage of the anterior shoulder is obstructed by the symphysis pubis. It also results from an impaction of the posterior shoulder on the maternal sacral promontory (ACOG, 2017c). The anterior shoulder or, more rarely, both shoulders become impacted above the pelvic rim. The first sign is a retraction of the fetal head against the maternal perineum after delivery of the head, sometimes referred to as turtle sign. This impaction of the fetal shoulders may lead to a prolonged delivery time of more than 60 seconds. Because shoulder dystocia is an unpredictable obstetrical emergency that can result in serious fetal morbidity and even mortality, it must be readily recognized and successfully managed. Several techniques that have been proven to assist delivery exist, and there is evidence that a systematic approach can improve outcomes (ACOG, 2017b).

Neonatal morbidity includes brachial plexus injuries, clavicle fracture, neurological injury related to asphyxia, and even death. Reduction in the interval of time from delivery of the head to the body is crucial to fetal outcome. Most experts note that more than a 5-minute delay in head-to-body interval may result in fetal hypoxemia and acidosis. It is estimated that a newborn can survive for approximately 6 minutes before irreversible brain and organ damage occurs. The incidence of shoulder dystocia ranges from reports of 0.2% to 3% (ACOG, 2017c). Studies have found that prepregnancy, antepartum, and intrapartum risk factors fail to accurately predict the possibility of shoulder dystocia. Additionally, no clear evidence supports the use of prophylactic maneuvers to prevent shoulder dystocia (Athukorala et al., 2006).

Risk Factors Associated With Shoulder Dystocia

- Fetal macrosomia (weight greater than 4,500 grams)
- Maternal diabetes
- History of shoulder dystocia
- Protracted labor or prolonged second stage
- Excessive weight gain

Risks Associated With Shoulder Dystocia for the Mother

- Maternal complications include severe perineal lacerations, including fourth-degree lacerations, maternal symphyseal separation and peripheral neuropathy, sphincter injuries, infection, bladder injury, or postpartum hemorrhage (ACOG, 2017c).

Risks Associated With Shoulder Dystocia for the Neonate

- Delay in delivery of the shoulders results in compression of the fetal neck by the maternal pelvis. This impairs fetal circulation and results in possible increased intracranial pressure, anoxia, asphyxia, and neurological injury. Although infrequent, some cases of shoulder dystocia may result in neonatal encephalopathy and even death. The duration of the shoulder dystocia alone has not been shown to be an accurate predictor of neonatal asphyxia or death (ACOG 2017c).
- A greater than 5-minute head-to-body interval may result in acid–base deterioration in a fetus whose condition was normal before the onset of shoulder dystocia.
- If fetal status was compromised before the shoulder dystocia, the fetus may have less physiological reserve; for example, prolonged pushing with recurrent late and variable decelerations can result in fetal oxygen desaturation, fetal metabolic acidemia, and risk of fetal hypoxic and ischemic injuries. In this situation, they have less ability to tolerate an additional insult such as shoulder dystocia (Simpson & O'Brien-Abel, 2021).
- Most shoulder dystocia cases are alleviated without injury to the fetus. Brachial plexus injuries and fractures of the clavicle and humerus can occur and usually resolve without long-term complications. However, the presence of a brachial plexus injury is not evidence that shoulder dystocia has occurred (ACOG 2017c).

Assessment Findings

- The first sign is a retraction of the fetal head against the maternal perineum after delivery of the head, sometimes referred to as the turtle sign.
- Delay in delivery of the shoulders may occur after delivery of the head.

Medical Management

When shoulder dystocia is suspected, the first intervention that should be attempted is the McRoberts maneuver because it is a simple, logical, and effective technique. This is performed by two assistants, each grasping a maternal leg and then sharply flexing the thigh back against the maternal abdomen, which causes cephalad rotation of the symphysis pubis and flattening of the lumbar lordosis that can free the impacted shoulder. Pressure is applied above the pubic bone with the palm or fist; then the pressure is directed on the anterior shoulder both downward (to below the pubic bone) and laterally (toward the fetus's face or sternum) to abduct and rotate the anterior shoulder. Fundal pressure should be avoided, as it may further complicate the impaction of the shoulder and also may cause uterine rupture.

If both the McRoberts maneuver and suprapubic pressure are unsuccessful, delivery of the posterior arm may be considered as the next maneuver to manage shoulder dystocia (ACOG, 2017c). The Woods corkscrew maneuver progressively rotates the posterior shoulder 180 degrees to disimpact the anterior shoulder. Episiotomy as an intervention for shoulder dystocia is controversial. Because shoulder dystocia is considered a "bony dystocia" and therefore not caused by obstructing soft tissue, its use may not be helpful (ACOG, 2017c).

Nursing Actions

- Explain the situation to the woman and the family, including the interventions to resolve dystocia and the importance of the woman's assistance with maneuvers. Request that the mother not push.

- The time of shoulder dystocia diagnosis and completion of delivery should be noted.
- Additional nursing, obstetric care provider, and anesthesia assistance should be requested.
- The patient should be positioned so that the health-care provider has adequate access for performing maneuvers.
- Insert a straight catheter into the woman to empty the bladder if it is distended to make more room for the fetus.
- A variety of techniques may free the impacted shoulder from beneath the symphysis pubis (ACOG, 2017c); pressure can be applied above the pubic bone or laterally to the pubic bone to dislodge the anterior shoulder and push it beneath the symphysis (Fig. 10–15).
- The mother should not push except when instructed to and only when it is believed the shoulder has been released.
- The McRoberts maneuver consists of sharply flexing the thigh onto the maternal abdomen to straighten the sacrum (Fig. 10–15).
- The Gaskin all-fours maneuver, in which the woman is placed on her hands and knees, can facilitate delivery.
- Fundal pressure is controversial and not indicated in shoulder dystocia.

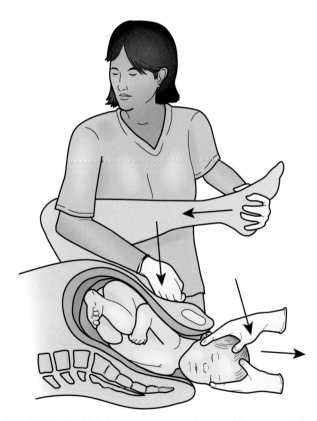

FIGURE 10–15 McRoberts maneuver and suprapubic pressure. When fetal shoulders become impacted under the maternal symphysis pubis, the nurse should initiate the McRoberts maneuver by hyperextending the birthing woman's legs onto her abdomen and simultaneously providing suprapubic pressure to assist the fetus in adducting the arms closer to the body in an attempt to release the impacted shoulders.

- More aggressive approaches may be warranted in cases of severe shoulder dystocia that are not responsive to commonly used maneuvers. The Zavanelli maneuver (cephalic replacement followed by cesarean delivery) has been described for relieving catastrophic cases but is rarely implemented (ACOG, 2017c).
- Notify the neonatal team and prepare for neonatal resuscitation.
- Document the series of interventions and clinical events with time intervals (Simpson & O'Brien-Abel, 2021).

Support and communication with the woman and family is important after a birth complicated by shoulder dystocia. They will be concerned about the condition of the baby and have questions about what occurred. Debriefing with the family soon after the shoulder dystocia can maximize communication and provide support (Simpson & O'Brien-Abel, 2021).

Prolapse of the Umbilical Cord

Prolapse of the umbilical cord occurs when the cord lies below the presenting part of the fetus (Fig. 10–16A–C). The cord may prolapse in front of the presenting part, into the vagina, or through the introitus. Occult prolapse is when the cord is palpated through the membranes but does not drop into the vagina. When cord prolapse occurs, it is typically with AROM or SROM, when the presenting part is not engaged in the pelvis. The cord becomes entrapped against the presenting part and circulation is occluded, resulting in FHR bradycardia. A loop of cord may be palpated or visualized in the vagina. An emergency cesarean birth is typically done to improve neonatal outcomes with a prolapsed cord.

A significant percentage of umbilical cord prolapse cases are diagnosed at the time of amniotomy (24%) or SROM (35%). Be aware of the potential for umbilical cord prolapse associated with these diagnoses, especially when abnormal FHR tracings follow membrane rupture. Iatrogenic umbilical cord prolapses (up to 50% of cases) can occur in procedures such as amniotomy, fetal blood sampling, and insertion of a cervical ripening balloon. The perinatal outcome largely depends on the location where the prolapse occurred and the gestational age or birth weight of the fetus. When diagnosed, delivery should be expedited. Usually, cesarean section is the delivery mode of choice, but vaginal or instrumental delivery could be tried if deemed quicker, particularly in the second stage of labor (Sayed Ahmed & Hamdy, 2018). The overall incidence of umbilical cord prolapse ranges from 0.1% to 0.6% (ACOG, 2014a). Although an uncommon obstetric emergency, with umbilical cord prolapse, the initial response can greatly impact the quality of maternal and infant outcomes (Phelan & Holbrook, 2013).

Risk Factors for Prolapse of the Umbilical Cord Related to the Fetus

- Malpresentation of the fetus (such as breech), fetal anomalies, intrauterine growth restriction and small for gestational age (IUGR/SGA), unengaged presenting part

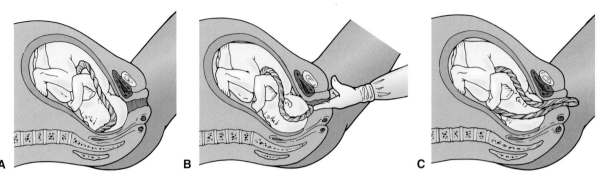

FIGURE 10–16 Prolapsed cord. (A) Occult. The cord cannot be seen or felt during a vaginal examination. (B) Complete. During a vaginal examination, the cord is felt as a pulsating mass. (C) Frank. The cord precedes the fetal head or feet and can be seen protruding from the vagina.

Risk Factors Related to Pregnancy

- The primary iatrogenic cause is AROM.
- Polyhydramnios, multiple gestation, SROM, preterm ROM, and grand multiparity

Risks Associated With Prolapse of the Umbilical Cord

- Total or partial occlusion of the cord, resulting in rapid deterioration in fetal perfusion and oxygenation, causes fetal hypoxia; if not treated swiftly, it can lead to long-term sequela, disability, or death (Phelan & Holbrook, 2013).

Assessment Findings

Umbilical cord prolapse can be occult or overt. Occult prolapse is neither visible nor palpable and occurs when the cord passes through the cervix alongside the presenting part of the fetus (Fig. 10–16A). With overt prolapse, the cord presents before the fetus and is visible or palpable within the vagina or even past the labia (Fig. 10–16B–C). Prolapse of the umbilical cord can lead to compression, causing FHR decelerations including severe sudden deceleration. This often occurs with prolonged bradycardia or recurrent moderate-to-severe variable decelerations.

Medical Management

- Vaginal birth or operative vaginal delivery is used.
- May be attempted if birth is imminent.
- Perform emergency cesarean section.

Nursing Actions

- Elevation of the presenting part. Occlusion of the cord may be partially relieved by lifting the presenting part off the cord with a vaginal exam. The examiner's hand remains in the vagina, lifting the presenting part off the cord until delivery by cesarean (Fig. 10–17).
- Notify the health-care provider and request immediate bedside evaluation and assistance.
- Explain to the woman and family that interventions are necessary to expedite delivery. Ensure the woman understands the importance of her assistance.
- Continue to monitor the fetus.

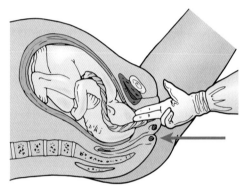

FIGURE 10–17 Vaginal examination with prolapsed cord, lifting the presenting part off the cord.

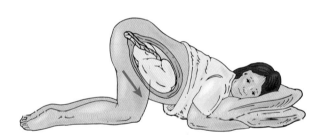

FIGURE 10–18 Knee-chest position with prolapsed cord.

- Recommend position changes such as knee–chest position or Trendelenburg to try to relieve pressure on the occluded cord (Fig. 10–18), administer O_2 at 10 L/min by mask, and give IV fluid hydration bolus.
- Discontinue oxytocin and consider tocolytic agent to decrease uterine activity.
- Move toward emergency delivery. If birth is imminent, the provider may proceed with vaginal delivery. If birth is not imminent, anticipate and prepare for emergency cesarean.
- Because a significant percentage of umbilical cord prolapse cases are diagnosed at the time of amniotomy or SROM, FHR should be evaluated immediately following membrane rupture.

Vasa Previa or Ruptured Vasa Previa

Vasa previa occurs when fetal vessels unsupported by the placenta or umbilical cord traverses the membranes over the cervix.

Vasa previa is defined as abnormal fetal blood vessels that run through the fetal membranes, over or near the endocervical os, unprotected by the placenta or umbilical cord. It is uncommon and occurs in 1 in 2,500 to 5,000 pregnancies. Vasa previa can be categorized as one of two types:

● Type I: Velamentous cord insertion and fetal vessels that run freely within the amniotic membranes overlying the cervix or in close proximity of it (2 cm from os). (Pregnancies with low-lying placentas or resolved placenta previas are at risk.)
● Type II: Succenturiate lobe or multilobe placenta (bilobed) and fetal vessels connecting both lobes course over or are in close proximity of the cervix (2 cm from os).

The condition usually results from velamentous insertion of the cord into membranes rather than the placenta or from vessels running between lobes of the placenta with one or more accessory lobes (Fig. 10–19A, B). If undiagnosed, it is associated with perinatal mortality of 60% (Oyelese, 2007). Pressure on unprotected vessels by the presenting part can lead to fetal asphyxia and death.

Ruptured vasa previa refers to the rupture of the unprotected fetal vessels running through the membranes and over the cervix. ROM frequently leads to rapid fetal exsanguination (Cunningham et al., 2018). This results from fetal-neonatal hemorrhage if fetal vessels tear during SROM or AROM or labor itself. Because the entire fetal blood volume is usually less than 100 mL/kg, emergent bleeding is often rapid. There is a theoretical risk of compromised blood flow to the fetus from the compression and subsequent occlusion of these compromised vessels by the presenting part of the fetus (Silver, 2015). A recent report with very few documented cases of vasa previa ($N = 19$) demonstrated some improved neonatal outcomes and survival (Dunn et al., 2017). Although not common, 1 in 2,500 deliveries; perinatal mortality rate for pregnancies complicated by vasa previa is relatively high at around 10% (Sinkey et al., 2015).

Risk Factors for Vasa Previa

● Low-lying placenta or a placenta previa
● Pregnancies in which the placenta has accessory lobes
● Multiple gestation
● Pregnancies resulting from in vitro fertilization

Risks Associated With Vasa Previa

● Fetal asphyxia from cord compression
● Fetal death from exsanguination

Assessment Findings

● Vasa previa is most commonly diagnosed when ROM is accompanied by vaginal bleeding or fetal distress or death, but increasingly it is diagnosed by antenatal ultrasonography.

Medical Management

● If diagnosed prenatally with ultrasound, cesarean birth before labor and ruptured membranes improves neonatal outcomes. Recommendations include planned cesarean birth at

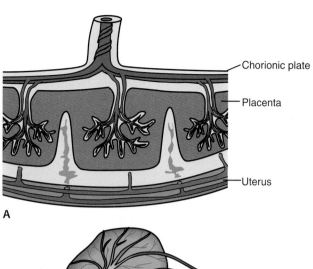

A

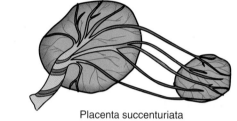

Placenta succenturiata

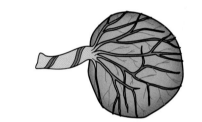

Marginal insertion of the cord

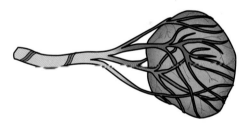

B   Velamentous insertion of the cord

FIGURE 10–19 (A) Normal insertion of umbilical cord into chorionic plate. Normally the umbilical cord inserts near the center of the chorionic plate, which stabilizes the fetal vessels as they leave the umbilical cord. Similar to the roots of a tree, the fetal vessels branch over the surface of the chorionic plate and then dive into the placental parenchyma. (B) Illustration depicting abnormalities of umbilical cord insertion into the placenta. With a velamentous insertion of the umbilical cord into the membranes or with a succenturiate lobe, fetal vessels, within the chorionic membranes and unprotected by the placenta, may course across the cervix and result in a vasa previa.

35 weeks, which improves neonatal survival to 95% (ACOG, 2018; Nahum, 2016; Oyelese, 2007). It is generally accepted that delivery be performed by cesarean before the onset of labor or ROM (Silver, 2015).
● Consider antenatal corticosteroids at 28 to 32 weeks of gestation in case of emergent delivery.

(Labels on Figure A: Chorionic plate, Placenta, Uterus)

- Decision for prophylactic hospitalization should be individualized and based on the presence or absence of symptoms (e.g., preterm contractions, vaginal bleeding); history of spontaneous preterm birth; logistics (distance from hospital); and balancing of the risks that are associated with bedrest and activity restriction (Sinkey et al., 2015).
- If diagnosed in labor, urgent cesarean delivery should be undertaken in cases of vaginal bleeding with suspected vasa previa.

Nursing Actions

- If a woman is diagnosed by ultrasound during pregnancy, she may be admitted to the hospital for surveillance, given corticosteroids to promote fetal lung maturity, and scheduled for planned cesarean birth at 35 weeks. Nursing care related to antenatal hospitalization for high-risk pregnancy is detailed in Chapter 7.
- If bleeding occurs with SVE by the nurse, an immediate bedside evaluation by the provider is indicated because urgent cesarean delivery should be accomplished in cases of vaginal bleeding with suspected vasa previa.
- Vasa previa should be suspected when vaginal bleeding is accompanied with a sinusoidal pattern in FHT tracing (Sinkey et al., 2015).

Rupture of the Uterus

Uterine rupture is typically a catastrophic event for the woman and fetus. Uterine rupture refers to the actual separation of the uterine myometrium or previous uterine scar, with rupture of the membranes and possible extrusion of the fetus or fetal parts into the peritoneal cavity. Dehiscence refers to separation of the old scar with the uterine serosa remaining intact; the fetus remains inside the uterus. This can occur from rupture of a uterine scar from prior uterine surgery, tachysystole, trauma, or, rarely, spontaneously (Salera-Vieira, 2021). Excessive bleeding usually occurs with rupture, whereas bleeding is generally minimal with dehiscence.

Uterine rupture occurs most frequently in women with a previous uterine incision through the myometrium and usually occurs during labor, although it can occur in the antepartum period. Hyperstimulation or hypertonus of the uterus by oxytocin or prostaglandin administration can cause uterine rupture even in the unscarred uterus. The use of misoprostol is contraindicated for third trimester use in patients with a previously scarred uterus from cesarean section, myomectomy, or other uterine surgeries (ACOG, 2017d). Invasive or blunt trauma, seen in women after a car accident, battery, fall, or knife or gunshot wound, is an additional cause.

From 1976 to 2012, 25 peer-reviewed publications described the incidence of uterine rupture, and these reported 2,084 cases among 2,951,297 pregnant women, yielding an overall uterine rupture rate of 1 in 1,146 pregnancies (0.07%) (Nahum, 2016). Studies show a 0.7% incidence of uterine rupture in women attempting TOLAC (Parfitt, 2016). The uterus with no surgical history that is spontaneously contracting is not likely to rupture. Therefore, avoiding induction of labor may substantially decrease risk of uterine rupture in mothers attempting a TOLAC or VBAC (Parfitt, 2016).

Signs and symptoms of uterine rupture are related to internal hemorrhage and reflected in the maternal and fetal status in relation to the extent of the rupture. The condition usually becomes evident because of signs of fetal compromise and maternal hypovolemia related to hemorrhage. If the fetal presenting part is in the pelvis, loss of station may occur, detected with a vaginal exam. Maternal and fetal outcomes and survival depend on prompt identification and surgical intervention. Fetal mortality with uterine rupture is reported at 5% to 7% and maternal mortality is as low as 1% in developed countries (Nahum, 2016). Common sequelae associated with uterine rupture include excessive hemorrhage requiring surgery; need for hysterectomy or blood product transfusion; hypovolemia; hypovolemic shock; injury to the bladder or ureters; bowel laceration; extrusion of any part of the fetus, umbilical cord, or placenta through the disruption; emergent cesarean birth for suspected rupture; emergent cesarean birth for indeterminate or abnormal fetal status; and general anesthesia (ACOG, 2010). Risk of rupture depends on the number, type, and location of the previous incisions (ACOG, 2017d).

Risk Factors Associated With Rupture of the Uterus

- Potential effects on the woman and fetus include hypovolemic shock, infection, hypoxemia, acidosis, neurological damage, and possible death.
- Maternal complications are primarily due to hypovolemia as a result of hemorrhage.
- Complications to the fetus may be due to uteroplacental insufficiency, placental abruption, cord compression, asphyxia, or hypovolemia.

Assessment Findings

- The clinical presentation of the woman experiencing a uterine rupture depends on the specific type of rupture. It may develop over several hours or suddenly. Impending rupture may be preceded by increasing uterine hypertonus or tachysystole (Salera-Vieira, 2021).
- Severe tearing sensation, burning or stabbing pain, and contractions may occur.
- Uterine tachysystole or hypertonus and vaginal bleeding may occur.
- Maternal assessment findings may include signs and symptoms of hypovolemic shock, such as hypotension, tachypnea, tachycardia, and pallor.
- Fetal response is related to hemorrhage and placental separation and may include sudden fetal bradycardia or prolonged late or variable decelerations present even before the onset of abdominal pain or vaginal bleeding (Parfitt, 2016).
- Ascending station of the fetal presenting part is observed.

Medical Management

- Treatment includes maternal hemodynamic stabilization and immediate cesarean birth. If possible, the uterine defect is repaired, or hysterectomy is performed.
- Perform emergency cesarean birth and control maternal hemorrhage. Transfusions may be needed.

Nursing Actions

- Explain to the woman and her family the interventions that will expedite delivery and the importance of their assistance for the best possible outcome.
- Notify the medical provider and request immediate bedside evaluation and assistance.
- Gain or maintain large-bore IV access. Stabilize the woman with O$_2$, IV fluids, and blood products.
- Maintain the woman in the lateral position to maximize urine blood flow (Parfitt, 2016).

CLINICAL JUDGMENT

Nursing Assessments and Interventions for Abnormal Bleeding and Hemorrhage

Abnormal bleeding leading to hemorrhagic complications during pregnancy is a significant causative factor of adverse maternal and fetal outcomes. Major blood loss places the woman at increased risk of hypovolemia, anemia, infection, preterm labor and birth, and even death. The fetus is also at risk for complications because significant maternal blood loss can negatively alter maternal hemodynamic status and decrease oxygen-carrying capacity potential, resulting in progressive physiologic deterioration (Salera-Vieira, 2021). This risk is directly related to the amount and duration of blood loss.

Initial Nursing Interventions

- Notify the physician or nurse-midwife and anesthesia providers.
- Secure airway; start oxygen via nonrebreather mask at 10 L/min.
- Establish intravenous (IV) access if there is not an existing IV line: Infuse lactated Ringer's solution (or normal saline) wide open, then start another IV with a 16-gauge catheter. (Do not infuse IV solutions containing glucose.)
- Obtain complete blood count (CBC), fibrinogen, prothrombin time (PT), partial thromboplastin time (PTT), and other laboratory tests as ordered.
- Draw 5 mL of the patient's blood in a red-top tube and observe frequently. If no clot forms within 5 to 10 minutes, suspect coagulopathy.
- Type and cross-match 4 units of packed red blood cells (PRBCs).
- Administer blood products as ordered. Institute massive transfusion protocol if available.

Secondary Nursing Interventions

- Insert Foley catheter with urometer; assess for output of at least 30 mL/hr.
- Apply oxygen saturation monitor.
- Assess maternal vital signs per hospital policy.
- Call for additional nursing help so that one nurse can be responsible for patient care and another nurse is available for obtaining necessary medications, administering IV fluids, and monitoring intake and output if possible.
- Obtain CBC, PT, PTT, fibrinogen, ionized calcium, and potassium after 5 to 7 units of PRBCs.
- Anticipate surgical intervention such as indicated.

- Prepare for emergency cesarean birth.
  - Insert Foley catheter, as bladder rupture is associated with uterine rupture (Parfitt, 2016).

Amniotic Fluid Embolism and Anaphylactic Syndrome

Amniotic fluid embolism (AFE), also known as anaphylactic syndrome, is a rare but life-threatening complication that can occur during pregnancy, labor, birth, or the first 24 hours postbirth. AFE affects 1.2 to 7.7 women per 100,000 pregnancies (Sultan et al., 2016). Though rare, it is among the leading five causes of pregnancy-related deaths in the United States (Farsight et al., 2017), with a maternal mortality rate of over 30%. Most patients who survive (85%) have permanent neurological injury (Thongrong et al., 2013).

This obstetric emergency is both unpreventable and unpredictable (Stanley Sundin & Bradham Mazac, 2017). Amniotic fluid is made up of maternal extracellular fluid, fetal urine, fetal squamous cells, lanugo, vernix caseosa, mucin, meconium, arachidonic acid metabolites, and, late in pregnancy, increased concentrations of prostaglandins. This fluid and the surrounding sac provide an important protective mechanism for the developing fetus. Before labor, amniotic fluid does not normally enter the maternal circulation, because it is sealed within the amniotic sac. It has been postulated that amniotic fluid may enter the maternal circulation in one of three ways: (1) through the endocervix following rupture of amniotic membranes; (2) at the site of placental separation; or (3) at the site of uterine trauma, often lacerations that occur during normal labor, fetal descent, and birth. In addition, amniotic fluid may be introduced into maternal circulation from placental abruption and accompanying clinical or subclinical disruption of fetal membranes (Drummond & Yeomans, 2019). Once this barrier is ruptured, alteration of the pressure gradient may allow amniotic fluid to enter uterine vessels and maternal venous circulation.

The pathophysiology of AFE disrupts the maternal-placental interface, allowing entry of fetal and amniotic components into the maternal circulation. These antigens likely provoke a massive release of mediators, which causes a proinflammatory and procoagulant reaction (Sultan et al., 2016). The anaphylactoid reaction leads to acute pulmonary hypertension and right ventricular failure, acute respiratory failure, disseminated intravascular coagulopathy (DIC), and left ventricular failure. Despite the term *embolism,* there is no vascular obstruction by amniotic or fetal components (Viau-Lapointe & Filewod, 2019).

Understanding of AFE is incomplete; however, AFE classically consists of hypoxia from acute lung injury and transient pulmonary hypertension, hypotension, and cardiac arrest and coagulopathy (Roth, 2021). Clinically useful risk factors and preventive measures remain elusive, and perinatal morbidity and mortality continue to be significant. Symptoms of sudden dyspnea, hypotension, and cardiac arrest, with evidence of fetal hypoxia during labor, are the classic presentation of AFE, followed by massive fibrinolysis (Roth, 2021). Presentation of AFE is often catastrophic, with sudden hypoxemia and shock that evolves rapidly into cardiorespiratory collapse. Early right ventricular failure followed by left ventricular failure can occur. AFE can also present as postpartum hemorrhage with severe DIC. It can lead to maternal hypoxic encephalopathy and fetal morbidity or mortality. Reported mortality is high, between 19% and 37% (Benson, 2017; Viau-Lapointe & Filewod, 2019).

Fetal or newborn outcomes of AFE are directly related to the time between maternal cardiac arrest and birth; however, the relationship is inconsistent due to the variability in onset and intensity of uterine hypoperfusion and maternal decompensation. In the presence of viable fetal gestational age, maternal resuscitative efforts should follow standard cardiac life support with the addition of consideration of birth (Roth, 2021).

Signs and symptoms of anaphylactoid syndrome are related to anaphylactic shock and cardiopulmonary collapse. This syndrome is discussed more completely in Chapter 14.

- The diagnosis is considered unmistakable with the signs and symptoms of sudden dyspnea, hypotension, and DIC that present during labor or immediately after birth (Clark, 2014).
- Symptoms of sudden dyspnea, hypotension, and cardiac arrest, with evidence of fetal hypoxia during labor, are the classic presentation of AFE, followed by massive fibrinolysis.
- AFE can result in acute lung injury by causing pulmonary vascular endothelial damage, complement activation, and direct platelet aggregation effects of amniotic fluid.
- Maternal mortality is a potential complication; if concomitant with cardiac arrest, chances of survival are less than 10% (Clark, 2014; Roth, 2021).

Risk Factors Associated With AFE

Risk factors include older maternal age, multiple pregnancy, placenta previa, labor induction, cesarean delivery, instrumental vaginal delivery, cervical or uterine trauma, and eclampsia.

Risks Associated With Anaphylactoid Syndrome

- Adult respiratory distress syndrome
- Heart failure
- DIC
- Multisystem organ failure

Assessment Findings

- Rapid onset of respiratory distress that occurs during labor, delivery, or 30 minutes postdelivery (Parfitt, 2016) with severe hypoxia; hypotension; cyanosis; loss of consciousness; foaming at the mouth; pulmonary edema; or uncontrolled bleeding from the uterus, IV sites, or any other incisions due to coagulopathy, seizures, cardiac arrest, and prolonged late decelerations or bradycardia resulting from fetal hypoxia.

Medical Management

- Treatment is mainly supportive with careful monitoring for the development of acute respiratory distress syndrome (ARDS) and coagulopathy. Basic, advanced, and obstetric cardiac life support protocols are generally followed in initial treatment and resuscitative efforts.

- Manage cardiopulmonary arrest, hypotension, and coagulopathy.
- Management goals:
  - Improve oxygenation.
  - Optimize cardiac output.
  - Correct coagulopathy.
  - Deliver fetus if undelivered.

Nursing Actions

- Perform careful assessment, monitor maternal pulse oximetry, maintain patent IV access, review left uterine displacement, notify OB team, implement advanced cardiac life support (ACLS) protocols, and documentation.
- Recognize life-threatening diagnosis. Ask for help and an immediate bedside evaluation. Activate labor and delivery (L&D) code team.
- Because DIC often complicates AFE, guidelines suggest early assessment of coagulation and massive transfusion in the context of significant bleeding.
- Prepare for emergent interventions such as rapid sequence intubation. Stabilize woman with O_2 and IV fluids and blood products (Parfitt, 2016; Roth, 2021).
- Maintain continuous FHR monitoring.
- Prepare for emergency delivery.

Disseminated Intravascular Coagulation

Disseminated intravascular coagulation (DIC) is a syndrome that occurs when the body is breaking down blood clots faster than it can form a clot. This quickly depletes the body of clotting factors, leading to hemorrhage, and can rapidly lead to maternal death. DIC is always a result of another pathological process or injury and is the final common pathway of coagulation dysregulation (DeLoughery, 2015). DIC can be triggered by a myriad of adverse obstetric events that include placental abruption, AFE, sepsis syndrome, acute fatty liver of pregnancy, severe preeclampsia, hemolysis, elevated liver enzymes, low platelet count syndrome, and massive obstetric hemorrhage (Cunningham & Nelson, 2015).

Risk factors for DIC include (Salera-Vieira, 2021):

- Abruptio placentae
- Hemorrhage
- Preeclampsia or eclampsia
- AFE
- Saline termination of pregnancy
- Sepsis
- Dead fetus syndrome
- Cardiopulmonary arrest
- Massive transfusion therapy

During pregnancy, maternal leukocytes are in a higher state of activation than in nonpregnant women and have characteristics akin to sepsis. However, they are well-controlled during pregnancy, and it has been proposed that the trophoblast plays a role in the maintenance of the balanced systemic maternal inflammation during pregnancy. Nevertheless, in cases of sepsis caused by an infectious agent or septic abortion and at least in some of the cases of AFE, this equilibrium is disturbed and the mother develops DIC (Erez et al., 2015). DIC is a dire obstetrical emergency that is a significant cause of maternal morbidity and mortality and is associated with up to 25% of maternal deaths (Cunningham & Nelson, 2015; Salera-Vieira, 2021). Prompt recognition and understanding of the underlying mechanisms of disease leading to this complication is essential for successful management and positive outcome (Erez et al., 2015). Women who experience DIC are transferred to the critical care unit and a perinatologist manages the care. This is discussed more completely in Chapter 14.

CRITICAL CARE IN PERINATAL NURSING

Critical care intrapartum nursing may be required when a woman has a preexisting condition or a maternal or fetal complication develops during pregnancy. The ability of a hospital to deliver this high level of care may vary; because high-risk and critically ill women may be encountered in any setting, all intrapartum nurses should be prepared to identify and participate in stabilizing critically ill women for transport to a tertiary care center or intensive care unit (AWHONN, 2008). Intrapartum nurses who care for critically ill women receive additional education and undergo didactic training and verification of learning and clinical skills beyond the scope of this chapter.

Most critically ill pregnant women are cared for in adult intensive care units or specialized obstetric critical care units. No matter where care is delivered, a comprehensive plan of care should address the woman's unique physiological needs. It is essential that when indicated, critical care and perinatal nurses collaborate to coordinate care for this unique population. Women who have any of the disorders or diseases presented in the high-risk didactic content have the potential to become critically ill if their condition deteriorates.

Nurses are often the first members of the health-care team to detect subtle signs and symptoms of developing complications; thus, their contribution to the rescue process is crucial. A nurse's role in alerting the team and mobilizing its response has a direct impact on the ultimate outcome. Women considered low-risk can become acutely ill with little warning, requiring rapid assessment, emergent mobilization of the team, and intervention to support the optimal outcomes (Behling & Renaud, 2015).

Women may have obstetric or nonobstetric conditions that can be complicated by the presence of a fetus and a myriad of potential comorbidities.

The maternal code protocol was developed in accordance with the American Heart Association's (AHA) ACLS algorithms (Jeejeebhoy et al., 2015; Panchal et al., 2020; Vanden Hoek et al., 2010).

Sudden cardiac arrest in pregnant women is a dangerous and complex condition because of the presence of two patients (mother and fetus) as well as the need for immediate treatment. The newly released 2020 American Heart Association Cardiopulmonary Resuscitation & Emergency Cardiovascular Care guidelines provide a framework to optimize resuscitation for in-hospital maternal cardiac arrest victims. The guidelines use existing research to generate an algorithm for maternal resuscitation that highlights the importance of concurrent intervention, meaning that advanced life support professionals responding to maternal cardiac arrest must simultaneously perform maternal and obstetric treatments per the published algorithm. Alongside the emphasis on simultaneous treatment, the guidelines emphasize collaborative obstetric, neonatal, emergency, anesthesiology, intensive care, and cardiac arrest services that focus care on oxygenation and ventilation, left lateral uterine displacement, and stabilization of the mother (Panchal et al., 2020). Mock code drills utilizing the maternal code protocol have assisted in keeping nurses' skills current in performing ACLS steps that are rarely implemented.

The leading causes of ICU admission during pregnancy and postpartum are hypertensive disorders and obstetric hemorrhage. Additional diagnoses that result in ICU admission include sepsis, trauma, respiratory conditions, cardiovascular disorders, diabetic ketoacidosis, gastrointestinal disorders (pancreatitis, appendicitis, bowel obstruction), overdose or poisoning, and neurological disorders (ACOG, 2019b). Most are postpartum admissions (ACOG, 2019b.)

When unexpected crises occur on the OB unit, nurses and other clinicians must act quickly and take appropriate steps to ensure best health outcomes. Use of protocols during mock emergency drills can assist in educating staff on critical steps that must be taken while maintaining a calm, collected setting, thus creating a positive learning environment. In the event these drills become reality, preparation that has occurred through use of these protocols can promote a controlled atmosphere with optimal results for both the women experiencing a health crisis and the health-care staff caring for them (Roth et al., 2015).

CONCEPT MAP |

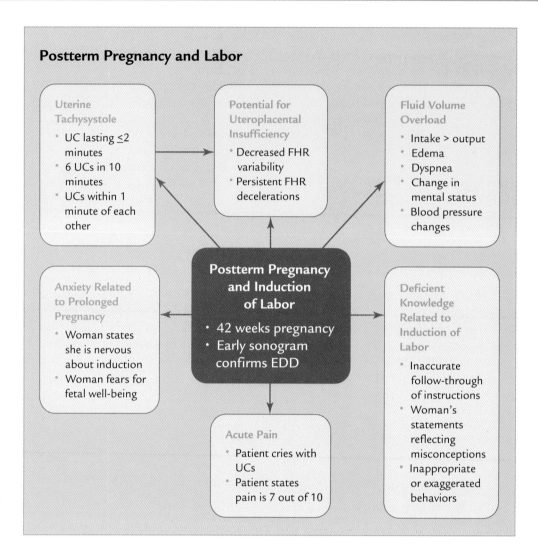

Postterm Pregnancy and Labor

Uterine Tachysystole
- UC lasting ≤2 minutes
- 6 UCs in 10 minutes
- UCs within 1 minute of each other

Potential for Uteroplacental Insufficiency
- Decreased FHR variability
- Persistent FHR decelerations

Fluid Volume Overload
- Intake > output
- Edema
- Dyspnea
- Change in mental status
- Blood pressure changes

Anxiety Related to Prolonged Pregnancy
- Woman states she is nervous about induction
- Woman fears for fetal well-being

Postterm Pregnancy and Induction of Labor
- 42 weeks pregnancy
- Early sonogram confirms EDD

Deficient Knowledge Related to Induction of Labor
- Inaccurate follow-through of instructions
- Woman's statements reflecting misconceptions
- Inappropriate or exaggerated behaviors

Acute Pain
- Patient cries with UCs
- Patient states pain is 7 out of 10

CARE PLANS

Problem 1: Uterine tachysystole

Goal: Decreased uterine activity

Outcome: Patient will have decreased contractions.

Nursing Actions
1. Evaluate UC strength, frequency, and resting tone duration by palpation or IUPC.
2. Evaluate uterine resting tone by palpation or IUPC pressure above 25 mm Hg.
3. Assess FHR in response to UCs.
4. Turn oxytocin down or off in the event of uterine tachysystole or indeterminate or abnormal FHR.
5. Assist with maternal position change.
6. Offer IV bolus of at least 500 mL of lactated Ringer's.
7. Administer O₂ by mask at 10 L/min.
8. If no response, consider terbutaline.
9. Notify provider.

Problem 2: Knowledge deficit related to induction of labor

Goal: Patient understands indication and process of labor induction.

Outcome: Patient states she understands indication and process of induction of labor.

Nursing Actions
1. Explain all procedures.
2. Encourage verbalization of questions.
3. Practice active listening.
4. Provide emotional support.
5. Make needed referrals to social services and mental health specialists if needed.

Problem 3: Anxiety related to prolonged pregnancy

Goal: Decreased anxiety

Outcome: Patient verbalizes that she feels less anxious.

Nursing Actions

1. Explain all information and procedures in lay language and repeat information prn.
2. Provide autonomy and choices.
3. Encourage patient and family to verbalize their feelings regarding prolonged pregnancy by asking open-ended questions.
4. Be calm and reassuring in interactions with the patient and her family.
5. Explore past coping strategies.

Problem 4: Fluid volume overload related to prolonged oxytocin

Goal: Fluid balance

Outcome: Patient maintains fluid balance.

Nursing Actions

1. Auscultate the lung sounds.
2. Assess I&O.
3. Maintain IV fluids as ordered.
4. Calculate intake of all fluids.
5. Measure output including emesis and urine.
6. Assess edema.

Problem 5: Acute pain related to UCs

Goal: Decreased pain

Outcome: Patient will state that pain is improved.

Nursing Actions

1. Assess level, location, and type of pain.

2. Sustain physical presence, eye contact.
3. Provide verbal encouragement, reassurance, and praise.
4. Provide comfort measures such as ice chips, fluids, food, and pain medications.
5. Provide hygiene, including mouth care, pericare, and changing underpads.
6. Assist with position changes.
7. Provide reassuring touch and massage.
8. Apply heat and cold.
9. Encourage hydrotherapy via shower or tub if no ROM.
10. Provide environment that is conducive to relaxation, such as low lights and decreased noise.
11. Teach the patient relaxation and breathing techniques.

Problem 6: Potential for uteroplacental insufficiency Category II or III FHR

Goal: Maintain normal FHR

Outcome: FHR pattern is Category I; baseline is normal with moderate variability and accelerations.

Nursing Actions

1. Assess FHR baseline variability and for decelerations.
2. Change the mother's position.
3. Provide IV bolus of at least 500 mL of lactated Ringer's.
4. Provide O_2 at 10 L/min by mask.
5. Turn oxytocin down or off.
6. Notify the provider.
7. Request bedside evaluation if the FHR is Category III.

Case Study

As an L&D nurse, this is your second shift caring for Mallory Polk. She is a 42-year-old, single, Black attorney whom you admitted yesterday at 32 weeks' gestation with the diagnosis of preterm labor. She was treated with magnesium sulfate and betamethasone. Tonight, when you come on your shift at 7:00 p.m., she remains on magnesium sulfate but is contracting regularly and at 3:20 a.m. has SROM for clear fluid. At 4:00 a.m. her cervix is 5 cm/90%/+1. At this time, the magnesium sulfate is discontinued and normal spontaneous vaginal birth anticipated because of advanced preterm labor. Over the next hour Mallory is contracting every 2 to 3 minutes and coping well with UCs. Her sister, Allison, is at the bedside providing labor support. The FHR baseline is 140s, with average variability, occasional accelerations, and no decelerations. At 5:15 a.m., Mallory feels the urge to have a bowel movement and you do an SVE. Her vaginal examination reveals that she is 10 cm/100%/+1.

Who needs to be notified of your significant assessment findings?

What would you report?

Within 15 minutes of your report, her physician arrives, confirms your assessment that Mallory is completely dilated, and wants her to start pushing. You coach Mallory to begin pushing with her next contraction.

What are your priorities in nursing care for Mallory?

Discuss the rationale for the priorities.

State nursing diagnosis, expected outcome, and interventions related to this problem.

What would you anticipate as Mallory's teaching needs?

Over the next hour, Mallory's contractions slow to every 7 minutes. She is open-glottis pushing and feels the urge to bear down with the peak of contractions. An SVE reveals descent of the fetal head is +2 station. You request the physician to come to the bedside to evaluate fetal descent. After her physician evaluates Mallory, she requests oxytocin augmentation to increase the frequency of contractions. You initiate oxytocin augmentation at 1 mU/min per physician orders.

Discuss the risk associated with oxytocin augmentation.

Outline nursing actions when caring for a patient with oxytocin augmentation.

Continued

What teaching would you include related to oxytocin augmentation?

Within 30 minutes of starting oxytocin, Mallory is having UCs every 1 to 2 minutes lasting 45 to 55 seconds, moderate to palpation with relaxed uterus between contractions. FHR baseline is 140s with variable decelerations to 90s for 40 seconds with UCs. FHR variability is moderate.

What are your priorities in nursing care?

Discuss the rationale for the priorities and nursing actions.

What are your nursing actions based on your assessment?

State the nursing diagnosis and expected outcomes.

Over the next hour, Mallory's contractions are every 3 to 4 minutes. She is pushing with contractions and has a strong urge to bear down with contractions. The FHR is 140s with moderate variability and variable decelerations to 100 bpm for 30 seconds with contractions and open-glottis pushing. Her SVE reveals fetal descent to +3 station.

What are your immediate priorities in nursing care for Mallory?

Discuss the rationale for the priorities.

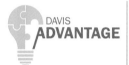

Go to Davis Advantage to complete your learning: strengthen understanding, apply your knowledge, and prepare for the Next Gen NCLEX®.

REFERENCES

Adams, E. D., Stark, M. A., & Low, L. K. (2016). A nurse's guide to supporting physiologic birth. *Nursing and Women's Health, 20*(1), 76–85. http://nwhjournal.org

Agency for Healthcare Research and Quality. (2001). *Reducing and preventing adverse drug events to decrease hospital costs.* Publication No. 01-0200. Author.

American Academy of Pediatrics & American College of Obstetricians and Gynecologists. (2017). *Guidelines for perinatal care* (8th ed.). Authors.

American College of Obstetricians and Gynecologists. (2009a, reaffirmed, 2019). Induction of labor. ACOG Practice Bulletin No. 107. *Obstetrics & Gynecology, 114*(2 Pt 1), 386–397. https://doi.org/10.1097/AOG.0b013 e3181b48ef5

American College of Obstetricians and Gynecologists. (2015). Informed consent. ACOG Committee Opinion No. 439. *Obstetrics & Gynecology, 114*(2 Pt. 1), 401–408. https://doi.org/10.1097/AOG.0b013 e3181b48f7f

American College of Obstetricians and Gynecologists. (2009c). Management of stillbirth. Practice Bulletin No. 102. *Obstetrics & Gynecology, 113*(3), 748–761.

American College of Obstetricians and Gynecologists. (2010). *Vaginal birth after previous cesarean delivery.* Practice Bulletin No. 115. Author.

American College of Obstetricians and Gynecologists. (2011). *Optimizing protocols for obstetrics: Oxytocin for induction.* Author.

American College of Obstetricians and Gynecologists. (2014a). Preparing for clinical emergencies in obstetrics and gynecology. Committee Opinion No. 590. *Obstetrics & Gynecology, 123*, 722–725.

American College of Obstetricians and Gynecologists. (2014b). Management of late-term and post-term pregnancies. Practice Bulletin No. 146. *Obstetrics & Gynecology, 124*, 390–396.

American College of Obstetricians and Gynecologists. (2014c). Safe prevention of the primary cesarean delivery. Obstetric Care Consensus No. 1. *Obstetrics & Gynecology, 123*, 693–711.

American College of Obstetricians and Gynecologists. (2016). Multifetal gestations: Twin, triplet, and higher-order multifetal pregnancies. Practice Bulletin No. 169. *Obstetrics & Gynecology, 128*, e131–e146.

American College of Obstetricians and Gynecologists. (2017a). Delivery of a newborn with meconium-stained amniotic fluid. Committee Opinion No. 689. *Obstetrics & Gynecology, 129*, e33–e34.

American College of Obstetricians and Gynecologists. (2017b). Intrapartum management of intraamniotic infection. Committee Opinion No. 712. *Obstetrics & Gynecology, 130*, e95–e101.

American College of Obstetricians and Gynecologists. (2017c). Shoulder dystocia. Practice Bulletin No. 178. *Obstetrics & Gynecology, 129*, e123–e133.

American College of Obstetricians and Gynecologists. (2017d). *Vaginal birth after previous cesarean delivery.* Practice Bulletin No. 184. Author.

American College of Obstetricians and Gynecologists. (2018). Placenta accreta spectrum. Obstetric Care Consensus No. 7. *Obstetrics & Gynecology, 132*, e259–e75.

American College of Obstetricians and Gynecologists. (2019a). Approaches to limit intervention during labor and birth. ACOG Committee Opinion No. 766. *Obstetrics & Gynecology, 133*, e164–e173.

American College of Obstetricians and Gynecologists. (2019b). Critical care in pregnancy. ACOG Practice Bulletin No. 211. *Obstetrics & Gynecology, 133*, e303–e319.

American College of Obstetricians and Gynecologists. (2019c). Ethical considerations for the care of patients with obesity. ACOG Committee Opinion No. 763. *Obstetrics & Gynecology, 133*. e90–e96.

American College of Obstetricians and Gynecologists. (2019d). Vaginal birth after cesarean delivery. ACOG Practice Bulletin No. 205. *Obstetrics & Gynecology, 133*, e110–e127.

American College of Obstetricians and Gynecologists. (2020a). External cephalic version. ACOG Practice Bulletin No. 221. *Obstetrics & Gynecology, 135*, e203–e212.

American College of Obstetricians and Gynecologists. (2020b). Macrosomia. ACOG Practice Bulletin No. 216. *Obstetrics & Gynecology, 135*, e18–e35.

American College of Obstetricians and Gynecologists. (2020c). *Management of stillbirth.* OB Care Consensus No. 10, March. Author.

American College of Obstetricians and Gynecologists. (2020d). Operative vaginal birth. ACOG Practice Bulletin No. 219. *Obstetrics & Gynecology, 135*, e149–e159.

American College of Obstetricians and Gynecologists. (2021). Obesity in pregnancy. ACOG Practice Bulletin No. 230. *Obstetrics & Gynecology, 137*, e128–e144. https://doi.org/10.1097/AOG.0000000000004395

American College of Obstetricians and Gynecologists & Society for Maternal-Fetal Medicine. (2014). Safe prevention of the primary cesarean delivery (Obstetric Care Consensus No. 1). *Obstetrics & Gynecology, 123*(3), 693–711. https://doi.org/10.1097/01.AOG.0000444441.04111.1d

Association for Women's Health, Obstetric and Neonatal Nurses. (2008). *Basic high risk and critical care intrapartum nursing clinical competencies and education guide* (4th ed.). Author.

Association for Women's Health, Obstetric and Neonatal Nurses. (2014). *Position statement: Nonmedically indicated induction and augmentation of labor.* Author.

Association for Women's Health, Obstetric and Neonatal Nurses. (2019). Elective induction of labor (Position Statement). *Nursing for Women's Health, 23*(2), 177–179. https://doi.org/10.1016/j.nwh.2019.03.001

Athukorala, C., Middleton, P., & Crowther, C. A. (2006). Intrapartum interventions for preventing shoulder dystocia. *Cochrane Database of Systematic Reviews, 4.* https://doi.org/10.1002/14651858.CD005543.pub2

Behling, D. J., & Renaud, M. (2015). Development of an obstetric vital sign alert to improve outcomes in acute care obstetrics. *Nursing for Women's Health, 19*(2), 128–141.

Benson, M. D. (2017). Amniotic fluid embolism mortality rate. *The Journal of Obstetrics and Gynaecology Research, 43*(11), 1714–1718. https://doi.org/10.1111/jog.13445

Bishop, E. H. (1964). Pelvic scoring for elective induction. *Obstetrics & Gynecology, 24*, 266–268.

Bowers, N. A. (2021). Multiple gestation. In K. Simpson, P. Creehan, N. O'Brien-Abel, C. Roth, & A. Rohan (Eds.), *Perinatal nursing* (5th ed., pp. 249–294). Wolters Kluwer.

Bricker, L., & Luckas, M. (2000). Amniotomy alone for induction of labour. *Cochrane Database of Systematic Reviews, 4.* https://doi.org/10.1002/14651858.CD002862

Centers for Disease Control and Prevention. (2017a). *Pregnancy mortality surveillance system.* https://www.cdc.gov/reproductivehealth/maternalinfanthealth/pmss.html

Centers for Disease Control and Prevention. (2017b). *Severe maternal morbidity in the United States.* Division of Reproductive Health, National Center for Chronic Disease Prevention and Health Promotion. https://www.cdc.gov/reproductivehealth/MaternalInfantHealth/SevereMaternalMorbidity.html

Centers for Disease Control and Prevention. (2019). *About natality 2007–2017.* Author.

Centers for Disease Control and Prevention. (2021). *Maternal mortality.* https://www.cdc.gov/nchs/maternal-mortality/index.htm

Clark, S. L. (2014). Amniotic fluid embolism. *Obstetrics & Gynecology, 123*(2 pt 1), 337–348. https://doi.org/10.1016/j.ajog.2019.07.036

Clark, S. L., Simpson, K., Knox, G., & Garite, T. (2009). Oxytocin: New perspectives on an old drug. *American Journal of Obstetrics & Gynecology, 200*(1), 35.e1–35.e6.

Cunningham, F. G., & Nelson, D. B. (2015). Disseminated intravascular coagulation syndromes in obstetrics. *Obstetrics & Gynecology, 126*(5), 999–1011. https://doi.org/10.1097/AOG.0000000000001110

Cunningham, F. G., & Wells, C. E. (2017). *Patient education: Vaginal birth after cesarean delivery (VBAC) (beyond the basics).* https://www.uptodate.com/contents/vaginal-birth-after-cesarean-delivery-vbac-beyond-the-basics

Cunningham, F. G., Leveno, K., Bloom, S., Dashe, J., Hoffman, B., Casey, B., & Spong, C. (2018). *Williams obstetrics* (25th ed.). McGraw-Hill.

DeLoughery, T. G. (2015). Disseminated intravascular coagulation. In DeLoughery, T. G. (Eds.), *Hemostasis and thrombosis* (3rd ed., pp. 39–42). Springer International Publishing. https://doi.org/10.1007/978-3-319-09312-3_8

Drummond, S., & Yeomans, E. (2019). Amniotic fluid embolism. In Troiano, N., Witcher, P., & McMurtry Baird, S. (Eds.), *High-risk & critical care obstetrics* (4th ed., pp. 286–295). Wolters Kluwer.

Dunn, T., Nassr, A., Moaddab, A., Eppes, C., & Shamshirsaz, A. (2017). Vasa previa: Maternal and early neonatal outcomes in the new era of obstetrical care [13K]. *Obstetrics & Gynecology, 129*(5), 1155. https://doi.org/10.1097/01.AOG.0000514606.70935.d2

Erez, O., Mastrolia, S. A., & Thachil, J. (2015). Disseminated intravascular coagulation in pregnancy: Insights in pathophysiology, diagnosis and management. *American Journal of Obstetrics & Gynecology, 213*(4), 452–463. https://doi.org/10.1016/j.ajog.2015.03.054

Farsight, A. Y., Jaimez-Carranza, N. M., & Coleman, C. R. (2017). Multidisciplinary response to amniotic fluid embolism. *Journal of Obstetric, Gynecologic & Neonatal Nursing, 46*(3), S56–S57.

Finucane, E. M., Murphy, D. J., Biesty, L. M., Gyte, G. M. L., Cotter, A. M., Ryan, E. M., . . . Devane, D. (2020). Membrane sweeping for induction of labour. *Cochrane Database of Systematic Reviews, 2,* CD000451. https://doi.org/10.1002/14651858.CD000451.pub3.

Geis, G. M. (2017). Meconium aspiration syndrome. *Medscape.* https://emedicine.medscape.com/article/974110-overview

Gilbert, E. (2011). Labor and delivery at risk. In S. Mattson & J. Smith (Eds.), *Core curriculum for maternal-newborn nursing* (4th ed.). Sage.

Gregory, E. C. W., Drake, P., & Martin, J. A. (2018). *Lack of change in perinatal mortality in the United States, 2014–2016.* NCHS Data Brief, No. 316. National Center for Health Statistics.

Grobman, W. A., Rice, M. M., Reddy, U. M., Tita, A. T., Silver, R. M., Mallett, G., . . . Macones, G. A. Labor induction versus expectant management in low-risk nulliparous women. Eunice Kennedy Shriver National Institute of Child Health and Human Development Maternal–Fetal Medicine Units Network. *New England Journal of Medicine, 379,* 513–523.

Gülmezoglu, A. M., Crowther, C. A., & Middleton, P. (2006). Induction of labour for improving birth outcomes for women at or beyond term. *Cochrane Database of Systematic Reviews, 4.* https://doi.org/10.1002/14651858.CD004945.pub2

Higgins, R. D., Saade, G., Polin, R. A., Grobman, W. A., Buhimschi, I. A., Watterberg, K., . . . Tse, N. K. for the Chorioamnionitis Workshop Participants. (2016). Evaluation and management of women and newborns with a maternal diagnosis of chorioamnionitis: Summary of a workshop. *Obstetrics & Gynecology, 127*(3), 426–436. https://doi.org/10.1097/AOG.0000000000001246

Hoyert, D. L., & Gregory, E. C. W. (2020). *Cause-of-death data from the fetal death file, 2015–2017. National Vital Statistics Reports, 69*(4). National Center for Health Statistics.

Institute for Healthcare Improvement. (2007). *Prevent harm from high alert medications: How to guide.* Author.

Institute for Safe Medication Practices. (2007). *High-alert medications.* Author.

Jacobson, C. H., Zlatnik, M. G., Kennedy, H. P., & Lyndon, A. (2013). Nurses' perspectives on the intersection of safety and informed decision making in maternity care. *Journal of Obstetric, Gynecologic & Neonatal Nursing, 42*(5), 577–587.

Jeejeebhoy, F. M., Zelop, C. M., Lipman, S., Carvalho, B., Joglar, J., Mhyre, J. M., . . . & American Heart Association Emergency Cardiovascular Care Committee, Council on Cardiopulmonary, Critical Care, Perioperative and Resuscitation, Council on Cardiovascular Diseases in the Young, and Council on Clinical Cardiology. (2015). Cardiac arrest in pregnancy: A scientific statement from the American Heart Association. *Circulation, 132,* 1747–1773. https://doi.org/10.1161/CIR.0000000000000300

Jonsson, M., Norden-Lindeberg, S., & Hanson, U. (2007). Analysis of malpractice claims with a focus on oxytocin use in labour. *Acta Obstetricia et Gynecologica, 86,* 315–319.

Jozwiak, M., Bloemenkamp, K., Kelly, A., Mol, B., Irion, O., & Boulvain, M. (2012). Mechanical methods for induction of labour. *Cochrane Database of Systematic Reviews, 3.* https://doi.org/10.1002/14651858.CD001233.pub2

Kelly, A. J., Alfirevic, Z., Hofmeyr, G. J., Kavanagh, J., Neilson, J. P., & Thomas, J. (2009). Induction of labour in specific clinical situations: Generic protocol. *Cochrane Database of Systematic Reviews, 2.* https://doi.org/10.1002/14651858.CD003398.pub2

Kelly, A. J., Kavanagh, J., & Thomas, J. (2013). Castor oil, bath and/or enema for cervical priming and induction of labour. *Cochrane Database of Systematic Reviews, 7,* CD003099. https://doi.org/10.1002/14651858.CD003099.pub2

Kunz, M. K., Loftus, R. L., & Nichols, A. M. (2013). Incidence of uterine tachysystole in women induced with oxytocin. *Journal of Obstetric, Gynecologic & Neonatal Nursing, 42,* 12–18. https://doi.org/10.1111/j.1552-6909.2012.01428.x

Lyndon, A., & Ali, L. U. (Eds.). (2008). *Fetal heart rate monitoring: Principles and practice* (4th ed.). Kendall Hunt.

Lyndon, A., Johnson, M. C., Bingham, D., Napolitano, P. G., Joseph, G., Maxfield, D. G., & O'Keeffe, D. F. (2015). Transforming communication and safety culture in intrapartum care. A multi-organization blueprint. *Journal of Obstetric, Gynecologic, & Neonatal Nursing, 44,* 341–349. https://doi.org/10.1111/1552-6909.12575

Lyndon, A., Zlatnik, M. G., Maxfield, D. G., Lewis, A., McMillan, C., & Kennedy, H. P. (2014). Contributions of clinical disconnections and unresolved conflict to failures in intrapartum safety. *Journal of Obstetric, Gynecologic & Neonatal Nursing, 43*(1), 2–12. https://doi.org/10.1111/1552-6909.12266

Macones, G. A., Hankins, G. D. V., Spong, C. Y., Hauth, J., & Moore, T. (2008). The 2008 National Institute of Child Health and Human Development workshop report on electronic fetal monitoring: Update on definitions, interpretation, and research guidelines. *Journal of Obstetric, Gynecologic and Neonatal Nursing, 37,* 510–515. https://doi.org/10.1111/j.1552-6909.2008.00284.x

Maher, M. A. (2021). Obesity in pregnancy. In K. Simpson, P. Creehan, N. O'Brien-Abel, C. Roth, & A. Rohan (Eds.), *Perinatal nursing* (5th ed., pp. 295–313). Wolters Kluwer.

Malone, F. D., & D'Alton, M. E. (2014). Multiple gestation: Clinical characteristics and management. In R. K. Creasy, R. Resnik, J. D. Iams, C. J. Lockwood, T. R. Moore, & M. F. Green (Eds.), *Creasy & Resnik's maternal-fetal medicine: Principles and practice* (7th ed., pp. 756–784). Elsevier/Saunders.

Martin, J. A., Hamilton, B. E., Osterman, M. J. K., & Driscoll, A. K. (2021). *Births: Final data for 2019. National Vital Statistics Reports, 70*(2). National Center for Health Statistics. 2021. https://doi.org/10.15620/cdc:100472

Martin, J. A., Hamilton, B. E., Osterman, M. J., Driscoll, A. K., & Mathews, T. J. (2017). Births: Final data for 2015. National Vital Statistics Reports: From the Centers for Disease Control and Prevention, National Center for Health Statistics. *National Vital Statistics System, 66*(1), 1. https://www.cdc.gov/nchs/data/nvsr/nvsr67/nvsr67_08-508.pdf

Martin, J. A., Hamilton, B. E., Osterman, M. J. K., & Driscoll, A. K. (2019). Births: Final data for 2018. *National Vital Statistics Reports, 68*(13), 1–47. https://www.cdc.gov/nchs/data/nvsr/nvsr68/nvsr68_13-508.pdf

Nahum, G. G. (2016). Uterine rupture in pregnancy. *Medscape.* https://reference.medscape.com/article/275854-overview

National Institutes of Health. (2010). Consensus development conference statement: Vaginal birth after cesarean: New insights March 8–10, 2010. *Obstetrics & Gynecology, 115,* 1279–1295. https://doi.org/10.1053/j.semperi.2010.05.001

Norwitz, E. R. (2017). Patient education: Post-term pregnancy (beyond the basics). *Up To Date.* https://www.uptodate.com/contents/postterm-pregnancy-beyond-the-basics

Oyelese, Y. (2007). Placenta previa, placenta accreta and vasa previa. In J. Queenan (Ed.), *High risk pregnancy.* American College of Obstetricians & Gynecologists.

Panchal, A. R., Bartos, J. A., Cabañas, J. G., Donnino, M. W., Drennan, I. R., Hirsch, K. G., . . . Berg, K. M.; on behalf of the Adult Basic and Advanced Life Support Writing Group. (2020). Part 3: Adult Basic and Advanced Life Support: 2020 American Heart Association guidelines for cardiopulmonary resuscitation and emergency cardiovascular care. *Circulation, 142*(suppl 2), S366–S468. https://doi.org/10.1161/CIR.0000000000000916

Parfitt, S. (2016). Labor and delivery at risk. In S. Mattson & J. E. Smith (Eds.), *AWHONN, core curriculum for maternal newborn nursing* (6th ed.). Elsevier.

Phelan, S. T., & Holbrook, B. D. (2013). *Umbilical cord prolapse.* Royal College of Obstetricians and Gynaecologists.

Roth, C. K. (2021). Pulmonary complications in pregnancy. In K. Simpson, P. Creehan, N. O'Brien-Abel, C. Roth, & A. Rohan (Eds.), *Perinatal nursing* (5th ed.. pp. 220–247). Wolters Kluwer.

Roth, C. K., Parfitt, S. E., Hering, S. L., & Dent, S. A. (2015). Developing protocols for obstetric emergencies. *Nursing for Women's Health, 18*(5), 378–390. https://doi.org/10.1016/j.jogn.2015.12.010

Salera-Vieira, J. (2021). Bleeding in pregnancy. In K. Simpson, P. Creehan, N. O'Brien-Abel, C. Roth, & A. Rohan (Eds.), *Perinatal nursing* (5th ed., pp. 123–140). Wolters Kluwer.

Sayed Ahmed, W. A., & Hamdy, M. A. (2018). Optimal management of umbilical cord prolapse. *International Journal of Women's Health, 10,* 459–465. https://doi.org/10.2147/IJWH.S130879

Silver, R. M. (2015). Abnormal placentation: Placenta previa, vasa previa, and placenta accreta. *Obstetrics & Gynecology, 126*(3), 654–668.

Simpson, K. R. (2020). *Cervical ripening labor induction and labor augmentation of labor* (54th ed.). AWHONN.

Simpson, K. R. (2021). Perinatal patient safety and quality. In K. R. Simpson, P. Creehan, N. O'Brien-Abel, C. Roth, & A. Rohan (Eds.), *Perinatal nursing* (5th ed., pp. 1–16). Wolters Kluwer.

Simpson, K. R., & Atterbury, J. (2003). Trends and issues in labor induction in the United States: Implications for clinical practice. *Journal of Obstetric, Gynecologic & Neonatal Nursing, 32,* 767–779.

Simpson, K. R., & Knox, G. (2009). High-alert medication: Implications for perinatal patient safety. *Maternal Child Nursing, 34*(1), 8–15.

Simpson, K. R., & James, D. C. (2008). Effects of oxytocin-induced uterine hyperstimulation during labor on fetal oxygen status and fetal heart rate patterns. *American Journal of Obstetrics & Gynecology, 199*(1), 34.e1–34.e5. https://doi.org/10.1016/j.ajog.2007.12.015

Simpson, K. R. & O'Brien-Abel, N. (2021). Labor and birth. In K. R. Simpson, P. Creehan, N. O'Brien-Abel, C. Roth, & A. Rohan (Eds.), *Perinatal nursing* (5th ed., pp. 325–411). Wolters Kluwer.

Sinkey, R. G., Odibo, A. O., & Dashe, J. S. (2015). Diagnosis and management of vasa previa. Society for Maternal–Fetal Medicine Consult Series #37. *American Journal of Obstetrics & Gynecology, 213*(5), 615–619. https://doi.org/10.1016/j.ajog.2015.08.031

Smith, C. A., Armour, M., & Dahlen, H. G. (2017). Acupuncture or acupressure for induction of labour. *Cochrane Database of Systematic Reviews, 10,* CD002962. https://doi.org/10.1002/14651858.CD002962.pub4

Sousou, J., & Smart, C. (2015). Care of the childbearing family with intrauterine fetal demise. *Nursing for Women's Health, 19*(3), 236–247.

Spong, C. Y., Berghella, V., Wenstrom, K. D., Mercer, B. M., & Saade, G. R. (2012). Preventing the first cesarean delivery: Summary of a joint Eunice Kennedy Shriver National Institute of Child Health and Human Development, Society for Maternal-Fetal Medicine, and American College of Obstetricians and Gynecologists workshop. *Obstetrics & Gynecology, 120*(5), 1181–1193. https://doi.org/10.1097/AOG.0b013e3182704880

Stanley Sundin, C., & Bradham Mazac, L. (2017). Amniotic fluid embolism. *American Journal of Maternal Child Nursing, 42*(1), 29–35.

Sultan, P., Seligman, K., & Carvalho, B. (2016). Amniotic fluid embolism: Update and review. *Current Opinion in Anaesthesiology, 29*(3), 288–296. https://doi.org/10.1097/ACO.0000000

Thongrong, C., Kasemsiri, P., Hofmann, J. P., Bergese, S. D., Papadimos, T.J., Gracias, V. H, . . . Stawicki, S. P. (2013). Amniotic fluid embolism. *International Journal of Critical Illness and Injury Science, 3*(1), 51–57. https://doi.org/10.4103/2229-5151.109422

Vanden Hoek, T. L., Morrison, L. J., Shuster, M., Donnino, M., Sinz, E., Lavonas, E. J., . . . Gabrielli, A. (2010). Part 12: Cardiac arrest in special situations: 2010 American Heart Association guidelines for cardiopulmonary resuscitation and emergency cardiovascular care. *Circulation, 122*(18 Suppl 3), S829–S861. https://doi.org/10.1161/CIRCULATIONAHA.110.971069.

Viau-Lapointe, J., & Filewod, N. (2019). Extracorporeal therapies for amniotic fluid embolism. *Obstetrics & Gynecology, 134*(5), 989–994. https://doi.org/10.1097/AOG.0000000000003513

Wegner, E., & Bernstein, I. (2021). Operative vaginal delivery. *Up To Date.* https://www.uptodate.com/contents/operative-vaginal-delivery

Wei, S., Wo, B. L., Qi, H. P., Xu, H., Luo, Z. C. Roy, C., & Fraser, W. D. (2013). Early amniotomy and early oxytocin for prevention of, or therapy for, delay in first stage spontaneous labour compared with routine care. *Cochrane Database of Systematic Reviews,* 8. https://doi.org/10.1002/14651858.CD006794.pub4

Wojcieszek, A. M., Shepherd, E., Middleton, P., Lassi, Z. S., Wilson, T., Murphy, M. M., . . . Flenady, V. (2018). Care prior to and during subsequent pregnancies following stillbirth for improving outcomes. *Cochrane Database of Systematic Reviews, 12,* CD012203. https://doi.org/10.1002/14651858.CD012203.pub2

Intrapartum and Postpartum Care of Cesarean Birth Families

11

Roberta F. Durham, RN, PhD
Diana Cortez, RN, BSN

LEARNING OUTCOMES

Upon completion of this chapter, the student will be able to:

1. Identify factors that place a woman at risk for cesarean birth.
2. Discuss preoperative nursing care and medical and anesthesia management for cesarean births.
3. Describe the intraoperative nursing care and medical and anesthesia management for cesarean births.
4. Discuss the postoperative nursing care of cesarean birth with women and their families.
5. Identify potential intraoperative and postoperative complications related to cesarean birth and nursing actions to reduce risk.
6. Describe safety measures to promote quality outcomes for pregnant women needing surgical care.
7. Provide discharge education after cesarean birth for the woman and her family

CONCEPTS

Caring
Clinical Judgment
Collaboration
Comfort
Communication
Elimination
Evidence-Based Practice
Family
Grief and Loss
Health Promotion
Infection
Mobility
Mood and Affect
Oxygenation
Perfusion
Safety
Self
Self-Care
Stress and Coping
Teaching and Learning
Thermoregulation
Tissue Integrity

Nursing Diagnosis

- At risk for low self-esteem related to perceived failure of life event
- At risk for injury related to surgical procedure and effects of anesthesia

Nursing Outcomes

- The woman expresses satisfaction with her birth experience.
- Parents will verbalize understanding of factors that contributed to the need for cesarean birth.

Continued

Nursing Diagnosis—cont'd

- At risk for fluid volume deficit related to blood loss and oral fluid restriction
- At risk for acute pain related to surgical incision
- At risk for infection related to surgical incision, tissue trauma, or prolonged rupture of membranes (PROM)
- At risk for altered parent–infant attachment related to surgical intervention

Nursing Outcomes—cont'd

- The woman will experience an uncomplicated intraoperative period and postoperative recovery.
- The woman will have adequate urinary output and normal amounts of lochia.
- The woman will verbalize a pain level she finds acceptable on a pain scale of 0 to 10.
- The woman will be afebrile and the abdominal incision site will be free of infection.
- The parents will hold the infant close to the body and demonstrate appropriate attachment behavior and care for infant needs.
- The woman will understand her postoperative care and discharge teaching.

INTRODUCTION

Cesarean birth, also referred to as cesarean section, C-section (C/S), or surgical birth, is an operative procedure in which the fetus is delivered through an incision in the abdominal wall and the uterus. All hospitals offering labor and birth services should be able to perform a cesarean birth. The consensus has been that hospitals should have the capacity of beginning a cesarean birth within 30 minutes of the decision to operate in an emergency (American Academy of Pediatrics [AAP] & American College of Obstetricians and Gynecologists [ACOG], 2017). Approximately one-third of pregnant women experience a cesarean birth. In 2018, the cesarean delivery rate decreased to 31.9% from 32.0% in 2017 (Martin et al., 2019). The percentage of cesarean births has increased from 20.7% in 1996 to 31.9% in 2016 and reflects a 54% increase over a 19-year period (Hamilton et al., 2011, 2017).

Recent data from California indicated Black women were significantly more likely to have a cesarean in nearly all hospital types, settings, and volume with a relative risk (RR) ranging from 1.1- to 1.3-fold higher than the rate for White women (Teal et al., 2020). Another large population-based study demonstrated Black, Asian, and Hispanic women all experience greater likelihood of cesarean delivery than White women, even after accounting for sociodemographic and clinical differences, and that indications for cesarean delivery vary by maternal race and ethnicity. These findings suggest that labor management strategies to promote vaginal delivery are not differentially applied by maternal race and ethnicity (Yee et al., 2017).

Understanding whether and how maternal race and ethnicity influence the complex decision-making processes that occur in obstetric care is critical to improving quality of care for all women. Although women of minority racial and ethnic status experience greater likelihood of cesarean delivery as well as differences in indications for cesarean delivery, current data suggest these differences are not clearly attributed to unequal application of labor management strategies intended to promote safe vaginal deliveries. Although these findings may offer some reassurance about equity in care provision, racial and ethnic disparities in cesarean delivery and other maternal and neonatal health outcomes remain and the reasons for these differences continue to require exploration.

High rates of cesarean births are partially attributed to these factors:

- The VBAC rate, which measures vaginal births among women with a previous cesarean delivery, remains relatively low. In 2019, fewer than 15% of women (13.8%) with a previous cesarean delivered vaginally. The rate has increased modestly every year since 2016 when national data became available (Martin et al., 2019).
- There has been a decrease of vacuum and forceps-assisted births.
- There has been an increase in the number of fetuses in breech position delivered by cesarean, as well as an increase in the number of cesarean deliveries on maternal request (CDMR). CDMR refers to elective delivery by maternal request in the absence of maternal or fetal medical indications. An estimated 2.5% of births in the United States are CDMR (ACOG, 2019a).
- There has been an increase in the labor inductions, especially for nulliparous women or women with an unfavorable cervix.
- There has been an increase in the average maternal age at delivery. Cesarean delivery continued to remain higher among older women compared with younger mothers; women aged 40 and over (48.0%) were more than twice as likely to deliver by cesarean as women under age 20 (19.8%) (Martin et al., 2019).
- An increase in malpractice litigation is perceived as contributing to the cesarean rate.

The needs and experiences for a cesarean birth are distinctly different from those of women who experience a vaginal birth. These differences include increased length of hospitalization, longer period of physical recovery, increased pain, and increased negative emotional responses to the childbirth experience. Women who experience a planned cesarean birth versus an unplanned cesarean birth often face additional challenges. Women who experience an unplanned cesarean birth may have feelings of guilt and failure for not achieving a vaginal birth. Reports of these feelings have decreased as cesarean births have become more common.

CLASSIFICATION OF CESAREAN BIRTHS

Cesarean births are classified as either scheduled (planned) or unscheduled (unplanned). Unscheduled cesarean births include emergent, urgent, and nonurgent cesarean births.

Scheduled Cesarean Births

Scheduled cesarean births occur before the onset of labor. Typically, the woman is admitted to the labor and birthing unit the day of surgery (Fig. 11–1). Diagnostic laboratory work, such as complete blood count (CBC), platelet count, urinalysis, blood type, and cross match, may be completed a few days before admission.

Common reasons for a scheduled cesarean birth are:

- Previous cesarean birth
- Maternal or fetal health conditions that place the woman or fetus at risk during labor or vaginal birth
- Malpresentation, such as breech presentation, diagnosed before labor
- CDMR

Unscheduled Cesarean Birth

Unscheduled cesarean births usually have an urgent or emergent cause, such as fetal intolerance of labor or placental problems. The woman and her family are usually highly anxious and have fears that either the woman's or infant's health is in danger. Due to the urgency of the cesarean birth, there may not be time to fully explain the reasons for the procedure. Therefore, the woman and her partner or support person need an opportunity during the immediate postpartum period to review the events leading up to the cesarean birth. Arrest of labor and abnormal or indeterminate fetal heart tracing characteristics are the most common indications for primary cesarean birth (ACOG, 2014). Less common indications include fetal malpresentation, suspected macrosomia, maternal infection, and multiple gestation.

Labor is not without risk. Maternal morbidity is increased the longer the woman is in labor before the transition to cesarean birth. Emergency cesarean births are associated with greater risk of anesthetic complications, accidental injury to the fetus and

nearby organs, and severe hemorrhage (Association of Women's Health, Obstetric and Neonatal Nurses [AWHONN], 2019a). Additionally, women with unplanned cesarean births reported poor communication by health-care teams, distrust of clinical team or the clinical diagnosis, fear of surgery, and loss of control (Burcher et al., 2016). Because all hospitals offering labor and birth services should be equipped to perform an emergency cesarean birth within 30 minutes, some clinical situations require more expeditious birth because they can directly or indirectly cause fetal death or other adverse maternal-fetal outcomes. These include hemorrhage from placenta previa, placental abruption, umbilical cord prolapse, uterine rupture, and an abnormal electronic fetal monitoring (EFM) tracing (AAP & ACOG, 2017).

- **Emergent cesarean birth** indicates an immediate need to deliver the fetus (e.g., prolapse of umbilical cord, rupture of uterus, or abnormal fetal heart rate [FHR] patterns).
- **Urgent cesarean birth** indicates a need for rapid delivery of the fetus, such as malpresentation diagnosed after onset of labor or placenta previa with mild bleeding and FHR with Category I FHR.
- **Nonurgent cesarean birth** indicates a need for cesarean birth related to complications such as failure to progress (cervix does not fully dilate) and failure to descend (fetus does not descend through the pelvis) with Category I FHR.

CRITICAL COMPONENT

Cesarean Delivery on Maternal Request

CDMR is defined as elective cesarean delivery for singleton pregnancy at the request of the woman in the absence of any medical or obstetric indications. After exploring the reasons behind the woman's request and discussing the risks and benefits, if a woman decides to pursue CDMR, the following is recommended by ACOG: in the absence of other indications for early delivery, CDMR should not be performed before a gestational age of 39 weeks. Given the high repeat cesarean delivery rate, patients should be informed that the risks of placenta previa, placenta accreta spectrum, and gravid hysterectomy increase with each subsequent cesarean delivery. CDMR is not recommended for women desiring several children, as the risks of placenta previa, placenta accreta, and gravid hysterectomy rise with each cesarean delivery.

- CDMR should not be performed prior to 39 weeks' gestation because of the significant danger of neonatal complications that include respiratory distress, hypothermia, hypoglycemia, and NICU admission.
- In the absence of maternal or fetal indications for cesarean delivery, a plan for vaginal delivery is safe and appropriate and should be recommended.
- If a woman's main motivation to elect a cesarean delivery is a fear of pain in childbirth, care providers should discuss and offer the patient analgesia for labor, as well as prenatal childbirth education and emotional support in labor.
- There is insufficient evidence to fully evaluate the benefits and risks of CDMR as compared with planned vaginal delivery; more research is needed (ACOG, 2019a).

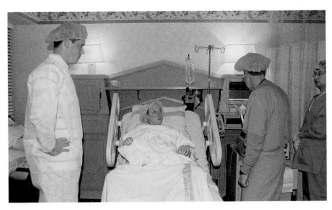

FIGURE 11–1 Couple awaiting scheduled cesarean section.

INDICATIONS FOR CESAREAN BIRTH

Cesarean births are performed for maternal or fetal reasons. The most common indications for primary (first) cesarean birth include, in order of frequency, labor dystocia, abnormal or indeterminate (Category II or III) FHR tracing, fetal malpresentation, multiple gestation, and suspected fetal macrosomia (ACOG, 2014). The major maternal medical indications for a cesarean birth are:

- Previous cesarean birth
- Placental abnormalities
- Mechanical impediment of the progress of labor or arrest of active labor
- Cephalopelvic disproportion, which occurs when ineffective uterine contractions lead to prolonged first stage of labor, when the size, shape, or position of the fetal head prevents it from passing through the maternal pelvis, or when the maternal bony pelvis is not large enough or appropriately shaped to allow for fetal descent.
- Previous uterine surgery (surgeries that involve incision through myometrium of the uterus)
- Preexisting, pregnancy-related preexisting, or pregnancy-related maternal medical conditions. such as cardiac disease, severe diabetes mellitus, severe hypertension, or preeclampsia.
- Increasing maternal age and obesity rates have led to an increase in maternal medical conditions that may impact the outcome of pregnancy and birth.
- Fetal indications affecting the method of delivery include malpresentation, abnormal FHR patterns, and maternal failure to progress through labor (ACOG, 2010, 2017; AWHONN, 2019a).

Preventing the First Cesarean Birth

The primary cesarean delivery rate, which measures cesarean deliveries among women who have not had a previous cesarean delivery, was 21.7%, very slightly down from 21.9% in 2017 (Martin et al., 2019). One in three infants born in the United States is delivered by cesarean birth. The leading driver of both the rise and variation is first-birth cesarean deliveries performed during labor. With the large increase in primary cesarean deliveries, repeat cesarean delivery has emerged as the largest single indication. There has been recent evidence of strategies that exhibited success in reducing cesarean deliveries. These interventions include training health-care providers and enhancing a maternity unit culture that values vaginal birth, educating patient and family of healthy labor experience, developing standardized admission criteria and triage management, offering adequate pain management to promote labor progress, having an in-house labor provider, and providing public reporting and tracking of cesarean deliveries from all institutions (Bell et al., 2017; Lagrew et al., 2018; Javernick & Dempsey, 2017).

Reserving labor induction primarily for medical indication is key to reducing cesarean delivery rates. If an induction is done for nonmedical indications, the gestational age should be at least 39 weeks or more and the cervix should be favorable, especially in the nulliparous woman. Review of the current literature demonstrates the importance of adhering to appropriate definitions for failed induction and arrest of labor progress. The diagnosis of failed induction should only be made after an adequate attempt. Adequate time for normal latent and active phases of the first stage and for the second stage should be allowed as long as the maternal and fetal conditions permit. The adequate time for each of these stages appears to be longer than traditionally estimated by the well-known Friedman curve. The risk of cesarean birth is not increased with the initiation of early neuraxial analgesia when compared with IV opioid analgesia (ACOG, 2019c). Operative vaginal delivery with forceps or vacuum extractor are acceptable when indicated and in the appropriate situations can be used to avoid a cesarean delivery (ACOG, 2020).

Main and colleagues (2012) concluded that national attention to the problem of unnecessary cesarean deliveries is a public health concern in the search for value and quality in U.S. health care. There is currently no evidence to demonstrate that a 31.9% cesarean delivery rate is beneficial to women or their infants. Rather, this rate exposes women and infants to unnecessary risks in the perinatal period and in the long-term results in considerable unnecessary health-care costs. Quality improvement projects aimed at reducing cesarean deliveries that demonstrated success included promotion of multidisciplinary in-house labor coverage, a multidisciplinary team approach, cultural transformation, standardized triage and admission guidelines, and support of normal physiological birth (AWHONN, 2019a). Outstanding evidence-based resources are readily available, including the California Maternal Quality Care Collaborative Toolkit (2016) and BirthTOOLS.org (American College of Nurse-Midwives [ACNM], 2017), which aggregate several practical resources for institutions and health-care providers to assist in implementing the bundle. These open-access materials are available to all birthing facilities, which reduces the burden of creating them at the local level. To successfully reduce the rate of primary cesarean birth, every organization will have to (1) make the appropriate commitment to the effort, (2) require quality improvement leadership from multiple types of health-care providers, and (3) obtain strong administrative support and proper funding to support changes (Simpson & O'Brien-Abel, 2021).

Research demonstrates nurses have an important influence on whether a woman has a cesarean or vaginal birth. In one study, nurses reported these aspects of care that they routinely offered to avoid a cesarean birth: emotional support, labor support (including ambulation, hydrotherapy, birthing ball, passive fetal descent in second-stage labor, safe titration of oxytocin for induction and augmentation of labor), sharing adequate and accurate information about what to expect, advocating on behalf of women, encouraging women to advocate for themselves,

CRITICAL COMPONENT

Interventions and Strategies for Preventing Primary Cesarean Births

1. Implement the ACOG and the Society for Maternal-Fetal Medicine's definition and management of labor dystocia. For example, define an arrest of labor in the first stage as 6-cm dilation with rupture of membranes (ROM) and 4 or more hours of adequate uterine contractions without cervical change (ACOG, 2014).
2. Develop standardized FHR interpretation and management.
3. Use cervical ripening agents when labor is induced in women with an unfavorable cervix.
4. If the maternal and fetal status allow, cesarean deliveries for failed induction of labor in the latent phase can be avoided by allowing longer durations of the latent phase (up to 24 hours or longer) and requiring that oxytocin be administered for at least 12 to 18 hours after membrane rupture before deeming the induction a failure (ACOG, 2014; AWHONN, 2019a; Caughey et al., 2014; Lagrew et al., 2018). Use nonmedical interventions such as continuous labor support by nurse or doula.
5. Use external cephalic version for breech presentation.
6. No elective inductions until 39 weeks.
7. In addition to greater expectant management of the second stage, two other practices could potentially reduce cesarean deliveries in the second stage: (1) operative vaginal delivery and (2) manual rotation of the fetal occiput for malposition.
8. Trial labor for women with twin gestations when first twin is in a vertex presentation.

and communicating with the health-care team on labor progress (Simpson & Lyndon, 2017).

Trial of Labor After Cesarean Section

Trial of labor after cesarean (TOLAC) refers to a planned attempt to deliver vaginally by a woman who has had a previous cesarean delivery, regardless of the outcome. This method provides women who desire a vaginal delivery the possibility of achieving a vaginal birth after cesarean delivery (VBAC). In addition to fulfilling a woman's preference for vaginal delivery, at an individual level, VBAC is associated with decreased maternal morbidity and a decreased risk of complications in future pregnancies as well as a decrease in the overall cesarean delivery rate at the population level. Women who had a previous cesarean section and want more than two children are encouraged to attempt a VBAC section. Although this comes with risks of its own, it avoids the risks of abdominal surgery, future abnormal placental implantation, and infection. The labor process in this situation is called a TOLAC section. This is discussed in more detail in Chapter 10.

RISKS RELATED TO CESAREAN BIRTH

Maternal deaths related to cesarean birth have decreased in the United States due to improved surgical techniques, anesthetic care, and the availability of blood transfusions and antibiotic therapy, but this procedure still poses a risk to both the woman and her fetus. Women who experience cesarean births are at higher risk for postpartum infection, hemorrhage, thromboembolic disease, and maternal death. Maternal death is most often related to intrapartum or postpartum hemorrhage (PPH). Neonates are at higher risk for fetal injury during surgery, low Apgar scores, and respiratory distress.

CLINICAL JUDGMENT

Obesity and Cesarean Births

Women with obesity may be affected by bias among health-care professionals, which may result in disrespectful or inadequate care (ACOG, 2019b). Nurses play an integral role in implementing best care practices and optimizing outcomes for women with obesity. Pregnant women with a body mass index (BMI) of 40 or higher have an almost 50% risk of cesarean birth and an increased risk of intrapartum complications, including cesarean delivery, failed trial of labor, endometritis, wound rupture or dehiscence, and venous thromboembolism (VTE; ACOG, 2015). Facilities should ensure their ability to accommodate women with a BMI greater than 50 with appropriate equipment and supplies (ACOG, 2015). Using a multidisciplinary team approach when preparing pregnant women with obesity for a cesarean birth improves care and outcomes. Staff need to anticipate the need for increased operative time and possible need for additional instruments and staff resources because surgery can be more challenging in women with obesity and usually takes longer.

Obese pregnant women are at increased risk for cesarean delivery, failed trial labor, endometritis, wound rupture or dehiscence, and venous thrombosis (ACOG, 2015). Obesity also increases a woman's risk of complications related to anesthesia. These include:

- Difficult intravenous (IV) access
- Difficulty in placement of spinal or epidural anesthesia related to loss of landmarks due to increased body size
- Impaired respirations for 2 hours following placement of spinal anesthesia
- Difficulty in placement of endotracheal tube due to increased tissue and edema
- Aspiration

Recommendations include:

- Early anesthesia consult
- Administration of broad-spectrum antimicrobial prophylaxis to decrease risk of infection.
- Use of pneumatic compression devices and low-molecular-weight heparin to decrease the risk of venous thrombosis (ACOG, 2015; AWHONN, 2019a).

Risks Related to Repeat Cesarean Birth

The most significant long-term complication of repeat surgical birth is placenta accreta. The spectrum of placenta accreta includes:

- Accreta: The placenta does not penetrate the entire thickness of the uterine muscle.
- Increta: The placenta extends farther into the myometrium.
- Percreta: The placenta extends fully through the uterine wall and may attach to other internal organs, such as the intestine or bladder.

In all forms of placenta accreta, the placenta fails to separate from the uterine wall after delivery, potentially leading to excessive hemorrhage, disseminated intravascular coagulopathy (DIC), organ failure, and, in severe cases, death. Typically, a hysterectomy is needed to control a massive hemorrhage.

Enhanced Recovery After Surgery

Enhanced Recovery After Surgery (ERAS) pathways enhance maternal recovery time and reduce short-term maternal morbidity. ERAS programs represent a comprehensive bundle of interventions for women undergoing elective cesarean birth. Although ERAS has not been universally adopted in the obstetric arena, various organizations have developed clinical pathways for enhanced recovery following cesarean delivery. Based on minimal interruption of oral intake, mitigation of intraoperative hypothermia, provision of fluids and food in recovery, thromboprophylaxis, scheduled postoperative nonopioid oral analgesia, early removal of indwelling catheters, and early mobilization, these pathways result in earlier discharge with a rapid return to normal activities following surgery (ACOG, 2018a; AWHONN, 2019a).

PERIOPERATIVE CARE

Perioperative perinatal nursing incorporates the skills of the specialties of obstetrics, surgery, and post-anesthesia care to provide safe and comprehensive care to women who have had cesarean births. In most hospitals, cesarean births are performed in an operating room in the obstetrics department and labor and delivery (L&D) nurses care for the family throughout the perioperative experience. Preoperative care may vary based on the urgency of the cesarean birth.

Preoperative Care

The preoperative period is a time to provide care to the woman and her family and includes both physical and psychological care. Supporting a family-centered environment helps decrease the woman's fear and anxiety. Reviewing the prenatal history and involving the woman in the plan of care provides valuable information that will be used to individualize the care that is needed for successful postoperative outcomes (AWHONN, 2019a).

CRITICAL COMPONENT

Evidence-Based Practice Guidelines

Nursing specialty organizations such as the AWHONN facilitate the use of research findings in clinical practice through the development of evidence-based practice guidelines. One such guideline is AWHONN's (2019a) perioperative care of the pregnant woman. This guideline describes evidence-based practice to ensure the following:

1. Patient safety measures for perioperative care of the pregnant woman
2. Family-centered education and care practices
3. Assessment and interventions appropriate during preoperative, intraoperative, and postoperative periods for women undergoing cesarean birth

---

Individualize care to meet the needs of the woman and her family. Include the family members and support persons in decisions, as applicable. Allow at least one support person to be present during the entire surgical time frame. Actively engage with support persons as partners in care. Promote a trusting relationship with a focus on open communication.

Medical Management

- Preoperatively, the surgeon will explain the reason for the cesarean birth and what it involved, as well as obtain surgical consent.
- Presurgical diagnostic laboratory tests, such as CBC, blood type, and Rh, are ordered.
- Education is provided about which current medications the woman should take or eliminate on the day of surgery.
- To prevent postoperative infection, many providers recommend the woman take at least one preoperative shower at home, using an antiseptic agent on the night prior for a scheduled cesarean.

Anesthesia Management

- The anesthesia provider (anesthesiologist or certified registered nurse anesthetist) meets with the family generally before the woman is transferred to the operating room.
- The anesthesia provider reviews the prenatal record.
- The anesthesia provider completes an anesthesia history and physical, discusses anesthesia options with the couple, and answers their questions regarding anesthesia and the procedure. This includes screening for anesthesia and analgesia alternatives for women diagnosed with chronic pain, opioid use disorder, or opioid dependence.
- Anesthesia care for cesarean birth may be performed using spinal, epidural, combined spinal and epidural, or general anesthesia. Neuraxial techniques are preferred over general anesthesia for most cesarean births; however, the selection of anesthetic technique should be individualized and based on

maternal and fetal risk factors, anesthesia provider judgment, and the preference of the woman.

- The anesthesia provider determines the need for a platelet count.

Nursing Actions

- Complete the appropriate admission assessments (including baseline vital signs) and required preoperative forms.
- Individualize care to meet the needs of the woman and her family. Include the family members and support persons in decisions, as applicable. For example, we typically allow at least one support person to be present during the entire surgical time frame.
- Promote a trusting relationship with a focus on open communication.
- Obtain laboratory testing per orders, such as CBC, platelets, and type and screen. A delay in laboratory results can result in a delay in surgery.
- Obtain a baseline FHR monitor strip of at least 20 minutes before and after administration of regional anesthesia, if possible.
- Review the prenatal chart for factors that place the woman at risk during or after cesarean birth and ensure that the physician and anesthesia provider are aware of risk factors such as low platelet count.
- Document last solid and liquid intake; last solid intake should be 6 to 8 hours before the procedure and last liquids should be clear liquids up to 2 hours before surgery.
- Ensure that all required documents, such as prenatal record, current laboratory reports, and consent forms, are in the woman's chart.
- Assess the woman's knowledge and educational needs and provide preoperative teaching that includes what she and her partner can expect before, during, and after the cesarean birth.
- Identify and respect the cultural values, choices, and preferences of the woman and her family and individualize care to meet the needs of the woman and her family.
- Start an IV line with 18G IV in case of blood transfusion due to increased risk of bleeding with cesarean section and administer an IV fluid preload as per orders. An IV fluid preload of 500 to 1,000 mL is given before administration of spinal or epidural anesthesia to increase fluid volume and decrease risk of hypotension related to the effects of the anesthetic agent (AWHONN, 2019a; Cunningham et al., 2018).
- Empty the urinary bladder before a cesarean while considering maternal preference and provider order. Methods may include indwelling urinary catheter, ambulation to bathroom, or intermittent catheterization before surgery.
- Insert a Foley catheter if ordered. Insertion is preferably done in the operating room after placement of the spinal or epidural and before the prep.
- Administer medications to reduce the risk of aspiration according to anesthesia orders and facility guidelines. This might include sodium citrate and sodium bicarbonate to reduce the acidity of stomach acids. H2 receptor antagonists such as famotidine to inhibit secretion of acid or metoclopramide may be used to reduce the incidence of nausea or vomiting and increase gastric motility.

- Collaborate with the primary health-care provider to determine the need for intrapartum prophylaxis in the case of unplanned cesarean birth or planned cesarean birth with ROM.
- Prepare the partner or the support person who plans to be present for the birth for the experience by providing appropriate surgical attire to wear in the operating room.
- Instruct the partner or the support person as to where they will sit and what they can anticipate regarding sights, sounds, and smells typical of an operating room.
- Provide emotional support for the couple as they wait to be transferred to the operating room.
- Complete the surgery checklist, which includes removal of jewelry, eyeglasses or contact lenses, and dentures. Eyeglasses can be given to the support person to bring into the operating room so the woman can use them to see her newborn baby.

Anesthesia care for cesarean birth may be performed using spinal, epidural, combined spinal and epidural, or general anesthesia. Neuraxial techniques are preferred over general anesthesia for most cesarean births. Women who are transitioning from an anticipated vaginal birth to a cesarean may already have an epidural in place. Women with a scheduled cesarean birth commonly have a spinal placed in the OR but practices vary. Nursing care when neuraxial anesthesia (AWHONN, 2020) is placed includes:

- Provide 1:1 registered-nurse-to-patient staffing ratios during initiation of regional analgesia or anesthesia and for a minimum of 30 minutes after the procedure is completed.
- Assess fetal status and maternal baseline blood pressure, pulse, respiratory rate, temperature, oxygen status, and labor progress before the administration of regional analgesia or anesthesia.
- Administer an intravenous fluid bolus (20 mL/kg or 1 to 2 L) as a preload, coload, or both according to anesthesia care provider orders and facility guidelines.
- Conduct a time-out before the administration of regional analgesia or anesthesia.
- Assist the woman into the appropriate position during the administration of regional analgesia or anesthesia, which may be the lateral, sitting, or pendant position.
- Initiate pharmacological hypotension prophylaxis based on maternal response and as ordered by the anesthesia care provider, including ephedrine and phenylephrine.
- Assess for severe adverse maternal reactions during and immediately after the administration of the test dose of regional analgesia or anesthesia. Initiate interventions to resolve maternal hypotension according to provider orders and facility, such as lateral positioning and administering non-glucose-containing crystalloid fluid boluses or vasopressors.
- Assess uterine activity and FHR patterns every 5 minutes for the first 15 minutes after the initiation.

Intraoperative Care

Nursing care during the intraoperative period is multifaceted and dynamic, relying heavily on the clinical knowledge, critical thinking, and judgment of the circulating registered nurse.

CRITICAL COMPONENT

Antibiotic and Venous Thromboembolic Prophylaxis

- Administer prophylactic antibiotics before surgery according to provider orders. Prophylactic antibiotics should be administered to all women undergoing cesarean birth to prevent infection. Identify women at higher risk for postoperative infection. For example, increasing the dose to 2 g for patients weighing 80 kg or more is recommended (ACOG, 2018b). Administration of prophylactic antibiotics should occur within 60 minutes before the skin incision (AWHONN, 2019a). A narrow spectrum first-generation cephalosporin, such as cefazolin, or for women with penicillin and cephalosporin allergy, clindamycin with an aminoglycoside, may be given (AAP & ACOG, 2017). Otherwise, antibiotics may be administered during the procedure, after cord clamp, or immediately after the procedure.
- Women undergoing unscheduled cesarean delivery may have an additional antibiotic ordered such as adding extended-spectrum prophylaxis with adjunctive azithromycin, reducing the risk of postoperative infection (AWHONN, 2019a).
- Perform an assessment for risk of VTE and classify the woman based on VTE classification guidelines. Preoperative anticoagulant therapy may be necessary for women classified as moderate or high-risk or with a history of recurrent thrombosis.
- Apply sequential compression devices before surgery.
- Using an antiseptic solution for vaginal cleansing preoperatively has shown to reduce surgical site infection (SSI); consider vaginal cleansing, especially for women with ruptured membranes or those who have labored before surgery (AWHONN, 2019a).

Complete these nursing actions for an urgent or emergent cesarean birth:

- Prioritize the care needed to facilitate delivery.
- Notify anesthesia, L&D team, and neonatal personnel of impending cesarean birth.
- Initiate continuous electronic FHR monitoring.
  - Expected findings: Category II or Category III FHR pattern when the cesarean section is related to fetal intolerance of labor.
- Administer oxygen when indicated (i.e., signs of fetal intolerance of labor).
- Assess the woman's vital signs.
  - Expected findings:
    - The woman's blood pressure is slightly elevated related to anxiety level.
    - There is a potential increase in temperature and pulse rate due to infection or dehydration related to prolonged labor and ROM.
- If pubic hair must be removed, wet clipping with a suction device is recommended in emergency.
- Facilitate the transition to unscheduled surgical birth in a timely manner. Guidelines in all hospitals that provide obstetric (OB) care should have the capability of responding to obstetrical emergencies within 30 minutes; hence, the 30-minute "decision to incision rule."
- Assess the couple's emotional response to the need for a cesarean birth.
  - Expected findings:
    - Woman and family may experience high levels of anxiety based on fear of injury to the woman or unborn child.
    - Woman is not emotionally or mentally prepared for cesarean birth.
    - Woman and family have a knowledge deficit regarding cesarean birth and anesthesia options.
    - Woman and family ask questions regarding cesarean birth and anesthesia options.
- Help ensure the woman and her support person(s) receive information appropriate to the circumstances. Reinforce the reason for the cesarean section and address questions.
- Provide emotional support during the transitional process from labor to preparation for surgery.
- Facilitate the woman and family's communication with the entire health-care team to decrease fear, anxiety, and distress.
- Facilitate the presence of a woman's support person during preoperative preparation and surgical procedure because emotional support decreases anxiety.
- Prepare the partner or support person who plans to attend the birth regarding what to anticipate in the operating room and provide proper surgical garb to wear in the operating room.

However, it is important to continue including the woman and her family in the plan of care. The circulating nurse will be attending many aspects of care, including providing maternal and family support during procedures, maternal positioning, skin antisepsis, assistance with anesthesia, and urinary catheter care. The complete intraoperative team includes a surgeon, an anesthesia provider, a surgical first assist, a circulating nurse, and neonatal staff. The circulating nurse is responsible for patient safety. This generally includes responsibility for positioning the woman safely, assuring time-outs and consents are completed appropriately, confirming the presence of newborn care providers at the birth, maintaining a correct count of surgical sponges, and labeling surgical specimens correctly and confirming their disposition to pathology or medical waste.

The woman and her family will be anxious about the cesarean birth, whether it is a scheduled or an unscheduled procedure. It is often the woman's first surgical experience, which can increase the anxiety level for both the woman and her partner. To help decrease anxiety, it is best if the nurse who admitted the woman for a scheduled cesarean section or the nurse who cared for the couple during labor continues to care for them during the surgery as the circulating nurse.

Anesthesia Management

● Ensure basic and advanced life support equipment and appropriately trained personnel are available to assist the anesthesia care provider as indicated.

- Determine the method of anesthesia based on the following factors:
  - Which one is the safest and most comfortable for the woman?
  - Which has the least effect on the fetus or neonate?
  - Which provides the optimal conditions for the surgery?
- Methods of anesthesia
  - Spinal anesthesia is the preferred method for scheduled cesarean sections or for laboring women who do not have an epidural in place (Fig. 11–2). Spinal anesthesia, which is faster than an epidural to place, provides a full sensory and motor block.
  - Epidural anesthesia is used for laboring women who have an epidural in place for labor pain management and who then require a cesarean birth (see Fig. 11–2). Women with epidurals may feel tugging and pulling during the procedure because epidurals are not as dense and do not provide full sensory and motor block.
  - General anesthesia, which is rarely used and carries increased risks, is indicated in situations such that rapid delivery is imperative because of severe hemorrhage, seizures, or a failed spinal.
    - Recognize potential complications with general anesthesia.
    - Assist with proper positioning for intubation, and may assist with cricoid pressure as required by the anesthesia provider; if failed intubation, the anesthesia provider may ask the nurse to help with laryngeal mask ventilation, if indicated.
- Contraindications for epidural or spinal anesthesia
  - Low platelet count, which is the most common contraindication, especially with women who have preeclampsia or HELLP (hemolysis, elevated liver enzymes, and low platelets) syndrome
  - Infection or dermatological issues of concern at the proposed site of needle insertion
  - Uncorrected maternal hypovolemia
  - The woman's refusal or inability to cooperate with the procedure
  - Spine abnormalities, injuries, or surgeries
  - Sepsis

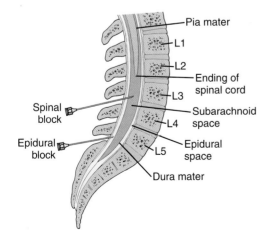

FIGURE 11–2 Spinal and epidural placements.

- Administration of anesthesia
  - Bupivacaine is the preferred anesthetic agent for spinal and epidural blocks.
  - Preservative-free morphine or fentanyl is administered intrathecally to provide postoperative analgesia.
  - Epidural or spinal anesthesia may be administered with the woman sitting on the operating room table or lying on her side. When the woman is lying down, position her with a hip tilt to maintain uterine displacement before, during, and after administration of anesthesia. This will decrease the risk of aortocaval compression related to compression on the aorta and inferior vena cava by the gravid uterus.
- Monitor vital signs and oxygen saturation.
  - Expected findings:
    - Vital signs and oxygen saturation within normal limits with potential mild increase in blood pressure due to anxiety
    - Hypotension following administration of the anesthetic agent
    - Spinal anesthesia may affect ability to maintain maternal normothermia
- Monitor level of anesthesia, effectiveness of anesthesia, and complications.
  - Gastric aspiration: Aspiration of gastric contents can lead to pneumonitis. This is a potential complication of general anesthesia. Additional conditions that may increase the risk of aspiration include:
    - Morbid obesity
    - Diabetes
    - Gastroesophageal reflux
    - Opioid analgesia
    - Difficult airway
    - Administer preload or colloid according to anesthesia provider orders and facility guidelines.
    - Administer preload approximately 20 to 30 minutes before initiation of anesthesia to ensure optimal prophylactic efficacy.
    - Administer colloid immediately after the initiation of regional anesthesia.
    - If indicated, administer medications to improve spinal-induced hypotension according to anesthesia provider orders and facility guidelines. Medications may include ephedrine, phenylephrine, or 5-HT3 receptor antagonist.
- Monitor blood loss, accomplished when the circulating nurse weighs lap sponges for a quantified blood loss (QBL) and reports findings to the surgical team. A QBL of up to 1,000 mL is expected in a cesarean birth.
- Administer antibiotics when indicated, generally within 1 hour of the incision time.
- Administer oxytocin after the delivery of the placenta to minimize bleeding.

Medical Management

- Two primary operative techniques are used for cesarean births. Most often, a Pfannenstiel incision, or "bikini cut," is the skin incision. This is a transverse skin incision made at the level of the pubic hairline (Fig. 11–3A). Typically, a lower uterine

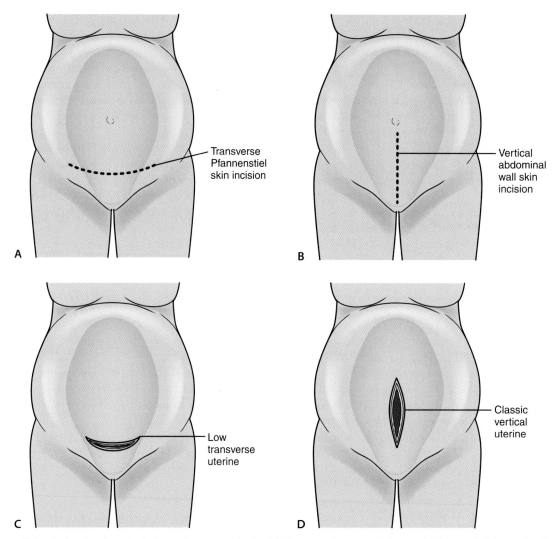

FIGURE 11–3 Abdominal wall and uterine incisions for cesarean births. (A) Pfannenstiel incision ("bikini cut"). (B) Vertical abdominal wall skin incision. (C) Low transverse uterine incision. (D) Classic vertical uterine incision.

segment incision is performed on the uterus (Fig. 11–3C). The second operative technique, the classical cesarean delivery, is a vertical abdominal wall skin incision and vertical incision in the body of the uterus (Fig. 11–3B and D). This technique is rare and is used in emergent cesarean births when immediate delivery is critical.

● The neonate is delivered through the uterine and abdominal incisions (Fig. 11–4). Following the delivery of the neonate, the placenta is manually removed. The uterus may be lifted out of the abdominal cavity or left in place while the uterine incision is repaired. The abdominal tissues and incision are repaired.

● Despite the prevalence of cesarean birth, data regarding many aspects of the preferred surgical technique are sparse. Skin closure is an integral step and influences postoperative pain, wound healing, cosmetic outcome, and surgeon and patient satisfaction. There is currently no definite evidence regarding the best method for skin closure after cesarean delivery; staples, Dermabond® glue, or monofilament epidermal sutures may be used. Studies identified that closing the transverse

skin incision with subcuticular suture decreases wound separation—despite the slightly longer surgical time it requires compared with staple closure (Pergialiotis et al., 2017). This may lead to a decrease in SSI.

Nursing Actions

● Conduct a pre-procedure informational process according to facility policy. Include assessments, comments, and lab work.

● Assist the mother into the appropriate position for administration of regional anesthesia, which may include sitting, pendant position, or side lying with head elevation.

● Assess women having scheduled cesarean birth for preoperative skin cleansing by bathing or showering.

● Cleanse the lower abdomen to clear the surgical site of soil, debris, and exudate if needed. Consider using preoperative skin cleansing wipes before OR transfer.

● Use a safe, effective, antiseptic agent for preoperative abdominal preparation according to health-care provider orders and facility guidelines.

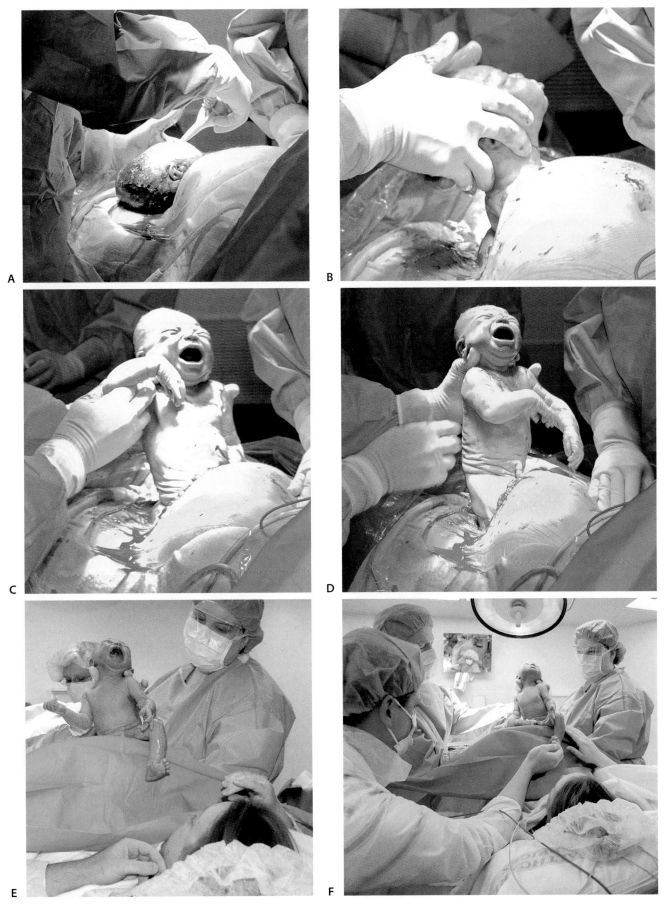

FIGURE 11–4 Cesarean birth. (A) Delivery of head. (B) Delivery of shoulders. (C, D) Delivery of body. (E, F) Mom and Dad meeting their daughter.

- Remove hair if it will interfere with the surgical incision. If hair must be removed, use hair clippers before moving into the operative suite or, in an emergency situation, wet clipping with the use of a suction device is recommended.
- Implement safety measures to protect the skin and prevent injury from skin preparation agents, such as positioning equipment from dripping or pooling of antiseptic agents, remove excess lines if pooling is present, and allow skin antiseptics and fumes to dissipate before application of surgical drapes. Remove alcohol-based soaked antiseptic materials from the room because they are a fire hazard.
- For scheduled cesarean births, document fetal status (baseline heart rate, presence of regular versus irregular rhythm, presence of increases or decreases in rate) before the scheduled procedure and according to facility guidelines.
- Monitor and document FHR before and after administration of regional anesthesia.
- Monitor fetal heart tones during initiation of anesthesia as indicated and whenever possible.
- In an emergency, continue external FHR monitoring until abdominal preparation is initiated. Remove the fetal scalp electrode (FSE) after abdominal surgical preparation is done and before delivery.
- Conduct a time-out before administering anesthesia and before initial incision for validating correct patient, site, and procedure.
- Recognize that intraoperative hypothermia may lead to an increase in maternal morbidity, including cardiac events, delayed surgical wound healing, SSIs, increased blood loss, and increased length of stay.
- Individualize active (conductive or convective) and passive (insulative) hypothermia prevention measures for the pregnant woman before the administration of anesthesia and throughout surgery whenever possible.
- Assess FHR after anesthesia placement.
- Apply the grounding device to the woman's thigh.
- Insert Foley.
- Perform abdominal skin prep using sterile technique.
- Secure the woman to the operating room table with a strap over her upper legs. Ensure a left lateral tilt when positioned to avoid supine hypotension.
- Perform the duties of the circulating nurse, including instrument count, needle count, and sponge count.
- Check equipment used for the newborn to ensure it is in working order and all supplies are readily available for care of the neonate.
- Assess the couple's response to the cesarean birth.
  - Expected findings:
    - Anxiety levels increase related to operating room environment and impending surgery.
    - Couples may have concerns related to potential injury to the woman from anesthesia or surgery.
    - The woman may feel abdominal pressure as the neonate is being delivered.
- Position the partner or support person on a stool next to the woman's head. Instruct the partner or support person to remain seated on the stool. This may prevent falling if the person feels faint.

- Instruct the partner or support person as to what they can and cannot touch.
- Provide emotional support to the woman and her partner or support person.
- Facilitate care for the neonate. Neonatal care is usually performed by the neonatal personnel (neonatal nurse, nurse practitioner, or neonatologist) who are present for the birth.
  - At least one person skilled in neonatal resuscitation should be available whose only responsibility is to receive and care for the baby.
  - Expected finding: The neonate's 1- and 5-minute Apgar scores are 7 or above unless there is fetal intolerance of labor before the birth.
- Record the time of delivery of the neonate and delivery of the placenta.
- Whenever possible, the newborn should remain in the operative suite with the mother.
- Complete identification bands and place on the neonate and parents before the neonate leaves the operating room.
- Ensure that new parents have an opportunity to see and hold their newborn. In many birthing units, the neonate, if stable, remains in the operating room and skin-to-skin contact is initiated. The neonate is then transferred to the L&D recovery room with the woman and her partner or support person.
- Transfer the unstable neonate to the nursery and encourage the partner or support person to accompany the newborn to the nursery. Neonatal personnel are responsible for transferring unstable neonates.
- Address parents' questions regarding the health of their newborn.
- Complete intraoperative documentation.

Intraoperative Complications

Intraoperative complications are rare because of advances in obstetrical anesthesia and surgical techniques. Women who are healthy during pregnancy are at low risk for complications. Intraoperative complications may include:

- Hemorrhage: Increased morbidity and mortality rates are associated with intraoperative and PPH, which can result in hypovolemic shock, DIC, renal or hepatic failure, and possibly the need for emergency hysterectomy.
- Bladder, ureter, and bowel trauma
- Maternal respiratory depression related to anesthesia
- Maternal hypotension related to anesthesia, which increases the risk for fetal acidemia
- Inadvertent injection of the anesthetic agent into the maternal bloodstream; the woman may experience ringing in her ears, metallic taste in her mouth, and hypotension that can lead to unconsciousness and cardiac arrest.

Postoperative Care

The recovery time following a cesarean birth is longer than for vaginal delivery due to the tissue trauma related to surgical intervention. The usual hospital stay is 3 days, with full recovery from

Evidence-Based Practice

Skin-to-Skin Contact During Cesarean Birth

Newborns who are born by cesarean receive the same benefits from skin-to-skin contact as those born vaginally (AWHONN, 2019a). Ideally, uninterrupted skin-to-skin contact should begin at birth and continue through the completion of the first breastfeeding. With its extensive list of benefits to both newborns and parents, skin-to-skin contact has been recommended by many national organizations for all healthy, term newborns. Although skin-to-skin has become more common during vaginal birth, women undergoing cesarean birth experience less opportunity to have this experience immediately following birth. Women's perceptions of early skin-to-skin contact during scheduled cesarean delivery are associated with decreased maternal anxiety and greater maternal satisfaction. A retrospective analysis was conducted to determine if immediate skin-to-skin contact during cesarean birth influenced the proportion of newborns transferred to the NICU for observation. Data was collected for the 2 years before implementing skin-to-skin contact immediately during cesarean birth (in the operating room) and for the first 3 years following implementation.

Inclusion criteria: Scheduled and nonemergent cesarean births between 37 and 42 weeks' gestation that occurred within 2 years preceding implementation and the first 3 years following implementation.

Sample: The sample included 2,841 newborns; 1,070 were born before implementation and 1,771 were born after implementation. The mean gestational age was 39 weeks and the mean birth weight was 3,401 g.

Results: The proportion of newborns transferred to NICU for observation was significantly lower after implementing skin-to-skin contact immediately following the birth. Before implementation, 5.6% of newborns were transferred to the NICU for observation; after implementation, 1.75% were transferred.

Nursing implication: Early and continuous contact with the newborn facilitates parent–infant bonding and attachment. Skin-to-skin contact in the operating room significantly decreases the percentage of newborns separated from parents due to transfers to the NICU for observation.

CRITICAL COMPONENT

Sudden Unexpected Postnatal Collapse

Sudden unexpected postnatal collapse (SUPC) is a rare event when a healthy-appearing, full-term infant suddenly experiences respiratory and cardiac arrest. Infants are at greatest risk during the first few hours of life. To decrease the risk of SUPC during skin-to-skin contact, proper positioning of the neonate with the mother is paramount. The nurse should place the infant prone on the mother's chest; head upright turned to the side, neck midline and erect, mouth and nares visible, extremities flexed; confirm that the mother is in a semi-upright and supported position (AWHONN, 2019a).

surgery taking 6 weeks or longer. The maternal morbidity rate is increased twofold with cesarean delivery compared with vaginal delivery (Cunningham et al., 2018). Principal sources of complications are infection, hemorrhage, and thromboembolism. Rehospitalization increases twofold. Rates of complications vary based on the status of cesarean and emergency versus planned. Infection rates with emergency cesarean are reported at 12%, wound complications at 1.2%, and operative injury at 0.5% (Cunningham et al., 2018). Wound infection presents with erythema, discharge, and induration of the incision; complicates 2% to 7% of patients; and generally develops 4 to 7 days after a cesarean. When wound infection develops within 48 hours, offending organisms usually are groups A or B hemolytic streptococcus (Kawakita & Landy, 2017).

Complications

Women who enter pregnancy in a healthy state and have experienced a healthy pregnancy are at low risk for complications. In contrast, women who experience a prolonged labor, multiple interventions such as internal monitoring, or prolonged ROM are at higher risk for postoperative complications. These include:

- Hemorrhage: PPH is most often identified in the intraoperative period or within the first few hours post-op.
- Anemia related to blood loss
- Deep vein thrombosis
- Pulmonary embolism (PE)
- Paralytic ileus
- Hematuria related to bladder trauma
- Infections of the bladder, endometrium, and incision
- Severe headache related to method of anesthesia

CLINICAL JUDGMENT

Maternal Early Warning Criteria

Abnormalities in physiological parameters usually precede a clinical decline. Therefore, strict monitoring of physical parameters in the postoperative period may help identify women who may have a rapid decline in the early phase of an acute illness. Earlier identification and interventions may help to decrease overall morbidity. Use evidence-based criteria (Maternal Early Warning Criteria [MEWC]) to monitor for signs of complications and deteriorating maternal conditions, including the following:

- Systolic blood pressure less than 90 or more than 160 mm Hg
- Diastolic blood pressure above 100 mm Hg
- Heart rate less than 50 or more than 120 beats per minute
- Respiratory rate less than 10 or more than 30 breaths per minute
- Oxygen saturation less than 95% in room air (sea level)
- Oliguria less than 30 mL/hour for 2 hours
- Maternal agitation, confusion, or unresponsiveness
- Women with hypertension who have persistent headache or shortness of breath

CRITICAL COMPONENT

Postoperative Complications

A multidisciplinary team approach is needed to provide care to women experiencing postoperative complications. Nurses have a key role in recognizing deteriorating conditions in the postoperative period. The most common preventable errors related to cesarean births are failure to recognize and act upon changes in vital signs and failure to act on PPH (Alliance for Innovation on Maternal Health, 2017).

- The most common etiologies for PPH include uterine atony, genital tract lacerations, retained placental tissue, and, less commonly, placental abruption (ACOG, 2017). In women with ongoing bleeding totaling 1,500 mL or more and women experiencing abnormal vital signs (tachycardia and hypotension), immediate preparation for blood transfusion should be made. Because large volumes of blood loss deplete coagulation factors, it is common for these women to develop DIC (ACOG, 2017).
- Given that estimation of blood loss is often inaccurate, determination of hematocrit or hemoglobin concentrations may not accurately reflect current hematologic status, and signs and symptoms may not occur until blood loss exceeds 15%, the decision for blood transfusion should be based on the amount of blood loss by quantified measurement (AAP & ACOG, 2017).
- The risk of VTE is four times greater after cesarean birth compared with vaginal birth. The incidence of VTE, including deep-vein thrombosis (DVT) (80%) and pulmonary embolism (PE) (20%), is 2.6 per 1,000 cesarean births, with the highest risk occurring in the first few weeks postpartum. Thromboembolic disease is a leading cause of maternal mortality; 9% of maternal deaths are attributed to embolism. Therefore, vigilance in risk assessment and prophylactic measures are indicated for all pregnant and postpartum women (AWHONN, 2019a).
- PE presents as an acute event. Signs and symptoms are dyspnea, tachypnea, chest tightness, shortness of breath, hypotension, and decreasing oxygen saturation levels.
- Cesarean birth is the single most important factor associated with postpartum infection and carries a fivefold to 20-fold increased risk of infection when compared with vaginal delivery (AWHONN, 2019a). Despite significant advances in infection control practices, including surgical safety checklists, improved operating room ventilation, sterilization methods, barriers, surgical technique, and antimicrobial prophylaxis, postoperative infections remain a substantial cause of prolonged hospitalization and maternal morbidity and mortality.
- Signs of SSIs include serous or purulent drainage, erythema, fever, pain, and wound dehiscence. Wound infection complicates 2% to 7% of patients and generally develops 4 to 7 days after cesarean. Endometritis is usually diagnosed within the first few days after delivery. Fever is the most common sign. Other signs include chills, uterine tenderness, and foul-smelling lochia (AWHONN, 2019a).

Immediate Postoperative Care

Postpartum monitoring is dictated by the mode of delivery, complications, and type of anesthesia or analgesia a woman receives (AAP & ACOG, 2017). All women who received general anesthesia, regional anesthesia, or monitored anesthesia care should be admitted to a post-anesthesia care unit (PACU) or equivalent, with care guided by approved policies and procedures, with a provider capable of managing anesthetic complications remaining readily available (AAP & ACOG, 2017). The woman's condition should be evaluated continuously in the immediate postoperative care period. Pain management and discharge from the recovery area should be guided by guidelines established by the obstetric provider and anesthesia personnel.

The woman and her newborn are transferred from the operating room to the L&D PACU or to her labor room following the cesarean birth. Immediate assessment and monitoring of maternal and newborn status is influenced by the type of anesthesia and preoperative or intraoperative complications. It focuses on maternal and fetal oxygenation, ventilation, circulation, level of consciousness, and body temperature. The purpose of PACU care is to stabilize vital signs, control bleeding, manage pain, itching, and nausea, and to monitor anesthesia level. One RN should be assigned solely to the care of the mother and one nurse assigned to her newborn until the critical elements are completed, such as report, assessments, and stable vital signs. Equipment comparable with that in the main PACU should be available for the care of post-op OB patients. Assess maternal status according to facility and professional organization guidelines. Assessments include but are not limited to:

- Level of consciousness
- Blood pressure and pulse (every 15 minutes for 2 hours)
- Color
- Oxygen saturation
- Cardiac monitoring for rate and rhythm
- Pain
- Dressing condition
- Intake and output
- Sensory and motor function
- Temperature at least hourly; if hypothermic, every 15 minutes
- Fundal height and lochia
- Assess the woman for side effects of anesthesia and provide interventions, if indicated. Side effects may include nausea and vomiting, pruritus, and shivering.
- Active warming measures are used to prevent hypothermia.
- If an indwelling urinary catheter was used, remove it in a timely manner during the postoperative period according to assessment of the woman's condition, health-care provider orders, and facility guidelines. Increasingly, the urinary catheter is removed in the immediate postoperative period.
- Implement standardized recommendations for VTE prevention during each perioperative phase based on the woman's identified risks.
- Facility-based scoring system is used to determine the appropriate timing for discharge from the recovery room.

First 24 Hours After Birth

After immediate recovery, the woman and family are transferred to a postpartum unit for care and recovery. Nursing actions are similar to those when caring for a woman who had a vaginal birth, with emphasis on monitoring and recovery from surgery and management of pain. Pain can obstruct a woman's ability to care for herself and her newborn (ACOG, 2018a). Routine monitoring and assessment of pain during the postoperative recovery period optimizes outcomes and detects complications. Evidence-based, individualized, multimodal postoperative pain management is essential in enhanced recovery after cesarean birth (AWHONN, 2019a). Post-cesarean pain consists of both visceral pain from the uterine incision and somatic pain related to the surgical wound. Given the variation in both intensity and type, a stepwise approach can enable obstetric care providers to effectively individualize postpartum pain management for women (ACOG, 2018a).

Medical Management

- Postoperative cesarean pain may be managed using oral and parenteral analgesics, including regimens designed to minimize the use of opioids that integrate nonsteroidal anti-inflammatory agents (NSAIDs), acetaminophen, and opioids, using a shared decision-making model (ACOG, 2018a). The use of parenteral or oral opioids should be reserved for breakthrough pain in the presence of other modes of pain management.
- Although multimodal analgesia principles have enabled reduction in opioid analgesia use, opioids continue to demonstrate the ability to achieve optimal pain relief, with neuraxial opioids remaining the most reliable option for post-cesarean birth relief.
- Assess for involutional changes and signs of potential complications.
- Assess pulmonary function: assess for atelectasis and pneumonia.
- Assess for ileus, cholecystitis, persistent nausea and vomiting, and intestinal obstruction.
- Medical orders are usually standardized. These orders include:
  - IV therapy
  - Medications such as analgesics and stool softeners
  - Antibiotic therapy for the woman at risk for infection related to prolonged ROM, prolonged labor, or elevated temperature during labor
  - Progression of diet
  - Removal of the Foley in the immediate postoperative period
  - Activity level
- Immediate care of the newborn is the same as for vaginal delivery and is detailed in Chapters 8 and 15.

Anesthesia Management

- When intrathecal morphine is used for postoperative pain management, the anesthesia provider manages the woman's pain for the first 24 hours and administers medications to counteract the side effects of intrathecal opioids.

SAFE AND EFFECTIVE NURSING CARE:
Understanding Medication

Preservative-Free Morphine

- Indication: Severe pain
- Action: Alters perception of and response to painful stimuli and produces generalized CNS depression
- Common side effects: Respiratory depression, itching, hypotension, nausea and vomiting, and urinary retention
- Route and dose: Administered intrathecally by anesthesiologist or CRNA; 5 to 10 mg (Vallerand & Sanoski, 2017)

CRITICAL COMPONENT

Maternal Respiratory Depression Related to Intrathecal Morphine

Severe respiratory depression (3% occurrence) is a life-threatening adverse reaction to intrathecal morphine.

- Naloxone and resuscitative equipment must be available whenever intrathecal morphine is administered and during the 24 hours postoperative after injection.
- Respiratory rate and level of sedation are monitored for the first 24 hours postoperative after administration. Normal respiratory rate is 12 to 20 breaths per minute.
- An initial dose of 0.4 to 2 mg of naloxone is administered intravenously for severe respiratory depression. Dose can be repeated every 2 to 3 minutes for a total of 10 mg.
- Respiratory resuscitation is initiated immediately and continued until normal respiratory function returns.

Nursing Actions

After a cesarean birth, most women recover in the labor and birthing recovery PACU instead of the PACU of the main OR. After immediate recovery, the woman and her family are transferred to a postpartum unit for care and further recovery. Nursing actions are similar to those when caring for a woman who had a vaginal birth, and emphasize the following for postoperative recovery:

- Monitor vital signs as per protocol.
  - Monitor respiratory rate, heart rate, blood pressure, pain, pulse oximetry, and level of sedation every hour for the first 24 hours after administration of intrathecal morphine.
  - Monitor for hemorrhage (increased bleeding, increased pulse, decreased blood pressure).
- Assess the fundus and lochia per protocol.
- Assess abdominal dressing for signs of bleeding.
- Surgical wounds heal by primary intention when the wound edges are brought together and secured, often with sutures,

glue, staples, or clips. Dressings are often applied to provide physical support, protect the wound, and absorb exudate. Routine postoperative wound care includes changing dressings and assessing wounds. Postoperative dressing types vary by facility and provider.

- Assess woman's level of pain and use pharmacological and nonpharmacological interventions for pain management. Evaluate the effectiveness of pain management interventions.
- Although multimodal analgesia principles have enabled reduction in opioid analgesia use, opioids continue to demonstrate the ability to achieve optimal pain relief, with neuraxial opioids remaining the most reliable option for post-cesarean birth relief (AWHONN, 2019a).
- Be aware of risks associated with pain management medications.
- Ensure analgesics are safe for women who choose to breastfeed. Breastfeeding is not recommended for mothers taking codeine or tramadol (AWHONN, 2019a).
- Consider rounding every 30 minutes and at least hourly.
- Review prenatal, labor, and intrapartal records for risk factors.
- Monitor for side effects of intrathecal morphine and provide appropriate interventions. The primary side effects and interventions are:
  - Pruritus: Administer medication as ordered, such as naloxone or diphenhydramine.
  - Nausea or vomiting: Administer medication as ordered, such as naloxone or metoclopramide.
  - Urinary retention: Occurs after removal of a catheter: Administer naloxone or catheterize as ordered.
  - Respiratory depression: Administer oxygen as needed and/or naloxone as ordered.
- Monitor the level of sensation.
- Monitor for seizures, spinal headache, and neurological deficits (e.g., prolonged decreased sensation in legs).
- Auscultate lungs, encourage coughing and deep breathing, and assist woman in using incentive spirometry.
- Monitor intake and urinary output (per Foley catheter and for the first 24 hours following catheter removal).
- If an indwelling urinary catheter was used, remove it in a timely manner during the postoperative period according to assessment of the woman's condition, health-care provider orders, and facility guidelines. Increasingly, the urinary catheter is removed in the immediate postoperative period.
- Assess for urinary output and bladder distention at least every 4 to 6 hours after removal of the urinary catheter. Encourage the woman to void spontaneously. Consider the use of a bladder scanner to detect bladder distention and assess for potential damage to the bladder or ureters demonstrated by inability to void.
- Initiate interventions according to facility protocols and provider orders to prevent potential gastrointestinal complications in the postoperative period; for example, early oral nutrition within 2 hours of birth and gum chewing during the first 12 hours of the postoperative period. Advance diet as tolerated.
- Regulate IV fluids as ordered.
- Oxytocin is added to IV fluids initially to reduce the risk of PPH related to uterine atony.

- Implement standardized recommendations for VTE prevention during each perioperative phase based on the woman's identified risks.
- Nurse should assist with ambulation as soon as possible, per protocol and orders, and continue to encourage ambulation every few hours.
- Facilitate skin-to-skin contact with parents and infant.
- Assist the woman into a comfortable position for infant feeding. Be aware that a cesarean birth is a risk factor for failed breastfeeding.
- Assist with infant care and provide teaching as indicated.
- Implement measures to recognize and prevent newborn falls. Risk factors leading to newborn falls are cesarean birth, maternal use of pain medication within 4 hours, and breastfeeding.
- Provide emotional support by actively listening to the couple recall their birth experience and addressing their questions and concerns.

Expected Assessment Findings

- Vital signs are within normal limits.
- Lochia is moderate to scant.
- The fundus is firm and midline and generally 1 to 2 cm above the umbilicus initially, moving down throughout the woman's hospital stay.
- The abdominal dressing is dry.
- The catheter is draining clear or yellow urine. A small amount of blood in the urine may be present when there has been trauma to the bladder during the procedure.
- The IV site is free of signs of infiltration or inflammation.
- The pain level is below 3 on a pain scale of 0 to 10, or within the woman's chosen number.
- The woman gradually regains full motor and sensory function as the effects of the anesthetic agent decrease.
- The woman sits at the bedside for short periods of time and ambulates with assistance when stable.
- The woman may experience itching, nausea, or decreased respirations related to side effects of morphine. Itching and nausea are most common. Itching varies from facial rash to a full-body rash. Antihistamines are given to promote comfort.
- The woman feeds her newborn with or without assistance.
- The partner and family assist in care of the newborn.
- The couple may be tired and need time to rest.
- Women with unplanned cesarean births may experience guilt or a sense of failure or disappointment.
- Couples with unplanned cesarean births may ask questions about the cesarean birth and the events leading up to it.
- The couple will want time alone with their newborn.
- The couple will call family and friends, informing them of the birth.

24 Hours Postoperative to Discharge

The following medical management and nursing actions take place before the mother and baby are discharged.

Medical Management

- Assess the woman for involutional changes and signs of potential postoperative complications.
- Administer antibiotic therapy for women who experienced a prolonged labor or prolonged ROM or who are febrile.
- Remove abdominal dressing and assess for signs of dehiscence and infection (redness, tenderness, swelling). The dressing is usually removed on the first postoperative day. Dressings are often applied to provide physical support, protect the wound, and absorb exudate. Routine postoperative wound care includes changing dressings and assessing wounds. Postoperative dressing types and skin care vary by facility and provider.
- Provide discharge instructions.

Nursing Actions

A comprehensive approach to address the complex care needs of all surgical patients is needed to achieve positive patient outcomes (AWHONN, 2019a). Because of rising maternal morbidity and mortality rates and the significant number of women who may not attend postpartum visits, it is critical that discharge education bridge the transition from intrapartum to postpartum care by addressing post-birth risks and warning signs (Suplee et al., 2016). In addition, social and ethnic disparities in the United States continue to result in adverse outcomes and maternal deaths (Suplee et al., 2016). Optimizing care with a woman-centered focus during the weeks following birth is essential to the long-term health and well-being of women (ACOG, 2018a). Nursing actions are similar to those when caring for a woman who had a vaginal birth with addition to or emphasis on the following:

- Monitor vital signs as per protocol, generally every 4 hours.
- Assess breath sounds.
- Instruct the woman to take deep breaths and cough every 2 hours.
- Instruct the woman on the use of an incentive spirometer if ordered.
- Assess postoperative pain and medicate as indicated.
- Use nonpharmacological pain management strategies.
- Assess the fundus and lochia per protocol. Use gentle pressure when assessing the fundus, as the woman's abdomen will be tender.
- Monitor for signs of hemorrhage and infection.
- Assess the abdominal dressing or surgical wound for drainage and signs of infection.
- Administer antibiotics as ordered.
- Remove the Foley catheter according to assessment of the women's condition, provider orders, and facility guidelines. This generally occurs in the immediate postoperative period or up to 12 hours post-surgery. Ensure the woman voids at least 200 to 300 mL after urinary catheter removal and inform the provider if she cannot. Avoid overdistention of the bladder to reduce risk of subinvolution and hemorrhage.
- Assist the woman with ambulation. The nurse should assist with ambulation as soon as possible, per protocol and orders, and continue to encourage ambulation every few hours.
- Encourage oral fluid intake to assist in hydration.

- Discontinue IV fluids as ordered, generally when the woman can take adequate fluids by mouth without nausea.
- Assess bowel sounds and allow the woman early oral nutrition within 2 hours of birth and gum chewing during the first 12 hours of the postoperative period; this has shown an earlier return of bowel function (AWHONN, 2019a).
- Provide information on nutrition to promote tissue healing.
- Assist the woman into a comfortable position for infant feeding. Breastfeeding mothers may be more comfortable in a side-lying position or football hold, which prevents pressure on the abdomen.
- Assist the woman with infant care.
- Facilitate mother–infant attachment by bringing the infant to the woman and ensuring the woman's comfort.
- Instruct the family that they need to assist the woman with infant care and housework, as she needs 6 weeks to recover from surgery.
- Provide opportunities for the family to ask questions about their cesarean birth experience.
- Provide teaching on infant care, postoperative care, and postpartum care.
- If present, remove staples before discharge per protocol. Instruct the woman to make an appointment at her provider's clinic or office for staple removal, if staples are not removed in the hospital.

Expected Assessment Findings

- Vital signs and laboratory results are within normal limits. Temperature elevations may signify infection.
- Lung sounds are clear bilaterally.
- The woman deep breathes and coughs every 2 hours while awake.
- Pain level is 3 or below or reflects the woman's chosen number on a pain scale of 0 to 10 with the use of nonpharmacological and pharmacological interventions.
- The fundus is firm and midline at one finger-breadth below the umbilicus.
- Lochia is moderate to scant.
- The abdominal incision is clean, intact, approximated, and free of redness, edema, ecchymosis, and drainage.
- The time the woman spontaneously voids may vary from 2 to 6 hours of Foley removal.
- The woman ambulates to the bathroom and in the hallways.
- Bowel sounds are present and the woman reports passing gas.
- The woman is able to tolerate oral fluids and food.
- The woman is able to feed her newborn with or without assistance.
- The couple cares for the needs of their newborn.
- The woman may remain in the taking-in phase longer, as her focus is on pain control and integration of the birthing experience.
- Couples talk about their cesarean birth experience with staff, family, and friends.
- Assess maternal readiness for discharge by reviewing the following:
  - Physical examination
  - Mood and anxiety disorder screen determined by a facility-approved screening tool
  - Laboratory findings

- Woman's ability to care for herself
- Woman's ability to care for her newborn
- Regardless of length of stay, the woman should meet these minimum criteria for discharge:
  - Normal vital signs
  - Firm uterine fundus
  - Adequate urinary output
  - Appropriate amount and color of lochia
  - Apparent healing of surgical repair or wound and no evidence of infection
  - Absence of abnormal emotional or physical findings
  - Ability to ambulate
  - Adequate pain control
  - Ability to eat and drink without difficulty
  - Demonstrated readiness to care for herself and her newborn (AAP & ACOG, 2017)
- Provide education about normal postpartum events and maternal self-care after discharge, including the following:
  - Pain management
  - Lochia pattern
  - Incision care
  - Urogenital care
  - Breast care

- Nutrition
- Physical activity
- Provide education related to post-birth maternal warning signs:
  - Abnormal vaginal bleeding
  - Infection
  - DVT or PE
  - Unexplained pain (e.g., headache, incisional pain, chest pain, leg pain)
  - Postpartum depression
- Encourage women to share negative emotions and discuss childbirth-related fears. Provide them with education related to mood and anxiety disorders. Recognize that cesarean birth increases the risk for postpartum depression. Provide information about post-discharge available resources and mental health treatment referrals.

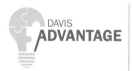

Go to Davis Advantage to complete your learning: strengthen understanding, apply your knowledge, and prepare for the Next Gen NCLEX®.

Clinical Pathway for Scheduled Cesarean Birth

Focus of Care	Preoperative and After Initial Transfer to the OR	Intraoperative	Immediate Postoperative First 2 hours	First 24 Postoperative Hours	Postoperative 24 Hours to Discharge
Assessments	Review prenatal record for risk factors. Complete admission assessments per protocol. Assess the couple's emotional responses.	Vital signs are monitored by the anesthesia provider. Apgar score on neonate by neonatal personnel. Assess the neonate per protocol. Conduct time-out.	Assess per protocol level of consciousness (orientation to time, place, person). Assessments to be done every 15 minutes for the first 2 hours, or as ordered: VS, color, cardiac monitoring, O2 sat, sensory motor function, presence or absence of oozing on dressing, fundal height, tone, location, and lochia. Assessments every hour for the first 4 hours or per protocol: urinary output, and bladder distention, I&O. Newborn assessments per protocol usually every 30 minutes for the first 2 hours.	Monitor VS as ordered, usually every hour × 4, then every 4 hours until stable, and then every 8 hours until discharge. Monitor respirations and sedation level as per post-intrathecal morphine administration protocol—usually every hour for the first 24 hours. Assess the level and location of pain. Assess abdominal dressing for bleeding or drainage. Monitor I&O. Monitor ability to void. Monitor for signs of potential PPH. Review laboratory test reports such as H&H, CBC.	Assess as per protocol, usually every 4 hours. Assess incisional site for drainage and signs of infection.

Clinical Pathway for Scheduled Cesarean Birth—cont'd

Focus of Care	Preoperative and After Initial Transfer to the OR	Intraoperative	Immediate Postoperative First 2 hours	First 24 Postoperative Hours	Postoperative 24 Hours to Discharge
				Monitor for signs of potential infections. Complete post-anesthesia assessments. Assess for adverse reaction related to intrathecal morphine, such as decreased respirations, itching, and vomiting, and intervene as per protocol.	
Activity Level	Ambulatory until bladder emptied or Foley inserted and sequential compression devices are placed on her legs.	Bedrest Maintain maternal uterine displacement	Bedrest	Bedrest until complete return of motor and sensory sensation or function (generally 6 to 12 hours). Following return of motor and sensory sensation, the woman is assisted on short walks and may sit in a chair for short periods. Assistance may be required for pericare and ADLs.	Up independently Encourage the woman to ambulate to encourage bowel activity and reduce risk of blood clots. May require minimal assistance with pericare and ADLs.
Education	Provide information on surgical procedure, anesthesia, and what to expect during cesarean birth and postoperatively. Keep the couple and their family informed on surgical time.	Provide information to the woman and her support person on the woman's and neonate's condition.	Provide information to the woman and her support person on woman's and neonate's condition. Emphasize importance of skin-to-skin contact with neonate.	Begin teaching on care of the neonate and of the woman's needs during the postpartum period. Emphasize importance of skin-to-skin contact with neonate. Educate on risk factors leading to newborn falls or drops.	Continue teaching and preparing the couple for discharge. Provide postoperative discharge teaching. Emphasize importance of skin-to-skin contact with neonate Educate on risk factors leading to newborn falls or drops.
Elimination	After the spinal anesthesia is completed, insert the Foley catheter and connect to continuous drainage if ordered.	Foley catheter connected to continuous drainage.	Monitor I&O.	Remove the Foley catheter as ordered, generally 12 hours after surgery. Assist the woman to the bathroom and measure voiding.	Assist the woman to the bathroom and measure voiding at least 2 times after the catheter is removed, if sufficient quantity.

Continued

Clinical Pathway for Scheduled Cesarean Birth—cont'd

Focus of Care	Preoperative and After Initial Transfer to the OR	Intraoperative	Immediate Postoperative First 2 hours	First 24 Postoperative Hours	Postoperative 24 Hours to Discharge
Emotional Needs	The couple may be anxious and excited. Provide emotional support and address questions and concerns. Patient desires and patient safety should guide practice.	The couple may be anxious and excited. Address the couple's concerns and questions. Patient desires and patient safety should guide practice Provide skin-to-skin immediately after the birth, for as long as possible, generally at least 1 hour. If the neonate is transferred to the nursery before surgery is over, encourage the partner or support person to accompany the neonate to the nursery.	The couple may be anxious and excited. Address the couple's concerns and questions. Patient desires and patient safety should guide practice Provide an opportunity for the family to be with their neonate.	Couples may be excited and tired. Address the couple's concerns regarding cesarean birth and the woman's and neonate's condition. Patient desires and patient safety should guide practice. Provide opportunities for the couple to share their experience and emotional responses to the birth.	Provide opportunities for the couple to share their thoughts and feelings regarding taking on care of the neonate or breastfeeding. Patient desires and patient safety should guide practice.
Medications	Administer preoperative medications per protocol. This may include IV or oral antacids, antiemetics, or antibiotics. Administer antibiotics ideally 60 min before skin incision. • Women undergoing unscheduled cesarean delivery may have an additional antibiotic ordered such as adding extended-spectrum prophylaxis with adjunctive azithromycin reducing the risk of postoperative infection. Consider vaginal cleansing immediately before the cesarean birth.	The anesthesia provider administers oxytocin and other medications as needed throughout surgery.	Administer medications as ordered by the anesthesia provider, including medications for treatment of intrathecal morphine side effects such as pruritus and nausea or vomiting.	Administer medications as ordered (i.e., stool softeners, Rhogam for Rh-negative women if indicated, Rubella for nonimmune women, prophylactic anticoagulant for those women identified as a moderate-to-high risk for VTEs, etc.).	Administer medications as ordered (i.e., stool softeners, etc.).

Clinical Pathway for Scheduled Cesarean Birth—cont'd

Focus of Care	Preoperative and After Initial Transfer to the OR	Intraoperative	Immediate Postoperative First 2 hours	First 24 Postoperative Hours	Postoperative 24 Hours to Discharge
Nutrition	Last solid intake should be 6 to 8 hours before the procedure and clear liquids up to 2 hours. Insert IV. Administer IV fluid preload.	NPO IV fluids	Ice chips, clear fluids, IV fluids Assist mother to breastfeed the neonate.	Advance to regular diet as ordered, or as woman tolerates. Assist with breastfeeding if indicated.	Diet as tolerated. Provide information on the role of nutrition in postpartum recovery and breastfeeding. Assist with breastfeeding if indicated.
Pain Management	Anesthesia provider meets with the couple to discuss anesthesia options.	Anesthesia provider inserts the epidural or spinal catheter and administers anesthetic agents. Anesthesia provider, or nurse, removes the epidural catheter.	Anesthesia provider is responsible for prescribing medication for pain management in PACU.	Administer oral pain medications as ordered by the surgeon. Intrathecal morphine is administered via epidural catheter by pump after the birth of the neonate. Anesthesia provider is responsible for prescribing medication for pain management and treatment of intrathecal morphine side effects for the first 24 hours post-op.	Per MD orders.

ADL, activities of daily living; CBC, complete blood count; H&H, hemoglobin and hematocrit; I&O, intake and output; IV, intravenous; NPO, nothing by mouth; OR, operating room; PACU, post-anesthesia care unit; VS, vital signs

Adapted from Association of Women's Health, Obstetric and Neonatal Nurses. (2019b). *Perioperative care of the pregnant woman* (Evidence-Based Clinical Practice Guideline, 2nd ed.). Author; and Simpson, K. R., & O'Brien-Abel, N. (2021). Labor and birth. In K. Simpson, P. Creehan, N. O'Brien-Abel, C. Roth, & A. Rohan (Eds.), *Perinatal nursing* (5th ed., pp. 325-411). Wolters Kluwer.

Case Study

Repeat Cesarean Birth

You are assigned to care for a couple scheduled to have a repeat cesarean birth. Lisa is a gravida 2 para 1, 25-year-old woman. Her husband, Joe, is 27 years old and plans to accompany Lisa into the operating room. Their first cesarean birth was due to cephalopelvic disproportion. Lisa and Joe have a healthy 3-year-old daughter, Sara, who is excited about having a baby brother.

Describe the nursing action for the preoperative period.

You transfer the couple to the operating room on the labor and birthing unit. You will be the circulating nurse. Spinal anesthesia is used for the cesarean birth.

Describe the major nursing action during the intraoperative period.
Describe the anesthesia management during this period of time.

Lisa experiences an uncomplicated cesarean birth and delivers a 3,800-gram baby boy with Apgar scores of 9 and 9. Lisa and her son are transferred to the OB recovery room where you continue to care for the family. Lisa plans to breastfeed her son.

Describe the major nursing actions during the immediate postoperative recovery period.

The following day you are assigned to Lisa and her family in the postpartum unit. The shift report indicates that Lisa's lungs are clear; bowel sounds are present, fundus firm at 1 above U. Lisa's Foley catheter was removed at 10:00 the night before. During the night, she ambulated to the bathroom twice and voided 450 mL each time. She is tolerating fluids and wants scrambled eggs for breakfast. Her H&H are 30 and 10.2. She is having difficulty with breastfeeding. She complained her pain was a 6 on a 10-point pain scale.

List the expected assessment findings for this period of time.

Discuss the nursing actions based on the shift report.

Discuss the major nursing action for couples and their newborn in preparation for discharge.

REFERENCES

Alliance for Innovation on Maternal Health. (2017). *Maternal safety bundles.* Author. https://safehealthcareforeverywoman.org/aim/patient-safety-bundles/maternal-safety-bundles/safe-reduction-of-primary-cesarean-birth-aim/

American Academy of Pediatrics & American College of Obstetricians and Gynecologists. (2017). *Guidelines for perinatal care* (8th ed.). American Academy of Pediatrics.

American College of Nurse Midwives. (2017). *Tools for optimizing the outcomes of labor safely.* Author.

American College of Obstetricians and Gynecologists. (2010). Vaginal birth after previous cesarean delivery. Committee Opinion No. 115. *Obstetrics & Gynecology, 116*(2 Pt 1), 450–463. https://doi.org/10.1097/AOG.0b013e3181eeb251

American College of Obstetricians and Gynecologists. (2014). Safe prevention of the primary cesarean delivery. Obstetric Care Consensus No. 1. *Obstetrics & Gynecology, 123*, 693–711.

American College of Obstetricians and Gynecologists. (2015). Obesity in pregnancy. Practice Bulletin No. 156. *Obstetrics & Gynecology, 126*, e112–e126. https://doi.org/10.1097/AOG.0000000000001211

American College of Obstetricians and Gynecologists. (2017). Postpartum hemorrhage. Practice Bulletin No. 183. *Obstetrics & Gynecology, 130*, e168–e186. https://doi.org/10.1097/AOG.0000000000002351

American College of Obstetricians and Gynecologists. (2018a). Postpartum pain management. Committee Opinion No. 742. *Obstetrics & Gynecology, 132*, 252–253. https://doi.org/10.1097/AOG.0000000000002711

American College of Obstetricians and Gynecologists. (2018b). Use of prophylactic antibiotics in labor and delivery. ACOG Practice Bulletin No. 199. *Obstetrics & Gynecology, 132*, e103–e119.

American College of Obstetricians and Gynecologists. (2019a). Cesarean delivery on maternal request. ACOG Committee Opinion No. 761. *Obstetrics & Gynecology, 133*, e73–e77. https://doi.org/10.1097/AOG.0000000000002833

American College of Obstetricians and Gynecologists. (2019b). Ethical considerations for the care of women with obesity. *Obstetrics & Gynecology, 133*, e90–e96. https://doi.org/10.1097/AOG.0000000000003015

American College of Obstetricians and Gynecologists. (2019c). *Obstetric analgesia and anesthesia.* Practice Bulletin No. 209. Author.

American College of Obstetricians and Gynecologists. (2020). Operative vaginal birth. ACOG Practice Bulletin No. 219. *Obstetrics & Gynecology, 135*, e149–e159. https://doi.org/10.1097/AOG.0000000000003764

Association of Women's Health, Obstetric and Neonatal Nurses. (2019a). *Evidence-based clinical practice guideline: Perioperative care of the pregnant woman second edition.* Author.

Association of Women's Health, Obstetric and Neonatal Nurses. (2019b). *Perioperative care of the pregnant woman* (Evidence-Based Clinical Practice Guideline, 2nd ed.). Author.

Association of Women's Health, Obstetric and Neonatal Nurses. (2020). *Analgesia and anesthesia in the intrapartum period evidence-based clinical practice guideline.* Author.

Bell, A. D., Joy, S., Gullo, S., Higgins, R., & Stevenson, E. (2017). Implementing a systematic approach to reduce cesarean birth rates in nulliparous women. *Obstetrics & Gynecology, 130*, 1082–1089. https://doi.org/10.1097/AOG.0000000000002263

Burcher, P., Cheyney, M. J., Li, K. N., Hushmendy, S., & Kiley, K. C. (2016). Cesarean birth regret and dissatisfaction: A qualitative approach. *Birth, 43*, 346–352. https://doi.org/10.1111/birt.12240

Caughey, A., Cahill, A., Guise, J., & Rouse, D. (2014). ACOG/SMFM obstetric care consensus safe prevention of the primary cesarean delivery. *American Journal of Obstetrics & Gynecology, 210*, 179–193.

Cunningham, F., Leveno, K., Bloom, S., Dashe, J., Hoffman, B., Casey, B., & Spong, C. (2018). *Williams obstetrics* (25th ed.). McGraw-Hill.

Hamilton, B., Martin, J., Osterman, M., Driscoll, A., & Rossen, L. (2017). *Births: Provisional data for 2016.* http://www.cdc.gov/nchs/data/vsrr/report002.pdf

Hamilton, B., Martin, J., & Ventura, S. (2011). Births: Preliminary data for 2010. *National Vital Statistics Reports, 60*(2), 1–29.

Javernick, J. A., & Dempsey, A. (2017). Reducing the primary cesarean birth rate: A quality improvement project. *Journal of Midwifery & Women's Health, 62*, 477–483. https://doi.org/10.1111/jmwh.12606

Kawakita, T., & Landy, H. J. (2017). Surgical site infections after cesarean delivery: Epidemiology, prevention and treatment. *Maternal Health, Neonatology and Perinatology, 3*, 12. https://doi.org/10.1186/s40748-017-0051-3

Lagrew, D., Kane Low, L., Brennan, R., Corry, M., Edmonds, J., Gilpin, B., . . . Jaffer, S. (2018). National partnership for maternal safety: Consensus bundle on safe reduction of primary cesarean births—supporting intended vaginal births. *Journal of Obstetric, Gynecologic & Neonatal Nursing, 47*(2), 214–226. https://doi.org/10.1016/j.jogn.2018.01.008

Main, E. K., Morton, C. H., Melsop, K., Hopkins, D., Giuliani, G., & Gould, J. B. (2012). Creating a public agenda for maternity safety and quality in cesarean delivery. *Obstetrics & Gynecology, 120*, 1194–1198. https://doi.org/10.1097/AOG.0b013e31826fc13d

Martin, J. A., Hamilton, B. E., Osterman, M. J. K., & Driscoll, A. K. (2019). *Births: Final data for 2018. National Vital Statistics Reports, 68*(13). National Center for Health Statistics.

Pergialiotis, V., Prodromidou, A., Perrea, D. N., & Doumouchtsis, S. K. (2017). The impact of subcutaneous tissue suturing at caesarean section on wound complications: A meta-analysis. *British Journal of Obstetrics and Gynaecology, 124*, 1018. https://doi.org/10.1111/1471-0528.14593

Simpson, K. R., & Lyndon, A. (2017). Labor nurses' views of their influence on cesarean birth. *MCN. The American Journal of Maternal Child Nursing, 42*(2), 81–87. https://doi.org/10.1097/NMC.0000000000000308

Simpson, K. R., & O'Brien-Abel, N. (2021). Labor and birth. In K. Simpson, P. Creehan, N. O'Brien-Abel, C. Roth, & A. Rohan (Eds.), *Perinatal nursing* (5th ed., pp. 325–411). Wolters Kluwer.

Suplee, P. D., Kleppel, L., & Bingham, D. (2016). Discharge education on maternal morbidity and mortality provided by nurses to women in the postpartum period. *Journal of Obstetric, Gynecologic & Neonatal Nursing, 45*, 894–904. https://doi.org/10.1016/j.jogn.2016.07.006

Teal, E. N., Anudokem, K. B., Baer, R. J., Rand, L., Jelliffe-Pawlowski, L. L., & Mengesha, B. M. (2020). *Racial disparities in cesarean delivery rates: Do hospital type, setting, and volume matter?* Society for Maternal Fetal Medicine Poster presentation 2020

Vallerand, A., & Sanoski, C. (2017). *Davis's drug guide for nurses* (15th ed.). F.A. Davis.

Yee, L. M., Constantine, M. M., Rice, M. M., Bailit, J., Reddy, U. M., Wapner, R. J., . . . Eunice Kennedy Shriver National Institute of Child Health and Human Development (NICHD) Maternal-Fetal Medicine Units (MFMU) Network. (2017). Racial and ethnic differences in utilization of labor management strategies intended to reduce cesarean delivery rates. *Obstetrics and Gynecology, 130*(6), 1285–1294. https://doi.org/10.1097/AOG.0000000000002343

The Postpartal Period

Postpartum Physiological Assessments and Nursing Care

12

Tara Loghry, MSN-ED, RNC-OB, C-EFM

LEARNING OUTCOMES

Upon completion of this chapter, the student will be able to:
1. Describe the physiological changes that occur during the postpartum period.
2. Identify critical elements of assessment and nursing care during the postpartum period.
3. Discuss safe and effective nursing care during the postpartum period.
4. Outline the critical elements of discharge teaching.

CONCEPTS

Clinical Judgment
Comfort
Elimination
Evidence-Based Practice
Family
Health Promotion
Infection
Mood and Affect
Nutrition
Reproduction and Sexuality
Self-Care
Stress and Coping
Tissue Integrity

Nursing Diagnosis

- Pain related to tissue trauma secondary to vaginal delivery
- Pain related to uterine involution secondary to vaginal delivery
- Pain related to congestion, increased vascularity, and milk accumulation secondary to breast engorgement
- At risk for infection related to perineal tissue trauma
- At risk for infection (mastitis) related to altered skin integrity and milk stasis
- At risk for fluid volume deficit related to hemorrhage from uterine atony
- At risk for impaired urinary elimination related to decreased sensation and tissue trauma
- At risk for constipation related to hormonal effects on smooth muscles
- At risk for knowledge deficit regarding health promotion postbirth related to lack of information

Nursing Outcomes

- The postpartum woman will report adequate pain control.
- The postpartum woman will remain free from symptoms of infection.
- The postpartum woman will have a firm fundus with scant to moderate lochia.
- The postpartum woman will spontaneously void within 2 to 4 hours postbirth.
- The postpartum woman will eat a nutritious diet high in fiber and roughage and drink at least 10 glasses of fluid per day (80 ounces).
- The postpartum woman will verbalize an understanding of major components of health promotion.
- The postpartum woman will identify signs of complications that must be reported to the health-care provider.
- The postpartum woman will verbalize a plan for postpartum follow-up care.

INTRODUCTION

The postpartum period, the 6-week period after childbirth, is a time of rapid physiological changes as the woman's body returns to a prepregnant state. Women who are healthy at conception and experience a low-risk pregnancy, labor, and birth are at low risk for postpartum complications. After birth, a woman and her family must adapt to many physical, social, and psychological changes, influenced by childbirth, changing hormones, and caring for the baby. The postpartum period is a time of joy and excitement, but this "fourth trimester" also presents considerable challenges for women due to lack of sleep, fatigue, pain, breastfeeding difficulties, stress, depression, and adapting to the new role of motherhood. The focus of this chapter is the physiological aspects of postpartum nursing care (Box 12-1) and includes information regarding the following:

- Assessment of postpartum physiological changes
- Providing comfort and restoring physiological functions affected by childbirth
- Assessing for early signs of potential complications
- Promoting health and education

Psychological adaptations in the postpartum period are presented in detail in Chapter 13. Perinatal mood and anxiety disorders in their most severe forms can be tragic and preventable causes of maternal and infant mortality. Perinatal mood and anxiety disorders and their sequelae can be addressed by actively screening women, following up on preexisting mental health disorders, having a plan for treatment or referral for those who screen positive, and actively engaging women, their families, and supporters in recognizing symptoms and seeking care in a timely manner (Suplee & Janke, 2020). Screening should occur in the immediate postpartum period with standardized tools such as the Edinburgh Postnatal Depression Scale. However, screening alone does not improve perinatal outcomes. Systems must be in place to ensure consistent screening with appropriate assessment tools, interventions, and monitoring of follow-up care for women with identified perinatal mood and anxiety disorders.

MATERNAL MORTALITY

Maternal mortality is the death of a woman from complications of pregnancy and childbirth occurring up to a year postpartum. In a federal report from 2017, the United States ranked 129th out of 184 countries for maternal mortality (Central Intelligence Agency, 2021) and displayed a rising maternal mortality rate nationwide in recent years. The most current U.S. pregnancy-related mortality rate shows a slight increase from 16.9 maternal deaths per 100,000 live births in 2016 to 17.3 deaths per 100,000 live births in 2017 (Centers for Disease Control and Prevention [CDC], 2020b). This rate is more than double the 1987 rate of 7.2 deaths per 100,000 births. Increased rates may be related to improvements in reporting, but the number is still high for a country with readily available medical care. The CDC and the Department of Health and Human Services Office of Disease Prevention and Health Promotion have set national health goals published in *Healthy People 2030,* several of which relate to the postpartum period (Table 12-1).

THE REPRODUCTIVE SYSTEM

The reproductive system, which includes the uterus, cervix, vagina, and perineum, undergoes dramatic changes after childbirth. Women are at risk for hemorrhage and infection. Nursing assessments and interventions are aimed at reducing these risks; see "Clinical Pathway for Uncomplicated Vaginal Delivery" for more details.

Uterus

After delivery of the placenta, the uterus begins the process of involution to return to its nearly prepregnant size, shape, and location as the placental site heals. This occurs through uterine contractions, atrophy of the uterine muscle, and a decrease in the size of uterine cells. Involution of the uterus takes between 6 and 8 weeks postdelivery (Cunningham et al., 2018; Smith, 2018). Primiparous women usually do not experience discomfort related to uterine contractions during the postpartum period because the uterus remains contracted. Multiparous women or women who are breastfeeding may experience "afterpains" caused by strong intermittent uterine contractions during the first few postpartum days. Afterpains are moderate to severe cramp-like pains related to the uterus working to remain contracted or the increase of oxytocin released in response to infant suckling. The intensity of afterpains will typically decrease after the third postpartum day. The uterus must be contracted during the postpartum period to decrease the risk of postpartum hemorrhage. The contracted uterine muscle compresses the open

BOX 12-1 | Overview of the Postpartum Assessment

The following should be assessed per the health-care provider's order or unit protocol:

- Vital signs, pain, breath and heart sounds
- Laboratory findings, such as CBC, rubella status, and Rh status
- Vaccination status, including tetanus, diphtheria, and acellular pertussis (Tdap); influenza; pneumococcal; and COVID-19 vaccine
- Breasts
- Uterus
- Bladder
- Bowel
- Lochia
- Episiotomy, lacerations, perineum, hemorrhoids
- Lower extremities
- Emotions, bonding with infant, fatigue, psychosocial factors

TABLE 12-1 *Healthy People 2030* Objectives Related to the Postpartum Period

OBJECTIVE	BASELINE	TARGET
Reduce maternal deaths.	17.4 maternal deaths per 100,000 live births	15.7 maternal deaths per 100,000 live births
Reduce severe maternal complications identified during delivery hospitalizations.	68.7 per 10,000 delivery hospitalizations	61.8 per 10,000 delivery hospitalizations
Increase the proportion of infants that are breastfed: Exclusively through age 6 months At 1 year	24.9% 35.9%	42.4% 54.1%
Increase the proportion of women who get screened for postpartum depression.	No baseline data provided	No target provided
Reduce the proportion of unintended pregnancies.	43.0%	36.5%
Reduce the proportion of pregnancies conceived within 18 months of a previous birth.	33.8%	26.9%
Reduce pregnancies among adolescent females	43.4% per 1,000	31.4% per 1,000

U.S. Department of Health and Human Services, Office of Disease Prevention and Health Promotion, 2020.

vessels at the placental site and decreases the amount of blood loss (Cunningham et al., 2018).

Nursing Actions

- Assess the uterus for location, position, and tone of the fundus.
  - After the third stage of labor, assess the uterus:
    - Every 15 minutes for the first hour
    - Every 30 minutes for the second hour
    - Every 4 hours for the next 22 hours
    - Every shift after the first 24 hours or as stated in hospital or unit protocols
    - More frequently if the assessment findings are not within normal limits
  - Frequent assessment of uterine tone and placement allows identification of complications such as uterine atony (decreased uterine muscle tone) that may cause postpartum hemorrhage.
    - The risk for postpartum hemorrhage is the greatest within the first hour following delivery.
    - Primary (early) postpartum hemorrhage occurs in the first 24 hours after birth.
    - Secondary (late) postpartum hemorrhage may occur from 24 hours to 12 weeks postdelivery but is most prevalent during the first 7 to 14 days following birth (Cunningham et al., 2018).
    - See Chapter 14 for more information on the care of the woman with postpartum hemorrhage.
- Before assessment, inform the woman that you will be palpating her uterus to evaluate for normal involution and bleeding.
- Explain the procedure.

- Instruct the woman to void.
  - Rationale: An overdistended bladder can result in uterine displacement and atony (James & Suplee, 2020). Encouraging the woman to void before uterine assessment will allow for an accurate assessment of uterine placement and tone.
- Provide privacy.
- Lower the head and foot of the bed so that the woman is in a supine position and flat.
- Remove her peripads to evaluate lochia at the same time the fundus is palpated.
- Support the lower uterine segment by placing one hand just above the symphysis pubis (Fig. 12–1).
  - Rationale: Pregnancy stretches the ligaments that hold the uterus in place. Fundal pressure could result in uterine inversion (James & Suplee, 2020). Supporting the lower uterine segment may prevent uterine inversion during fundal assessment or massage.
- Locate the fundus with the other hand using gentle downward pressure and assess the position, tone, and location of the fundus.
- Give oxytocin as per the physician's or midwife's postpartum orders. Refer to Safe and Effective Nursing Care: Oxytocin (Pitocin) Administration.
  - Rationale: Oxytocin promotes contraction of the uterus by stimulating its smooth muscle, which prevents and controls postpartum hemorrhage (Wilson et al., 2020).
- Notify the physician or midwife if the uterus does not respond to massage and postpartum orders have been implemented.
  - Lack of response to fundal massage and oxytocin administration may indicate complications such as retained placental tissue or birth trauma. Continued uterine atony can

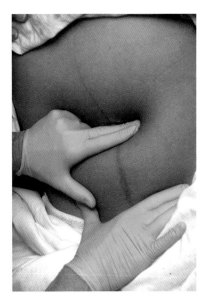

FIGURE 12–1 Nurse supporting lower uterine segment while assessing the postpartum uterus.

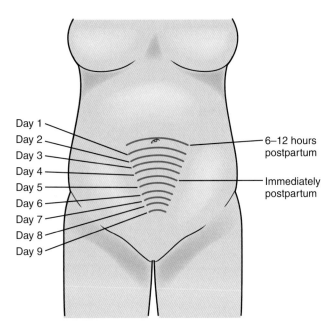

Day 1
Day 2
Day 3
Day 4
Day 5
Day 6
Day 7
Day 8
Day 9

6–12 hours postpartum

Immediately postpartum

FIGURE 12–2 Location of fundus at 6 to 12 hours postpartum and 1 to 9 days postpartum.

lead to postpartum hemorrhage and requires assessment and potentially further treatment by the woman's healthcare provider.

- Determine the position of the uterus.
  - Rationale: A uterus that is shifted to the side may indicate a distended bladder. This interferes with uterine contractibility, which places the woman at risk for uterine atony and increases her risk of hemorrhage (James & Suplee, 2020).
  - If the uterus is deviated, soft, or elevated above the umbilicus, the immediate action is to explain to the patient the need for her to void and to assist her to the bathroom. Reassess the uterine position after the woman has voided and returned to her bed. If the patient is unable to void, urinary catheterization may be necessary.
- Measure the distance between the fundus and umbilicus with your fingers. Each finger-breadth equals 1 cm (see Fig. 12–2).

Expected assessment findings include the following:

- Immediately after birth, the uterine fundus is palpated midway between the umbilicus and symphysis pubis and is firm and midline. In the next few hours, it is palpated at the umbilicus.
- Within 12 hours after birth of the placenta, the fundus is located at the level of the umbilicus or 1 cm above the umbilicus and is firm and midline.
- 24 hours after birth of the placenta, the fundus is located at 1 cm below the umbilicus and is firm and midline.
- The uterus descends 1 cm per day; by day 14, the fundus has descended into the pelvis and is not palpable.
- Subinvolution is the failure of the uterus to involute or descend as expected. Causes include retained placental fragments, infection, and overdistended uterus (e.g., from a large baby). Subinvolution may lead to prolonged or excessive bleeding during the postpartum period (Cunningham et al., 2018).

CRITICAL COMPONENT

Uterine Atony (Boggy Uterus)

Uterine atony is the most common cause of postpartum hemorrhage. Because hemostasis associated with placental separation depends on myometrial contraction, atony is treated initially by uterine massage, followed by drugs that promote uterine contraction.

- A boggy uterus is a sign that the uterus is not contracted.
- Risk of excessive blood loss or hemorrhage is increased.
- The immediate action is to massage the fundus with the palm of your hand in a circular motion until firm and reevaluate within 5 to 10 minutes.
- If the uterus does not respond to massage, follow the standing order for oxytocin and notify the physician or midwife.

SAFE AND EFFECTIVE NURSING CARE: Understanding Medication

Oxytocin (Pitocin) Administration

Oxytocin stimulates the upper segment of the myometrium to contract rhythmically, which constricts spiral arteries and decreases blood flow through the uterus. Oxytocin is an effective first-line treatment for postpartum hemorrhage. As a high-alert medication, IV oxytocin premixed bags should be administered on an infusion pump in a standardized concentration as per facility protocol. The bag should also be prominently and clearly labeled and stored separately and use a bar code scanning technology (Association of Women's Health, Obstetric and Neonatal Nurses [AWHONN], 2021a).

Oxytocin Given as a Component of Active Management of Third Stage of Labor

- Increase IV oxytocin rate, 500 mL/hour of 10 to 40 units/500 to 1,000 mL solution.
- Indication: Reduction of blood loss.
- Action: Stimulates uterine smooth muscle to produce uterine contraction.
- Adverse reactions with IV use include coma, seizures, hypertension, hypotension, and water intoxication.
- Administer via IV infusion using an IV infusion pump, or via the intramuscular (IM) route if the patient does not have IV access. For patients without IV access, administer 10 units of oxytocin IM.
- Premixed bags of IV fluid containing oxytocin should be clearly marked with bright labels and stored in a different area than plain IV fluid bags.
- Bolus at a rate of 1,000 mL/hr for 30 minutes (10 units of oxytocin), immediately after birth followed by a maintenance dose of 125 mL/hr for 3.5 hours.
- Women who have a cesarean birth or are at high risk for postpartum hemorrhage may require continuation of oxytocin administration for greater than 4 hours. Duration and dosage are based on assessment of fundal tone and amount of vaginal bleeding (AWHONN, 2021a).
- Nursing actions and implications include the following: Monitor vital signs frequently; assess fundal position, tone, and location; assess lochia color amount and odor; assess for signs of water intoxication (drowsiness, headache, anuria); and teach patient that oxytocin will cause uterine cramping.
- Have other uterotonics on hand such as methylergonovine (Methergine), misoprostol (Cytotec), and carboprost (Hemabate) (AWHONN, 2021a).

The nurse should also provide information regarding afterpains, uterine cramps caused by the contraction, and relaxation of the uterus as it decreases in size.

- Afterpains occur within the first few days and typically decrease 3 days after delivery.
  - They occur more commonly with multiparous women and increase with each additional pregnancy or birth.
  - They may increase when breastfeeding during the first few postpartum days.
- Comfort measures include the following:
  - Encourage her to void frequently, as a distended bladder can increase afterpains.
  - Apply a warm blanket to the abdomen.
  - Relaxation techniques and warm compresses can interfere with the transmission and sensation of pain.
  - Analgesics such as ibuprofen and acetaminophen are effective in relieving uterine cramping.

The Endometrium

The endometrium, the mucous membrane that lines the uterus, exfoliates and regenerates after the birth of the placenta through necrosis of the superficial layer of the decidua and regeneration of the decidua basalis into endometrial tissue. Lochia is a bloody discharge from the uterus that contains red blood cells (RBCs), sloughed-off decidual tissue, epithelial cells, and bacteria (Cunningham et al., 2018). The placental site heals by exfoliation, which involves sloughing of necrotic endometrial tissue and regeneration of the endometrium at the placental site (Cunningham et al., 2018; Smith, 2018). This prevents scarring of the endometrial tissue (James & Suplee, 2020). Changes in lochia reflect the healing stages of the uterine placental site (Table 12-2).

- Lochia is described as scant, light, moderate, or heavy (Fig. 12–3).
  - Scant is less than 1 inch on the pad.
  - Light is less than 4 inches on the pad.
  - Moderate is less than 6 inches on the pad.
  - Heavy is when the pad is saturated within 1 hour; excessively heavy is when a pad is soaked within 15 minutes.

Uterine contractions constrict the vessels around the placental site and decrease blood loss. A primary complication is metritis, an infection of the endometrial tissue (see Chapter 14). Frequent assessment of lochia in the early postpartum period allows the nurse to monitor blood loss and identify excessive bleeding, determine clot presence, and assess for signs of infection.

Nursing Actions

Assess lochia at the same time the uterus is assessed. Document the lochia stage, amount, presence of odor, and interventions.

- Assess lochia color (stage of lochia)
  - Initial lochia for the first 3 days is rubra, which is red and bloody.
  - The next stage of lochia is serosa, which is pink or brown.
  - The final stage is alba, which is clear or whitish.
- Assess lochia amount, documented as scant, light, moderate, or heavy (see Fig. 12–3).
- Assess lochia for odor. Lochia has a fleshy odor and smells similar to menstrual blood.
- Assess for clots, which occur when the lochia has been pooling in the lower uterine segment.
  - Small clots should be noted in the patient chart.
  - A clot the size of an egg or larger should be weighed and findings reported to the physician or midwife as large clots can interfere with uterine involution.
    - 1 g in weight equals 1 mL of blood loss.
  - Clots should be examined for the presence of tissue.
    - Retained placental tissue can interfere with uterine involution and lead to excessive bleeding.

Expected assessment findings are further described in Table 12-2.

Patient Education

- Teach the woman how to assess the fundus and explain the normal process of involution.

TABLE 12-2   Stages and Characteristics of Lochia

STAGE	TIME FRAME	EXPECTED FINDINGS	DEVIATIONS FROM NORMAL
Lochia rubra	Days 1–3	Bloody with small clots Moderate to scant amount Increased flow on standing or breastfeeding Fleshy odor	Large clots Heavy amount; saturates pad within 1 hour (sign of possible hemorrhage), excessively heavy, saturates a pad in 15 minutes Foul odor (sign of infection) Placental fragments
Lochia serosa	Days 4–10	Pink or brown color Scant amount Increased flow during physical activity Fleshy odor	Continuation of rubra stage after day 4 Heavy amount; saturates pad within 1 hour (sign of possible hemorrhage), excessively heavy; saturates pad within 15 minutes Foul odor (sign of infection)
Lochia alba	Day 10	Yellow to white in color Scant amount Fleshy odor	Bright red bleeding, saturates pad within 1 hour (sign of possible late postpartum hemorrhage) Foul odor (sign of infection)

Scant: Blood only on tissue when wiped or 1- to 2-inch stain

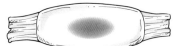

Light: 4-inch or less stain

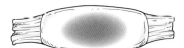

Moderate: Less than 6-inch stain

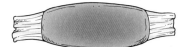

Heavy: Saturated pad

FIGURE 12–3 Comparison of heavy, moderate, light, and scant lochia on pads.

- Teach the woman how to massage her uterus if boggy and instruct her to notify the nurse while in the hospital and healthcare provider after discharge.
  - Rationale: Secondary hemorrhage often occurs after the patient has been discharged. To prevent serious complications, women should understand the normal progression of lochia and uterine involution and report abnormal amounts of bleeding. Potential causes of secondary hemorrhage include placental site subinvolution, infection, retained placental tissue, and von Willebrand disease.

- Provide information on the normal stages of lochia.
- Explain that the flow of lochia can increase when getting up in the morning or after sitting for prolonged periods due to vaginal pooling of lochia, or from excessive physical activity.
  - Instruct the woman to notify the nurse, physician, or midwife if she experiences an increase in the amount of lochia, if the color of lochia changes back to bright red after the rubra stage is over, or if the lochia has a foul odor.
  - Rationale: Lochia should decrease in amount every day. Foul-smelling lochia could indicate the development of an infection. An increase in lochia or the return of bright red bleeding may be signs of secondary hemorrhage (Cunningham et al., 2018).
- Provide information for reducing the risk of infection such as instructing the patient to change the peripad frequently, wash hands before and after changing pads, and use a peri-bottle to keep the area clean.
  - Rationale: Lochia is a medium for bacterial growth. Frequent pad changes and hand washing are actions aimed at preventing infection.

CLINICAL JUDGMENT

Excessive Bleeding and Early Warning Signs

The leading cause of maternal mortality in the United States is postpartum hemorrhage, accounting for 10.7% of maternal deaths between 2014 to 2017. Inaccurate measure of blood loss is attributed to visual estimation of blood loss (EBL), leading to delays in timely recognition and intervention of obstetric hemorrhage. Quantification of blood loss (QBL), a more accurate and objective measurement, is completed by weighing blood-saturated items and blood clots. Weight of 1 gram is equal to 1 mL (AWHONN, 2021b). Scale access is recommended for every room, along with a postpartum hemorrhage cart containing postpartum hemorrhage treatment algorithms. Electronic charting systems should be set to automatically deduct dry weights from wet weights whenever possible.

Immediate nursing actions for postpartum hemorrhage include the following:

- Assess the position, tone, and location of the fundus.
- If the uterus is boggy, massage it.
- If the uterus is boggy and displaced to the side, instruct the patient to void and reevaluate.
  - Ambulate the patient to the bathroom and measure void. Use a bladder scanner when available.
- Quantify blood loss (QBL) by weighing all blood-soaked peripads and materials.
  - 1 g equals 1 mL of fluid.
  - Realtime completion of QBL reduces delay in interventions and may reduce the need for additional interventions such as administration of uterotonic medication, unnecessary procedures, and blood transfusions.
  - QBL promotes team awareness improving response time for additional resources and improves patient outcomes.
  - A scale with an attached laminated card with the dry weights of peripads or chux should be available on units providing care to postpartum patients (AWHONN, 2021b).
- Notify the health-care team of excessive bleeding and QBL.
- If uterine atony continues, utilize health-care's staging algorithm to guide interventions (for more information, see Chapter 14).

Continued heavy bleeding with firm fundal tone may indicate the presence of a genitourinary tract laceration or hematoma of the vulva or vagina. Be alert to early warning signs. Verify isolated abnormal measurements, particularly for blood pressure, heart rate, respiratory rate, and oxygen saturation. Urgent bedside evaluation is usually indicated if any of these values persist for more than one measurement, present with additional abnormal parameters, or recur more than once (Box 12-2).

While awaiting arrival of the evaluating clinician, the bedside nurse should follow basic resuscitation principles:

- Achieve free-flowing appropriate venous access
- Increase frequency of vital signs
- Provide supplemental oxygen therapy
- Ensure indwelling catheter, uterotonic drugs, and laboratory supplies are at bedside
- Consider the activation of the rapid response team

Vagina and Perineum

- The vagina and perineum experience changes related to the birthing process that may include edema, mild stretching, minor lacerations, major tears, or episiotomy.
- A first-degree laceration involves the vaginal mucous membranes and the perineal skin.

BOX 12-2 | The Maternal Early Warning Criteria

MEASURE	VALUE
Systolic blood pressure (mm Hg)	<90 or >160
Diastolic blood pressure (mm Hg)	>100
Heart rate (bpm)	<50 or >120
Respiratory rate (breaths per min)	<10 or >30
Oxygen saturation on room air, at sea level %	<95
Oliguria, mL/hr for ≥2 hrs	<35
Maternal agitation, confusion, or unresponsiveness	
Woman with preeclampsia reporting a nonremitting headache or shortness of breath	

- A second-degree laceration involves the vaginal mucous membranes, perineal skin, and the fascia of the perineal body.
- A third-degree laceration involves the perineal skin, vaginal mucous membranes, fascia of the perineal body, and the rectal sphincter.
- A fourth-degree laceration involves the perineal skin and fascia, vaginal mucous membranes, rectal sphincter, and the rectal mucosa and lumen.
- A midline episiotomy is an incision that is midline on the perineum. This type of incision tends to heal more quickly and cause less pain than a mediolateral episiotomy.
- A mediolateral episiotomy is an incision that is made at a 45-degree angle to the perineum.

See Chapter 8 for further discussion of lacerations and episiotomy.

The woman may experience mild to severe pain, depending on the degree and type of vaginal or perineal trauma. Women who have a third- or fourth-degree laceration, an episiotomy, or hemorrhoids may require a stool softener or laxative to facilitate bowel movements. The primary complication is infection at the laceration or episiotomy site. Lacerations can tear posteriorly toward the rectum, causing difficulty with bowel movements. Lacerations can also tear anteriorly toward the urethra, causing swelling and difficulty with urination. The vagina and perineum undergo healing and restoration during the postpartum period. Immediately after delivery, the vaginal walls are smooth, but rugae are reestablished within 3 weeks (James & Suplee, 2020).

Nursing Actions

- The perineum is assessed when the fundus and lochia are checked in the postdelivery period. After that, the perineum is assessed every shift using the acronym REEDA (redness, edema, ecchymosis, discharge, approximation of edges of episiotomy or laceration).
  - Rationale: Frequent assessment of the perineum using the REEDA scale will allow identification of potential complications, such as excessive swelling, infection, hematoma,

and excessive bleeding. See Chapter 14 for more information about lacerations and hematoma.

- Explain the procedure.
- Provide privacy.
- Lower the head and foot of the bed so that the woman is in a supine position and flat.
- Remove her peripads to evaluate labia and perineum anteriorly.
- Assist the woman to her side and separate her buttocks to expose the perineum and rectum for assessment.
  - Rationale: Assess the perineum anteriorly, then place the woman in the side-lying position to inspect the perineal area and assess the amount of lochia present on the entire peripad. While the woman is in the side-lying position, assess the rectal area for hemorrhoids.
- Expected assessment findings:
  - Mild edema
  - Minor ecchymosis
  - Approximation of the edges of the episiotomy or laceration if visible; most lacerations are internal and not visible.
  - Mild to moderate pain
- Assess for discomfort and provide comfort measures.
  - Apply ice to the perineum or encourage the use of cold sitz baths for the first 24 to 48 hours to manage swelling.
    - Rationale: Ice causes local vasoconstriction, which decreases edema and provides an anesthetic effect (Cunningham et al., 2018).
  - Instruct the woman to take warm sitz baths, starting 24 hours after delivery twice a day for 20 minutes.
    - Rationale: Warm sitz baths promote circulation, healing, and comfort.
  - Encourage the woman to lie on her side.
    - Rationale: The side-lying position decreases pressure on the perineum.
  - Instruct the woman to tighten her gluteal muscles as she sits down and to relax muscles after she is seated.
    - Rationale: This helps cushion the perineum and increases comfort when assuming a sitting position.
  - Instruct the woman to wear peripads snugly to prevent rubbing.
  - Administer a topical anesthetic per the physician's or midwife's order.
    - Rationale: Topical anesthetics may relieve localized discomfort.
  - Administer analgesia per the physician's or midwife's order and assess adequacy of pain relief within 30 minutes. Note the patient's acceptable pain level, as sometimes we cannot achieve 0 pain. Analgesics such as ibuprofen or acetaminophen are effective in treating perineal pain.
- Reduce the risk for infection.
  - Instruct the woman to use a peri-bottle with warm water and rinse the perineum after elimination.
  - Instruct the woman to change the peripad frequently.
  - Instruct the woman to properly dispose of soiled pads and to wash her hands.
    - Rationale: Lochia is a medium for bacterial growth. Frequent pad changes and hand washing before and after a pad change will reduce the risk for infection.

CLINICAL JUDGMENT

Assessment and Management of Pain in the Postpartum Period

Pain in the postpartum period may result from uterine contractions or afterpains, perineal trauma, lacerations, episiotomy, surgical incision after cesarean delivery, nipple pain caused by improper infant latch, breast engorgement, hemorrhoids, and general soreness related to the work of labor and birth.

Pain should be assessed routinely when doing vital signs, when the patient complains of pain, before and after a painful procedure, and before and after implementation of a pain management intervention. Assess pain using an appropriate pain scale per agency protocol. Many scales measure pain intensity, duration, quality, location, factors that make pain better or worse, and acceptable level of pain. The woman's culture influences her response to pain, and pain behaviors are culturally bound. Sometimes pain measurement tools that rely on numbers or any kind of linear format, such as a row of faces, do not work well across cultures. Through careful listening and probing, nurses can uncover what is really happening with each patient's pain.

Examples of nonpharmacological interventions include:

- Ice packs
- Warm compresses
- Aromatherapy
- Sitz baths
- Repositioning
- Walking
- Showering
- Topical treatments, such as witch hazel pads and anesthetic sprays applied to localized perineal discomfort

Pharmacological interventions may include:

- NSAIDs such as ibuprofen (for mild to moderate pain):
  - Ibuprofen (Motrin) may be administered with food or milk to decrease GI upset. Give with a full glass of water.
  - Patients with asthma, nasal polyps, or who are allergic to aspirin are at risk for hypersensitivity to ibuprofen.
  - Route and dose for ibuprofen: PO; 400 to 600 mg every 4 to 6 hours PRN, maximum 24-hour dose 3,200 mg/day. Assess pain before and 30 minutes after administration.
- Acetaminophen 650 mg every 4 hours PRN
- Opioid analgesics are reserved for moderate to severe pain that persists after the previously listed interventions have been conducted with the patient. The medications should be used in combination with a nonopioid medication for added analgesic effect. The duration of use of opiate medications should be limited to the least amount of reasonable time to reduce the risk for constipation and persistent use of opioids.

Breasts

During pregnancy, the breasts undergo changes to prepare for lactation. After delivery, estrogen and progesterone decrease and prolactin increases (Cunningham et al., 2018). Prolactin stimulates breast milk production. When the infant suckles, the posterior pituitary releases oxytocin, resulting in the milk ejection reflex (let-down reflex; Cunningham et al., 2018). Immediately after delivery, breast fullness is normal. Although breast tissue may be swollen, it is soft and nontender (James & Suplee, 2020). Around the third postpartum day, both breastfeeding and nonbreastfeeding women experience some degree of primary breast engorgement, an increase in the vascular and lymphatic system of the breasts that precedes milk production. The woman's breasts become larger, firm, warm, and tender, and she may feel a throbbing pain in the breasts. Primary engorgement subsides within 24 to 48 hours. Engorgement can also happen later in breastfeeding mothers due to missed feedings or inadequate removal of milk from the breast. Mothers should be encouraged to pump or express breasts as they become firm and uncomfortable if not with the infant to breastfeed.

Colostrum, a yellowish fluid, precedes milk production and is secreted after delivery. It is higher in protein and lower in carbohydrates than breast milk and contains immunoglobulins G and A, which provide protection for the newborn during the early weeks of life. Colostrum continues for 5 days to 2 weeks postdelivery, during which time transition to mature milk occurs (Cunningham et al., 2018). Mature milk contains proteins, carbohydrates, fat, minerals, vitamins, hormones, and immunological substances such as secretory IgA, lymphocytes, and growth factor (Cunningham et al., 2018). The composition of breast milk changes during the feeding and throughout the course of feedings during the day.

A primary complication associated with breastfeeding is mastitis, an infection of the breast. Breastfeeding, lactation, and nipple assessment are discussed in more detail in Chapter 16. Highlights of breast care and assessment are provided in Box 12-3.

Nursing Actions for the Breastfeeding Woman

- Inspect and palpate the breasts for signs of engorgement: Tenderness, firmness, warmth, or enlargement
- Expected assessment findings:
  - During the first 24 hours postpartum, the breasts are soft and nontender.
  - On postpartum day 2, the breasts are slightly firm and nontender.
  - On postpartum day 3, the breasts are firm, tender, and warm to touch.
- Assess the nipples for signs of irritation and nipple tissue breakdown.
  - Rationale: Signs of irritation and tissue breakdown are cracked, blistered, or reddened areas. Skin breakdown of the nipples is often associated with an improper infant latch. Nipple soreness is a primary reason that women stop breastfeeding, so this complaint should be addressed (Janke, 2020). Additionally, skin breakdown can be an entry point for bacteria. See Chapter 16 for interventions to prevent and treat nipple irritation and breakdown.

Nursing Actions for the Nonbreastfeeding Woman

- Assess the breasts for primary engorgement.
- Inspect and palpate the breasts for signs of engorgement: Tenderness, firmness, warmth, or enlargement.

BOX 12-3 | Breast Care and Assessment

Common findings include:

- Breast engorgement: Caused by an increase in the vascular and the lymphatic systems within the breast and milk accumulation.
- Physiological engorgement:
  - Breasts are swollen.
- Pathological engorgement:
  - Breasts are hard, swollen, red, and tender or painful.
  - Breasts feel warm to the touch.
  - Woman may feel a throbbing sensation in the breasts.
  - Woman may have an elevated temperature.
  - Infant may have difficulty latching on if severe engorgement.
- Treatment for breastfeeding women:
  - Frequent feedings to empty the breasts and to prevent milk stasis
  - Warm compresses to the breast and breast massage to facilitate the flow of milk before feeding sessions
  - Express milk by breast pump or manually if the infant is unable to nurse (i.e., preterm infant)
  - Ice packs after feedings to reduce inflammation and discomfort
  - Analgesics for pain management
  - Wear a supportive bra
- Prevention and treatment for nonbreastfeeding women:
  - Wear a supportive bra
  - Avoid stimulating the breast
  - Ice packs to breast
  - Analgesics for pain management
  - Subsides within 48 to 72 hours
- Plugged milk ducts are associated with inadequate emptying of the breasts and stasis of the milk.
- Symptoms: Palpation of tender breast lumps the size of peas
- Treatments:
  - Frequent feedings
  - Changing infant feeding positions
  - Application of warm compresses to breast or taking a warm shower before feeding session
  - Massaging the breasts before feeding session
- Continued milk stasis or unresolved plugged milk ducts can lead to mastitis and potential breast abscess.
- Patient education
  - Encourage the woman to wear a supportive but nonconstrictive bra.

Continued

BOX 12-3 | Breast Care and Assessment—cont'd

- Instruct the woman to examine her nipples before feedings for signs of irritation.
- After feeding, the woman should expose her nipples to air.
- Improper latch should be adjusted to decrease nipple tissue breakdown.
- Instruct the woman to feed her infant frequently on demand or express milk if she is experiencing breast engorgement.
- Encourage the woman to wash her hands frequently and to keep her breasts clean to prevent infection.
- Provide information on mastitis.
  - Mastitis typically occurs at 3 to 4 weeks postbirth.
  - The infection may be caused by bacterial entry through cracks in the nipples and is associated with milk stasis, engorgement, long intervals between feedings, stress, and fatigue.
  - Symptoms include fever, chills, malaise, flu-like symptoms, unilateral breast pain, and redness and tenderness in the infected area.
  - The woman needs to report symptoms to her health-care provider.
  - A culture of breast milk may be ordered before starting antibiotics.
  - Treatment: Empty the affected breast, antibiotic therapy, analgesia, rest, adequate nutrition, and hydration.
  - The woman should continue to breastfeed or pump her breasts as per the physician's or midwife's recommendation.
  - The woman should apply moist heat to the affected breast before breastfeeding.
  - Document findings, interventions, and evaluation.

James & Suplee, 2020; Janke, 2020.

- Rationale: In women who do not breastfeed, milk leakage, breast pain, and engorement may occur between 1 and 4 days postdelivery (James & Suplee, 2020).
- Expected assessment findings:
  - During the first 24 hours postpartum, the breasts are soft and nontender.
  - On postpartum day 2, the breasts are slightly firm and nontender.
  - On postpartum day 3, the breasts are firm and tender.

Patient Education

- Instruct the woman to wear a supportive bra or sports bra 24 hours a day until her breasts become soft. Teach the woman to avoid expressing milk or stimulating the breasts.
  - Rationale: Atrophy in milk-secreting cells of the breasts can be caused by back pressure in the milk ducts that occurs when the breasts are not emptied (Janke, 2020).

- Instruct the woman who is experiencing engorgement to:
  - Apply ice packs to the breasts.
  - Not express milk because this stimulates milk production.
  - Avoid heat to the breast because this can stimulate milk production.
  - Take an analgesic for pain.
- Document findings, interventions, and evaluation.

THE CARDIOVASCULAR SYSTEM

Women experience an average blood loss of 200 to 500 mL through vaginal birth. This has a minimal effect on a woman's system due to pregnancy-induced hypervolemia. Stroke volume and cardiac output increase during the first few postpartum hours as blood that was shunted through the uteroplacental unit returns to the maternal system. Cardiac output is elevated for 24 to 48 hours after delivery and returns to prepregnant levels within 10 days (Cunningham et al., 2018). After delivery, plasma volume initially decreases due to blood loss, then increases due to shifts from the extracellular to vascular space (Isley, 2020). Along with a decrease in the total blood volume, this often results in a transient anemia that typically resolves by 8 weeks after delivery (Isley, 2020). White blood cell (WBC) levels may increase to 30,000/mm within a few hours of birth as the result of the stress of labor and birth and return to normal levels within 7 days (Cunningham et al., 2018).

Women are at risk for thromboembolism related to the increase of circulating clotting factors during pregnancy (Isley, 2020). Clotting factors slowly decrease after delivery of the placenta and return to normal ranges within the first 2 postpartum weeks. A potentially life-threatening complication of thrombus formation is pulmonary emboli (James & Suplee, 2020).

Risk of orthostatic hypotension, which is a sudden drop in the blood pressure with standing, increases during the first postpartum week due to decreased vascular resistance in the pelvis. Most women experience an episode of feeling cold and shaking during the first few hours following birth. This phenomenon, called postpartum chills, is related to vascular instability.

Nursing Actions

- Assess pulse and blood pressure:
  - Every 15 minutes for the first hour after delivery
  - Every 30 minutes for the second hour
  - Every 4 hours for the next 22 hours
  - Every shift after the first 24 hours or as stated in hospital or unit protocols
    - Rationale: Hemodynamic changes occur during labor and delivery and in the postpartum period, including rapid changes in blood volume and cardiac output. Assessment of pulse and blood pressure is important to identify potential complications such as excessive blood loss, orthostatic hypotension, infection, and gestational hypertension or preeclampsia. An elevated pulse may

indicate excessive blood loss, fever, or infection (James & Suplee, 2020).

- Assess for excessive blood loss. Expected findings include:
  - Pulse and blood pressure within normal ranges. However, after delivery systolic and diastolic blood pressure may show a transient 5% elevation (Isley, 2020).
  - Bradycardia may occur postdelivery and in the early postpartum period, and is considered normal (James & Suplee, 2020).
- Assess lower extremities for venous thrombosis.
  - Rationale: Increased coagulability associated with pregnancy continues into the postdelivery period. Additionally, venous stasis may occur when there is limited mobility in the immediate postpartum period. These factors lead to an increased risk of venous thrombosis (Isley, 2020).
- Assess the calves and the groin area for tenderness, edema, and sensation of warmth each shift. Compare pulses in both extremities. Measure the calf width if thromboembolism is suspected (James & Suplee, 2020).
  - Rationale: Symptoms of deep vein thrombosis include muscle pain; tenderness; redness or increased warmth to touch; palpation of a hard, cord-like vessel; swelling of veins; edema; and decreased blood circulation to the affected area.
- Expected assessment findings:
  - No tenderness or sensation of warmth.
- Assess for orthostatic hypotension. Women are at risk for orthostatic hypotension during the first postpartum week when standing from a seated or prone position.
  - Explain the cause and incidence of orthostatic hypotension.
  - Instruct the woman to rise slowly to a standing position.
  - Assist the woman when ambulating during the first 24 hours postbirth.
  - Assist the woman to a sitting or supine position if she becomes dizzy or faint.
  - Use an ammonia ampule if the woman faints.
  - Check laboratory values such as a complete blood count (CBC), if ordered.
    - Rationale: Components of the CBC, such as the hematocrit and hemoglobin, are assessed in cases where excessive blood loss has occurred. The hematocrit measures the concentration of RBCs in the blood (Kee, 2018). Hemoglobin decreases by 1 to 1.5 g/dL and hematocrit decreases 3% to 4% per 500 mL of blood loss (James & Suplee, 2020).
  - Expected assessment findings:
    - Blood loss is within normal ranges.
    - Hemoglobin and hematocrit are within normal ranges.
    - Anemia is not unusual during the postpartum period and is diagnosed with hemoglobin less than 11 g/dL and hematocrit less than 32%. Women may receive an oral iron supplement (ferrous sulfate) to treat postpartum anemia.
    - Pulse rate should be within normal limits; however, some women have bradycardia. Blood pressure should be within normal limits. Increased pulse rate may indicate excessive blood loss or infection (James & Suplee, 2020).
- Assess for postpartum chills.
  - Assess temperature.
  - Women who are experiencing chills with temperature within normal ranges may be offered a warm blanket and reassurance that it is normal.
  - Women who are experiencing chills with elevated temperature should be evaluated further for possible infection, and the physician or midwife needs to be notified.

Patient Education

- Instruct the woman on ways to reduce the risk of orthostatic hypotension. Women should be accompanied by the nurse during ambulation in the early postpartum period.
  - Rationale: Orthostatic hypotension places the patient at risk for fainting and falls.
- Encourage frequent ambulation.
  - Rationale: Early and frequent ambulation prevents deep vein thrombosis by preventing stasis of blood in the lower extremities (Cunningham et al., 2018).
- Instruct the woman not to cross her legs (James & Suplee, 2020).
- Apply compression stockings per provider orders for women with a history of blood clots (James & Suplee, 2020).

THE RESPIRATORY SYSTEM

Chest wall compliance returns after the birth of the infant as diaphragm pressure is reduced. The respiratory system returns to a prepregnant state by the end of the postpartum period.

Nursing Actions

- Assess the respiratory rate:
  - Every 15 minutes for the first hour
  - Every 30 minutes for the second hour
  - Every 4 hours for the next 22 hours
  - Every shift after the first 24 hours or as stated in hospital or unit protocols
- Assess breath sounds.
  - Rationale: Women who received oxytocin, large amounts of IV fluids, or tocolytics such as magnesium sulfate or terbutaline; had multiple birth, infection, or preeclampsia; or who were on bedrest are at risk for pulmonary edema (James & Suplee, 2020).
- Expected assessment findings:
  - Within normal limits. The respiratory rate in the postpartum period is typically in the range of 12 to 20 breaths per minute (bpm). The Pao$_2$ should be 95% or higher (James & Suplee, 2020).
  - Breath sounds clear.
- Document findings and intervention.

THE IMMUNE SYSTEM

The immune system, which is suppressed during pregnancy, returns to normal in the postpartum period (Isley, 2020). It is common for the postpartum woman to experience mild temperature elevations during the first 24 hours postbirth related to muscular exertion, exhaustion, dehydration, or hormonal changes. A temperature greater than 100.4°F (38°C) after the first 24 hours on two occasions may be indicative of postpartum infection and requires further evaluation.

Women who are rubella nonimmune should be immunized for rubella before discharge (Cunningham et al., 2018). Women may be required to sign a consent form before vaccine. Women may also receive vaccinations such as Tdap (tetanus, diphtheria, and pertussis), hepatitis B, varicella, and influenza in the postpartum period (CDC, 2020c; Suplee & Janke, 2020).

Rh isoimmunization occurs when an Rh-negative woman develops antibodies to Rh-positive blood related to exposure either by blood transfusion or during pregnancy with an Rh-positive fetus. Women who are sensitized produce IgG anti-D (antibody), which crosses the placenta and attacks the fetal RBCs, causing hemolysis. Rh isoimmunization is preventable.

SAFE AND EFFECTIVE NURSING CARE:
Understanding Medication

Rubella Immunization

- Women who contract rubella during the first trimester have a 90% chance of transmitting the virus to their fetuses.
- Fetuses exposed to rubella during the first trimester are at risk for birth defects that include deafness, blindness, heart defects, and mental retardation.
- Postpartum women who are rubella-nonimmune should be immunized for rubella before discharge. The measles, mumps, and rubella vaccine is often given.
- Women who are immunized should avoid pregnancy for 4 weeks, although the risk of the fetus developing birth defects from the vaccine is extremely low.

CDC, 2020c; Suplee & Janke, 2020.

SAFE AND EFFECTIVE NURSING CARE:
Understanding Medication

Prevention of Rh Isoimmunization

Rho immune globulin is given to Rh-negative women at 28 weeks' gestation. Rh-negative women who gave birth to an Rh-positive neonate are screened for anti-Rh antibodies (Coombs' test). A second injection of Rho immune globulin is given to the woman in the postpartum period if her baby is Rh positive and she is Coombs' negative.

Medication

Rh (D) immune globulin (RhoGAM, Rhophylac)
- Indication: Administered to Rh-negative women who have an Rh-positive neonate

- Action: Prevents production of anti-Rh (D) antibodies
- Adverse reactions: Pain at the injection site, anemia, allergic reaction
- Route and dose: 300 mcg RhoGAM IM only, or Rhophylac, 300 mcg IV or IM within 72 hours postbirth. Do not confuse IM and IV formulations.
- Nursing actions: Confirm that the mother is Rh negative and the infant is Rh positive before administration.

Nursing Actions

- Assess temperature:
  - Every 15 minutes for the first hour
  - Every 30 minutes for the second hour
  - Every 4 hours for the next 22 hours
  - Every shift after the first 24 hours or as stated in hospital or unit protocols
    - Rationale: Assessing the postpartum patient's temperature allows health-care providers to monitor for complications such as infection.
- For temperature elevations of less than 100.4°F (38°C) during the first 24 hours postbirth:
  - Encourage the woman to drink 8 to 10 glasses of fluid, or at least 64 ounces a day.
  - Promote relaxation and rest.
  - Reassess 1 hour after intervention.
    - Rationale: Slight temperature elevations during the first 24 hours postpartum are likely associated with dehydration.
- For temperature elevations of 100.4°F (38°C) or higher after 24 hours postbirth:
  - Encourage the woman to drink a minimum of 64 ounces of fluids a day
  - Notify the physician or midwife of the elevated temperature and anticipate further evaluation. Notify the nursery of the maternal temperature elevation.
    - Rationale: Temperature of 100.4°F (38°C) on two different occasions after the first 24 hours postdelivery signifies infection (James & Suplee, 2020).
- Administer rubella vaccine as indicated.
- Administer other needed vaccines as ordered.
- Administer Rho(D) immune globulin (Rhophylac or RhoGAM) as indicated.
- Document findings and interventions.

THE URINARY SYSTEM

Women are at risk for urinary complications after birth. Transient stress incontinence associated with impaired pelvic muscle function involving the urethra may occur in the first 6 weeks postpartum (Isley, 2020). Many factors are associated with stress urinary incontinence, including pregnancy, multiparity, perineal trauma, infant size, length of second-stage labor, and pushing techniques that increase pressure on the pelvic floor (James & Suplee, 2020). Primary complications are bladder distention and cystitis.

Bladder Distention

Bladder distention, rapid bladder filling, incomplete emptying, and inability to void are common during the first few days postbirth (Cunningham et al., 2018). These are related to administration of intravenous fluids in the postdelivery period, decreased sensation of the urge to void due to anesthesia or analgesia, edema around the urethra, perineal lacerations or episiotomy, operative vaginal delivery, or bladder trauma (Cunningham et al., 2018). Diuresis caused by decreased estrogen levels occurs within 12 hours after birth and aids in the elimination of excess tissue fluids. During this time urine output may be 3,000 mL or more per day (James & Suplee, 2020).

Nursing Actions

- Assist the woman to the bathroom and encourage her to void within 2 to 4 hours postbirth.
  - Rationale: Early voiding decreases the risk of cystitis and prevents bladder distention, which could lead to uterine atony and postpartum hemorrhage (James & Suplee, 2020).
- Assess for urinary disturbances.
- Measure urinary output postbirth. The woman should be able to void at least 300 mL within 2 to 4 hours of delivery.
  - Rationale: Various birth-related factors, such as the stretching of the urethra, displacement of the bladder, birth trauma-associated neural dysfunction, and anesthesia, may interfere with the return of urinary function. Rapid filling of the bladder associated with the administration of IV fluids during labor and delivery and postpartum diuresis can lead to overdistention of the bladder (James & Suplee, 2020). Measuring urinary output allows the nurse to identify inadequate output and problems with urinary elimination.
  - If the patient is voiding less than 150 mL, the nurse must palpate for bladder distention, as this is indicative of urinary retention. Signs of bladder distention include uterine atony, displacement of the uterus above the umbilicus to the right, increased lochia, and fullness in the suprapubic area (James & Suplee, 2020). Incomplete emptying of the bladder can lead to uterine atony and postpartum hemorrhage. Urinary retention may also lead to cystitis.
  - A bladder scanner using ultrasound technology may be used to assess for urinary retention or to measure bladder residual volume after a void of less than 150 mL.
  - If the woman is unable to spontaneously void and has an overdistended bladder postbirth, she will need to be catheterized. An indwelling urinary catheter left in place for 24 hours is recommended when inability to void is related to edema (Cunningham et al., 2018).
    - A straight or "in and out" catheterization may be done if there is little or no edema present and repeated catheterizations are not needed.
  - An integrative and less invasive method when a woman is unable to void is the use of peppermint oil. That entails saturating a cotton ball with peppermint oil and placing it in the "hat" (urine-collection container) with a small amount of water and placing the "hat" on the toilet. Instruct the woman to sit on the toilet. The vapors of the peppermint oil have a relaxing effect on the urinary sphincter.
    - The woman should be able to void within 2 to 4 hours of delivery.
- Assess for frequency, urgency, and burning on urination.
  - Notify the physician or midwife if the patient reports frequency, urgency, or burning on urination.
    - Rationale: These are signs of possible cystitis.
  - Expected assessment findings:
    - The woman spontaneously voids within 2 to 4 hours postbirth.
    - Each voiding is at least 300 mL.
    - The woman does not have frequency, urgency, and burning on urination.
  - Instruct the woman to increase fluid intake to a minimum of 10 glasses per day.
- Document findings and interventions.

Evidence-Based Practice: Urinary Incontinence

Woodly, S. J., & Hay-Smith, E. J. C. (2021). Narrative review of pelvic floor muscle training for childbearing women—why, when, what, and how. *International Urogynecology Journal, 32*(7), 1977–1988. https://doi.org/10.1007/s00192-021-04804-z

Urinary incontinence is experienced by approximately one-third of women during the first 3 months postpartum, with a decrease in prevalence during the first postpartum year. Urinary incontinence impacts women's abilities to engage in their usual activities and alters behaviors to avoid symptoms. The purpose of this narrative review was to summarize quantitative and qualitative evidence on the effectiveness of pelvic floor muscle training (PFMT) in preventing and treating urinary incontinence in pregnant and postpartum women. The data collected in the author's previously published Cochrane Review is the primary source on the effectiveness of PFMT. It was a review of 38 studies, including randomized controlled trials and quasi-experimental studies, that compared voluntary pelvic floor muscle exercises that were taught and supervised by health professionals with usual prenatal or postpartum care, which may have included advice on pelvic floor exercises.

Results:

- Targeting continent antenatal women early in pregnancy and offering a structured PFMT program may prevent onset of urinary incontinence in late pregnancy and postpartum. PFMT can also prevent prolapse and improve sexual function and labor and delivery outcomes.

- When PFMT was initiated in early pregnancy by primiparous women, it was effective in reducing the incidence of urinary incontinence in late pregnancy and up to 6 months postpartum. Childbearing women should be asked at every appointment if they are continent.

- When PFMT began during the antenatal or postpartum period to treat urinary incontinence, it was effective in treating urinary incontinence up to 1 year postdelivery.

- All women need clear, accurate instructions in how to do PFMT. A program comprised of doing eight contractions (8-second holds), three times a day, 3 days a week, for at least 3 months is a reasonable minimum prescription.

Cystitis

Cystitis is a bladder inflammation or infection.

- Symptoms: Frequency, urgency, pain or burning on urination, suprapubic tenderness, hematuria, and malaise
- Treatment: Antibiotic therapy, increased hydration, rest

THE ENDOCRINE SYSTEM

Abrupt changes occur in the endocrine system after delivery of the placenta. For example, estrogen, progesterone, and prolactin levels decrease. Estrogen levels begin to rise after the first week postpartum. For nonlactating women, prolactin levels decline throughout the first 3 postpartum weeks. Menses begins 7 to 9 weeks postbirth. The first menses is usually anovulatory. Ovulation usually occurs by the fourth cycle. The average time for women who are not breastfeeding to return to ovulation is 10 weeks postpartum (James & Suplee, 2020). In women who are lactating, prolactin levels increase in response to the infant's suckling. Lactation suppresses menses, likely due to hormonal changes, including elevated prolactin levels (James & Suplee, 2020). Return of menses depends on the length and amount of breastfeeding. Ovulation is suppressed longer for lactating women than for nonlactating women. The mean time to return to ovulation for women who breastfeed is 17 weeks postdelivery (James & Suplee, 2020).

Both lactating and nonlactating women should be advised to use contraception when they resume sexual intercourse, as ovulation can precede the return of menses. Breastfeeding is not an effective contraceptive method.

Diaphoresis

Diaphoresis occurs during the first few postpartum weeks in response to decreased estrogen levels. This profuse sweating, which often occurs at night, assists the body in excreting the increased fluid accumulated during pregnancy.

Nursing Actions

- Assess for diaphoresis.
  - If present, assess for infection by taking the woman's temperature.
  - Expected assessment findings:
    - Diaphoresis with temperature within normal ranges

Patient Education

- Instruct the woman regarding the cause of diaphoresis.
- Discuss comfort measures such as wearing cotton nightwear.
- Discuss that feelings of warmth, sweating, and chills are signs of fever, a cardinal sign of infection. Women with these symptoms need to differentiate between fever and diaphoresis, the latter of which is a normal physiological process.
- Document findings, interventions, and evaluation.

THE MUSCULAR AND NERVOUS SYSTEMS

After birth, the abdominal muscles experience reduced tone and the abdomen appears soft and flabby. Some women experience a separation of the rectus muscle, which is noted as diastasis recti abdominis (Fig. 12–4). This separation becomes less apparent as the body returns to a prepregnant state. Women may experience muscular soreness related to the labor and birth experience. Lower body nerve sensation may be diminished for women who have received an epidural during labor. Delay ambulation until full sensation returns.

Nursing Actions

- Assess for diastasis recti abdominis.
  - The nurse can feel the separation of the rectus muscle when assessing the fundus.
  - Reassure the woman that this is normal and will diminish over time.
- Assess for muscle tenderness.
  - Rationale: Muscle soreness may result from positioning during labor and delivery, and generalized muscle use during second-stage labor or pushing.
  - Expected assessment findings:
    - Mild to no muscle soreness
  - Comfort measures for muscle soreness:
    - Ice pack to area for 15 minutes
    - Heat to area: Applying heat increases circulation, which facilitates healing. Cold packs result in vasoconstriction and decreased swelling. These interventions may alter the woman's perception of pain according to the gate control theory of pain modulation (Wilkinson et al., 2020). Analgesics alter a patient's perception of pain.
    - Warm shower
    - Analgesia

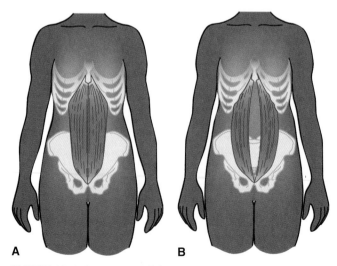

FIGURE 12–4 Diastasis recti abdominis. (A) Normal location of rectus muscles of the abdomen. (B) Diastasis recti. There is separation of the rectus muscles.

- Assess for decreased nerve sensation.
  - Rationale: Epidural or spinal anesthesia causes lack of sensation that may last several hours into the early postpartum period. Regional anesthesia may interfere with urinary elimination and mobility until the effects wear off.
  - Expected assessment findings:
    - Full sensation of lower extremities for women who did not receive an epidural during labor
    - Diminished lower body sensation for women who received an epidural during labor with full sensation returning within a few hours postbirth
    - Delay ambulation or assist the woman when ambulating until full sensation has returned.
      - Rationale: Women who have received spinal or epidural anesthesia are at risk for falls until full sensation has returned.
- Assess for headache.
  - If the woman complains of headache, assess its location and quality.
  - Notify the woman's health-care provider if the headache is associated with signs and symptoms of preeclampsia, or if a postepidural or spinal headache is suspected.
    - Rationale: Women who have had spinal or epidural anesthesia may develop headaches related to dural puncture and subsequent leakage of cerebrospinal fluid (CSF) leading to decreased levels of CSF. Headaches related to epidural or spinal anesthesia tend to be worse when the patient is in an upright position and improved when the patient is lying down. Headache may also be associated with preeclampsia (James & Suplee, 2020).
- Assess for fatigue
  - Rationale: Fatigue is a common complaint among women during the postpartum period. Discomfort and lack of sleep related to newborn care activities contribute to feelings of fatigue.
- Promote rest and sleep.
  - Provide teaching about the importance of sleep and rest.
  - Encourage the woman to sleep or nap while the baby is sleeping and to prioritize activities with a focus on self- and infant care.
  - Cluster nursing care such as assessments, interventions, and medication administration.
    - Rationale: This minimizes disruptions to the woman's sleep or naps.
  - Medicate the woman for pain as per orders or offer non-pharmacological interventions if appropriate.
    - Rationale: Pain interferes with sleep.
- Document findings and interventions.

THE GASTROINTESTINAL SYSTEM

Gastrointestinal (GI) muscle tone and motility decrease postbirth with a return to normal bowel function by the end of the second postpartum week.

- Constipation
  - Women are at risk for constipation due to decreased GI motility from the effects of progesterone; decreased physical activity; dehydration and fluid loss from labor; fear of having a bowel movement after perineal lacerations or episiotomy; and perineal pain and trauma.
- Hemorrhoids
  - Women commonly develop hemorrhoids during pregnancy or the birthing process. Hemorrhoids often slowly resolve but can be painful. Sometimes hemorrhoids persist postpartum.
- Appetite
  - Women are hungry after the birthing experience and can be given a regular diet, unless they are on a prescribed diet such as for pregestational diabetes. Women are exceptionally hungry during the first few postpartum days and may require snacks between meals.
- Weight loss
  - Most women will experience significant weight loss during the first 2 to 3 weeks postpartum. Immediately after birth, women lose approximately 11 to 12 pounds as the result of delivery and blood loss.
  - Diuresis results in the loss of approximately another 5 to 8 pounds postdelivery (Cunningham et al., 2018).
  - The average American woman at the end of 6 months postpartum is approximately 3 pounds above prepregnancy weight (Cunningham et al., 2018).

Nursing Actions

- Assess bowel sounds at each shift.
- Notify the physician or midwife if bowel sounds are faint or absent.
  - Rationale: Decreased motility can lead to diminished peristalsis and intestinal obstruction.
- Assess for constipation.
- Ask the woman if and when she had a bowel movement.
  - Rationale: Constipation is common in the postpartum period. Bowel function usually returns in 2 to 3 days (James & Suplee, 2020). Decreased frequency of bowel movements and passage of hard, dry stools indicate constipation.
- Instruct the woman to increase fluid intake and increase fiber and roughage in the diet to decrease risk of constipation. Bring her water and prune juice. Remind her to drink often.
  - Rationale: A diet that includes fiber-rich foods (i.e., fruits, vegetables, whole grains, and legumes) promotes intestinal peristalsis. Adequate fluid intake is necessary when women are encouraged to increase dietary fiber to prevent constipation. Intake of 3,000 mL of fluids a day will soften bowel movements and provide adequate mucus to lubricate the colon (James & Suplee, 2020).
- Ask the woman what she did for constipation during pregnancy or in the past and implement these strategies.
- Encourage ambulation.
  - Rationale: Ambulation promotes intestinal peristalsis and reduces the risk for constipation.
- Administer a stool softener or laxative as per the health-care provider's orders.
  - Rationale: Stool softeners prevent constipation by increasing water in the stool, promoting stool softening and elimination. Laxatives are effective in relieving constipation and

work by adding bulk to the stools or stimulating the nerves that irritate the intestinal wall (Vallerand & Sanoski, 2021).

- Docusate sodium (Colace) is a stool softener that helps incorporate water into the stool and can be administered to prevent constipation.
  - Route and dose: PO; 100 mg twice a day.
  - Nursing actions and implications: Administer with a full glass of water or juice; do not administer within 2 hours of other laxatives, such as mineral oil. Effectiveness may take 1 to 3 days after administration.
- Assess for hemorrhoids.
  - Rationale: Hemorrhoids may increase in size during labor and cause discomfort in the postpartum period (James & Suplee, 2020).
  - Instruct the woman to lie on her side, then separate her buttocks to expose the anus.
  - If hemorrhoids are present:
    - Encourage the woman to avoid sitting for long periods of time by lying on her side.
    - Witch hazel pads or topical anesthetics reduce discomfort (Isley, 2020).
    - Sitz baths are helpful in promoting circulation and reducing pain.
- Assess appetite.
  - Assess the amount of food eaten during meals.
  - Ask the woman if she is hungry.
    - Rationale: In most cases, after a vaginal delivery women can resume eating a regular diet (James & Suplee, 2020).
- Ask the woman if she is nauseous or has vomited.
  - Rationale: Nausea and vomiting may occur during labor. Nausea is also a common side effect of opioid analgesics commonly used for pain management during labor and delivery.

Patient Education

- Instruct the woman to increase fluid intake and increase fiber and roughage in the diet to decrease the risk of constipation.
- Provide nutritional education. This is especially important for lactating women and women who had a cesarean birth. Women who are breastfeeding need to increase their caloric intake by 500 to 1,000 calories a day (James & Suplee, 2020).
- Encourage the woman to ambulate to increase GI motility and decrease the risk of gas pains.
- Instruct the woman to increase fluid intake to a minimum of 10 glasses per day.

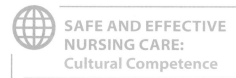

SAFE AND EFFECTIVE NURSING CARE: Cultural Competence

Food Preferences Across Cultures

- Foods and their preparations can be significant to women of different cultures. Certain foods may be encouraged to promote healing or restore health, whereas other foods may be prohibited because they are thought to cause illness, either immediately or in the future. The nurse should ask women about foods they prefer to eat based on their cultural beliefs; if not available in the hospital, encourage patients to have family members bring homemade dishes. In-service training should be provided to staff about cultures that are common to that unit.

FOLLOW-UP CARE

Guidelines recommend that women see their maternal care provider within the first 3 weeks postpartum to determine if additional care is needed before their follow-up visit 4 to 6 weeks after birth (Suplee & Janke, 2020). However, as many as 40% of women do not attend a postpartum visit. Attendance rates are lower among populations with limited resources (American College of Obstetricians and Gynecologists [ACOG], 2018).

The comprehensive postpartum visit includes a full assessment of physical, social, and psychological well-being, with screening for postpartum depression using a validated instrument such as the Edinburgh Postnatal Depression Scale. Birth spacing recommendations and reproductive life plans should be reviewed and a commensurate contraceptive method provided. Systems should be in place to ensure that women who desire long-acting reversible contraception (LARC) or another form of contraception can receive it during the comprehensive postpartum visit if placement wasn't done immediately after birth. Vaccination history should be reviewed and immunizations provided as needed. Women should be asked about common postpartum concerns, including perineal or cesarean wound pain, incontinence, dyspareunia, fatigue, depression, anxiety, and infant feeding problems, and identified concerns should be addressed. Suggested topics for anticipatory guidance include newborn feeding, expressing breast milk if returning to work or school, postpartum weight retention, sexuality, physical activity, and nutrition. Smoking and substance use cessation also should be addressed and are discussed in the following section.

DISCHARGE TEACHING

Nurses are the health-care providers who perform most postpartum education in the United States, so it is critical that they work to improve discharge education with information that is efficient, timely, and evidence-based. When women are discharged after birth, nurses play a vital role in providing them with education on self-care, transitioning home, and caring for a newborn. Many women are unaware of their health needs after giving birth. Therefore, it is important to help them understand how to differentiate signs and symptoms that are normal from those that are not. Women also need to know why it is necessary and appropriate to proactively seek and obtain care when they are not feeling well and how urgently they should obtain this care based on the types of symptoms they are experiencing. Armed with information about and understanding the postbirth warning signs, women can be empowered to act immediately rather than wait and suffer potentially devastating consequences.

Although the window of opportunity for discharge planning and teaching postpartum women is small and the volume of information to be relayed substantial, the necessity of providing this critical information cannot be overstated. Nurses can work together within their maternity services to develop best practices to accomplish essential maternal and newborn discharge teaching in the most efficient and effective manner possible. For example, plan discharge teaching over the course of the woman's postpartum stay rather than waiting for the day of discharge. Another strategy is to include this information as part of prenatal education. Incorporating a checklist and patient education tool (such as the AWHONN tools) into hospital electronic health record systems and the discharge education process will provide nurses with a resource handout to use when providing evidence-based care education.

The lack of follow-up care for the 40% of women who do not attend these visits represents missed opportunities to improve the health of women who have recently given birth. This poor rate of attendance at postpartum visits further supports the need to take full advantage of the limited postpartum hospital stay by providing consistent discharge education on postbirth warning signs of potentially life-threatening conditions that require immediate medical attention. Discharge teaching for the woman and her family should focus on:

- Signs of complications that need to be reported to the physician or midwife:
  - Heavy lochia (saturating a pad in 1 hour) indicates possible secondary postpartum hemorrhage.
  - The return of bright red, heavy bleeding after lochia has diminished or that becomes serosa or alba, or the passage of clots the size of an egg or larger indicates possible secondary postpartum.
  - Foul-smelling lochia indicates possible infection.
  - Increased temperature (100.4°F [38°C] or higher) indicates possible infection.
  - Pelvic or abdominal tenderness or pain indicates possible infection.
  - Frequency, urgency, or burning on urination indicates possible cystitis.
  - Unilateral breast tenderness, warm reddened area, and chills and fever indicate possible mastitis, which often occurs 3 to 4 weeks after delivery.
  - Blurry vision, severe headaches, epigastric abdominal pain, and fluid retention may be associated with preeclampsia.
  - Leg pain, swelling, and redness may indicate venous thrombosis. Chest pain and difficulty breathing may be associated with pulmonary embolism.
  - Thoughts of harming the infant or self, difficulty caring for self or the infant, difficulty sleeping or sleeping too much, and persistent feelings of depression and sadness are associated with postpartum depression.
- Expected physical changes
  - Uterine involution, afterpains, progression of lochia
  - Breast changes, engorgement
  - Diaphoresis and diuresis
  - Weight loss
  - Women can expect to lose approximately 12 pounds immediately after delivery, and an additional 5 to 8 pounds due to fluid losses associated with uterine involution and diuresis (Cunningham et al., 2018).
- Self-care
  - Hygiene
  - Perineal care; continue to change pad frequently and use peri-bottle until lochia has stopped
  - Breast care for lactating and nonlactating women
  - Pharmacological and nonpharmacological pain control measures

SAFE AND EFFECTIVE NURSING CARE:
Patient Education

AWHONN Postpartum Discharge Teaching Project: Warning Signs

Call 911 for:

Pain in the chest
Obstructed breathing or shortness of breath
Seizures
Thoughts of hurting yourself or baby

   Call your provider for:

Bleeding soaking though one pad/hour or passing a clot the size of an egg
Incision that is not healing
Red or swollen leg that is warm or painful to touch
Temperature of 100.4°F (38°C) or higher
Headache that does not get better even after taking medicine, or bad headache with changes in vision

   If you cannot reach your provider, go to an emergency room.
AWHONN, 2018.

HEALTH PROMOTION

Health promotion topics for new mothers are as follows:

- Explain all discharge medications, including dose, frequency, action, and side effects.
- Stress the importance of following through with postpartum follow-up visits to her physician or midwife as previously discussed.
- Schedule a postpartum visit before discharge to facilitate attendance.

Nutrition and Fluids

The nurse must provide instruction about nutritional needs for lactating and nonlactating women.

- Lactating women should increase their caloric intake by 500 to 1,000 calories per day and have a fluid intake of approximately 2 to 3 liters per day (see Chapter 16).

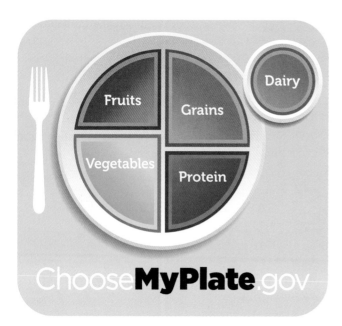

FIGURE 12–5 MyPlate illustrates the five food groups using a familiar mealtime visual, a place setting.

- Teach the woman how to use MyPlate (www.ChooseMyPlate .gov) and how this can assist in meeting her nutritional needs (Fig. 12–5).
- Women who are anemic should increase consumption of leafy green vegetables, beans, red meat, poultry, iron-fortified cereal, breads, pasta, and dried fruits such as raisins.
- To prevent constipation, women who have hemorrhoids, perineal lacerations, or episiotomy should consume foods with roughage such as fruits, vegetables, beans, and whole grains.

Activity and Exercise

Physical activity is good for the overall health of postpartum women with no other medical problems. For example, moderate-intensity physical activity, such as brisk walking, keeps the heart and lungs healthy after pregnancy. Physical activity also helps improve mood throughout the postpartum period. Exercise helps maintain a healthy weight, and when combined with eating fewer calories helps with weight loss.

Healthy women should get at least 150 minutes (2.5 hours) per week of moderate-intensity aerobic activity such as brisk walking (CDC, 2020a). Although 150 minutes each week seems to be a lot of time, women can break it into smaller chunks throughout the week. In fact, it is best to spread activity out during the week, as long as you exercise with moderate or vigorous effort for at least 10 minutes at a time.

- Explain the importance of activity to decrease risk of constipation and to promote circulation and a sense of well-being.
- Instruct the woman about appropriate exercises in the postpartum period, such as walking.
- Encourage the woman to do Kegel exercises to strengthen the pelvic floor.

Evidence-Based Practice: Weight Loss in Women After Childbirth

Wiser, D., & Boisvert, J. (2019). What lifestyle interventions are most effective for promoting postpartum weight loss? *Evidence-Based Practice, 22*(10), 13–14. https://doi.org/10.1097/EBP.0000000000000388

Gaining weight during pregnancy is normal. Postdelivery retention of weight gained during pregnancy is common and linked to long-term weight problems and obesity in women. Overweight and obesity may lead to chronic disease and lifelong negative health effects. A Cochrane Review of 12 mostly nonblinding randomized controlled trials measured postpartum weight loss after changes in diet, exercise, or both and found that:

- Diet alone and exercise plus diet are both effective for postpartum weight loss.
- Self-monitoring using exercise logs, diaries, heart rate monitors, or pedometers may enhance postpartum weight loss.
- Breastfeeding may be beneficial for postpartum weight loss.

Rest and Comfort

- Teach the woman the importance of rest in promoting healing and lactation.
- Problem-solve with the woman about ways to increase rest time (e.g., nap when the baby is napping, prioritize activities).
- Encourage the woman to take medications as ordered by the physician or midwife (e.g., vitamins, iron, pain medications).

Sexual Activity

- Instruct the couple to discuss with the provider when they can resume sexual intercourse.
- General guidelines are to resume sexual intercourse when the lochia has stopped, perineum has healed, and the woman is physically and emotionally ready.
- Explain that an artificial vaginal lubricant might be needed to increase comfort during intercourse due to changes in hormone levels that result in vaginal dryness.
- Explain the importance of using contraception when the couple resumes sexual activity.

Contraception

- Assess the couple's desire for future pregnancies.
- Assess satisfaction with the previous method of contraception.
- Encourage the patient to discuss contraceptive options with the health-care provider. Immediate placement of LARC, such as intrauterine devices and contraceptive implants, is an option during the postpartum period. LARC is highly effective in preventing unwanted pregnancy and short intervals between pregnancies (ACOG, 2019).
- Provide information on various methods of contraception (see Table 12-3).

TABLE 12-3   Methods of Contraception

METHOD	FAILURE RATE	AVAILABILITY	ADVANTAGES	DISADVANTAGES
Natural Methods				
Abstinence	0%	Readily available	No contraindications Prevents exposure to STIs Readily available	Must be consistently practiced or it is not effective
Natural family planning	24%	Handouts and information from care provider Internet access of information Fertility monitoring devices now available	No contraindications or side effects	Must have a regular menstrual cycle and have knowledge or willingness to frequently monitor body functions: Temperature, as well as vaginal mucus production and consistency Does not protect against STIs
Withdrawal	22%		No cost or contraindications	Does not protect against STIs Disrupts sexual intercourse
Lactational amenorrhea method (LAM)			No cost or contraindications	Requires exclusive breastfeeding or infant suckling Using a barrier method with LAM increases effectiveness
Barrier Methods				
Condoms (male and female)	18% male condom 21% female condom	Over-the-counter (OTC) purchase	Readily available Protects against STIs No systemic effects	Allergic reactions may occur Barrier methods have higher rate of protection when combined with spermicides Must be applied at time of coitus and may be considered disruptive
Vaginal sponges	12% if no prior births 24% if previous births	OTC Limited availability No fitting needed Spermicide is added, but must be activated with addition of fluid before insertion	One-time use May be placed before intercourse May leave in for up to 30 hours Protects repeated acts of intercourse	Must be left in place for at least 6 hours postintercourse Irritation, discomfort, and allergic reaction may occur May increase risk for infections, including STIs
Cervical caps	14% if no prior birth 29% in women with prior birth	Provider determines fit based on OB history; no examination needed Limited availability Spermicide must be added before each insertion	No systemic effects Fits snugly over cervix May leave in for up to 48 hours for repeated intercourse No systemic effects	Must be left in place for 6 hours after coitus Does not protect against STIs

Continued

TABLE 12-3   Methods of Contraception—cont'd

METHOD	FAILURE RATE	AVAILABILITY	ADVANTAGES	DISADVANTAGES
Diaphragms	12%	Limited availability Must be fitted by provider and must be refitted after birth or a large weight gain	No systemic effects May be placed in anticipation of intercourse Fits over cervix May leave in place for 24 hours for repeated intercourse	Need additional doses of spermicide for repeated intercourse Leave in place for 6 hours after intercourse May increase risk of yeast infection, cystitis, and toxic shock syndrome if use is prolonged
Spermicidal gels, cream suppository, or foam	28%	OTC	No systemic effects Foam may be used for an immediate emergency contraceptive	Allergic reaction Irritation Frequent use contraindicated for individuals at risk for HIV
Hormonal Methods				
Combination estrogen and progesterone oral contraception	9%	Prescription only Many options available; 12-week pill cycle with menses only four times per year	Suppresses ovulation Take one pill a day Many noncontraceptive benefits include reduced risk for: endometrial and ovarian cancer, benign breast disease, anemia, may improve acne	Contraindications to hormonal methods: History of deep vein thrombosis, pulmonary emboli, hypertension, heart disease Women aged 35 or older, who smoke Active cancer Genetic clotting disorders, liver disease May have multiple side effects (nausea, headache, spotting, weight gain, breast tenderness, chloasma) Increased risks for blood clots, heart disease, and strokes Do not provide protection against STIs
Emergency contraceptives (not to be used as regular form of birth control)	9%	Postcoital ingestion of hormones Must take within 72 to 120 hours of incident OTC for women aged 17 years or older Prescription only for women younger than 17 years old	Reduces risk of pregnancy for one-time unprotected intercourse by suppressing ovulation	Side effects include headache, nausea, vomiting, abdominal pain Heavier or lighter menstrual bleeding, fatigue, diarrhea Does not protect against STIs

TABLE 12-3   Methods of Contraception—cont'd

METHOD	FAILURE RATE	AVAILABILITY	ADVANTAGES	DISADVANTAGES
Progestin only	6%	Prescription only	Take one pill at the same time every day Can be used during lactation	Weight gain Irregular bleeding May have minor side effects: nausea, mood changes Does not protect against STIs
Depo-Provera	3%	Injectable every 3 months Prescription only	One injection four times a year; can be used during lactation	Weight gain, decreased bone density Delayed fertility Bleeding abnormalities Headache, mood changes, breast tenderness Does not protect against STIs
Contraceptive patch	9%	Prescription only	Place a new patch weekly for 3 weeks, then remove for 1 week	Risk similar to those for oral contraceptives, including increased risk for thrombotic event Possibly less effective for larger women Possible skin irritation Does not prevent STIs
Vaginal ring	9%	Prescription only	Flexible hormone-filled ring inserted and left in the vagina for 3 weeks, then removed for 1 week Ring can be left in for 28 days, with immediate placement of new ring	Side effects similar to oral contraceptives Vaginal irritation and discharge may occur Does not protect against STIs
Long-Acting Reversible Contraceptives Intrauterine contraceptives (IUCs), copper material or hormone releasing (Levonorgestrel)	0.8% 0.2%	Prescription Inserted during office visit May also be placed in the hospital during the immediate postpartum period	May be used with lactation Can be used by teens, as well as women with medical problems or contraindications to other hormonal methods Highly effective Long-term contraceptive method; good for 1 to 10 years Copper-releasing IUC can be used as an emergency contraceptive; must be inserted within 7 days of intercourse	Low risk of uterine perforation Contraindicated in women diagnosed and treated for pelvic inflammatory disease (PID) within the prior 3 months Increase of cramping and bleeding in the first few cycles Does not protect against STIs

Continued

TABLE 12-3   Methods of Contraception—cont'd

METHOD	FAILURE RATE	AVAILABILITY	ADVANTAGES	DISADVANTAGES
Hormone implants	0.05%	One rod implanted in the arm Office procedure May be placed during the immediate postpartum period in the hospital setting	Once in place, there is minimal discomfort Lasts for several years Can be used during lactation	Side effects similar to oral contraceptives Irregular bleeding Skin irritation at site Does not protect against STIs Must be removed
Sterilization Vasectomy	0.15%	Surgical procedure done under local anesthesia in the office or clinic	High rate of effectiveness	Discomfort for 2 to 3 days Difficult to reverse Need to use alternative contraceptive method until two postsurgery sperm tests indicate procedure is effective
Tubal ligation	0.5%	Surgical procedure done under general anesthesia	High rate of effectiveness	Bleeding or pain at incision site Difficult to reverse
Sterilization implant	0.03%	Office procedure	Implants placed in the fallopian tubes, which cause scar tissue that eventually blocks the tubes	Another contraceptive method needs to be used until blockage is confirmed, usually 3 months

Suplee & Janke, 2020.

CRITICAL COMPONENT

AWHONN Position Statement: Insurance Coverage for Contraceptives

AWHONN supports the inclusion of all contraceptive drugs, devices (including device insertion), and related services that are approved by the U.S. Food and Drug Administration as covered health insurance benefits in public and private plans. AWHONN considers access to widespread, affordable, and acceptable health care, which includes safe and reliable contraceptives, to be a basic human right (AWHONN, 2020).

Smoking Cessation and Relapse Prevention

- Ask women about tobacco use.
- Teach women about the dangers of smoking (e.g., cancer, lung problems such as chronic obstructive pulmonary disease, osteoporosis).
- Teach women to never allow smoking around their infant or children, as secondhand smoke is associated with problems such as ear infections and respiratory issues.
- Encourage women who quit smoking for pregnancy to remain abstinent. Most women who quit smoking during pregnancy relapse after delivery.
- Advise women who currently smoke to quit. Provide information about resources to assist with cessation, such as counseling services or classes, cessation help lines, and medications.

Clinical Pathway for Uncomplicated Vaginal Delivery

Focus of Care	Postpartum: Admission	Postpartum: First 4 Hours	Postpartum: Greater Than 4 Hours Discharge	Expected Outcomes and Discharge Criteria
Diagnostic tests	RPR, hepatitis B surface antigen, rubella, blood type and Rh status documented or drawn if no prenatal record available GBS status documented with appropriate interventions Urine toxicology screenings per policy	Fetal Rh study as indicated (woman Rh-negative and neonate Rh-positive)	CBC as ordered Notify CNM/MD of abnormal results or if the woman is symptomatic.	Rubella status known and MMR vaccine given if indicated. Rh status known—Rh immune globulin given if indicated. CBC is within normal ranges. Needed vaccinations are given as ordered (flu shots, Tdap, varicella, etc.).
Activity and safety	Moves legs Lifts bottom off bed Needs assistance with initial ambulation Infant security and safety reviewed	Women who received an epidural for labor or birth will need assistance with ambulation until the return of sensory and motor sensation.	Able to stand and walk with minimal assistance	Ambulates without assistance
Treatments and patient care	Assess vital signs. Assess level of consciousness. Assess fundus, lochia, and perineum. Apply ice to perineum. Assess lower extremities for edema, pain, and pulses. Assess Foley catheter if in place. Assess IV site and fluids if in place. Assess breast for potential breastfeeding problems.	Vital signs as per orders Postpartum physical assessment as per orders or unit protocol Pericare with each voiding Ice to perineum Input and output while Foley catheter or IV in place. Measure first 2 voidings; notify CNM/MD if urine output <30 mL/hr. If patient is unable to void or voids less than 150 mL, and uterus is above the umbilicus and deviated to the side, consider catheterization.	Vital signs as per orders Postpartum physical assessment as per orders Pericare with each voiding Ice to perineum for first 24 hours Assess breast for signs of engorgement and nipple irritation.	Vital signs stable and within normal limits Fundus firm, midline, and descending by 1 cm per day Lochia moderate to scant Perineum healing without signs of infection Breasts exhibit physiological changes of lactation. Breastfeeding without difficulty Bowel and bladder function within normal limits.

Continued

Clinical Pathway for Uncomplicated Vaginal Delivery—cont'd

Focus of Care	Postpartum: Admission	Postpartum: First 4 Hours	Postpartum: Greater Than 4 Hours Discharge	Expected Outcomes and Discharge Criteria
Medications	Maintain IV patency if indicated.	IV is discontinued if fundus firm and lochia within normal limits.	Analgesics or comfort measures as indicated for pain management	Mild to moderate pain relieved with comfort measures or PO analgesia
	Oxytocin as indicated to reduce risk of or treat postpartum hemorrhage	Oxytocin is discontinued if fundus firm and lochia within normal limits.	Rubella vaccine administered, if indicated, at least 30 minutes before discharge	Rubella vaccine administered when indicated
	Analgesics or comfort measures as indicated for pain management	Analgesics or comfort measures as indicated for pain management	Rh(D) immune globulin administered as indicated	Rh(D) immune globulin administered as indicated
			Stool softener as ordered	Discharge medication teaching provided
Nutrition	Regular diet as tolerated PO fluids	Regular diet as tolerated PO fluids	Regular diet as tolerated PO fluids	Maintains adequate diet and fluid intake.
Discharge planning and evaluation of social support	Evaluate need for referrals such as social worker, lactation specialist, and dietitian.	Continue to evaluate need for referrals.	Review discharge preparation with the woman and her family.	The woman and her family have appropriate support on discharge.
	Explain physical changes.	Initiate referrals as indicated.	Explain physical and emotional changes.	The woman can provide appropriate self-care.
	Teach self-care and health promotion.	Explain physical changes.	Teach self-care and health promotion.	The woman and her family verbalize the importance of follow-up care for both the woman and infant.
		Teach self-care and health promotion.		
Patient and family education	Initiate discharge teaching by assessing immediate learning needs.	Continue discharge teaching based on the woman's and family's learning needs.	Complete discharge teaching.	The woman and her family verbalize understanding of the infant's needs and the woman's needs.
	Assist with breastfeeding.			The woman and her family demonstrate basic well-baby care skills.
				The woman and her family verbalize understanding of signs and symptoms that warrant contact with the healthcare provider.

CBC, complete blood count; CNM/MD, certified nurse-midwife/medical doctor; GBS, group B strep; MMR, measles, mumps, and rubella; RPR, rapid plasma reagin.

CONCEPT MAP |

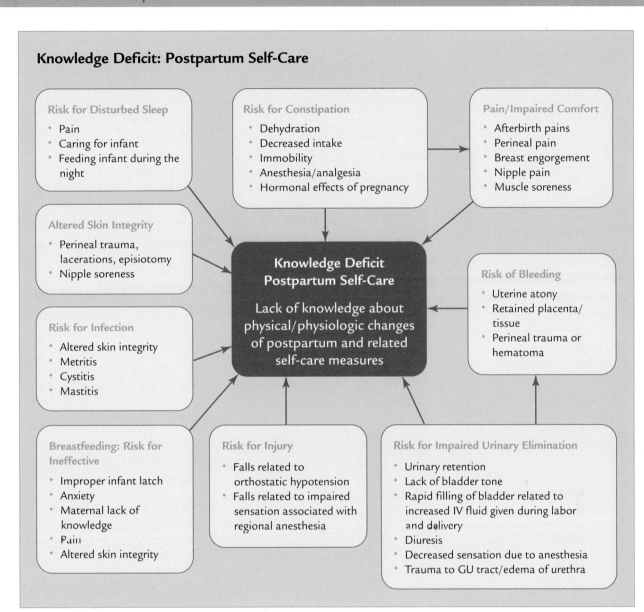

Knowledge Deficit: Postpartum Self-Care

Risk for Disturbed Sleep
* Pain
* Caring for infant
* Feeding infant during the night

Risk for Constipation
* Dehydration
* Decreased intake
* Immobility
* Anesthesia/analgesia
* Hormonal effects of pregnancy

Pain/Impaired Comfort
* Afterbirth pains
* Perineal pain
* Breast engorgement
* Nipple pain
* Muscle soreness

Altered Skin Integrity
* Perineal trauma, lacerations, episiotomy
* Nipple soreness

Knowledge Deficit Postpartum Self-Care

Lack of knowledge about physical/physiologic changes of postpartum and related self-care measures

Risk of Bleeding
* Uterine atony
* Retained placenta/tissue
* Perineal trauma or hematoma

Risk for Infection
* Altered skin integrity
* Metritis
* Cystitis
* Mastitis

Breastfeeding: Risk for Ineffective
* Improper infant latch
* Anxiety
* Maternal lack of knowledge
* Pain
* Altered skin integrity

Risk for Injury
* Falls related to orthostatic hypotension
* Falls related to impaired sensation associated with regional anesthesia

Risk for Impaired Urinary Elimination
* Urinary retention
* Lack of bladder tone
* Rapid filling of bladder related to increased IV fluid given during labor and delivery
* Diuresis
* Decreased sensation due to anesthesia
* Trauma to GU tract/edema of urethra

CARE PLANS

Problem 1: Risk for bleeding
Goal: The amount of vaginal bleeding will be within normal limits.
Outcome: The woman's lochia amount will be moderate to small; the woman's fundus is firm and midline. The woman's vital signs will be within normal limits. Urine output will be within normal limits. The woman will verbalize when to notify the provider if bleeding is excessive.

Nursing Actions
1. Teach the woman the purpose of fundal checks.
2. Teach the woman to palpate her fundus and massage it if soft.
3. Teach the woman about the normal progression of lochia; what to expect regarding amount, color, and flow.

4. Instruct the woman to notify the nurse or provider if she soaks more than one pad an hour or passes clots.
5. Instruct the woman about the purpose of oxytocin administration; provide information about afterpains.
6. Teach the woman the importance of emptying her bladder every 3 to 4 hours.

Problem 2: Risk for impaired urinary elimination
Goal: Spontaneous voids of a sufficient quantity (at least 300 mL per void)
Outcome: The woman will spontaneously void at least 300 mL per void. The woman will state the importance of voiding frequently and adequately. The woman will identify that she will notify the nurse or provider of burning, frequency, or urgency with voiding.

Continued

CONCEPT MAP | —cont'd

Nursing Actions

1. Explain to the woman that urine output will be measured after delivery.
2. Encourage the woman to void within 2 to 4 hours of delivery and to empty her bladder.
3. Explain to the woman that if she is unable to void, she will need to have a catheter placed to empty her bladder.
4. Instruct the woman to notify the nurse or health-care provider if she experiences frequency, burning, or urgency during urination.
5. Encourage the woman to drink 10 glasses of fluids a day (80 ounces) and bring water to the bedside.
6. Teach the woman that diuresis is a normal process and often begins within 12 hours of delivery.

Problem 3: Pain or impaired comfort

Goal: Pain or discomfort is adequately controlled.

Outcome: The woman will identify nonpharmacological and pharmacological methods to treat pain and discomfort. The woman's pain or discomfort is adequately controlled.

Nursing Actions

1. Teach the woman to report pain by providing information about the intensity, location, and quality of her discomfort.
2. Provide the patient with nonpharmacological methods of pain control:
   a. Ice packs for 24 to 48 hours
   b. Sitz baths or warm compresses
   c. Peri-bottle
   d. Repositioning
   e. Deep breathing and relaxation
   f. Warm shower
3. Inform the woman about medications ordered and administered for pain (action, dose and frequency, potential side effects).
4. Educate the woman about nonpharmacological methods of pain control.

Problem 4: Risk for infection

Goal: Reduce risk of infection.

Outcome: The woman will remain free from signs of infection. The woman will identify ways to prevent infection and when to call the nurse or health-care provider for signs of infection.

Nursing Actions

1. Explain the importance of monitoring vital signs and monitor them per protocol.
2. Instruct the woman to call the provider if she has signs of infection such as temperature over 100.4°F (38°C); chills; pain in her abdomen, perineum, or breasts; burning, frequency, or urgency with urination; or foul-smelling lochia.
3. Teach the woman the importance of hand washing before and after pericare and after pad changes.
4. If indicated, teach the woman about immunizations that will be given before discharge.

Problem 5: Risk for injury

Goal: Reduce risk for injury.

Outcome: The woman will call for assistance with ambulation until sensation returns to her lower extremities (postepidural) and her blood pressure and pulse are within normal limits. The woman will remain free from injury associated with falls.

Nursing Actions

1. Explain orthostatic hypotension and the importance of requesting assistance in the initial postpartum period.
2. Instruct the woman to rise slowly to a standing position.
3. Advise the woman to ambulate with assistance the first few times up after birth.
4. Instruct the woman to return to bed or the sitting position if she becomes dizzy and to call for help.

Problem 6: Altered skin integrity

Goal: Regain skin integrity through healing

Outcome: The woman will identify perineal care and comfort measures. She will identify signs of perineal infection and notify her health-care provider if she experiences signs of infection.

Nursing Actions

1. Teach the woman that her perineal area will be assessed for redness, bruising, swelling, and drainage. Explain the procedure and position the woman on her side to better visualize the area.
2. Teach the woman about comfort measures for perineal lacerations or episiotomy such as ice packs during the first 24 to 48 hours and warm sitz baths after the first 24 hours.
3. Instruct the woman on topical treatments that may be ordered by the health-care provider.
4. Teach the woman to rinse the perineum with a peri-bottle using warm water after each elimination.
5. Encourage the woman to change peripads frequently, and to wash her hands before and after pad changes to reduce the risk of infection.
6. Teach the woman to lie on her side to decrease pressure on her perineum.
7. Instruct the woman to take ordered analgesics as directed to decrease perineal pain.
8. Teach the woman to report signs of perineal infection such as drainage, swelling, pain, and fever to the health-care provider.

Problem 7: Risk for constipation

Goal: The woman will have regular, soft bowel movements.

Outcome: The woman will state ways to promote regular, soft bowel movements. The woman will not develop constipation.

Nursing Actions

1. Provide fluid, water, and prune juice to facilitate hydration.
2. Teach the woman the importance of a diet high in fruits, vegetables, and whole grains.
3. Teach the woman the importance of drinking 2,000 to 3,000 mL of fluids daily.

4. Teach the woman the importance of ambulating several times daily.

5. Instruct the woman to have a bowel movement when she feels the urge.

6. If ordered, teach the woman about stool softeners, laxatives, and so on. Discuss the action, dose and frequency, and potential side effects.

Problem 8: Risk for disturbed sleep

Goal: Adequate sleep and rest

Outcome: The woman will report adequate sleep patterns, and report feeling rested. The woman will identify strategies for getting enough rest and sleep.

Nursing Actions

1. Attempt to cluster care to decrease interruptions.

2. Teach the woman the importance of sleep and rest in healing and recovery from childbirth.

3. Encourage the woman to identify strategies to get enough sleep, such as sleeping when the baby sleeps and naps, prioritizing activities to focus on self- and infant care, and occasionally delegating infant care and feeding to other family members if possible so she can rest.

4. Teach the woman ways to treat pain and discomfort to facilitate rest and sleep.

Problem 9: Breastfeeding—risk for ineffective feeding

Goal: Effective breastfeeding

Outcome: The woman will identify how to tell if the baby is breastfeeding effectively. She will demonstrate proper positioning and technique for breastfeeding her infant. The baby will latch to the mother's nipple properly and demonstrate signs of adequate feedings. The woman will identify community resources to contact for support and assistance with breastfeeding.

Nursing Actions

1. Teach the woman to recognize cues that the baby is hungry.

2. Assist the woman to prepare for a feeding by getting into a comfortable position.

3. Assist the woman in positioning the infant for breastfeeding (cradle hold, cross-cradle hold, football hold, etc.).

4. Teach the woman how to get the infant latched to the nipple, and signs of correct latch-on.

5. Teach the woman about the frequency and duration of feedings.

6. Teach the woman how to remove the baby from the breast and how to burp the baby.

7. Teach the woman how to recognize that the baby is receiving adequate feedings.

8. Provide the woman with information about lactation consultant services and community resources available to support breastfeeding after discharge.

Nursing Care Plan

Problem *(Check Appropriate Line)*	Actual or Potential	Action *(Initial Care Provided)*	Expected Outcome or Discharge Criteria *(Initial Outcomes Obtained)*
Potential or actual postpartum hemorrhage related to: _____ Uterine atony _____ Retained placenta _____ Laceration _____ Hematoma _____ Full bladder _____ Other _____	Initiated by: RN: _____ Date/time _____ ☐ Actual ☐ Potential Change in status: Date/time _____ RN: _____ ☐ Actual ☐ Potential Resolved: Date/time _____ RN: _____	_____ Monitor and assess vital signs, including blood pressure and woman's mental status, lochia flow, and uterine tone per policy. _____ Encourage voiding every 2 to 3 hours. _____ Massage fundus as needed and instruct the woman on self-assessment. _____ Notify CNM/MD for heavy bleeding or saturation of one pad in less than 1 hour. _____ Give medications such as oxytocin, Methergine, or Hemabate per CNM/MD order. _____ Assist with activity PRN. _____ Notify the provider if the woman has continued excessive bleeding or dizziness.	_____ Lochia scant to moderate rubra _____ Fundus firm and at midline _____ No signs or symptoms of postpartum hemorrhage

Continued

Nursing Care Plan—cont'd

Problem	Actual or	Action	Expected Outcome

Problem
(Check Appropriate Line)

Actual or Potential

Action
(Initial Care Provided)

Expected Outcome or Discharge Criteria
(Initial Outcomes Obtained)

Potential or actual alteration in comfort related to:

_____ Uterine cramping

_____ Incision

_____ Perineal or rectal pain

_____ Breast discomfort

_____ Other_____

Potential or actual alteration in effective breastfeeding related to:

_____ Poor latch

_____ Previous breast surgery

_____ Twins or higher-order multiples

_____ Infant with cleft lip or palate

_____ Nearly term infant

_____ Infant in NICU

_____ Patient's health status

_____ Other _____

Potential or actual impaired parent–infant bonding related to:

_____ Adolescent parents

_____ Substance abuse

_____ Domestic violence

_____ Social risk factors

_____ Infant's health status

_____ Mother's health status

_____ Other _____

Initiated by:

RN: _____

Date/time _____

☐ Actual

☐ Potential

Change in status:

Date/time _____

RN: _____

☐ Actual

☐ Potential

Resolved: _____

Date/time

Initiated by:

RN: _____

Date/time _____

☐ Actual

☐ Potential

Change in status:

Date/time _____

RN: _____

☐ Actual

☐ Potential

Resolved:

Date/time _____

RN: _____

Initiated by:

RN: _____

Date/time _____

☐ Actual

☐ Potential

Change in status:

Date/time _____

RN: _____

☐ Actual

☐ Potential

Resolved:

Date/time _____

RN: _____

_____ Pain assessment

_____ Provide or assist with nonpharmacological comfort measures for relief.

_____ Provide analgesics as ordered.

_____ Assess breastfeeding by observing breastfeeding sessions each shift.

_____ Assess latch score.

_____ Assess the breasts or nipples for pain and skin breakdown.

_____ Assess for psychosocial factors that may interfere with parental bonding with infant.

_____ Assess parental bonding and caretaking behaviors.

_____ Assess the parent's support system.

_____ Pain will be adequately controlled by analgesics and nonpharmacological comfort measures.

_____ The mother will demonstrate proper positioning of the infant during feedings.

_____ The baby will latch properly during feedings.

_____ The mother will remain comfortable during breastfeeding.

_____ No signs of skin breakdown or trauma on mother's nipples.

_____ Parents will demonstrate signs of bonding with infant:

_____ Attentive to infant cues and needs

_____ Holds infant en face

_____ Cuddles infant

_____ Talks to infant

_____ Calls baby by name

_____ Breastfeeds/bottle feeds baby

Problem (Check Appropriate Line)	Actual or Potential	Action (Initial Care Provided)	Expected Outcome or Discharge Criteria (Initial Outcomes Obtained)
Potential or actual postpartum infection related to: _____ Perineum _____ Uterus _____ Breast _____ GBS _____ Other _____	Initiated by: RN: _____ Date/time _____ ☐ Actual ☐ Potential Change in status: Date/time _____ RN: _____ ☐ Actual ☐ Potential Resolved: Date/time _____ RN: _____	_____ Vital signs monitored per policy. _____ CNM/MD notified immediately if any signs or symptoms of infection are present. _____ Woman instructed in self-care, including pericare, incisional care, and breast care. _____ Woman instructed in signs and symptoms of infection.	_____ Woman will exhibit no signs or symptoms of infection (i.e., temperature less than 100.4°F [38°C], no abnormal discharge, incision clean and dry if present, breasts without redness). _____ Woman will verbalize understanding of signs and symptoms of infection and is aware of when to notify CNM/MD.
Potential or actual alteration in elimination related to: _____ Loss of bladder or bowel sensation or function following childbirth _____ Other _____	Initiated by: Date/time _____ ☐ Actual ☐ Potential Change in status: Date/time _____ RN: _____ ☐ Actual ☐ Potential Resolved: Date/time _____ RN. _____	_____ Assess and monitor for bladder distention as needed. _____ Assess and document initial voidings after delivery to ensure >30 mL/hr without retention in first 6 to 12 hours. _____ If unable to void, catheterize per CNM/MD order. _____ Provide instructions on Kegel exercises. _____ Encourage early ambulation, adequate fluid intake, and diet with roughage to prevent constipation. _____ Provide stool softener as ordered.	_____ Woman is voiding without difficulty. _____ Fundus is firm and midline. _____ Woman is able to verbalize methods of avoiding constipation and to notify CNM/MD if no stool in 4 days.

CNM/MD, certified nurse-midwife/medical doctor; GBS, group B strep.

Case Study

As the nurse, you admit Margarite Sanchez to the postpartum unit at 10:50 a.m. and receive the transfer report from labor and delivery stating the following:

- Patient is a 28-year-old G3 P2 Hispanic woman who gave birth at 8:39 a.m., vaginal delivery with a second-degree perineal laceration.
- She received two doses of Nubain in labor at 2:15 a.m. and at 4:40 a.m. for pain relief in active labor.
- Both mother and newborn are stable.
- The mother's bleeding during recovery in labor and delivery was moderate, the fundus was firm at the umbilicus and midline.
- VS are 120/68-72-20-98.2.

- Ms. Sanchez did not void after delivery in labor and delivery.
- Ms. Sanchez nursed her baby for 15 minutes on each breast after the birth.

José, her husband, has accompanied her to the unit.

Detail the aspects of your initial assessment.

As part of the physical assessment, you discover her fundus is 2 cm above the umbilicus and deviated to the right; her lochia is moderate, saturating one-third of the pad during transfer; and her perineum is swollen.

What are your immediate priorities in nursing care for Margarite Sanchez?

Discuss the rationale for the priorities.

What should your initial teaching for Margarite Sanchez include?

At 5 hours postpartum, Margarite rates her perineal pain at 6 on a scale of 0 to 10.

State the nursing diagnosis, expected outcome, and interventions related to this problem.

The next day you are assigned to care for the Sanchez family. Your report from the previous shift indicated that:

• Her vital signs were within normal limits.
• She had voided once during the night.
• Her fundus was 1 cm below the umbilicus.
• Lochia was scant to mild.
• She breastfed her infant twice.

Margarite informs you that she experienced night sweats.

Discuss your nursing actions, including rationales.

You are anticipating that she will be discharged in the afternoon.

Discuss your plan for discharge teaching, indicating the priority needs with rationales.

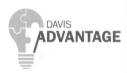

Go to Davis Advantage to complete your learning: strengthen understanding, apply your knowledge, and prepare for the Next Gen NCLEX®.

REFERENCES

American College of Obstetricians and Gynecologists. (2018). Optimizing postpartum care. Committee Opinion No. 736. *Obstetrics & Gynecology, 131,* e140–e150. https://doi. 10.1097/AOG.0000000000002633

American College of Obstetricians and Gynecologists. (2019). Interpregnancy care. Committee Opinion No. 8. *Obstetrics & Gynecology, 133,* e51–e72. https://doi: 10.1097/AOG.0000000000003025

Association of Women's Health, Obstetric and Neonatal Nurses. (2018). *Save your life: Get care for these POST-BIRTH warning signs.* https://www.awhonn.org/education/hospital-products/post-birth-warning-signs-education-program/

Association of Women's Health, Obstetric and Neonatal Nurses. (2020). *Insurance coverage for contraception.* www.awhonn.org

Association of Women's Health, Obstetric and Neonatal Nurses. (2021a). Guidelines for active management of the third stage of labor using oxytocin: AWHONN Practice Brief Number 12. *Journal of Obstetric, Gynecologic & Neonatal Nursing, 50*(12), 499–502. https://doi.org/10.1111/1552-6909.12528.

Association of Women's Health, Obstetric and Neonatal Nurses. (2021b). Quantification of blood loss: AWHONN Practice Brief Number 13. *Journal of Obstetric, Gynecologic & Neonatal Nursing, 50*(4), 503–505. https://doi: 10.1016/j.jogn.2021.04.007

Centers for Disease Control and Prevention. (2020a). *Healthy pregnant or postpartum women.* https://www.cdc.gov/physicalactivity/basics/pregnancy/

Centers for Disease Control and Prevention. (2020b). *Pregnancy surveillance system.* https://www.cdc.gov/reproductivehealth/maternal-mortality/pregnancy-mortality-surveillance-system.htm

Centers for Disease Control and Prevention. (2020c). Use of tetanus toxoid, reduced diphtheria toxoid, and acellular pertussis vaccines: Updated recommendations of the advisory committee on immunization practices—United States, 2019. *Morbidity and Mortality Weekly Report, 69,* 77–83.

Central Intelligence Agency. (2021). *The world factbook.* http://www.cia.gov/library/publications/resources/the-world-factbook/rankorder/2223rank.html

Cunningham, F. G., Leveno, K. J., Bloom, S. L., Dashe, J. S., Spong, C. Y., Hoffman, B. L., & Casey, B. M. (2018). *Williams obstetrics* (25th ed.). McGraw Hill Medical.

Isley, M. (2020). Postpartum care and long-term health considerations. In M. B. Landon, H. L. Galan, E. R. M. Jauniaux, D. A. Driscoll, V. Berghella, W. A. Grobman, S. J. Kilpatrick, & A. G. Cahill (Eds.), *Obstetrics: Normal and problem pregnancies* (8th ed., pp. 459–474). Elsevier.

James, D., & Suplee, P. (2020). Postpartum care. In K. Simpson & P. Creehan (Eds.), *AWHONN: Perinatal nursing* (5th ed., pp. 509–561). Lippincott, Williams & Wilkins.

Janke, J. (2020). Newborn nutrition. In K. Simpson & P. Creehan (Eds.), *AWHONN: Perinatal nursing* (5th ed., pp. 609–643). Lippincott, Williams & Wilkins.

Kee, J. (2018). *Laboratory and diagnostic tests with nursing implications* (10th ed.). Pearson.

Smith, R. (2018). Normal postpartum changes. In R. P. Smith & F. H. Netter's (Eds.), *Netter's obstetrics and gynecology* (3rd ed., pp. 440–442). Elsevier.

Suplee, P., & Janke, J. (Eds.). (2020). *AWHONN Compendium of postpartum care* (3rd ed.). Association of Women's Health, Obstetric, and Neonatal Nurses.

U.S. Department of Health and Human Services, Office of Disease Prevention and Health Promotion. (2020). *Healthy People 2030 topics and objectives.* https://www.healthypeople.gov/

Vallerand, A. H., & Sanoski, C. A. (2021). *Davis's drug guide for nurses* (17th ed.). F.A. Davis.

Wilkinson, J., Treas, L., Barnett, K., & Smith, M. (2020). *Fundamentals in nursing* (4th ed.). F.A. Davis.

Wilson, B., Shannon, M., & Shields, K. (2020). *Pearson nurse's drug guide.* Pearson.

Wiser, D., & Boisvert, J. (2019). What lifestyle interventions are most effective for promoting postpartum weight loss? *Evidence-Based Practice, 22*(10), 13–14. https://doi.org/10.1097/EBP.0000000000000388

Woodly, S. J., & Hay-Smith, E. J. C. (2021). Narrative review of pelvic floor muscle training for childbearing women—Why, when, what, and how. *International Urogynecology Journal, 32*(7), 1977–1988. https://doi:10.1007/s00192-021-04804-z

Transition to Parenthood

13

Linda Chapman, RN, PhD

LEARNING OUTCOMES

Upon completion of this chapter, the student will be able to:

1. Describe the process of "becoming a mother."
2. Identify factors that influence women and men in their role transitions to mother and father.
3. Discuss bonding and attachment.
4. Identify factors that affect family dynamics.
5. Describe nursing actions that support couples during their transition to parenthood.

CONCEPTS

Evidence-Based Practice
Grief and Loss
Growth and Development
Health and Promotion
Self
Self-Care
Stress and Coping
Teaching and Learning

Nursing Diagnosis

- Knowledge deficit related to role of parent due to being a first-time parent
- At risk for situational self-esteem disturbance due to new parenting role
- At risk for altered family processes related to incorporation of a new family member
- At risk for altered parent–infant attachment related to anxiety of being a new parent

Nursing Outcomes

- Parents will verbalize an understanding of parental role expectations and responsibilities.
- Parents will verbalize stressors of new role.
- Parents will demonstrate positive comments and actions when interacting with family members.
- Parents will hold the infant close to the body, attend to the infant's needs, and interact with the infant.

INTRODUCTION

The postpartum period is a time of both physiological and psychological adjustments. As the woman adjusts to the numerous physiological changes within her body, she and her partner are adjusting to their new roles as parents and the effect these new roles have on their relationship and the family unit (Fig. 13–1). This chapter focuses on the psychological, emotional, and developmental changes that take place during the transition to parenthood.

TRANSITION TO PARENTHOOD

The transition to parenthood is a dynamic developmental process that begins with the knowledge of pregnancy and continues throughout the postpartum period as the couple takes on their new or expanded roles of mother and father. Whether this is the first child or tenth child, this transition is a major life event that is both exciting and stressful, producing developmental challenges

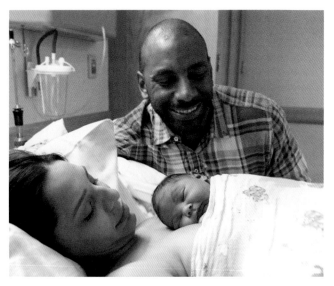

FIGURE 13–1 Family time.

for the individual, the couple's relationship, and family members. New parents may experience:

● Increased stress related to learning the role of mother or father, childcare tasks, financial concerns, work–family conflict, and chronic fatigue
● Decreased satisfaction within their couple relationship
● Decrease in sexual and intimate activities

Evidence-Based Practice: Challenges for First-Time Parents

Levesque, S., Bisson, V., Charton, L. & Fernet, M. (2020). Parenting and relational well-being during the transition to parenthood: Challenges for the first-time parents. *Journal of Child and Family Studies, 29,* 1938–1956.

The aim of this qualitative study was to examine new parents' experiences and perceptions of the challenges in assuming the parenting role and maintaining relational well-being. The sample included 23 first-time parents with a child aged 6 to 18 months. Nineteen couples identified as heterosexual and four identified as same-sex couples. Couples were recruited from Montreal, Quebec. Each couple was interviewed together and then individually.

Three central challenges were identified:

1. Loss of individuality and couplehood as parenthood became the primary role

2. Parental role equality in terms of childcare and related tasks: A significant source of irritation

3. Managing expectations: The influence of social norms, judgment, and pressures on parental self-development.

Factors that impeded adjustment were identified:

1. Fatigue and lack of sleep

2. Social isolation and feelings of solitude

3. Financial precariousness and discrimination at work

4. Balancing work

Implications:

1. Expectant parents need to be informed of the challenges they might experience as new parents and they should be encouraged to discuss how these challenges might affect them and ways to decrease the effects.

2. Health-care providers postbirth need to be aware of these challenges and address these during women and infant care.

Each individual deals with the growth, realization, and preparation of becoming a parent in different ways. Personal values, societal expectations, and cultural beliefs influence how an individual takes on the role of parent. Transition to parenthood is fostered or hampered by many factors, some of which include:

● Previous life experiences: Previous experiences caring for infants and children can foster a smoother transition to parenthood.
● How they were parented: A positive feeling of how they were parented can enhance the transition to parenthood.
● Length and strength of the relationship between partners: A strong relationship between the couple can foster a smoother transition to parenthood.
● Financial considerations: Financial concerns can cause stress and hamper the transition to parenting.
● Educational levels: Decreased ability to read and comprehend information regarding child care may hamper the couple's ability to gain knowledge in the care of the infant.
● Support systems: A lack of positive support in the care of the woman and infant can increase stress and hamper the transition to parenting.
● Desire to be a parent: A lack of desire to be a parent can hamper the transition to parenting.
● Age of parents: Adolescent parents may have a more difficult transition to parenthood.

The transition to parenthood involves taking on the role of mother or father, viewing the child as an individual with a unique personality, and incorporating the new child into the family system.

Parental Roles

Individuals have many roles throughout their lifetimes. Children take on the roles of son or daughter, sister or brother, grandchild, and student. Additional roles are acquired with age, and roles change over time as the individual matures and new roles are added. The role of mother or father evolves and changes over time as the child grows and additional children are added to the family. Each new role has expectations and responsibilities that the individual must learn in order to be successful in the role.

Couples are given the title of mother and father with the birth of their child but must learn the expectations and responsibilities of these roles.

● Examples of parental role expectations are that others will acknowledge the person as being a parent or that the child will obey the parents.

- Examples of responsibilities are that the parents will love and protect their child.

Knowledge of these expectations and responsibilities is acquired through intentional learning (formal instructions) and incidental learning (observing others in the role). Most individuals have little intentional or instructional learning regarding the role of mother or father and must rely on incidental learning of these expectations and responsibilities. Examples of incidental learning of the parental role are:

- Observing other individuals who are mothers and fathers
- Recalling how they were parented
- Watching movies or television programs that have mothers or fathers as characters

The process of learning and developing parental roles should start during the pregnancy. Partners who learn together during the pregnancy have better outcomes when they take on the role of parents. Providing couples with written information regarding different styles of parenting roles allows the expectant couple to learn about parenting behaviors. The expectant couple can then discuss parenting issues and mutually agree on expectations and responsibilities for their new roles.

Expected Findings

- Parents identify changing roles and are willing to make lifestyle changes to accommodate the new roles.
- Parents identify with the parental roles.
- Parents discuss what the roles mean to them.
- Couples incorporate a third person, the infant, into their relationship.
- Couples support each other in mutual caregiving tasks.

Nursing Actions

Nursing actions are directed at supporting the couple as they take on their role of mother or father. Nursing actions include:

- Providing an environment that is conducive to rest, such as uninterrupted periods of time so that parents can sleep
  - Adequate rest can increase the couple's ability to take in new information and develop new skills.
- Providing culturally sensitive care
  - Mother and father role expectations and responsibilities vary based on cultural backgrounds.
- Active listening; encourage the parents to talk about their expectations of each other in their respective role of mother or father.
  - Having realistic and mutually agreed-upon expectations decreases the level of stress within the relationship.
- Providing parental education on infant care with a variety of educational strategies such as handouts, videos, and demonstrations of procedures (burping, swaddling, entertaining, and stimulating the infant)
  - Information needs to be appropriate and relevant for the couple.

- Providing positive feedback for parents' infant care behaviors
  - New parents are insecure regarding infant care and need to know they are correctly interacting with and caring for their infant.
- Providing information on community parenting classes and support groups
  - This will provide parents opportunities for both intentional and incidental learning.

MOTHERHOOD

Becoming a mother is a phrase used to describe the process that women undergo in their transition to motherhood and establishment of their maternal identity (Mercer, 2004). Mercer describes four stages through which women progress in the transition to motherhood:

- Commitment, attachment, and preparation for an infant during pregnancy
- Acquaintance with and increasing attachment to the infant, learning how to care for the infant, and physical restoration during the early weeks after birth
- Moving toward a new normal during the first 4 months
- Achievement of a maternal identity around 4 months (Mercer, 2006)

The process of becoming a mother begins during pregnancy but can occur before pregnancy. Some women begin preparing for this role as children when they fantasize about being mothers and role-play motherhood with dolls. Others actively improve their health in preparation for the pregnancy before conceiving (Mercer, 2006). These factors influence the process:

- How the woman was parented
- Her life experiences
- Her unique characteristics
- Her cultural beliefs
- The pregnancy experience
- The birth experience
- Support from partner, family, and friends
- The woman's willingness to assume the role of mother
- The infant's characteristics such as appearance and temperament (Mercer, 1995, 2006)

Nursing Actions

- Review prenatal and labor records for risk factors such as complications during pregnancy and labor and birth.
  - Pregnancy and birth experiences can either enhance or impede the process of becoming a mother.
- Assess the stages of "becoming a mother."
  - Assessment data assists in developing individualized nursing actions.
  - Expected assessment findings:
    - Positive feelings toward being pregnant
    - Positive health behaviors
    - Nurturing behaviors toward the infant

- Protective feelings toward the infant
- Increasing confidence in knowing and caring for the infant
- Establishment of new family routines (Mercer, 2006)

- Provide rooming-in or couplet care to facilitate bonding and attachment.
- Provide private time for the parents to interact with their infant.
- Provide comfort measures for the woman to promote rest and healing.
- Listen to the woman's concerns in order for her to process the incorporation of the infant into her life.
- Provide information on the care of infants.
- Praise the woman for the care she provides her infant.

Evidence-Based Practice

Maternal Adaptation During the Early Postpartum Period

In the 1960s, Reba Rubin conducted qualitative research studies focusing on maternal adaptation during the early postpartum weeks. Her research is the foundation of our understanding of the psychosocial experience of women during the postpartum period. Two concepts identified through her research are "maternal phases" and "maternal touch." Rubin (1984) refined and modified the process as more evidence was linked to maternal adjustments and behaviors and identified areas of development that women progress through to "becoming a mother."

Ramona Mercer, a student and colleague of Rubin, added to and expanded this body of nursing knowledge through numerous research studies that focused on the maternal role. Based on these studies, Mercer (1995) developed the theory of "maternal role attainment," which describes and explains the process women progress through as they become a mother. Based on her previous research and the research of others, Mercer (2004) supports replacing the term *maternal role attainment* with *becoming a mother*. The term *becoming a mother* reflects that the process is not stagnant but continually evolving as the woman and her child are changing and growing.

The theories generated by Rubin's and Mercer's research agendas are the cornerstone of evidence-based knowledge used in establishing nursing guidelines for the care of postpartum women and families.

Maternal Phases

As defined by Rubin (1961, 1967), a three-phase maternal process occurs during the first few weeks of the postpartum period (Table 13-1). Rubin's theory, developed in the 1960s, is still relevant today, but women move through the phases more rapidly than when the initial research was conducted and the theory formalized. At that time, women were heavily sedated during labor and birth and often could not recall the birth experience. Additionally, women had limited interactions with their newborns during their 5-day postpartum stay. Newborns typically remained in the central nursery and were brought to their mothers every 4 hours for feedings. The effects of the sedation during labor and birth and the limited interactions with their newborns slowed down the progression through these phases.

A delay in transitioning through the phases may indicate that the woman is experiencing difficulty in becoming a mother.

Factors that can affect the woman's transition through the maternal phases are:

- Medications (e.g., magnesium sulfate or analgesics) that depress the central nervous system (CNS), leading to tiredness and a slow response to stimuli.
- Complications during pregnancy, labor and birth, or postpartum (e.g., preterm labor, chronic illness, difficult birth, or cesarean birth) can cause the woman's focus to shift to her health and well-being, or to resolving feelings of disappointment.
- Cesarean births can cause increased discomfort that interferes with the woman's ability to care for her infant. Pain causes a shift of maternal attention from focusing on caring for the baby to seeking pain relief for self.
- Preterm infants or infants who experience complications can cause additional stress on the woman and delay her transition through the phases.
- Mood disorders such as depression cause the woman's focus to be more on self and less on the infant.
- Lack of support from the partner or support system may lead to maternal exhaustion.
- Adolescent mothers are more focused inwardly and on peer relationships than on care of the infant.
- Lack of financial resources forces the woman to focus on obtaining basic needs rather than on her infant.
- Cultural beliefs can influence the woman's behavior and the amount of time she spends in each phase. In some cultures, for example, women are expected to rest rather than be actively involved in care or decision making during the first months of the infant's life.

Nursing Actions

- Review prenatal and labor records for factors that might delay progression through the maternal phases.
- Assess for maternal phases.
  - Assessment data assists in developing individualized nursing actions.
  - Expected assessment findings:
    - Taking-in behaviors during the first 24 to 48 hours
    - Taking-hold behaviors from 24 to 48 hours through the first few weeks
  - Nursing care during the taking-in phase is directed by the nurse because the woman is more dependent during this phase and has difficulty making decisions.
  - Nursing care during the taking-hold phase is directed more by the woman, as she is becoming more independent and has an increased ability to make decisions.
- Provide comfort measures such as backrubs, uninterrupted periods of rest, and analgesics.
- Adapt teaching to reflect the maternal phase.
  - During the taking-in phase, teaching is directed to immediate learning needs and is provided in short sessions, as the woman's focus is on self versus learning about the care of the infant.
  - During the taking-hold phase, praise the woman for her learning, as she is eager to learn but can become frustrated with not being able to master a new task quickly.

TABLE 13-1   Maternal Phases

TAKING-IN PHASE	TAKING-HOLD PHASE	LETTING-GO PHASE
The taking-in phase, a period of dependent behaviors, occurs during the first 24 to 48 hours after birth and includes the following maternal behaviors: • The woman is focused on her personal comfort and physical changes. • The woman relives and speaks of the birth experience. • The woman adjusts to psychological changes. • The woman is dependent on others for her and her infant's immediate needs. • The woman has a decreased ability to make decisions. • The woman concentrates on personal physical healing (Rubin, 1961, 1967).	The taking-hold phase, the movement between dependent and independent behaviors, follows the taking-in phase. It can last weeks and includes the following maternal behaviors: • The focus moves from self to the infant. • The woman begins to be independent. • The woman has an increased ability to make decisions. • The woman is interested in the infant's cues and needs. • The woman gives up the pregnancy role and initiates taking on the maternal role. • The woman is eager to learn; it is an excellent time to initiate postpartum teaching. • The woman begins to like the role of "mother." • The woman may have feelings of inadequacy and being overwhelmed. • The woman needs verbal reassurance that she is meeting her infant's needs. • The woman may show signs and symptoms of baby blues and fatigue. • The woman begins to let more of the outside world in (Rubin, 1961, 1967).	In the letting-go phase, the movement from independence to the new role of mother is fluid and interchangeable with the taking-hold phase. Maternal characteristics during this phase are: • Grieving and letting go of old relationship behaviors in favor of new ones. • Incorporating the infant into her life whereby the baby becomes a separate entity from her. • Accepting the infant as the child really is. • Giving up the fantasy of what it would or could have been. • Independence returns; may go back to work or school. • May have feelings of grief, guilt, or anxiety. • Reconnection and growth in relationship with partner (Rubin, 1961, 1967).

CLINICAL JUDGMENT

The Nurse Role During the Taking-In Phase

Women in the taking-in phase are in a more dependent state and may have difficulty making decisions and initiating self-care and infant care. The nurse needs to be more directive in her patient care (i.e., remind the woman to take a shower or to change her newborn's diapers and then assist her in initiating the action).

FATHERHOOD

Men's preparation for the role of father is vastly different from women's preparation for motherhood. In general, men do not fantasize about being a father, nor do they role-play being a father during childhood. During pregnancy, men mentally evaluate how they were fathered and how they want to father, but the reality of becoming a father may not occur until the child is born (May, 1982). Additionally, expectant fathers often picture themselves parenting older children rather than infants (Dayton et al., 2016).

The meaning of "father" varies based on the man's interpretation of the role and its expectations and responsibilities. This is influenced by:

● How he was fathered
● How his culture defines the role
   ● In some cultures, men are not expected to be involved in the birthing process or care of the infant.
● By friends and family and by his partner

Evidence-Based Practice: Expectant Fathers' Beliefs and Expectations

Dayton, C., Buczkoski, R., Murik, M., Goletz, J., Hicks, L., Walsh, T., & Bocknek, E. (2016). Expectant fathers' beliefs and expectations about fathering as they prepare to parent a new infant. *Social Work Research, 40*, 225–237.

The purpose of this qualitative study was to gain a deeper understanding of expectant fathers' experiences as they prepared to parent a new infant. Forty-four expectant fathers were interviewed during their partner's third trimester. Five major themes emerged from the data:

1. Being there: Men talked about the importance of being present in their child's life.

2. Fathering older children: Men talked more frequently about parenting older children versus infants. They focused on father roles with children beyond infant and toddler periods.

3. Preparation for life in society: Men talked about the importance of fathers preparing their children to be successful in their community and society. They identified their father roles as educator and life coach, providing emotional support to their children in dealing with life's challenges, serving as a positive role model, and facilitating their children's engagement within the community.

4. Heaviness of the fathering role: Men described fathering as an extremely difficult task that included being responsible for another life and the importance of providing financial and concrete support to their children.

5. Parenting support: Men indicated that they relied on women versus men for support in their role as father. The women were usually their partner, their mother, or other female relatives.

Implications:

1. This provides opportunities for expectant fathers to talk about their preparation and feelings regarding their new and emerging role of father.

2. Father involvement that begins in pregnancy is associated with positive maternal and infant outcomes. The provision of prenatal and post-partum education interventions can assist men in understanding the importance of early father involvement in the care of their infant and its effect on the infant's development. Early parenting behaviors include rocking, soothing, and carrying their infant.

The man's partner has a major influence on the degree of the man's involvement in infant and child care. For the man to be an involved father, his partner needs to share this desire and be supportive.

Becoming a father evolves over time as the man has increasing contact with his infant, increasing knowledge of the infant and infant care, and increasing experiences in infant care. Factors that influence the man's transition to fatherhood are:

- Developmental and emotional age
- Cultural expectations
- Relationship with his partner
- Knowledge and understanding of fatherhood
- Previous experiences as a father
- The way he was fathered
- Financial concerns
- Support from partner, friends, and family

Nursing Actions

- Provide information on infant care and infant behavior.
- Demonstrate infant care such as diapering, feeding, and holding.
  - Providing information and demonstrating infant care skills enhances the father's comfort in caring for his infant.
- Praise the father for his interactions with his infant.
  - Praising can encourage continued interactions with his infant.
- Provide opportunities for the father to talk about the meaning of fathering.
  - Talking about the meaning of fathering assists in identifying beliefs about the role.
- Facilitate a discussion with the father and his partner to identify mutual expectations of the fathering role.
  - Mutually agreed-upon expectations can decrease the stress level within the relationship.

ADOLESCENT PARENTS

Adolescence is the transition between childhood and adulthood. This is a very challenging time, as the individual experiences many physiological, psychological, and social changes.

Adolescent parenting is a stressful life experience in that the adolescent is taking on the role responsibilities of being a mother or father while at the same time working through the developmental tasks of being a teenager. Additionally, adolescent parents have few life experiences that prepare them for the role conflicts and strain experienced by first-time parents.

Adolescent mothers and fathers come from every social and racial group and may or may not feel support from their families and friends. It is not uncommon for them to experience financial and educational challenges. Becoming a parent will be challenging but can also be rewarding and a positive life experience. Adolescent mothers have reported that they found parenting to help them mature and become more focused and responsible (Cox et al., 2021).

Adolescent fathers need to be recognized as an important part of their child's life. In a qualitative study focused on adolescent fathers, the researchers emphasized the importance of including the expectant fathers in the prenatal care (Florsheim et al., 2020). They also explained the importance of providing opportunities for the young fathers to talk about how they feel about becoming a father.

Nursing Actions

Nursing actions are directed at supporting the adolescent parents in developing childcare behaviors and learning to cope with the stress of parenting, as well as increasing the adolescent father's involvement in the support, care, and nurturing of his child. These nursing actions include the following:

- Assess level of knowledge.
  - Information needs to be appropriate and relevant for the individual or couple for learning to occur.
- Present information at an age-appropriate level.
  - Learning styles and teaching strategies are different for young teens and older teens. Information needs to be provided in a manner that will engage the adolescent parent in the learning process.
- Include the adolescent father in infant care teaching sessions.
  - Adolescent fathers need to be recognized as fathers and they need information and encouragement in developing care behaviors.
- Involve the maternal grandparent in teaching sessions focused on infant care.
  - Grandparents need a review of infant care because teen mothers might live with their parents during the first years or rely on their mother for assistance and information.
- Discuss with adolescent parents expectations of each other regarding child care and support.
  - Realistic and mutually agreed-upon expectations decrease the level of stress within the relationship.
- Involve adolescent fathers in prenatal care based on the adolescent mother's comfort level.
  - Adolescent fathers who are involved during the prenatal period have greater involvement with infants following the birth.

Evidence-Based Practice

Adolescent Mothers
Cox, S., Lashley, C., Hensen, L., & Hans, S. (2021). Making meaning of motherhood: Self and life transition among African American adolescent mothers. *American Journal of Orthopsychiatry, 91,* 120–131. https://doi.org/10.1037/ort0000521

The aim of this qualitative study was to describe the experience of first-time African American mothers across the first 2 years of motherhood. The study included 179 urban African American women who at the time of enrollment in study were between the ages of 13 and 19 years. Interviews were completed at 4, 12, and 24 months postbirth. The interviews focused on maternal and child health, education, work, parenting, and family relationships. Eighteen themes emerged from the content analysis of the responses to the questions on how the mother and her life have changed since giving birth. Twelve of these themes were focused on positive changes related to the parenting role, whereas six were focused on challenges related to the parenting role.

The five most common themes under positive changes were:

- Becoming more responsible
- Making room for the baby in their life
- Becoming mature
- Becoming more serious and cautious in their behavior
- Being motivated to succeed

The five challenges related to the parenting role were:

- Limited in being able to go out or see friends
- Feeling busy and burdened
- Lacking sleep
- Experiencing financial challenges
- Challenged to protect the child

This study expands the understanding of Black adolescent mothers and identifies positive growth in the young women and the challenges as they transition through motherhood and adolescence.

SAME-SEX PARENTS

In the United States, 5.1% of female adults and 3.9% of male adults identify as lesbian, gay, bisexual, or transgender (LBGT) (Newport, 2018). The number of millennials, the present childbearing generation, who identify themselves as LGBT is 8.1% (Newport, 2018). The percentage of Americans' satisfaction with acceptance of gays and lesbians in the United States has risen from 51% in 2002 to 72% in 2019, and the percentage of dissatisfied Americans has decreased from 42% in 2002 to 21% in 2019 (Poushter & Kent, 2020). These statistics indicate an increasing acceptance of the homosexual lifestyle and an increasing number of lesbian women of childbearing age.

Before conception, lesbian couples have discussions similar to those of heterosexual couples regarding parenting philosophies, child care, and work arrangements. However, unlike heterosexual couples, lesbian couples must decide which woman will become the child's biological mother. This decision is based on which woman desires to be pregnant and may be influenced by the age and health of each partner, career goals, and which woman's insurance covers the cost of reproductive technology and the pregnancy and childbirth medical care (Amato & Jacob, 2010; Wojnar & Katzenmeyer, 2014). In some cases, both women want to conceive a child and decide that one will conceive the first child and the other will conceive the second child.

Once the couple has decided who will conceive, they must decide how they will conceive. Most lesbian couples use artificial insemination (AI) and thus must decide whether they want a known or unknown sperm donor. Lesbian couples share similar feelings as heterosexual couples who are using AI. They often find the process to be stressful due to the monitoring of ovulation and the timing of insemination, and the process becomes more stressful when pregnancy does not occur within the first few months of AI (Amato & Jacob, 2010; Gregg, 2018; Wojnar & Katzenmeyer, 2014).

During postpartum hospitalization, the couple needs information regarding care of their infant and of the postpartum woman. The postpartum couple often views themselves as coparents and plans to equally share in the care of their child. It is important to include both women in teaching sessions regarding infant care. Most lesbian mothers breastfeed their infants; in fact, it is not uncommon for both mothers to breastfeed their infant. It is important for nurses to ask the mothers if they both plan to breastfeed and, if so, assist both in breastfeeding and providing information on induction of lactation and use of lactation supplementation. The initiation of lactation for the non-birthing woman can be difficult and challenging but is also often successful and rewarding.

SAFE AND EFFECTIVE NURSING CARE:
Patient Education

Induction of Lactation

Several methods can be used to induce lactation for non-birthing mothers. These include hormonal therapy, manual or electric pumping of the breast, use of an at-breast supplementation device, or a combination of these methods. The non-birthing mother should begin preparing her breasts for lactation several months before the birth of the baby. The La Leche League International Web site provides additional information for non-birthing women who desire to breastfeed.

Lesbian couples take on the role of birth mother and co-mother during their transition to parenting. They will experience similar stress-producing issues as heterosexual couples as they take on their new roles, but research findings indicate that lesbian parents report less parental stress than heterosexual couples (Borneskog et al., 2014).

Lesbian couples report lower parental stress related to feelings of incompetence as a parent and social isolation compared with heterosexual couples (Borneskog et al., 2014). Most lesbian couples are egalitarian in their roles and equally share in the care of their infant (Borneskog et al., 2014). These relationship traits might influence the lower levels of parental stress.

The non-childbearing mother, who is not visibly pregnant, might experience stress related to "invisibility and lack of support from their work or social community" (McManus et al., 2006). The non-childbearing mother can also experience stress related to parental rights, as rights for the nonbirth mother vary from state to state. Even when the couple is legally married, the non-childbearing mother may not automatically have parental rights. It is recommended that the non-childbearing mother seek legal advice in regards to her legal rights.

Children raised by lesbian parents are well-adjusted and have similar emotional, social, and cognitive development as children of heterosexual parents. A longitudinal study by Farr (2017) compared adoptive children of same-sex couples and heterosexual couples, collecting data when the children were preschool age and then 5 years later. The results from this study indicated no difference between the children of same-sex parents and heterosexual parents. Same-sex-parented children were well adjusted at each data collection point. The same-sex parents were capable in their parenting role and satisfied with their couple relationship (Farr, 2017).

Nursing Actions

- Self-assessment of the nurse's attitudes, beliefs, and knowledge of homosexuality
  - Personal beliefs, attitudes, and knowledge can have a positive or negative influence on patient–nurse interactions and nursing care.
  - Nurses need to be respectful of people with diverse lifestyles.
- Assess the couple's knowledge of infant care and parenting roles.
  - It is important to evaluate the couple's knowledge level and then reinforce and add to the knowledge base.
- Include both mothers in teaching sessions that focus on infant care.
  - Lesbian couples tend to be egalitarian in their roles and equally share the care of their infant (Lindsey, 2015).
- Clarify if both mothers are planning to breastfeed their infant; if so, provide breastfeeding teaching and support to each mother.
  - Often both mothers will breastfeed their infant and both need assistance.
- Encourage both mothers to hold the infant and engage in infant care.
  - Bonding and attachment are important for each parent's mother–child relationship.

Evidence-Based Practice

Lesbian Women and Motherhood

Gregg, I. (2018). The health care experience of lesbian women becoming mothers. *Nursing for Women's Health, 22,* 40–50. https://doi:10.1016/j.nwh.2017.12.003

The purpose of this review was to explore how lesbian women experienced the health-care system during prenatal, labor and delivery, and the postpartum period. The review included 10 studies. Three themes were identified:

- Making the decision to become pregnant
- Access to care
- Stigma in the health system

The women reported a strong desire and need to start a family with their partner. Women expressed that their desire to go through the experience of pregnancy, birth, and breastfeeding was more relevant than the desire to have biologically related children. Women expressed fear of informing their care provider of their sexual identity. All of the women experienced some degree of homophobia in their care. Four categories of homophobia were identified: exclusion, heterosexual assumptions, inappropriate questioning, and refusal of service.

Nursing Implications

- Develop skills and reflect on cultural assumptions as the nurse works toward caring for all minorities and cultural groups in a positive manner.
- Develop intake form and questions that use gender-neutral terms.
- Attend educational training about LGBTQ health.

BONDING AND ATTACHMENT

Bonding and attachment between parents and children are critical factors in the transition to parenting and parental role attainment. Bonding is defined as the emotions that begin during pregnancy or shortly after birth between the parent and the infant (Klaus & Kennell, 1982). Bonding is unidirectional from parent to infant. Attachment is an emotional connection that forms between infants and their parents (Bowlby, 1969). It is bidirectional from parent to infant and from infant to parent. Attachment has a lifelong impact on the developing individual. The quality of this attachment influences the person's physical and emotional development and is the foundation for the formation of future relationships. With each interaction, the parent and infant become more acquainted with each other, recognizing and becoming sensitive to each other's behaviors. This leads to reciprocal behaviors and emotional bonds between the parent and infant over time (Table 13-2).

Bonding and Attachment Behaviors

Bonding and attachment are affected by time, proximity of parent and infant, whether the pregnancy is planned or wanted, and the ability of the parents to process through the necessary development tasks of parenting. Other factors that influence bonding and attachment include:

- The knowledge base of the couple
- Past experience with children
- Maturity and educational levels of the couple
- Type of extended support system
- Maternal or paternal expectations of the pregnancy
- Maternal or paternal expectations of the infant
- Cultural expectations

TABLE 13-2   Bonding and Attachment Behaviors

BONDING BEHAVIORS UNIDIRECTIONAL: PARENT → INFANT	ATTACHMENT BEHAVIORS BIDIRECTIONAL: PARENT ↔ INFANT
En face	Parents respond to the infant's cry.
Calls the baby by name	The infant responds to the parents' comforting measures.
Cuddles the baby close to their chest	Parents stimulate and entertain the infant while awake.
Talks or sings to the baby	Parents become "cue sensitive" to the infant's behavior.
Kisses the baby	
Breastfeeds the baby or holds the baby close when bottle-feeding	

Risk Factors for Delayed Bonding or Attachment

- Maternal illness during pregnancy or the postpartum period that interferes with the woman's ability to interact with her infant
- Neonatal illness such as prematurity that necessitates separation of the infant from the parents
- Prolonged or complicated labor and birth that exhausts both the woman and her partner
- Fatigue during the postpartum period related to lack of rest and sleep
- Physical discomfort experienced by women postbirth
- Age and developmental age of the woman, such as adolescent or developmentally challenged
- Outside stressors not related to pregnancy or childbirth (e.g., concerns with finances, poor social support system, or need to return to work soon after the birth)

Nursing Actions

- Review the prenatal and labor record for risk factors that place the woman or couple at risk for delayed bonding or attachment.
- Assess for risk factors that could delay bonding and attachment.
  - Early identification of couples at risk can lead to early interventions to enhance bonding or attachment.
- Assess cultural beliefs.
  - Type of interactions between parents and infants can vary based on cultural beliefs.
- Assess for bonding and attachment by observation of parent–infant interaction.
  - Assessment data provides information for individualizing nursing actions.
  - Expected assessment findings:
    - Parents hold the infant close.
    - Parents refer to the infant by name or proper sex.
    - Parents respond to the infant's needs.
    - Parents speak positively about the infant.
    - Parents appear interested in learning about the infant.
    - Parents ask appropriate questions about infant care.
    - Parents appear comfortable holding and caring for the infant.
  - Maladaptive assessment findings:
    - Parents call the infant "it."

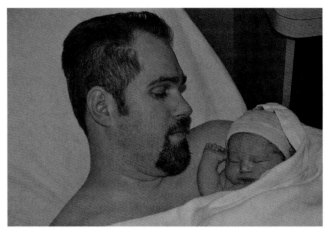

FIGURE 13-2 Skin-to-skin contact can enhance bonding and attachment.

- Parents avoid eye contact with the infant (this can be viewed as adaptive based on culture).
- Parents do not respond to the infant's cries.
- Parents are emotionally unavailable to the infant.
- Parents allow others to care for the infant, showing no interest (this can be viewed as adaptive based on culture).
- Parents demonstrate poor feeding techniques such as propping bottles, not burping the infant, or seeming uncomfortable or irritated when nursing.
- Teach parents about bonding and attachment and the importance of these to the child's development of future relationships.
  - Understanding why it is important enhances the likelihood of increased bonding and attachment behaviors by parents.
- Instruct parents regarding the importance of parents responding to the infant's cues such as crying, cooing, and movement.
  - Attachment is bidirectional.
- Promote bonding and attachment by:
  - Initiating early and prolonged contact between the parent and infant (Fig. 13–2)
  - Initiating rooming-in or couplet care
  - Providing positive comments to parents regarding their interactions with the infant
  - Encouraging mothers to breastfeed
  - Encouraging the woman and her partner to talk about their birth experience and feelings regarding becoming parents

- Promote attachment between mothers and infants separated due to either maternal illness or neonatal complications by:
  - Recommending that family members take pictures of the infant and bring them to the mother to keep in her room
  - Assisting parents to the NICU or nursery so that they can see and touch their infant
  - Providing opportunities for parents to care for the infant in the NICU or nursery
  - Instructing the woman on breast milk pumping and encouraging her to bring breast milk to the NICU for use with her infant
  - Informing parents that they can call the NICU or nursery any time of the day or night and talk with the nurse caring for their infant

PARENT–INFANT CONTACT

Early contact between the parents and their infant fosters the development of attachment and integration of the infant into the maternal and paternal relationship. Continued contact and interaction provide the avenue for the parents and infant to learn more about each other. As they interact and perform their roles, they find themselves becoming more aware of the cues that make them respond to each other. This interaction cycle of behavior is called reciprocity, a biorhythmic or inherent rhythm that exists between the parents and infant and becomes stronger with each interaction and the passing of time. This sequence of events strengthens the bonding and attachment processes that are the foundation for all the child's future relationships.

Maternal Touch

New mothers begin to progress through the transition of maternal touch with the first physical contact with their infants (Rubin, 1963). New mothers will progress through three stages before feeling comfortable holding the infant close to the body. In the earlier stages, the breastfeeding woman can feel awkward in holding her infant close to feed. Progression through the stages usually occurs over a few hours when a mother has early and continuous contact with her infant. It can take several days if the mother has limited contact with her infant, which can occur if the infant is ill and admitted to an intensive care nursery. These stages, as described by Rubin, are:

- Initial stage: The woman touches her infant tentatively with her fingertips.
- Second stage: The woman, as she becomes more comfortable with herself as a mother, uses her hand to stroke her infant's head or body.
- Final stage: The mother holds her infant in her arms and brings her infant close to her body.

Rubin's maternal touch is a component of the acquaintance process through which mothers and infants transition. Mothers go through multiple stages of awareness during early contact with their infants. The first time the new mother touches and meets her infant, she is excited about her infant's features and

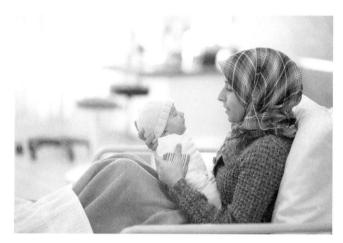

FIGURE 13–3 En face position.

verbally responds to sounds and expressions the baby makes. Later, after the new mother enters the final stage of maternal touch, she will hold her infant en face, a position in which the mother and infant are face-to-face with eye contact (Fig. 13–3). The en face position provides a positive connection that facilitates the bonding process.

Paternal–Infant Contact

In the 1980s, studies provided data that promoted and supported fathers' involvement in the birth of their infants. When expectant fathers participated in the labor and birth of their children in roles that were comfortable for them, they had a greater sense of belonging, which led to deeper engagement in the father role. Reinforcement of this type of involvement has had positive benefits to the family unit and strengthened early and positive parental involvement in the bonding and attachment process. Early physical contact with the infant provides an opportunity for the new father to become comfortable touching and holding, which fosters a more active role in caring for his infant.

New fathers experience an intense preoccupation about and interest in their infants. Greenberg and Morris (1974) identified these behaviors as engrossment (Fig. 13–4). These behaviors can vary based on the cultural beliefs of the couple.

Evidence-Based Practice: The Infant's Impact on the Father

Greenberg, M., & Morris, N. (1974). Engrossment: The infant's impact upon the father. *American Journal of Orthopsychiatry, 44*, 520–531.

In their research of new fathers, Greenberg and Morris identified the concept of engrossment that new fathers experience during the postpartum period in relationship to their infants. They defined engrossment as an absorption, preoccupation, and interest with their infants. New fathers can be observed gazing at their infants for prolonged periods of time as if they are in a hypnotic trance. Greenberg and Morris described seven characteristics of engrossment:

- A visual awareness of the infant: Seeing their infant as attractive

- A tactile awareness of the infant: Having a desire to touch the infant
- An awareness of and positive comments about their infant's distinct features
- A perception that their infant is perfect
- A strong attraction to their infant
- A feeling of strong elation
- An increase of self-esteem

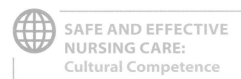

SAFE AND EFFECTIVE NURSING CARE: Cultural Competence

How Cultural Beliefs Impact Postpartum Care

Cultural beliefs influence the ways parents relate to and care for infants, including the role of fathers during the postpartum period and care of infants. Awareness of variations across cultural practices is an important component in providing appropriate care. Cultural beliefs can influence:

- The degree of the father's involvement in infant care
- The role extended family members have in the care of the infant and new mother
- The method of infant feeding
- Foods that are eaten and foods that are avoided during the postpartum period
- When a woman can bathe and wash her hair
- When the baby is named and who names the baby

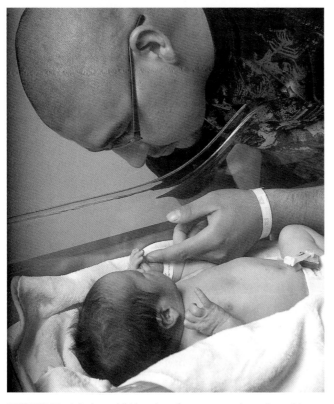

FIGURE 13–4 Father exhibiting sign of engrossment by gazing at his son.

Nursing Actions for Parent–Infant Contact

- Assess for stages of maternal touch.
  - Assessment data assists in developing individualized nursing care.
  - Expected findings (varies based on cultural beliefs):
    - Tentatively touching her infant's extremities with her fingertips
    - Progressing to fuller touch and examination of the infant
    - Verbalizing positive comments about the infant
    - Snuggling and providing comfort to the infant
    - En face positioning to interact with the infant
- Assess paternal-infant interactions.
  - Expected findings (varies based on cultural beliefs)
    - Spends prolonged periods of time gazing at the infant.
    - Assists with infant care.
    - Holds the infant close to the body.
    - Expresses delight in his infant's features.
    - Verbally and physically expresses love and joy for both his infant and partner.
- Maladaptive findings (may be viewed as adaptive based on cultural beliefs)
  - Displays little or no interest in the infant.
  - Makes negative comments about or to the infant.
  - Ignores the infant's needs and cues.
  - Displays sadness or anger to the partner or infant.
  - Does not spend time with the infant or is emotionally absent.
  - Experiences mood swings.
  - Has conflict between family members over the infant.
- Provide early, continuous, and uninterrupted periods of time for parents to see, hold, and interact with their infant.
  - Bonding and attachment occur over time and with continued contact.
- Facilitate rooming-in, which provides the opportunity for the infant and father to stay in the mother's room throughout the hospital stay.
- Promote parental interaction with the infant by delaying unnecessary procedures.
- Provide adequate rest periods for the parents. This ensures they have the stamina and rest to take care of and provide emotional support to each other.
- Provide comfort measures to assist the parents in feeling rested and relaxed.
- Explain to new parents that they may not feel comfortable holding the infant close and that these feelings will decrease with increasing contact with their infant.
- Role model en face positioning.
- Role model appropriate behaviors by calling the infant by name and identifying normal infant behaviors.
- Use therapeutic listening and provide positive feedback to parents when they are verbalizing their feelings about their infant.
- Educate parents about the infant's unique behaviors and temperament.
  - Educate and give information to both parents using multiple models of learning.

● Teaching strategies need to fit the learning style of the parents.
  ● Provide culturally sensitive care to the family unit.
● The way parents interact with their infant can vary based on cultural beliefs.

COMMUNICATION BETWEEN PARENT AND CHILD

Communication is a bidirectional process that involves a sender and a receiver. People communicate through verbal and written words and through their eyes, ears, faces, and body gestures. Infants can see, hear, and smell; respond to their environments; and display displeasure. They engage in behaviors designed to evoke a response from individuals in their environments. They rely on vocal noises such as crying and cooing, as well as facial expressions and body movements to participate actively in relationship-building with other humans. The challenge to parents is learning the cues infants use to communicate their needs and pleasures.

Nurses are in the unique position to provide information about the infant's ability to communicate. They can help parents identify infant behaviors and offer appropriate interventions to promote positive interactions. These are examples of infant communication styles and cues:

● Crying
● Cooing
● Facial expressions
● Eye movements
● Smelling
● Cuddling
● Arm and leg movements
● Entrainment, a phenomenon in which the infant moves their arms and legs in rhythm with the speech patterns of an adult.

Responding to and encouraging infant communication assists the infant in developing communication and language skills. The parents' ability to recognize their infant's positive response cues fosters their confidence in their parenting skills. Teaching parents how to identify their infant's unique cues and behaviors promotes a positive relationship that empowers the dyad to continue to grow and learn as the infant matures and adds new skills and insights into the relationship.

Parents who are aware of and start to understand infant behaviors by becoming cue-sensitive will be able to identify:

● The best times to communicate with their infant
● Ways to comfort
● Methods to help infant self-comfort
● When the infant is overstimulated and how to provide quiet times during fussy periods

Infants have very acute senses when interacting with their parents. Infants who are placed on their mothers' abdomens will crawl to the breast. Infants also interact with their parents by responding to voices and touch. They look en face and root when stimulated. These initial interactions and ongoing interactions lead to synchrony events, which are reciprocal actions between parents and infants that show mutual expressions of

contentment. These interactions are very pleasurable for parents and infants. Examples of synchrony events are:

● The mother holding the infant in an en face position. The response to this action is that they gaze into each other's eyes and talk, coo, or smile at each other.
● The father placing his finger in the infant's hand. The infant grabs the father's finger and they gaze at each other.

CRITICAL COMPONENT

Positive Interactions Between Parents and Infants

Infants have the ability to communicate, to interact, and to be stimulated by early interactions. Depending on the state of awareness, infants can respond positively by becoming more alert or can respond negatively by crying. Nurses who understand infant behaviors, infant states of awareness, and communication cues can identify and promote positive interactions between parents and caregivers and their infants through role modeling and parent education (Table 13-3).

TABLE 13-3　Infant States

STATES	BEHAVIORS	ACTIONS
Deep sleep	Minimal body twitches and eye movement; cycles between deep and light sleep	Do not try to wake up or feed infant.
Light sleep	More active body movement; may smile	More easily aroused and stimulated
Drowsy	Awakens easily; can be rocked back to sleep or made more awake	May enjoy being held and cuddled Responds to gentle stimuli May self-comfort by sucking
Quiet alert	Eyes open; quiet and attentive	Best time for interacting
Active alert	More sensitive to stimuli, active body movement; may be tired or hungry or need changing	Decrease stimuli. Provide a quiet environment. Provide comfort measures. The infant may attempt to self-comfort.
Crying	Grimaces, cries, or whimpers	The infant may self-comfort. Meet infant needs.

Nursing Actions

- Review prenatal, labor and birth, and postpartum records for factors that might delay or hinder parent–infant communication and provide early interventions.
- Assess parent–infant interactions.
  - Expected findings:
    - Parents gently touch their infant and hold the infant close to the body.
    - Parents talk to or sing to their infant.
    - Parents, when culturally acceptable, hold their infant en face.
    - Parents respond to their infant's cues for interaction and care.
    - The infant responds to their parents' touch and voice.
- Role model communication with the infant.
  - Parents learn through incidental and intentional learning.
- Praise parents for their interactions with their infant.
- Provide teaching on infant communication:
  - The infant's ability and need to communicate
  - Eye contact, when culturally appropriate
  - Synchronized interactions
  - Recognizing and interpreting the infant's cues
  - Entrainment
  - Infant alertness states

FAMILY DYNAMICS

Family dynamics are the unique ways in which family members interact and participate within the family. Adaptation to these dynamics determines the cohesiveness, or lack thereof, in the family unit.

There are several types of relationships and family compositions. The family structure can be as small as the mother and infant, or as large as two or more generations plus extended family members. Each has its own unique dynamics and structure that present challenges and offer rewarding experiences to nurses who come into contact with these various family compositions. Examples of family compositions include:

- Married or nonmarried male–female couples
- Married and nonmarried same-sex couples
- Adoptive couples
- Adolescent women with partner, mother, or grandmother as support system
- Adolescent women without support system
- Single adult women with no partner
- Blended families

The time immediately after childbirth is filled with emotional changes for the partners and family members. Family members are redefining who they are as individuals and their roles within the family. Adjustments within the couple's relationship and family unit occur as the couple and family members incorporate and make room for the newest family member. Couples make adjustments within their relationship and learn how to support each other in their roles as parents. They reprioritize their other

responsibilities and roles to fit their new roles and responsibilities. Siblings take on the role of older brother or sister and adjust to the decreased amount of time the parents have to interact with and care for them.

The family unit is affected and influenced by changes both within and outside the family. Outside influences, such as friends and relatives, may have positive or negative effects on the family. The couple needs to determine which resources are helpful and which are stressful, and from whom they can seek positive assistance. Nursing care is directed at assisting families in identifying their needs and adjustment during this period of transition.

Coparenting

Coparenting is "a conceptual term that refers to the ways that parents and/or parental figures relate to each other in the role of parents" (Feinberg, 2003, p. 96). Coparenting:

- Occurs when the parents have shared responsibilities in child rearing.
- Consists of support for each other and coordination they exhibit in child rearing.
- Does not imply that parenting roles are or should be equal in responsibilities or authority (Feinberg, 2003).
- Develops during the transition to parenthood and is influenced by:
  - The parent's beliefs, values, desires, and expectations
  - The individual's cultural background and the dominant culture of the society (Feinberg, 2003)
  - The infant's temperament

Multiparas

The maternal role changes and becomes more complex with each additional child. Multiparas may have more knowledge and practice regarding the care of infants, but they usually experience more exhaustion and have less help than with their first child. In a classic 1979 article, Ramona Mercer described the unique concerns of multiparas:

- Concerns for her other children
  - Will her other children feel abandoned?
- Concerns about being able to love the new child
  - Does she have the capacity to love this new child as she does her other child?
- Concerns for her ability to care for more than one child
  - Does she have the time and energy to care for an additional child?
- Concerns about her ability to get rest and sleep
  - Will she be able to find time for sleep and rest?
- Concerns about having help at home to care for her and her expanding family
  - Will family members and friends be willing to help her with a second child?

It is important that nurses who care for multiparous women provide them with opportunities to express their concerns, fears, and doubts in caring for and loving another child. Nurses can facilitate this transition by providing reassurance and suggesting strategies in caring for an additional child. Strategies for caring include:

- Spending quality time with the older child when the infant is sleeping
- Carrying the infant in a sling to free hands for doing things with the older child
- Having prepared meals ready to use during the day
- Encouraging the partner to take on more responsibility for cleaning, cooking, and caring for the older child

Sibling Rivalry

The addition of a new family member can be a stressful life event for siblings within the family unit. They will need to adjust in their young lives in response to the incorporation of the infant within the family. Depending on the age of the siblings and birth order, children experience varying degrees of feeling displaced. Younger children experience a sense of loss over no longer being the "baby" of the family, whereas older children may have a sense of increased responsibility due to their parents' expectation that they assist in caring for younger children.

Preparing for the family addition should begin during pregnancy as the parents talk about the expected new baby. Providing opportunities for children to feel the fetus move and hear the fetal heartbeat are concrete ways to assist children in understanding the upcoming event. Discussion on what it will mean to have a new baby in the family can also help in adjustment.

Siblings should be introduced to their new brother or sister as soon as possible and spend time with the mother and baby during the postpartum hospitalization. They should be allowed to hold and touch the new baby with supervision (Fig. 13–5).

CRITICAL COMPONENT

Sibling Adjustment

The addition of a new member to the family can be stressful for siblings. Actions that can facilitate their adjustment include the following:

- Spending time during the prenatal period talking about the upcoming arrival of a new baby
- Providing opportunities for siblings to feel the baby move and hear the heartbeat during pregnancy
- Providing opportunities for siblings to spend time with their new brother or sister during the hospital stay
- Encouraging siblings to lie in bed with their mother during hospital visits
- Giving siblings a present from their new brother or sister
- Understanding the importance of quality time with other children, such as sitting and reading books with them, playing games, and listening to them
- Taking siblings on a special outing while the infant stays at home with a babysitter
- Explaining why babies cry and how they communicate

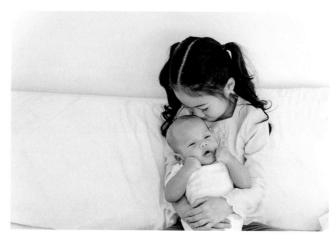

FIGURE 13–5 Big sister and her new brother.

Nursing Actions for Family Dynamics

Introducing a new member into the family can be stressful for each member of the family. The majority of nursing actions are aimed at reducing stress within the family and on family members. Nursing actions include the following:

- Review the records for relationship issues, pregnancy history, and delivery summary.
  - Complications encountered during pregnancy or labor and birth can have a negative effect on family dynamics.
- Assess for prior experiences with infants.
- Assess for maladaptive behaviors and make referrals to social services or the community health nurse as indicated.
- Respect cultural beliefs and incorporate them in the nursing care.
  - How an individual interacts within the family unit is influenced by their cultural beliefs.
- Provide information of the potential adjustments parents, couples, and siblings will encounter as they incorporate the infant into the family.
- Assist parents in identifying ways to assist their other children in their adjustments to the new family member.
- Provide positive verbal reinforcement for their family interactions.
- Provide opportunities for family members to talk about the adjustments within the family.
  - Increased communication can decrease misunderstanding.
- Provide opportunities for couples to talk about the adjustments within their couple relationship and ways to enhance their relationship.

POSTPARTUM BLUES

Postpartum blues, also known as baby blues, occur during the first few postpartum weeks, last for a few days, and affect the majority of women. During this period, the woman feels sad and cries easily but is still able to take care of herself and her infant. (Postpartum psychological complications are discussed in Chapter 14.)

Possible causes of postpartum blues include:

- Changes in hormonal levels
- Fatigue
- Stress from taking on the new role of mother

Signs and symptoms of postpartum blues are:

- Anger
- Anxiety
- Mood swings
- Sadness
- Weeping
- Difficulty sleeping
- Difficulty eating

Nursing Actions

- Provide information to the couple regarding postpartum blues. The nurse should:
  - Explain that this occurs in the majority of postpartum women.
  - Explain the importance of rest in reducing stress.
  - Explain to the woman's partner the importance of emotional and physical support during this period of time.
  - Explain that the woman or family should seek assistance from the health-care provider if the symptoms persist beyond 4 weeks or if symptoms concern the woman or her family, as she may be experiencing postpartum depression.

PARENTS WITH SENSORY IMPAIRMENTS

Parents with sensory impairments such as vision or hearing loss present challenges to nurses and other health-care professionals. These challenges can turn into opportunities to creatively adapt nursing care to meet the needs of these parents. It is important that health-care professionals be aware of the rights of individuals with disabilities, provide information in ways they can understand, and provide care that is sensitive to their needs.

Visual impairment and auditory impairment vary in degree. Visual impairment ranges from visual loss, where the person can read large print, to complete blindness, where the person has no usable vision. Auditory impairment ranges from mild to profound hearing loss. Those with mild hearing loss have enough

---

CRITICAL COMPONENT

Parents With a Sensory Impairment

It is important to treat parents with sensory impairments as people and not as disabilities. They have the same capacity to love and nurture their infant. They have the same need for information and assistance in learning to care for their infant. They are aware of their limitation due to their impairment and, in most cases, have already developed strategies for caring for the infant. Nurses need to assess parents for their knowledge level and their plans for caring for their infants and then modify nursing care to meet the needs of the new parents.

---

hearing to carry on a conversation under ideal conditions. However, people with profound hearing loss usually rely on sign language to communicate and will not be able to converse orally with hearing people.

Nursing Actions

For visually impaired parents, nursing actions are as follows:

- When reporting, use the person's name. Do not call her the "blind woman in room 211."
- When entering a room, address the person by name and introduce yourself and anyone else who is in the room.
- When leaving a room, announce your departure and indicate if others are staying or leaving.
- Speak directly to the person in a clear manner. Do not exaggerate word pronunciation or speak in a loud voice.
- Keep doors, cabinets, and closets closed to prevent injury.
- Use sighted-guide when assisting with ambulation (the visually impaired person holds the elbow of the sighted person when walking). Avoid shoving, pushing, or grabbing unless in an emergency.
- Do not pull on the person's cane to direct her.
- Do not play with a seeing-eye dog while it is in a harness. Ask permission to touch the dog.
- Orient the person to the area of the room or new location after you have guided her to this new area.
  - At a given point (the door or bed), orient the room by describing its contents in logical sequence of progressive order (e.g., "To the right as you lie in the bed is the nightstand with the phone and call button; beside that is the bed curtain and then a chair. Next to the chair is the door to the bathroom").
- Describe the location of food on a plate according to the clock face (e.g., "Potatoes are at 2:00, meat is at 5:00"). Ask the woman if she needs assistance.
- Offer to read printed material or ask for the preferred manner for receiving information that is in printed form.
- Provide space for Braillers (Braille typewriters) and other special equipment.
- Provide teaching in a manner the parents can understand. Example of teaching instructions:
  - Instruct the parents in diapering by having them diaper their child while you explain the steps.
- Provide discharge teaching and instructions in Braille or on audiotape.

For Hearing-Impaired Parents:

- Face the parents when speaking to them.
- Be articulate but do not exaggerate pronunciation.
- Speak in a normal voice volume.
- Be within 6 to 8 feet of the parents when speaking to them. Make sure that light from windows is behind the parents.
- Avoid putting your hand over your mouth or turning your back to the parents when speaking.
- When communicating information with the use of illustrations, provide time for parents to study the illustrations.

- If there is more than one speaker, take turns speaking with clear indication who is speaking.
- Minimize background noises (e.g., turn off the volume of the TV, close the door to the room).
- If there is misunderstanding, do not repeat words louder; instead, use synonyms or other words that mean the same thing.
- Provide discharge teaching and information in written form that parents can easily understand.
- Use graphics and visuals when available.
- Ensure a registered interpreter for the deaf person is present when discussing medical information and teaching. When using an interpreter:
  - Allow sufficient time for the interpreter to complete a thought.
  - Speak directly to the patient and not to the interpreter.
  - Avoid saying, "Tell them . . ."
  - Check the parent for understanding or if they are getting too much information.
  - Allow time for questions and concerns.
- A head nod by the parent may have different meanings, such as "yes" or "continue"; it may not mean that the parent understands.
- Flick lights on and off to get the attention of the parent. Do not shout, wave, or touch to get their attention.
- Be aware that hearing aids amplify sound 6 to 10 times, so shouting and loud noises can be uncomfortable.
- Provide a closed-captioned TV, writing pad, and implements.

- Discuss with the parents how they have adapted their home for the infant.
  - Some parents will use a device that causes a light to flash in response to the infant's cry, alerting parents to check on their infant.
  - Some parents might use closed-circuit TV to monitor the infant from another room.

CRITICAL COMPONENT

Assisting Parents With a Sensory Impairment
Nurses can best assist parents who have sensory impairments by exploring, identifying, and implementing techniques, tools, and alternative ways to:

- Facilitate bonding and attachment.
- Teach parents about infant care.
- Promote a safe environment for the infant.
- Enhance the family dynamics.

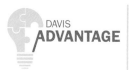

DAVIS
ADVANTAGE

Go to Davis Advantage to complete your learning: strengthen understanding, apply your knowledge, and prepare for the Next Gen NCLEX®.

Clinical Pathway for Transition to Parenthood

Focus of Care	Postpartum Admission	Postpartum 4 to 24 Hours	Postpartum 24 to 48 Hours	Discharge Criteria
Emotional status	Taking-in phase	Progressing toward the taking-hold phase	Taking-hold phase. The woman shows more independence in managing her own and the infant's care.	The woman is able to provide self-care. The woman demonstrates increased confidence in infant care.
Nursing action	Provide care and comfort to the woman. Provide positive reinforcement of appropriate behaviors. Discuss the infant's unique capabilities. Provide early and consistent contact with the infant to facilitate bonding.	Encourage the woman and her family to participate in self- and infant care. Encourage extended infant contact. Observe for bonding and attachment behaviors. Begin discharge education.	Observe for bonding and attachment behaviors, noting any signs of maladaptive behaviors. Provide written or visual information on infant behaviors and characteristics. Teach methods for comforting the infant.	Positive bonding and attachment behaviors are noted. Parents express understanding of infant behaviors and cues. Parents express positive understanding of how to care for the infant. Provide resources for parents to call as needed.
Family dynamics	Parents demonstrate beginning bonding behaviors. Parents begin introducing the infant to the extended family.	Parents demonstrate positive bonding and attachment behaviors. Extended family demonstrate positive and supportive behaviors toward the infant.	Parents continue to demonstrate bonding and attachment behaviors. Extended family demonstrates positive behaviors toward the infant and parents.	Parents demonstrate positive adaptive behaviors.

CONCEPT MAP |

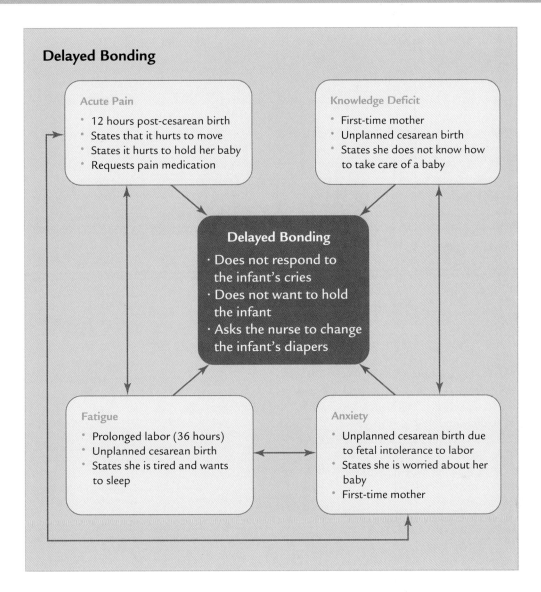

Delayed Bonding

Acute Pain
- 12 hours post-cesarean birth
- States that it hurts to move
- States it hurts to hold her baby
- Requests pain medication

Knowledge Deficit
- First-time mother
- Unplanned cesarean birth
- States she does not know how to take care of a baby

Delayed Bonding
- Does not respond to the infant's cries
- Does not want to hold the infant
- Asks the nurse to change the infant's diapers

Fatigue
- Prolonged labor (36 hours)
- Unplanned cesarean birth
- States she is tired and wants to sleep

Anxiety
- Unplanned cesarean birth due to fetal intolerance to labor
- States she is worried about her baby
- First-time mother

CARE PLANS

Problem 1: Acute pain

Goal: Minimal pain

Outcome: Woman reports that her pain is controlled at a level at or below 2 on a 10-point scale.

Nursing Actions

1. Assess level, location, and type of pain.
2. Assist woman into a comfortable position.
3. Administer pain medications based on assessment data as per orders.
4. Provide an environment that is conducive to relaxation (i.e., low lights, decreased noise, and uninterrupted rest periods).
5. Teach woman relaxation techniques.
6. Demonstrate position when holding infant that promotes maternal comfort (i.e., woman lying on her side with infant next to her, avoiding external pressure on the woman's abdomen).

Problem 2: Knowledge deficit

Goal: Improved knowledge of infant care

Outcome: By time of discharge, mother will state she feels comfortable caring for her infant.

Nursing Actions

1. Assess woman's level of knowledge regarding infant care and cesarean births to identify learning needs and level of understanding.
2. Provide information at woman's level of understanding.
3. Create an environment that is conducive of learning (i.e., turn off TV, close door to room, help mother into a comfortable position).
4. Medicate for pain, if needed, before teaching sessions to promote comfort.
5. Provide information on infant care, bonding and attachment, and post-cesarean birth recovery during several short teaching sessions.

Continued

6. Assist woman with infant care (i.e., bring infant to her so she can change diaper).
7. Praise mother for infant care behaviors.

Problem 3: Fatigue
Goal: Increased level of energy
Outcome: Woman states that she feels rested.

Nursing Actions

1. Assess level of fatigue.
2. Create an environment that is conducive to rest and sleep by:
   a. Assisting woman into comfortable position
   b. Clustering nursing activities to increase the amount of uninterrupted time
   c. Providing pain management techniques (e.g., pain medications, back rubs)
   d. Closing door to room and dimming lights
3. Explain the importance of rest in the healing process.
4. Provide information on high-energy foods.

Problem 4: Anxiety
Goal: Decreased level of anxiety
Outcome: Woman states that she feels comfortable holding and caring for infant.

Nursing Actions

1. Assess the woman's beliefs, attitudes, concerns, and questions regarding infant care and mothering.
2. Discuss with the woman her labor and birth experience and clarify reasons for cesarean birth and any misconceptions.
3. Discuss with the woman the health of her infant and address her concerns.
4. Encourage the woman to hold the infant by:
   a. Explaining the importance of mother–infant contact
   b. Helping her into a comfortable position
   c. Bringing the infant to her
5. Praise the woman for her infant care behaviors.

Case Study

As the nurse in the postpartum unit, you are caring for the Sanchez family. Margarite gave birth to a healthy boy 5 hours ago. Both she and her son are stable. She breastfed her son for 15 minutes after the birth.

You notice that she is lightly touching the top of her infant's head with her fingertips. She comments that she does not feel comfortable holding her baby close to her body for breastfeeding.

Discuss your nursing actions that are based on your knowledge of maternal touch.

List the maternal phase and expected maternal behaviors for this period of time.

List five expected bonding behaviors for this period of time.

The next day you are again assigned to care for the Sanchez family. Mom and baby are stable. José, Margarite's husband, is present during the shift. Margarite and José voice concern about integrating their infant into the family.

Discuss your nursing actions that reflect an understanding of the couple's transition to parenthood.

Discuss specific strategies to decrease sibling rivalry.

Margarite tells you that she thinks she experienced postpartum depression with her first baby. She tells you that she cried a lot during the first week at home but was able to care for herself and her infant.

Discuss the appropriate nursing actions in response to her concerns.

REFERENCES

Amato, P., & Jacob, M. (2010). Can two eggs make a baby? Fertility options for lesbians. In S. Dibble & P. Robertson (Eds.), *Lesbian health 101.* UCSF Nursing Press.

Borneskog, C., Lampic, C., Sydsjo, G., Bladh, M., & Svanberg, A. (2014). How lesbian couples compare with heterosexual in vitro fertilization and spontaneous pregnant couples when it comes to parenting stress? *ACTA Paediatrica, 103,* 537–545. https://doi:10.1111/apa.12568

Bowlby, J. (1969). *Attachment and loss. Vol. 1. Attachment.* Basic Books.

Cox, S., Lashley, C., Hensen, L., & Hans, S. (2021). Making meaning of motherhood: Self and life transition among African American adolescent mothers. *American Journal of Orthopsychiatry, 91,* 120–131. https://doi.org/10.1037/ort0000521

Dayton, C., Buczkoski, R., Murik, M., Goletz, J., Hicks, L., Walsh, T., & Bocknek, E. (2016). Expectant fathers' beliefs and expectations about fathering as they prepare to parent a new infant. *Social Work Research, 40,* 225–237.

Farr, R. (2017). Does parental sexual orientation matter: A longitudinal follow-up of adoptive families with school-aged children. *Developmental Psychology, 53,* 252–264. https://doi.org/10.1037/dev0000228

Feinberg, M. (2003). The internal structure and ecological context of coparenting: A framework for research and intervention. *Parenting: Science and Practice, 3,* 95–131.

Florsheim, P., Moore, D., & Burrow-Sanchez, J. (2020). Helping young fathers across the transition to parenthood. *Zero to Three, 40*(6), 12–19.

Greenberg, M., & Morris, N. (1974). Engrossment: The newborn's impact upon the father. *American Journal of Orthopsychiatry, 44,* 520–531.

Gregg, I. N. (2018). The health care of lesbian women becoming mothers. *Nursing of Women's, Health, 22,* 40–50. https://doi:10.1016/j.nwh.2017.12.003

Klaus, M., & Kennell, J. (1982). *Parent–infant bonding.* C. V. Mosby.

Levesque, S., Bisson, V., Charton, L., & Fernet, M. (2020). Parenting and relational well-being during the transition to parenthood: Challenges for the first-time parents. *Journal of Child and Family Studies, 29,* 1938–1956.

Lindsey, L. (2015). *Gender roles: A sociological perspective* (6th ed.). Routledge.

May, K. (1982). Three phases of father involvement in pregnancy. *Nursing Research, 31,* 337–342.

McManus, A., Hunter, L., & Renn, H. (2006). Lesbian experiences and needs during childbirth: Guidance for health care providers. *Journal of Obstetric, Gynecologic, & Neonatal Nursing, 1,* 13–23.

Mercer, R. (1979). Having another child: "She's a multip—she knows the ropes." *Journal of Maternal Child Nursing, 4,* 301–304.

Mercer, R. (1995). *Becoming a mother: Research from Rubin to the present.* Springer.

Mercer, R. (2004). Becoming a mother versus maternal role attainment. *Journal of Nursing Scholarship, 36,* 226–232.

Mercer, R. (2006). Nursing support of the process of becoming a mother. *Journal of Obstetric, Gynecologic & Neonatal Nursing, 35,* 649–651.

Newport, F. (2018). *U.S. estimate of LGBT population to 4.5%.* https://news.gallup.com/poll/234863/estimate-LGBT-population-rises.aspxpolitics

Poushter, J., & Kent, N. (2020). *The global divide on homosexuality.* http://www.pewresearch.org/global/202/06/25/global-divide-on-homosexuality-persists

Rubin, R. (1961). Puerperal change. *Nursing Outlook, 9,* 753–755.

Rubin, R. (1963). Maternal touch. *Nursing Outlook, 11,* 828–831.

Rubin, R. (1967). Attainment of the maternal role. Part 1. Processes. *Nursing Research, 16,* 237–346.

Rubin, R. (1984). *Maternal identity and the maternal experience.* Springer.

Wojnar, D., & Katzenmeyer, A. (2014). Experiences of preconception, pregnancy, and new motherhood for lesbian nonbiological mothers. *Journal of Obstetric, Gynecologic, & Neonatal Nursing, 45,* 50–60. https://doi: 10.1111/1552-6909.12270

Postpartum Complications and Nursing Care

14

LaShea Haynes, RNC, MEd, MSN, AGCNS-BC
Paulina Van, RN, PhD, CNE
Roberta F. Durham RN, PhD

LEARNING OUTCOMES

Upon completion of this chapter, the student will be able to:

1. Describe the primary causes of postpartum hemorrhage (PPH) and the related nursing actions and medical care.
2. Describe the primary postpartum infections and the related nursing actions and medical care.
3. Describe the primary postpartum psychological complications and the related nursing actions and medical care.
4. Describe the primary postpartum cardiovascular complications and the related nursing actions and medical care.
5. Describe how social determinants of health affect maternal outcomes.

CONCEPTS

Caring
Clinical Judgment
Collaboration
Comfort
Communication
Elimination
Evidence-Based Practice
Family
Fluid and Electrolytes
Grief and Loss
Health Promotion
Infection
Mobility
Mood and Affect
Nutrition
Oxygenation
Perfusion
Person-Centered Concepts
Physiological Concepts
Psychosocial Concepts
Safety
Self-Care
Stress and Coping
Teaching and Learning

Nursing Diagnosis

- At risk for hemorrhage related to uterine atony, lacerations, retained placental tissue, or hematoma
- At risk for infection related to tissue trauma or prolonged rupture of membranes (PROM)
- At risk for mood disorders related to stress, hormonal changes, lack of rest, or lack of social support
- At risk for increased maternal morbidity or mortality related to health equity and social determinants of health

Nursing Outcomes

- The woman's fundus will remain firm, and lochia will be within normal range.
- The woman will remain asymptomatic of infection.
- The woman indicates she feels respected, listened to, and her needs are being met.

INTRODUCTION

The postpartum period is a critical time to ensure women and their newborns are healthy. It is important to closely monitor a woman's health during recovery—especially if she experienced complications during pregnancy or childbirth—as over half of maternal deaths occur during the first days, weeks, and months after birth. Even healthy women who give birth are at risk for these complications. The most common yet preventable causes of severe maternal morbidity (SMM) and maternal mortality include obstetric hemorrhage, infection, perinatal mood and anxiety disorders (PMADs), hypertensive disorders of pregnancy, and venous thromboembolism (VTE). Each of these will be addressed in this chapter.

Most women do not experience complications during the postpartum period, but when they do, it can be life-threatening and disrupt the family unit. Most complications occur after discharge and may require readmission to the hospital. Many hospitals do not allow the infant to be readmitted with the mother, so readmission for treatment of complications can interfere with the attachment process and increase stress within the family.

A focus of postpartum nursing care is to reduce women's risks for complications related to childbirth and identify complications early for prompt interventions. Women need to be evaluated by their health-care provider when a complication is suspected. Pregnancy can create conditions that may cause problems as long as a year after delivery. Patient teaching and support should include instruction regarding the signs for concern and the importance of seeking medical care immediately. These signs include:

- Persistent or worsening headache
- Vision changes
- Breathing difficulty
- Excessive swelling of hands or face
- Fever

CRITICAL COMPONENT

Risk Reduction for Postpartum Complications

Reducing a woman's risk for postpartum complications is a major component of postpartum nursing care. Nursing actions to reduce risk are:

- Reviewing the prenatal and intrapartum records for risk factors such as anemia, long labor, and operative vaginal delivery and addressing these risk factors in planning care
- Assessing for signs of a postpartum complication and intervening appropriately
  - Early identification and treatment decrease the impact of the complication.
- Assisting the woman with ambulation or appropriate activity for women with disabilities
  - Ambulation and activities based on the woman's abilities decrease risk of VTE.
- Preventing overdistended bladder
  - Overdistended bladder can place the woman at risk for uterine atony, neurogenic bladder, or cystitis.
- Using good hand washing techniques by health-care workers, patients, and visitors
- Promoting health with appropriate diet, fluids, activity, and rest
- Assessing for psychological complications
- Providing culturally appropriate care for women of color, women with disabilities, women with same-sex partners, and patients who identify as lesbian, gay, bisexual, transgender, and queer (LGBTQ).

SEVERE MATERNAL MORBIDITY

SMM includes unexpected perinatal outcomes that result in significant short- or long-term consequences to a woman's health. It is not entirely clear why SMM is increasing, but hospitals can take action steps and implement interventions to improve response, recognition, interventions, and care of their patients. The California Maternal Quality Care Collaborative (CMQCC) has a toolkit with clear, well-researched steps and interventions that can improve outcomes in national high-risk populations (CMQCC, 2015).

Documented contributing factors of SMM in the literature include lack of access to appropriate level of care, health inequities, social determinants of health, lack of transportation, preexisting chronic medical conditions, and cesarean deliveries. Over the past decade, SMM in the United States has increased by 75% for complications associated with delivery, specifically for postpartum hemorrhage (PPH). More than 50,000 women experienced

SMM, with a mortality rate of 18.0 per 100,000, higher than in many other developed countries (Callaghan et al., 2012; D'Alton et al., 2019). As noted in Chapter 10, identifying potential problems early, developing written protocols that outline a clear plan of response for common emergencies, and using mock drills to train staff in protocol responses can help ensure that no tasks are redundant or omitted and ultimately create a more controlled environment that promotes positive health outcomes. Communication and teamwork are an essential part of safety and enhanced patient outcomes. Effective, patient-centered communication facilitates interception and correction of harmful conditions and errors. All team members, including women, their families, physicians, midwives, and nurses, have roles in identifying potential harm during labor and birth (Lyndon et al., 2015).

A review in action's report from nine maternal morbidity and mortality review committees estimated 63.2% of the pregnancy-related deaths were preventable (Building U.S. Capacity to Review and Prevent Maternal Deaths, 2018; Jackson & Haynes, 2020). A current national initiative to improve outcomes is the Safe Motherhood Initiative (Box 14-1), focused on the following measures:

- Early opportunities exist to assess risk for, anticipate chances of, and plan for an obstetric hemorrhage (ensuring inductions of high-risk patients are done on optimal dates and times for a multidisciplinary approach, utilizing a risk assessment tool on every patient; every time, ensuring staff have proper education and competency to care for high-risk moms during emergencies) (James & Suplee, 2021).
- Multidisciplinary coordination and preparation, particularly with the blood bank, is critical to provide safe obstetrical care.
- A standardized approach to obstetric hemorrhage includes a clearly defined, staged checklist of appropriate actions to take in an emergency that can help improve patient outcomes.
- Women of color experience higher rates of postpartum complications, including death, as compared with White women (Altman et. al., 2020; Centers for Disease Control and Prevention [CDC], 2019b; Davis et al., 2019). These adverse outcomes can be attributed to a history of racism, discrimination, and exclusion; lack of adequate access to care; structural determinants of health; institutional implicit bias and barriers;

BOX 14-1 | Maternal Safety Bundle: Obstetric Hemorrhage

A leading cause of maternal morbidity and mortality is failure to recognize excessive blood loss during childbirth. Women die from obstetric hemorrhage because effective interventions are not initiated early enough. Hemorrhage is the most frequent cause of SMM and preventable maternal mortality and therefore is an ideal topic for the initial national maternity patient safety bundle. These safety bundles outline critical clinical practices that should be implemented in every maternity unit (ACOG, 2015; 2022; Main et al., 2015). Obstetric Hemorrhage: Patient Safety Bundle from the Alliance for Innovation on Maternal Health, the National Partnership for Maternal Safety, Council on Patient Safety in Women's Health Care.

Readiness — Every Unit/Team

- Develop processes for the management of patients with obstetric hemorrhage including: a designated interdisciplinary rapid response; a facility-wide, hemorrhage management plan; massive transfusion protocols including patients who decline blood products; and review of policies to identify and address organizational root causes of racial and ethnic disparities in outcomes of obstetric hemorrhage.
- Maintain a hemorrhage cart and ensure immediate access to first- and second-line hemorrhage medications.
- Conduct interprofessional and interdepartmental team-based drills

Recognition and Prevention — Every Patient

- Assess and communicate hemorrhage risk to all team members as clinical conditions change or high-risk conditions are identified; at admission, during labor and birth and postpartum.
- Measure and communicate cumulative blood loss to all team members, using quantitative approaches and actively manage the third stage of labor per department-wide protocols.
- Provide ongoing education to all patients on obstetric hemorrhage

Response — Every Event

- Utilize a facility-wide obstetric hemorrhage emergency management plan
- Provide trauma-informed support for patients.

Reporting and Systems Learning — Every Unit

- Establish a culture of multidisciplinary planning, huddles, and post-event debriefs
- Perform multidisciplinary reviews of serious complications per established facility criteria to identify system issues.
- Monitor outcomes and process measures related to obstetric hemorrhage.
- Establish processes for data reporting and the sharing of data with the obstetric team.

Respectful, Equitable, and Supportive Care — Every Unit/Provider/Team Member

- Include each patient that experienced an obstetric hemorrhage and their identified support network as respected members of and contributors to the multidisciplinary care team and as participants in patient-centered huddles and debriefs.
- Engage in open, transparent, and empathetic communication with pregnant and postpartum people and their identified support network to understand diagnoses, options, and treatment plans, including consent regarding blood products and blood product alternatives.

Summarized from American College of Obstetrics and Gynecologists. (2022). *Patient safety bundle: Obstetric hemorrhage. Council on Patient Safety in Women's Health Care.* American College of Obstetrics and Gynecologists. Available at https://safehealthcareforeverywoman.org/patient-safety-bundles/obstetric-hemorrhage. Retrieved 2022.

inadequate relationship building; and communication barriers with health-care providers (Altman et al., 2019; Howell et al., 2018; Rogers et al., 2020).

- The family structure has evolved, yet health-care providers' knowledge and care models for parents who identify as same-sex and transgender has not kept pace (Gregg, 2018; Ruud, 2018). These parents may experience similar obstacles and interactions as those described among women of color (Smith & Turell, 2017).
- A systematic review reported that women with physical, sensory, or intellectual and developmental disabilities were at increased risk for postpartum complications (Tarasoff et al., 2020). Consider culturally sensitive models of care, strategies to foster authentic interpersonal interactions that nurture and recognize their individualized life experiences, as you support and guide them as parents of their newborns.

HEMORRHAGE

PPH is typically defined as blood loss greater than 500 mL for vaginal deliveries and greater than 1,000 mL for cesarean deliveries with a 10% drop in hemoglobin or hematocrit (H&H; Griffith-Gilbert & Rousseau, 2020). The American College of Obstetricians and Gynecologists (ACOG) defines *hemorrhage* as cumulative blood loss of 1,000 mL or greater or blood loss accompanied by symptoms of hypovolemia within 24 hours following the birth process (includes intrapartum loss) (ACOG, 2014).

Patients with PPH are treated using a two-pronged approach: (1) resuscitation and management of obstetric hemorrhage and potential hypovolemic shock and (2) identification and management of the underlying cause(s) of the hemorrhage. Hemorrhagic and hypovolemic shock are emergent situations in which perfusion of body organs may become severely compromised and death may ensue. Aggressive treatment is necessary to prevent adverse sequelae (e.g., cellular death, fluid overload, acute respiratory distress syndrome [ARDS], or oxygen toxicity).

Common clinical symptoms of inadequate intravascular volume (i.e., hypovolemia) that necessitate blood replacement include evidence of hemorrhage (i.e., loss of a large amount of blood externally or internally in a short period of time), evidence of hypovolemic shock (i.e., increasing pulse; cool, clammy skin; rapid breathing; restlessness; and reduced urine output), or a significant decrease in H&H. Signs and symptoms of maternal hypovolemia may include tachycardia, hypotension, tachypnea, low oxygen saturation (less than 95%), oliguria, pallor, dizziness, or altered mental status (ACOG, 2014). Excessive bleeding immediately postpartum can cause a number of symptoms beyond hypovolemia such as pallor, light-headedness, weakness, palpitations, diaphoresis, restlessness, confusion, air hunger, and syncope. Clinical signs and symptoms such as hypotension, dizziness, pallor, and oliguria do not occur until blood loss is substantial (James & Suplee, 2021).

The primary source of blood loss is from the placental site. The increase of blood volume and red blood cells (RBCs) during pregnancy normally compensates for the blood loss that occurs following the detachment of the placenta. Additionally, physiological changes during pregnancy and immediately after expulsion of the placenta decrease the amount of blood loss

---

CRITICAL COMPONENT

Quantification of Blood Loss After Birth

Normal blood loss for a vaginal birth is approximately 500 mL within 24 hours. Visual estimation of blood loss (EBL) is common practice in obstetrics; however, the inaccuracy of EBL has been well-established and blood loss can be underestimated by up to 50% (Association of Women's Health, Obstetric and Neonatal Nurses [AWHONN], 2021b). AWHONN recommends that cumulative blood loss be formally measured or quantified after every birth. Inaccurate measurement of postpartum blood loss has the following implications:

- Visual EBL has long been established as an inaccurate measure that can lead to delays in timely recognition.
- Overestimation can lead to costly, invasive, and unnecessary treatments such as blood transfusions that expose women to unnecessary risks.
- Direct measurement of blood loss can be accomplished by two complementary approaches.
  - The easiest method is to collect blood in calibrated, under-buttocks drapes for vaginal birth.
  - The second approach is to weigh blood-soaked items and clots. These items can be collected in a single bag and weighed using a gravimetric method. By using this method, the weight of dry pads is subtracted from the total weight to obtain an estimate of blood loss. Weigh all blood-soaked materials and clots to determine cumulative volume.

AWHONN, 2021b.

---

from the placental site. These physiological changes include the following:

- Hypercoagulability
- Factor VIII complex increases during pregnancy.
- Factor V increases following placental separation.
- Platelet activity increases during pregnancy.
- Fibrin formation increases during pregnancy.
- Contractions of the uterine myometrium
- Blood vessels that supply the placental site pass through the myometrium, an interlacing network of smooth muscle fibers.
- Contractions of the myometrium compress the blood vessels at the placental site, thus decreasing the amount of blood loss.

An estimated 2% to 6% of women who have a vaginal birth will have a PPH (Salera-Vieira, 2021). Worldwide, PPH is among the top five causes of maternal mortality (Belfort, 2018). The term PPH describes an event, not a diagnosis. Major complications include hemorrhagic shock related to hypovolemia, disseminated intravascular coagulation (DIC), organ failure, and death. The primary causes of PPH in descending order of frequency are the "4 Ts":

- Tone: Uterine atony
- Tissue: Retained placental fragments
- Trauma: Lower genital tract lacerations
- Thrombin disorders: DIC (Table 14-1).

PPH is classified as primary (early) and secondary (late) hemorrhage. Primary or early PPH occurs within the first 24 hours after

TABLE 14-1   Precipitating Factors for Hemorrhage—the 4 Ts

	MEDICAL FACTORS	SIGNS AND SYMPTOMS	NURSING ACTIONS
Tone (uterine atony)	• Large baby • High parity • Rapid labor • Fever • Fibroids	• Bleeding may be slow and steady, or profuse • Large, boggy uterus • Clots	• Assist the uterus to contract via massage or medications. • Monitor bleeding—weigh pads and Chux (1 gm = 1 mL). • Maintain fluid balance (may need second IV, Foley catheter). • Monitor vital signs and laboratory results; blood type and screen if ordered. • Administer oxygen 10–12 L via face mask. • Keep patient warm.
Tissue	• Retained or abnormal placenta	• In addition to the previously noted items, uterus may not respond to interventions. • Uterus may remain larger than normal. • Strings of tissue may be seen in the blood.	• Call provider to assess; D&C may be needed. • Monitor for signs of shock. • Administer oxygen if indicated.
Trauma	• Lacerations	• Firm uterus with continued bleeding • Steady trickle of unclotted, bright red blood	• Call provider to evaluate, locate, and repair laceration. • Monitor vital signs and lochia. • Weigh pads and Chux to monitor blood loss.
	• Hematoma (may be vulvar, vaginal, cervical, or retroperitoneal)	• Firm uterus • Sudden onset of painful perineal pressure • Bulging area just under the skin • Difficulty voiding or sitting	• Assess for visible hematoma. • Call provider to assess. • Anticipate possible excision and ligation if greater than 3 cm. • Consider indwelling catheter. • Continue to assess vital signs, blood loss, and fluid maintenance. • Provide pain management, including ice to the area.
Thrombin disorders	• Preeclampsia • Stillbirth	• Disseminated (systemic) intra-vascular coagulopathy (DIC) • Oozing from IV sites • Nosebleeds • Petechiae • Bleeding gums • Hypotension and other signs of shock • Abnormal clotting laboratory values	• Early recognition is a key factor in survival. • Confirm accurate blood loss estimates. • Monitor laboratory values, vital signs, and intake and output. • Manage systemic manifestations such as volume replacement, platelets IV, and oxygen by mask at 10 L/min.

childbirth and is caused by uterine atony, lacerations, or hematomas. The greatest risk for early PPH is during the first hour after birth because large venous areas are exposed after placental separation. Late or secondary PPH occurs 24 hours to 6 weeks postdelivery and is caused by hematomas, subinvolution, or retained placental tissue.

Risk Factors

Preexisting risk factors for PPH include the following:

● High parity
● Previous PPH
● Previous uterine surgery
● Coagulation defects or medical disorders of clotting

Current pregnancy risk factors for PPH include the following:

● Antepartal hemorrhage
● Uterine overdistention (macrosomia, multiple gestation, or polyhydramnios)
● Chorioamnionitis or intra-amniotic infection
● Placental abnormality (succenturiate lobe, placenta previa, placenta accreta, abruptio placentae, hydatidiform mole)
● Fetal death

Risk factors for PPH associated with labor and birth include the following:

- Rapid or prolonged labor
- Use of tocolytic or halogenated anesthetic agents
- Large episiotomy
- Operative vaginal birth
- Cesarean birth
- Abnormally located or attached placenta
- Inversion of uterus

Nursing Actions

The following assessments and interventions are included in comprehensive care during PPH based on the individual clinical situation (James & Suplee, 2021):

- Plan for care and assessment to ensure early recognition of hemorrhage.
- Ask for help.
- Packed RBCs should be typed and cross-matched if excessive blood loss is anticipated (American Academy of Pediatrics [AAP] & ACOG, 2017; James & Suplee, 2021).
- Accurately assess blood loss.
- Weigh peripads or Chux dressing (1 g = 1 mL) (keep a gram scale on unit). Quantification of blood loss assessment is superior to estimated blood loss.
- Assess excessive bleeding, which is defined as one perineal pad saturated within 15 minutes.
- Look for severe loss that may occur with steady, slow seepage.
- Assess vital signs at least every 15 minutes, or more often if indicated. Mean arterial pressure (MAP), which is the mean blood pressure (BP) in arterial circulation, should be assessed because the first BP response to hypovolemia may be a pulse pressure decreased to 30 mm Hg or less (Cunningham et al., 2018).
- Assess for tachypnea and tachycardia, which may occur while BP is constant or slightly lowered.
- Assess for shock. Keep in mind that normal vital signs do not mean the woman is not in shock. Common signs of hypovolemic shock are not evident until 10% to 30% of the total blood volume is lost. This is because pregnancy-induced hypervolemia that accounts for the 30% to 70% increase in blood volume (an additional 1 to 2 L) prevents symptoms with the typical 500 mL blood loss (ACOG, 2017b). Remember the initial response of vasoconstriction shunts blood to vital organs to maintain their function and viability.
- Maintain accurate measurements of intake and output.
- Ensure large-bore (14, 16, or 18 gauge) needle intravenous (IV) access (two sites preferably).
- Replace volume with crystalloid (normal saline or lactated Ringer's) 1:3 or colloid (Hespan or albumin) 1:1 while waiting for blood or deciding on transfusion. The goal is to produce at least 30 mL/hour of urine output and hematocrit values of 30% (Cunningham et al., 2018).
- Draw blood for H&H (compare with prenatal or admission values), type and cross-match, perform coagulation studies (i.e., fibrinogen, prothrombin time, partial thromboplastin time (PTT), fibrin split products, and fibrin degradation products), and blood chemistry. The blood bank should be notified that transfusion may be necessary.
- Arterial blood may be drawn for blood gas determinations.
- If blood transfusion is necessary, each unit of packed RBCs (240 mL is the usual volume of 1 U) can be expected to increase hematocrit 3 percentage points and hemoglobin by 1 g/dL. Packed RBCs contain RBCs, white blood cells (WBCs), and plasma (ACOG, 2017c).
- Deficits in clotting factors may necessitate cryoprecipitate (i.e., for fibrinogen deficiency), recombinant activated factor VII, or fresh frozen plasma (FFP) (i.e., for decreased levels of clotting factors) (AAP & ACOG, 2017).
- Use correct uterine massage to avoid ligament damage and potential uterine inversion and massage with only the force needed to effect contraction or expulsion of clots. Overaggressive uterine massage may tire muscle fibers and contribute to further atony.
- Anticipate pain management needs for fundal massage and uterotonic medications for treatment of hemorrhage.
- Insert a Foley catheter to empty the bladder and allow accurate measurement of output. A full bladder can impede complete uterine contraction.
- Administer prescribed medication per hemorrhage protocol. Labor and birth units should have the following pharmacologic agents available: oxytocin, methylergonovine, ergot alkaloids, 15-methyl-prostaglandin F2α, prostaglandin F2α, misoprostol, and dinoprostone (AAP & ACOG, 2017; ACOG, 2017c).
- Apply pulse oximeter and administer oxygen according to unit protocol. This is usually accomplished with a nonrebreather facemask at 10 to 12 L/min.
- Continuous electrocardiographic monitoring may be indicated for hypotension, continuous bleeding, tachycardia, or shock.
- Elevate the legs to a 20- to 30-degree angle to increase venous return.
- Prepare for additional interventions if the situation does not resolve. These include packing the uterus with gauze or using a balloon tamponade, dilatation and curettage, exploratory laparotomy, bilateral uterine artery ligation, arterial embolization, and other surgical techniques. In some cases, PPH may require a transfer or return to the surgical suite. The surgical team should be notified that they may be needed.

CLINICAL JUDGMENT

Examples of Threshold Parameters

Clinical situations such as PPH or infection mandate further actions by the health-care team according to protocol, such as bringing the attending physician to the patient's bedside immediately. Some clinical emergencies are preceded by a period of instability during which timely intervention may help avoid disaster. Obstetric (OB) emergency teams, sometimes referred to as an OB stat team for obstetrical emergencies, are rapid response teams in the perinatal department. Perinatal nurses need to recognize that certain changes in a patient's condition can indicate an emergency that requires immediate intervention. A "red" trigger typically mandates an immediate bedside evaluation, whereas a "yellow" trigger indicates the need for further clinical evaluation (ACOG, 2014).

Careful assessment and interpretation of maternal vital signs are critical inpatient care during active bleeding. Remember, normal signs of hypovolemic shock are sometimes not evident until 10% to 30% of the total blood volume is lost. This is due to the pregnancy-induced hypervolemia. The initial response of vasoconstriction shunts blood to vital organs to maintain their function and viability (James & Suplee, 2021). Signs and symptoms of maternal hypovolemia may include tachycardia, hypotension, tachypnea, low oxygen saturation (less than 95%), oliguria, pallor, dizziness, or altered mental status (ACOG, 2014). Excessive bleeding immediately postpartum can cause several symptoms beyond hypovolemia such as pallor, lightheadedness, weakness, palpitations, diaphoresis, restlessness, confusion, air hunger, and syncope. Clinical signs and symptoms such as hypotension, dizziness, pallor, and oliguria do not occur until blood loss is substantial.

	RED TRIGGER	YELLOW TRIGGER
Temperature; °C	<35 or >38	35–36
Systolic BP; mm Hg	<90 or >160	150–160 or 90–100
Diastolic BP; mm Hg	>100	90–100
Heart rate; beats/min	<40 or >120	100–120 or 40–50
Respiratory rate; breaths/min	<10 or >30	21–30
Oxygen saturation; %	<95	

BP, blood pressure.

CRITICAL COMPONENT

Indications of Primary Postpartum Hemorrhage

- A 10% decrease in the hemoglobin or hematocrit postbirth
- Saturation of the peripad within 15 minutes
- A fundus that remains boggy after fundal massage
- Tachycardia (late sign)
- Decrease in BP (late sign)

Because failure to recognize and intervene related to obstetric hemorrhage can result in SMM and even mortality, protocols are used to stage obstetric hemorrhage and outline a protocol and standard line of care. Box 14-2 presents the elements of common obstetric hemorrhage protocols.

Blood transfusion or cross-matching is warranted for certain obstetric events (Box 14-3). In cases of severe obstetric hemorrhage, at least 4 units of blood products may be necessary to save the life of a maternity patient. Hospitals are encouraged to coordinate efforts with their laboratories, blood banks, and quality improvement departments to determine the appropriateness of transfusion and quantity of blood products necessary for these patients.

Uterine Atony

Uterine atony, or decreased tone in the uterine muscle, is the major cause of primary PPH. Uterine contractions constrict the open vessels at the placental site and assist in decreasing blood loss. When the uterus is relaxed, the vessels are less constricted

---

BOX 14-2 | Staging Obstetric Hemorrhage: Elements of Common Protocols

Stage 1 May Be Labeled Mild Hemorrhage

Hemorrhage: Blood loss greater than 500 mL to 1,000 mL vaginal OR blood loss greater than 1,000 mL cesarean with normal vital signs and laboratory values

Initial Steps

Ensure 16G or 18G IV access.

Increase IV fluid (crystalloid without oxytocin).

Insert indwelling urinary catheter.

Perform fundal massage.

Medications

Increase oxytocin, additional uterotonics

Oxytocin (Pitocin), 10 to 40 units per 500 to 1,000 mL solution

Methylergonovine (Methergine), 0.2 mg IM (may repeat)

15-methyl PGF2α (Hemabate, Carboprost), 250 mcg IM (may repeat in q15 minutes, maximum 8 doses)

Misoprostol (Cytotec), 800 to 1,000 mcg PR 600 mcg PO or 800 mcg PL

Blood Bank

Type and cross-match two units RBCs

Action

Determine etiology and treat. Consider the 4 Ts—tone (i.e., atony), trauma (i.e., laceration), tissue (i.e., retained products), and thrombin (i.e., coagulation dysfunction).

Prepare the operating room, if clinically indicated (optimize visualization and examination).

Stage 2 Moderate Hemorrhage

Hemorrhage: Continued bleeding EBL up to 1,500 mL OR greater than 2 uterotonics with normal vital signs and laboratory values

May see some hypotension, tachycardia, and anxiety

Initial Steps

Mobilize additional help

Place second IV (16G to 18G)

Draw STAT labs (CBC, coagulation studies, fibrinogen)

Prepare OR

Continued

BOX 14-2 | Staging Obstetric Hemorrhage: Elements of Common Protocols—cont'd

Medications

Continue Stage 1 medications

Blood Bank

Obtain 2 units RBCs (DO NOT wait for labs. Transfuse per clinical signs and symptoms). Thaw 2 units FFP.

Action

Escalate therapy with goal of hemostasis.

Huddle and move to Stage 3 if continued blood loss or abnormal vital signs.

Stage 3 or Severe Hemorrhage

Hemorrhage: Continued bleeding with EBL greater than 1,500 mL or greater than 200 mL OR greater than 2 units RBCs given OR patient at risk for occult bleeding or coagulopathy OR any patient with abnormal vital signs, labs, or oliguria

Typically see hypotension; tachycardia; tachypnea; decreased urine output; cool, pale skin; restlessness; or anxiety.

With hemorrhage of greater than 2,500 mL, patient has lost 40% of blood volume and may be in shock.

Initial Steps

Mobilize additional help.

Move to operating room.

Announce clinical status (vital signs, cumulative blood loss, etiology).

Outline and communicate plan.

Medications

Continue Stage 1 medications

Blood Bank

Initiate massive transfusion protocol (if clinical coagulopathy, add cryoprecipitate, and consult for additional agents).

Action

Achieve hemostasis, interventions based on etiology

Stage 4

Hemorrhage: Cardiovascular collapse (massive hemorrhage, profound hypovolemic shock, or AFE)

Initial Steps

Mobilize additional resources

Medications

ACLS

Blood Bank

Simultaneous aggressive massive transfusion

Action

Immediate surgical intervention to ensure hemostasis (hysterectomy)

ACOG, 2015; Main et al., 2015.

BOX 14-3 | Massive Transfusion Protocol

Blood Bank: Massive Transfusion Protocol

To provide safe obstetric care, institutions must:

- Have a functioning massive transfusion protocol (MTP).
- Have a functioning emergency release protocol (a minimum of 4 units of O-negative or uncross-matched RBCs).
- Have the ability to obtain 6 units PRBCs and 4 units FFP (compatible or type-specific) for a bleeding patient.
- Have a mechanism in place to obtain platelets and additional products in a timely fashion.

Example of a Blood Bank: Massive Transfusion Protocol

I. Patient Currently Bleeding and at Risk for Uncontrollable Bleeding

  1. Activate MTP—call (add number) and say, "Activate massive transfusion protocol."

  2. Nursing and anesthesia draw stat labs

     a. Type and cross-match

     b. Hemoglobin and platelet count, PT(INR)/PTT, fibrinogen, and ABG (as needed)

II. Immediate Need for Transfusion (type and cross-match not yet available)

  Give 2 to 4 units O-negative PRBCs ("OB emergency release")

III. Anticipate Ongoing Massive Blood Needs and Obtain Massive Transfusion Pack

  Administer as needed in the following ratio 6:4:

  6 units PRBCs

  4 units FFP

  1 apheresis pack of platelets

IV. Initial Lab Results

  If normal → anticipate ongoing bleeding → repeat massive transfusion pack → bleeding controlled → deactivate MTP

  If abnormal → repeat massive transfusion pack → repeat laboratory tests → consider cryoprecipitate and consultation for alternative coagulation agents (prothrombin complex concentrate, recombinant Factor VIIa, tranexamic acid)

ABG, arterial blood gas; FFP, fresh frozen plasma; PRBC, packed red blood cells; PT, prothrombin time; PTT, partial thromboplastin time; RBC, red blood cell.

ACOG, 2015.

and the woman experiences increased blood loss from the placental site. Uterine atony often occurs in women:

- Whose uterus was overdistended by a multiple pregnancy or large fetus
- Who have given birth more than five times
- Who had prolonged or dysfunctional labor with or without oxytocin augmentation

Assessment Findings

- Soft (boggy) fundus versus firm fundus
- Saturation of the peripad within 15 minutes
- Slow and steady or sudden and massive bleeding
- Presence of blood clots
- Pale color and clammy skin
- Anxiety and confusion
- Tachycardia
- Hypotension

Medical Management

- Medications used for active bleeding: oxytocin, methylergonovine, misoprostol, and carboprost to stimulate uterine contractions
    - After expulsion of the placenta, oxytocin may be given intramuscularly (IM) or in an IV solution titrated as indicated.
- Bimanual compression of the uterus per provider (Fig. 14–1)
- IV therapy initially to reduce risk of hypovolemia
    - Isotonic, non-dextrose crystalloid solutions (normal saline or lactated Ringer's)
    - A ratio of 3 to 1, 3 liters of IV solution replacement per liter of estimated blood loss
    - Blood replacement to reduce risk for hemorrhagic shock
- Platelets, FFP, and cryoprecipitate replacement in management of massive obstetric hemorrhagic shock
- Nonsurgical interventions such as uterine packing with gauze or uterine tamponade
    - Uterine tamponade: A catheter device with a 300-mL balloon is inserted into the uterus via the vagina. The catheter balloon is filled with approximately 300 mL saline, enough to exert pressure on vessels at the placental site and stop the bleeding.

- Surgical interventions such as dilation and curettage (D&C) or hysterectomy may be indicated when all other treatments have failed to contract the uterus.

Nursing Actions

In addition to nursing actions for hemorrhage if indicated, nursing actions for uterine atony include the following:

- Review prenatal and intrapartum records for PPH risk factors and closely monitor women who are at risk for uterine atony.
- Assess for a displaced uterus; it will generally be to the patient's left. An overdistended bladder can displace the uterus and cause it to relax. When the uterus is displaced to the side during fundal examination:
    - Assist the woman to void in the bathroom, bedside commode, or bedpan, then reassess location and firmness of fundus and amount and characteristics of lochia.
    - Catheterize the woman if she cannot void or experiences small, frequent voiding.
    - Use a bladder scanner to assess urine volume.
- Assess the fundus for degree of firmness. If boggy:
    - Massage the uterus and reassess every 5 to 15 minutes (Fig. 14–2).
    - Put baby to breast to initiate release of oxytocin.
- Assess lochia for amount and clots.
    - Express clots, which can interfere with uterine contraction.
    - Weigh bloodied pads and linens to obtain an accurate amount of blood loss: 1 g = 1 mL of blood.
- Review laboratory tests such as H&H.
- Notify physician or midwife of abnormal assessment findings or test results.
    - Establish IV site with large-bore IV catheter.
    - Administer oxytocin, methylergonovine, misoprostol, or carboprost (Hemabate) to stimulate uterine contractions as ordered.
    - Start and monitor blood transfusions as ordered and per protocol.
- Provide emotional support and teaching to both the woman and partner, because PPH can increase the anxiety and stress levels of the patient and her family.

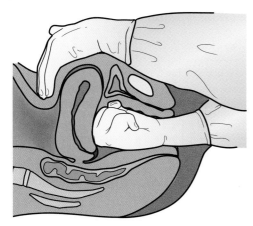

FIGURE 14–1 Bimanual compression of the uterus.

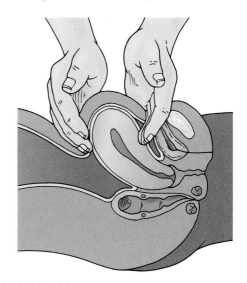

FIGURE 14–2 Fundal massage.

SAFE AND EFFECTIVE NURSING CARE: Understanding Medication

Uterotonics and Medication for Postpartum Hemorrhage

Labor and birth units should have pharmacologic agents for proper management of PPH (James & Suplee, 2021). Oxytocin, the recommended uterotonic drug to prevent PPH, should be used to manage the third stage of labor for all births (ACOG, 2017c; AWHONN, 2021a; Suplee & Janke, 2020).

Oxytocin (Pitocin)

- Classification: Hormone or oxytocic
- Route: Oxytocin should be administered only by the IM or IV route, not by IV push. As a high-alert medication, IV oxytocin premixed bags should be infused via an IV infusion pump to control administration.
- Prominently and clearly label with bright-colored labeling.
- Store separately to prevent a 1,000-mL IV bag with oxytocin being mistaken for a plain 1,000-mL bag used for IV fluid resuscitation bolus.
- Administer IV oxytocin by providing a bolus dose followed by a total minimum infusion time of 4 hours after birth. For women who are at high risk for a PPH, continuation beyond 4 hours is recommended. Rate and duration should be titrated according to uterine tone and bleeding.
- Common dosing is 20 units oxytocin in 1 L normal saline or lactated Ringer's solution with an initial bolus rate of 1,000 mL/hour bolus for 30 minutes (equals 10 units) followed by a maintenance rate of 125 mL/hour over 3.5 hours (equals remaining 10 units).
- Give oxytocin 10 units IM in women without IV access.
- Actions: Stimulates uterine smooth muscle that produces intermittent contractions. Has vasopressor and antidiuretic properties.
- Indications: Control of postpartum bleeding after placental expulsion.

Methylergonovine (Methergine)

- Classification: Oxytocic or ergot alkaloids
- Route or dosage: PO 200 to 400 mcg (0.4 to 0.6 mg) every 6 to 12 hours for 2 to 7 days. IM 200 mcg (0.2 mg) every 2 to 4 hours up to 5 doses. IV (for emergencies only) same dosage as IM.
- Actions: Directly stimulates smooth and vascular smooth muscles causing sustaining uterine contractions.
- Indications: Prevent or treat postpartum hemorrhage, uterine atony, or subinvolution. Contraindicated in hypertensive patients.

Carboprost—Tromethamine (Hemabate)

- Classification: Prostaglandin
- Route or dosage: IM 250 mcg injected into a large muscle or the uterus

- Actions: Contraction of uterine muscle
- Indications: Uterine atony

Misoprostol (Cytotec)

- Classification: Antiulcer or prostaglandins
- Route or dosage: PO or rectally 200 to 1,000 mcg
- Actions: Acts as a prostaglandin analogue; causes uterine contractions
- Indications: To control postpartum hemorrhage. This medication is used off label and is not yet approved by the U.S. Food and Drug Administration (FDA) for this use.

Tranexamic Acid (TXA) (not a uterotonic)

- Classification: Antifibrinolytic agent
- Considerations: This drug should be given within 3 hours from the time of delivery.
- Route or dosage: IV or PO 1 gram IV over 10 minutes (add 1 gram vial to 100 mL non-saline solution and give over 10 minutes); may be repeated once after 30 minutes

AWHONN, 2021a; James & Suplee, 2021).

Lacerations

Lacerations of the cervix, vagina, labia, and perineum can occur during childbirth and are the second-most common cause of primary PPH. Lacerations often occur in women who:

- Give birth to large babies (fetal macrosomia).
- Experience an operative vaginal delivery, such as use of forceps or vacuum extraction.
- Experience a precipitous labor and birth.

Assessment Findings

- A firm uterus that is midline with heavier-than-normal bleeding
- Bleeding that is usually a steady stream without clots
- Tachycardia
- Hypotension

Medical Management

- Visual inspection of cervix, vagina, perineum, and labia
- Surgical repair of laceration

Nursing Actions

- Review labor and birth records for risk factors and frequently monitor women at high risk for lacerations.
- Monitor vital signs.
- Monitor blood loss.
  - Weigh bloodied pads and linens to obtain accurate amount of blood loss: 1 g = 1 mL of blood.
- Notify the physician or midwife of increased bleeding with a firm fundus.
- Administer medications for pain management as ordered.
- Prepare the woman for a pelvic examination.
- Provide emotional support to the woman and her family.

Hematomas

Hematomas occur when blood collects within the connective tissues of the vagina or perineal areas related to a vessel that ruptures and continues to bleed (Fig. 14–3). It is difficult to determine the degree of blood loss because the blood is retained within the tissue; thus, PPH may not be diagnosed until the woman is in hypovolemic shock. Trauma caused by episiotomies, use of forceps, and prolonged second stage of labor is the most common cause of hematomas.

Assessment Findings

- Women express severe pain in the vaginal or perineal area, and the intensity of pain cannot be controlled by standard postpartum pain management.
- Presence of tachycardia and hypotension is observed.
- Hematomas in the vagina cannot be visualized by the nurse. However, affected women will express severe pain, a heaviness or fullness in the vagina, or rectal pressure.
- Hematomas in the perineal area present with swelling, discoloration, and tenderness.

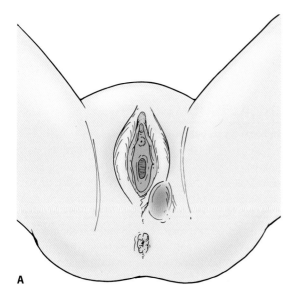

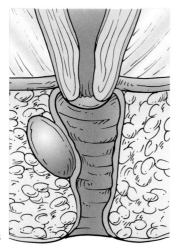

FIGURE 14-3 (A) Vulvar hematoma. (B) Vaginal wall hematoma.

- Hematomas can become large enough to displace the uterus and cause uterine atony, which can increase the degree of blood loss even though the blood is not visible externally.

Medical Management

- Small hematomas are evaluated and monitored without surgical intervention.
- Large hematomas are surgically excised and the blood evacuated. The open vessel is identified and ligated.
  - Women experience immediate relief from pain once the blood has been evacuated.

Nursing Actions

- Review the chart for risk factors and closely monitor women at risk for a hematoma.
- Apply ice to the perineum for the first 24 hours to decrease the risk of hematoma.
- Assess the degree of pain by using a pain scale.
  - Severe vaginal or perineal pain is a primary symptom of hematoma.
  - Ask women who verbally or nonverbally indicate increased pain if they are experiencing any heaviness or fullness in their vaginal or rectal areas.
- Monitor for decrease in BP and increase in pulse rate, signs that indicate shock.
- Administer prescribed analgesia for pain management.
- Review laboratory reports such as H&H, as a decrease in H&H may be an indication of blood loss.
- Notify the physician or midwife of nursing assessment findings for further evaluation.
- Provide emotional support and teaching to the patient, as increasing pain can increase anxiety and stress levels.

Subinvolution of the Uterus

Subinvolution of the uterus means the uterus does not decrease in size and does not descend into the pelvis (arrest or delay of involution). This usually occurs later in the postpartum period. Subinvolution can occur in women who have fibroids, endometritis, or retained placental tissue.

Assessment Findings

- The uterus is soft and larger than normal for the days postpartum.
- Lochia returns to the rubra stage and can be heavy.
- Back pain is present.

Medical Management

- Ultrasound evaluation is used to identify intrauterine tissue or subinvolution of the placental site (ACOG, 2017b).
- Medical intervention depends on the cause of the subinvolution.
  - A D&C is performed for retained placental tissue.
  - Methergine PO is prescribed for fibroids.
  - Antibiotic therapy is initiated for endometritis.

Nursing Actions

- Review prenatal and labor records for risk factors.
- Monitor women who are at risk for subinvolution of the uterus more frequently.
- Patient education is the primary action, as PPH from subinvolution usually occurs post-discharge.
  - Provide education on involution and signs to report, such as increased bleeding, clots, or a change in the lochia to bright red bleeding.
  - Provide education on ways to reduce the risk for infection, such as changing peripads frequently, hand washing, nutrition, adequate fluid intake, and adequate rest.
  - Explain to women who have fibroids that they are at risk for subinvolution. Provide instruction on the proper use of discharge medication, because these women are usually discharged with an order for Methergine PO.

Retained Placental Tissue

Retained placental tissue, which is the primary cause of secondary PPH, occurs when small portions of the placenta called cotyledons remain attached to the uterus during the third stage of labor. Manual removal of the placenta increases the risk of retained placental tissue. The retained placental tissue can interfere with involution of the uterus, potentially leading to endometritis and subinvolution of the uterus.

Assessment Findings

- Profuse bleeding that suddenly occurs after the first postpartum week
- Subinvolution of the uterus
- Elevated temperature and uterine tenderness if endometritis is present
- Pale skin color (patients with white or light skin pigmentation)
- Blue discoloration of skin or mucous membranes (patients with brown or dark skin pigmentation) (Hadjiliadis & Harron, 2019)
- Tachycardia
- Hypotension

Medical Management

- D&C is performed to remove retained placental tissue.
- IV antibiotic therapy may be prescribed because of the increased risk for endometritis.

Nursing Actions

- Patient education is a primary intervention, as PPH from retained placental fragments usually occurs after discharge.
  - Instruct women to report to their health-care provider any sudden increase in lochia, bright red bleeding, elevated temperature, or uterine tenderness.

Nursing Actions Following a Postpartum Hemorrhage

- Because failure to recognize and intervene related to obstetric hemorrhage can result in SMM and even mortality, protocols

are used to stage obstetric hemorrhage and outline a protocol and standard line of care. See Box 14-2 for the elements of common obstetric hemorrhage protocols.

- Assess the fundus and lochia every hour for the first 4 hours and then PRN.
- Instruct the woman on how to assess the fundus, how to do fundal massage, and the signs of PPH that should be reported to the health-care provider.
- Increase oral and IV fluid intake to decrease the risk of hypovolemia.
- Explain the importance of preventing bladder distention to reduce the risk for further PPH.
- Assist with ambulation or transfers because there is an increase of orthostatic hypotension related to blood loss.
- Anticipate the risk of fatigue related to blood loss.
- Provide uninterrupted rest periods while in the hospital.
- Provide an opportunity for the woman and her support to talk about their experiences with PPH, as they may have related feelings of fear, anxiety, and stress.
- Provide information on foods high in iron and the importance of eating a high-iron diet to decrease the risk of anemia.
- Review the H&H laboratory report. Notify the physician or certified nurse-midwife (CNM) of abnormal results.

CLINICAL JUDGMENT

Alternatives to Whole Blood

Some patient populations such as Jehovah's Witnesses may decline whole blood (RBCs, WBCs, platelets, or plasma) because of religious practices or beliefs but want to receive blood component therapy. Most often, patients and families want information on any alternative blood component options. The CMQCC PPH toolkit has an entire section dedicated to bloodless medicine and alternative options that can be used to develop protocols and policies for this population. Ensure an appropriate plan of care has developed before patient delivery. Be sure to inquire about an advanced directive so that early planning with the blood bank, pharmacy, health-care provider, and the nursing team can be completed before delivery (CMQCC, 2015). Alternative options to receiving whole blood may include:

- Cryoprecipitate: Clotting factors for those with bleeding disorders are removed from the plasma, processed, and then banked.
- Albumin: Proteins to use as fluid expanders or in the treatment of burns are removed from the plasma, processed, and then banked.
- Erythropoietin: This human-derived product stimulates erythropoiesis, or RBC production.
- Cell saver or salvage: This involves collecting, washing, and filtering the patient's own blood and then returning it to the patient.

COAGULATION DISORDERS

Various complications can occur during the postpartum period related to alterations in the clotting mechanisms, including DIC, anaphylactoid syndrome of pregnancy (sometimes referred to as amniotic fluid embolism [AFE]), and thrombosis.

Disseminated Intravascular Coagulation

DIC is a syndrome in which coagulation pathways are hyperstimulated. When this occurs, the woman's body breaks down blood clots faster than it can form them, quickly depleting the body of clotting factors and leading to hemorrhage and death (McGovern et al., 2019).

- DIC is a complication of an underlying pathological process called anaphylactoid syndrome of pregnancy.
- DIC may present on a wide spectrum from hemorrhage to thrombosis. It has been suggested that there are four types of obstetric DIC depending on the degree of hypercoagulation and hyperfibrinolysis that is present.
  - Asymptomatic type (limited coagulation and fibrinolysis)
  - Bleeding type (fibrinolysis dominant)
  - Massive bleeding type (hypercoagulation and hyperfibrinolysis)
  - Organ failure type (hypercoagulation dominant)
- Women who experience DIC are transferred to critical care units, and a perinatologist, when available, manages their care.

Predisposing Conditions to Disseminated Intravascular Coagulation

- Placental abruption (the most frequent cause of death from DIC)
- Preeclampsia with severe features or eclampsia
- HELLP (hemolysis, elevated liver enzymes, and low platelets) syndrome
- Anaphylactoid syndrome of pregnancy
- Massive obstetric hemorrhage
- Sepsis
- Retained intrauterine fetal demise [IUFD] or demise of twin

Assessment Findings

- Prolonged, uncontrolled uterine bleeding
- Bleeding from the IV site, incision site, gums, and bladder
- Purpuric areas at pressure sites, such as BP cuff site
- Abnormal clotting study results, such as low platelets and activated PTT
- Increased anxiety
- Signs and symptoms of shock related to blood loss:
  - Pale and clammy skin (patients with white or light skin pigmentation)
  - Blue discolored clammy skin (patients with brown or dark skin pigmentation)
  - Tachycardia
  - Tachypnea
  - Hypotension

Medical Management

Medical management focuses on optimizing hemodynamic function and improving overall tissue oxygenation while identifying and eliminating underlying pathology (Sisson & Hamner, 2019).

- Laboratory tests (e.g., fibrinogen levels, prothrombin time [PT], PTT, and platelet count) to assess for abnormal clotting
- Identification of the primary cause of bleeding and intervention based on this knowledge
- IV therapy
- Blood replacement
- Platelet transfusion
- FFP
- Cryoprecipitate
- Oxygen therapy

Nursing Actions

- Reduce the risk of DIC.
  - Review prenatal and labor records for risk factors.
  - Monitor women more frequently who are at risk for DIC: maternal vital signs as well as urine output should be assessed hourly to determine if she has adequate renal perfusion (Sisson & Hamner, 2019).
  - Assess for PPH and intervene appropriately. Early intervention can decrease the risk of DIC.
  - Monitor vital signs and immediately report to the MD or CNM abnormal findings, such as increased heart rate, decreased BP, and change in quality of respirations.
- Obtain IV site with large-bore intracatheter as per orders.
  - Administer IV fluids as ordered.
- Administer oxygen as ordered.
- Obtain laboratory specimens as ordered.
- Review laboratory results and notify the physician of results.
- Start blood transfusion as ordered.
- Provide emotional support and information to the woman and family to decrease the level of anxiety.
- Facilitate transfer to ICU.

Anaphylactoid Syndrome of Pregnancy

Anaphylactoid syndrome of pregnancy, also referred to as AFE, is a rare but often fatal complication that can occur during pregnancy, labor and birth, or the first 24 hours postbirth. AFE classically consists of hypoxia from (Roth, 2021):

- Acute lung injury
- Transient pulmonary hypertension
- Hypotension
- Cardiac arrest
- Coagulopathy

Historically, AFE was thought to be the infusion of amniotic fluid cells and other debris into maternal circulation. Now researchers theorize that a shift of a systemic inflammatory response syndrome occurs with inappropriate release of endogenous inflammatory mediators (Roth, 2021). AFE should be suspected if a pregnant patient develops the following symptoms with, during, or immediately after birth (Roth, 2021):

- Dyspnea
- Coagulopathy
- Hypotension
- Cyanosis
- Cardiopulmonary arrest
- Severe hypoxemic respiratory failure
- Cardiac and respiratory arrest

Medical Management

- Treatment is mainly supportive with monitoring for the development of ARDS and coagulopathy.
- Hypoxia is treated with supplemental oxygen or perhaps mechanical ventilation.
- Complete blood count (CBC), platelet count, arterial blood gases, fibrinogen, and PT are a few of the laboratory tests that might be ordered.
- Check blood type and screen for possible transfusion.
- Perform a chest x-ray
- Utilize blood replacement, packed RBCs, and platelets.
- Transfer to the critical care unit.
- A heart–lung bypass machine, when available, may be used to help stabilize the woman.

Nursing Actions

- Notify the physician immediately of assessment data so early interventions can be initiated.
- Optimize hemodynamic function, cardiac output, and oxygen transport.
- Establish two IV sites with large-bore intracatheters, one for IV fluid replacement and one for blood replacement.
- Maintain systolic BP at 90 mm Hg or greater, urine output at 30 mL/hr or greater, Sao_2 at 90% or greater, and arterial Po_2 at 60 mm Hg or greater.
- Correct coagulation abnormalities.
- Provide emotional support to the woman and her support system. Call code and initiate CPR when indicated.
- Facilitate transfer to the ICU.

Venous Thromboembolic Disease

VTE, a blood clot that starts in a vein, is the third-leading vascular diagnosis after heart attack and stroke, affecting about 300,000 to 600,000 Americans each year. There are two types of VTE: deep vein thrombosis (DVT), which is a clot in a deep vein, usually in the leg but sometimes in the arm or other veins, and pulmonary embolism (PE), which occurs when a DVT clot breaks free from a vein wall, travels to the lungs, and blocks the blood supply. Blood clots in the thigh are more likely to break off and travel to the lungs than blood clots in the lower leg or other parts of the body.

Thromboembolism is a blood clot that can potentially block blood flow and damage the organs, which is a leading cause of maternal morbidity and mortality in the United States. The risk of VTE and PE in otherwise healthy women is considered highest during pregnancy and the postpartum period (Cunningham et al., 2018, Griffith-Gilbert & Rousseau, 2020). Pregnancy is a hypercoagulable state with increased fibrin generation, increased coagulation factors, and decreased fibrinolytic activity. Venous stasis in the lower extremities, increased blood volume, and compression of the inferior vena cava and pelvic veins with advancing gestation all combine to increase risk five times over that of nonpregnant women. About 80% of thromboembolic events during pregnancy are venous, with PE and VTE responsible for 1.1 deaths per 100,000 deliveries, or 9.2% of all pregnancy-related deaths in the United States (AWHONN, 2020).

Physiological and anatomical changes during pregnancy increase the risk for thromboembolism during the postpartum period. Overall, the risk of VTE is greatest during the antepartum period, but extends through the 12-week postpartum period and significantly decreases by 6 weeks postpartum (Griffith-Gilbert & Rousseau, 2020). Hypercoagulability, increased venous stasis, decreased venous outflow, uterine compression of the inferior vena cava and pelvic veins, reduced mobility, and changes in levels of coagulation factors normally regulating hemostasis result in an increased thrombogenic state. Risk factors for VTE unrelated to pregnancy include personal history of VTE, thrombophilia, obesity, cancer, smoking, immobility, trauma, and infection (Griffith-Gilbert & Rousseau, 2020). Medical conditions such as diabetes, heart disease, hypertension, renal disease, sickle-cell disease, smoking, or serious infections increase the risk for VTE (AAP & ACOG, 2017).

Classic signs of DVT are dependent edema, abrupt unilateral leg pain, erythema, low-grade fever, and positive Homan's sign (i.e., pain with dorsiflexion of the foot). A PE may present with shortness of breath, tachypnea, tachycardia, dyspnea, pleural chest pain, fever, and anxiety.

Objective tests for DVT include Doppler ultrasound, magnetic resonance venography, and pulsed Doppler study. Chest x-ray, CT, and electrocardiography are used to diagnose PE. The ACOG (2018d) recommends preventive treatment with anticoagulant medication for women who have had an acute VTE during pregnancy, a history of thrombosis, or those at significant risk for VTE during pregnancy and postpartum, such as women with high-risk acquired or inherited thrombophilias. Women with a history of thrombosis should be evaluated for underlying causes to determine whether anticoagulation medication is appropriate during pregnancy. Most women who take anticoagulation medications before pregnancy will need to continue during pregnancy and postpartum. Treatment goals include prevention of further clot propagation, prevention of PE, and prevention of further VTE.

- Anticoagulation therapy is required for women experiencing a DVT during pregnancy with heparin compounds titrated to achieve a PTT of 1.5 to 2.5 times control values. IV anticoagulation should be maintained for at least 5 to 7 days, after which treatment is converted to subcutaneous heparin (Cunningham et al., 2018).
- Early reviews concluded that low-molecular-weight heparins (LMWH) are safe and effective for use throughout pregnancy.

LMWH have less risk of bleeding and lower incidence of severe thrombocytopenia and osteoporosis than other anticoagulants. They do not appear in significant amounts in breast milk and do not cross the placenta (Witcher & Hamner, 2019).

- Treatment of PE is to stabilize a woman with a life-threatening PE and transfer to the ICU. Thromboembolic therapy and catheter or surgical embolectomy may be done.

Nursing Actions

These assessments and interventions are included in comprehensive nursing care of thrombophlebitis:

- Apply a supportive bandage or antiembolic support stockings.
- Apply warm packs to the affected area.
- Slightly elevate the involved leg.
- Perform serial measurements of the circumferences of the calves; a circumference difference of more than 2 cm is classified as leg swelling.
- Monitor vital signs every 4 hours; there may be a slight increase in temperature.
- Compare pulses in both extremities, which may show decreased venous flow to the affected area.
- Heparin anticoagulation therapy may be ordered.
- Bedrest with elevation of the involved extremity until swelling is reduced and anticoagulation therapy are effective (promote venous return and decrease edema).
- As soon as symptoms allow, ambulation is encouraged as bedrest can increase venous stasis.
- Administer anticoagulation therapy with IV heparin, followed by oral warfarin
- Carefully assess unusual bleeding. Heavy vaginal bleeding, generalized petechiae, bleeding from the mucous membranes, hematuria, or oozing from venipuncture sites should be reported to the physician. The heparin antidote protamine sulfate should be readily available.
- Educate and prepare women for diagnostic testing.
- Begin ambulation or body movements according to the woman's abilities after symptoms dissipate (Cunningham et al., 2018; Griffith-Gilbert & Rousseau, 2020).
- Administer elastic stockings.
- Manage pain, administering pain medication as needed.
- Teach the patient how to administer heparin subcutaneously to her abdomen.
- Instruct the woman to report side effects such as bleeding gums, nosebleeds, easy bruising, or excessive trauma at the injection site.
- VTE bundle is discussed in detail in Chapter 7.

INFECTIONS

Postpartum infections comprise a wide range of entities that can occur after vaginal and cesarean births or during breastfeeding. In addition to trauma sustained during the birth process or cesarean procedure, physiological changes during pregnancy contribute to the development of postpartum infections (Wong, 2017).

An estimated 6% of postpartum women will experience a postpartum infection (Wong, 2017), causing an estimated 12.7% of maternal deaths (Building U.S. Capacity to Review and Prevent Maternal Deaths, 2018). Common sites for infections during the postpartum period are the uterus, bladder, breast, and incision site. Most infections can be easily treated when identified at an early stage. Infections that are not identified and treated early can lead to serious complications such as abscess formation, cellulitis, thrombophlebitis, and septic shock. The following are risk factors for postpartum infections:

- History of cesarean delivery
- Premature ROM
- Frequent cervical examination
  - Sterile gloves should be used in examinations. Other than a history of cesarean delivery, this risk factor is most important in postpartum infection.
- Internal fetal monitoring
- Preexisting pelvic infection, including bacterial vaginosis
- Diabetes
- Nutritional status
- Obesity

Complications of postpartum infection may include:

- Scarring
- Infertility
- Sepsis
- Septic shock
- Death

Endometritis

Endometritis, also referred to as metritis, is an infection of the endometrium, myometrium, or parametrial tissue decidua (uterine lining). It is the most common cause of postpartum fever (Suplee & Janke, 2020) and usually starts at the placental site and spreads to encompass the entire endometrium. Approximately 2% of women who experience a vaginal birth and 15% of women who experience a cesarean birth develop endometritis; in addition, a high prevalence of postpartum infections is reported among women who had a history of chronic infections (e.g., chronic urinary tract infections [UTIs], chronic respiratory tract infections, cervicitis) when they became pregnant (Barinov et al., 2020). The uterine cavity is usually sterile until rupture of the amniotic sac. During labor, delivery, and associated manipulations, anaerobic and aerobic bacteria can contaminate the uterus. Endometritis is an infection of the uterus characterized by postpartum fever, midline lower abdominal pain, and uterine tenderness. Purulent lochia, chills, headache, malaise, or anorexia may be present.

Risk Factors

- Cesarean birth, which is a primary risk factor
- Prolonged labor or ROM
- Use of invasive procedures: Internal monitoring, amnioinfusion
- Poor nutrition
- Smoking

- Anemia
- Multiple cervical examinations during labor
- Pyelonephritis or diabetes

Assessment Findings

- Elevated temperature greater than 100.4°F (38°C) with or without chills
- Midline lower abdominal pain or discomfort
- Uterine tenderness
- Tachycardia
- Subinvolution
- Malaise
- Headache
- Chills
- Lochia heavy and foul-smelling when anaerobic organisms are present
  - Foul-smelling lochia is a later sign when the entire endometrium is involved.
  - Lochia is scant and odorless when beta-hemolytic streptococcus is present.

Medical Management

Endometritis is usually treated with broad-spectrum IV antibiotics and rest. Blood cultures to identify the causative organism of endometritis are done if the patient does not respond to empiric therapy. WBC counts are monitored.

- CBC to assess for leukocytosis (WBC count greater than 20,000/mm^3)
- Endometrial cultures
- Blood cultures
- Urinalysis to rule out UTI, which can present with similar symptoms
- Antibiotic therapy
  - Mild cases: Oral antibiotic therapy
  - Moderate to severe cases: IV antibiotic therapy, which is discontinued after the woman is afebrile for 24 hours.
  - Improvement should be noted within 72 hours of initiation of antibiotic therapy.

Nursing Actions

- Reduce risk of endometritis.
  - Educate regarding proper hand washing techniques to reduce spread of bacteria.
  - Instruct the woman in proper pericare and to wipe perineum front to back.
  - Instruct the woman to change her peripad every 3 to 4 hours or sooner because lochia is a medium for bacterial growth.
  - Encourage early ambulation by explaining how ambulation reduces the risk of infection by promoting uterine drainage. Provide alternative movement options for women with disabilities or limitations.
  - Encourage intake of fluids to rehydrate by explaining to the woman that maintaining adequate hydration can reduce

her risk for infections. Women should have a minimum fluid intake of 3,000 mL/day (James & Suplee, 2021).
  - Educate the woman on a diet high in protein and vitamin C to aid tissue healing.

The following assessments and interventions are included in comprehensive nursing care for postpartum infections:

- Fever occurring about the third postnatal day is the most important finding.
- Observe for tachycardia (rise of 10 bpm for every degree Celsius).
- Assess and evaluate lower abdominal pain and assess uterine tenderness on palpation (extending laterally) and slight abdominal distention.
- Determine cause of foul-smelling lochia (if organism is anaerobic).
- Obtain order for urinalysis to rule out UTIs.
- Assess leukocytosis (WBC count greater than 20,000/mm^3 with increased neutrophils or polymorphonuclear leukocytes).
- Obtain blood cultures; however, blood cultures are positive in about 10% of women and endometrial cultures may have limited value because of contamination of the specimen.
- Anticipate parenteral broad-spectrum antibiotic therapy is promptly initiated when postpartum endometritis is diagnosed.
  - Treatment continues until the woman has been afebrile for 48 hours.
  - A common treatment regimen is a combination of clindamycin and an aminoglycoside such as gentamicin, with ampicillin added in refractory cases.
  - Women usually respond rapidly (48 to 72 hours) to antibiotic therapy.
  - Occasional complications include pelvic abscesses, septic pelvic thrombophlebitis, persistent fever, and retained infected placenta (AAP & ACOG, 2017).
- Increase fluid intake and encourage adequate nutrition.
  - Encourage intake of 2,000 mL fluids.
  - Encourage intake of at least 1,800 to 2,000 calories daily if lactating and 1,500 calories if not lactating.
  - Encourage the woman to eat a varied diet, with representation of foods from all food groups, that is high in protein and vitamin C to promote wound healing.
  - Ensure adequate output (30 mL/hour) because renal toxicity can occur with antibiotic therapy.
- Provide comfort through meeting the woman's personal hygiene needs. Cool compresses, linen changes, massage, and positioning may enhance comfort.
- Assess maternal vital signs every 4 hours or every 2 hours if her temperature is elevated.
- Use a semi-Fowler position, ambulation, or both, to promote uterine drainage.
- Administer oxytocics as ordered to promote uterine contraction and drainage.
- Observe for signs of septic shock: tachycardia (greater than 120 bpm), hypotension, tachypnea, changes in sensorium, and decreased urine output (i.e., oliguria) (Cunningham et al., 2018).
  - If septic shock develops, increase the frequency of obtaining vital signs and other assessments, depending on the clinical situation.

- Provide pain management measures.
- Provide emotional support to the woman and her family.
- Discharge teaching
  - Provide information on discharge medications.
  - Provide information on signs and symptoms to report to the health-care provider.

Urinary Tract Infection

UTIs are common during the postpartum period. A woman's urethra and bladder are often traumatized during labor and birth due to intermittent or continuous catheterizations and the pressure of the infant as it passes through the birth canal. Additionally, the bladder and urethra lose tone after delivery, making the retention of urine and urinary stasis common. Women may develop a UTI due to epidural anesthesia or vaginal procedures. Bacteria most frequently found in UTIs are normal bowel flora, including *Escherichia coli, Klebsiella, Proteus,* and *Enterobacter* species. Diagnosis and treatment of bacteriuria can prevent the development of pyelonephritis and places the fetus at increased risk for preterm birth or low birth weight (James & Suplee, 2021). Patients with UTIs may complain of frequent, urgent, and painful urination with suprapubic pain. Low-grade fever and hematuria may be present. UTIs are treated with antibiotics, but the patient must drink adequate fluids to flush bacteria from the system.

Risk Factors

- Epidural anesthesia, which decreases the woman's ability to feel the urge to void, leading to an increased risk for an overdistended bladder
- Overdistended bladder or incomplete emptying of the bladder, which can cause an increase of bacterial growth in the bladder
- Operative vaginal deliveries, forceps, or vacuum extractor, which can cause edema around the urethra
- Intrapartum vaginal exams, urinary catheter placement, genital tract injury, and cesarean birth

Assessment Findings

- Low-grade fever (101.3°F [38.5°C])
- Burning on urination
- Suprapubic pain
- Urgency to void
- Small, frequent voiding of less than 150 mL per voiding

Medical Management

- Urinalysis, CBC, and urine culture and sensitivity
- Antibiotics (usually PO) started before culture results

Nursing Actions

- Risk reduction for UTI
  - Assist the woman to the bathroom to void within a few hours after birth to flush bacteria out of the urethra. For women who have disabilities, offer their preferred appropriate options to void.
  - Catheterize the woman if she is unable to void within 2 to 3 hours postbirth.
  - Remind the woman to void every 3 to 4 hours; she may not feel the urge to void during the first 24 to 48 hours following birth.
  - Measure voiding for the first 24 hours, assessing for complete emptying of the bladder. Each voiding should be equal to or greater than 150 mL.
  - Change peripads at least every 3 to 4 hours. Soiled peripads can encourage growth of bacteria that can enter the urethra.
  - Encourage hydration, mainly water (at least 2,000 mL/day)
  - Encourage foods that increase urine acidity, such as cranberry juice, apricots, and plums.
- Monitor for signs and symptoms of UTI.
  - Report findings of possible UTI to the physician or CNM for further evaluation.
- Obtain laboratory specimens as ordered.
- Administer antibiotics as ordered.
- Encourage oral hydration and good nutrition.
- Discharge teaching
  - Provide information on proper use of discharge medications, and the importance of taking the medication until it's complete, appearance of urine, proper perineal care (wiping from front to back), and wearing cotton underwear.
  - Provide information on signs and symptoms of pyelonephritis and cystitis and report these changes to the health-care provider.

Mastitis

Mastitis is an inflammation or infection of the breast tissue common among lactating women. It usually occurs in just one breast, most often in the upper outer breast quadrant. Although it usually develops in the first 3 to 6 months of breastfeeding, it can happen at any time. Between 2% and 10% of women develop mastitis within the first 3-month postpartum period (Suplee & Janke, 2020). The most common organism reported in mastitis is *Staphylococcus aureus,* usually from the breastfeeding infant's mouth or throat. Patients with mastitis have very tender, engorged, erythematous breasts, and infection is frequently unilateral. Mastitis is generally self-limiting, and continued breastfeeding can help clear up the infection and condition. It does not harm the baby. If antibiotic therapy is indicated, the infection generally resolves within 24 to 48 hours of antibiotic therapy. Abscess formation can occur in 10% of women who develop mastitis.

Contributing Factors

- History of mastitis with a previous infant or partial plugged duct
- Cracked or sore nipples
- Oversupply of milk
- Infrequent or missed feedings
- Using only one position for breastfeeding, which may reduce emptying of the breast
- Wearing a tight-fitting bra
- Rapid weaning

Assessment Findings

- Breast tenderness or warmth to the touch
- Generally feeling ill (malaise) or muscle ache
- Breast swelling and hardness
- Pain or a burning sensation continuously or while breastfeeding
- Skin redness, often in a wedge-shaped pattern
- Fever of 101°F (38.3°C) or greater

Medical Management

- Oral antibiotics therapy for 10 to 14 days
- Culture of expressed milk from affected breast if infection does not resolve

Nursing Actions

- Risk reduction:
  - Mastitis is less likely to occur with complete emptying of the breasts and good breastfeeding technique. Postpartum nurses must teach breastfeeding patients proper latch-on technique and stress regular breastfeeding and complete emptying of both breasts. Breastfeeding patients are also encouraged to avoid missing feedings, which causes the breasts to become engorged.
  - Treatment for mastitis typically involves antibiotic therapy and regular breastfeeding or pumping the breast. Nurses can encourage these patients to apply cold or warm compresses to ease discomfort and to take analgesics as needed. Mastitis usually resolves quickly if patients continue to breastfeed or pump regularly.
  - Explain to the woman the importance of washing her hands before feeding to decrease the spread of bacteria.
  - Proper hand washing technique is encouraged by hospital personnel.
  - Teach the woman methods to decrease nipple irritation and tissue breakdown, such as correct infant latch-on and removal from the breast, more than one breastfeeding position, and air-drying nipples after feedings (see Chapter 16 for more information).
  - Teach the woman the importance of a healthy diet and adequate fluids to decrease risk for any infection.
  - Recommend that the patient consider a larger bra size as breast size changes.
  - Recommend massaging the breast during breastfeeding, especially over tender areas and under the armpit, which is a common location of engorgement.
  - Empty both breasts fully during breastfeeding.
- Palpate and inspect the breasts for signs of mastitis.
  - Report assessment data of possible mastitis to the physician or CNM.
- Administer antibiotics as ordered.
- Administer analgesia as ordered.
- Apply warm compresses to the affected area for comfort and promotion of circulation.
- Instruct the woman to continue to breastfeed or to massage and express milk from the affected breast to promote continuation of milk flow.
- Explain to the woman that it is very common for lactating women to experience mastitis and that it is easily treated when identified early.

Wound Infections

Wound infections can occur at the laceration site, episiotomy site, and cesarean incision site. Aseptic technique throughout childbirth and postpartum is critical in decreasing the woman's risk for wound infections. Most often, the etiologic organisms associated with perineal cellulitis and episiotomy site infections are *Staphylococcus* or *Streptococcus* species and gram-negative organisms, as in endometritis. Postpartum patients with wound infections typically have wounds that exhibit redness, warmth, poor wound approximation, tenderness, and pain. If untreated, these patients may develop a fever and other symptoms of an infection, such as malaise. Blood cultures may be obtained to isolate the causative organism. Antibiotics will typically be administered, and drainage of the wound may be necessary.

Patients must be taught about proper hand washing and encouraged to maintain adequate fluid intake and increased protein intake to assist in wound healing. Wound infections can be intensely painful, especially in the perineum. Therefore, the nurse assists these patients in managing pain with analgesics and positioning.

Risk Factors

- Obesity
- Diabetes
- Malnutrition
- Long labor
- Prolonged operative time during cesarean section
- Premature ROM
- Preexisting infection, including chorioamnionitis
- Immunodeficiency disorders
- Corticosteroid therapy
- Poor suturing technique

Assessment Findings

- Erythema
- Swelling
- Tenderness
- Purulent drainage
- Low-grade fever
- Increased pain at incision or laceration site

Medical Management

- Obtain a culture specimen from the wound or laceration if indicated.
- For mild to moderate wound infections that do not have purulent drainage:
  - Administer oral antibiotic therapy.
  - Apply warm compresses to the area.
- Wound infections with purulent drainage:
  - Open and drain the wound.
  - IV antibiotic therapy.

Nursing Actions

- Assess perineum or surgical incision for REEDA (redness, edema, ecchymosis, discharge, approximation of edges of episiotomy or laceration) (Griffith-Gilbert & Rousseau, 2020).
- Inform the physician or midwife of abnormal assessment data.
- Assess vital signs.
- Obtain laboratory specimens such as cultures as ordered.
- Review laboratory reports and notify the physician or midwife of abnormal results.
- Administer antibiotics as ordered.
- Pain management
  - Administer analgesia for fever and discomfort as ordered.
  - Apply hot packs for abdominal wounds or sitz bath for perineal wounds to promote comfort and circulation.
- Use proper hand washing technique before and after contact with the wound.
- Provide education on proper diet, fluids, good hygiene, and rest that can decrease the risk for infection and assist in the healing process.
- Provide information on proper use of discharge medications.

MANAGEMENT OF PREGNANCY COMPLICATIONS IN THE POSTPARTUM PERIOD

The postpartum period is a critical time to ensure women and their newborns are recovering from birth, adapting, and healthy. It is important to closely monitor a woman's health during this recovery time, particularly if she experienced complications during pregnancy. It is also critical health-care providers and delivery facilities provide education to patients and families on the severity of her condition. Additionally, our Consensus Bundle on Severe Hypertension During Pregnancy and Postpartum reported that many of these deaths were preventable and resulted from lack of knowledge of specific symptoms (stomach pain, severe headaches, feeling nauseous, swelling in the hands and face, seeing spots and shortness of breath) that ultimately led to a delay in seeking care (Bernstein et al., 2017).

Educating women on hypertensive disorders in pregnancy and ensuring they understand symptoms can last up to 6 weeks postpartum can improve follow-up care and compliance with short- and long-term medical management. Educational websites provide resources, support groups, education (in the patient's preferred language using Google Language), and volunteer opportunities for growth and mentoring.

Finally, patients with hypertensive disorders, especially those placed on new BP medications or adjustments made shortly before discharge according to ACOG's Optimizing Care in the Postpartum Period, should be seen postdischarge in 3 to 10 days for BP check and follow-up care because of a high-risk condition (ACOG, 2017b).

Acute Onset of Severe Hypertension Postpartum

Women in the postpartum period with acute-onset, severe systolic (greater than or equal to 160 mm Hg) hypertension; severe diastolic (greater than or equal to 110 mm Hg) hypertension; or both; require urgent antihypertensive therapy. Treatment with first-line agents should be expeditious and occur as soon as possible within 30 to 60 minutes of confirmed severe hypertension to reduce the risk of maternal stroke, seizure, or death. Establishing lifesaving emergent protocols and order sets allows faster response to severe hypertension or preeclampsia. Additionally, standardized treatment plans and proper escalation measures have been documented as strategies that have improved maternal outcomes (Main et al., 2015).

IV labetalol and hydralazine have long been considered first-line medications for the management of acute-onset, severe hypertension in pregnant women and women in the postpartum period. Immediate-release oral nifedipine also may be considered as a first-line therapy, particularly when IV access is not available. It is important to note differences in recommended dosage intervals between these options, which reflect differences in their pharmacokinetics. Protocols should be followed for maternal monitoring of BP every 5 to 15 minutes. None of the recommended drugs require cardiac monitoring.

Although all three medications are appropriately used for the treatment of hypertensive emergencies in pregnancy, each agent can be associated with adverse effects. For example, parenteral hydralazine may increase the risk of maternal hypotension (systolic BP 90 mm Hg or less). Parenteral labetalol may cause neonatal bradycardia and should be avoided in women with asthma, heart disease, or congestive heart failure. Nifedipine has been associated with an increase in maternal heart rate, and with overshoot hypotension (ACOG, 2017a). Extensive discussion of preeclampsia is found in Chapter 7.

Management of Diabetes Postpartum

Diabetes is a complex disorder caused by various pathological mechanisms in secretion of or response to insulin. The result is hyperglycemia, which damages organ systems. Hyperglycemia affects 7% to 18% of all pregnant women (ACOG, 2018a). Diabetes can incur significant morbidity and mortality for the mother, fetus, and the newborn into adulthood. Diabetes in all forms is the most common metabolic disease complicating pregnancy and postpartum. More than almost any other disease or condition, it requires patient collaboration and partnership to ensure successful management and follow-up (AWHONN, 2016).

Women who have diabetes can provide information about their food choices, activity, compliance with blood glucose (BG) monitoring, and medication administration that health-care professionals need to make collaborative decisions about course and treatment. However, not all women are aware of the importance of this information. Further, many women with diabetes may lack understanding of their role and influence on

BG management. Therefore, education and empowerment are critical from the outset, and appropriate postpartum follow-up is essential (AWHONN, 2016). Women with chronic medical conditions such as diabetes should be counseled about the importance of timely follow-up with their primary care provider for ongoing care coordination. This can be a challenge for women who only have emergency Medicaid, which provides follow-up only at 6 weeks postdelivery in most states, further exacerbating the problems of diet, medical management, and her ability to receive nutritional counseling. Without proper management, women have a higher lifetime risk of maternal cardiometabolic disease.

Pregestational Diabetes

Insulin requirements for the pregestational diabetic woman decrease in the immediate postpartum period. With oral intake, subcutaneous insulin doses can resume, typically at prepregnancy normal glucose tolerance postpartum doses (Daley, 2014). Women with diabetes are at higher risk for complications such as infection and should be closely monitored for mastitis, endometritis, and wound infections. Breastfeeding is highly encouraged. Benefits include a reduction in the risk of developing type 2 diabetes mellitus (T2DM) for women with gestational diabetes mellitus (GDM).

Gestational Diabetes

Most women with gestational diabetes return to normal glucose tolerance postpartum (Daley, 2014; Roth, 2021). Although carbohydrate intolerance of GDM frequently resolves after delivery, up to one-third of affected women will have diabetes or impaired glucose metabolism at their postpartum screening. It has been estimated that 15% to 50% develop type 2 diabetes later in life (ACOG, 2018a; CDC, 2019a). Postpartum screening at 6 to 12 weeks is recommended for women who had GDM to identify diabetes mellitus (DM), impaired fasting glucose levels, or impaired glucose tolerance. Follow-up is essential to ensure normal fasting glucose values.

Nursing Actions

The nurse must counsel women with a history of GDM that they have a sevenfold increased risk of developing type 2 diabetes compared with women with no GDM history (ACOG, 2018a). Counseling can be provided to modify risk factors such as obesity with weight reduction and exercise. Women should also be informed that they are at high risk for developing GDM with subsequent pregnancies. For women who may have subsequent pregnancies, more frequent screening can detect abnormal glucose metabolism before pregnancy and provides an opportunity to ensure preconception glucose control (ACOG, 2018a). Women should be encouraged to discuss their GDM history and need for screening with their health-care providers.

Exercise or increased activity is recommended for women with a high risk of diabetes, such as those with a history of GDM. Exercise independent of weight loss has a role in preventing or delaying the development of overt diabetes, due to the resulting decrease in insulin resistance. Additionally, inactivity is a risk factor for the development of T2DM (AWHONN, 2016).

Explore challenges related to the prevention of overt diabetes. Strategies include:

- Assessing knowledge, risk perception, self-efficacy, current prevention behaviors, and intention to change behavior
- Identifying barriers to health-promoting behaviors and solutions to promote behavior change such as access to health-care providers, access to nutritional foods in the community, access to safe and affordable exercise facilities, or access to outside areas conducive to exercise such as parks and walking paths
- Identifying social support (including family and support system) in education, counseling, and problem-solving of nutritional diet, food portions, and food group choices
- Designing interventions that are individualized and easily accessible, such as phone counseling and computer-based education
- Providing information about resources such as affordable exercise classes and diet advice
- Providing links as needed to dietitians, primary care providers, and mental health professionals to ensure ongoing support
- Breastfeeding, which is strongly recommended after delivery for all women with pregestational diabetes mellitus or gestational diabetes mellitus
- Scheduling a follow-up appointment 2 to 6 weeks postdischarge with the provider who managed the patient's diabetes during pregnancy (Ensure pregnant patients on Medicaid are seen as early as possible because traditionally those benefits end in 6 weeks postdelivery in most states.)

Maternal Obesity Postpartum

Mothers who are obese are at risk for complications postpartum regardless of method of birth, including increased incidence of infection and wound complications. Maternal obesity, defined by a body mass index (BMI) of 30 or higher, has long been recognized as a risk factor in pregnancy. Being overweight or obese during pregnancy is associated with many adverse outcomes, including impaired glucose tolerance and gestational diabetes, hypertension, and sleep apnea (Opray et al., 2015). Obesity during pregnancy increases the risk of morbidity and mortality for the mother and baby and is a well-established risk factor for the development of comorbid conditions such as preeclampsia, gestational and type 2 diabetes, and thrombosis (ACOG, 2021). These complications are associated with future metabolic dysfunction.

Forty-six percent of obese pregnant women have gestational weight gain that exceeds the Institute of Medicine pregnancy weight gain guidelines. Excess gestational weight gain is a significant risk factor for postpartum weight retention, further increasing the risk of metabolic dysfunction and pregravid obesity in future pregnancies. Pregravid obesity is associated with early termination of breastfeeding, postpartum anemia, and depression (ACOG, 2021). Obesity is a risk factor for VTE in the general medical population. For prevention of VTE in very-high-risk groups, pharmacological thromboprophylaxis should be considered in addition to pneumatic compression devices.

Nursing Actions

- Precisely assess the uterus. Tone and lochia may be difficult due to maternal size, so turning the woman on her side will assist with better visibility of her perineum and bleeding.
- Reinforce information on maternal complications postpartum and postop associated with obesity such as increased risk for type 2 diabetes, DVT, and chronic hypertension.
- Because the postpartum period presents an ideal time during which to initiate simple healthy behaviors, such as walking and proper diet that can be maintained after birth, offer suggestions and encouragement for lifestyle changes (Farpour-Lambert et al., 2018).
- According to ACOG's most recent 2021 bulletin on obesity, all women who have obesity should be provided with or referred for behavioral counseling interventions focused on improving diet and exercise to achieve a healthier weight before another pregnancy (ACOG, 2021). Interpregnancy weight loss in obese women may decrease the risk of a large-for-gestational-age neonate in a subsequent pregnancy. Behavioral interventions employing diet and exercise improve postpartum weight reduction more than exercise alone (ACOG, 2021). Research programs that offer services to patients with and without private insurance.
- Women with increased BMI may need additional support while breastfeeding. Utilizing the football hold may be beneficial and allow for better visualization of the baby during the feeding. She may also benefit from additional blankets or washcloths rolled under the feeding breast for additional support and visualization of both her areola and the baby's mouth.
- Encourage the woman to sleep in a sitting position; this may help, as effects of obesity on the respiratory system are decreased in this position.
- Make appropriate environmental changes to accommodate the larger patient, such as assuring that patient beds and chairs can support at least 400 pounds.

POSTPARTUM FOLLOW-UP

At discharge from maternity care, the woman should receive contact information for her postpartum care team and written instructions about the timing of follow-up postpartum care. Women are recommended to have a comprehensive postpartum visit within the first 6 weeks after birth (if they have high-risk health conditions, it could be sooner, perhaps as early as 3 to 10 days after delivery; ACOG, 2018b). This visit will include a full assessment of physical, social, and psychological well-being and a discussion of the desired form of contraception. At the conclusion of the postpartum visit, the woman and her provider determine who will assume primary responsibility for her ongoing care. If responsibility is transferred to another primary care provider, the obstetric care provider is responsible for ensuring that communication continues with the primary care provider so they can understand the implications of any pregnancy complications for the woman's future health and maintain continuity of care. Postpartum patients and families are instructed to call the health-care provider if the woman experiences:

- Fever
- Foul-smelling lochia
- Large blood clots (golf ball–sized or bigger) or bleeding that saturates a pad in 1 hour
- Discharge, erythema, or severe pain from incisions or stitched areas
- Hot, red, painful areas on the breasts or legs
- Bleeding or severe pain in the nipples or breasts
- Severe headaches that will not go away or blurred vision
- Chest pain or dyspnea without exertion
- Frequent, painful urination
- Signs of depression

A postpartum care plan should be reviewed, updated, and discussed with women after the birth. Women are often uncertain about whom to contact for postpartum concerns. Up to one in four postpartum women did not have a phone number for a health-care provider to contact for concerns about themselves or their infants (ACOG, 2018b). The care plan includes contact information and written instructions on the timing of follow-up postpartum care. Just as a health-care professional or

SAFE AND EFFECTIVE NURSING CARE: Patient Education

Post-Birth Warning Signs

An excellent acronym developed by AWHONN to help patients with postbirth warning signs is POST BIRTH:

- Pain in chest
- Obstructed breathing or shortness of breath
- Seizures
- Thoughts of hurting yourself or someone else
- Bleeding, soaking through one pad per hour, or blood clots the size of an egg or bigger
- Incision that is not healing
- Red or swollen leg that is painful or warm to touch
- Temperature of 100.4°F (38°C) or higher
- Headache that does not get better, even after taking medicine, or bad headache with vision changes (AWHONN, 2018)

Educate women to see their health-care provider if they notice any of these signs.

health-care practice leads the woman's care during pregnancy, a primary maternal care provider should assume responsibility for her postpartum care.

The comprehensive postpartum visit is typically scheduled between 4 and 6 weeks after delivery. However, recommendations for the timing of postpartum visits considerably vary. Early follow-up is recommended for women with hypertensive disorders of pregnancy, with BP evaluation no later than 7 to 10 days postpartum; other experts have recommended follow-up at 3 to 5 days. Early follow-up also may be beneficial for women at high risk of complications, such as postpartum depression (PPD), cesarean or perineal wound infection, lactation difficulties, or chronic conditions (ACOG, 2018b). These visits, which may be conducted through home nursing evaluations, are essential for follow-up.

The postpartum visit provides an opportunity for women to ask questions about labor, childbirth, and complications. Complications should be discussed with respect to risks for future pregnancies, and recommendations made to optimize maternal health during the interconception period. Resources such as the AWHONN postbirth warning signs can be beneficial tools in communicating warning signs that birthing families must know (AWHONN, 2018). It is important that women with gestational diabetes, hypertensive disorders of pregnancy, or preterm birth be counseled that these disorders are associated with a higher lifetime risk of maternal cardiometabolic disease (ACOG, 2018b).

POSTPARTUM PSYCHOLOGICAL COMPLICATIONS

Childbirth has been recognized as one of the most powerful possible triggers of psychiatric illness during a woman's lifetime (C. T. Beck et al., 2018). A women's psychological state is affected during the postpartum period by hormonal changes, lack of sleep, and stress of integrating a new person into the woman's life and the family unit. Most women experience short-term postpartum blues, which do not require medical intervention (see Chapter 13 and Table 14-2). About 15% of women experience major mood disorders that profoundly affect the ability to care for themselves or their infants. PMADs can occur during the first year after childbirth and have a negative effect on the mother–infant relationship (Milgrom & Holt, 2014).

Two major mood disorders are PPD and postpartum psychosis, which require management by mental health professionals.

PMADs are among the most common mental health conditions among women of reproductive age. When left untreated, these disorders can have profound adverse effects on women and their children, such as poor adherence to medical care, exacerbation of medical conditions, loss of interpersonal and financial resources, smoking and substance use, suicide, and infanticide. PMADs are associated with increased risks of maternal and infant mortality and morbidity and are recognized as a significant patient safety issue. In 2015, the Council on Patient Safety in Women's Health Care convened an interdisciplinary workgroup to develop an evidence-based patient safety bundle to address maternal mental health. Its focus is PMADs (Box 14-4). Modeled after other bundles released by the Council on Patient Safety in Women's Health Care, it provides broad direction for incorporating PMAD screening, intervention, referral, and follow-up into maternity care practice across health-care settings (Kendig et al., 2017).

The primary role of the perinatal nurse is assessing for early signs of potential mood disorders and reporting these findings to the woman's health-care provider for further evaluation and treatment. Assessing for postpartum mood disorders and anxiety disorders should be included in the nurse's postpartum assessments (AWHONN, 2015).

Postpartum Depression

Major depressive disorder with peripartum onset is the official diagnosis for PPD, according to the *Diagnostic and Statistical Manual of Mental Disorders,* Fifth Edition *(DSM-5).* There is also a specifier called "with peripartum onset" (Beck, 2020). About 10% to 20% of women have depression or anxiety during pregnancy or in the postpartum period, making this the most common complication of childbirth (ACOG, 2018c).

Perinatal depression and other mood disorders, such as bipolar disorder and anxiety disorders, can have devastating effects on women, infants, and families. During the pregnancy and 1 year after delivery, maternal suicide is the leading cause of death (Beck, 2020). Maternal suicide exceeds hemorrhage and hypertensive disorders as a cause of pregnancy-associated maternal mortality. Perinatal depression often goes unrecognized because changes in sleep, appetite, and libido may be attributed to normal pregnancy and postpartum changes. In addition to clinicians not recognizing such symptoms, women may be reluctant to report changes in their mood (ACOG, 2016). Data indicates

TABLE 14-2 Major Differences Between Postpartum Blues and Postpartum Depression	
POSTPARTUM BLUES	**POSTPARTUM DEPRESSION**
Symptoms disappear without medical intervention.	Requires psychiatric interventions.
Occurs within the first 2 weeks postpartum.	Occurs within the first 12 months postpartum.
Able to safely care for self and baby.	Unable to safely care for self or baby.

BOX 14-4 | Maternal Safety Bundle: Depression and Anxiety

Maternal Mental Health: Perinatal Depression and Anxiety Patient Safety Bundle, Council on Patient Safety in Women's Health Care

PMADs in their most severe forms can be tragic and preventable causes of maternal and infant mortality. PMADs and their sequelae can be addressed by actively screening women, having a plan in place for treatment or referral for those who screen positive, and actively engaging women, their families, and supporters in recognizing symptoms and seeking help in a timely manner. Everyone must work together to remove the stigma that still surrounds mental health disorders. The elements of the bundle are general so that they can be adapted for a variety of settings. The purpose is to provide a consistent approach to recognition and treatment of PMADs.

Readiness (Every Clinical Care Setting)

- Identify mental health screening tools to be made available in every clinical setting (outpatient obstetric clinics and inpatient facilities).
- Establish a response protocol and identify screening tools for use based on local resources.
- Educate clinicians and office staff on use of the identified screening tools and response protocol.
- Identify an individual who is responsible for driving adoption of the identified screening tools and response protocol.

Recognition and Prevention (Every Woman)

- Obtain individual and family mental health history (including past and current medications) at intake, with review and updates as needed.
- Conduct validated mental health screening during appropriately timed patient encounters, to include both during pregnancy and in the postpartum period.

- Provide appropriately timed perinatal depression and anxiety awareness education to women and family members or other support persons.

Response (Every Case)

- Initiate a stage-based response protocol for a positive mental health screening result.
- Activate an emergency referral protocol for women with suicidal or homicidal ideation or psychosis.
- Provide appropriate and timely support for women as well as family members and staff as needed.
- Obtain follow-up from mental health-care providers on women referred for treatment (this should include release of information forms).

Reporting and Systems Learning (Every Clinical Care Setting)

- Establish a nonjudgmental culture of safety through multidisciplinary mental health rounds.
- Perform a multidisciplinary review of adverse mental health outcomes.
- Establish local standards for recognition and response to measure compliance, understand individual performance, and track outcomes.

Reprinted with Permission from American College of Obstetricians and Gynecologists. (2016). *Patient safety bundle: Maternal mental health: Perinatal depression and anxiety. Council on Patient Safety in Women's Health Care.* American College of Obstetricians and Gynecologists. Available at http://safehealthcareforeverywoman.org/patient-safety-bundles/maternal-mental-health-depression-and-anxiety/. Retrieved 2021.

---

that fewer than 20% of women eventually diagnosed with PPD had reported their initial symptoms to a health-care provider. Therefore, it is important for clinicians to ask the pregnant or postpartum patient about her mood.

PPD is a mood disorder characterized by severe depression that occurs within the first 6 to 12 months postpartum and affects about 11.5% of postpartum women (Ko et al., 2017). PPD affects the woman, her partner, and other children within the family unit. Women who identify as lesbian or bisexual have a higher prevalence of PPD as compared with women who identify as heterosexual (Flanders et al., 2015; Maccio & Pangburn, 2011).

PPD is classified as a major depressive disorder when the woman has a depressed mood or a loss of interest or pleasure in daily activities for at least 2 weeks in addition to four of the following symptoms:

- Significant weight loss or gain: a change of more than 5% of body weight in a month
- Insomnia or hypersomnia
- Changes in psychomotor activity: agitation or retardation
- Decreased energy or fatigue

- Feelings of worthlessness or guilt
- Decreased ability to concentrate; inability to make decisions
- Decreased interest in normal activities

Risk Factors or Predictors of Postpartum Depression

- History of depression before pregnancy
- Depression or anxiety during pregnancy
- Inadequate social support
- Poor quality relationship with partner
- Life and childcare stresses
- Complications of pregnancy or childbirth
- Low level of support from mother or mother figure
- Low socioeconomic status
- History of childhood sexual abuse
- Domestic or intimate partner violence

Assessment Findings

- Sleep and appetite disturbance
- Fatigue greater than expected when caring for a newborn

- Despondency
- Uncontrolled crying
- Anxiety, fear, or panic
- Inability to concentrate
- Feelings of guilt, inadequacy, or worthlessness
- Inability to care for self or baby
- Decreased affectionate contact with the infant
- Decreased responsiveness to the infant
- Thoughts of harming baby
- Thoughts of suicide

Medical and Psychiatric Management

- Mild PPD
  - Interpersonal psychotherapy
- Moderate PPD
  - Interpersonal psychotherapy
  - Antidepressants
- Severe PPD or suicidal ideation
  - Intense psychiatric care
  - Crisis interventions
  - Interpersonal psychotherapy
  - Antidepressants
  - Electroconvulsive therapy

An appraisal of the systematic reviews of therapeutic options for women with PPD over the past 20 years concluded that research is of low to moderate quality and has remained unchanged over time. Based on the systematic reviews with the highest methodological quality, use of antidepressants and telecommunication therapy are the most effective interventions for PPD. Traditional Chinese herbal medicine was effective in the management of PPD and thus could provide a useful therapeutic alternative for women who prefer natural options over conventional therapies. The efficacy of physical exercise, hormonal therapies, and CBT for the treatment of PPD remain equivocal (Chow et al., 2021).

Nursing Actions

- Review prenatal record for risk factors.
- Monitor mother–infant interactions more closely for women at risk for PPD.
- Anticipatory guidance: Teach the woman and her partner signs of PPD that should be reported to her health-care provider.
- Be supportive and encouraging in interactions.
- Provide the woman with information regarding postpartum support groups and other community resources to assist her with parenting issues and to provide support.
- Postpartum support by health-care professionals can mitigate the onset of postpartum mood disorders (AGOG, 2016; Yonkers et al., 2011).
- For women who want to avoid pharmacological therapies, explore complementary and alternative approaches to treatment (e.g., massage therapy, exercise, acupuncture) or use them as an adjunct to her overall treatment plan (Beck, 2020).
- Educate the birth mother about the possibility of depression in a non-birth mother or partner.

Postpartum Psychosis

According to the *DSM-5,* brief psychotic disorder with peripartum onset is the official diagnosis for postpartum psychosis (Beck, 2020). Postpartum psychosis is relatively rare, with prevalence in the general population of 0.1% to 2.6% per 1,000 births (Beck, 2020; VanderKruik et al., 2017). The onset of symptoms is rapid and can occur as early as 2 to 3 days after childbirth.

Diagnostic criteria include the presence of at least one or more of the following symptoms: delusions, hallucinations, disorganized speech, and grossly disorganized or catatonic behavior (C. T. Beck et al., 2018). Women who have PPD require immediate medical attention and acute inpatient psychiatric treatment because maternal suicide and infanticide are major concerns. Women with preexisting bipolar disorder have the highest risk for developing postpartum psychosis. Because this can occur as early as 3 days after delivery postpartum, nurses may be the first to identify these symptoms in mothers before discharge.

Risk Factors

- Women who have known bipolar disorder
- Personal or family history of bipolar disorder or affective disorder (Jones et al., 2014).

Assessment Findings

- Paranoia, as well as grandiose or bizarre delusions, usually associated with the baby
- Mood swings
- Extreme agitation
- Depressed or elated moods
- Distraught feelings about ability to enjoy infant
- Confused thinking
- Strange beliefs, such as that the mother or her infant must die
- Disorganized behavior

Medical and Psychiatric Management

- Hospitalization to the psychiatric unit
- Psychiatric evaluation
- Antidepressant and antipsychotic drug treatment
- Psychotherapy
- Electroconvulsive therapy

Nursing Actions

AWHONN recommends that health-care facilities caring for childbearing women provide education to professional nurses on symptoms of postpartum depressive disorders. Patients should be screened for this potentially disabling condition. In addition, nurses should be aware of the treatment options for women suffering from postpartum depressive disorders so these patients can obtain treatment as early as possible when the condition occurs (Beck, 2020).

- Review the prenatal record for risk factors or psych history, including affective disorders or bipolar disorder.

- Educate the birth mother and non-birth mother or partner at risk and their support system of early signs of PPD, such as mood swings, hallucinations, and strange beliefs, and instruct them to contact the health-care provider if symptoms are present.
- Early detection and treatment can prevent a major episode (Wesseloo et al., 2016).
- Utilize resources such as www.postpartum.net, a national non-profit organization with resources including online support groups, loss and grief resources, and local support coordinators available 24-7.
- Provide current information that indicates the use of antidepressants and telecommunication therapy are the most effective interventions for PPD.

Father, Non-Birth Mother, or Partner Postnatal Depression

Postnatal depression may be experienced by the non-birth parent in heterosexual couples or same-sex couples (J. Beck, 2014; Engqvist & Nilsson, 2011; Flanders et al., 2015; Maccio & Pangburn, 2011). Most new fathers, non-birth mothers, and partners experience feelings of happiness and excitement, but some experience depression. Paternal postnatal depression (PPND) is estimated to occur in 1% to 8% of new fathers during the first 6 months following childbirth. Because current data regarding experiences of same-sex couples is lacking, the following narratives are presented within the context of male experiences within heterosexual relationships. During the first few months postpartum, the man's testosterone levels decrease and estrogen levels increase. Lower levels of testosterone are linked with depression in men. PPND can have a negative effect on the couple's relationship and on the father–child relationship, and it can have a long-term negative effect on the mental well-being of the child (Melrose, 2010).

Signs and Symptoms

Signs and symptoms of PPND are not as apparent as they are with maternal PPD.

- The man may withdraw from social interactions.
- The man may be cynical in his interactions and experience irritable moods.

- The man may demonstrate avoidance behaviors such as spending more time away from family.
- The man's affect may appear anxious or mad rather than sad.

Risk Factors

- Maternal PPD, which is the primary risk factor.
- Depressive symptoms during partner's pregnancy
- Unplanned or unexpected pregnancy
- Baby with health or feeding problems
- Lack of social support
- Excessive stress about becoming a father
- Preexisting mental health disorder
- Stressful life event (e.g., death of his parent)

Assessment Findings

- Irritable
- Overwhelmed
- Frustrated
- Indecisive
- Avoidance of social situations
- Cynical
- Increased alcohol consumption
- Drug use
- Domestic violence

Medical Management

- Interpersonal psychotherapy
- Antidepressant medications

Nursing Actions

- Provide information on PPND to the man and his partner.
- Stress the importance of seeking professional help for symptoms of PPND.
  - Explain that PPND can have negative long-term effects on his child.

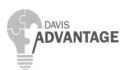

Go to Davis Advantage to complete your learning: strengthen understanding, apply your knowledge, and prepare for the Next Gen NCLEX®.

CONCEPT MAP

Postpartum Hemorrhage

Altered Tissue Perfusion
- Increased capillary refill—greater than 3 seconds
- Cold hands and feet
- Pale and clammy skin
- Dehydration
- Blood loss

Fluid Volume Deficit (Isotonic)
- Hypotension— B/P 90/60
- Tachycardia— HR 110
- Decreased urinary output—50 mL in 4 hours
- Increased lochia
- Boggy uterus

Postpartum Hemorrhage
Boggy uterus, heavy lochia, clots, decrease in hematocrit and hemoglobin

Acute Pain
- Fundal massage
- Oxytocin
- Afterpains
- Woman states her pain is 8 on the pain scale
- Analgesia

Anxiety
- Woman states she is afraid
- Woman is crying
- Blood loss

Impaired Gas Exchange/ Oxygenation
- Hemoglobin 9 g/dL
- Dyspnea
- Hypoxia
- Restlessness

Delay in Mother-Infant Attachment
- Unable to care for newborn
- Fatigue

CARE PLANS

Problem 1: Fluid volume deficit (isotonic)

Goal: Increase fluid volume

Outcome: The woman's BP and heart rate will be within normal ranges, and intake and output will be within 200 mL of each other by the end of the shift.

Nursing Actions

1. Assess fundus for firmness: massage if boggy.
2. Assess lochia for amount, color, and clots.
3. Instruct and remind the woman to drink lots of fluids.
4. Initiate IV therapy as ordered.
5. Initiate oxytocin therapy as ordered.
6. Assess intake and output.
7. Assist the woman to the bathroom every 3 to 4 hours.
8. Monitor BP and pulse every 2 hours.
9. Assess skin turgor and mucous membranes every 4 hours.

Problem 2: Altered tissue perfusion

Goal: Normal tissue perfusion

Outcome: BP and pulse within normal limits; capillary fill less than 3 seconds.

Nursing Actions

1. Every 2 hours, monitor vital signs, capillary refill, and motor and sensory status.
2. Compare post-hemorrhage H&H with results on admission to labor.
3. Administer oxygen as per orders and monitor oxygen saturation levels.

Problem 3: Anxiety

Goal: Decreased anxiety

Outcome: The woman verbalizes that she feels less anxious.

Nursing Actions

1. Be calm and reassuring in interactions with the woman and her family. Direct eye contact, warm touch, a smile, getting to know them, and reassuring them of the plan of care are also helpful when patients are anxious about being hospitalized.
2. Explain all procedures.
3. Teach the woman relaxation breathing techniques.
4. Encourage the woman and family to verbalize their feelings regarding recent hemorrhage by asking open-ended questions.

Problem 4: Delay in mother–infant attachment

Goal: Positive mother–infant attachment

Outcome: The woman will hold the infant close, respond to the infant's needs, and state she enjoys her baby.

Nursing Actions

1. Support skin-to-skin immediately after delivery to initiate bonding.
2. Support the mother with breastfeeding immediately after delivery (if she desires to breastfeed).
3. Encourage rooming in.
4. Assist the patient with infant care as needed.
5. Encourage holding of the infant by assisting the woman parent into a comfortable position and placing the infant in her arms.
6. Praise the woman and family for positive parent–infant interactions.
7. Provide information on infant care.

Problem 5: Acute pain

Goal: Decreased pain

Outcome: The woman will state that pain is within her chosen numerical level on the pain scale.

Nursing Actions

1. Assess level, location, and type of pain.
2. Prevent overdistention of the bladder by reminding the woman to void every 3 to 4 hours.
3. Administer pain medications based on assessment data as ordered.
4. Provide an environment that is conducive to relaxation, such as low lights, decreased noise, and uninterrupted rest periods.
5. Teach the woman relaxation techniques.

Problem 6: Impaired gas exchange or oxygenation

Goal: Maintain oxygenation

Outcome: Oxygen saturation is 98% and respiratory rate and pattern are within normal limits.

Nursing Actions

1. Monitor respirations, breath sounds, and oxygen saturation.
2. Provide oxygen by mask as ordered.
3. Instruct and assist the woman with deep breathing and coughing to decrease the risk of pneumonia.
4. Initiate iron replacement therapy as ordered.
5. Provide nutritional information on foods high in iron such as green leafy vegetables.

Case Study

You are a nurse working in the postpartum unit. You are assigned Mallory Polk, a 42-year-old Black woman. (Refer to the Case Studies in Chapters 7 and 10 for antepartum and intrapartum data.)

Summary of Labor and Delivery Record

Mallory was admitted 2 days ago at 31 weeks' gestation for preterm labor. She was given magnesium sulfate to delay delivery and provide fetal neuroprotection and received two doses of betamethasone for lung maturity. She spontaneously delivered a 1,559-gram boy with Apgar scores of 5/7 at 1 and 5 minutes, respectively. Her baby is experiencing mild signs of respiratory distress and is in the NICU.

Postpartum Report

Mallory is 4 hours postbirth and has an IV of 500 mL lactated Ringer's solution with 30 units of oxytocin at 100 mL/min in her left arm. She voided in the recovery unit 2 hours postbirth.

Assessment Findings

Vital signs: Temperature 98.6°F (37°C); pulse 106 bpm; respirations 14 breaths/min; BP 110/70 mm Hg.

Fundus is at the umbilicus and boggy.
Lochia is heavy.

Based on assessment findings and Mallory's history, what are your immediate nursing actions?

Discuss the rationale for your nursing actions.

You reevaluate Mallory 10 minutes after your initial nursing actions. Her fundus is firm, midline, and 1 finger-breadth below the umbilicus with scant lochia. You continue to monitor Mallory and 15 minutes later her fundus is boggy with heavy lochia. The fundus becomes firm after massage. You increase the rate of oxytocin to 150 mL/min. Her pulse is 118 bpm and BP is 100/60 mm Hg. You notify her CNM and report your findings.

Detail the aspects of your assessment findings that you will report to the CNM.

The CNM orders an injection of Methergine 0.2 mg IM now.

Discuss your nursing actions and rationale for actions.

Discuss the assessment data needed to determine the effectiveness of medical and nursing actions.

You note that in her prenatal chart she has a diagnosis of fibroids.

Discuss the implications of the diagnosis as it relates to your nursing care and discharge teaching plan.

REFERENCES

Altman, M. R., McLemore, M. R., Oseguera, T., Lyndon, A., & Franck, L. S. (2020). Listening to women: Recommendations from women of color to improve experiences in pregnancy and birth care. *Journal of Midwifery & Women's Health, 65*(4), 466–473. https://doi.org/10.1111/jmwh.13102

Altman, M. R., Oseguera, T., McLemore, M. R., Kantrowitz-Gordon, I., Franck, L. S., & Lyndon, A. (2019). Information and power: Women of color's experiences interacting with health care providers in pregnancy and birth. *Social Science & Medicine, 238,* 112491. https://doi.org/10.1016/j.socscimed.2019.112491

American Academy of Pediatrics and the American College of Obstetricians and Gynecologists. (2017). *Guidelines for perinatal care* (8th ed.). Author.

American College of Obstetricians and Gynecologists. (2014). *reVITALize: Obstetric data definitions (version 1.0).* Author.

American College of Obstetricians and Gynecologists. (2015). *Maternal safety bundle: Obstetric hemorrhage: Safe motherhood initiative.* Author.

American College of Obstetricians and Gynecologists. (2016). *Patient safety bundle: Maternal mental health: Perinatal depression and anxiety.* http://safehealthcareforeverywoman.org/patient-safety-bundles/maternal-mental-health-depression-and-anxiety/

American College of Obstetricians and Gynecologists. (2017a). Emergent therapy for acute-onset, severe hypertension during pregnancy and the postpartum period. Committee Opinion No. 692. *Obstetrics & Gynecology, 129,* e90–e95. https://doi: 10.1097/AOG.0000000000003075

American College of Obstetricians and Gynecologists. (2017b). *Postpartum hemorrhage from vaginal delivery.* Patient Safety Checklist Number 10. https://www.acog.org/Clinical-Guidance-and-Publications/Patient-Safety-Checklists-Li

American College of Obstetricians and Gynecologists. (2017c). Postpartum hemorrhage. Practice Bulletin. *Obstetrics & Gynecology, 108,* 1039–1046.

American College of Obstetricians and Gynecologists. (2018a). Gestational diabetes mellitus. Practice Bulletin No. 190. *Obstetrics & Gynecology, 131*(2), e49–e64. https://doi:10.1097/AOG.0000000000002501

American College of Obstetricians and Gynecologists. (2018b). Optimizing postpartum care. ACOG Committee Opinion No. 763. *Obstetrics & Gynecology, 131,* e140–e150.

American College of Obstetricians and Gynecologists. (2018c). Screening for perinatal depression. Committee Opinion No 757. *Obstetrics & Gynecology, 132,* 5. https://doi.org/10.1097/AOG.0000000000002927

American College of Obstetricians and Gynecologists' Committee on Practice Bulletins—Obstetrics (2018d). ACOG Practice Bulletin No. 196: Thromboembolism in Pregnancy. *Obstetrics and gynecology, 132*(1), e1–e17.

American College of Obstetricians and Gynecologists. (2021). Obesity in pregnancy. Practice Bulletin No. 230. *Obstetrics & Gynecology, 137*(6), 128–144. https://doi.org/10.1097/AOG.0000000000004395

Association of Women's Health, Obstetric and Neonatal Nurses. (2015). Position statement mood and anxiety disorders in pregnant and postpartum women. *Journal of Obstetric, Gynecologic, and Neonatal Nursing, 44,* 687–689.

Association of Women's Health, Obstetric and Neonatal Nurses. (2016). *The nursing care of the woman with diabetes in pregnancy: Evidence-based clinical practice guideline.* Evidence-Based Clinical Practice Guideline Development Team.

Association of Women's Health, Obstetric and Neonatal Nurses. (2018). *SAVE YOUR LIFE: Get care for these POST-BIRTH warning signs.* Author.

Association of Women's Health, Obstetric and Neonatal Nurses. (2020). Position Statement: Standardized practices to address maternal venous thromboembolism: AWHONN Practice Brief 7. *Journal of Obstetric, Gynecologic, and Neonatal Nursing, 49,* 1. https://doi.org/10.1016/j.jogn.2019.11.002

Association of Women's Health, Obstetric and Neonatal Nurses. (2021a). Guidelines or oxytocin administration after birth. Practice Brief No. 12. *Journal of Obstetric, Gynecologic, & Neonatal Nursing, 50,* 4. https://doi.org/10.1016/j.jogn.2021.04.006

Association of Women's Health, Obstetric and Neonatal Nurses. (2021b). Quantification of blood loss: AWHONN Practice Brief No. 13. *Journal of Obstetric, Gynecologic, & Neonatal Nursing, 25,* 4. https://doi.org/10.1016/j.nwh.2021.04.005

Barinov, S. V., Tirskaya, Y. I., Kadsyna, T. V., Lazareva, O. V., Medyannikova, I. V., & Tshulovski, Y. I. (2020). Pregnancy and delivery in women with a high risk of infection in pregnancy. *The Journal of Maternal-Fetal & Neonatal Medicine,* 1–6. https://doi.org/10.1080/14767058.2020.1781810

Beck, C. T., Watson, S., & Gable, R. K. (2018). Traumatic childbirth and its aftermath: Is there anything positive? *The Journal of Perinatal Education, 27*(3), 175–184. https://doi.org/10.1891/1058-1243.27.3.175

Beck, J. (2014, April 21). Postpartum depression can happen to any parent. *The Atlantic.* https://www.theatlantic.com/health/archive/2014/04/postpartum-depression-can-happen-to-any-parent/360918/

Beck C. T. (2020). Postpartum Depression: A Metaphorical Analysis. *Journal of the American Psychiatric Nurses Association,* 1078390320959448. Advance online publication. https://doi.org/10.1177/1078390320959448

Belfort, M. A. (2018, May 18). *Postpartum hemorrhage: Medical and minimally invasive management.* UpToDate: Evidence-Based Clinical Decision Support. https://www.uptodate.com/contents/overview-of-postpartum-hemorrhage?topicRef=6714&source=see_link

Bernstein, P. S., Martin, J. N., Jr., Barton, J. R., Shields, L. E., Druzin, M. L., Scavone, B. M., . . . Menard, M. K. (2017). Consensus bundle on severe hypertension during pregnancy and the postpartum period. *Journal of Midwifery & Women's Health, 62*(4), 493–501. https://doi.org/10.1111/jmwh.12647

Building U.S. Capacity to Review and Prevent Maternal Deaths. (2018). *Report from nine maternal mortality review committees.* https://stacks.cdc.gov/view/cdc/51660

California Maternal Quality Care Collaborative. (2015). *Improving health care response to obstetric hemorrhage.* Center for Academic Medicine Neonatology.

Callaghan, W. M., Creanga, A. A., & Kuklina, E. V. (2012). Severe maternal morbidity among delivery and postpartum hospitalizations in the United States. *Obstetrics & Gynecology, 120*(5), 1029–1036. https://doi.org/10.1097/aog.0b013e31826d60c5

Centers for Disease Control and Prevention. (2019a). *Gestational diabetes.* https://www.cdc.gov/diabetes/basics/gestational.html

Centers for Disease Control and Prevention. (2019b). *Racial and ethnic disparities continue in pregnancy-related deaths.* https://www.cdc.gov/media/releases/2019/p0905-racial-ethnic-disparities-pregnancy-deaths.html

Chow, R., Huang, E., Li, A., Li, S., Fu, S. Y., Son, J. S., & Foster, W. G. (2021). Appraisal of systematic reviews on interventions for postpartum depression: Systematic review. *BMC Pregnancy and Childbirth, 21*(1), 1–11. https://doi.org/10.1186/s12884-020-03496-5

Cunningham, F., Leveno, K., Bloom, S., Dashe, J., Hoffman, B., Casey, B., & Spong, C. (2018). *Williams obstetrics* (25th ed.). McGraw-Hill.

D'Alton, M. E., Friedman, A. M., Bernstein, P. S., Brown, H. L., Callaghan, W. M., Clark, S. L., . . . Foley, M. R. (2019). Putting the "M" back in maternal-fetal medicine: A 5-year report card on a collaborative effort to address maternal morbidity and mortality in the United States. *American Journal of Obstetrics and Gynecology, 221*(4), 311.e1–317.e1. https://doi.org/10.1016/j.ajog.2019.02.055

Daley, J. (2014). Diabetes in pregnancy. In K. Simpson & P. Creehan (Eds.), *Perinatal nursing* (4th ed.). Lippincott, Williams & Wilkins.

Davis, N. L., Smoots, A. N., & Goodman, D. A. (2019). Pregnancy-related deaths: Data from 14 U.S. maternal mortality review committees, 2008–2017. *Maternal Mortality Review Information App.* https://www.cdc.gov/reproductivehealth/maternal-mortality/erase-mm/MMR-Data-Brief_2019-h.pdf

Engqvist, I., & Nilsson, K. (2011). Men's experience of their partners' postpartum psychiatric disorders: Narratives from the internet. *Mental Health in Family Medicine, 8*(3), 137–146.

Farpour-Lambert, N. J., Ells, L. J., Martinez de Tejada, B., & Scott, C. (2018). Obesity and weight gain in pregnancy and postpartum: An evidence review of lifestyle interventions to inform maternal and child health policies. *Frontiers in Endocrinology, 9.* https://doi.org/10.3389/fendo.2018.00546

Flanders, C. E., Gibson, M. F., Goldberg, A. E., & Ross, L. E. (2015). Postpartum depression among visible and invisible sexual minority women: A pilot study. *Archives of Women's Mental Health, 19*(2), 299–305. https://doi.org/10.1007/s00737-015-0566-4

Gregg, I. (2018). The health care experiences of lesbian women becoming mothers. *Nursing for Women's Health, 22*(1), 40–50. https://doi.org/10.1016/j.nwh.2017.12.003

Griffith-Gilbert, L., & Rousseau, J. B. (2020). Assessment and care in postpartum women. In P. D. Suplee & J. Janke, J. (Eds.), *AWHONN Compendium of postpartum care* (3rd ed., pp. 1–34). Association of Women's Health, Obstetric and Neonatal Nurses.

Hadjiliadis, D., & Harron, P. F. (2019, May 16). Blue discoloration of the skin: MedlinePlus Medical Encyclopedia. *MedlinePlus*. https://medlineplus.gov/ency/article/003215.htm

Howell, E. A., Brown, H., Brumley, J., Bryant, A. S., Caughey, A. B., Cornell, A. M., . . . Grobman, W. A. (2018). Reduction of peripartum racial and ethnic disparities. *Obstetrics & Gynecology, 131*(5), 770–782. https://doi.org/10.1097/aog.0000000000002475

Jackson, A., & Haynes, L. (2020). *A blueprint for medium fidelity postpartum hemorrhage simulations, 2020*. AWHONN. https://doi.org/10.1016/j.nwh.2020.07.008

James, D., & Suplee, P. (2021). Postpartum care. In K. Simpson, P. Creehan, N. O'Brien-Abel, C. Roth, & A. Rohan (Eds.), *Perinatal nursing* (5th ed., pp. 508-562). Wolters Kluwer.

Jones, I., Chandra, P. S., Dazzan, P., & Howard, L. M. (2014). Bipolar disorder, affective psychosis, and schizophrenia in pregnancy and the post-partum period. *Lancet, 384*(9956), 1789–1799. https://doi.org/10.1016/S0140-6736(14)61278-2

Kendig, S., Keats, J. P., Hoffman, M. C., Kay, L. B., Miller, E. S., Moore Simas, T. A., . . . Lemieux, L. A. (2017). Consensus bundle on maternal mental health: Perinatal depression and anxiety. *Journal of Obstetric, Gynecologic & Neonatal Nursing, 46*(2), 272–281.

Ko, J. Y., Rockhill, K. M., Tong, V. T., Morrow, B., & Farr, S. L. (2017). Trends in postpartum depressive symptoms—27 states, 2004, 2008, and 2012. *MMWR Morbidity and Mortality Weekly Report, 66,* 153–158. https://doi.org/10.15585/mmwr.mm6606a1

Lyndon, A., Lagrew, D., Shields, L., Main, E., & Cape, V. (2015). *Improving health care response to obstetric hemorrhage. California Maternal Quality Care Collaborative Toolkit to Transform Maternity Care*. California Maternal Quality Care Collaborative.

Maccio, E. M., & Pangburn, J. A. (2011). The case for investigating postpartum depression in lesbians and bisexual women. *Women's Health Issues, 21*(3), 187–190. https://doi.org/10.1016/j.whi.2011.02.007

Main, E. K., Goffman, D., Scavone, B. M., Low, L. K., Bingham, D., Fontaine, P. L., . . . Levy, B. S. (2015). National partnership for maternal safety: Consensus bundle on obstetric hemorrhage. *Journal of Obstetric, Gynecologic & Neonatal Nursing, 44,* 462–470. https://doi.org/10.1111/1552-6909.12723

McGovern, B., Bingham, D., & Dildy, G. (2019). Obstetric hemorrhage. In N. Troiano, P. Witcher, & S. McMurtry Baird (Eds.), *High risk & critical care obstetrics* (4th ed., pp. 258–285). Wolters Kluwer.

Melrose, S. (2010). Parental postpartum depression: How can nurses help? *Contemporary Nurse, 34,* 199–210.

Milgrom, J., & Holt, C. (2014). Early intervention to protect the mother–infant relationship following postnatal depression: Study protocol for a randomised controlled trial. *Trials, 15,* 385. https://doi.org/10.1186/1745-6215-15-385

Opray, N., Grivell, R. M., Deussen, A. R., & Dodd, J. M. (2015). Directed preconception health programs and interventions for improving pregnancy outcomes for women who are overweight or obese. *Cochrane Database of Systematic Reviews, 7,* CD010932. https://doi.org/10.1002/14651858.CD010932.pub2

Rogers, H. J., Hogan, L., Coates, D., Homer, C. S., & Henry, A. (2020). Responding to the health needs of women from migrant and refugee backgrounds—Models of maternity and postpartum care in high-income countries: A systematic scoping review. *Health & Social Care in the Community, 28*(5), 1343–1365. https://doi.org/10.1111/hsc.12950

Roth, C. (2021). Pulmonary complications in pregnancy. In K. Simpson, P. Creehan, N. O'Brien- Abel, C. Roth, & A. Rohan (Eds.), *Perinatal nursing* (5th ed., pp. 220–247). Wolters Kluwer.

Ruud, M. (2018). Cultural humility in the care of individuals who are lesbian, gay, bisexual, transgender, or queer. *Nursing for Women's Health, 22*(3), 255–263. https://doi.org/10.1016/j.nwh.2018.03.009

Salera-Vieira, J. (2021). Bleeding in pregnancy. In K. Simpson, P. Creehan, N. O'Brien-Abel, C. Roth, & A. Rohan (Eds.), *Perinatal nursing* (5th ed., pp. 123–140). Wolters Kluwer.

Sisson, M., & Hamner, L. (2019). Disseminated intravascular coagulation in pregnancy. In N. Troiano, P. Witcher, & S. McMurtry Baird (Eds.), *High risk & critical care obstetrics* (4th ed., pp. 286–295). Wolters Kluwer.

Smith, S., & Turell, S. (2017). Perceptions of healthcare experiences: Relational and communicative competencies to improve care for LGBT people. *Journal of Social Issues, 3,* (3), 637–657. https://doi.org/10.1111/josi.12235

Suplee, P. D., & Janke, J. (Eds.). (2020). *AWHONN Compendium of postpartum care* (3rd ed.). Association of Women's Health, Obstetric and Neonatal Nurses.

Tarasoff, L. A., Ravindran, S., Malik, H., Salaeva, D., & Brown, H. K. (2020). Maternal disability and risk for pregnancy, delivery, and postpartum complications: A systematic review and meta-analysis. *American Journal of Obstetrics and Gynecology, 222*(1), 27.e1–27.e32. https://doi.org/10.1016/j.ajog.2019.07.015

VanderKruik, R., Barreix, M., Chou, D., Allen, T., Say, L., Cohen, L., and on behalf of the Maternal Morbidity Working Group. (2017). *BMC Psychiatry, 17,* 272. https://doi.org/10.1186/s12888-017-1427-7

Wesseloo, R., Kamperman, A. M., Munk-Olsen, T., Pop, V. J. M., Kushner, S. A., & Bergink, V. (2016). Risk of postpartum relapse in bipolar disorder and postpartum psychosis: A systematic review and meta-analysis. *American Journal of Psychiatry, 173*(2), 117–127. https://doi.org/10.1176/appi.ajp.2015.15010124

Witcher, P., & Hamner, L. (2019). Venous thromboembolism in pregnancy. In N. Troiano, P. Witcher, & S. McMurtry Baird (Eds.), *High risk & critical care obstetrics* (4th ed., pp. 176–193). Wolters Kluwer.

Wong, A. (2017). Pregnancy, postpartum infections. *eMedicine*. http://emedicine.medscape.com/article/796892-overview

Yonkers, K., Vigod, S., & Ross, L. (2011). Diagnosis, pathophysiology, and management of mood disorders in pregnancy and postpartum women. *Obstetrics & Gynecology, 117,* 961–977.

The Neonatal Period

Nursing Care of the Neonate and Family

15

Sharon C. Hitchcock, DNP, RNC-MN
Connie S. Miller, DNP, RNC-OB, CNE

LEARNING OUTCOMES

Upon completion of this chapter, the student will be able to:

1. Identify changes that occur during the transition from intrauterine to extrauterine life and the related nursing actions.
2. List critical elements of a neonatal assessment.
3. Delineate critical elements of a neonatal gestational age assessment.
4. Discuss methods used in neonatal pain management.
5. Formulate a plan of nursing care for neonates during the first week of life.
6. Explain common laboratory and diagnostic tests for neonates.
7. Outline nursing actions that support parents in the care of their newborn.
8. Describe common therapeutic and surgical procedures used for neonates and the related nursing care.
9. Demonstrate the importance of incorporating knowledge of cultural beliefs, values, customs, and newborn variations in the care of the parents and newborn.
10. Educate parents on newborn care.

CONCEPTS

Comfort
Culture
Elimination
Family
Immunity
Infection
Metabolism
Nutrition
Oxygenation or Gas
   Exchange
Perfusion
Safety
Teaching and Learning
Thermoregulation

Nursing Diagnosis

- At risk for altered body temperature, hypothermia, related to decreased amounts of subcutaneous fat or large body surface
- At risk for infections related to tissue trauma or poor hand washing techniques by health-care providers and parents
- At risk for impaired gas exchange related to transitioning from fetal to neonatal circulation, cold stress, or excessive mucus production
- At risk for knowledge deficit related to first-time parenting or limited learning resources

Nursing Outcomes

- The neonate's temperature will be within normal limits, and the skin will be pink and feel warm to the touch.
- The neonate will not exhibit signs or symptoms of infection.
- The neonate's respiratory and heart rate will be within normal ranges and the airway will remain clear.
- The neonate will void a minimum of three times daily by day 3 and stool a minimum of three times daily by day 3.
- The parents will demonstrate proper care of their newborn.
- The parents will convey they are comfortable with caring for their newborn.
- The parents will list signs of potential infant illness they must report to the health-care provider.

INTRODUCTION

The neonatal period is from birth through the first 28 days of life. During these few weeks, the neonate transitions from intrauterine to extrauterine life and adapts to a new environment. Most term neonates whose mothers experienced an uncomplicated pregnancy and birth accomplish this transition with relative ease (Fig. 15–1).

The focus of nursing care during the transition to extrauterine life is to assess, monitor, and support neonates as they undergo numerous physiological changes. This is accomplished by:

- Maintaining respiratory and cardiac function
- Maintaining body heat
- Decreasing the risk for infection
- Assessing for signs of complications
- Assisting parents in providing appropriate nutrition
- Educating parents in caring for their newborn

TRANSITION TO EXTRAUTERINE LIFE

The transition to extrauterine life begins with the neonate's first breaths and clamping of the umbilical cord. These events initiate a sequence of changes within the neonate's respiratory and cardiovascular systems and are the most critical and immediate changes necessary for the transition from fetus to neonate. These initial events include fluid clearance from the lungs, lung expansion with air, circulatory changes, and shunt closures, which ultimately transfer gas exchange from the placenta to the lungs (Fernandes, 2019). Other systems that undergo significant changes are the thermoregulatory, metabolic, hepatic, gastrointestinal (GI), renal, and immune systems (Blackburn, 2018).

The Respiratory System

The establishment of respirations is the first physiological change that must occur after birth. Respirations, combined with cessation

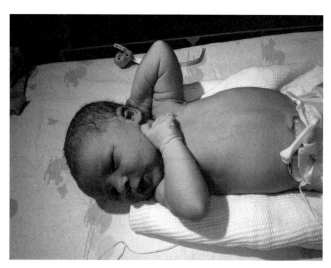

FIGURE 15–1 Neonate 15 minutes after birth transitioning to extrauterine life.

of blood flow through the placenta (umbilical cord clamping), cause the fetus to transition to the neonatal circulatory pattern. Chemical, mechanical, and sensory stimuli, such as from temperature changes, sounds, lights, and touch, are involved in causing these first respirations (Fig. 15–2) (Blackburn, 2018).

Preparation for extrauterine respirations starts in utero during labor with compression of the fetal thorax during contractions and while passing (being squeezed) through the birth canal. This assists with clearing some alveolar fluid from the lungs. Once through the birth canal, the lungs re-expand, and passive inspiration occurs. Because of mild hypoxia that all fetuses experience during the birthing process, the respiratory center in the brain is stimulated, causing the diaphragm to contract immediately after birth. Sensory stimuli, including drying the infant, sounds, lights, temperature change, and skin-to-skin contact on the mother, also play a role in stimulating and maintaining respirations. The neonate crying increases intrathoracic pressure, further stimulating respirations and clearing of the lung fluids. With these first breaths, most lung fluid is cleared from the alveoli and replaced with air. Lung fluids are cleared in most term newborns within the first 4 hours and oxygen levels quickly rise to greater than 90% saturation within 5 to 15 minutes in healthy term neonates (Blackburn, 2018). Improved oxygenation leads to further pulmonary vasodilation and a decrease in pulmonary vascular resistance (PVR). As pulmonary vessels relax, gas exchange improves in the alveoli and blood flow is maximized throughout the lungs (Blackburn, 2018; Fernandes, 2019).

The presence of **surfactant,** a phospholipid, within the alveoli assists in the establishment of **functional residual capacity** and is necessary to keep the alveoli open. This residual capacity (volume of air left in the alveolar sacs at the end of expiration) helps keep the sacs partially open, which decreases the amount of pressure and energy required on inspiration (see Chapter 17).

Two factors that negatively affect the transition to extrauterine respirations are:

- Decreased surfactant levels related to immature lungs
- Severe or persistent hypoxemia and acidosis that lead to continued ↑PVR and failure of the pulmonary vessels to fully dilate

Approximately 10% of neonates require some degree of assistance with respirations at the time of delivery, and 1% require extensive resuscitation (American Academy of Pediatrics [AAP] & American College of Obstetrics and Gynecologists [ACOG], 2017; Blackburn, 2018).

CRITICAL COMPONENT

Signs of Neonatal Respiratory Distress
- Central cyanosis
- Tachypnea
- Apnea
- Grunting
- Flaring of nostrils
- Retractions of the chest wall
- Hypotonia (late sign)

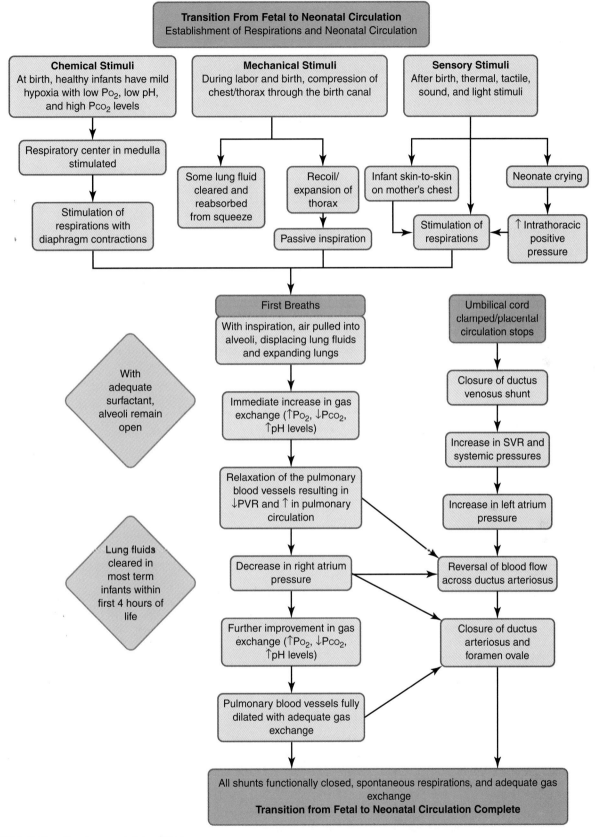

FIGURE 15-2 Transition to neonatal circulation.

The Circulatory System

The transition from fetal circulation to neonatal circulation begins within seconds of initiation of the first breaths and clamping of the umbilical cord. The transition to neonatal circulation is dependent on changes within the respiratory system and pressure changes within the cardiovascular system. With cessation of blood flow through the umbilical cord, an immediate rise in systemic vascular resistance (SVR) and systemic pressures occurs. These dramatic changes in systemic and pulmonary pressures improve gas exchange in the lungs and close the fetal shunts. Fetal circulation is discussed in Chapter 3 (Fig. 15–3).

The three major fetal circulatory structures (shunts) that undergo changes are the ductus venosus (DV), foramen ovale (FO), and the ductus arteriosus (DA). During fetal life, these structures shunt oxygenated blood coming from the placenta away from the lungs and liver and into systemic circulation. After birth, these shunts are no longer needed and must close as part of the intrauterine to extrauterine transition.

- The **ductus venosus** (DV), which connects the umbilical vein to the inferior vena cava, diverts most of the blood away from the liver. The DV closes with cessation of blood flow through the placenta and umbilical cord. The DV is permanently closed within 2 weeks and becomes a ligament (Blackburn, 2018).
- The **foramen ovale** (FO), an opening between the right atrium and the left atrium, closes when left atrial pressure exceeds right atrial pressure as PVR decreases and SVR increases. Significant neonatal hypoxia and increase in PVR can cause reopening of the FO. This shunt functionally closes within 1 to 2 hours of birth, and permanently by 30 months (Blackburn, 2018).
- The **ductus arteriosus** (DA), which connects the pulmonary artery with the aorta, usually closes within 15 hours in most term infants, and by 96 hours in nearly all neonates (Blackburn, 2018). Permanent closure occurs within 3 months. The DA can remain open or reopen when the lungs fail to expand, hypoxia occurs, or PVR increases.

The Thermoregulatory System

The fetus is surrounded in amniotic fluid that maintains a fairly constant environmental temperature based on the maternal body temperature. Once the neonate enters the extrauterine world, the child must adapt to changes in the environmental temperatures. The neonate's responses to temperature changes during the first few weeks are often delayed and place the neonate at risk for hypothermia and cold stress. A **neutral thermal environment** (NTE) is needed to support the infant during this transition. NTE maintains body temperature with minimal oxygen consumption and decreased metabolic rate (Blackburn, 2018). NTE decreases possible complications of the neonate's limited ability to respond to environmental temperature changes.

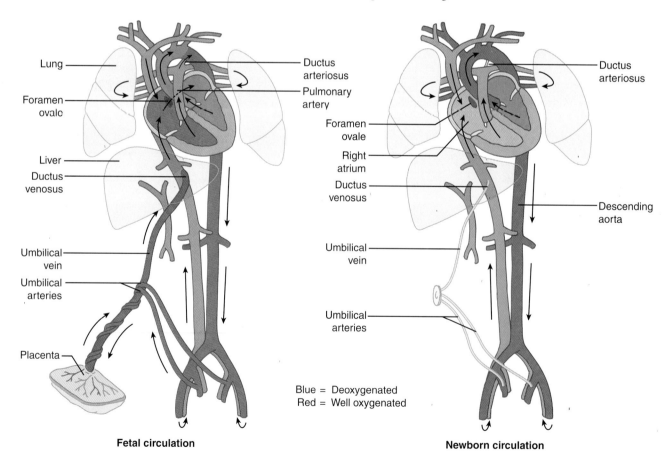

Fetal circulation   **Newborn circulation**

Blue = Deoxygenated
Red = Well oxygenated

FIGURE 15–3 Fetal and neonatal circulation.

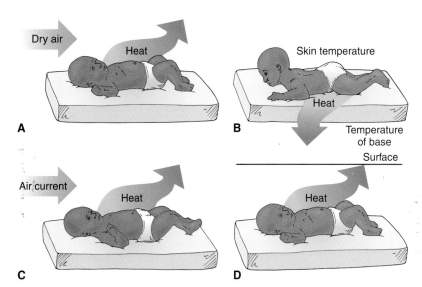

FIGURE 15–4 The four mechanisms of heat loss in the newborn. (A) Evaporation. (B) Conduction. (C) Convection. (D) Radiation.

The neonate responds to cold by:

- An increase in metabolic rate and oxygen consumption
- An increase of muscle activity (i.e., restlessness or crying) and flexed positioning
- Peripheral vascular constriction (mottling, acrocyanosis, or pallor)
- Metabolism of **brown adipose tissue (BAT)**

BAT metabolism is also called **nonshivering thermogenesis.** BAT is a highly dense and vascular adipose tissue. Full-term neonates possess large amounts of BAT, whereas preterm neonates, children, and adults have smaller amounts (Blackburn, 2018). BAT is located in the neck, thorax, axillary area, intrascapular areas, and around the adrenal glands and kidneys. BAT reserves are rapidly depleted during periods of cold stress.

BAT metabolism promotes:

- Heat production through intense lipid metabolism
- Heat transfer to the peripheral system (Blackburn, 2018)

Neonates are at higher risk for thermoregulatory problems related to:

- Higher body-surface-area-to-body-mass ratio
- Limited subcutaneous fat
- Higher metabolic rate
- Limited thermoregulatory abilities and inability to shiver

Factors that negatively affect thermoregulation are:

- Decreased subcutaneous fat
- Decreased BAT in preterm neonates
- Loss of body heat from evaporation, conduction, convection, or radiation (Fig. 15–4):
  - Evaporation: Loss of heat that occurs when moisture on the neonate's skin is converted to vapors, such as during bathing or directly after birth
  - Conduction: Transfer of heat to cooler surface by direct skin contact, such as cold hands of caregivers or cold equipment
  - Convection: Loss of heat from the neonate's warm body surface to cooler air currents, such as air conditioners or oxygen masks

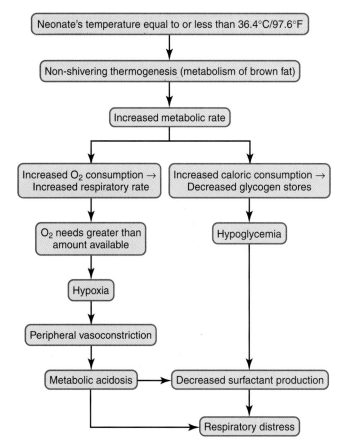

FIGURE 15–5 Cold stress.

- Radiation: Transfer of heat from the neonate to cooler objects that are not in direct contact with the neonate, such as cold walls of the isolette or cold equipment near the neonate

Cold Stress

Cold stress is a term to describe excessive heat loss that results in the utilization of compensatory mechanisms to maintain the neonate's body temperature (Fig. 15–5). Cold stress occurs when there is a decrease in environmental temperature that causes a decrease in the neonate's body temperature, which can lead to respiratory distress and other serious outcomes.

Possible consequences of cold stress are:

- Hypoglycemia
- Hypoxia
- Metabolic acidosis
- Decreased surfactant production
- Respiratory distress that can lead to delayed or return to fetal circulatory patterns
- Increased bilirubin and jaundice
- Poor feeding and weight loss
- Apnea
- Neonatal death

Risk Factors

- Prematurity
- Small for gestational age (SGA)
- Hypoglycemia
- Prolonged resuscitation efforts
- Sepsis
- Neurological, endocrine, or cardiorespiratory problems (Blackburn, 2018)

Signs and Symptoms

- Axillary temperature below 97.7°F (36.5°C)
- Cool skin
- Restlessness or crying
- Pale or mottled skin
- Acrocyanosis
- Tachypnea
- Grunting
- Hypoglycemia
- Hypotonia
- Lethargy
- Jitteriness
- Weak suck

Nursing Actions

Preventive actions should include the following:

- Dry the neonate thoroughly immediately after birth.
- Remove wet blankets from the neonate's direct environment.
- Place a stocking cap on the neonate's head (Fig. 15–6).
- Provide skin-to-skin contact with the mother or partner with a warm blanket over both.
- Use prewarmed blankets and clothing.
- Prewarm radiant warmers and heat shields.
- Warm stethoscope with hands before use.
- Delay initial bath until the neonate's temperature is stable.
- Bathe baby under a radiant heat source.
- Place the neonate away from air vents, open windows, or drafts.
- Place the neonate away from outside walls and windows.

(Blackburn, 2018; Simpson et al., 2021)

Actions when the neonate displays signs or symptoms of cold stress include the following:

- Monitor temperature as per institutional protocol.
- Place a stocking cap on the neonate's head.

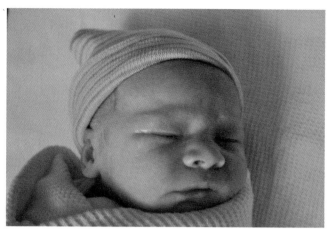

FIGURE 15–6 Stocking cap is placed on the neonate's head to reduce heat loss due to radiation and convection.

- Arrange for skin-to-skin contact with the mother or partner with a warm blanket over both.
- Swaddle in warm blankets.
- Assess for and correct environmental conditions that might worsen cold stress in the neonate.
- Reassess temperature as per institutional protocol, generally every 30 minutes until stable.
- Obtain a heel stick to assess for hypoglycemia (glucose below 40 to 45 mg/dL) and treat for hypoglycemia based on glucose level and hospital protocol.
- Place the undressed (diaper-only) neonate under a preheated radiant warmer.
  - Rewarm neonate under radiant warmer as per institutional protocol or manufacturer guidelines.
  - Attach the servo-controlled probe on the neonate's abdomen or other body surface that is closest to the radiant source, and as per institutional protocol.
  - Monitor the neonate's temperature, respiratory rate, and heart rate every 5 minutes when rewarming.

The Metabolic System

Large quantities of glycogen and fat are stored by the fetus during the third trimester of pregnancy to meet energy requirements for the transition from intrauterine to extrauterine life. Immediately after birth, the neonate becomes independent of the mother's metabolism and must balance the increase in energy demands with glucose and glycogen availability (Blackburn, 2018). Glucose values normally are lower the first few hours after birth and slowly rise during the first 12 hours (AAP & ACOG, 2017). Newborn glucose levels on the first day and after the first 4 hours range between 40 and 60 mg/dL, and after the first day between 50 and 90 mg/dL (Lo, 2020)

Hypoglycemia (blood glucose levels below 40 to 45 mg/dL in the neonate) is common during the transitional time, especially in neonates with complications. During intrauterine life, neonates of diabetic mothers produce high levels of insulin in response to high levels of circulating maternal glucose. After birth, the neonate's insulin level remains higher than normal, leading to hypoglycemia.

CRITICAL COMPONENT

Hypoglycemia

Hypoglycemia is defined as a blood glucose level below 40 to 45 mg/dL in the neonate.

Risks for Hypoglycemia
- Neonates of diabetic mothers
- Large-for-gestational-age (LGA) neonates
- Post-term neonates
- Late preterm neonates
- Preterm neonates
- SGA neonates
- Hypothermia
- Neonatal infection
- Respiratory distress
- Neonatal resuscitation
- Birth trauma

Signs and Symptoms
- Jitteriness, tremors
- Irritability
- Tachypnea, grunting
- Seizures
- Apnea
- Hypotonia
- Lethargy
- Hypothermia
- Cyanosis
- Poor feeding

(Blackburn, 2018; Simpson et al., 2021)

Nursing Actions

- Monitor for signs and symptoms of hypoglycemia.
- Assess blood glucose level with use of a glucose monitor.
- Assist the woman to either breastfeed or formula feed her infant. Buccal dextrose gel can be used if the mother does not want to use formula or when hypoglycemia persists.
- IV infusion of a dextrose solution can be given but necessitates admission to a neonatal intensive care unit (NICU).
- Maintain an NTE to decrease the risk of cold stress.

The Hepatic System

The liver is an extraordinary organ with multiple functions that include involvement in the metabolism of carbohydrates, proteins, and lipids; storage of fat-soluble vitamins and iron; synthesis of coagulation factors; bilirubin production and excretion; and detoxification and elimination of waste products. The neonatal liver is immature at the time of birth; thus, many functions are depressed or slowed. The following are several liver functions that can create risks for the neonate after birth (Costanzo, 2018; Simpson et al., 2021).

- Carbohydrate metabolism:
  - The liver regulates the blood glucose levels by converting excessive glucose to glycogen (insulin and cortisol facilitate this process) and converting glycogen to glucose when glucose levels are low. Preterm, post-term, SGA, and other at-risk neonates may not have enough glucose or glycogen stores to maintain normal glucose levels. Early feeding may contribute to stabilization of blood glucose levels in infants experiencing hypoglycemia (Simpson et al., 2021).
- Blood coagulation:
  - Neonates are at risk for delayed clotting and hemorrhage due to a temporary vitamin K deficiency after birth. This disorder, called *vitamin K deficiency bleeding,* can occur in some neonates due to liver immaturity, short half-life of maternal-acquired vitamin K, and lack of needed intestinal flora. Vitamin K is synthesized in the intestinal flora, which is absent at birth. The intestinal flora develops after the introduction of microorganisms, which usually occurs with the first feedings. Coagulation factors II, VII, IX, and X are synthesized in the liver and vitamin K is needed in the activation of these factors (Blackburn, 2018).
  - A single dose of vitamin K is given prophylactically to all neonates within the first hour of birth to decrease the risk of bleeding (Blackburn, 2018).
- Conjugation of bilirubin
  - The neonate's red blood cell (RBC) turnover (shorter RBC life span) and RBC count increase at birth. These (and other) factors contribute to a proportionally greater amount of bilirubin production after birth (see Chapter 17). There are two forms of bilirubin: indirect and direct.
    - **Indirect bilirubin** (unconjugated bilirubin), a fat-soluble substance, is produced from the breakdown of RBCs. It is converted to **direct bilirubin** (conjugated bilirubin), a water-soluble substance, by liver enzymes. Bilirubin must be conjugated (made water soluble) before it can be excreted in the urine and stool.
    - **Hyperbilirubinemia** is a condition characterized by a high level of unconjugated bilirubin in the neonate's blood related to the immature liver function, high RBC count common in neonates, and increased hemolysis caused by the shorter life span of fetal RBCs.
      - Hyperbilirubinemia is categorized into physiological jaundice and pathological jaundice (see Chapter 17). **Jaundice** is the yellowing of the skin and sclera that can be seen as the bilirubin levels rise.
      - Hyperbilirubinemia is very common, occurring in most term and nearly all preterm infants (Flaherman et al., 2017; Simpson et al., 2021). Although most jaundice is benign (mild or physiological), pathological jaundice can lead to permanent neurological damage if untreated. The AAP recommends screening all neonates for hyperbilirubinemia before discharge (AAP & ACOG, 2017).
- Storage of fat-soluble vitamins A, D, E, and K and iron
  - The formation of new RBCs is suppressed during the first few weeks postbirth. During this time, the liver stores iron from destroyed RBCs. This iron is used when RBC formation is resumed (Blackburn, 2018).
- Detoxification
  - The liver produces enzymes that detoxify harmful substances such as medications. Because the neonate's liver is

immature at birth, they sometimes do not have the capacity to synthesize the enzymes needed to detoxify medication, increasing the risk of toxic effects from medications (Blackburn, 2018).

SAFE AND EFFECTIVE NURSING CARE: Understanding Medication

Phytonadione (Vitamin K, Mephyton)
- Indication: Prevention of vitamin K deficiency bleeding (previously called hemorrhagic disease in neonate).
- Action: Vitamin K is required for the hepatic synthesis of blood coagulation factors II, VII, IX, and X.
- Common side effects: Erythema, pain, and swelling at the injection site
- Route and dose: intramuscularly (IM); 0.5 to 1 mg within 1 hour of birth

Vallerand & Sanoski, 2021.

The Gastrointestinal System

The neonate's GI system is not fully mature at birth but can rapidly adapt to demands for growth and development through ingestion, digestion, and absorption of nutrients, as well as eliminations of waste. Bowel sounds can normally be heard within the first hour of life due to the neonate swallowing air and peristalsis (Simpson et al., 2021). The gastric size of a newborn is approximately 6 mL/kg or 15 to 24 mL for most term infants (Blackburn, 2018). Newborn intake of colostrum is approximately 2 to 10 mL/feed the first 24 hours and increases to 30 to 60 mL/feed by day 4 (Kellmans et al., 2017). Stomach emptying time is 2 to 4 hours. Breast milk is digested faster than formula, so breastfed infants feed every 2 to 3 hours, whereas formula-fed infants feed every 3 to 4 hours. Neonates may appear uninterested in feeding during the first few days.

The characteristics of stools and stool patterns vary depending on type, frequency, and amount of feeding and age of the neonate (Table 15-1). Breastfed neonates tend to have more stools per day than formula-fed neonates, and stool is thinner in consistency. Some neonates may pass three to eight stools per day, whereas others will stool less. The types of stools are:

- Meconium stool begins to form in the fetus during the fourth gestational month and is the first stool eliminated by the neonate. It is sticky, thick, greenish-black, and odorless. It is first passed within 24 to 48 hours.
- Transitional stool begins around the third day and can continue for 3 or 4 days. The stool transitions from black to greenish black to greenish brown or yellow. This phase of stool characteristics occurs in both breastfed and formula-fed neonates.
- Breastfed stool is yellow and semiformed. Later it becomes a golden yellow with a pasty consistency, "seedy" appearance, and sour odor.
- Formula-fed stool is firmer and more formed than breastfed stools. It is a paler yellow or brownish yellow and has an unpleasant odor.
- Diarrheal stool is loose, watery, and green.

The Renal System

Two major functions of the kidneys are control of fluid and electrolyte balance, and excretion of metabolic waste. During fetal life, these functions are assumed by the placenta. Initially the kidneys are immature. This places neonates, especially preterm or sick neonates, at risk for:

- Overhydration: The glomerular filtration rate (GFR) is initially low in the neonate but doubles by 2 weeks of age (Blackburn, 2018).
  - Decreased GFR → ↓ ability to excrete water → ↑ risk of overhydration and water intoxication

TABLE 15-1	Minimum Number of Wet Diapers and Stools During the First Month		
NEONATE'S AGE	**NUMBER OF WET DIAPERS**	**NUMBER OF STOOLS**	**TYPE OF STOOL**
Day 1	1–2	1	Meconium—sticky, thick, and greenish black
Day 2	2–3	2	Meconium—sticky, thick, and greenish black
Day 3	3–4	3–4	Transitional—looser, lighter, greenish black or greenish brown
Day 4	4–5	3–4	Yellow, soft, and watery
Day 5	4–5	3–4	Breastfed stool or formula-fed stool
Day 6	6–8	3+	
Day 7	8+	3+	

AAP & ACOG, 2017.

- Dehydration: This can occur due to the neonatal kidneys' limited ability to concentrate urine.
- Electrolyte disorders: Examples include hyponatremia and hypernatremia in the preterm neonate. Increased sodium loss can occur in increased water loss, which increases the risk of hyponatremia. Dehydration related to excessive sodium intake increases the risk for hypernatremia (Blackburn, 2018).
- Drug toxicity: The limited abilities of the kidneys can affect the excretion of drugs from the neonate's systems and increase the risk of side effects and toxicity (Blackburn, 2018).

Full-term neonates excrete 15 to 60 mL/kg of urine per day for the first few days of life. Urinary output increases to 250 to 400 mL by the end of the first month (Blackburn, 2018). Neonates usually lose 5% to 10% of birth weight during the first week of life due in part to diuresis, which can lead to dehydration. Delayed or decreased urinary output can occur in neonates whose mothers received magnesium sulfate during labor, causing urinary retention (Blackburn, 2018).

The Immune System

The immune system protects the body from invasion by foreign materials such as bacteria and viruses. In utero, fetuses have some ability to respond to pathogenic antigens, peaking by 32 to 33 weeks, but rely heavily on **passive immunity (immunoglobulins)** from the maternal immune system for protection (Blackburn, 2018). After birth, neonates begin the process of developing normal microbial flora in the gut and its immunoglobulins (antibodies secreted by lymphocytes) through **active immunity** in response to pathogenic organisms. Establishment of gut flora helps provide protection against GI infections (Blackburn, 2018). Cell-mediated immunity including the lymphocytic response (white blood cells [WBCs]), is also present but immature at birth (Simpson et al., 2021). Because of the immature immune system, neonates have a slower inflammatory response, limiting their ability to recognize, isolate, and destroy organisms. Signs and symptoms of infection in the newborn are often subtle and non-specific. Typically, the sick newborn will become hypothermic instead of having a fever (Blackburn 2018). Although fetuses can be exposed to pathogens in utero, generally neonates are first exposed to organisms (both healthy and pathogenic) from the maternal genital tract during the birthing process. The maternal genital tract may contain group B streptococcus and *Escherichia coli,* which can result in neonatal infection and sepsis (see Chapter 17).

Neonates are at risk for infections related to:

- Immature immune system defense mechanisms and slower response to threats
- Lack of experience with and exposure to organisms (and thus lack of specific immunoglobulins needed)
- Exposure to dangerous organisms in utero that can cross the placenta
- Exposure to dangerous organisms during the birthing process
- Breakdown of skin and mucous membranes after birth, which provides a portal of entry (Blackburn, 2018)

Humoral immunity is the process in which B cells detect antigens and produce specific *immunoglobulins* (antibodies) against them. Maternal immunoglobulins provide *passive* immunity to the fetus through the placenta, which is not permanent. *Active* (long-term) immunity is developed by the neonate after exposure to an antigen (naturally or from vaccination).

Key immunoglobulins responsible for immunity in the neonate are IgG, IgA, and IgM.

- Maternal IgGs can cross the placenta and provide passive immunity for the neonate. These antibodies temporarily protect the neonate from bacterial and viral infections for which the mother has developed antibodies (Simpson et al., 2021).
- Maternal IgAs do not cross the placenta but are found in colostrum and breast milk. These antibodies provide passive immunity to breast-fed babies. These immunoglobulins also have anti-inflammatory properties and play a role in development of the immune system (Blackburn, 2018).
- Fetal IgMs are the primary antibodies produced in utero by the fetus in response to exposure to pathological organisms. Maternal IgMs do not cross the placenta. Common intrauterine infections (traditionally called "TORCH" infections) are toxoplasmosis, rubella, cytomegalovirus, syphilis, varicella virus, herpes, and the Zika virus.

NEONATAL ASSESSMENT

A neonate is assessed starting at birth with Apgar scores, vital signs, and a general survey. Head-to-toe (complete) assessment is typically done within 2 hours of birth. These initial assessments provide baseline data for the neonate, evaluate the transition to extrauterine life, and assist in determining the course of nursing and medical care. Other assessment components include pain assessment, weight and length measurements, behavioral assessment, neonatal reflexes, and gestational age assessment if indicated or per organizational policy (Simpson et al., 2021).

CLINICAL JUDGMENT

Methods of Reducing Heat Loss During Assessments

Thermoregulatory systems of neonates respond slower to external temperature changes than those of adults. Prevention of heat loss is critical when doing assessments. To maintain NTE and reduce heat loss during assessment:

- Ensure the room is warm and free of air drafts.
- Place the neonate under a radiant warmer or assess the neonate in the mother's arms. Skin-to-skin contact between the mother and neonate can decrease the amount of heat loss.
- Keep the neonate wrapped and expose only the body area that is being checked when doing assessments in an open crib or in a parent's arms.

Preparation for Assessment

- Review the prenatal record and birth record for factors that could place the neonate at risk for complications. Examples of risk factors are:
  - Late, inadequate, or no prenatal care
  - Maternal alcohol or substance use
  - Maternal age younger than 16 or older than 35
  - Chronic maternal illnesses such as diabetes and hypertension
  - Hypertensive disorders of pregnancy
  - Birth before 37 weeks' gestation
  - Operative delivery: Use of forceps or vacuum extractor
  - Medications during labor that affect the central nervous system (CNS), such as magnesium sulfate and analgesia or anesthesia
  - Prolonged rupture of membranes (ROM; longer than 24 hours)
  - Meconium-stained amniotic fluid
  - Placental abnormalities, such as placenta previa, placental abruption, or abnormal placentations
  - Apgar score 7 or below at 5 minutes
- Gather the equipment needed for the assessment: Gloves, measuring tape, stethoscope, thermometer, scale for weighing, and documentation records.
- Ensure that assessment is done in an NTE (i.e., close doors to prevent drafts, regulate room temperature, consider a radiant warmer for small or preterm infants).
- Inform the parents of the assessment and invite them to watch. This is especially helpful for the woman's partner and first-time parents.

General Survey

- A general survey of the neonate is completed before the physical assessment. This survey is best completed while the neonate is quiet.
- Observe the respiratory pattern and auscultate lung and heart sounds. It can be difficult to assess cardiac and respiratory systems once the neonate responds to being handled (cries) during the physical assessment.
- Assess the skin for color, signs of hypoxia (central cyanosis), and birth trauma.
- Observe the level of alertness and activity.
- Assess muscle tone and posture.

Physical Assessment

Typically, the physical assessment starts with the head and ends with legs and feet. However, the sequence of the physical assessment will depend on the cooperation of the infant and personal preferences of the nurse, and typically will begin with the most noninvasive assessments first (Simpson et al., 2021). Refer to Table 15-2 for neonatal assessment by area or system, Table 15-3 for common newborn characteristics, and Table 15-4 for newborn reflexes.

Gestational Age Assessment

Gestational age of the neonate can be established from the mother's menstrual history (last menstrual period [LMP]), prenatal ultrasonography, or a neonatal gestational age assessment. The calculation of gestational age by assessment tools such as the New Ballard Score (NBS) assists in estimating gestational age, predicting potential problems, and establishing a plan of care. The NBS tool is commonly used and evaluates both physical and neuromuscular characteristics. It can estimate gestational age down to approximately 20 weeks and is accurate to within 2 weeks of gestation (Simpson et al., 2021). Most hospitals have policies guiding which neonates should be assessed for gestational age, and who will do the assessment. Gestational age assessment is commonly completed on:

- Neonates of mothers who had no or inadequate prenatal care
- Preterm neonates, born before 37 weeks based on LMP dates
- Post-term neonates, born after 42 weeks by dates
- Neonates who weigh less than 2,500 g or more than 4,000 g
- Neonates of diabetic mothers
- Neonates whose condition requires admission to a NICU.

The NBS gestational age assessment is calculated by assessing six physical and six neuromuscular characteristics of the neonate (Table 15-5). The examination determines weeks of gestation and classifies the neonate as preterm (less than 37 weeks), term (37 to 42 weeks), or post-term (older than 42 weeks). The score from these examinations provides a gestational age based on weight, length, and head circumference to determine if the neonate is average for gestational age (AGA), SGA, or LGA (Fig. 15–7).

- SGA is a term used for neonates whose weight is below the 10th percentile for gestational age.
- LGA is a term used for neonates whose weight is above the 90th percentile for gestational age.

Pain Assessment

Neonates are subjected to a variety of painful stimuli during their transition to extrauterine life (e.g., injections, heel sticks for blood samples, and circumcision). In the past, health-care providers believed neonates did not experience pain because of their immature CNSs, so little attention was given to assessing and treating pain. Researchers now recognize that neonates do experience and react to pain, and often are hypersensitive to painful stimuli. Pain left untreated can lead to short- and long-term negative consequences. Goals of pain management include identification, prevention, and treatment interventions (AAP Committee on Fetus and Newborn and Section on Anesthesiology and Pain Medicine, 2016; Perry et al., 2018).

Pain management is part of the routine nursing care of neonates (Box 15-1). Several pain assessment scales, such as Premature Infant Pain Profile (PIPP) and Neonatal Infant Pain Scale (NIPS), have been developed to assess for neonatal pain. Pain assessment tools commonly look at the state of arousal, cry, motor activity, respiratory pattern, and facial expressions. Some

(text continues on p. 505)

TABLE 15-2   Neonatal Assessment by Area or System

AREA OR SYSTEM	TECHNIQUE AND ASSESSMENT	EXPECTED FINDINGS FOR TERM NEONATE	DEVIATIONS FROM NORMAL
Posture	Unwrap the newborn and observe posture when the neonate is quiet.	Extremities are flexed with symmetrical movements. Hands are clenched.	Limp or floppy, or extension of extremities often related to prematurity; effects of medications given to mother during labor such as magnesium sulfate and analgesics or anesthesia; birth injuries; hypothermia; hypoglycemia; or hypoxia (late sign).
Head circumference	Measure by placing tape around the head just above the ears and eyebrows. Measurement is usually recorded in centimeters.	32–36 cm (12.5–14 in.)	Microcephaly: Head circumference is below the 10th percentile of normal for newborn's gestational age. This is often related to congenital malformation, maternal drug or alcohol ingestion, or maternal infection during pregnancy. Macrocephaly: Head circumference is >90th percentile. This can be related to hydrocephalus.
Chest circumference	Measure by placing tape around the chest over the nipple line.	30.5–33 cm (12–13 in.) or 2–3 cm less than head circumference	
Length	Measure the length of body by securing tape on a flat surface. Place the top of the neonate's head at the top of the tape. Extend the body and one leg. Measurement is taken from the top of the head to the bottom of the heel.	46–52 cm (18–20.5 in.)	Molding may interfere with accurate assessment of length. Neonates whose length is below the 10th percentile should be further assessed for causes such as intrauterine growth restriction or prematurity.

Continued

TABLE 15-2   Neonatal Assessment by Area or System—cont'd

AREA OR SYSTEM	TECHNIQUE AND ASSESSMENT	EXPECTED FINDINGS FOR TERM NEONATE	DEVIATIONS FROM NORMAL
Weight	Clean scale before use. Place clean paper on the scale. Set the scale at zero. Place the naked neonate on the scale. Record the neonate's weight. Do not leave the neonate unattended while weighing.	2,500–4,100 g (5.5 to 9.0 lb) Weight loss of 5%–10% of birth weight during the first week is normal. This is due to fluid loss through urine, stools, and lungs; and inadequate caloric and fluid intake the first days of life. The neonate will regain birth weight within 10–14 days.	Weight above the 90th percentile is common in neonates of diabetic mothers. Weight below the 10th percentile may be due to prematurity, intrauterine growth restriction, or malnutrition during the pregnancy. Neonate should be evaluated for feeding problems if weight loss exceeds 7%.
Temperature	Place a clean temperature probe in the axillary area. Axillary temperatures are preferred in the hospital setting but rectal temperatures may also be done. Rectal temperatures are considered the most accurate.	97.7°F–99°F (36.5°C–37.2°C) Axillary	Hypothermia or hyperthermia is related to infection, environmental extremes, or neurological disorders.
Respirations	Assess respiratory rate by auscultating and observing the rise and fall of the chest and abdomen (without clothing) for 1 full minute.	30–60 breaths per minute Unlabored Irregular with pauses up to 15 seconds (periodic breathing), with no color change Diaphragmatic and abdominal breathing Rate increases when crying and decreases when sleeping.	Periods of apnea >20 seconds, especially if associated with color change. Tachypnea that may be related to sepsis, pain, hypothermia, hypoglycemia, or respiratory distress syndrome. Respirations <30; may be related to maternal analgesia or anesthesia during labor.
Pulse	Assess apical pulse rate by auscultating for 1 full minute. Assess rate and rhythm. Use of a stethoscope designed for neonates is recommended.	110–160 bpm Rate may increase (to 180 bpm) with crying and may decrease (to 90 bpm) when asleep. Murmurs may be heard, especially in the first 24 hours as shunts are closing; most are not pathological and disappear by 6 months.	Tachycardia (>160 bpm) indicates possible sepsis, pain, respiratory distress, or congenital heart abnormality. Bradycardia (<100 bpm) indicates possible sepsis, increased intracranial pressure, or hypoxemia.
Blood pressure	Blood pressure is not a routine part of neonatal assessment. Requires the use of specially designed equipment for neonates. The blood pressure is obtained from either the arm or leg of the neonate.	50–75/30–45 mm Hg	

TABLE 15-2   Neonatal Assessment by Area or System—cont'd

AREA OR SYSTEM	TECHNIQUE AND ASSESSMENT	EXPECTED FINDINGS FOR TERM NEONATE	DEVIATIONS FROM NORMAL
Pulse oxygen saturation levels (pulse oximetry)	Pulse oximetry is not routinely done with vital signs but may be done when there is respiratory distress or other concerns. Also used in screening for CCHD. Requires a neonatal-specific sensor.	Oxygen saturation levels are low at birth and rise over the first 10 minutes. >95% (Goyal, 2020)	
Integumentary or skin	Inspect the skin for color, intactness, bruising, birth marks, dryness, rashes, warmth, texture, and turgor. Inspect nails. Stork bite	Skin is pink and warm with acrocyanosis (cyanosis of hands and feet). Milia are present on the bridge of the nose and chin (see Table 15-4). Lanugo is present on the back, shoulders, and forehead, which decreases with advancing gestation (see Table 15-4). Peeling or cracking is often noted on infants >40 weeks' gestation. Slate gray patches (previously called Mongolian spots; see Table 15-4) Hemangiomas such as salmon-colored patch (stork bites), nevus flammeus (port-wine stain), and strawberry hemangiomas are developmental vascular abnormalities. Stork bites are found at the nape of the neck, on the eyelid, between the eyes, or on the upper lip. They deepen in color when the neonate cries. They disappear within the first year of life. Nevus flammeus are purple- to red-colored flat areas that can be located on various portions of the body. These do not disappear. Strawberry hemangiomas are raised bright red lesions that develop during the neonatal period. They spontaneously resolve during early childhood. Erythema toxicum, newborn rash (see Table 15-4).	Central cyanosis after the first 10 minutes of life is caused by reduced oxygen saturation and hypoxia. Circumoral cyanosis with pink mucous membranes may be benign. Jaundice within the first 24 hours is pathological (see Chapter 17). Pallor occurs with anemia, hypothermia, shock, or sepsis. Greenish or yellowish vernix indicates passage of meconium during pregnancy or labor. Persistent ecchymosis or petechiae occurs with thrombocytopenia, sepsis, or congenital infection. Abundant lanugo is often seen in preterm neonates. Thin and translucent skin, and increased amounts of vernix caseosa, are common in preterm neonates. Nails are longer in neonates >40 weeks' gestation. Pilonidal dimple: A small pit or sinus in the sacral area at the top of the crease between the buttocks; the sinus can become infected later in life.

Continued

TABLE 15-2　Neonatal Assessment by Area or System—cont'd

AREA OR SYSTEM	TECHNIQUE AND ASSESSMENT	EXPECTED FINDINGS FOR TERM NEONATE	DEVIATIONS FROM NORMAL
Head	Note the shape of the head. Inspect and palpate fontanels and suture lines. Inspect and palpate the head for caput succedaneum or cephalohematoma (see Table 15-4). 	Molding present (see Table 15-4). Fontanels are open, soft, intact, and slightly depressed. They may bulge with crying. The anterior fontanel is diamond shaped, approximately 2.5–4 cm (closes by 18 months of age). The posterior fontanel is a triangle shape that is approximately 0.5–1 cm (closes between 2 and 4 months). May be difficult to palpate due to excessive molding. There are overriding sutures when there is increased molding.	Fontanels that are firm and bulging and not related to crying are a possible indication of increased intracranial pressure. Depressed fontanels are a possible indication of dehydration. Bruising and laceration are observed at the site of the fetal scalp electrode or vacuum extractor. Presence of caput succedaneum or cephalohematoma is observed (see Table 15-4).
Neck	Lift the chin to assess the neck area. 	The neck is short with skin folds. Positive tonic neck reflex may be present (see Table 15-5).	Webbing or large thick skin folds at the back of the neck is a possible indication of genetic disorders. Absent tonic neck reflex is an indication of nerve injury.
Eyes	Assess the position of the eyes. Open the eyelids and assess the color of sclera and pupil size. Assess for blink reflex, red light reflex, and pupil reaction to light. 	Eyes are equal and symmetrical in size and placement. The neonate is able to follow objects within 12 inches of the visual field. Edema may be present due to pressure during labor and birth or reaction to eye prophylaxes. The iris is blue-gray or brown. The sclera is white or bluish white. Subconjunctival hemorrhage may be present due to pressure during labor and birth. Pupils are equally reactive to light.	Absent red-light reflex indicates cataracts. Unequal pupil reactions indicate neurological trauma. Blue sclera is a possible indication of osteogenesis imperfecta.

TABLE 15-2   Neonatal Assessment by Area or System—cont'd

AREA OR SYSTEM	TECHNIQUE AND ASSESSMENT	EXPECTED FINDINGS FOR TERM NEONATE	DEVIATIONS FROM NORMAL
		Positive red light reflex and blink reflex are observed. No tear production (tear production begins at 2 months). Transient strabismus and nystagmus are related to immature muscular control.	
Ears	Inspect the ears for position, shape, lesions, skin tags, dimples, or drainage. Hearing test is done before discharge.	Top of the pinna is aligned with the external canthus of the eye. Pinna is without deformities, well-formed and flexible. The neonate responds to noises with positive startle signs. Hearing becomes more acute as Eustachian tubes clear. Neonates respond more readily to high-pitched vocal sounds.	Low-set ears are associated with genetic disorders such as Down syndrome. Absent startle reflex is associated with possible hearing loss. Skin tags, dimpling, or other lesions may be associated with kidney or other abnormalities.
Nose	Observe the shape of the nose. Inspect the opening of the nares.	The nose may be flattened or bruised related to the birth process. Nares should be patent. Small amount of mucus is present. Neonates primarily breathe through their noses.	Large amounts of mucus drainage can lead to respiratory distress. A flat nasal bridge is seen with Down syndrome. Nasal flaring is a sign of respiratory distress.
Mouth	Inspect the lips, gums, tongue, palate, and mucous membranes. Open the mouth by placing gentle pressure on the lower lip. Test for rooting, sucking, swallowing, and gag reflexes (see Table 15-5).	Lips, gums, tongue, palate, and mucous membranes are pink, moist, and intact. Reflexes are positive. Dry lips are common after birth. Epstein's pearls are present (see Table 15–4).	Cyanotic or bluish mucous membranes are a sign of hypoxia. Dry mucous membranes are a sign of dehydration Natal teeth, which can be benign or related to congenital abnormality (see Table 15-4). Thin philtrum may be indicative of fetal alcohol syndrome. Cleft lip or palate, which is a congenital abnormality in which the lip or palate does not completely fuse (see Chapter 17).

Continued

TABLE 15-2   Neonatal Assessment by Area or System—cont'd

AREA OR SYSTEM	TECHNIQUE AND ASSESSMENT	EXPECTED FINDINGS FOR TERM NEONATE	DEVIATIONS FROM NORMAL
Chest and lungs	Inspect shape, symmetry, and chest excursion. Inspect the breast for size and drainage. Auscultate breath sounds.	The chest is barrel-shaped and symmetrical. Breast engorgement may be present in both male and female neonates related to maternal hormones and resolves within a few weeks. Clear or milky fluid from nipples related to maternal hormones. Lung sounds are clear and equal. Scattered crackles may be detected during the first few hours after birth. This is due to retained lung fluid, which will be absorbed through the lymphatics.	Pectus excavatum (funnel chest) is a congenital abnormality. Pectus carinatum (pigeon chest) can obstruct respirations. Chest retractions are a sign of respiratory distress. Persistent crackles, wheezes, stridor, grunting, paradoxical breathing, decreased breath sounds, or prolonged periods of apnea (>15–20 seconds) are signs of respiratory distress. Decreased or absent breath sounds are often related to meconium aspiration or pneumothorax.
Cardiac	Auscultate heart sounds; listen for at least 1 full minute. Palpate brachial and femoral pulses.	Point of maximal impulse (PMI) at the third or fourth intercostal space. S_1 and S_2 are present. Regular rhythm with some variability related to activity and respiratory changes. Murmurs in 30% of neonates, which disappear within 2 days of birth. Brachial and femoral pulses are present and equal.	Dextrocardia: Heart on the right side of the chest. Displaced PMI occurs with cardiomegaly. Persistent murmurs indicate persistent or return to fetal circulation (opening of shunts with blood flow through them), or CHDs. Femoral pulses that feel weaker than brachial pulses may indicate a CHD.

TABLE 15-2   Neonatal Assessment by Area or System—cont'd

AREA OR SYSTEM	TECHNIQUE AND ASSESSMENT	EXPECTED FINDINGS FOR TERM NEONATE	DEVIATIONS FROM NORMAL
Abdomen	Inspect size and shape of the abdomen. Palpate the abdomen, assessing for tone, hernias, and diastasis recti. Auscultate for bowel sounds. Inspect the umbilical cord and surrounding skin. 	The abdomen is soft, round, protuberant, and symmetrical. Bowel sounds are present but may be hypoactive for the first few days. Passage of meconium stool within 48 hours postbirth. The cord is opaque or whitish blue with two arteries and one vein, and covered with Wharton's jelly. Skin around the umbilical cord should be assessed for infection and have no redness, swelling, drainage, or foul smell. The cord becomes dry and darker in color within 24 hours postbirth and detaches from the body within 2 weeks.	Asymmetrical abdomen indicates a possible abdominal mass. Hernias or diastasis recti are more common in Black neonates and usually resolve on their own within the first year. One umbilical artery and vein is associated with heart or kidney malformation. Failure to pass meconium stool is often associated with imperforated anus or meconium ileus.
Rectum	Inspect the anus.	The anus is patent. Passage of stool within 24 hours.	Imperforated anus requires immediate surgery. Anal fissures or fistulas may be present.
Genitourinary: female	Place thumbs on either side of the labia and gently separate tissue to visually inspect the genitalia. Assess for the presence and position of the clitoris, vagina, and urinary meatus. 	Labia majora covers the labia minora and clitoris. Labia majora and minora may be edematous. Blood-tinged vaginal discharge is related to the abrupt decrease of maternal hormones (pseudomenstruation). Whitish vaginal discharge is observed in response to maternal hormones. Urine may appear dark with urate crystals that appear as a red or rust-colored stain on the diaper ("brick dust"). This is normal the first few days of life. The neonate urinates within 24 hours. The urinary meatus is midline.	Prominent clitoris and small, visible labia minora are often present in preterm neonates. Ambiguous genitalia; may require genetic testing to determine sex. No urination in 24 hours may indicate a possible urinary tract obstruction, polycystic disease, or renal failure.

Continued

TABLE 15-2   Neonatal Assessment by Area or System—cont'd

AREA OR SYSTEM	TECHNIQUE AND ASSESSMENT	EXPECTED FINDINGS FOR TERM NEONATE	DEVIATIONS FROM NORMAL
Genitourinary: male	Inspect the penis, noting the position of the urinary meatus. Inspect and palpate the scrotum to assess for testicles. With the thumb and forefinger of one hand, palpate each testis while the other thumb and forefinger are placed over the inguinal canal to prevent the ascent of testes during assessment. Start at the upper aspect of the scrotum and move away from the body.	The urinary meatus is at the tip of the penis. The scrotum is large, pendulous, and edematous with rugae (ridges or creases) present. Both testes are palpated in the scrotum. The neonate urinates within 24 hours with an uninterrupted stream. Urine may appear dark with urate crystals ("brick dust") that appear as a red, orange, pink, or rust-colored stain on the diaper. This is normal the first few days of life. 	Hypospadias: The urethral opening is on the ventral (under) surface of the penis. Epispadias: The urethral opening is on the dorsal (upper) side of the penis. Undescended testes (cryptorchidism): testes are not palpated in the scrotum. Hydrocele is enlarged scrotum due to excess fluid. No urination in 24 hours may indicate possible urinary tract obstruction, polycystic disease, or renal failure. Ambiguous genitalia may require genetic testing to determine sex. Inguinal hernia.
Musculoskeletal Assessing range of motion for arm is especially important if there was shoulder dystocia during the birthing process.	Inspect extremities, spine, and gluteal folds. Palpate the clavicles. Perform the Barlow and Ortolani maneuvers.	Arms are symmetrical in length and equal in strength. Legs are symmetrical in length and equal in strength. 10 fingers and 10 toes. Full range of motion is observed of all extremities. No clicks at joints. Equal gluteal folds. C-shaped spine with no openings is felt or observed in vertebrae. No dimpling or sinuses are observed.	Polydactyly: Extra digits may indicate a genetic disorder. Syndactyly: Webbed digits may indicate a genetic disorder. Unequal gluteal folds or positive Barlow and Ortolani maneuvers are associated with congenital hip dislocation. Decreased range of motion or muscle tone indicates possible birth injury, neurological disorder, or prematurity. Swelling, crepitus, or neck tenderness indicates possible broken clavicle, which can occur during the birthing process in neonates with large shoulders. Simian creases, short fingers, wide space between big toe and second toe are common with Down syndrome. Vertebrae openings may indicate spina bifida. Dimpling or sinuses may indicate pilonidal cyst or a more serious neurological disorder.

TABLE 15-2   Neonatal Assessment by Area or System—cont'd

AREA OR SYSTEM	TECHNIQUE AND ASSESSMENT	EXPECTED FINDINGS FOR TERM NEONATE	DEVIATIONS FROM NORMAL
Neurological	Assess posture. Assess tone. Test newborn reflexes (see Table 15-5). 	Flexed position Rapid recoil of extremities to the flexed position Positive newborn reflexes	Hypotonia: Floppy, limp extremities indicate possible nerve injury related to birth, depression of CNS related to maternal medication received during labor or to fetal hypoxia during labor, prematurity, or spinal cord injury. Hypertonia: Tightly flexed arms and stiffly extended legs with quivering indicate possible drug withdrawal. Paralysis indicates possible birth trauma or spinal injury. Tremors are possibly due to hypoglycemia, drug withdrawal, or cold stress.

Blackburn, 2018; Jarvis, 2016; Simpson et al., 2021.

TABLE 15-3   Common Newborn Characteristics

CHARACTERISTIC	APPEARANCE	SIGNIFICANCE
Acrocyanosis 	Hands or feet are blue or pale.	Response to cold environment Immature peripheral circulation
Central cyanosis	Blue discoloration of skin around the mouth, mucous membranes, or torso	Due to reduced oxygen saturation and perfusion, and often present during the early transitional period (first 10 minutes). May be related to failure to transition to adult circulatory pattern, or cardiopulmonary abnormality. Central cyanosis should never be assumed to be normal.
Mottling	A benign transient pattern of pink and white blotches on the skin.	Response to cold environment

Continued

TABLE 15-3 Common Newborn Characteristics—cont'd

CHARACTERISTIC	APPEARANCE	SIGNIFICANCE
Harlequin sign	One side of the body is pink and the other side is white.	Related to vasomotor instability
Slate gray patches (previously called Mongolian spots)	Flat, bluish discolored area on the lower back or buttock. Seen more often in Black, Asian, Hispanic, and American Indian infants.	Might be mistaken for bruising. Need to document size and location. Resolves on own by school age.
Erythema toxicum	A rash with red macules and papules (white to yellowish-white papule in center surrounded by reddened skin) that appear in different areas of the body, usually the trunk area. Can appear within 24 hours of birth and up to 2 weeks.	Benign Disappears without treatment
Milia	White papules on the face; more frequently seen on the bridge of the nose and chin.	Exposed sebaceous glands that resolve without treatment. Parents might mistake these for acne or whiteheads. Inform parents to leave them alone and let them resolve on their own.
Lanugo	Fine, downy hair that develops after 16 weeks' gestation. The amount of lanugo decreases as the fetus approaches full term. Often seen on the neonate's back, shoulders, and forehead.	Gradually falls out The presence and amount of lanugo assist in estimating gestational age. Abundant lanugo may be a sign of prematurity or genetic disorder.

TABLE 15-3   Common Newborn Characteristics—cont'd

CHARACTERISTIC	APPEARANCE	SIGNIFICANCE
Vernix caseosa	A protective substance secreted from sebaceous glands that covered the fetus during pregnancy. It looks similar to a whitish, cheesy substance. May be noted in auxiliary areas and genital areas of full-term neonates.	The presence and amount of vernix assists in estimating gestational age. Full-term neonates usually have none or small amounts of vernix.
Jaundice	Yellow coloring of skin. First appears on the face and extends down the trunk (cephalocaudal) and eventually the entire body. It is best assessed in natural lighting. When jaundice is suspected, the nurse can apply gentle pressure to the skin over a firm surface such as the nose, forehead, or sternum. The skin blanches to a yellowish hue.	Liver is not fully mature at birth and is the primary organ involved in the clearance of bilirubin. Jaundice within the first 24 hours is considered pathological; usually related to blood type incompatibility or sequestered blood (see Chapter 17). Jaundice occurring after 24 hours is usually physiological jaundice and is related to increased amount of unconjugated bilirubin in the system (see Chapter 17).
Molding	Elongation of the fetal head as it adapts to the birth canal	Resolves within 1 week.

Continued

TABLE 15-3   Common Newborn Characteristics—cont'd

CHARACTERISTIC	APPEARANCE	SIGNIFICANCE
Caput succedaneum Suture line Scalp Edema Periosteum Skull Brain	This is a localized soft tissue edema of the scalp. It feels "spongy" and can cross suture lines.	Results from prolonged pressure of the head against the maternal cervix during labor. Resolves within the first week of life.
Cephalhematoma Suture line Scalp Periosteum Blood Skull Brain	Hematoma formation between the periosteum and skull with unilateral swelling. It appears within a few hours of birth and can increase in size over the next few days. It has a well-defined outline. It does not cross suture lines.	Related trauma to the head due to prolonged labor, forceps delivery, or use of vacuum extractor. Can contribute to jaundice due to the large amounts of RBCs being hemolyzed. Resolves within 3 months.
Epstein's pearls	White, pearl-like epithelial cysts on gum margins and palate	Benign and usually disappears within a few weeks.
Natal teeth	Immature caps of enamel and dentin with poorly developed roots Usually only one or two teeth are present.	They are usually benign but can be associated with congenital defects. Natal teeth are often loose and are removed to decrease the risk of aspiration.

Blackburn, 2018; Jarvis, 2016; Simpson et al., 2021.

TABLE 15-4   Newborn Reflexes

REFLEX	HOW ELICITED	EXPECTED RESPONSE	ABNORMAL RESPONSE
Moro (startle) Present at birth; disappears by 6 months	Jar the crib, make a loud sound, or, from a supine position, lift the baby's shoulders slightly off the mattress and release, letting the shoulders drop back. 	Symmetrical abduction and extension of arms and legs, and then legs flex up against the trunk. The neonate makes a "C" shape with the thumb and index finger.	A slow response might occur with preterm infants or sleepy neonates. An asymmetrical response may be related to temporary or permanent birth injury to the clavicle, humerus, or brachial plexus. Possible neurological deficit or deafness is observed if unresponsive to loud noise.
Tonic neck Present between birth and 6 weeks; disappears by 4–6 months	With the neonate in a supine position, turn the head to the side so that the chin is over the shoulder. 	The neonate assumes a "fencing" position with arms and legs extended in the direction in which the head was turned.	Response after 6 months may indicate cerebral palsy.
Rooting Present at birth; Disappears between 3 and 6 months	Brush the side of a cheek near the corner of the mouth. 	The neonate turns the head toward the direction of the stimulus and opens the mouth. Instruct mothers who are lactating to touch the corner of the neonate's mouth with a nipple and the infant will turn toward the nipple for feeding.	May not respond if recently fed. Prematurity or neurological defects may cause weak or absent response.
Sucking Present at birth; disappears at 10–12 months	Place a gloved finger or nipple of a bottle in the neonate's mouth. 	Sucking motion occurs.	May not respond if recently fed. Prematurity or neurological defects may cause weak or absent response.

Continued

TABLE 15-4   Newborn Reflexes—cont'd

REFLEX	HOW ELICITED	EXPECTED RESPONSE	ABNORMAL RESPONSE
Palmar grasp Present at birth; disappears at 3–4 months	The examiner places a finger in the palm of the neonate's hand.	The neonate grasps fingers tightly. If the neonate grasps the examiner's fingers with both hands, the child can be pulled to a sitting position.	Absent or weak response indicates a possible CNS defect, or nerve or muscle injury.
Plantar grasp Present at birth; disappears at 3–4 months	Place a thumb firmly against the ball of the infant's foot.	Toes flex tightly down in a grasping motion	Weak or absent may indicate possible spinal cord injury.
Babinski Present at birth; disappears at 1 year	Stroke the lateral surface of the sole in an upward motion.	Hyperextension and fanning of toes	Absent or weak may indicate a possible neurological defect.
Stepping or dancing Present at birth; disappears at 3–4 weeks	Hold the neonate upright with feet touching a flat surface.	The neonate steps up and down in place.	Diminished response may indicate hypotonia.

Blackburn, 2018; Eichenwald, 2020; Jarvis, 2016; Simpson et al., 2021.

tools also include respiratory and heart rate, blood pressure, and oxygen saturation levels. Assessment tools vary based on hospital provider preferences.

BOX 15-1 | CCHD Screening: What Do Preductal and Postductal Mean and What Are We Looking for?

Preductal refers to blood from the left atrium located in the aorta *before* the area of the DA and supplies blood to the right arm via the brachiocephalic artery.

Postductal refers to blood from the left atrium that is in the aorta *past* the area of the DA and supplies blood to the lower body via the descending aorta.

The pulse oximetry screening can detect differences in preductal versus postductal oxygen saturations as well as mild hypoxemia in otherwise asymptomatic neonates. Some CCHDs are difficult to detect after birth with typical physical examination components including auscultation of the heart, palpation of pulses, blood pressure, and visual assessment for cyanosis. Some CCHDs that can be identified with this screening include hypoplastic left heart syndrome, pulmonary atresia, tetralogy of Fallot, and transposition of the great arteries. CCHD screening will also identify many pulmonary abnormalities.

Sources: AAP, 2021b; AAP & ACOG, 2017; Texas Department of State Health Services, n.d.

CRITICAL COMPONENT

Prevention and Treatment of Pain in the Neonate: Nonpharmacological and Pharmacological Strategies

Combinations of the following interventions are more effective than singular use:

- Swaddling
- Facilitated tucking (holding infant in a flexed position close to the caregiver's body)
- Non-nutritive sucking (NNS; pacifier)
- Infant massage
- Skin-to-skin contact
- Breastfeeding
- Sensory stimuli such as gentle talking to the infant while stroking or touching the face or back
- Use of heel warmers before blood draws
- Oral sucrose or glucose solutions
- Opioids (i.e., morphine, fentanyl), benzodiazepines (i.e., lorazepam, midazolam)
- Acetaminophen, nonsteroidal anti-inflammatory drugs (NSAIDs), local or regional anesthetics (i.e., lidocaine)

(Perry et al., 2018)

BEHAVIORAL CHARACTERISTICS

The neonate is a biosocial being with unique behavioral characteristics that affect parent–infant attachment (see Chapter 13). Infant temperament has a major influence on the parent–infant relationship and can range from an infant being an "easy" baby to a "fussy" baby. Most infants vacillate between the two extremes of temperament. Some infants are more sensitive to stimulus and are difficult to comfort, but most infants respond to parents' efforts to console. Infant temperaments that match parent expectations foster parent–infant attachment, but those who do not match parent expectations can hamper attachment (see Chapter 13).

Periods of Reactivity

Neonates experience predictable behavior during the first 6 to 8 hours of extrauterine life, referred to as periods of reactivity. Neonates transition through two periods of activity with one period of inactivity between. Each period is characterized by predictable behaviors (Desmond et al., 1966; Olsson, 2020).

Initial Period of Reactivity

This period of reactivity occurs in the first 30 to 40 minutes post-birth. The neonate is alert and active and vigorously responds to external stimuli. During this period, the newborn is ready to interact and will often breastfeed. This period, sometimes referred to as the "golden hour," is an important time for the nurse to help the mother with skin-to-skin positioning and breastfeeding (Fig. 15–8). It is also a critical time for cardiopulmonary transition, which requires frequent and careful nursing assessments.

- Respirations are irregular and rapid and can be as high as 80 breaths per minute; the heart rate is rapid and can be as high as 180 beats per minute (bpm).
- The neonate may have increased oral secretions and crackles in the lungs. The child may exhibit transient grunting, flaring, and retractions as fluids are being cleared from the lungs.
- The neonate may experience brief periods of central cyanosis.
- Bowel sounds are typically absent

Period of Relative Inactivity

This period of relative inactivity (deep sleep) begins approximately 30 to 40 minutes after birth and lasts 2 to 4 hours. Respiratory rate and heart rate decrease and can fall slightly below the normal range. Oral secretions decrease and bowel sounds can now typically be heard.

Second Period of Reactivity

The second period of reactivity lasts 2 to 8 hours. Neonates vacillate between active alert and quiet alert states and are more responsive to external stimuli. Periods of rapid respirations and

TABLE 15-5   Ballard Gestational Age Assessment

NEUROMUSCULAR MATURITY	PHYSICAL MATURITY
Posture Assess the position the neonate assumes while lying quietly on the back. The more mature, the greater the degree of flexion in the legs and arms.	**Skin** The examiner inspects the neonate's chest and abdominal skin areas for texture, transparency, thickness, and peeling or cracking. A preterm neonate's skin is smooth, thin, and translucent (numerous veins visible). A full-term neonate's skin is thicker and more opaque with some degree of peeling.
Square Window Assess the degree of the angle created when the examiner flexes the neonate's hand toward the forearm. The more mature, the greater the flexion, with the hand almost able to lie on wrist.	**Lanugo** The examiner assesses the amount of lanugo on the neonate's back. Lanugo begins to form around 24 weeks' gestation. It is abundant in preterm neonates and decreases in amount as the neonate matures.
Arm Recoil With the neonate in a supine (back) position, the examiner fully flexes the forearm against the neonate's chest for 5 seconds. The examiner extends the arms and releases them. The more mature, the faster the arms return to the flexed position (recoil).	**Plantar Creases** The examiner inspects the bottom of the feet for location of creases. The more creases over the greater proportion of the foot, the more mature the neonate. Plantar creases develop from the ball of the foot to the heel.
Popliteal Angle With the neonate in a supine position and pelvis flat, the examiner flexes the neonate's thigh to the abdomen. The leg is then extended. The angle at the knee is estimated. The lesser the angle, the greater the maturity.	**Breast Tissue** The examiner assesses the degree of nipple formation. The size of the breast bud is measured by gently grasping the tissue with thumb and forefinger and measuring the distance (in millimeters) between the thumb and forefinger. The greater the degree of nipple formation and size of the breast bud, the greater the maturity.
Scarf Sign With the neonate in a supine position, the examiner takes the neonate's hand and moves the arm across the chest toward the opposite shoulder. The examiner notes where the elbow is in relationship to the midline of the chest. The more preterm, the more the elbow crosses the midline.	**Eye and Ear Formation** Very preterm infants will have eyelids that are fused closed. The examiner assesses the ear for shape, thickness, and firmness. The more defined the ear is and the firmer it is, the more mature the neonate.
Heel to Ear With the neonate in a supine position, the examiner takes the neonate's foot and moves it toward the ear. The lesser the flexion (the farther the heel is from the ear), the greater the maturity.	**Genitalia** *Male:* The examiner palpates the scrotum for the presence of testes and inspects the scrotum for appearance. The greater the descent of the testes and the greater degree of rugae (creases), the greater the maturity. *Female:* The examiner moves the neonate's hip one-half abduction and visually inspects the genitalia. The more the labia majora covers the labia minora and clitoris, the greater the maturity.

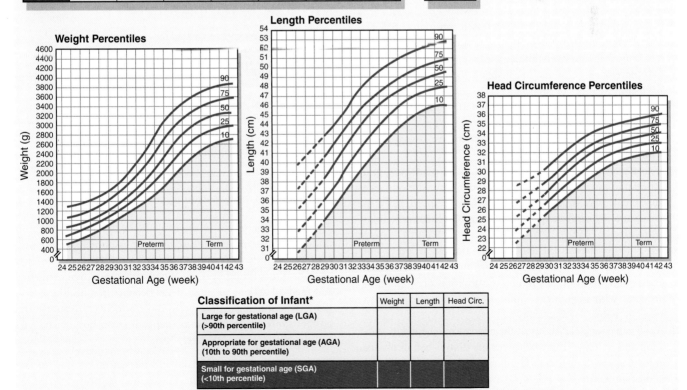

FIGURE 15–7 Ballard Gestational Age Assessment Tool.

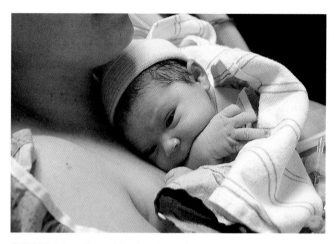

FIGURE 15–8 The "golden hour": Newborn is 30 minutes old. Awake, skin-to-skin, and interested in sucking.

increased heart rate occur in response to stimuli and activity. This period is another ideal time for breastfeeding as the neonate is interested in feeding and sucking.

Brazelton Neonatal Behavioral Assessment Scale

The Brazelton Neonatal Behavioral Assessment Scale (BNBAS) evaluates the neonate's responses to the environment. The BNBAS was originally developed as a research tool and has been adapted for use in the clinical setting, primarily to help educate families and facilitate the parent–infant relationship. The BNBAS is not routinely performed on healthy neonates. It consists of 28 behavior items and 18 reflex items in six categories (Nugent, 2013; Tedder, 1991):

● Habituation: Development of decreased sensitivity to a repeated stimulus such as light, sound, or heel stick, a protective mechanism against overstimulation. Habituation may not be fully developed in premature neonates or in neonates with CNS abnormalities or injuries.

● Orientation: The ability of the neonate to focus on visual or auditory stimuli. The neonate will turn their head in the direction of sound or will follow a visual stimulus. This response is diminished in premature neonates.

● Motor maturity: The ability of the neonate to control and coordinate motor activity. Normal findings are smooth, free movement with occasional tremors. Movement is jerky in premature neonates or in neonates with CNS abnormalities or injuries.

● Self-quieting ability: The ability of the neonate to quiet and comfort self. It is accomplished by sucking on the fist or hand or attending to external stimuli. The ability is diminished in neonates with neurological injuries or in those exposed to drugs in utero.

● Social behaviors: The ability of the neonate to respond to cuddling and holding. These behaviors are diminished or absent in neonates with neurological injuries or in neonates exposed to drugs in utero.

● Sleep and awake states: These are also referred to as infant states or behavior states. There are two sleep states and four awake states.

  ● Deep sleep: During this state, there is no body movement except an occasional startle reflex. External stimuli are less likely to awaken the infant. No eye movements occur.

  ● Light sleep: This state makes up the largest portion of sleep. During this state, the neonate may easily startle, may smile or make brief fussy sounds, or have random body movements and display rapid eye movement (REM). The neonate will be much easier to wake up than while in a deep sleep.

  ● Drowsy: During this state, intermittent body movement occurs. Eyes open and close and have a dull, heavy-lidded appearance. External stimuli will most likely wake the neonate.

  ● Quiet Alert: During this state, the neonate's eyes are wide open with a bright look. The infant is relaxed and most attentive to the environment and caregivers present. Providing visual or other pleasurable stimuli often can maintain this state.

  ● Active Alert: During this state, there is a considerable body movement with periods of fussiness or irritability. The neonate responds to disturbing stimuli (such as excessive noise or activity, cold, fatigue, or hunger) with increased motor activity and fussiness. Consoling or correcting interventions may settle the infant back to a quiet alert state.

  ● Crying: During this state, there is high motor activity and the neonate is difficult to calm. Eyes are opened or tightly closed and there is an extreme response to unpleasant stimuli. Crying is the neonate's communication signal that limits have been reached. Self-consoling can occur, whereas at other times the caregiver will need to intervene (Simpson et al., 2021).

NURSING CARE OF THE NEONATE

Nursing care of the neonate during hospitalization is divided into two time frames. The first is the fourth stage of labor, from birth through the first 4 hours of extrauterine life. The second is from 4 hours of age to discharge.

Nursing Actions During the Fourth Stage of Labor

The changes that occur in the neonate's body during the transition to extrauterine life require frequent assessments and monitoring to identify early signs of physiological compromise. Early identification of complications allows earlier initiation of nursing and medical actions to support the neonate in a healthy transition. These nursing actions occur in labor/delivery/recovery and postpartum/couplet care units, depending on hospital policies and the health of the neonate.

● Before birth, review prenatal and intrapartal records for factors that place the neonate at risk, such as prolonged ROM (risk of infection), meconium-stained fluid (risk of respiratory distress), and diabetes (risk of hypoglycemia).

● Immediately after birth, dry and stimulate by rubbing the neonate's back with towels.

● Support respirations by clearing the mouth and nose of excessive mucus with a bulb syringe when indicated.

● Obtain Apgar score at 1 and 5 minutes and initiate appropriate actions based on the score (see Chapter 8).

● Assess vital signs.
  ● Usually done within 30 minutes of birth, 1 hour after birth, and every hour for the remainder of the recovery period.
  ● Vital signs are assessed every 5 to 15 minutes for neonates with signs of distress.
  ● The frequency of assessments may vary based on institutional policies and the health of the neonate.
  ● Administer O$_2$ per institutional protocol if the heart rate is below 100 bpm, oxygen saturation levels are low, central cyanosis is present, or apnea occurs.

● Prevent hypothermia or cold stress by:
  ● Drying the neonate immediately after birth
  ● Discarding wet blankets and placing the neonate on dry, warm blankets or sheets
  ● Placing a stocking cap on the neonate's head
  ● Placing the neonate skin-to-skin on the mother's chest with a warm blanket over the mother and baby or placing the neonate under a preheated radiant warmer

● Use universal precautions. Wear gloves until after the neonate has been bathed to decrease exposure to pathogens from amniotic fluid, maternal blood, and other secretions.

● Assist with cord clamping and cutting.

● Inspect the clamped cord for number of vessels and for bleeding.

● Complete and place identifying bands on the neonate and parents before the neonate is separated from the parents (e.g., taken to the nursery or NICU).

● Weigh and measure the neonate.

● Complete a full neonatal assessment within 2 hours of birth.

● Complete a gestational age assessment if indicated as per hospital policy.

● Obtain blood glucose levels on symptomatic neonates or infants at risk for hypoglycemia per hospital policy.

● To prevent ophthalmic neonatorum (gonorrhea or chlamydial eye infections), administer erythromycin ophthalmic ointment within 1 hour of birth.

● Administer phytonadione IM within 1 hour of birth.

● Support breastfeeding by assisting the mother and providing a relaxing environment for the woman and her newborn (Fig. 15–9).

● Promote parent–infant attachment by creating a relaxing environment:
  ● Cluster nursing activities to allow for periods of uninterrupted time for new parents to spend with their newborn.
  ● Dim the lights and close the room door.

● Notify the neonate's physician or nurse practitioner of the neonate's date and time of birth and assessment findings.

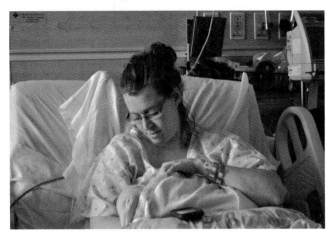

FIGURE 15–9 Newborn breastfeeding during the fourth stage of labor.

SAFE AND EFFECTIVE NURSING CARE: Understanding Medication

Erythromycin Ophthalmic Ointment (0.5%)

● Indication: Prophylaxis treatment for gonococcal or chlamydial eye infections
● Action: Prevents bacterial growth by suppressing protein synthesis within bacterial ribosome
● Common side effects: Edema and inflammation of eyelids
● Route and dose: Apply a 1 cm bead of ointment to lower eyelid of each eye.
● Precaution: Prevent the applicator tip from directly touching the eye by holding the application tube ½ inch from the eye.

Vallerand & Sanoski, 2021.

CRITICAL COMPONENT

Promoting Parent–Infant Attachment

The promotion of parent–infant attachment is a critical component of nursing care and needs to occur as soon as possible after birth. Often, nurses allow other nursing actions to take priority over parent–infant attachment or find it is easier to do assessments under the warming unit. Assessments and monitoring of vital signs can be performed in the parent's arms when the neonate is full-term, the Apgar score is 8 or higher, and no signs of fetal distress occurred during labor or at birth. Parent–infant interaction is influenced by the parent's cultural beliefs. It is important for nurses to demonstrate cultural awareness in their nursing care.

Nursing Actions

• Initiate skin-to-skin contact with a warm blanket over the neonate and parent.

Continued

CRITICAL COMPONENT—cont'd

- Point out and explain expected neonatal characteristics such as molding, milia, and lanugo.
- Provide alone time for the couple and their neonate by organizing care that allows for uninterrupted time.
- Delay administration of eye ointment until parents have had an opportunity to hold the baby. Once ointment is administered, the neonate is less likely to open their eyes and make eye contact with parents.
- Provide nursing care that reflects respect for the parents' cultural beliefs.

CRITICAL COMPONENT

Danger Signs

The following signs may be an indication of a serious abnormality or complication. Document these signs in the neonatal record and report them to the physician or nurse practitioner:

- Tachypnea (greater than 60 breaths per minute)
- Grunting
- Nasal flaring
- Retractions of chest wall
- Abdominal distention
- Seizures
- Lethargy
- Jaundice within first 24 hours of birth
- Temperature, either abnormally high or low
- Jitteriness
- Persistent hypoglycemia
- Persistent temperature instability
- Failure to pass meconium stool within 48 hours of birth
- Failure to void within 24 hours of birth

Nursing Actions From 4 Hours of Age to Discharge

The second stage of neonatal care focuses on monitoring the neonate's adaptation to extrauterine life and helping parents learn about their newborns and how to care for them. The nursing actions listed are for neonates who do not exhibit signs of distress or potential complications.

- Assess vital signs as per hospital policy.
  - Neonates continue to have difficulty in regulating their body temperature during this period. Vital signs for stable term neonates are assessed at least once per shift. The physician or nurse practitioner should be notified when the temperature decreases persist (see Critical Component: Hypothermia and Cold Stress).
- Complete neonatal assessment at least once per shift. The type of assessment varies based on institutional policies. Late preterm infants may be assessed more frequently.

CRITICAL COMPONENT

Hypothermia and Cold Stress

Neonates with temperatures below 97.7°F (36.5°C) are at risk for hypothermia and cold stress.
   Nursing actions include the following:

- Place the infant skin-to-skin on the mother (or partner) with a warm blanket over both the neonate and the adult or wrap the neonate in warm blankets. Ensure the infant's hat is on.
- If the temperature remains below 97.7°F (36.5°C), place the neonate under a preheated radiant warmer. Unwrap the neonate so that skin is exposed to the radiant heat. Attach an electronic skin probe. The warmer is set at 34.7°F (1.5°C) above the neonate's temperature. Continue to adjust the temperature in relationship to the neonate's temperature.
- Monitor the blood glucose level per institutional policies, as hypothermia can cause hypoglycemia.
- Notify the physician or nurse practitioner if the neonate's temperature does not return to normal ranges after rewarming.
- Document the temperature and actions taken.
- Delay bathing until 6 to 24 hours after birth and until the temperature is stable and at least 98.2°F (36.8°C). For the late preterm infant (LPI), wait 12 to 24 hours after birth.

- Follow the institution's policy on newborn bathing and timing of the first bath.
- Bathe the neonate following the institution's policy on newborn bathing and timing of the first bath. Delay the bath for at least 6 to 24 hours as feasible as delayed bathing is associated with decreased rates of hypothermia and hypoglycemia and higher rates of exclusive breastfeeding (see Evidence-Based Practice: Delayed Newborn Bathing).
- See discharge teaching section at end of chapter for more information on bathing newborn.

Evidence-Based Practice: Delayed Newborn Bathing

Warren, S., Midodzi, W. K., Newhook, L. A., Murphy, P., & Twells, L. (2020). Effects of delayed newborn bathing on breastfeeding, hypothermia, and hypoglycemia. *Journal of Obstetric, Gynecologic, and Neonatal Nursing, 49*(2), 181–189. https://doi.org/10.1016/j.jogn.2019.12.004

- The aim of this retrospective cohort study was to determine if delaying the newborn bath by 24 hours from birth in healthy newborns would increase the prevalence of initiating breastfeeding and exclusive breastfeeding at discharge. The relationship between delayed newborn bathing and incidences of hypothermia and hypoglycemia was also examined.

- Study participants included a random sampling of 1,225 healthy full-term and late preterm newborns (34 0/7 to 36 6/7 weeks' gestation) on a mother–baby unit. Newborns bathed before 24 hours after birth ($n = 680$) were compared with newborns bathed after 24 hours ($n = 545$).

- Hypoglycemia was defined as a glucose level less than 47 mg/dL and hypothermia was defined as a temperature less than 97.7°F (36.5°C).

- Among newborns in this study, delaying bathing by 24 hours resulted in higher prevalence of exclusive breastfeeding (no formula or other supplementation) at the time of discharge; however, no statistically significant increase in initiation of breastfeeding was found.
- Decreased incidence of hypothermia and hypoglycemia occurred in those bathed at least 24 hours after birth; however, incidence was low and neither difference was statistically significant.
- Researchers conclude that delaying the initial bath by at least 24 hours in healthy term and late preterm newborns may provide optimal conditions for breastfeeding, newborn thermoregulation, and glycemic control.

- Promote parent–infant attachment by providing uninterrupted time with their newborn.
- Promote sibling attachment by providing opportunities for interactions with the newborn, such as having older siblings assist with newborn care or listen to the newborn's heart (see the Newborn Care Parent Education section at the end of the chapter for more information).
- Follow hospital policies and procedures to prevent infant abductions. Common practices include:
  - Taking footprints and photo of the infant for identification purposes.
  - Placing armbands on the mother, her partner, and the neonate that contain the same identification number. The bands of neonates should be checked with the bands of parents at the beginning of each shift and when taking or returning neonates from or to the mother's room.
  - Placing infant security tags (typically connected to an angle band or cord clamp) and using hospital abduction systems that trigger an alarm, lock doors, and freeze elevators if the infant comes within 4 feet of an exit or elevator (Fig. 15–10).
  - Requiring personnel working in the maternal-newborn units to wear name tags specific to that unit.

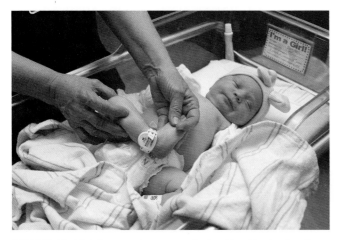

FIGURE 15–10 Infant security tag attached to identification band.

- Instructing parents to not allow anyone to take their newborn if the person does not possess the appropriate name tag specific to the maternity unit.
- Instructing parents not to leave their newborn in the mother's room unattended. This includes when she is taking a shower.
- Securing the maternal-newborn units by having all entrances locked, allowing only visitors with identification to enter.
- Assist parents with breastfeeding or formula feeding (see Chapter 16).
- Teach parents about sleep safety such as placing newborns on their backs to sleep and not bed-sharing.
- See the Newborn Care Parent Education section at the end of the chapter for additional teaching topics.

SKIN CARE

The skin of a term neonate is smooth, soft, and has less pigmentation than that of an older child (Blackburn, 2018). The neonate's skin is subjected to various stresses related to the birthing process and transition to extrauterine life. Causes of potential threats to skin integrity are:

- Pressure exerted on the presenting part of the fetus during the labor and birthing process from maternal structures such as the pelvis, causing bruising, edema, and hematomas
- Abrasions, bruising, and edema of the skin related to use of vacuum extractors, forceps, and internal fetal monitoring
- Use of adhesive tapes
- Drying out and flaking of skin and lips, a natural process that occurs during the first few weeks of life
- Diaper dermatitis

Nursing Actions

- Assess skin once per shift and the perineal area at each diaper change. Intact and healthy skin is a first-line defense against infection.
- Decrease risk of diaper dermatitis by changing diapers and cleaning the perineal area with water or disposable diaper wipes every 1 to 3 hours.
- Apply barrier products containing petrolatum or zinc oxide at each diaper change for infants at risk for diaper dermatitis. Complete removal of the skin barrier product is not necessary. Avoid vigorous rubbing of the skin when cleaning (Association of Women's Health, Obstetrics, and Neonatal Nurses [AWHONN], 2018).
- Use adhesive tape that causes the least amount of trauma. Slowly remove using moist gauze (AWHONN, 2018).
- See the Newborn Care Parent Education section at the end of the chapter for more information on skin care.

SCREENING TESTS

Before hospital discharge, screening tests are performed to assist the neonate's health-care provider to identify congenital and other common disorders not easily seen at birth. Newborn screening programs focus on disorders for which early detection and treatment improve health outcomes. Required screenings vary by state. Most states require a genetic disease screen (GDS), also called a blood spot test, hearing screen, hyperbilirubinemia screen, and critical congenital heart defect (CCHD) screen. Hypoglycemia screening is provided for high-risk (or symptomatic) infants, such as infants of diabetic mothers and SGA, LGA, preterm, and post-term infants (AAP & ACOG, 2017).

Genetic Disease Screen

The GDS blood test screens for infections, genetic diseases, and metabolic disorders and is performed on all babies born in the United States. This screening began in the 1960s when all babies were screened for phenylketonuria (PKU); today, newborns are screened for approximately 30 disorders. Each state has regulations on what is included in the GDS, and the degree of screening varies from state to state. Specific information on each state's requirements can be accessed online such as babysfirsttest.org. Most GDS tests are done within the first 24 to 48 hours of birth and again at around 5 days. Information pertaining to the test and follow-up is given to the parents. The blood is obtained from a heel stick (Fig. 15–11).

CRITICAL COMPONENT

Phenylketonuria

PKU is an inborn error of metabolism. Neonates with PKU cannot metabolize phenylalanine, an amino acid found in many foods including breast milk and formula. This leads to a buildup of phenylpyruvic and phenylacetic acids, which are abnormal metabolites of phenylalanine. This accumulation can cause permanent brain damage and death, but is preventable with early detection and dietary management.

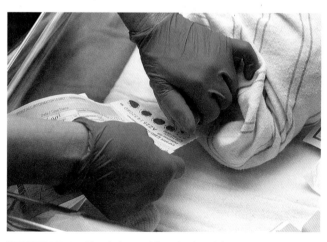

FIGURE 15–11 Blood obtained from heel stick for GDS.

CRITICAL COMPONENT

Heel Stick

The heel stick is a common procedure performed on neonates. Blood is collected to assess blood glucose, hematocrit, and serum bilirubin and to conduct the GDS.

Procedure

1. Review the orders for the test being done.
2. Provide parents with information on the test.
3. Warm the neonate's foot for 5 to 10 minutes by wrapping it in a commercial heel-warmer or warm, moist washcloth. This helps facilitate circulation to the peripheral area. Heel warming may be unnecessary for tests that require a very small amount of blood (such as blood glucose).
4. Put on gloves.
5. With the nondominant hand, hold the neonate's foot in a dorsiflexed position. The nurse or technician should have a firm grasp of the foot, but the foot should not be tightly squeezed.
6. Clean the heel with alcohol and allow to dry.
7. Puncture the skin in the lateral or medial aspect of the heel to decrease the risk of nerve damage.

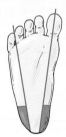

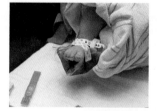
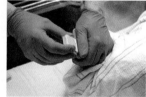

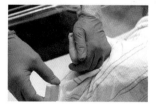

8. Wipe off the first drop of blood.
9. Allow large drops of blood to form and scoop them into the collection container or place them on the testing material.
10. Clean the puncture area and place a small bandage or dressing over it.

Document that blood was collected, type of test, site of puncture, and response of the neonate.

Hearing Screening

Language development begins at birth as neonates are exposed to sounds and voices in their environment. Hearing loss is a common congenital abnormality with a prevalence of 1.6 per 1,000 screened infants. Early detection of hearing loss provides parents with the opportunity to seek interventions that foster language development. In 1993, the National Institutes of Health (NIH) recommended that all newborns be screened for hearing loss before hospital discharge (NIH & National Institute on Deafness and Other Communication Disorders [NIDCD], 2020). All states have established early hearing detection and intervention programs that mandate newborn hearing loss screening, usually in the hospital before discharge.

The screening test relies on physiological measures instead of behavioral responses but does not provide information on the type or degree of hearing impairment. The test must be conducted in a quiet room when the newborn is calm or asleep. Vernix, blood, and amniotic fluid in the ear can interfere with accurate screening. Neonates who fail the screening are rescreened in 1 month. Diagnostic testing is recommended for neonates who fail the second screening (Fig. 15–12).

Hyperbilirubinemia (Jaundice) Screen

Hyperbilirubinemia occurs in most newborns (60% of term and 80% of preterm) and is usually physiological and benign. However, extreme (pathological) levels of bilirubin can be toxic and cause acute bilirubin encephalopathy or kernicterus. Kernicterus causes severe and permanent neurological damage (Blackburn, 2018). The AAP recommends universal screening of bilirubin levels on all neonates before discharge, and levels are interpreted according to the infant's age in hours using an established nomogram (such as the Bhutani curve). Use of a transcutaneous bilirubin meter is acceptable (Fig. 15–13) as is measuring the total serum bilirubin level in a blood sample. Visual estimations, although helpful, are not recommended for

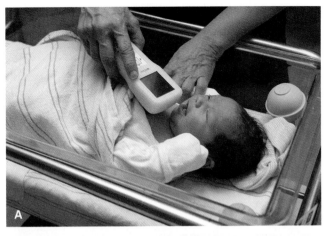

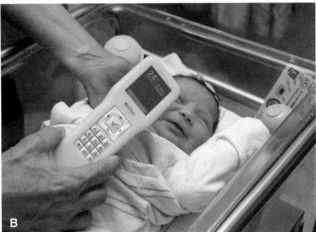

FIGURE 15–13 Screening for hyperbilirubinemia with a transcutaneous bilirubin (TcB) meter. (A) The TcB meter is pressed lightly on the neonate's sternum. (B) The TcB level is indicated on the screen.

this screening and can be especially inaccurate in darkly pigmented neonates (AAP & ACOG, 2017)

Critical Congenital Heart Defect Screen

Almost 3% of neonates are born with a birth defect, most often caused by congenital heart defects (CHDs). CCHDs make up a small portion of all CHDs. Certain CCHDs go undetected during the prenatal and immediate postnatal period as the neonate shows no signs or symptoms the first days after birth. Therefore, these neonates are thought to be healthy and are sent home where they may quickly deteriorate. CCHD screening is a simple pulse oximetry test that compares preductal and postductal oxygen saturation levels as well as the overall oxygenation levels. This screening is now recommended to be done universally on all neonates after 24 hours of age (when the DA is typically closed). A pulse oximetry reading is taken on both the right hand (preductal) and either foot (postductal; AAP, 2021b). A "passing" test is typically when oxygen saturation levels are 95% or greater in either extremity, and there is 3% or less difference between the preductal and postductal readings.

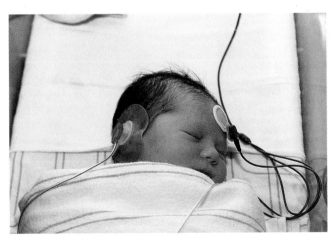

FIGURE 15–12 Newborn hearing screening.

THERAPEUTIC AND SURGICAL PROCEDURES

Therapeutic and surgical procedures that healthy newborns may encounter include immunizations and elective male circumcisions.

Immunizations

Hepatitis B, spread through contact with blood of an infected person or sexual contact with an infected person, causes inflammation of the liver. The Centers for Disease Control and Prevention (CDC) recommends that all neonates be vaccinated for hepatitis B before hospital discharge. The CDC also recommends that neonates who may have been exposed to hepatitis B during birth be given both the hepatitis B vaccine and hepatitis B immune globulin (HBIg) within 12 hours of birth. The second dose of hepatitis B vaccine is given at 1 to 2 months of age. The third dose is given at 6 to 18 months of age (see https://www.cdc.gov/vaccines/schedules/hcp/imz/child-adolescent.html).

CRITICAL COMPONENT

Intramuscular Injections

Procedure

1. Review the written orders for the newborn.
2. Inform parents of the reason for the medication or vaccine and invite them to participate as feasible, such as by holding the infant.
3. Obtain written consent when required.
4. Follow the medication rights before administration.
5. Draw up medication or vaccine in a 1-mL syringe with a 25-gauge 5/8 needle.
6. Put on gloves.
7. Identify the injection site. The preferred site is the vastus lateralis.
8. Clean the area with an alcohol swab and let it dry. It is important to remove all maternal blood and amniotic fluid from the injection site to prevent transmission of blood-borne pathogens.
9. Stabilize the knee with the heel of the hand. Grasp the tissue of the injection site with thumb and forefinger.
10. Insert the needle at a 90-degree angle with a darting motion, then aspirate to check for blood and inject the fluid. Immunizations do not require aspiration.

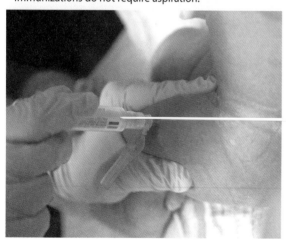

11. Withdraw the needle and apply gentle pressure.
12. Properly cap the needle and dispose.
13. Document the date, time, and location of injection.

Circumcision

Male circumcision is the elective surgical removal of the foreskin of the penis, commonly performed during the neonatal period. Multiple health benefits are associated with newborn male circumcision, and the most recent evidence suggests these benefits outweigh the risk of the procedure (AAP & ACOG, 2017). The decision to circumcise is made by the parents based on cultural, religious, and personal beliefs, as well as knowledge of the procedure. Parents considering circumcision need to be educated on the potential health benefits and risks involved. Although the AAP does not recommend routine newborn circumcisions for all newborns, they do support providing access to all families that desire it. Circumcisions can be done in the hospital before discharge or later in the pediatric clinic.

Benefits of newborn circumcision (over the lifetime) include:

● Reduced risk of urinary tract infections in the first year of life
● Reduced risk of HIV and other sexually transmitted infections
● Reduced risk of balanitis, phimosis, and paraphimosis
● Reduced risk of some cancers, including of the penis and prostate (Morris et al., 2017)

Contraindications for circumcision include:

● Preterm neonates
● Neonates with a genitourinary defect
● Neonates at risk for bleeding problems
● Neonates with compromising disorders such as respiratory distress syndrome

Risks related to circumcision include:

● Hemorrhage
● Infection
● Adhesions
● Pain

Three common devices used for circumcisions are the Gomco clamp, Mogen clamp, and Plastibell (Fig. 15–14). The Mogen clamp is commonly used by mohels (a rabbi or person who performs ritual Jewish circumcisions) when performing ceremonial circumcisions.

Surgical Procedure

Preoperative care measures are as follows:

● Provide information regarding the benefits and risks of circumcisions, and ensure the procedure is provided by the health-care provider.
● Obtain written consent from the parents.

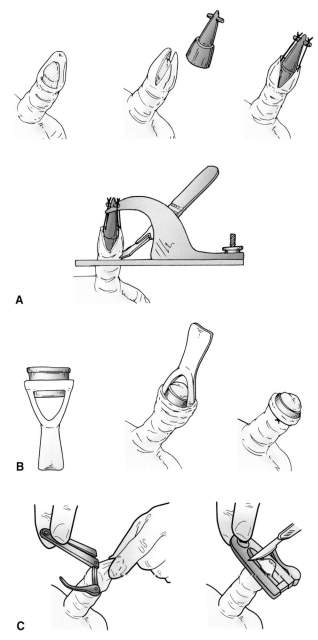

FIGURE 15-14 Removal of the prepuce during circumcision. (A) Gomco clamp. (B) Plastibell. (C) Mogen clamp.

- The physician administers a penile nerve block.
- A sucrose-dipped pacifier is offered during the nerve block and procedure for pain management (see Evidence-Based Practice feature).
- The physician surgically removes the foreskin with a scalpel, using either a Gomco clamp, Mogen clamp, or Plastibell device (see Fig. 15–14).

Evidence-Based Practice: Sucrose as Analgesia for Minor Procedural Pain Management in Neonates

Thakkar, P., Arora, K., Das, B., Javadekar, S., & Panigrahi, S. (2016). To evaluate and compare the efficacy of combined sucrose and non-nutritive sucking for analgesia in newborns undergoing minor painful procedure: A randomized controlled trial. *Journal of Perinatology, 36,* 67–70. https://doi-org.ezproxy1.library.arizona.edu /10.1038/jp.2015.122

The aim of this randomized controlled study was to evaluate and compare the effectiveness of combined sucrose and NNS for pain management for neonatal heel-stick procedures. The sample consisted of 180 full-term neonates with birth weight greater than 2,200 g who were older than 24 hours. The neonates were randomized into one of four groups with intervention administered 2 minutes before the procedure.

- Group 1 received 30% sucrose solution PO by sterile syringe.
- Group 2 received NNS, in which sterile gauze was held gently in the neonate's mouth and the palate tickled to stimulate sucking.
- Group 3 received both 30% sucrose and NNS.
- Group 4 received no interventions.

Two minutes before the intervention(s), baseline heart rate and oxygen saturation were recorded. Continuous video recording of the procedure, including heart rate and oxygen saturations, were done throughout the procedure. The PIPP, which is used on both full-term and preterm infants, was used to evaluate neonates' pain during the procedure.

Results:
The median PIPP score significantly decreased in groups 1, 2, and 3 compared with the non-intervention group (group 4). The combined intervention (group 3) of sucrose and NNS significantly decreased the medium PIPP score compared with groups 1 and 2.

Conclusion:
Use of sucrose and NNS are effective methods of pain management for full-term infants undergoing heel-stick procedures with combined use of sucrose and NNS being more effective.

- Verify that the neonate has voided and has no anatomical abnormalities that might contraindicate circumcision.
- Administer acetaminophen, if desired, 1 hour before the procedure per the provider's order for pain management.
- Assemble equipment and obtain anesthetic to be used by the provider during the procedure.

During intraoperative care:

- The neonate is positioned and secured on a specially designed plastic board, often referred to as a circumcision board.
- A bulb syringe is placed near the neonate to use in case of vomiting or increased mucus.
- The penis is cleaned and a sterile drape designed for circumcision is placed over the trunk.

Postoperative care includes the following:

- Gomco or Mogen clamp:
  - Petroleum-impregnated gauze may be wrapped around the end of the penis, or a large amount of petroleum ointment may be placed directly on the penis to prevent friction and sticking of the penis to the diaper.
  - Apply a protective lubricant over the circumcision site after each diaper change for the first week or two. The protective lubricant helps keep the area clean and keeps the wound from adhering to the diaper.
  - The circumcised area heals within 2 weeks.

- Plastibell method:
  - Do not apply lubricants on the penis when a Plastibell has been used. Lubricants can increase the risk of displacement of the plastic ring.
  - The plastic ring falls off in a few days to a week. Parents should not pull it off.
- The penis is assessed every 15 minutes for the first hour for bleeding, then every 2 to 3 hours according to hospital policies. The physician is notified when excessive bleeding is present (spots larger than the size of a quarter).
- Acetaminophen PO may be administered every 4 to 6 hours.
- Voiding is assessed and documented. The neonate should void within 24 hours of the procedure.

Circumcision Care Parent Education

- Inform parents that the circumcised glans penis (tip of the penis) will appear red and form yellow crusted areas as it heals; these areas should not be washed off.
- Parents should check for bleeding every 4 hours for the first 24 hours postprocedure and notify the health-care provider of bleeding at the circumcised area.
- Inform parents that the gauze, if used, will fall off on its own and they should not pull it off.
- If petroleum without gauze is used, the ointment should be placed directly on the penis, with enough ointment provided to coat the inside front of the diaper, not just the tip of the penis.
- Instruct parents how to fasten the diaper; ensure it is not too loose to allow rubbing when the baby moves, but not too tight to cause pain on the surgical site.
- Instruct parents to notify their health-care provider if:
  - Bleeding is present (larger than the size of a quarter).
  - The entire penis is red, warm, and swollen or there is drainage from the surgical site (signs of infection).
  - The neonate has not voided within 24 hours.

NEWBORN CARE PARENT EDUCATION

Caring for a newborn and raising a child to adulthood are among the most important roles parents will assume in their lifetimes, yet little formal education exists for these responsibilities. Couples' knowledge of newborn care varies based on past experiences with children, cultural beliefs, information from friends and relatives, and books read or classes attended.

It is the responsibility of the nursing staff to ensure parents have adequate knowledge of newborn care to safely care for their child. A teaching plan is developed based on an assessment of knowledge level and cultural beliefs. Some require minimal teaching whereas others need intensive education.

Discharge planning and parent education usually begin during pregnancy, when couples are encouraged to read about infant care and attend infant care classes in preparation for their emerging role as parents. They also receive educational information from their health-care provider. Throughout the postpartum hospital stay, teaching is provided in short sessions to the woman, her partner, and other family caregivers of the newborn. Most hospitals or birthing centers have standard discharge teaching forms that can be individualized for each patient based on specific learning needs. These forms are completed and signed by the mother and discharge nurse with a written copy of key points of newborn care given to parents on discharge. Before discharge, the mother's physicians or midwife will identify care needs for her and the infant and schedule a follow-up appointment within 48 hours or up to 2 weeks based on assessed needs. The following newborn care educational topics are presented in alphabetical order for reference.

Bathing

The first few bathing experiences can be stressful for parents, but over time it typically becomes a very pleasurable experience for both the parents and the infant (Fig. 15–15). Immersion (in a tub) or swaddled immersion bathing (loosely swaddled in a towel and immersed in water) are acceptable as is bathing with a sponge. Immersion or swaddled immersion bathing are ideal as the infant experiences less heat loss and cold stress, and maintains a calmer state (AWHONN, 2018). Daily bathing with soap is not necessary and can cause skin irritation. Bathing every few days is sufficient. Use of a mild preservative-free soap that has neutral pH is recommended to decrease the risk of skin irritation. The use of soap on the face is not recommended. Genital and rectal areas should be cleaned at each diaper change with water or diaper wipes.

Gather all items for bathing (e.g., soap, towels, washcloth, clean clothing, diapers, blankets) before the bath so they are in easy reach. Never leave the infant unattended while in the bath. To maintain the infant's body temperature, bathe in a warm room free of drafts. The bath water temperature should be between 100°F and 104°F (37.7°C to 40°C). Keep bath time short (5 to 10 minutes) to reduce heat loss (AWHONN, 2018).

Immerse the infant in warm water deep enough to cover the shoulders to ensure even temperature distribution and decreased heat loss due to evaporation. The bathing procedure is as follows:

- Support the infant's head and neck during the bath.
- Start from the cleanest area (eyes) and end with the dirtiest area (buttock).
- Cleanse eyes from the inner to outer aspects using a clean corner of the washcloth per eye to reduce the risk of transfer of infection from one eye to the other. Wring out excess water from the washcloth before washing the eyes and face.
- Wash hair by massaging the scalp with a hand, soft brush, or washcloth. Rinse with water. Dry hair immediately (or wash hair last) as the infant can lose significant heat from a wet head.
- Lift the chin to clean neck folds, where milk often collects.
- Cleanse the upper body with your hands or soft cloth and rinse.
- Cleanse the lower body.
- Clean female genitals by washing from front to back to decrease the risk of cystitis.
- Elevate the scrotum and cleanse the area.
- Dry the infant by patting the skin with a towel. Move from the damp towel to dry towel or blanket. Once dry, dress the infant in a clean diaper and clean clothes.

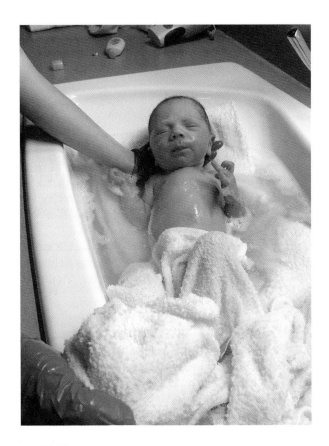

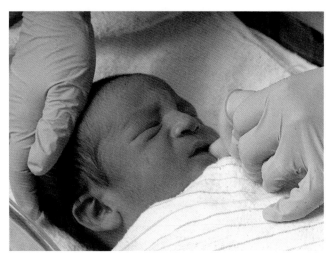

FIGURE 15–16 A bulb syringe in used to remove mucus.

- Only suction the nose if mucus or secretions are seen. Care should be taken as trauma can occur if suction is applied to the tissue, resulting in swelling.
- Release pressure from the syringe and allow it to slowly expand.
- Remove drainage from the syringe by compressing it and forcing the contents into a tissue.
- Repeat until the newborn is clear of mucus.

Clothing

The amount of clothing needed varies depending on whether the infant is inside or outside and the temperature of the environment. The amount and type of clothing can be influenced by cultural beliefs. Newborns are usually comfortable wearing a diaper, T-shirt, and loose-fitting outfit when inside. When outside, the infant's skin must be protected from the sun. Add additional layers of clothing or heavier blankets and a hat when outside in cooler weather. However, newborns and infants can become overheated with too many clothes or blankets, so it is important to explore what parents know and believe about infant dressing and educate them on risks of overheating and overbundling. Remind parents to avoid overbundling the infant at bedtime. An overheated infant has an increased risk of sudden unexpected infant death (SUID) during sleep. Signs of overheating are:

- Sweating
- Damp hair
- Reddened skin or heat rash
- Rapid breathing
- Restlessness

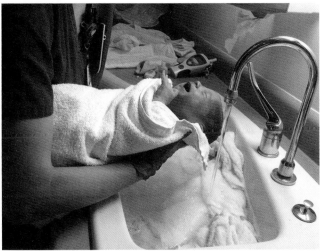

FIGURE 15–15 Newborn's first bath.

Bulb Syringe

A bulb syringe is used to assist the infant in clearing mucus from the nasopharynx. It is important for parents to learn how to properly use a bulb syringe and they should be given opportunities to practice before discharge. Newborns should have their own bulb syringe that is cleaned with soapy water and rinsed after each use. The procedure for bulb syringe use is as follows:

- Compress the syringe and insert it into either the nose or the mouth.
  - When using in the mouth, the syringe is placed in each side of the mouth, the roof of the mouth, and the back of the mouth (Fig. 15–16).

Cord Care

The umbilical cord begins to dry once the cord is clamped and cut. The cord clamp can be removed 24 hours after birth; however, some cord clamps contain an infant security device and remain on until discharge (Fig. 15–17). Over the next few days, the cord becomes dry, hard, and black, then falls off. The site subsequently heals within 2 weeks. Cord care includes these measures:

- The diaper is placed below the cord to facilitate drying of the cord.

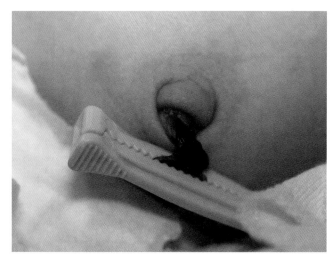

FIGURE 15–17 Normal dry cord with slight erythema on surrounding skin.

- If the cord becomes dirty, clean it with plain water and pat dry with a clean, absorbent cloth.
- Use of alcohol for cord care is not necessary.
- Parents should contact the health-care provider if there is bleeding from the cord site, foul-smelling drainage, redness in the surrounding skin, or fever.

Crying and Colic

Crying is how infants communicate, including when they experience hunger, pain, sickness, fatigue, or sensory overload. The type, duration, and intensity of the cry varies depending on the reason and temperament of the child. Intensity ranges from gentle fussing to high-pitched screams. On average, most newborns cry very little during the first 2 weeks of life. Crying generally increases to about 2 to 3 hours per day by week 6, but some infants cry less and some more. By 12 weeks, infants average 1 hour of crying per day (Marcdante & Kliegman, 2019).

Colic is a term used for excessive, inconsolable crying for no apparent reason in an otherwise healthy infant. Healthy infants who cry for at least 3 hours a day, for 3 or more days a week, for at least 3 weeks are considered colicky. The cause of colic is unknown and is a diagnosis of exclusion made only after a thorough examination by a health-care provider. Symptoms of a colicky infant include:

- Cry is louder and with a higher pitch, sounding similar to a scream.
- Cry is paroxysmal: Infant suddenly changes from happy to crying.
- Infant appears in pain or with facial grimacing.
- Infant flexes legs up or arches their back when crying.
- Infant is more irritable when placed in a crib.
- Infant is difficult to soothe or console.

Parents should keep a diary of when their infant is awake, asleep, eating, and crying. This will assist the pediatrician or nurse practitioner to determine if crying is related to a medical cause (AAP, 2015) and offer specific methods for soothing the infant. Methods for soothing colicky infants include the following:

- Hold the infant and sway from side to side or walk around with the infant.
- Give the infant a pacifier.
- Swaddle the infant.
- Place the infant (abdomen facing down) over the knees and gently rub or pat the back.
- Place the infant in a baby bouncer.
- Place the infant in a car seat and go for a ride in the car.
- Place the infant in a car seat and place near (but not on) a running clothes dryer or by a running vacuum cleaner.
- Place the infant in a stroller and go for a walk.
- If the parent begins to feel frustrated or anxious, it is appropriate to place the infant alone in a safe crib in the bedroom and allow the child to cry, checking on them every 10 minutes.

Caring for an infant with colic can be an emotionally and physically draining experience for the parents and can lead to **pediatric abusive head trauma** (AHT; see section that follows) or other injuries if the baby is shaken out of frustration or anger. Parents can become increasingly frustrated as their efforts to calm their infant do not seem to work. During these periods of feeling frustrated and overwhelmed, the parents need to take a break from their infant and seek support.

CRITICAL COMPONENT

Colic

The AAP has the following advice for parents and caregivers who are feeling frustrated when caring for infants with colic:

- Take a deep breath and count to 10.
- Place your baby in a safe place, such as a crib or playpen without blankets and stuffed animals; leave the room and let your baby cry alone for about 10 to 15 minutes.
- While your baby is in a safe place, consider some actions that may help calm you down:
  - Listen to music for a few minutes.
  - Call a friend or family member for emotional support.
  - Do simple household chores, such as vacuuming or washing the dishes.
- If you have not calmed down after 10 to 15 minutes, check on your baby but do not pick up your baby until you have calmed down. When you have calmed down, go back and pick up your baby. If your baby is still crying, retry soothing measures.
- Call your doctor. There may be a medical reason why your baby is crying.
- Call a family member or friend and ask for help.
- Try to be patient. Keeping your baby safe is the most important thing you can do. It is normal to feel upset, frustrated, or even angry, but it is important to keep your behavior under control. Remember, it is never safe to shake, throw, or hit a child—it never solves the problem and can cause permanent injury or death.

AAP, 2016b.

Diaper Dermatitis (Diaper Rash)

Diaper dermatitis is common and can occur when diapers are not changed frequently or the area is not cleaned thoroughly at each diaper change. It can also occur with a change in the infant's diet, with teething, or when the infant is taking medications that can change the chemistry of the urine and stools. Methods to reduce the risk of and treat diaper dermatitis include:

- Change diapers frequently; every 1 to 3 hours during the day and at least once during the night.
- Consider using superabsorbent disposable diapers instead of cloth diapers (AWHONN, 2018).
- Cleanse the infant's bottom with water or disposable diaper wipes during each diaper change. Avoid vigorous rubbing of the skin.
- Use petroleum-based or zinc oxide ointments during diaper changes (at the first sign of a rash). Complete removal of the skin barrier product during diaper change is not necessary
- Avoid use of baby (talcum) powders, cornstarch, and antibiotic ointments. These products can increase the risk of bacterial and candida growth, and powders can cause respiratory irritation (AWHHON, 2018).
- If diaper rash does not resolve with these interventions, the parent should consult with their health-care provider before using other products.
- Some evidence indicates that topical human milk can effectively treat diaper dermatitis, especially if commercial products are unavailable or in low-resource settings. A small amount of breast milk can be rubbed into the diaper area after each breastfeeding (AWHONN, 2018).

Diapering

Most parents use disposable diapers that come in various sizes based on infant weight; others use cloth diapers, such as all-in-one diapers that contain a cotton diaper, nylon cover, and Velcro or snap fasteners. Some parents use a combination of both—cloth at home and disposable when away. Diapers must be changed when they become wet or soiled to prevent skin irritation. Parents should check diapers every few hours to see if they need changing. It is recommended to change diapers every 1 to 3 hours during the day and at least once at night (AAP, 2021a). Take the following steps when changing diapers:

- Gather supplies (e.g., clean diaper, clean clothing, and wet washcloth or diaper wipes) before placing the infant on a flat surface such as a changing table.
- Unfasten the diaper and lower the front of the diaper.
- Lift the infant's bottom using an ankle hold (both ankles). Wipe the buttocks with a clean portion of the diaper (if stool is present) before tucking underneath the buttocks.
- Use water or commercial diaper wipes to clean the genital and rectal areas, wiping from front to back for female infants. For male infants, lift the scrotum and wash under it. The foreskin of the uncircumcised male should not be retracted during cleaning.
- Do not vigorously scrub the skin.

- Lift the bottom of the infant using the ankle hold, remove the soiled diaper, and then place a clean diaper under the infant.
- Fasten both sides of the diaper so that there is a snug fit. The front of the diaper should be folded over to avoid covering the umbilical cord.
- Properly dispose of the diaper.
- Wash hands and document the output.

Elimination

The frequency and characteristics of infant stools and urination are important for parents to track during the first few weeks after birth. An infant's stool and urination reflect feeding and hydration. Providing guidelines for what is normal and what to expect can assist parents in early identification of potential feeding and dehydration problems. The teaching plan should include:

- Instruct parents on the stages of newborn stools (see Table 15-1).
- Explain that newborns should pass several stools per day and have at least six wet diapers per day by day 6 of life.
- Inform parents that a newborn's diapers may have a pink or rust stain ("brick dust") related to urates, which is a normal occurrence in the first few days of life.
  - Urates persisting in more than two diapers may suggest dehydration and weight loss. Parents need to report a continued presence of urates to the health-care provider.
- Inform parents that blood may occur on the diaper of female newborns related to a withdrawal of maternal hormones. This is referred to as pseudomenstruation.
- Instruct parents to notify the health-care provider if stools are runny and green or if the infant has fewer than six wet diapers per day after day 6.
- Instruct parents to notify the health-care provider if the infant becomes constipated. Constipation can signify inadequate fluid intake and must be evaluated.

Follow-Up Care

Routine follow-up care of the newborn is an essential component of safe infant care and health promotion. Typically, the pediatrician or nurse practitioner will want a newborn follow-up visit within 48 to 72 hours of discharge. The nurse can assist parents with scheduling the appointment and should reinforce the importance of well-child checkups. These visits provide an opportunity to:

- Assess the infant's growth.
  - Growth spurts occur at 14 days, 3 weeks, 6 weeks, 3 months, and 6 months. During these growth spurts, infants can be fussy and need to be fed more frequently.
- Assess the feeding pattern.
- Assess the developmental level.
- Assess for jaundice.
- Provide the appropriate immunizations (see https://www.cdc.gov/vaccines/schedules/hcp/imz/child-adolescent.html).
- Do follow-up GDS.
- Continue teaching parents about the care of their child and what to expect at each developmental milestone.

The AAP recommends the following:

- First visit within 2 to 4 days after hospital discharge
- Subsequent visits at 1, 2, 4, 6, 9, and 12 months of age

Jaundice

Jaundice is the yellow color that appears in the skin of 60% of newborns soon after birth. Jaundice is caused by elevated bilirubin levels (also called hyperbilirubinemia). Bilirubin is a substance in RBCs removed by the liver, which is typically immature at birth. Mild jaundice is harmless and common, but in rare cases extreme hyperbilirubinemia can cause permanent brain damage. To reduce the risk of extreme hyperbilirubinemia, parents need to be taught the following:

- Explain why their baby might be at risk of severe hyperbilirubinemia (such as from blood type differences, bruising, prematurity, or feeding difficulties).
- Explain how bilirubin levels are assessed in the hospital.
- Explain the importance of taking the infant to all follow-up visits
- Explain how to assess for jaundice and how the yellow color starts in the head and face, and progresses to the chest, abdomen, arms, legs, and sclera.
- Explain how to assess for jaundice in darker skinned babies by also checking the gums and inner lips. Parents may need to be instructed to call the provider sooner when color changes are difficult to assess.
- Explain to the parent to call the provider if the baby
  - Has become very jaundiced
  - Has become very sleepy or is hard to awaken
  - Is not feeding well, either by breastfeeding or by bottle
  - Is very fussy
  - Has a decrease in number of wet or dirty diapers
  - Has other signs of dehydration such as dry mucous membranes

(CDC, 2020)

Pediatric Abusive Head Trauma

Pediatric AHT, also referred to as shaken baby syndrome (SBS), is an injury to the skull or intracranial contents of an infant or child younger than 5 caused by inflicted blunt impact or violent shaking. Approximately 1,200 to 1,400 cases of pediatric AHT occur each year, mostly in children between ages 3 and 8 months. It is the number one cause of death in children under age 2; up to 25% of AHT cases are fatal. Neurological impairment affects 65% of children who survive AHT (Joyce et al., 2021).

Infant crying is usually the trigger that causes the parent or caretaker to shake or hit the infant's head. Infants are at higher risk for injury related to violent shaking due to their weak neck muscles and large, heavy heads. When the infant is violently shaken, the brain bounces back and forth against the skull, causing bruising, swelling, and bleeding within brain tissue. Pediatric AHT injuries can cause death or permanent and severe brain damage. It is important that parents receive AHT information

and strategies to use when their frustration levels are high. The teaching plan should include:

- How shaking causes injury to the infant's brain and eyes
- The long-term effects of AHT
- Information on the stages of infant and childhood development
- Information on infant crying (refer to the earlier Crying and Colic section).
- Information on stress reduction:
  - Assist parents in identifying ways to cope with their frustrations.
  - Explain it is normal to feel frustrated when efforts to calm a baby are not effective.
  - Explain to the parents that it is okay to place their infant in a crib and leave the room for 10 minutes while they regain composure.
- Information on what to do when feeling overwhelmed:
  - Ask for help—ask a friend or family member to care for the infant so they can have time to relax and regain composure.
  - Contact community resources such as the Parental Stress Line.

Pediatric AHT is preventable. Several prevention programs have been developed by health centers and organizations; these are an important component in decreasing the incidence of AHT.

Safe Infant Sleep

Parents and all caregivers should be educated on safe infant sleep. SUID is the broad term for the death of a sleeping infant younger than 1 year of age when the cause is not immediately known. After a full investigation, SUIDs are determined to be from either accidental suffocation, sudden infant death syndrome (SIDS), or an unknown cause (typically the baby is found in an unsafe environment, but suffocation cannot be determined). Most of these deaths are now considered preventable with safe sleep practices. In 1992 the AAP made its first safe sleep recommendation that all infants be placed only on their backs for all sleep (Fig. 15–18). Since then, the AAP has made other recommendations based on the research. SUIDs have decreased by almost 50% with safe sleep practices.

In 2011 and 2016, the AAP further expanded its recommendations which now focus on infant positioning as well as the sleep environment and preventive factors such as breastfeeding and pacifier use (AAP, 2016a). The National Institute of Child Health and Human Development supports AAP recommendations and instituted the Safe to Sleep public health campaign, which focuses on educating parents and the public on safe infant sleep. To reduce the risk of SUIDs, the AAP (2016a) recommends the following:

- Teach parents, grandparents, and all caregivers about sleep safety such as placing newborns on their backs to sleep, avoiding loose bedding, and not bed-sharing.
- Place infants on their back for all sleep. Side positioning is not safe. Once infants can turn on their own from back to front, it is safe to leave them in the position they assume. Infants

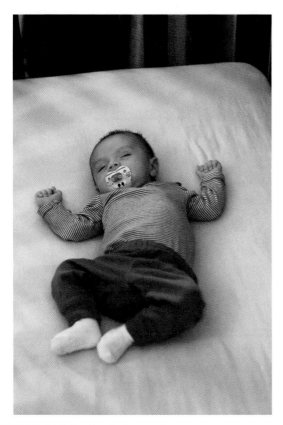

FIGURE 15–18 Infant in safe sleep environment.

should not be swaddled once they can move around and appear to be close to rolling over (usually around 2 months).

- Use a firm sleep surface made for infants, covered by a fitted sheet.
- Keep soft objects, toys, and loose bedding out of the infant's sleep area, including bumper pads. Use swaddle sacks, blanket sleepers, or footed pajamas instead of blankets.
- Cribs, bassinets, and portable cribs need to meet the safety standards of the Consumer Product Safety Commission.
- Infants should not sleep in an adult bed, on a couch, or in a lounge chair, whether alone or with anyone else. This is called bed-sharing.
- Infants should sleep in their own bed in the same room as the parent for at least the first 6 months of life. This is called room sharing.
- Women should get regular health care during pregnancy and should not smoke, drink alcohol, or use illegal drugs during pregnancy or after the baby is born.
- Parents should not smoke or allow smoking around their baby.
- Breastfeeding is protective against SIDS. Exclusive is best but any amount is helpful.
- Pacifiers are protective against SIDS and should be offered but not forced. Once the pacifier falls out, it does not need to be replaced. Allow breastfeeding to be established before introducing a pacifier.
- Do not allow infants to overheat during sleep. Do not overbundle.
- Immunizations and well-baby checks are protective against SIDS.

- Avoid products that claim to reduce the risk of SIDS and other sleep-related deaths.
- Provide "tummy time" when the infant is awake and supervised. Placing an infant on its stomach helps normal development and prevents plagiocephaly (flat spots on the back of head). This should start soon after birth and be done every day.

Safety

Parents are responsible for the safety of their children. Newborns and infants are at risk for injury related to falls, ingestion of harmful products, and accidents. An infant safety teaching plan should include education on the following topics.

Accident Prevention

- Keep small objects out of the reach of infants to prevent choking.
- Remove strings and ribbons from bedding, sleepwear, and pacifiers to prevent strangulation.
- Keep plastic bags out of reach.
- Keep all sharp objects in drawers or cabinets and out of the infant's reach.
- Check water temperature used for bathing. Water temperature should be 100°F to 100.4°F (37.8°C to 38°C).
- Set the water heater thermostat at 120°F or lower.
- Do not leave the infant in the bathtub unsupervised.
- Keep any guns unloaded and locked and out of the infant's reach.
- Install safety devices around swimming pools.
- Do not cook while holding the infant.
- Do not drink hot liquids when holding the infant.
- Supervise infants when pets are in the room.
- Ensure infant crib, highchair, and other furniture or play equipment meet current safety standards (i.e., all four sides of cribs are fixed and unmovable).
- Cover electrical outlets.

Car Seats

Car seats must be used for all infants and children when traveling in a motor vehicle, including on the day of discharge from the hospital. Infants and children at least until age 12 should be secured in the back seat. Rear-facing car seats are used until 2 to 3 years of age when the child has reached the weight or height limit allowed by the manufacturer of the infant seat (U.S. Department of Transportation, n.d.). Parents need to select a car seat that fits their vehicle and follow instructions to secure the seat to the vehicle's seat and properly position and secure the infant.

- Parents can contact a certified child passenger safety (CPS) technician for assistance in the installation and use of infant car seats before bringing the newborn home. Instruct parents to visit www.seatcheck.org to locate a CPS near their home.
- Each state has laws that govern the use of infant and child car seats. Laws for specific states can be viewed at www.seatcheck.org.
- Instruct parents to never leave their child in a car unattended.

Fall Prevention

- Instruct parents not to leave the infant on an elevated flat surface without supervision.
- Instruct parents not to leave the infant in an infant car seat on an elevated surface unattended.
- Install gates at stairwells.
- Select a highchair with a wide base to prevent tipping over.

Poisoning Prevention

- Place all cleaning materials in upper cabinets out of the infant's reach.
- Place all medications, including vitamins, in upper cabinets out of the infant's reach.
- Place safety latches on all lower cabinets and keep the cabinet doors closed.
- Remove lead paint from older cribs and infant furniture and walls.
- Never leave infants unattended in rooms or yards.

Sibling Attachment

There will be some degree of adjustment for siblings when a new baby is introduced into the family. Older children will feel the shift of attention from them to the new baby and may react negatively to this change. Toddlers may begin wetting themselves, wanting to use diapers, or crying to get attention. Others may want to drink from a bottle. Some children may hit or pinch their new sibling. Parents can decrease the degree of sibling rivalry using the following methods:

- Start preparing older children during pregnancy for the new family addition by talking to them about becoming an older brother or sister, having them feel the baby kick, and having them around newborn infants (see Chapter 5).
- Have older siblings attend sibling classes offered by some hospitals and agencies.
- Bring older children to the postpartum unit to meet their new sibling (Fig. 15–19)
- Give the older children a gift and tell them it is from their new brother or sister.

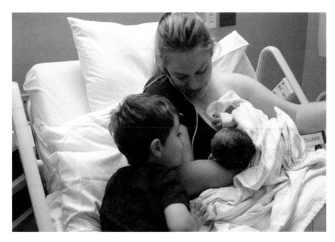

FIGURE 15–19 Toddler meeting new sibling on the postpartum unit.

- Spend quality time with older children such as reading or playing games.
- Take older children on special outings without the new sibling.
- Teach the older sibling about why babies cry and why mom or dad needs to attend to the baby's cry.

Skin Care

The newborn's skin is delicate and can be irritated easily. The skin should be inspected daily for signs of tissue irritation and breakdown. The following general skin care information should be included in the teaching plan:

- Avoid daily bathing with soap. Bathing every few days is generally adequate.
- Use mild cleansers that have neutral pH.
- Avoid use of adhesives. Removing adhesives can remove the epidermis layer of the skin and lead to a breakdown of the skin barrier.
- Apply petroleum-based ointments sparingly to dry skin and avoid the head and face.
- Avoid use of skin ointments with perfume, dyes, and preservatives.

Soothing Babies

Newborns and infants cry when they are hungry, uncomfortable, bored, exposed to new experiences, or sick (see the earlier sections on crying, colic, and AHT). The parents' task is to attempt to determine the cause of crying and then respond with appropriate soothing techniques. The parent should check to see if the infant is hungry or needs a diaper change. Parents should check for signs of illness or injury, such as rash, elevated temperature, or swollen gums. If the child appears ill or injured, contact the doctor or nurse practitioner. Techniques that can be used to soothe or calm the infant include the following:

- Feed if crying is related to hunger.
- Reposition the infant to a more comfortable position.
- Talk or sing to the infant.
- Swaddle the infant.
- Hold the infant close to the body so the child can feel the warmth of the parent's body and hear the parent's heartbeat.
- Hold the infant and rock back and forth or walk around the house or dance with the infant.
- Offer the infant a pacifier.
- Place the infant in a stroller and go for a walk.

Swaddling

Swaddling means to wrap the infant snugly in a blanket to provide warmth and a sense of security that can have a calming effect. Parents need to be instructed on the proper method of swaddling. Improper swaddling can increase the infant's risk for accidental suffocation and hip dysplasia. Swaddling should be discontinued around the second month or when the infant shows signs of trying to roll from the back to stomach position (AAP, 2017).

Swaddling Instructions

- Place the blanket on a flat surface.
- If using a square blanket, fold the top corner over.
- Place the infant on the blanket with the shoulders at the fold line.
- Bring the left arm down (also okay to leave the arm flexed so the hands are up by the face) and wrap the blanket across the arm and chest. Tuck the blanket under the infant's right side.
- Bring the right arm down (or leave the arm flexed) and wrap the blanket across the arm and chest. Tuck the blanket under the infant's left side.
- Loosely fold the bottom end of the blanket and tuck behind the infant.
  - The legs should be bent up and out, rather than extended.
  - Leave enough room for the hips to move.
- Check the tightness of swaddle. The parent should be able to get two to three fingers between the infant's chest and the swaddle, but not so loose that the baby can wiggle enough to become unwrapped (AAP, 2017).

Temperature Taking

There are two main methods for assessing an infant's temperature: axillary and rectal. It is important for parents to ask their infant's health-care provider their preferred method of assessing the infant's temperature. Rectal temperatures are considered the most accurate, but also the most invasive. Digital or temporal artery thermometers are recommended over mercury-filled ones. Parents should take the infant's temperature before calling the health-care provider if they feel that their child is sick. The teaching plan should include the following:

- Instruct parents to take an axillary temperature by placing the digital thermometer in the axillary region and holding the child's arm against their side until the thermometer beeps (Fig. 15–20).
- Instruct parents that if a temporal thermometer is used, instructions must be carefully followed as some are "no-touch" of the skin and some are not.
- Tympanic thermometers are not recommended for infants under 6 months of age.
- Teach parents how to take a rectal temperature:
  - Clean the end of the thermometer with alcohol or soapy water and rinse in cold water.
  - Lubricate the end of the thermometer with a lubricant such as petroleum jelly.
  - Place the child on their back and hold the legs in a flexed position.
  - Insert the thermometer no farther than 0.5 inches into the rectum.
  - Hold the thermometer in place until it beeps.
  - Remove the thermometer after it has beeped and check the digital reading.

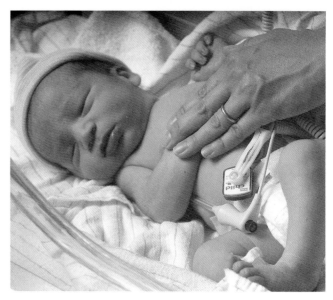

FIGURE 15–20 Placement of thermometer when taking an axillary temperature.

- Teach parents how to read a thermometer.
  - An elevated temperature might be related to overheating from too many blankets or clothing. Instruct parents to remove some clothing and retake the temperature after 15 to 20 minutes.

When to Call the Pediatrician or Nurse Practitioner

Parents should notify the infant's health-care provider if the infant:

- Has a rectal temperature above 100.4°F (38°C) or axillary temperature above 99°F (37.2°C)
  - Ask the health-care provider which method to use to assess the infant's temperature; this will vary based on the health-care provider's preferences or hospital's and clinic's policies.
- Has loss or change of appetite
- Refuses to eat
- Is lethargic
- Is sleepy and not as active as usual
- Does not wake on own for feedings or is not interested in feeding
- Does not cry or has a weak cry
- Has watery green stools
- Is vomiting
- Has a decrease in the number of wet diapers
- Has a skin rash
- Has sunken or bulging fontanels
- Is bleeding from the circumcision site or cord site
- Has a foul odor from the circumcision site or cord site

Clinical Pathway for Full-Term Low-Risk Neonate

Delivery Date and Time

Focus of Care	Birth to First Hour	1 to 4 Hours of Age	4 to 24 Hours of Age	24 Hours of Age to Discharge
Assessments	Obtain Apgar score at 1 and 5 minutes. Inspect the skin for abrasions or bruises.	Complete neonatal assessment by 2 hours of age. Complete gestational assessment as per hospital policy. Weigh and measure head, chest, and length.	Assess at the beginning of each shift or per hospital policies. Weigh the newborn each day per hospital policy.	Assess at the beginning of each shift or per hospital policies and before discharge. Weigh the newborn each day per hospital policy.
Thermoregulation	Close the doors to the birthing room. Dry the neonate thoroughly and place in a prewarmed crib or skin-to-skin on the mother's chest with a warm blanket over them. Place a stocking cap over top of the neonate's head. Assess axillary temperature every 30 minutes or per hospital policy.	Prevent heat loss by maintaining an NTE. Encourage skin-to-skin contact with either parent and with a warm blanket over both the neonate and parent. Wrap the neonate in blankets when in an open crib. Place a stocking cap on the head.	Prevent heat loss by maintaining an NTE. Wrap the neonate in blankets when in an open crib. Place a stocking cap on the neonate's head.	Prevent heat loss by maintaining an NTE. Assist the mother in dressing her infant for discharge in clothing and blankets that help maintain the neonate's normal body temperature.
Respiratory	Clear the nose and mouth of mucus with use of a bulb syringe. Assess respirations every 30 minutes. Assess lung sounds. Monitor for signs of respiratory distress: grunting, flaring, retractions.	Keep the nose and mouth free of mucus with use of a bulb syringe. Assess respirations every hour. Assess lung sounds. Monitor for signs of respiratory distress: grunting, flaring, retractions.	Assess respirations once per shift or per hospital policy. Assess lung sounds once per shift or per hospital policy. Monitor for signs of respiratory distress: grunting, flaring, retractions.	Assess respirations once per shift. Assess lung sounds once per shift and before discharge.
Cardiovascular	Assess skin color for cyanosis. Assess heart rate every 30 minutes.	Assess skin color for cyanosis. Assess heart rate every hour.	Assess the heart rate once per shift, or per hospital policy.	Assess heart rate once per shift and before discharge.
Activity	Assess the level of activity and compare with periods of reactivity. Monitor for signs of hypoglycemia (i.e., jitteriness).	Assess the level of activity and compare with periods of reactivity. Monitor for signs of hypoglycemia (i.e., jitteriness).	Assess the level of activity and compare with periods of reactivity. Monitor for signs of hypoglycemia (i.e., jitteriness).	Assess the level of activity.

Clinical Pathway for Full-Term Low-Risk Neonate—cont'd

Delivery Date and Time

Focus of Care	Birth to First Hour	1 to 4 Hours of Age	4 to 24 Hours of Age	24 Hours of Age to Discharge
Nutrition	Ideal time to introduce breastfeeding is when the neonate is in the first period of reactivity.	Breastfeed on demand.	The ideal time for feeding is when the neonate is in the second period of reactivity. Breastfeed or bottle feed on demand; feeding should be every 2–4 hours.	Breastfeed or bottle feed on demand; feeding should be every 2–3 hours for breastfed infants and every 3-4 hours for formula-fed infants.
Elimination	The neonate may or may not void or pass meconium stool.	The neonate may or may not void or pass meconium stool.	The neonate voids within 24 hours. The neonate may or may not pass meconium stool.	The neonate voids a minimum of two times on day 2 and three times on day 3. The neonate passes meconium or transitional stools two to four times a day.
Medications and immunizations	Inform the parents which medications are being administered and why. Administer vitamin K injection, hepatitis B vaccine, and eye ointment as per physician's order. Administer hepatitis B immune globulin vaccine when indicated per physician order.	Inform parents which medications are being administered and why. Administer vitamin K injection and eye ointment if not done during first hour as per physician order.	Administer vitamin K injection, hepatitis B vaccine, and eye ointment if not previously done, as per physician order. Administer hepatitis B immune globulin vaccine if not previously done per physician order.	
Special procedures	Heel stick to assess glucose levels as indicated (i.e., jitteriness), LGA, and SGA.	Heel stick to assess glucose levels as indicated (i.e., jitteriness), LGA, and SGA.		Newborn screening tests: GDS blood sample Hearing screening CCHD screening Hyperbilirubinemia screen Circumcision might be done after 24 hours or several hours before discharge.

Continued

Clinical Pathway for Full-Term Low-Risk Neonate—cont'd

Delivery Date and Time

Focus of Care	Birth to First Hour	1 to 4 Hours of Age	4 to 24 Hours of Age	24 Hours of Age to Discharge
Family attachment	Delay eye ointment until parents have had the opportunity to hold their newborn. Provide time for parents to see and touch or hold the newborn. Explain to partners they can stay with newborn while assessments are completed.	Complete necessary assessments as quickly as possible to provide uninterrupted time for parents to hold and be with their newborn. Complete assessments at bedside when possible.	Arrange nursing care to provide uninterrupted time for parents and their newborn. Teach parents about normal newborn characteristics and behavior.	Arrange nursing care to provide uninterrupted time for parents and their newborn.
Education	Point out normal newborn characteristics such as molding, lanugo, and vernix. Begin education on breastfeeding (e.g., positioning, latching on, releasing suction).	Teaching is kept to a minimum because parents are usually tired during this period of time or want to call family members to announce the birth.	Ideal time for teaching. Provide information on caring for a newborn (see Chapter 16).	Continue teaching parents about the care of their newborn (see Chapter 16). Complete the appropriate hospital discharge teaching forms. Give parents a copy of written discharge instructions. Explain the importance of follow-up well-child checkups and the importance of scheduling their first appointment as recommended by their pediatrician or pediatric nurse practitioner (PNP).
Safety	Place completed ID bands on the neonate, mother, and her partner. Attach infant safety tag. Keep the side of warmer up when not at crib side. Teach parents how to support the head and neck of their neonate. Use the five rights when administering medications. Wear gloves until after the first bath.	Teach parents abduction prevention protocol. Place the neonate on their back. Teach parents safe sleep strategies. Instruct parents not to leave the newborn unattended on a flat surface such as the mother's bed. Teach parents the importance of placing the neonate on back to sleep. Wear gloves if there is the possibility of exposure to body fluids.	Provide education on infant safety (see Chapter 16). Follow hospital policies to prevent infant abduction. Wear gloves if there is the possibility of exposure to body fluids.	Review infant safety before discharge. Follow hospital policies to prevent infant abduction. Wear gloves if there is the possibility of exposure to body fluids. Inform parents that a federally approved car seat will be needed to transport the infant home and that it will need to be properly placed in the car.

CCHD, critical congenital heart defect; LGA, large for gestational age; NTE, neutral thermal environment; SGA, small for gestational age.

CONCEPT MAP

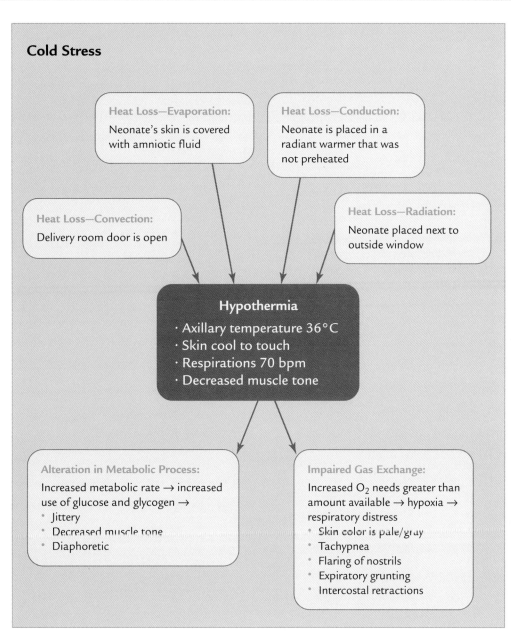

Cold Stress

Heat Loss—Evaporation:
Neonate's skin is covered with amniotic fluid

Heat Loss—Conduction:
Neonate is placed in a radiant warmer that was not preheated

Heat Loss—Convection:
Delivery room door is open

Heat Loss—Radiation:
Neonate placed next to outside window

Hypothermia
· Axillary temperature 36°C
· Skin cool to touch
· Respirations 70 bpm
· Decreased muscle tone

Alteration in Metabolic Process:
Increased metabolic rate → increased use of glucose and glycogen →
· Jittery
· Decreased muscle tone
· Diaphoretic

Impaired Gas Exchange:
Increased O_2 needs greater than amount available → hypoxia → respiratory distress
· Skin color is pale/gray
· Tachypnea
· Flaring of nostrils
· Expiratory grunting
· Intercostal retractions

CARE PLANS

Problem 1: Heat loss due to evaporation
Goal: Maintain an NTE.
Outcome: The neonate's temperature is within normal range.

Nursing Actions
1. Dry the neonate's body with a warm towel.
2. Remove wet bedding and clothing.
3. Monitor vital signs.

Problem 2: Heat loss due to conduction
Goal: Maintain an NTE.
Outcome: The neonate's temperature is within normal range.

Nursing Actions
1. Encourage skin-to-skin contact with the parent with a warm blanket over both the neonate and the parent.
2. Preheat the warmer before use.
3. Use warm blankets.
4. Warm hands before touching the neonate.
5. Warm equipment before contact with the neonate.
6. Monitor vital signs.

Problem 3: Heat loss due to convection
Goal: Maintain an NTE.
Outcome: The neonate's temperature is within normal range.

Continued

Nursing Actions

1. Close the doors to the room.
2. Place the neonate away from the air vent, windows, and doors.
3. Place a stocking cap on the neonate's head.
4. Warm O_2 when administering oxygen.
5. Monitor vital signs.

Problem 4: Heat loss due to radiation
Goal: Maintain an NTE.
Outcome: The neonate's temperature is within the normal range.

Nursing Actions

1. Preheat the radiant warmer before use.
2. Place the neonate away from cold walls and windows.
3. Keep cold objects away from the neonate.
4. Place a stocking cap on the neonate's head.
5. Monitor vital signs.

Problem 5: Alteration in metabolic processes—hypoglycemia
Goal: Manage an episode of hypoglycemia.
Outcome: The neonate's glucose level is within normal range.

Nursing Actions

1. Monitor for signs and symptoms of hypoglycemia.
2. Monitor glucose levels.
3. Assist the woman with breastfeeding or formula feeding.
   a. Assess glucose levels 30 minutes after feeding.
4. Maintain an NTE.

Problem 6: Impaired gas exchange—respiratory distress
Goal: Adequate gas exchange
Outcome: PaO_2 is 60 to 70 mm Hg; $PaCO_2$ is 35 to 45 mm Hg; skin color is pink; lung sounds are clear; and no signs of retractions, grunting, or nasal flaring.

Nursing Actions

1. Monitor vital signs, oxygen saturation, and arterial blood gases.
2. Maintain patent airway.
3. Suction airway as indicated.
4. Administer oxygen as per orders.
5. Maintain an NTE.

Case Study

You are assigned to the mother–baby couplet unit, where your patients for the day include the Sanchez family. Margarite is a 28-year-old G3 P2 Hispanic woman who gave birth to a healthy male, Manuel, at 0839. Margarite experienced an uncomplicated labor of 12 hours. Membranes ruptured 7 hours before delivery. She received two doses of Nubain during labor. The last dose was given at 0440.

Manuel weighs 3,800 g and is 50 cm in length. His 1- and 5-minute Apgar scores were 8 and 9, respectively. Manuel is 2 hours old. The Ballard score indicates that Manuel is 39 weeks. Margarite breastfed her son for 15 minutes on each breast immediately after the birth.

Your initial shift assessment findings are:

Vital signs: Axillary temperature, 97.2°F (36.2°C); apical pulse, 100 bpm; respirations, 30 breaths per minute.

Skin is warm and pink with acrocyanosis.

Fontanels are soft and flat.

Molding is present.

Lung sounds are clear.

There is mild nasal flaring.

Manuel is in a sleep state and unresponsive to external stimuli.

Based on the previously noted information, discuss the primary nursing diagnoses for baby Manuel.

Discuss the immediate nursing actions for baby Manuel. Provide rationales for your nursing actions.

Thirty minutes later, you note that Manuel is jittery and exhibits signs of hypoglycemia.

List the signs and symptoms of hypoglycemia and related nursing actions.

Several hours later, Manuel's father is present and holding Manuel.

List signs of parent–infant bonding.

Discuss nursing actions that will support parent–infant attachment.

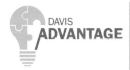
DAVIS **ADVANTAGE**

Go to Davis Advantage to complete your learning: strengthen understanding, apply your knowledge, and prepare for the Next Gen NCLEX®.

REFERENCES

American Academy of Pediatrics. (2015). *Colic relief tips for parents.* https://www.healthychildren.org/English/ages-stages/baby/crying-colic/Pages/Colic.aspx

American Academy of Pediatrics. (2016a). SIDS and other sleep-related infant deaths: Evidence base for 2016 update recommendations for safe infant sleeping environment. *Pediatrics, 138,* e20162940. DOI: 10.1542/peds.2016-2940

American Academy of Pediatrics. (2016b). *Why parents and caregivers need breaks from crying babies.* http://www.healthychildren.org/English/ages-stages/baby/crying-colic/Pages/Calming-A-Fussy-Baby.aspx

American Academy of Pediatrics. (2017). *Swaddling: Is it safe?* http://www.healthychildren.org/English/ages-stages/baby/diapers-clothing/Pages/Swaddling-Is-it-Safe.aspx

American Academy of Pediatrics. (2021a). *Changing diapers.* http://www.healthychildren.org

American Academy of Pediatrics. (2021b). *Newborn screening: Critical congenital heart defects.* AAP Advocacy & Policy. https://www.aap.org/en-us/advocacy-and-policy/aap-health-initiatives/PEHDIC/Pages/Newborn-Screening-for-CCHD.aspx

American Academy of Pediatrics, Committee on Fetus and Newborn and Section on Anesthesiology and Pain Medicine. (2016). Prevention and management of procedural pain in the neonate: An update. *Pediatrics, 137*(2), 1–13. https://doi.org/10.1542/peds.2015-4271

American Academy of Pediatrics & The American College of Obstetrics and Gynecologists. (2017). *Guidelines for perinatal care* (8th ed.). Authors.

Association of Women's Health, Obstetrics and Neonatal Nurses. (2018). *Neonatal skin care: Evidence-based clinical practice guideline* (4th ed.). AWHONN. https://www.awhonn.org/

Blackburn, S. T. (2018). *Maternal, fetal, neonatal physiology: A clinical perspective* (5th ed.). Elsevier.

Centers for Disease Control and Prevention. (2020). *What are jaundice and kernicterus?* https://www.cdc.gov/ncbddd/jaundice/facts.html

Costanzo, L. S. (2018). *Physiology* (6th ed.). Elsevier.

Desmond, M. M., Desmond, A. J., Rudolph, P., & Hitaksphraiwan, P. (1966). The transitional care nursery. A mechanism for preventive medicine in the newborn. *Pediatric Clinics of North America, 13*(3), 651–666. https://doi.org/10.1016/S0031-3955(16)31875-2

Eichenwald, E. C. (2020). *Overview of cyanosis in the newborn.* UpToDate. https://www.wolterskluwer.com/en/solutions/uptodate

Fernandes, C. J. (2019). *Physiologic transition from intrauterine to extrauterine life.* UpToDate. https://www.wolterskluwer.com/en/solutions/uptodate

Flaherman, V. J., Maisels, M. J., & Academy of Breastfeeding Medicine. (2017). ABM protocol #22: Guidelines for management of jaundice in the breastfeeding infant 35 weeks or more of gestation—revised 2017. *Breastfeeding Medicine, 12*(5), 250–257. https://doi.org/10.1089/bfm.2017.29042.vjf

Goyal, N. K. (2020). The newborn infant. In R. M. Kliegman, J. W. St Geme, J. Blum, S. S. Shaw, R. C. Tasker, K. M. Wilson, & R. E. Behrman (Eds.), *Nelson textbook of pediatrics* (21st ed., pp. 867–876). Elsevier.

Jarvis, C. (2016). *Physical examination & health assessment* (7th ed.). Elsevier.

Johnson, J. D., Cocker, K., & Chang, E. (2015). Infantile colic: Recognition and treatment. *American Family Physician, 92*(7), 577–582.

Joyce, T., Grossman, W., & Huecker, M. R. (2021). Pediatric abusive head trauma. *StatPearls.* https://www.ncbi.nlm.nih.gov/books/NBK499836/

Kellmans, A., Harrel, C., Omage, S., Gregory, C., Rosen-Carole, C., & Academy of Breastfeeding Medicine. (2017). ABM Clinical Protocol #3: Supplementary feedings in the healthy term breastfed neonate, revised 2017. *Breastfeeding Medicine, 12*(3), 1–11. https://doi.org/10.1089/bfm.2017.29038.ajk

Lo, S. F. (2020). Reference intervals for laboratory tests and procedures. In R. M. Kliegman, J. W. St Geme, N. J. Blum, S. S. Shah, R. C. Tasker, & K. M. Wilson (Eds.), *Nelson textbook of pediatrics* (21st ed., pp. e5–e14). Elsevier.

Marcdante, K. J., & Kliegman, R. M. (2019). Crying and colic. In *Nelson essentials of pediatrics* (8th ed., pp. 41–43). Elsevier.

Morris, B. J., Krieger, J. N., & Klausner, J. D. (2017). CDC's male circumcision recommendations represent a key public health measure. *Global Health: Science and Practice, 5*(1), 15–27. https://doi.org/10.9745/GHSP-D-16-00390

National Institutes of Health and National Institute on Deafness and Other Communication Disorders. (2020). *Your baby's hearing screening.* National Institutes of Health. https://www.nidcd.nih.gov/health/your-babys-hearing-screening

Nugent, J. K. (2013). The competent newborn and the neonatal behavioral assessment scale: T. Berry Brazelton's legacy. *Journal of Child and Adolescent Psychiatric Nursing, 26*(2013), 173–179. https://onlinelibrary.wiley.com/journal/17446171

Olsson, J. M. (2020). The newborn. In R. M. Kliegman, J. W. St Geme, N. J. Blum, S. S. Shah, R. C. Tasker, & K. M. Wilson (Eds.), *Nelson textbook of pediatrics* (21st ed., pp. 128–131). Elsevier.

Perry, M., Tan, Z., Chen, J., Weidig, T., Xu, W., & Cong, X. S. (2018). Neonatal pain: Perceptions and current practice. *Critical Care Nursing Clinics of North America, 30*(4), 549–561. https://doi.org/10.1016/j.cnc.2018.07.013

Simpson, K. R., Creehan, P. A., O'Brien-Abel, N., Roth, C. K., & Rohan, A. J. (Eds.). (2021). *Perinatal nursing* (5th ed.). AWHONN/Wolters Kluwer.

Tedder, J. L. (1991). Using the Brazelton Neonatal Assessment Scale to facilitate the parent–infant relationship in a primary care setting. *The Nurse Practitioner, 16*(3), 26–36. https://journals.lww.com/tnpj/pages/default.aspx

Texas Department of State Health Services. (n.d.). *Screening for critical congenital heart disease in the apparently healthy newborn* [PowerPoint PDF]. https://dshs.texas.gov/newborn/cchdtoolkit/

Thakkar, P., Arora, K., Das, B., Javadekar, S., & Panigrahi, S. (2016). To evaluate and compare the efficacy of combined sucrose and non-nutritive sucking for analgesia in newborns undergoing minor painful procedure: A randomized controlled trial. *Journal of Perinatology, 36,* 67–70. https://doi:10.1038/jp.2015.122

U.S. Department of Transportation. (n.d.). *Car seats and booster seats.* NHTSA. https://www.nhtsa.gov/equipment/car-seats-and-booster-seats

Vallerand, A. H., & Sanoski, C. A. (2021). *Davis's drug guide for nurses* (17th ed.). F.A. Davis.

Warren, S., Midodzi, W. K., Newhook, L. A., Murphy, P., & Twells, L. (2020). Effects of delayed newborn bathing on breastfeeding, hypothermia, and hypoglycemia. *Journal of Obstetric, Gynecologic, and Neonatal Nursing, 49*(2), 181–189. https://doi.org/10.1016/j.jogn.2019.12.004

Newborn Nutrition

Lyrae Perini, MSN, RN, IBCLC, RLC
Connie S. Miller, DNP, RNC-OB, CNE

16

LEARNING OUTCOMES

Upon completion of this chapter, the student will be able to:
1. Discuss the nutritional needs of the newborn.
2. Outline the benefits of breastfeeding for both mother and newborn.
3. Assess proper latch and positioning of the breastfed newborn.
4. Identify prevention and treatment strategies for common breastfeeding issues.
5. Teach signs of adequate intake and output for a breastfed newborn.
6. Explain how to select an appropriate formula and amount for a newborn.
7. Articulate preparation and needed supplies for a formula-fed newborn.

CONCEPTS

Elimination
Health Promotion
Infection
Nutrition
Teaching and Learning

Nursing Diagnosis

- Knowledge deficit related to infant feeding due to lack of experience or information.
- Anxiety related to breastfeeding due to lack of experience or information.
- Pain related to sore nipples due to improper latch.
- Alteration in comfort related to engorgement due to lack of information.
- Knowledge deficit related to signs and symptoms of mastitis due to lack of information.

Nursing Outcomes

- The postpartum mother will effectively breastfeed or bottle feed her newborn.
- The postpartum mother will identify how to establish and maintain an adequate milk supply.
- The postpartum mother will describe prevention and management of sore nipples.
- The postpartum mother will list signs and symptoms that need to be reported to the provider.
- The postpartum mother will discuss the safe preparation and feeding of formula.

INTRODUCTION

New parents have many important concerns, such as deciding how to feed their infants. Newborns are nourished by breast or bottle. Premature newborns and those who cannot suck or swallow are often gavage-fed (see Chapter 17). A mother's decision on how to feed her infant is influenced by previous feeding experience; cultural beliefs; support from her partner; and support from family or friends. Women who desire to breastfeed are encouraged to begin preparing during the prenatal period by reading information online or in books, participating in a breastfeeding class, or finding community support groups. Women planning to bottle feed are encouraged to prepare by gathering supplies before birth.

BREASTFEEDING

According to the Centers for Disease Control and Prevention (CDC), close to 85% of all newborns are breastfed after birth in the United States (CDC, 2021). The World Health Organization (WHO), American Academy of Pediatrics (AAP), and U.S. Department of Health and Human Services (HHS) all recommend exclusive breastfeeding for the first 6 months of life, meaning no other food or anything by mouth other than medication (Box 16-1). These agencies also recommend breastfeeding infants for up to 2 years in addition to complementary foods; however, only 47% of infants are still breastfed by 3 months of age (CDC, 2021). Sore nipples, low milk supply, lack of adequate support, mothers returning to the workforce, and anxiety related to breastfeeding are some issues that lead to early weaning.

Anxiety related to breastfeeding is common among new mothers. Concerns about adequate intake, positioning, latch techniques, and how to wake a sleepy newborn arise in the early postpartum period. Anxiety may also come from negative past breastfeeding experiences. Assessing previous experience will allow the nurse to determine essential educational needs. Emotional support and good listening skills are important to assess the mother's motivation or hesitation to breastfeed. Nurses play an important role in educating new mothers on prevention of these issues by evaluating proper breastfeeding technique, teaching management of common breastfeeding concerns, and providing resources for breastfeeding help after discharge.

A mother's decision to breastfeed is greatly influenced by the values, norms, beliefs, and established practices of her culture. Cultural sensitivity is essential when it comes to breastfeeding support as a woman's culture can affect rituals, beliefs, or practices she may follow.

BOX 16–1 | Position Statements on Breastfeeding

"AWHONN supports, protects and promotes breastfeeding as the optimal method of infant nutrition, including the provision of human milk for preterm and other vulnerable infants. Women should be encouraged and supported to exclusively breastfeed for the first 6 months of an infant's life and continue to breastfeed for the first year and beyond" (AWHONN, 2021).

"Exclusive breastfeeding—defined as the practice of only giving an infant breast-milk for the first 6 months of life (no food or water)—has the single largest potential impact on child mortality of any preventative intervention" (WHO, 2014).

"Breastfeeding is a natural and beneficial source of nutrition and provides the healthiest start for an infant. In addition to the nutritional benefits, breastfeeding promotes a unique and emotional connection between mother and infant" (AAP, 2012).

Benefits of Breastfeeding for the Newborn

Short-term benefits have shown a reduced risk of gastroenteritis, respiratory syncytial virus, otitis media, necrotizing enterocolitis, and sudden unexplained infant death (SUID). Decreased risk of asthma, atopic dermatitis, cardiovascular disease, celiac disease, inflammatory bowel disease, and obesity are some of the long-term benefits breastfeeding provides.

Benefits of Breastfeeding for the Mother

Mothers who breastfeed also experience health benefits associated with breastfeeding such as decreased blood loss, decreased infection, and increased weight loss following delivery. Long-term benefits include a decreased risk of diabetes, metabolic syndrome, osteoporosis, autoimmune diseases, and ovarian and breast cancers. The psychological impact of breastfeeding has been shown to reduce anxiety and stress in the mother (Krol & Grossmann, 2018).

Contraindications for Breastfeeding

While rare, a few contraindications to breastfeeding exist. In addition, mothers should not breastfeed or feed infants expressed breast milk if they:

- Have newborns diagnosed with galactosemia, a rare hereditary genetic metabolic disorder of carbohydrate metabolism
- Have active and untreated tuberculosis
- Have active herpes simplex lesions on a breast
- Receive treatment with radiation
- Receive treatment with antimetabolites or chemotherapeutic agents
- Use illicit drugs such as amphetamines, PCP, cannabis, or cocaine
- Are HIV-positive
  - In developing countries where clean water and formula may not be available, the risks associated with artificial feedings may outweigh the risks of acquiring HIV through breast milk; therefore, women who have HIV are encouraged to breastfeed (WHO, 2021).

In these cases, human milk or breastfeeding would not be recommended.

Composition of Breast Milk

Human milk is considered the gold standard to meet the newborn's nutritional needs. Breast milk is composed of fats, carbohydrates, proteins, lactose, vitamins, minerals, and hormones.

- Human milk contains 87% water, 1% protein, 3.8% fats, and 7% lactose.
- Fat content ranges from 3.5% to 4.5% and is considered the most important component of breast milk. Fats are a source of energy and help central nervous system development.

- Fats provide 50% of the total calories (energy) of breast milk and lactose provides 40%.
- A mother's milk is likely to provide all the essential nutrition for her newborn, even if her diet is inadequate.
- Human milk has all the essential vitamins except for vitamin D and K (Martin et al., 2016).

Breast Milk by Stage

Three stages of breast milk production occur during the lactation process.

- Stage 1: Colostrum—This is considered the first milk and is present in the breast beginning in the second trimester. Colostrum is a thick, clear to golden yellow fluid with higher levels of protein and lower levels of fats, carbohydrates, and calories than mature breast milk. It also contains high levels of immunoglobulins G and A. Colostrum is produced in small amounts; a typical newborn will consume 7 to 14 mL during a feeding the first day of life. This amount is ideal as a newborn's stomach capacity is approximately the size of a large marble. Colostrum also acts as a laxative to assist in the passage of meconium.
- Stage 2: Transitional milk—During this stage, the milk will gradually change from colostrum to mature milk, with decreasing levels of protein and increasing levels of fats, carbohydrates, and calories until the mature milk comes in around day 12 following birth.
- Stage 3: Mature milk—Arriving approximately 12 days after birth, mature milk is composed of 20% solids and 80% water and contains approximately 22 to 23 calories per ounce. Mature milk is whiter and thinner, appearing watery and often with a bluish cast.
  - Foremilk is the milk produced and stored between feedings and is released at the beginning of a feeding. It is more dilute and satisfies thirst.
  - Hindmilk, milk produced during a feeding session, is received toward the end of the feeding and has a higher fat content.

A mother's body produces breast milk specifically tailored to meet the needs of her newborn. For instance, if a mother delivers her newborn prematurely, her breast milk contains more protein and less fat and lactose than breast milk of mothers who delivered full-term newborns. Breast milk composition changes according to the gestational age of the newborn at birth to meet specific nutritional needs (Caldeo et al., 2020).

Breast Milk Production

- Mammogenesis refers to the breast changes that occur during pregnancy. This is a period of rapid breast growth and development (Fig. 16–1). The glandular system and milk ducts grow under the influence of two hormones, estrogen and progesterone.
- Lactogenesis I occurs from pregnancy until postpartum day 2. This period is the transition from pregnancy to lactation. The start of milk synthesis begins during this phase along with

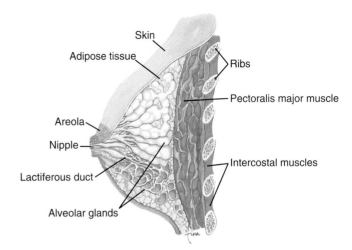

FIGURE 16–1 Mammary gland shown in midsagittal section.

divergence of the alveolar cells into secretory cells. Mammary secretory cells are stimulated by prolactin to produce milk.
- Lactogenesis II occurs from day 3 to 8 following birth, prompted by expulsion of placenta and rapid decrease in progesterone levels. Milk production changes from endocrine (hormonal) control, which occurs regardless of if a mother is breastfeeding, to autocrine (local) control, based on the process of supply and demand for breastfeeding mothers.
- Galactopoiesis starts on day 9 following birth until cessation of lactation. This is considered the maintenance period of lactation. Breast stimulation and milk removal are required for lactation to continue, and the amount of milk removed from the breast is the primary control mechanism for the amount of milk produced.
- Involution is the last phase of lactation as milk production decreases. This occurs when there is less demand for breast milk such as when the infant weans (Wambach & Genna, 2021).

CRITICAL COMPONENT

Lactogenesis and Supply and Demand

Lactogenesis is the transition from pregnancy to lactation. After delivery, milk production shifts from lactogenesis I to lactogenesis II and from endocrine (hormone-driven) to autocrine (driven by milk removal). Therefore, both breastfeeding mothers and mothers who have chosen not to breastfeed their newborn produce colostrum the first few days following birth. A mother's milk supply is dependent on two factors: stimulation of the breast and milk removal. Offering the breast every 2 to 3 hours and on demand is recommended to establish and maintain adequate milk supply. When the mother and newborn are separated or unable to breastfeed due to prematurity or illness, encourage the mother to initiate pumping as soon as possible after birth.

During pregnancy the breasts enlarge and prepare to lactate with the increase of progesterone and estrogen. An increase in estrogen during pregnancy is responsible for expanding the

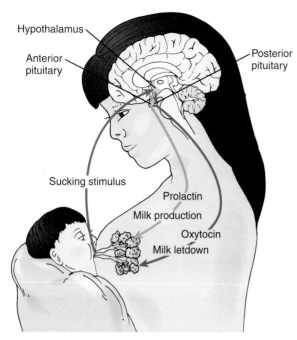

FIGURE 16–2 The role of prolactin in breastfeeding.

lactiferous ductal system into the adipose tissue of the breast. These ducts multiply and elongate as the adipose tissue decreases. The pituitary gland is also affected by estrogen and begins to produce elevated levels of prolactin. Prolactin is required for the cells of the alveoli to secrete milk. The increase in prolactin assures that the mammary glands are adequately developed and ready to produce breast milk by the 20th week of gestation (Alex et al., 2020). Progesterone and estrogen levels fall after delivery and prolactin levels increase, which allows for the production and secretion of breast milk. At the beginning of a feeding, prolactin increases due to stimulation of the breast. Prolactin levels also rise during the night into the early morning hours (Fig. 16–2).

The hormone oxytocin, released by the posterior lobe of the brain in response to breast or nipple stimulation, causes the myoepithelial cells of the alveoli to contract, ejecting the milk into the duct system. Milk travels through the ducts in the let-down reflex or milk ejection reflex, which forces milk into the lactiferous duct system. A let-down response is strongest at initiation of a feeding; however, let-down occurs multiple times during each feeding. The let-down reflex can be inhibited by stress, anxiety, pain, and fatigue and can be stimulated by hearing a newborn cry. Oxytocin also serves to relax the mother and initiate bonding with her newborn.

Skin-to-Skin

Skin-to-skin care (also referred to as kangaroo care) helps stabilize the newborn's body temperature and blood sugar levels. Additional benefits for the mother include:

- It stimulates production of oxytocin and prolactin, which plays an important role in breastfeeding and bonding between mother and newborn.
- It increases milk supply.
- It decreased stress.

Placing the newborn skin-to-skin as often as possible after delivery and especially before feeding times is beneficial in assisting to wake the newborn for feeds.

Evidence-Based Practice: The Effect of Skin-to-Skin on Success of First Breastfeeding

Karimi, F. Z., Sadeghi, R., Maleki-Saghooni, N., & Khadivzadeh, T. (2019). The effect of mother–infant skin to skin contact on success and duration of first breastfeeding: A systematic review and meta-analysis. *Taiwanese Journal of Obstetrics and Gynecology, 58*, 1–9. https://doi.org/10.1016/j.tjog.2018.11.002

Research shows that placing the newborn skin-to-skin with the mother immediately following birth can increase the success and duration of the first breastfeeding compared with routine nursing care. It is believed that the newborn displays innate behaviors such as searching and suckling during the first hour of life, a critical time to establish breastfeeding. Because newborns are sensitive to touch, warmth, and olfaction stimulation during this time, separation of the mother and newborn can disrupt this behavior.

- If the mother and newborn are stable after birth, initiate skin-to-skin.
- Place diapered newborn on mother's bare chest, facing mother with head turned to one side.
- As much surface area as possible of the newborn's skin should be touching the mother's chest.
- If the newborn shows feeding cues or rooting behavior, guide the newborn to the breast for feeding.

Conclusion: Implementing skin-to-skin as soon as possible after birth has been shown in this systematic review and meta-analysis to increase success and duration of the first breastfeeding.

Initiating Breastfeeding

A primary role of a nurse caring for a breastfeeding mother is to facilitate success by providing evidence-based education and techniques as well as support and encouragement (Fig. 16–3).

Breastfeeding should be initiated as soon as possible after birth. Newborns are born with a strong suck reflex following delivery, which usually only lasts a couple of hours before they transition to a recovery sleep phase. For the initial feeding, the nurse assists the mother with positioning that supports both the newborn's neck and the mother's breast. This bedside assistance is crucial in ensuring a deep latch to prevent sore nipples and stimulate milk production more efficiently. If not prevented, sore nipples can lead to early weaning.

Latching the Newborn

Latching is when the newborn grasps the areola and pulls the breast tissue deep into their mouth. A deep latch stimulates the suck-and-swallow reflex. To ensure a deep latch, the mother is encouraged to wait until the newborn opens their mouth wide (such as a yawn), then quickly brings the newborn to the breast.

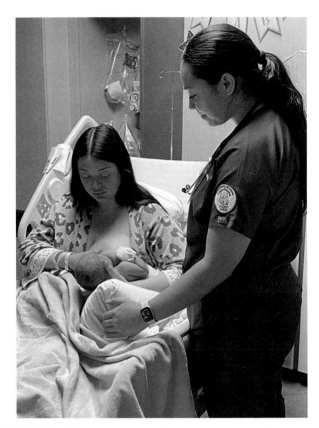

FIGURE 16-3 Student nurse assisting the new mother with positioning to breastfeed.

Feeding Cues

Teaching a mother to observe for newborn feeding cues will facilitate on demand feedings. Newborns will often demonstrate subtle hunger cues:

- Licking their lips
- Smacking their lips
- Extending their tongue
- Putting their hand to their mouth
- Sucking on their fingers
- Turning their head to their mother's voice
- Entering a quiet alert stage

These hunger cues may be present for up to 30 minutes. If cues are missed, a newborn may begin to cry or fall back asleep. Encourage mothers to observe for signs the infant is hungry and offer the breast accordingly. If the infant does not initiate a feeding, the mother is encouraged to gently awaken the infant and offer the breast every 2 to 3 hours until breastfeeding is established.

Positioning the Newborn at the Breast

The mother is encouraged to find a comfortable position. Pillows are essential for support. Proper positioning begins with the newborn facing the mother "tummy to tummy." The newborn's arms should form around the breast similar to a "hug." Breast support is important to maintain a proper latch. Because the newborn's neck is not strong at this time, it should be supported with the mother's hand, with her thumb and fingers resting below the newborn's ears. Two positions recommended when initiating breastfeeding are the football hold and the cross-cradle hold (Fig 16–4). Once breastfeeding is established, the cradle-hold or side-lying position to breastfeed can be used.

- Rather than leaning forward over the newborn, encourage the mother to bring the newborn to the breast when the newborn's mouth is wide open; this will assist with a deeper latch.
- It is important to start a feeding with a fully awake newborn. An awake newborn will open their mouth wide to facilitate a deep latch.
- Teach the mother to bring the newborn close to the breast with their chin touching the lower half of the breast (see Fig. 16–5A). The mother then brings the newborn up and over the nipple to achieve an asymmetrical latch with more areola visible at the top of the mouth than on the bottom (see Fig. 16–5B).
- With a deep latch, the newborn's mouth surrounds the areola with the nipple positioned in the back of the newborn's mouth (see Fig. 16–5C).
- When the nipple is pulled far into the newborn's mouth, it stimulates the suck-and-swallow reflex.
- To remove the newborn from the breast, gently slide a clean finger into the corner of the newborn's mouth to break suction (see Fig. 16–5D) before removing the newborn from the breast. Proper removal of the newborn from the breast is crucial to prevent nipple trauma.

SAFE AND EFFECTIVE NURSING CARE: Patient Education

Supporting the Breastfeeding Relationship

- Teach the mother to allow the newborn to finish nursing from one side before switching to the second breast. Encourage the mother to always offer the second breast. Depending on the infant's hunger, they may not nurse on the second breast every time. If the newborn nursed on both breasts the last feeding, the mother is encouraged to offer the breast the newborn finished on first at the next feeding. If the newborn only fed on one breast, she is encouraged to offer the opposite breast first. This ensures both breasts receive equal stimulation.
- Teach the mother to observe for a nutritive suck pattern, infant satiety cues, and softening of breasts once transitional milk is in to determine if the infant has fed well. When the infant is done nursing, they may come off the breast, fall asleep, or continue sucking in a non-nutritive pattern.
- Teach the mother to attempt to burp the newborn after each breast. Infants do not take in air at the breast, so they may not burp every time.

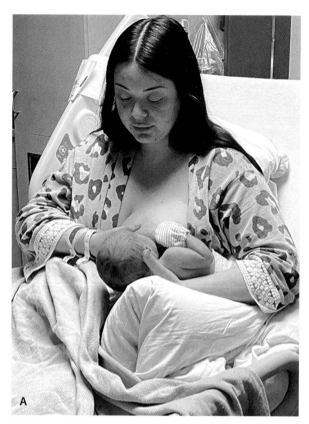 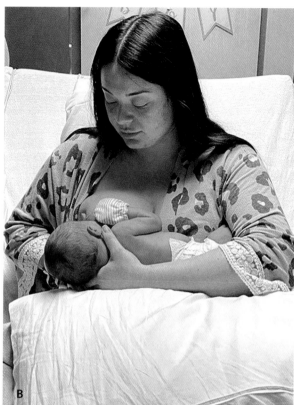

FIGURE 16–4 Positions for breastfeeding. (A) Football hold. (B) Cross-cradle hold.

It is recommended that during hospitalization, a feeding is observed by the nurse at least once a shift to determine the mother's ability to properly position and latch her newborn. This clinical assessment will ensure a successful start to breastfeeding and build confidence in the mother.

Nutritive Suck and Swallow

There are two types of suck patterns: Nutritive suck, which is a rhythmic suck pattern, and non-nutritive suck, also known as comfort sucking. A common concern for a breastfeeding mother is how to determine if her newborn is receiving adequate nutrition from the breast. The nurse can teach the mother to observe for a nutritive suck pattern. When a newborn is ingesting breast milk, the child will suckle at the breast until their mouth is full, pause and swallow and repeat this pattern over and over. During the colostrum phase, this pattern usually consists of four to six sucks, followed by a 5- to 10-second pause allowing the newborn to swallow. A soft sigh may be heard with a swallow.

Once the transitional milk is in, the newborn may only suck once or twice before swallowing due to the volume of milk during this phase. This type of suck differs from a comfort suck pattern, which is nonrhythmic and does not effectively transfer milk out of the breast. An indication of a good feeding is determined by at least 10 minutes of nutritive sucking. Most newborns nurse an average of 15 to 20 minutes, but some will continue longer. If the newborn is still on the breast after 30 minutes, encourage the mother to observe for the nutritive suck pattern to determine if the newborn is actually eating. Only remove the newborn from the breast if they are no longer in a nutritive suck pattern.

Adequate Output

Monitoring output indicates that an infant is breastfeeding well. Frequency and characteristics of stools indicate a healthy breastfed infant. The breastfed infant will stool more often than a formula-fed infant. It is not uncommon to see a stool with every feeding. Starting on day 3 to 4 of life, breast milk stools transition from dark, sticky meconium to a yellowish color with a seedy appearance. During this time, five to six wet diapers and two to three soiled diapers indicate adequate intake.

Determining Effective Feeding

A common tool used by nurses to assess and document breastfeeding is the LATCH assessment tool (Jensen et al., 1994). This five-item scoring tool evaluates effective breastfeeding with a numerical score (0, 1, or 2 points) given in each of these areas:

- "L" represents how well the newborn latches on the breast.
- "A" represents audible swallowing.
- "T" identifies the type of mother's nipple.
- "C" represents the mother's degree of comfort (breast or nipple).
- "H" describes the amount of assistance needed to hold or position the newborn at the breast to maintain an effective latch.

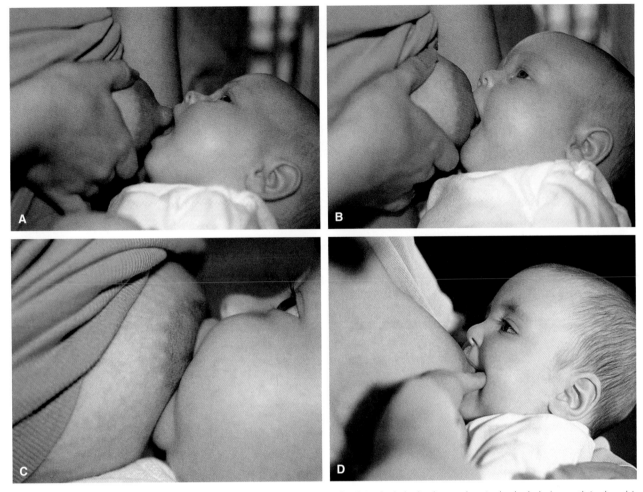

FIGURE 16–5 Infant latch-on. (A) Nipple is aligned with the baby's nose. (B, C) As the baby latches to the nipple, the baby's mouth is placed 1 to 2 inches beyond the base of the nipple. (D) To remove the baby from the breast, the woman inserts her finger into the corner of the baby's mouth to break the seal.

With 2 points the highest score for each area, a score of less than 2 points indicates areas where further support or assistance may be needed (Table 16-1).

SAFE AND EFFECTIVE NURSING CARE: Patient Education

Determining if the Newborn Is Latching Well

Teaching the mother how to determine if the newborn is latching well and feeding well is important to avoid newborn weight loss, dehydration, sore nipples, and milk supply issues:

- The latch should be comfortable, with as much of the areola in their mouth as possible.
- No clicking or smacking sounds should be heard.
- Nutritive sucking is observed with audible swallows.
- Absence of nipple pain and nipple trauma. The nipple should appear round and slightly elongated after a feeding.
- Newborn nurses at least 10 to 30 minutes before being offered the second breast.

- Newborn wakes and feeds at least every 2 to 3 hours or 8 to 12 times in 24 hours.
- Newborn appears satiated and relaxed following feeding.
- Newborn has minimum number of wet diapers and stools in 24 hours (see Table 15-1 in the previous chapter).
- Newborn regains to birth weight by 2 weeks of age.

Assessment of Nipples

Nipples have many variations (Fig. 16–6). They may be:

- Everted: Protrudes outward from the areola.
- Inverted: Drawn below the skin surface. A true inverted nipple does not evert with stimulation.
- Flat: Even in appearance with the areola.
- Retracted: Drawn inward but are usually easily stimulated to evert.

Contrary to popular belief, the mother's nipple size or shape does not determine a successful breastfeeding experience. A mother with flat or inverted nipples can breastfeed successfully if the areola is compressible enough for the infant to latch deeply.

TABLE 16-1   Latch Scoring System

	0	1	2
L: Latch	Too sleepy or reluctant No latch achieved	Repeated attempts Hold nipple in mouth Stimulate to suck	Grasps breast Tongue down Lips flanged Rhythmic sucking
A: Audible swallowing	None	A few with stimulation	Spontaneous and intermittent <24 hours old Spontaneous and frequent >24 hours old
T: Type of nipple	Inverted	Flat	Everted (after stimulation)
C: Comfort (breast and nipple)	Engorged Cracked, bleeding, large blisters, or bruises Severe discomfort	Filling Reddened or small blisters or bruises Mild or moderate pain	Soft Tender
H: Hold (positioning)	Full assist (staff holds infant at breast)	Minimal assist (i.e., elevate head of bed; place pillow for support) Teach one side; mother does the other side Staff holds and then mother takes over	No assist from staff. Mother is able to position and hold the infant.

Jensen et al., 1994.

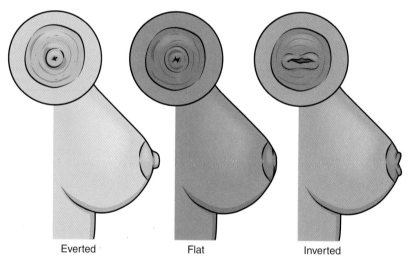

Everted   Flat   Inverted

FIGURE 16–6 Types of nipple variations

CLINICAL JUDGMENT

Prevention of Sore Nipples, Tissue Breakdown, and Mastitis

Sore nipples are a primary reason why women stop breastfeeding. Poor or shallow latch can lead to nipple soreness, redness, bruising, or skin breakdown. Preventing tissue breakdown keeps bacteria from entering through cracks or abrasions in the nipple and causing mastitis (see Critical Component: Mastitis). Nurses play an important role in assisting new mothers with education and the initiation of breastfeeding including the following measures to prevent sore nipples:

• Ensure proper technique for latching on and releasing suction.

• Express and apply colostrum to sore nipples after a feeding session to aid in healing.
• Begin the feeding session on the least sore breast first as sucking is more vigorous at the beginning of the feeding session.
• Change positions (e.g., from cross-cradle to football hold) to change pressure points on the areola.
• Wash breasts with water only. Avoid use of soaps and alcohol, which cause excessive dryness of the nipple.

If a newborn is having difficulties with latching or is unable to latch properly, due to prematurity, illness, physical anatomy of the mother, or any other reason, nursing staff can order a lactation consultation.

CRITICAL COMPONENT

Mastitis

Mastitis is an infection of the breast tissue and presents with redness on the breast, warmth, moderate to severe pain, and flu-like symptoms such as fever, chills, nausea, vomiting, body aches, and fatigue. The mother should be taught to contact her health-care provider immediately if she experiences any of these signs and symptoms of mastitis. The woman should be encouraged to continue breastfeeding, even on the affected breast, and seek treatment. The only effective way to treat mastitis is with antibiotics. Untreated mastitis can lead to a breast abscess that may require hospitalization or surgery.

The Lactation Consultant Role

Women who have trouble breastfeeding or latching the infant will benefit from additional support by the nurse or a consultation by an International Board-Certified Lactation Consultant (IBCLC), commonly referred to as a lactation consultant (LC). IBCLCs are employed by hospitals, birthing centers, and private practice to assist with breastfeeding. Although LCs are valuable members of the health-care team, they do not replace the nurse's responsibility to provide proper breastfeeding teaching and support. The nurse and LC work together to ensure a positive breastfeeding experience. Before discharge, the mother should be given community resources including information on LCs and resources she can contact if she has questions or needs assistance.

CRITICAL COMPONENT

Promoting Successful Breastfeeding

Hospital policies and lactation support from nursing staff can promote a successful start to breastfeeding by:

- Encouraging the mother to offer the breast immediately after birth if she and the newborn are stable
- Teaching the benefits of skin-to-skin in the early postpartum period and before feedings
- Encouraging unlimited feedings on demand or at least every 2 to 3 hours
- Having specially trained staff to assist with latch and identify concerns to be referred to an LC
- Avoiding use of pacifiers or formula
- Encouraging the mother to rest when the newborn is sleeping
- Keeping the mother comfortable and pain-free

A variety of tools and products are designed to assist with latching a newborn on the breast. Alternative feeding methods that may be implemented by the LC include:

- Nipple shield: A thin silicone shell that stretches over the areola and provides a firm nipple to assist with latch for a premature newborn or physical anatomy limitation of the mother.
- Supplemental nursing system: A thin tube that attaches to a bottle on one end fastened approximately ¼ inch beyond the mother's nipple to allow the newborn to receive a supplement while nursing. The infant must be able to suckle at the breast.
- Cup: A small soft flexible cup held up to the lips designed to give small amounts. The infant must be awake and held at an upright angle for this method.
- Spoon: Small spoon used to feed drops of colostrum if an infant is not nursing during the early postpartum period.

CRITICAL COMPONENT

Baby-Friendly Hospital Initiative

The Baby-Friendly Hospital Initiative (BFHI) is a global program started in 1991 as a combined effort between the WHO and the United Nations Children's Fund (UNICEF) to encourage global implementation of the Ten Steps to Successful Breastfeeding and the International Code of Marketing of Breast-Milk Substitutes. In 2007, fewer than 3% of births in the United States occurred in a Baby-Friendly designated facility. In 2019, more than 28% of births were documented in one of the 600 Baby-Friendly facilities (Baby-Friendly USA, 2021). To become designated as "Baby-Friendly," a facility must adhere to the Ten Steps of Successful Breastfeeding as outlined in the list that follows:

1. Have a written breastfeeding policy that is routinely communicated to all health-care staff.
2. Train all health-care staff in the skills necessary to implement this policy.
3. Inform all pregnant women about the benefits and management of breastfeeding.
4. Help mothers initiate breastfeeding within 1 hour of birth.
5. Show mothers how to breastfeed and how to maintain lactation, even if they are separated from their infants.
6. Give infants no food or drink other than breast milk unless medically indicated.
7. Practice rooming-in: Allow mothers and infants to remain together 24 hours a day.
8. Encourage breastfeeding on demand.
9. Do not give pacifiers or artificial nipples to breastfeeding infants.
10. Foster the establishment of breastfeeding support groups and refer mothers to them on discharge from the hospital or birth center (Baby-Friendly USA, 2021).

Milk Expression and Breast Pumps

Every breastfeeding mother will benefit from being taught how to express breast milk. Expressing can be done manually by hand or with a breast pump. In the early postpartum period, it is important to be able to manually express and supplement with colostrum if the newborn does not feed well. A breast pump may be used initially to stimulate the mother's breasts if circumstances prevent the newborn from nursing effectively. However, if the newborn is nursing well, using a breast pump can overstimulate the breasts.

Once breastfeeding is established and the newborn is back to birth weight (usually by 3 weeks postpartum) the mother can begin using a breast pump regularly to express her breast milk into a bottle.

To manually express breast milk:

- Wash hands before beginning.
- Massage each quadrant of the breast starting at the chest wall and working downward toward the nipple. A circular motion works well.
- Place the thumb and forefinger so they form the letter C with the thumb at the 12:00 position and the forefinger at the 6:00 position.
- Push the thumb and finger straight back toward the chest wall. Avoid spreading the fingers. It is important to get behind the milk ducts before pushing forward toward the nipple.
- Collect breast milk into a clean container.
- Repeat the process until the desired amount of milk is collected.
- Reposition the thumb and forefinger to the 3:00 and 9:00 positions and repeat the previous sequence.

The best time to pump breast milk for collecting and storing is in the morning as prolactin levels rise during the night and into the early morning hours. Encourage the mother to pump halfway between feeds to allow collection of the most milk. Pumping both breasts simultaneously increases the amount of milk. Pumping for 15 to 20 minutes is recommended. Breast pumps vary in efficiency at removing milk from the breast. It is important to educate the mother that a breast pump will not remove breast milk as efficiently as a newborn who is nursing well.

Selecting a Breast Pump

Choosing the right breast pump is important. There are many types of pumps available:

- Hospital-grade electric pumps are specifically designed to pump every 2 to 3 hours. These pumps have a more efficient design and motor than professional-grade breast pumps purchased at a retail store or online. They are intended to be used by mothers whose newborns are in the NICU so they can maintain their milk supply with frequent pumping.
- Professional-grade pumps are designed for the working mother who needs to pump four to five times a day while away at work. Most of these pumps can pump both breasts at once.
- Small electric and manual pumps are appropriate for mothers who only pump occasionally.

Storing Breast Milk

Expressed breast milk can be stored for use when the mother is not present to breastfeed. Breast milk can be stored in glass bottles, hard BPA-free plastic containers, or plastic bags designed for storage of breast milk. Write the date and time of milk expression and collection on a label placed on the container. Store frozen breast milk in the back of the freezer. Breast milk can safely be stored:

- At room temperature (77°F [25°C]) for up to 6 to 8 hours
- In the refrigerator 7 to 8 days
- In the freezer that is attached to a refrigerator for 6 months
- In a deep freezer for 6 to 12 months

Breast milk can be safely thawed in the refrigerator overnight or in a cup of warm water. Breast milk should not be heated in the microwave, which can heat the milk unevenly. Overheating by microwave or stovetop can destroy antibodies within the breast milk. Breast milk can be fed directly from the refrigerator and does not need to be warmed.

Engorgement

Following birth, women commonly experience increased fullness of the breasts known as engorgement. This is transitory and is associated with increased blood or lymph fluid congestion of late pregnancy or from large amounts of IV fluids administered during labor. Breast fullness is normal as transitional milk comes in around 3 to 5 days after birth and gradually diminishes as lactation is fully established. Engorgement can also happen later due to missed feedings or inadequate removal of milk from the breast. Mothers should be encouraged to pump or express breasts as they become firm and uncomfortable if not with the infant to breastfeed.

SAFE AND EFFECTIVE NURSING CARE: Understanding Medication

Medication and Nicotine Use in Breastfeeding Women

Although most medications and immunizations are safe to use during lactation, it is recommended that all breastfeeding women consult with their health-care provider before taking medications. This includes over-the-counter medications and herbal supplements. Medications that are contraindicated in breastfeeding include anticancer agents, antimetabolite agents, or radioactive drugs (Hale & Baker, 2018). Smoking cigarettes is discouraged for breastfeeding women, but benefits of breast milk outweigh risks of nicotine to the newborn. Women should never smoke while breastfeeding and be taught that smoking immediately after a feeding will result in lower levels of nicotine in the breast milk than smoking before a feeding.

SAFE AND EFFECTIVE NURSING CARE: Patient Education

Nutrition for Lactating Mothers

Encourage the lactating mother to consume a healthy diet while breastfeeding. Making healthy food choices and including light exercise is recommended in place of dieting, and the mother should avoid calorie-restricted diets during this time. Nutritional education includes the following:

- A nursing mother needs to consume an extra 500 calories a day to replace calories used to breastfeed her newborn.
- A mother's diet (what she eats or drinks) will not impact her ability to produce milk.
- Having a glass of water or juice while nursing will help to satisfy the thirst some mothers report while breastfeeding.
- It is also important to note that most foods, including spicy foods and caffeine, are fine to consume while breastfeeding.
- Questions regarding alcohol consumption should be discussed with her pediatrician.

Obtaining Breast Milk From Donors

Human breast milk from a donor milk bank is the preferred choice for adoptive or surrogate parents who have an infant with a medical need. An order from a prescribing physician is required. Many states now have at least one human milk bank, but costs to obtain the milk can be prohibitive for many families.

Induced lactation can be accomplished for an adoptive or surrogate mother willing to pump her breasts and use prescribed hormonal therapy to prepare the body to produce breast milk. If an adoptive or surrogate mother is unable or unwilling to complete the process required to induce lactation, she may seek breast milk in the community through mother's groups and social media. However, it is important for the mother to understand the potential risks of this practice. Disease transmission, contaminated milk by improper handling or storage, and milk from a mother using prescription or illicit drugs can harm an infant. There is no way to guarantee that breast milk shared in this manner is safe. Therefore, the role of the health-care provider or nurse is to provide information to the mother and allow her to make an informed decision.

FORMULA FEEDING

Although human breast milk is considered the "gold standard" and recommended form of newborn nutrition, some women do not breastfeed for personal reasons or newborn considerations. Commercially prepared formula is considered an acceptable alternative to breast milk and is fed to the newborn with a bottle (Fig. 16–7). Formula comes in many varieties, including cow's milk, soybean, higher calorie for preterm newborns, and hypoallergenic formulations. Formula is packaged as "ready-made," or available in a powder or concentrate to prepare with water. Whey-predominant formula is the most common milk-based formula, and formula companies routinely alter the ingredients in formula production to mimic the composition of breast milk.

Newborns and infants can be fed on demand or at least every 3 to 4 hours. Newborns consume 0.5 to 1 ounce (15 to 30 mL) per feeding during the first few days of life. This increases to 2 to 3 ounces (60 to 90 mL) per feeding by day 4 and gradually to

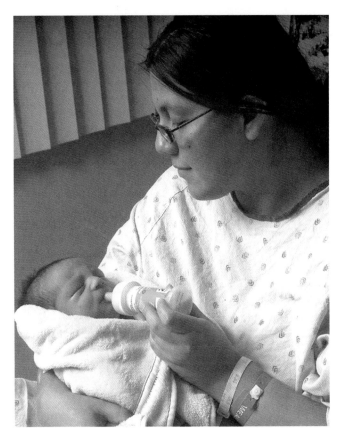

FIGURE 16–7 Mother bottle feeding newborn

32 daily ounces (950 mL). As a rule of thumb, feed 2.5 ounces of formula to every 1 pound of baby weight per day.

Advantages of Formula Feeding

- Provides an opportunity for the partner to assist with feedings.
- Allows the mother to leave the newborn to run errands or return to work without having to pump or adhere to a feeding schedule while away.
- Decreases frequency of feedings because digestion of formula is slower than of breast milk.

Disadvantages of Formula Feeding

- Increased cost to purchase formula, bottles, nipples, and cleaning supplies.
- Additional time required to prepare formula and clean bottles.
- Increased risk of infection due to lack of antibodies that are naturally present in breast milk.
- Increased risk of childhood illness, obesity, and insulin-dependent diabetes.

Intolerance to Formula

Some newborns cannot tolerate a milk protein called casein in formula. They may have difficulty digesting casein or another ingredient. Symptoms of formula intolerance or allergy include:

- Vomiting
- Diarrhea with mucus or blood present
- Weight loss or slow weight gain
- Colic

Hypoallergenic formulas are designed for infants with allergies or intolerance to standard milk-based formula. Encourage the mother to speak to her pediatrician if she suspects her newborn has an intolerance or allergy to formula.

SAFE AND EFFECTIVE NURSING CARE: Patient Education

Formula Feeding

- Parents should select bottles that are BPA-free and easy to clean.
- Parents can opt for either rubber or silicone nipples.
  - Silicone nipples retain fewer odors and last longer.
  - Rubber nipples are cheaper but tend to break down faster and retain odors.
  - Nipples need to be washed with soapy warm water and rinsed well.
  - The rate of flow from the nipples is controlled by either the shape of the hole or the size of the hole. There are three types of flow rates:
    - Slow: designed for newborn infants
    - Medium: designed for infants under 6 months
    - Fast: designed for older infants
- Formulas are available in powder, concentrated, and ready-to-use forms. It is important to instruct the parents to follow manufacturer directions when preparing formula.
- When feeding, hold the newborn close to the body in the crook of the arm, with the head higher than the body. This position will prevent formula from pooling in the newborn's mouth and flowing into the middle ear, increasing the risk of otitis media.
- Tilt the bottle so that the nipple is full of milk to decrease the amount of air swallowed.
- Do not prop bottles, as this places infants at higher risk for choking, otitis media, and tooth decay.
- Check the size of the nipple hole.
  - The hole may be too big if the infant has a sudden mouthful of formula and almost chokes, or when you turn the bottle upside down and the milk flows out of the nipple instead of dripping.
  - The hole may be too small if the infant seems to be working hard when sucking or the bottle is upside down and takes longer than a second per drip of formula.
- Burp the newborn halfway through and at the end of feeding by tapping or patting the back for a few minutes. Some infants may not burp with each feeding.
- Discard unused formula that remains in the bottle at the end of feeding to decrease the risk of bacterial contamination.

CRITICAL COMPONENT

Preparing Infant Formula
- Clean and disinfect the formula preparation area.
- Wash hands.
- Use bottles, nipples, and a can opener that have been washed in hot, soapy water and rinsed well or have been washed in a dishwasher.
- Check the expiration date on the formula packaging.
- Wash, rinse, and dry the top of the formula can.
- Mix boiled nonfluoride water or bottled water with concentrated or powdered formula.
  - Water should be cooled (room temperature) before mixing it with the formula.
- Follow the directions on the formula packaging for proper dilution of concentrate or amount of powder formula per ounce of water.
  - Prolonged overdilution of the formula can cause water intoxication; prolonged underdilution can cause dehydration.
  - Once bottles of formula have been prepared, they must be kept refrigerated and used within 24 hours to decrease the risk of bacterial contamination.
  - Opened cans or bottles of ready-to-use formula need to be kept refrigerated and used within 24 hours to decrease the risk of bacterial contamination.
- Mix the formula by gently shaking or swirling the bottle.
- Store mixed formula in airtight bottles in the refrigerator for up to 24 hours. Freezing mixed formula is not recommended.
- Store open containers of ready-to-use, concentrated formula or a prepared bottle in the refrigerator and discard after 24 hours if not used. Do not refrigerate unmixed powder.
- Warm a refrigerated bottle by placing it in a container filled with warm water. Do not microwave it as it can burn the baby.

Nutritional Needs Beyond the Newborn Period

During the first year of life, the infant experiences rapid growth, doubling birth weight by 5 months and tripling it by age 1. Caloric needs vary based on the infant's size, rate of growth, activity, and metabolic rate.

- Infants experience growth spurts at 3 to 5 days, 1 week, 6 weeks, 3 months, and 6 months and require more frequent feedings during these time periods.
- Adequate nutritional intake is determined by plotting the weight and length of the infant at each well-child checkup.

From 4 to 6 Months

Feeding breast milk or formula is continued. Introduction of semisolid foods is determined by the physician or nurse practitioner in collaboration with parents. The AAP and WHO guidelines recommend waiting to start solids until 6 months of age to reduce allergy risks. Before 4 to 6 months, the sucking reflex forces semisolid food out of the mouth versus to the back of the mouth. Parents should not introduce semisolid foods until recommended by the health-care provider. Infants are ready for semisolid foods when they:

● Can sit independently
● Can draw in the lower lip as a spoon is removed
● Indicate hunger by opening the mouth
● Refuse food by closing the mouth and turning away

Pureed fruits and vegetables and single-grain cereal such as rice and oats are the first food to be introduced. Cereal should not be given in bottles; this increases the risk of choking and aspiration.

Prevention of Dental Decay

Infants' teeth are susceptible to baby bottle tooth decay, which occurs when formula, juice, or other sweetened liquids are given in bottles to infants and allowed to remain in the mouth for a period of time. Within 20 minutes, the sugar from the sweetened liquid responds to mouth bacteria and forms acids that cause dental decay (American Dental Association [ADA], 2021). Infants who fall asleep with a bottle in their mouths or who receive several bottles of sweetened liquids during the day are at higher risk for tooth decay.

CRITICAL COMPONENT

Decreasing the Risk of Baby Bottle Tooth Decay
The ADA (2021) recommends the following to decrease risk of baby bottle tooth decay:

• Do not put infants to bed with a bottle of milk, juice, or sugar water.
• Do not give infants bottles with sugar water or soda.
• Clean the infant's gums with clean gauze after each feeding.
• Brush teeth once the first tooth erupts.
• Consult a dentist regarding fluoride treatments if the water supply does not contain it.
• Begin regular dental appointments by the first birthday.

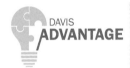

Go to Davis Advantage to complete your learning: strengthen understanding, apply your knowledge, and prepare for the Next Gen NCLEX®.

Clinical Pathway for the Stages of Milk Production

Three stages of breast milk production occur during the lactation process.

Stage	Stage 1: Colostrum	Stage 2: Transitional Milk	Stage 3: Mature Milk
Description	Considered first milk, thick clear to golden yellow color	Graduating changing and less yellow than colostrum	Watery appearance with slight bluish cast
Time frame	Present midpregnancy and available at birth to day 3	Present 3–5 days after birth up to 2 weeks	Approximately 10–12 days following birth
Volume	Small amounts	Onset of copious milk	Copious and based on supply and demand; maintained by frequent milk removal
	Acts as laxative to assist in passage of meconium. High concentration of protein	Gradually changes with decreasing levels of protein and decreasing levels of fats, carbohydrates, and calories	Foremilk—lower fat content
	Contains many antibodies to protect the newborn from pathogens		Hindmilk—higher fat and calories
Frequency of feeding	At least every 2–3 hours or on demand; wake the newborn for feedings as needed	Every 3 hours or on demand	Feeding 8–12 times in a 24-hour period
Newborn output	One soaking wet diaper and stool on day 1, two wet diapers and stools on the second day, three wet diapers and stools on the third day.	Three to five wet diapers and three to four stools per day	Six to eight wet diapers and three or more stools per day

CONCEPT MAP |

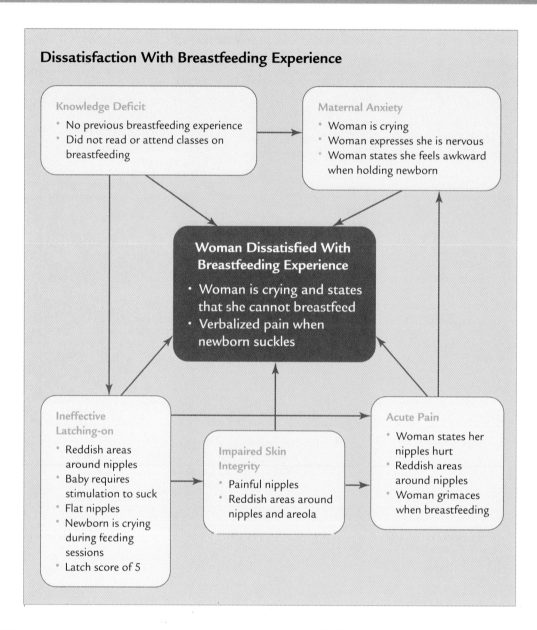

Dissatisfaction With Breastfeeding Experience

Knowledge Deficit
- No previous breastfeeding experience
- Did not read or attend classes on breastfeeding

Maternal Anxiety
- Woman is crying
- Woman expresses she is nervous
- Woman states she feels awkward when holding newborn

Woman Dissatisfied With Breastfeeding Experience
- Woman is crying and states that she cannot breastfeed
- Verbalized pain when newborn suckles

Ineffective Latching-on
- Reddish areas around nipples
- Baby requires stimulation to suck
- Flat nipples
- Newborn is crying during feeding sessions
- Latch score of 5

Impaired Skin Integrity
- Painful nipples
- Reddish areas around nipples and areola

Acute Pain
- Woman states her nipples hurt
- Reddish areas around nipples
- Woman grimaces when breastfeeding

CARE PLANS

Problem 1: Knowledge deficit

Goal: The mother will demonstrate proper breastfeeding techniques before discharge.

Outcome: Establishment of breastfeeding as evidenced by:
- How to wake the infant for feedings
- How to position the newborn at the breast
- Proper latch-on
- Nutritive suck pattern
- Absence of pain while nursing or sore nipples
- Mother states she feels comfortable breastfeeding without assistance

Nursing Actions

1. Teach feeding cues and encourage the mother to offer the breast if the infant is showing them. Demonstrate wake-up techniques and encourage the mother to wake the infant at least every 3 hours, or sooner for on-demand feeding.

2. Demonstrate different positions for positioning the newborn when breastfeeding, such as cross-cradle and football positions. Teach the cradle and side-lying holds to use later when the newborn's neck is stronger and breastfeeding is established.

3. Show placement of pillows in assisting the mother to a comfortable position.

4. Teach the mother how to align the baby's body to her body when breastfeeding, by assisting her and the baby in a proper position and explaining how this facilitates effective feeding.
5. Instruct the mother to support the newborn's neck while nursing.
6. Instruct the mother to bring the newborn to her breast and not her breast to the newborn.
7. Explain the importance of waiting until the newborn opens wide (such as a yawn) and quickly bring the child onto the breast deeply.
8. Explain that the mother should feel a tugging sensation as the newborn begins to suckle.
9. Explain that she should not experience pain when the newborn is suckling. Pain may be an indication that the baby has not properly latched on and needs to be repositioned.
10. Teach the mother to observe for a nutritive suck pattern and listen for soft audible swallowing.
11. Teach signs of good latch and that the nipple should appear round and elongated after a feeding.
12. Demonstrate how to properly remove the baby from her breast by placing a clean finger in the side of the baby's mouth to release the suction.
13. Provide written resources on LCs and breastfeeding support groups in the community.

Problem 2: Maternal anxiety
Goal: Decrease of anxiety level
Outcome: The mother expresses that she feels comfortable with breastfeeding.

Nursing Actions

1. Assess the mother's cultural beliefs, attitudes, concerns, and questions regarding breastfeeding to identify the source of anxiety and determine areas to address in the action plan.
2. Assess the mother's knowledge of breastfeeding and provide information to increase her knowledge level.
3. Assess the level of the partner's support for the woman's desire to breastfeed and explain how the partner can assist the mother with breastfeeding.
4. Assess the mother's comfort level and implement ways to promote comfort such as relaxation techniques, proper positioning for feeding, use of pillows to support the mother and her newborn, and ensuring adequate rest and sleep for the mother.
5. Establish a conducive environment for the mother to breastfeed with privacy and quiet.
6. Provide encouragement for the mother by praising her for her decision to breastfeed, for using proper breastfeeding techniques, and for responding to the baby's feeding cues.
7. Reevaluate the mother's level of anxiety by assessing verbal and nonverbal behaviors.

Problem 3: Ineffective latch
Goal: Effective latch

Outcome: The newborn will effectively latch as evidenced by:
● The newborn's mouth covering most of the mother's areola
● The mother's nipple drawn into the back of the newborn's mouth
● The newborn's lips creating a firm seal around the areola
● Nutritive suck pattern or audible swallowing
● Absence of soreness, reddened areas, or nipple trauma
● LATCH score of 8 or greater

Nursing Actions

1. Assess the mother's breastfeeding technique.
2. Assess the nipples and areola for signs of irritation.
3. Provide information on correct latch.
4. Assist the mother with proper positioning that facilitates a correct latch.
5. Instruct the mother to bring the newborn to the breast when the newborn's mouth is wide open.
6. Instruct the mother to delay use of a pacifier until breastfeeding is established, and newborn is latching well, which is usually by the third week postpartum.

Problem 4: Acute pain
Goal: Absence of pain
Outcome: The newborn will latch properly and the mother will report latch is comfortable.

Nursing Actions

1. Assess the level of pain using a pain scale.
2. Assess the breast for signs of irritation, such as reddened areas, blisters, or cracking, and encourage deeper latch and to apply colostrum to damaged areas.
3. Assess breastfeeding technique by observing the woman during a feeding session.
4. Provide information and assistance to facilitate latch.
5. Provide information on positions for holding the newborn during feeding.
6. Explain that cool compresses or breast milk applied to the nipple may decrease nipple pain and help heal the nipple.
7. Medicate with analgesia PRN.

Problem 5: Impaired skin integrity
Goal: Skin will remain intact.
Outcome: The tissue of the nipples and areola will be intact with no redness, cracks, or blisters.

Nursing Actions

1. Assess nipples and areolas for signs of irritation.
2. Instruct the mother to inspect her nipples and areolas after each feeding.
3. Assess the mother during feeding sessions for proper breastfeeding techniques.
4. Provide information on proper positioning of the newborn for breastfeeding.
5. Provide information on correct latch.
6. Instruct the mother to express and apply colostrum to nipples and areolas after each feeding.

Case Study

You are the nurse caring for Emma Patterson, a 32-year-old primipara who has been exclusively breastfeeding her son since delivery 24 hours ago. Emma tells you her nipples are sore and red. During your assessment you note bilateral, reddened nipples. Emma states she did not attend a breastfeeding class and has not had help with breastfeeding while in the hospital. You know that proper positioning and a deep latch is necessary to prevent sore nipples. How do you assist Emma? What positions do you recommend for her? How do you help her obtain a deep latch? What measures can you teach her to relieve her sore nipples?

Based on your knowledge of the Patterson family, list the priority learning needs and state the rationale for your selection of learning needs.

Describe your teaching plan based on the identified priority learning needs, including:
- Preparation of the learning environment
- Methods to assess their learning needs
- Information that will be shared with the couple
- Method for evaluating effectiveness of teaching

REFERENCES

Alex, A., Bhandary, E., & McGuire, K. P. (2020). Anatomy and physiology of the breast during pregnancy and lactation. *Advances in Experimental Medicine and Biology, 1252*, 3–7. https://doi.org/10.1007/978-3-030-41596-9_1

American Academy of Pediatrics. (2012). Breastfeeding and the use of human milk. Policy statement. *Pediatrics, 129*, e827–e835. https://doi:10.1542/peds.2011-3552

American Dental Association. (2021). *Baby bottle tooth decay.* https://www.ada.org/en/about-the-ada/ada-positions-policies-and-statements/statement-on-early-childhood-caries

Association of Women's Health, Obstetric and Neonatal Nurses. (2021). *AWHONN position statement: Breastfeeding and the use of human milk.* https://www.awhonn.org/news-advocacy-and-publications/awhonn-position-statements/

Baby-Friendly USA. (2021). *Ten steps to successful breastfeeding.* http://www.babyfriendlyusa.org

Caldeo, V., Downey, E., O'Shea, C., Affolter, M., Volger, S., Cortet-Comondu, M., . . . Kelly, A. (2020). Protein levels and protease activity in milk from mothers of pre-term infants: A prospective longitudinal study of human milk macronutrient composition. *Clinical Nutrition, 40*, 3567–3577. https://doi.org/10.1016/j.clnu.2020.12.013

Centers for Disease Control and Prevention. (2021). *Percentage of U.S. children who were breastfed, by birth year, national immunization survey, United States.* https://www.cdc.gov/breastfeeding/data/nis_data/results.html

Hale, T., & Baker, T. (2018). *Breastfeeding and the use of medications.* https://doi.org/10.21428/3d48c34a.ea40659a

Hale, T., & Rowe, H. (2017). *Medications & mothers' milk.* Springer.

Jensen, D., Wallace, S., & Kelsay, P. (1994). LATCH: A breastfeeding charting system and documentation tool. *Journal of Obstetric, Gynecologic, & Neonatal Nursing, 23*, 27–32. https://doi.org/10.1111/j.1552-6909.1994.tb01847.x

Karimi, F. Z., Sadeghi, R., Maleki-Saghooni, N., & Khadivzadeh, T. (2019). The effect of mother–infant skin to skin contact on success and duration of first breastfeeding: A systematic review and meta-analysis. *Taiwanese Journal of Obstetrics and Gynecology, 58*, 1–9. https://doi.org/10.1016/j.tjog.2018.11.002

Krol, K., & Grossman, T. (2018). Psychological effects of breastfeeding on children and mothers. *Bundesgesundheitsblatt—Gesundheitsforschung—Gesundheitsschutz, 61*(8), 977–985. https://doi.org/10.1007/s00103-018-2769-0

Martin, C., Ling, P., & Blackburn, G. (2016). Review of infant feeding: Key features of breast milk and infant formula. *Nutrients, 8*(5), 279. https://doi.org/10.3390/nu8050279

U.S. Department of Health and Human Services. (2017). *Healthy People 2020 topics and objectives.* https://www.healthypeople.gov/2020/topics-objectives

Wambach, K., & Genna, C. W. (2021). Anatomy and physiology of lactation. In K. Wambach & B. Spenser (Eds.), *Breastfeeding and human lactation* (6th ed., p. 55). Jones & Bartlett Learning.

World Health Organization. (2014). *Global nutrition targets 2025: Breastfeeding policy brief (WHO/NMH/NHD/14.7).* World Health Organization.

World Health Organization. (2021). *Infant and young child feeding.* https://www.who.int/news-room/fact-sheets/detail/infant-and-young-child-feeding

Complications of the Neonate and Nursing Care

17

Caroline Lambton, MSN, RN
Carolyn Mahaffey, MSN, RNC-NIC

LEARNING OUTCOMES

Upon completion of this chapter, the student will be able to:

1. Describe the physiology and pathophysiology associated with selected complications of the neonatal period.
2. Identify critical elements of assessment and nursing care of the neonate experiencing complications.
3. Develop a discharge plan for the neonate experiencing complications.
4. Describe the loss and grief process experienced by parents whose infant has died.

CONCEPTS

Addiction
Behaviors
Collaboration
Comfort
Evidence-Based Practice
Family
Fluid and Electrolytes
Grief and Loss
Growth and Development
Infection
Intracranial Regulation
Nutrition
Oxygenation
Thermoregulation
Tissue Integrity
Safety
Stress and Coping

Nursing Diagnosis

- Impaired gas exchange related to inadequate surfactant and immature lung tissue
- Risk for ineffective airway clearance related to meconium aspiration
- Ineffective thermoregulation related to prematurity, lack of subcutaneous fat, environmental temperature fluctuations, and heat loss mechanisms

Nursing Outcomes

- The neonate exhibits a breathing pattern within normal limits with respiratory rate between 30 and 60 breaths per minute with no signs of respiratory distress.
- The neonate maintains temperature within normal limits.
- The neonate gains weight, consumes adequate nutritional intake, has adequate output, and is free of signs of hypoglycemia or malnutrition.

Continued

Nursing Diagnosis—cont'd

- Imbalanced nutrition related to prematurity, inability to absorb nutrients, decreased perfusion to gastrointestinal tract, postnatal change from high glucose exposure to low glucose exposure and hyperinsulinism, and cleft lip or cleft palate
- Risk for infection related to prematurity, exposure to infectious agents, and maternal chorioamnionitis
- Pain related to procedures; birth trauma
- Risk for injury related to lack of oxygen to the brain, prolonged ventilation and oxygen administration, effects of drugs on fetal or neonatal growth and development, birth trauma, hypoglycemia, asphyxia, meconium aspiration, and kernicterus
- Risk for ineffective parent and family coping related to infant illness or death
- Grieving related to the infant with complications, loss of the dream of the perfect infant, and death of the infant
- Risk for impaired parent–infant attachment related to separation

Nursing Outcomes—cont'd

- The neonate remains free of signs of infection; the white blood cell (WBC) count is within normal limits and the blood, urine, and cerebrospinal fluid (CSF) cultures are negative.
- The neonate exhibits decreased signs of pain after receiving nonpharmacological or pharmacological pain-reduction interventions.
- The neonate is free of signs of injury.
- Parents communicate needs, state ability to cope, identify a support system, and ask for help and information when needed.
- Parents identify what to expect during the grieving process.
- Parents visit the neonate in the intensive care nursery, demonstrate caregiving behaviors, express interest in the newborn, and respond to the infant's behavioral cues.

INTRODUCTION

This chapter provides an overview of the critical components of neonatal intensive care unit (NICU) nursing. NICU nursing, a subspecialty of maternal-newborn nursing, focuses on caring for neonates and their families who are experiencing complications. Nurses who elect to work in a neonatal intensive care nursery will need to gain in-depth knowledge through additional readings and classes that focus on this unique population and their parents.

The infant mortality rate (IMR) in the United States in 2018 was 5.67 deaths per 1,000 live births and is the nation's lowest reported historic IMR (Ely & Driscoll, 2020). Infant mortality has been decreasing since 2005 and the current statistic represents a 17% decline compared with an IMR of 6.68 in 2005 as well as a 2% decline compared with an IMR of 5.79 in 2017 (Ely & Driscoll, 2020). Despite a significant and steadfast decrease over the last two decades, it indicates that in 2018, 21,498 infant deaths still occurred despite the available resources possessed by the United States (Ely & Driscoll, 2020).

A primary cause of illness and death in the neonate is complications related to prematurity. Causes unrelated to prematurity will be covered later in the chapter.

PRETERM NEONATES

The two most important predictors of an infant's health and survival are period of gestation and birth weight. Prematurity and low birth weight (LBW) are the leading causes of infant death in the United States after congenital malformations (Xu et al.,

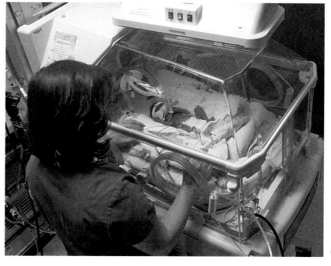

FIGURE 17–1 A very premature neonate born at 27 weeks' gestation.

2020). The premature birth rate in the United States rose to 10.02% in 2018, a 1% rise from 9.93% in 2017 and the fourth straight year of increase (Martin et al., 2019).

Prematurity is defined as any birth before 37 completed weeks of gestation and is further classified as:

- Extremely premature: Neonates born at less than 28 weeks' gestation (Fig. 17–1).
- Very premature: Neonates born between 28 and 31 6/7 weeks' gestation.
- Premature: Neonates born between 32 and 33 6/7 weeks' gestation.
- Late premature: Neonates born between 34 and 36 6/7 weeks' gestation (Stavis, 2019d).

TABLE 17-1 Risk Factors for Preterm Labor and Birth

NONMODIFIABLE RISK FACTORS	TREATABLE AND MODIFIABLE RISK FACTORS
Previous preterm birth	Age at pregnancy <17 or >35 years
Multiple gestation	Unplanned pregnancy
Uterine or cervical anomaly	Low socioeconomic status or poverty
Race or ethnic group	Low educational level
Pregnancy-induced hypertension	Domestic violence, unsafe environment
Short interval between pregnancies	Life stress
Premature rupture of membranes	In vitro fertilization (IVF) and pregnancy after IVF
Bleeding in the second or third trimester	Low pre-pregnancy weight or obesity
Family history of premature birth	Health problems that can be treated: hypertension, diabetes, clotting problems, anemia
	Sexually transmitted infections or other infections along the genitourinary tract
	Substance or alcohol use
	Cigarette smoking or exposure to secondhand smoke
	Long hours of employment or standing
	Late or no prenatal care
	Air pollution or exposure to other toxins such as lead or paint

March of Dimes, 2018.

Disparities exist in the percentage of premature births based on mother's race:

- Non-Hispanic Black: 13.8%
- American Indian or Alaska Native: 11.6%
- Hispanic: 9.6%
- Non-Hispanic White: 9.1%
- Asian or Pacific Islander: 8.7% (March of Dimes, 2020)

Prematurity is a primary reason for LBW. Classification of birth weight (regardless of gestational age) is as follows:

- Extremely LBW: Less than 1,000 grams at birth.
- Very LBW: 1,000 grams to 1,499 grams at birth.
- LBW: 1,500 grams to 2,500 grams at birth (Stavis, 2019d).

Often the reason for premature birth is unknown, but multiple factors place a woman at risk for preterm labor and birth. Some are modifiable, but many are not (Table 17-1). Common complications related to prematurity are respiratory distress syndrome (RDS), bronchopulmonary dysplasia (BPD), patent ductus arteriosus, intraventricular hemorrhage, necrotizing enterocolitis (NEC), and retinopathy of prematurity (ROP).

Assessment Findings

- Gestational age by Ballard score is at or below 37 weeks.
- Physical characteristics vary based on gestational age (Fig. 17–2).
  - Tone and flexion increase with gestational age. Early in gestation, resting tone and posture are hypotonic and extended.

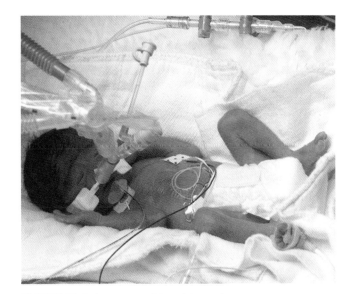

FIGURE 17–2 A neonate at 27 weeks' gestation.

- The skin is very thin, making it translucent and transparent. The color may be pale, red, or mottled.
- Subcutaneous fat is decreased.
- Lanugo is present between 20 and 28 weeks' gestation. At 28 weeks' gestation, lanugo begins to disappear on the face and the front of the trunk.
- Creases on the anterior part of the foot are not present until 28 to 30 weeks. As gestation increases, plantar creases spread toward the heel of the foot.

- Eyelids are fused in very preterm neonates. Eyelids open between 26 and 28 weeks' gestation.
- Overriding sutures are common among premature, low-birth-weight neonates.
- Before 34 weeks, the pinna of the ear has little cartilage and will stay folded on itself.
- The testes are not descended and are found in the inguinal canal. The clitoris is prominent with small, widely separated labia.
- Tremors and jittery movement may be noted.
- The cry is weak.
- Reflexes may be diminished or absent.
- Suck, swallow, and breathing reflexes remain immature until 34 weeks' gestation. These neonates are unable to take adequate oral feedings and require supplementation via feeding tube or parenteral nutrition.
- Apnea is commonly observed in premature infants. It is defined as the cessation of breathing for at least 20 seconds; or less than 20 seconds if complicated by cyanosis, pallor, hypotonia, or bradycardia [heart rate less than 100 beats per minute] (Churchman, 2021).
- Hypotension may occur from hypovolemia related to blood loss from delivery, infection, or result from immature cerebral autoregulation (Seattle Children's, 2019).
- Heart murmur may be present related to patent ductus arteriosus.
- Anemia is common due to frequent lab sampling and diminished erythropoietin (EPO) production (Diehl-Jones & Fraser, 2021).

Medical Management

- Information about the neonate's condition, treatment plan, and follow-up care is provided to parents.
- Lung maturity is determined with lecithin/sphingomyelin (L/S) ratio or phosphatidylglycerol (PG) before elective induction or cesarean birth and for women in preterm labor.
- Antenatal steroid administration is one of the most important interventions to improve newborn outcomes (Tsakiridis et al., 2020). Corticosteroids [betamethasone or dexamethasone] are administered to pregnant women who present in preterm labor or if preterm birth is anticipated within 7 days (Forest, 2021). Steroids accelerate the normal pattern of lung growth. Robust evidence demonstrates that they reduce the incidence of respiratory distress syndrome (RDS) and intraventricular hemorrhage (IVH), significantly decreasing neonatal morbidity and death over the last four decades (Forest, 2021; Tsakiridis et al., 2020).
- Monitoring is performed of cardiorespiratory status, oxygen saturation, blood gas values, and end CO_2.
- Respiratory support:
  - Low-flow nasal cannula (LFNC), high-flow nasal cannula (HFNC), nasal continuous positive airway pressure (NCPAP), or tracheal intubation depending on the gestational age and respiratory status of infant
- Laboratory tests:
  - Bilirubin level
  - Blood cultures based on risk factors
  - Blood gas
  - Blood glucose
  - Complete blood count (CBC) with manual differential
  - Electrolytes
  - Liver function tests
- Blood transfusion may be indicated for anemia caused by frequent laboratory testing or blood loss related to birth trauma (Lopriore, 2019).
- Intravenous fluids are provided as indicated.
- Parenteral (intravenous) nutrition is offered if indicated by the neonate's gestational age or clinical condition.
- Central line placement is used if long-term parenteral nutrition is required.
- Umbilical artery and umbilical vein catheters are considered central lines and can be used to administer medications, parenteral nutrition, and for hemodynamic monitoring.
- Medications:
  - Antibiotic therapy as indicated to decrease the risk of infection or treatment of infection
  - Dopamine or dobutamine for treatment of hypotension
  - EPO administration to stimulate production of red blood cells (RBCs) if indicated
    - The use of EPO reduces the need for RBC transfusions as well as decreases the incidence of IVH and NEC. Moreover, recent studies have found that administration of EPO does not increase the risk of ROP as was previously believed (Ohlsson & Aher, 2020).
  - Exogenous surfactant therapy for RDS, as indicated (Forest, 2021)
  - Opioids to treat pain associated with procedures that cause moderate to severe pain, such as with surgical procedures
  - Sodium acetate to treat metabolic acidosis (See Safe and Effective Nursing Care)

SAFE AND EFFECTIVE NURSING CARE: Understanding Medications

Sodium Bicarbonate

In its *Textbook of Neonatal Resuscitation,* the American Academy of Pediatrics (AAP) no longer recommends sodium bicarbonate in the treatment of metabolic acidosis. Because CO_2 is produced as bicarbonate is metabolized, the infant must be adequately ventilated to blow off the excess CO_2. Without adequate ventilation, the acidosis will worsen (AAP, 2016). Additionally, research indicates that a paradoxical worsening of intracellular acidosis may occur. Sodium bicarbonate administration in premature, LBW infants is also associated with cerebral blood flow fluctuations resulting in IVH (Massenzi et al., 2021).

Nursing Actions

- Review prenatal, intrapartum, and neonatal histories for any known risk factors that would potentially impact the neonate.
- Participate in resuscitation of the neonate as indicated.

- The NICU nurse, neonatologist, or neonatal nurse practitioner should be present at all births with pregnancy-related or intrapartum complications.
- Stabilize and transfer the neonate to the NICU for ongoing specialized care.
- Perform gestational assessment with Ballard score to determine the age of the neonate if the gestational age is unknown or unreliable.
  - Protocols of care differ with gestational age.
- Perform a physical assessment, evaluating for problems associated with prematurity.
  - Nursing care includes the immediate recognition and prioritization of problems to decrease neonatal morbidity and mortality.

CLINICAL JUDGMENT

Signs of Respiratory Distress

The most common life-threatening diseases in newborns are respiratory in origin and account for most admissions to the NICU. Neonatal nurses must be adept at assessing respiratory status and recognizing signs of respiratory distress in neonates.

- Audible expiratory grunting
  - Caused by air being forced past a partially closed glottis
- Nasal flaring
- Retracting
  - May be visualized at the sternum as well as the subcostal and intercostal spaces of the infant's chest
- Duskiness or cyanosis
- Tachypnea (RR greater than 60 breaths per minute) (Fraser, 2021)

- Provide respiratory support.
  - Maintain a patent airway.
  - Suction airway as needed to remove secretions. Neonates have a smaller airway diameter, which increases the risk of obstruction.
  - Administer oxygen to maintain oxygen saturation within ordered parameters.
    - Oxygen administration may be given using LFNC or HFNC, NCPAP, or a ventilator.
    - Oxygen is humidified and warmed to prevent drying of mucous membranes and dropping of body temperature.

CRITICAL COMPONENT

Maintaining a Neutral Thermal Environment

Premature neonates are unable to protect themselves against fluctuations in environmental temperatures due to thin, immature skin as well as minimal stores of subcutaneous brown fat. Nurses must enact interventions that support the maintenance of a neutral thermal environment (NTE) to prevent the development of cold stress.

- Dry the infant gently immediately after birth, removing the wet linen, and covering the infant's head with a hat to prevent heat loss from evaporation.

- Place plastic barriers made of polyethylene over preterm neonates (less than 32 weeks' gestation) after birth to prevent heat loss by decreasing water loss that can occur through the neonate's immature skin, known as transepidermal water loss (TEWL).
- Use of a chemical warming mattress during resuscitation and transport to the NICU improves thermal control in preterm and LBW infants. Be sure to place a blanket between the mattress and the infant's skin to prevent burns.
- Prewarm all supplies and equipment that will come into direct contact with the infant.
- Control environmental temperature with use of the servo control setting on transport equipment, radiant warmers, and incubators. A temperature-control probe should be placed on the neonate directly below the underarm, midaxillary line to assist in maintaining the neonate's temperature within the normal range (axillary 97.7°F to 99.5°F [36.5°C to 37.5°C]).
- Place the premature, LBW neonate in a double-walled incubator and add humidity to the environment to prevent heat loss and TEWL.
- Encourage kangaroo care (skin-to-skin care) once stable, which promotes thermoregulation in neonates of all gestational ages.
- Weaning from the incubator to an open crib can be considered once the infant is medically stable and weighs 1,600 g or greater (Brand & Shippey, 2021).

- Assess cardiovascular system.
  - Color
  - Heart rate and rhythm
  - Blood pressure
  - Murmurs
  - Pulses
  - Capillary refill
- Provide cardiovascular support.
  - Monitor heart rate and rhythm, blood pressure, oxygen saturation, and blood gases.
  - Obtain and monitor hemoglobin and hematocrit as per order.
  - Administer blood transfusion as per order.
- Assess responses to interventions. These responses may be changes in breathing, oxygen saturation, vital signs, laboratory results, or neonatal behavior.
- Maintain fluid and electrolyte balance.
  - Monitor input and output (I&O) by:
    - Weighing diapers to determine output
    - Assessing frequency, color, and amount of urine to determine hydration
    - Recording fluid I&O from IV fluids, feedings, chest tubes, urinary catheters, stomas, and laboratory draws
- Restrict fluid intake as per order.
  - Fluid restriction is commonly ordered for neonates with BPD and PDA or other complications that can lead to pulmonary edema.

- Monitor electrolyte levels as per order.
  - Hyperkalemia (elevated potassium levels), hyponatremia (low sodium level), and hypernatremia (high sodium level) may occur among preterm infants due to immaturity of the renal and integumentary systems (Chowdhury et al., 2019).
- Administer intravenous fluids as per order.
  - Monitor the site of intravenous access hourly for signs of infection, skin breakdown, infiltration, and extravasation.
- Add humidity to the neonate's environment.
  - Humidity decreases TEWL, which reduces fluid requirements as well as promotes electrolyte balance (Forest, 2021).
- Meet the neonate's nutrition requirements.
  - Obtain and monitor blood glucose levels as per order.
  - Administer parenteral nutrition if the neonate is unable to receive enteral feedings (via gastrointestinal tract) or is advancing slowly on feeding volumes.
    - Neonates less than 32 weeks' gestation and LBW infants:
      - Initially often require parenteral nutrition
      - May lack the ability to digest and absorb feedings due to an immature gastrointestinal tract
      - Have an immature suck, swallow, and breathe reflex and thus are at risk for aspiration (Parker, 2021)
  - Administer trophic feedings (small volume enteral feedings) as per order. They are not given for nutritional purposes but instead are often given while neonates are receiving parenteral feedings to ease the transition to full enteral feedings by promoting continued functional maturation of the gastrointestinal tract via stimulation of intestinal motor activity, colonization of normal flora in the GI tract, and secretion of GI hormones and peptides (Forest, 2021; Parker, 2021).
  - Administer enteral feedings orally or by gastric tube (gavage feedings), depending on the infant's gestational age and clinical condition. Most neonates who are older than 34 weeks' gestation usually receive oral feedings soon after birth.
    - Human milk (mother's own or donated breast milk) reduces the risk of NEC and therefore is preferred over formula for enteral feedings (Altobelli et al., 2020).
    - Human milk alone is insufficient in meeting the unique nutritional needs of preterm infants and requires fortification to provide adequate calories, protein, and minerals (Radmacher & Adamkin, 2017).
  - When the neonate is unable to breastfeed, instruct the mother in the use of a breast pump and storage of breast milk. Encourage the mother to bring breast milk to the NICU so that it can be used for enteral feedings for her infant.
- Administer gavage feedings as per order.
  - Before each feeding, assess for signs of feeding intolerance such as abdominal distention, emesis, blood in stools, apnea, and bradycardia (Parker, 2021).
  - Offer a pacifier during gavage feedings. Non-nutritive sucking eases the transition from gavage feeding to bottle feeding and results in decreased length of hospital stay for preterm neonates (Foster et al., 2016).
  - Monitor weight daily. Weight gain of 15 to 20 g/kg/day indicates appropriate growth and caloric intake for a preterm neonate (Parker, 2021).
- Monitor head circumference and length weekly. Changes in head circumference indicate brain growth; length is compared with weight to ensure proportional growth (Parker, 2021).
- Transition the neonate from gavage feedings to oral feedings.
  - Transitioning to oral feedings occurs when the neonate:
    - Has cardiorespiratory regulation.
    - Demonstrates a coordinated suck, swallow, and breathe reflex and a strong gag reflex, which occurs at approximately 34 weeks' corrected gestation.
    - Demonstrates hunger cues such as bringing hand to the mouth, sucking on fingers, and rooting.
    - Can maintain a quiet alert state.
  - Properly position the neonate for bottle feeding by holding the infant in a side-lying, semi-upright position.
  - Observe the neonate closely for respiratory status, apnea, bradycardia, oxygenation, and feeding tolerance.
  - Pace feeding and allow for breathing breaks because preterm neonates may become fatigued during feedings.
- Provide breastfeeding support.
  - Educate the mother about feeding cues, breastfeeding positions, correct latch, and how to evaluate the feeding.
    - Encourage and support breastfeeding as frequently as possible to establish successful latching. Mothers who are given ample breastfeeding support while in the NICU are more likely to establish breastfeeding and to continue with it after discharge (Cartwright et al., 2017).
  - Weigh the neonate before and after breastfeeding to monitor intake.
    - Many mothers are hesitant to breastfeed their premature or ill neonate because they are afraid the volume will not be adequate. Weighing the neonate before and after breastfeeding can be an accurate way to demonstrate successful breastfeeding (Juliano et al., 2019).
  - Refer to Chapter 16 for additional nursing actions to support breastfeeding.
- Administer medications as per order.
- Provide skin care as follows (Forest, 2021):
  - Assess overall skin condition using the Braden QT scale (Fig. 17-3) which is a tool to predict pressure-related skin injury in pediatric patients (Curley, et al., 2018).
  - Use adhesives sparingly and avoid their use on areas of skin breakdown.
  - Use extreme care with adhesive removal and avoid removers or solvents.
  - Change diapers frequently.
  - Change positions a minimum of every 4 hours.
  - Use hydrocolloid products as a protective layer under medical devices.
- Obtain laboratory tests as per orders.
- Assess for signs of jaundice.
- Manage pain to prevent potential long-term sensory disturbances and altered pain responses that may last into adulthood (Walden, 2021).
  - Frequently assess the neonate for signs of pain, especially during painful procedures. Instruments to measure neonatal

Braden QD Scale

Intensity and Duration of Pressure				Score
Mobility The ability to independently change & control body position	**0. No Limitation** Makes major and frequent changes in body or extremity position independently.	**1. Limited** Makes slight and infrequent changes in body or extremity position **OR** unable to reposition self independently (includes infants too young to roll over).	**2. Completely Immobile** Does not make even slight changes in body or extremity position independently.	
Sensory Perception The ability to respond meaningfully, in a **developmentally** appropriate way, to pressure-related discomfort	**0. No Impairment** Responsive **and** has no sensory deficits which limit ability to feel or communicate discomfort.	**1. Limited** Cannot always communicate pressure-related discomfort **OR** has some sensory deficits that limit ability to feel pressure-related discomfort.	**2. Completely Limited** Unresponsive due to diminished level of consciousness or sedation **OR** sensory deficits limit ability to feel pressure-related discomfort over most of body surface.	
Tolerance of the Skin and Supporting Structure				
Friction & Shear *Friction:* occurs when skin moves against support surfaces *Shear:* occurs when skin & adjacent bony surface slide across one another	**0. No Problem** Has sufficient strength to completely lift self up during a move. Maintains good body position in bed/chair at all times. Able to completely lift patient during a position change.	**1. Potential Problem** Requires **some** assistance in moving. Occasionally slides down in bed/chair, requiring repositioning. During repositioning, skin often slides against surface.	**2. Problem** Requires **full** assistance in moving. Frequently slides down and requires repositioning. Complete lifting without skin sliding against surface is impossible **OR** spasticity, contractures, itching, or agitation leads to almost constant friction.	
Nutrition *Usual* diet for age—assess pattern over the most recent 3 consecutive days	**0. Adequate** Diet for age providing **adequate** calories & protein to support metabolism and growth.	**1. Limited** Diet for age providing **inadequate** calories **OR** **inadequate** protein to support metabolism and growth **OR** receiving supplemental nutrition any part of the day.	**2. Poor** Diet for age providing **inadequate** calories **and** protein to support metabolism and growth.	
Tissue Perfusion & Oxygenation	**0. Adequate** Normotensive for age, & oxygen saturation ≥ 95%, & normal hemoglobin, & capillary refill ≤2 seconds.	**1. Potential Problem** Normotensive for age **with** oxygen saturation <95%, **OR** hemoglobin <10 g/dL, **OR** capillary refill >2 seconds.	**2. Compromised** Hypotensive for age **OR** hemodynamically unstable with position changes.	
Medical Devices				
Number of Medical Devices	**Score 1 point for each medical device* up to 8 (Score 8 points maximum)** **Any diagnostic or therapeutic device that is currently attached to or traverses the patient's skin or mucous membrane.*			
Repositionability/ Skin Protection	**0. No Medical Devices**	**1. Potential Problem** All medical devices can be repositioned **OR** the skin under each device is protected.	**2. Problem** Any one or more medical device(s) can**not** be repositioned **OR** the skin under each device is not protected.	
			Total **(≥13 considered at risk)**	

© Curley MAQ; Adapted with permission from B. Braden and N. Bergstrom, Braden Scale for Predicting Pressure Sore Risk (1987)

FIGURE 17–3 Braden QD Scale.

pain among preterm neonates are available and should be integrated into routine care.

- Administer sucrose and promote non-nutritive sucking during painful procedures.
- Administer opioids as per orders to treat pain associated with procedures that cause moderate to severe pain.
- Use nonpharmacological interventions such as swaddling, positioning, holding and kangaroo care, therapeutic touch, and decreasing environmental stimuli.
- Evaluate the effectiveness of nonpharmacological and pharmacological interventions.

- Provide developmentally appropriate care to decrease stress and enhance neurodevelopment (Spruill, 2021).
  - Maintain a quiet setting.
  - Physiological responses such as apnea and fluctuations in heart rate, blood pressure, and oxygen saturation may occur in response to loud noises.
  - Keep lighting dim.
  - At 32 weeks begin cycling the lighting in the infant's room to simulate night and day, which has been shown to improve normal circadian rhythm development and improve weight gain (Pineda et al., 2019).
  - Cluster nursing activities to provide for extended periods of sleep.
  - Avoid clustering painful interventions together.
  - Provide individualized care based on the neonate's responses and needs.
  - Allow a break in care or stimulation if the neonate becomes stressed.
  - Minimize handling for neonates in an unstable condition.
  - Position and swaddle
    - Change the neonate's position slowly and gently.
    - Reposition every 2 to 3 hours. Assess the neonate's response to repositioning.
    - Positioning the neonate in the side-lying or prone position enhances oxygenation and gastric emptying.
    - The head of the bed may be elevated 15 degrees.
    - Swaddle in flexion with arms and hands placed toward the infant's midline.
    - Create a nest with blankets and positioning aids to enhance containment.
- Encourage kangaroo care (skin-to-skin contact with the parents) for medically stable neonates. Benefits of kangaroo care include the following (Spruill, 2021):
  - Temperature stability
  - Modulates pain
  - Increases duration of quiet sleep
  - Improves daily weight gain
  - Improves mother–infant attachment
- Provide emotional support to parents and family members.
- Involve parents and family in all aspects of the infant's care. This helps to decrease anxiety and fears, thus allowing for an increase in parent–infant bonding.
  - Teach parents what to expect from their preterm infant and how to interpret behavioral cues.
  - Teach parents how to provide care for their infant (Fig. 17–4).

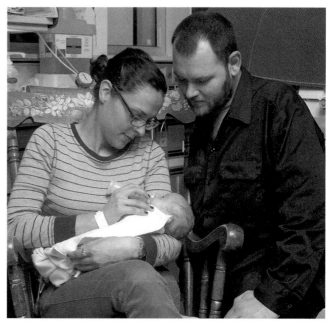

FIGURE 17–4 Parents bottle-feeding their baby.

- Facilitate parent–infant bonding by welcoming parents to the NICU, encouraging participation in the infant's care, and providing positive reinforcement often.
- Teach parents about the infant's condition and involve parents in the plan of care.

RESPIRATORY DISTRESS SYNDROME

RDS is a life-threatening lung disorder that results from small, underdeveloped alveoli and insufficient levels of pulmonary surfactant. These combined factors can cause an alteration in alveoli surface tension that eventually results in atelectasis. The incidences of RDS are inversely related to gestational age and birth weight, affecting 51% of neonates born weighing less than 1,000 g (Fraser, 2021). The effects of atelectasis are:

- Hypoxemia and hypercarbia
- Pulmonary artery vasoconstriction
- Right-to-left shunting through the ductus arteriosus and foramen ovale as the neonate's body attempts to counteract the compromised pulmonary perfusion
- Metabolic acidosis that occurs from a buildup of lactic acid that results from prolonged periods of hypoxemia
- Respiratory acidosis that occurs from the collapsed alveoli being unable to rid the body of excess carbon dioxide

Pulmonary surfactant is a substance composed of 90% phospholipids and 10% proteins. It reduces the surface tension within the lungs and increases the pulmonary compliance that prevents the alveoli from collapsing at the end of expiration. Type II alveolar cells within the lungs begin to produce pulmonary surfactant around 24 to 28 weeks and continue to term (Fraser, 2021). Tests used to evaluate fetal lung maturity are:

- PG:
  - PG is synthesized from mature lung alveolar cells.
  - It is present in the amniotic fluid within 2 to 6 weeks of full-term gestation.
  - The presence of PG indicates lung maturity, and a decrease indicates risk of RDS.
- L/S ratio:
  - Lecithin and sphingomyelin are two phospholipids that are detected in the amniotic fluid.
  - The ratio between two phospholipids provides information on the level of surfactant.
  - An L/S ratio greater than 2:1 in a nondiabetic woman indicates the fetus's lungs are mature.
  - An L/S ratio of 3:1 in a diabetic woman indicates the fetus's lungs are mature.

Complications of RDS

- PDA
- Pneumothorax
- BPD
- Pulmonary edema
- Hypotension
- Anemia
- Oliguria
- Hypoglycemia and altered calcium and sodium levels
- ROP
- Seizures
- IVH (Fraser, 2021)

Assessment Findings

- Respiratory distress varies based on degree of prematurity.
- Respiratory difficulty begins immediately or within a few hours after the delivery and the neonate must work progressively harder at breathing to maintain open terminal airways.
- Tachypnea
- Retractions and seesaw breathing patterns occur.
- Audible expiratory grunting
  - Used by the neonate in an attempt to prevent alveolar collapse
  - More pronounced with severe distress
- Nasal flaring
- Increased oxygen levels to maintain a Pao_2 and $Paco_2$ within normal limits.
  - The normal range of Pao_2 is 60 to 70 mm Hg.
  - The normal range of $Paco_2$ is 35 to 45 mm Hg.
- Skin color is gray or dusky.
- Breath sounds on auscultation are decreased and crackles are present as RDS progresses.
- The neonate is lethargic and hypotonic.
- X-ray examination shows a reticulogranular pattern of the peripheral lung fields and air bronchograms.
- Hypoxemia may occur (Pao_2 less than 50 mm Hg).

- Acidosis may result from sustained hypoxemia.
- Tachycardia
  - Heart rate greater than 160 beats per minute
  - More prevalent with acidosis and hypoxemia (Balest, 2019b; Fraser, 2021).

Medical Management

- Cardiorespiratory, oxygen saturation, and blood gas monitoring
- Exogenous surfactant as indicated for neonates at risk for or with RDS
- Respiratory support as indicated. The mode of ventilation and settings are based on the neonate's condition and arterial blood gas results. Methods of respiratory support include:
  - Continuous positive airway pressure (CPAP); this is used for neonates who are at risk for RDS or who have RDS. It can be administered by nasal cannula, nasal mask, nasal prongs, endotracheal tube, or nasopharyngeal route.
  - Endotracheal tube and mechanical ventilation; this is used when CPAP is not effective (use judiciously to avoid damage to lung tissue).
  - High-frequency oscillatory ventilation; this is used when mechanical ventilation has proven unsuccessful.
    - Delivers small volumes of gas at a high rate (greater than 300 breaths/minute)
    - Less traumatic on fragile lung tissue
- Diagnostic tests
  - Chest x-ray examination to assist in evaluation of RDS
- Laboratory tests
  - Arterial, venous, or capillary blood gases
  - Blood cultures if neonate is at risk for infection
- Medications
  - Antibiotics as indicated.

SAFE AND EFFECTIVE NURSING CARE: Understanding Medications

Surfactant Replacement Therapy Administration

Natural Surfactant

- Composed of calf, pig, or cow lung (minced) combined with lipids
- Examples: Survanta, Curosurf, Infasurf

Synthetic Surfactant

- Example: Exosurf

Action

- It reduces surface tension of the alveoli, thus preventing collapse during expiration.
- It enhances lung compliance to allow easier inflation, which decreases the work of breathing.
- It improves overall oxygenation of the infant.

Indications

- RDS

Route

- Administered via endotracheal tube
- Can also be administrated via a thin catheter or laryngeal mask if attempting to avoid intubation and mechanical ventilation

Dosing Regimen (Dose and Technique Vary by Product)

- Prophylaxis: Initiated within 15 minutes of birth, based on risk factors of RDS such as gestational age less than 27 to 30 weeks, especially if the mother did not receive antenatal steroids. Multiple doses can be given if indicated.
- Rescue therapy: Treatment of confirmed RDS. Treatment is typically initiated within 6 hours of birth for infants who have increased oxygen demands (Fio_2 greater than 40%) or need mechanical ventilation.

Adverse Effects

- Bradycardia, decreased oxygen saturation, tachycardia, reflux, gagging, cyanosis, blockage of the endotracheal tube, hypotension

Benefits of Surfactant Therapy

- Prophylactic therapy decreases the occurrence of RDS and mortality in preterm neonates.
- Decreased risk of pneumothorax
- Decreased risk of intraventricular hemorrhage
- Decreased risk of BPD
- Decreased risk of pulmonary interstitial emphysema (Fraser, 2021)

Nursing Actions

Nursing actions for neonates with RDS are similar to actions for preterm neonates, with additional emphasis on the following:

- Provide respiratory support.
  - Maintain a patent airway.
  - If the neonate is intubated, assess for correct placement of the endotracheal tube.
    - Listen for equal breath sounds bilaterally, assess for equal chest rise, and use a commercial end tidal CO_2 detector.
  - Administer oxygen as ordered to maintain oxygen saturation within ordered parameters.
    - Hypoxemia and acidosis may further decrease surfactant production.
  - Minimize oxygen demand by maintaining an NTE, clustering care to decrease stress, and treating acidosis as clinically indicated and ordered.
  - Suction the airway as needed for removal of secretions, as neonates have a smaller airway diameter, which increases the risk of obstruction.
    - Be aware that suctioning may stimulate the vagus nerve, causing bradycardia, hypoxemia, or bronchospasm.
- Monitor vital signs, oxygen saturation, and blood gas results.

- Maintain NTE to decrease the risk of cold stress.
  - Cold stress increases oxygen consumption, which promotes acidosis and may further impair surfactant production.
- Monitor I&O and daily weights.
  - Dehydration impairs ability to clear airways because mucus becomes thickened.
  - Overhydration may contribute to alveolar infiltrates or pulmonary edema.
  - Weight loss and increased urine output may indicate the diuretic phase of RDS.
- Promote rest by implementing calming measures or administering ordered sedation.
  - Minimizing stimulation and energy expenditure reduces metabolic rate and oxygen consumption.

BRONCHOPULMONARY DYSPLASIA

BPD is a chronic lung disease that affects neonates who have been treated with prolonged periods of mechanical ventilation and oxygen for problems such as RDS. The lungs of premature infants are more vulnerable to the inflammatory changes and thus neonates who are dependent on oxygen beyond 28 days of life or have been on mechanical ventilation are at risk for BPD (Balest, 2019a). This condition leads to decreased lung compliance and pulmonary function secondary to fibrosis, atelectasis, increased pulmonary resistance, and overdistention of the lungs (Bancalari & Walsh, 2015) (Fig. 17–5). Pulmonary edema results from the increased pulmonary vascular resistance. The prognosis for neonates with BPD is dependent on the severity of the disease and the infant's overall health status. Long-term outcomes may include prolonged hospitalization, long-term oxygen therapy that may be required after discharge, cerebral palsy, ROP, and hearing loss.

Risk Factors

- Lower gestational age and birth weight (less than 32 weeks and less than 1,500 g)
- RDS
- Oxygen toxicity
- Intubation
- Assisted ventilation with positive pressure
- Infection
- Excessive fluid intake
- Nutritional deficiencies
- Pulmonary vascular damage secondary to excessive fluid administration, right-to-left shunting associated with PDA, and increased airway resistance (Fraser, 2021).

Complications of BPD

- Intermittent bronchospasm
- Inability to be weaned from ventilator or oxygen supplementation
- Recurrent infections of pneumonia, upper respiratory infections, and otitis media

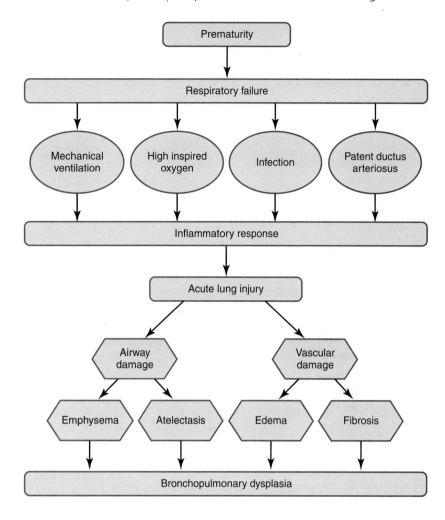

FIGURE 17-5 Bronchopulmonary dysplasia.

- Congestive heart failure
- Developmental delays and cerebral palsy
- Gastroesophageal reflux (Fraser, 2021)

Assessment Findings

- Chest retractions
- Audible wheezing, rales, and rhonchi
- Hypoxia
- Respiratory acidosis
- Bronchospasm
- Difficulty weaning from ventilator or increased requirements for ventilator
- Intolerance to fluids: edema, decreased urinary output, and weight gain
- Chest x-ray exhibiting multicystic or sponge-like appearance, with alternating areas of emphysema, pulmonary scarring, and atelectasis (Balest, 2019a; Fraser, 2021)

Medical Management

- Diagnostic tests
  - Chest x-ray examination
  - Echocardiogram if cardiac complications are suspected

- Laboratory tests
  - Electrolytes
  - Arterial blood gases
- Medications
  - Bronchodilators: Administered to reduce bronchoconstriction
  - Corticosteroids: Administered to reduce bronchospasm, edema, and inflammation of pulmonary tissue
  - Diuretics: Administered to treat fluid retention and decrease risk for pulmonary edema
- Prophylaxes against respiratory syncytial virus; infants with BPD are predisposed to RSV
- Chest physiotherapy
- Respiratory assistance and oxygen therapy
- Monitor I&O
- Determine the method of feeding to meet the neonate's nutritional and caloric needs

CRITICAL COMPONENT

Bronchopulmonary Dysplasia
Treatment for BPD is a regimen of support and time: time for the normal repair process within the lungs to improve functioning and time for the infant to grow and thrive.

Nursing Actions

Nursing actions for neonates with BPD are similar to actions for preterm neonates with additional emphasis on the following:

● Provide mechanical ventilation and oxygen administration as per orders.
● Gradually wean neonate from mechanical ventilation as per orders.
● Provide chest physiotherapy as per orders to clear secretions from the lungs.
● Provide fluids as ordered.
  ● Fluid restriction may help reduce pulmonary edema and right-sided heart failure (Fraser, 2021).
  ● Provide increased calories to compensate for increased work of breathing and fluid restriction (Fraser, 2021). Fortification of formula or breast milk may be needed to obtain optimal growth.
● Administer medications and monitor for adverse reactions.
● Monitor I&O and daily weights.
  ● Infants with BPD are at risk for fluid overload and pulmonary edema.

PATENT DUCTUS ARTERIOSUS

PDA occurs when the ductus arteriosus remains open after birth (Fig. 17–6). During fetal circulation, the ductus arteriosus connects the pulmonary artery with the descending aorta and shunts blood away from the lungs. Normally, the ductus arteriosus closes within a few hours of birth, but this can take as long as 96 hours. The incidence of PDA among term neonates is 1 in 2,000 live births (Sadowski & Verklan, 2021). Occurrence of PDA is greater among neonates of lower gestational age and birth weight, occurring in 45% of neonates who weigh less than

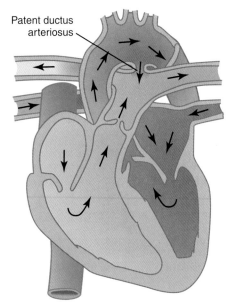

Patent ductus arteriosus

FIGURE 17–6 Patent ductus arteriosus.

1,750 g and 80% of neonates who weigh less than 1,200 g at birth (Beerman, 2020). Complications of PDA include congestive heart failure, chronic lung disease, renal insufficiency, feeding intolerance, NEC, and IVH (Beerman, 2020).

Assessment Findings

● Heart murmur heard at the upper left sternal border (some neonates with PDA may not have an audible murmur)
● Active precordium (visible movement of the heart contracting on the patient's left chest)
● Bounding pulses
● Widened pulse pressure with decreased diastolic blood pressure
● Tachycardia and tachypnea
● Recurrent apnea
● Increased work of breathing
● Increased demand for oxygen or ventilation
● Difficulty weaning from ventilator support
● The presence of a PDA confirmed by echocardiogram
● Chest x-ray examination may show prominence of the left atrium, left ventricle, and ascending aorta as well as increased pulmonary vascular markings (Beerman, 2020; Sadowski & Verklan, 2021).

Medical Management

The medical treatment of PDA includes managing symptoms with fluid restriction and diuretics.

● Diagnostic tests
  ● Echocardiogram to assist in evaluation of PDA
● Fluid restriction to less than 130 mL/kg/day (Sadowski & Verklan, 2021).
● Medications
  ● Diuretics
  ● Indomethacin and ibuprofen when indicated. These medications were frequently used in the past but rarely today due to side effects such as gastrointestinal bleeding, decreased glomerular filtration, and decreased urine output.
● Cardiology consult to determine treatment method and need for surgical intervention
● Surgical ligation (suture, clip, or coil) of PDA is indicated for neonates with a hemodynamically significant PDA who do not respond to medical management (Sadowski & Verklan, 2021).

Nursing Actions

Nursing actions for neonates with PDA are similar to actions for preterm neonates with additional emphasis on the following:

● Administer oxygen and mechanical ventilation as per orders.
● Administer medications as per orders.
● Monitor I&O for signs of fluid overload.
  ● Fluids may be restricted until PDA is resolved.
  ● Infant will be NPO during treatment and surgery.
● Prepare the neonate and family for surgery.

INTRAVENTRICULAR HEMORRHAGE

IVH occurs in the germinal matrix tissue surrounding the lateral ventricles of the developing brain. They occur primarily among premature, very LBW neonates and affect 40% to 60% of these infants. Because germinal matrix is not present in most infants beyond 36 weeks, IVH in full-term infants is rare (3.5% to 4.6%). Most hemorrhages occur in the first week of life, with 90% occurring within 72 hours of birth (Ditzenberger, 2021).

There are four grades of IVH based on the extent of involvement; the higher the grade, the more severe the hemorrhage and the higher the risk for long-term sequelae:

- Grade I: Hemorrhage in germinal matrix
- Grade II: IVH without ventricular dilatation
- Grade III: IVH with ventricular dilatation; clots fill more than 50% of the ventricle
- Grade IV: Extension of blood into cerebral tissue or parenchymal involvement (Ditzenberger, 2021)

Risk Factors

- Prematurity, birth at less than 34 weeks' gestation
- LBW
- Perinatal asphyxia or birth trauma
- RDS necessitating ventilatory support
- Rapid volume expansion
- Rapid administration of sodium bicarbonate
- Low 5-minute Apgar score
- Alteration of blood pressure, either hypotension or hypertension
- Acidosis, hypercarbia
- Low hematocrit
- Pneumothorax
- Ligation of PDA (Ditzenberger, 2021)

The long-term prognosis often depends on the severity of the hemorrhage with death rates of 5% for small hemorrhage, 10% for moderate hemorrhage, and 50% for severe hemorrhage. Neurological problems such as cerebral palsy and delayed mental development occur in 10% of neonates with a small hemorrhage, 40% with a moderate hemorrhage, and 80% with a severe hemorrhage. Approximately 50% of premature infants do not experience neurological problems, and 25% to 30% of very LBW neonates who had IVH do not exhibit neurodevelopment problems (Ditzenberger, 2021).

Assessment Findings

- Sudden deterioration in condition
- Oxygen desaturation
- Bradycardia
- Hypotonia
- Metabolic acidosis
- Shock
- Significant decrease in hematocrit
- Full or tense anterior fontanel

- Hyperglycemia
- Signs that bleeding is worsening include:
  - Apnea
  - Increased ventilatory support
  - Seizures
  - Full, tense fontanels
  - Diminished activity or level of consciousness (Ditzenberger, 2021)

Medical Management

- Diagnostic tests
  - Cranial ultrasounds on NICU neonates should be performed within the first week of life to assess for IVH.
  - Lumbar puncture is used to assist in evaluation of IVH. CSF is analyzed for RBCs, increased protein concentration, xanthochromia, and decreased glucose concentration.
- Laboratory tests
  - Hemoglobin and hematocrit are used to evaluate the extent of bleeding.
- Blood transfusions as indicated (Ditzenberger, 2021)

Nursing Actions

Nursing actions for neonates with IVH are similar to actions for preterm neonates, with additional emphasis on the following:

- Assess for changes in vital signs, behavior, and neurological status, which may indicate increased intracranial pressure.
- Reduce stress to the neonate by maintaining a quiet and dark environment.
- Administer fluid volume replacement slowly to minimize fluctuations in blood pressure.

Evidence-Based Practice
Nursing Strategies to Prevent IVH

Kaspar, A., & Rubarth, L. B. (2016). Neuroprotection of the preterm infant. *Neonatal Network, 35*(6), 391–395. https://doi.org/10.1891/0730-0832.35.6.391

Shifts in cerebral perfusion have been linked to the development of IVH, and many studies have evaluated the effects of routine nursing care on fluctuations in cerebral blood flow.

Based on the physiological data and the views of experts in the field, nursing strategies used to decrease cerebral blood flow fluctuations include:

- Ensure supine midline head positioning.
- Keep head of bed flat or slightly elevated.
- Keep hips below head level with diaper changes.
- Maintain temperature within the normal range.
- Minimize crying.
- Minimize environmental stimulation such as light and noise.

Conclusion: Implementing nursing strategies to decrease cerebral blood flow fluctuations can decrease the incidence of IVH, which promotes better outcomes for the premature infant.

NECROTIZING ENTEROCOLITIS

NEC is an acquired gastrointestinal disease and is the most common gastrointestinal emergency among neonates (Cochran, 2020). NEC is characterized by inflammation and necrosis of the bowel, most commonly the proximal colon or terminal ileum, and the majority (90% to 95%) of NEC cases occur following the initiation of enteral feeding (Bradshaw, 2021). Over 90% of cases of NEC occur in premature infants (Cochran, 2020). Preterm neonates are predisposed to NEC due to:

- Decreased immunological factors in the intestinal tract
- Increased gastric pH
- Immature intestinal barrier
- Decreased intestinal motility (Bradshaw, 2021)

Other Risk Factors

- Prolonged rupture of membranes with amnionitis
- Birth asphyxia
- Small for gestational age (SGA) infants
- Congenital heart disease
- Anemia
- Formula feeding (breast milk significantly lowers risk for NEC) (Cochran, 2020)

Assessment Findings

Symptoms of NEC typically begin between 3 and 10 days after birth but can occur up to several weeks of age:

- Lethargy
- Apnea and bradycardia
- Blood in the stool: occult or frank
- Temperature instability
- Hypotension, shock
- Diminished urinary output
- Abdominal distention, tenderness, bilious vomiting, increased gastric residuals, discoloration of abdomen, and visible bowel loops
- Abdominal x-ray films of neonates with NEC may show diffuse distention of the intestines with gas; gas in one part of the intestine, and lack of gas in other parts; air in the wall of the intestine or the portal venous system; dilated loops of bowel; and air in the abdomen (Bradshaw, 2021).

Medical Management

- Diagnostic tests
  - Abdominal x-ray examination to assist in the evaluation of NEC
  - Serial x-rays to determine worsening or improvement
- Laboratory tests
  - Blood cultures, CBC, C-reactive protein, stool cultures, electrolyte panel, arterial blood gases, and coagulation studies

- Medications
  - Antibiotics
  - Analgesia
  - Antihypertensives
- Discontinuation of oral feedings, NPO
- Intravenous fluids
- Gastric decompression (Bradshaw, 2021)

Surgical Management

- Surgical intervention for the removal of necrotic bowel, resection of bowel, or for perforation of bowel related to NEC. A temporary colostomy may be performed (Bradshaw, 2021).

Nursing Actions

Nursing actions for neonates with NEC are similar to actions for preterm neonates with additional emphasis on the following:

- Assess for abdominal distention, visible bowel loops, emesis, bloody stools, and abnormal vital signs.
  - Early recognition and prompt treatment increases the chances for medical management.
- Withhold feedings as per orders and obtain intravenous access.
- Perform gastric decompression as per orders by placing an orogastric tube and connecting it to low suction.
- Monitor I&O.
  - Maintain circulating blood volume.
  - Maintain adequate hydration.
- Prepare the neonate and family for surgery when indicated.

Long-Term Outcomes

- NEC is fatal in 20% to 30% of cases.
- Short bowel syndrome may occur in neonates who have had surgical treatment (Bradshaw, 2021).

RETINOPATHY OF PREMATURITY

ROP is common in premature neonates and those with LBW. ROP occurs because the retina is not completely vascularized, making it susceptible to stress or injury, which can interrupt the normal vascularization process. This is followed by vasoproliferation, an abnormal growth of vasculature within the retina or extending into the vitreous body. Ultimately, this abnormal vascularization can result in bleeding and fluid leakage that causes scar tissue. This tissue pulls and distorts the retina and displaces the macula. Retinal folds may occur and can lead to retinal detachment and blindness. The International Classification of Retinopathy of Prematurity provides a system of five stages to classify ROP based on the severity of the disease; stage 4 is partial retinal detachment, and stage 5, the most severe, is complete retinal detachment (Diehl-Jones & Fraser, 2021).

The incidence of ROP increases as gestational age and birth weight decrease. In neonates weighing less than 1,000 grams, the rate of ROP is up to 80%. Severe ROP occurs in 1% to 43% of these infants. Long-term outcome for this disease depends on the extent of its progression and ranges from normal vision to blindness (Khazaeni, 2020).

Risk Factors

- Prematurity and LBW
- Prolonged hyperoxia (exposure to high levels of oxygen) and duration of mechanical ventilation
- Hypoxia, hypercapnia, hypocapnia, and acidosis
- Steroid exposure
- Infection or sepsis
- Patent ductus arteriosus
- Multiple gestation
- Intraventricular hemorrhage
- Blood transfusion
- Maternal diabetes, bleeding, smoking, and hypertension (Diehl-Jones & Fraser, 2021)

Long-term outcomes are as follows:

- 90% of neonates with ROP experience recovery with no or minimal loss of vision.
- Complications such as glaucoma, strabismus, cataracts, amblyopia, retinal detachment, and blindness may occur.
- Corrective glasses may be needed to treat visual deficits (Diehl-Jones & Fraser, 2021).

Assessment Findings

- Retinal changes noted on ophthalmic examination.

Medical Management

- Eye evaluation for possible ROP completed by the pediatric ophthalmologist for all neonates born before 30 weeks' gestation, or with a birth weight of less than 1,500 g. Neonates who weigh between 1,500 g and 2,000 g at birth with medical complications should also receive an eye examination. The eye examination should occur at 4 to 6 weeks after birth.
- Neonates with immature or abnormal vessel development should have repeated eye examinations to monitor progression of the disease.
- The aim of medical treatment is to decrease the risk of blindness. Treatment is determined by the extent of abnormal vessel development and may include:
  - Laser photocoagulation: Laser is used to coagulate the avascular periphery of the retina to prevent vessel proliferation.
  - Cryotherapy: A supercooled probe is used to prevent vessel proliferation by freezing the avascular retina.
  - Vitreoretinal surgery: Done to reattach the retina (Diehl-Jones & Fraser, 2021).

Nursing Actions

- Reduce the risk for ROP.
  - Administer oxygen to maintain prescribed pulse oximetry parameters.
  - Use oxygen blenders and oxygen-calibrating systems to ensure exact concentration of oxygen.
  - Avoid bright lights by keeping lighting in the nursery at a low level and by covering isolettes with blankets.

SAFE AND EFFECTIVE NURSING CARE: Understanding Medications

Reducing ROP Risk

Decreasing risk of ROP when administering oxygen includes:

- Continuous monitoring of oxygen to maintain prescribed pulse oximetry parameters
- Careful use of oxygen during procedures such as suctioning
- Use of equipment such as oxygen blenders to ensure the exact concentration of oxygen
- Properly maintaining and calibrating oxygen systems (Diehl-Jones & Fraser, 2021)

POSTMATURE NEONATES

Post-term pregnancy is a pregnancy that lasts greater than or equal to 42 weeks' gestation (Stavis, 2019c). Although the cause is largely unknown, post-term pregnancy can result in a large for gestational age (LGA) infant, discussed later in the chapter. Sometimes, however, if the pregnancy continues past term, the placenta can no longer adequately support the developing fetus (Moldenhauer, 2020). The fetus is forced to use its subcutaneous fat and glycogen stores. This results in an SGA infant and is considered postmature.

Characteristics of postmaturity include dry peeling skin, long nails, marked creases, and a lack of fat deposition. The skin can be stained green or yellow from meconium. Inadequate nutrients and oxygen delivered by the placenta increase the risk for hypoxia to the fetus at the onset of labor and hypoglycemia following birth. Although placental insufficiency can occur at any gestational age, it is most common in post-term pregnancies (Stavis, 2019c).

When a pregnancy goes beyond term, there is a higher risk of morbidity and mortality for both mother and infant (Tappero, 2021). Post-term delivery at 42 weeks or greater is associated with significantly higher rates of perinatal mortality as well as higher rates of adverse perinatal outcomes (Maoz et al., 2018). Post-term pregnancies have higher rates of complications including oligohydramnios, macrosomia, meconium-stained amniotic fluid, shoulder dystocia, low Apgar scores, hysterectomy, and intrauterine fetal death (Maoz et al., 2018).

Risk Factors

- Anencephaly
- History of post-term pregnancies
- First pregnancy
- Grand multiparous women

Complications

- Meconium aspiration: The presence of meconium in the amniotic fluid related to fetal hypoxia places the neonate at risk for meconium aspiration syndrome (MAS), discussed later in this chapter. MAS may be exacerbated because of decreased amniotic fluid volume, which is less dilute when aspirated (Stavis, 2019c).
- Fetal hypoxia: This is related to placental insufficiency and a decrease in amniotic fluid, which increases the risk of cord compression.
- Neurological complications: This includes seizures related to fetal asphyxia during labor and birth due to alterations in oxygenation.
- Hypoglycemia: This is related to decreased glycogen stores and glucose production due to inadequate placental functioning.
- Hypothermia: This is related to loss of subcutaneous fat related to insufficient nutrient transport through the placenta.
- Polycythemia (hematocrit greater than 65% in neonate): Compensatory response caused by alteration in oxygenation from placental insufficiency (Stavis, 2019e; Walter, 2020).

Assessment Findings

- Dry, peeling, cracked skin
- Lack of vernix
- Profuse hair
- Long fingernails
- Thin, wasted appearance
- Meconium staining (green or yellow staining on skin, nail beds, or umbilical cord)
- Hypoglycemia
- Poor feeding behavior

Medical Management

- Oxygen therapy administered for perinatal depression or respiratory distress
- Hematocrit to assess for polycythemia
- Blood glucose monitoring for hypoglycemia

Nursing Actions

- Assess the prenatal record and intrapartum history including Apgar scores for risk factors.
- Assess the neonate for:
  - Gestational age with use of gestational age scoring system
  - Respiratory distress (e.g., grunting, nasal flaring, chest retractions, tachypnea)
  - Cyanosis
  - Oxygen saturation if respiratory distress or cyanosis is present
  - Signs of meconium staining
  - Blood glucose levels
  - Vital signs
  - Weight
  - Gross anomalies

- Monitor for signs of hypoglycemia.
  - Jitteriness, irritability, poor feeding, apnea, grunting, lethargy
- Provide early and frequent feedings if respiratory status is stable.
  - Early and frequent feedings reduce the risk of hypoglycemia.
- Monitor I&O.
  - Post-term infants may be poor feeders and thus at risk for inadequate fluid intake.

MECONIUM ASPIRATION SYNDROME

MAS is a cause of respiratory failure in term and post-term neonates. The term *meconium-stained amniotic fluid* (MSAF) is used when meconium stool is present in the amniotic fluid. This occurs when there is a relaxation of the fetus's anal sphincter in utero, usually due to fetal asphyxia. Deep gasping respirations, which are associated with fetal hypoxia, can occur, resulting in aspiration of the MSAF. The incidence of MSAF is between 8% and 20% of all deliveries. Of these infants, approximately 5% develop MAS (Gomella et al., 2020).

The presence of thick MSAF in the neonate's lungs can result in obstruction of the upper airways. If it progresses to the lower airways, air trapping and hyperinflation of the alveoli distal to the obstruction increases the risk of air leaks into the surrounding tissue, atelectasis, and hypoxia. MAS can also cause a chemical pneumonitis and inhibit surfactant action. Additionally, the neonate is at risk for pulmonary hypertension due to increased pulmonary vascular resistance and for pneumonia (Gomella et al., 2020).

Assessment Findings

- Meconium-stained amniotic fluid is observed.
- Greenish or yellowish discoloration of the skin, nail beds, and umbilical cord is visible.
- Respiratory depression is observed at the time of birth or within a few hours after birth.
- Low Apgar scores are viewed.
- There is a need for resuscitation after delivery due to perinatal depression.
- Signs of respiratory distress are observed such as nasal flaring, grunting, or chest retractions.
- Chest may appear barrel-shaped and overdistended.
- The expiration phase of breathing may be extended.
- Diminished air movement, and the presence of rales and rhonchi, is assessed on auscultation.
- Atelectasis and hyperinflated areas through the lungs are noted on chest x-ray.
- Arterial blood gas findings may include low PaO_2 despite administration of 100% oxygen, and respiratory and metabolic acidosis in serious cases (Fraser, 2021).

Medical Management

- Prevention of fetal distress by recognizing maternal factors that could lead to fetal hypoxia, monitoring for distress during labor, and amnioinfusion of isotonic fluid into the amniotic cavity in settings where perinatal surveillance is limited (Gomella et al., 2020).

- Immediate availability of a clinician with intubation skills when MSAF is present (AAP, 2016; Korioth, 2020).
- Oral suctioning for secretions or meconium with a bulb syringe from a nonvigorous infant, especially if positive pressure ventilation is anticipated. Avoid vigorous or deep oropharyngeal suctioning (AAP, 2016).
- Endotracheal intubation is indicated for tracheal suctioning and resuscitation if the airway is obstructed by thick secretions or meconium (AAP, 2016). Routine endotracheal suctioning is not indicated for vigorous or nonvigorous infants (AAP, 2016; Korioth, 2020).
- Arterial blood gases are used to determine respiratory status and guide treatment.
- Chest x-ray may be used.
- Blood glucose monitoring may be used.
- Oxygen therapy, conventional ventilation, or high frequency ventilation may be used, depending on the neonate's condition.
- Surfactant replacement is used to decrease the risk of need for extracorporeal membrane oxygenation (ECMO) and improve gas exchange (Gomella et al., 2020).
- Sedatives or paralytic agents are used to relax neonates who are receiving ventilation.
- Antibiotics are used to treat pneumonia.
- Cooling therapy, inhaled nitric oxide (iNO), or ECMO may be indicated (Gomella et al., 2020).
  - Therapeutic hypothermia reduces cerebral injury and improves neurological outcomes for neonates who experience a hypoxic event or asphyxia in utero or during the birthing process (Wassink et al., 2019).

Nursing Actions

- Assist with suctioning and resuscitation at the time of delivery.
- Assess neonate for:
  - Respiratory distress such as grunting, flaring, retracting, cyanosis, and tachypnea
  - Complications of MAS, such as acidosis, hypoglycemia, hypocalcemia, pneumonia, pneumothorax, BPD, and persistent pulmonary hypertension
  - Neurological problems secondary to asphyxia (Fraser, 2021)
- Administer oxygen or assisted ventilation as per order.
- Monitor blood glucose.
  - Complication of respiratory distress is an increased metabolic rate and thus a higher incidence of hypoglycemia.
- Manage neonates receiving cooling, iNO, or ECMO.

PERSISTENT PULMONARY HYPERTENSION OF THE NEWBORN

Normally after birth, the pulmonary vascular bed relaxes, allowing blood circulation to the lungs. Persistent pulmonary hypertension (PPHN) results when the normal vasodilation and relaxation of the pulmonary vascular bed does not occur. This leads to elevated pulmonary vascular resistance, high pulmonary artery pressure, right ventricular hypertension, and right-to-left shunting of blood through the foramen ovale and ductus arteriosus (Fraser, 2021). The result is hypoxemia, reduced cardiac output, systemic hypotension, impaired tissue oxygenation, and metabolic acidosis, which contributes to a cycle of worsening pulmonary vasoconstriction and clinical deterioration (Montasser & Patel, 2021). Affecting 2 to 6 infants per 1,000 live births (Gomella et al., 2020), PPHN is predominantly a problem among term or near-term neonates who experience hypoxia or asphyxia, RDS, meconium aspiration, sepsis, or congenital lung anomalies such as diaphragmatic hernia (Montasser & Patel, 2021).

Risk Factors

- Hypoxia and asphyxia, which are the most common risk factors for PPHN
- Low Apgar scores
- RDS, meconium aspiration, or pneumonia
- Bacterial sepsis
- Delayed circulatory transition at birth caused by factors such as delayed resuscitation, central nervous system (CNS) depression, or hypothermia
- Hypothermia or hypoglycemia leading to acidosis
- Polycythemia or hyperviscosity of the blood, which can cause blockages in the pulmonary vascular bed
- Prenatal pulmonary hypertension associated with premature closure of the ductus arteriosus, or fetal systemic hypertension
- Underdevelopment of pulmonary vessels associated with congenital anomalies of the lung or heart
- Maternal factors: Nonsteroidal anti-inflammatory drugs (NSAIDs) have been associated with premature closure of the fetal ductus arteriosus, and late trimester use of selective serotonin reuptake inhibitors (SSRIs) has been associated with PPHN (Fraser, 2021).

Assessment Findings

- Respiratory issues
  - Slow to breathe, difficult to ventilate
  - Symptoms evident within 12 hours of birth
  - Tachypnea
  - Chest retractions or grunting
  - Cyanosis
  - Low Pao_2, even with administration of high levels of oxygen
  - Chest x-ray with infiltrates (but may also be normal) (Fraser, 2021)
- Cardiac issues
  - Hypotension
  - Heart murmur
  - Echocardiogram shows pulmonary hypertension and enlarged right side of heart
  - Congestive heart failure
- Metabolic issues
  - Hypocalcemia
  - Hypoglycemia
  - Metabolic acidosis (Fraser, 2021)

- Hematological issues
  - Disseminated intravascular coagulation (DIC)
  - Thrombocytopenia
  - Possible kidney damage, leading to decreased urine output, proteinuria, and hematuria
- Long-term outcomes after PPHN include:
  - Hearing loss (sensorineural)
  - Neurological deficits
  - Chronic lung disease
  - Death (Fraser, 2021)

Medical Management

- Main goal is to correct hypoxia and acidosis.
- Preductal and postductal blood gases and continuous pulse oximetry:
  - Right-to-left shunting is suspected when there is a difference of 15 mm Hg or more between the preductal and postductal PaO_2, with preductal higher (Fraser, 2021).
  - Pulse oximetry will reveal a difference of 5% or greater between pre- and postductal oxygen saturation (Gomella et al., 2020).
- Echocardiogram is used to evaluate for cardiac anomalies, right-to-left shunting of blood, pulmonary resistance, and pulmonary artery pressures.
- Oxygen and conventional mechanical ventilation:
  - Oxygenation goal is to keep Pao_2 levels above 50 mm Hg (Fraser, 2021); weaning the oxygen level down should be done gradually to avoid hypoxia. The ventilation goal is to keep $Paco_2$ values normal (over 30 mm Hg) to prevent the vasoconstrictive action of hypercapnia. Hyperventilation should be avoided, as hypocapnia may cause poor neurodevelopmental outcomes (Gomella et al., 2020).
  - If conventional mechanical ventilation is ineffective, high-frequency oscillatory ventilation may be instituted.
  - ECMO is used if other treatments are not effective.
- Intravenous fluids
- Laboratory tests (CBC, glucose, electrolytes, calcium, arterial blood gases, blood cultures)
- Umbilical catheters: arterial (for blood gases and BP monitoring) and venous (to administer vasopressors as indicated)
- Surfactant therapy
- Nitric oxide therapy
  - Nitric oxide induces vasodilation and reduces pulmonary resistance.
  - Use of nitric oxide reduces the percentage of neonates with PPHN needing ECMO (Gomella et al., 2020).
- Medications
  - Vasopressors such as dopamine decrease right-to-left shunting by maintaining systemic vascular pressure above pulmonary vascular pressure (Gomella et al., 2020).
  - Vasodilators such as sildenafil and prostaglandins are used to promote pulmonary artery dilation.
  - Paralyzing agents for neonates who resist ventilation have become controversial and may increase pulmonary vascular resistance (Gomella et al., 2020).
- Sedatives and analgesics are used such as midazolam (Versed) and morphine (Gomella et al., 2020).
- Antibiotic therapy is used to decrease the risk of or treat infection.

Nursing Actions

- Review maternal prenatal, intrapartal, and neonatal histories.
- Assess the neonate for respiratory distress, meconium aspiration, and clinical manifestations of PPHN.
- Administer oxygen and mechanical ventilation as ordered.
- Monitor vital signs and pulse oximetry.
- Anticipate the placement of umbilical catheters.
  - Vasoconstriction makes peripheral intravenous access difficult.
  - Arterial blood gases and laboratory values are easily accessed via an umbilical catheter, thus preventing the infant from receiving painful heel sticks and venipunctures.
  - Multiple intravenous fluids and medications can be administered simultaneously via umbilical catheters.
- Administer IV fluids as per order.
- Administer medications as per order.
- Obtain and monitor results of laboratory tests.
  - Immediate intervention is required for abnormal laboratory results.
- Keep handling, treatments, suctioning, and stimulation to a minimum, as these can result in decreased PaO_2 levels and vasoconstriction.
- Provide emotional support for parents, incorporate them in care of their infant, and keep them informed of their infant's condition.

SMALL FOR GESTATIONAL AGE AND INTRAUTERINE GROWTH RESTRICTION

An SGA neonate is one whose weight is less than the 10th percentile for their gestational age. Intrauterine growth restriction (IUGR) occurs in utero and is a result of a uterine insult. It is an ultrasound finding, whereas SGA is a clinical finding (Gomella et al., 2020). There are two types of IUGR: symmetric and asymmetric.

- Symmetric IUGR, a generalized proportional reduction in the size of all structures and organs except for heart and brain, occurs early in pregnancy and affects general growth. When a complication occurs very early in pregnancy, fewer cells develop, leading to smaller organ size. Symmetric IUGR can be identified by ultrasound in the early part of the second trimester. Conditions that may result in symmetric IUGR include exposure to teratogenic substances, congenital infections, and genetic problems (Tappero, 2021).
- Asymmetric IUGR (also known as head sparing) is a disproportional reduction in the size of structures and organs, resulting from maternal or placental conditions that occur later in pregnancy and impede placental blood flow. Examples of

conditions that may result in asymmetric IUGR include pre-eclampsia, placental infarcts, or severe maternal malnutrition (Tappero, 2021).

Risk Factors

Risk factors contributing to IUGR are:

- Maternal
  - Chronic diseases (cardiac, asthma, hemoglobinopathies, lupus, diabetes, hypertension)
  - Anemia
  - Gestational diabetes
  - Malnutrition
  - Multiple gestation
  - Multiparity
  - Age (greater than 35, less than 16)
  - Unexplained stillbirth or miscarriage
  - History of IUGR infant
  - Preeclampsia
  - Low maternal pre-pregnancy BMI
  - Pregnancy weight gain
  - Ethnicity
  - Lack of adequate prenatal care
  - Single marital status
  - Low socioeconomic status or education level
  - Medications (i.e., beta blockers and thiazide diuretics)
  - Use of addictive drugs, tobacco, or alcohol (Gunatilake & Patil, 2021)
- Fetal
  - Congenital infections (TORCH)
  - Chromosomal abnormalities
  - Congenital malformations
- Placental anatomy and function
  - Infarction
  - Previa
  - Abruption
  - Anatomic malformations or abnormal cord insertion
  - Twin-to-twin transfusion
- Environmental
  - High altitude
  - Arsenic
  - Lead (Gomella et al., 2020; Tappero, 2021)

Outcomes

Neonates with IUGR are at risk for:

- Labor intolerance related to placental insufficiency and inadequate nutritional and oxygen reserves
- Meconium aspiration related to asphyxia during labor
- Hypoglycemia related to inadequate glycogen stores and reduced gluconeogenesis, and an increase in metabolic demands from heat loss, which diminishes glucose stores (Armentrout, 2021)
- Hypocalcemia, defined as serum calcium levels less than 7.5 mg/dL, related to birth asphyxia (Bell, 2021).
  - Signs of hypocalcemia are often similar to those of hypoglycemia and include jitteriness, tetany, and seizures.

Assessment Findings

- Physical characteristics of the IUGR neonate include:
  - Large head in relationship to the body
  - Long nails
  - Large anterior fontanel
  - Decreased amounts of Wharton's jelly present in the umbilical cord
  - Thin extremities and trunk
  - Loose skin due to a lack of subcutaneous fat
  - Dry, flaky, or meconium-stained skin
- Weight, head circumference, and length are all below the 10th percentile for gestational age in symmetric IUGR (Tappero, 2021).
- Head circumference and length are appropriate for gestational age, but weight is below the 10th percentile for the baby's gestational age in asymmetric IUGR (Tappero, 2021).
- RDS may occur in SGA neonates born prematurely or who have aspirated MSAF.
- Hypothermia is related to decreased subcutaneous fat and glucose supply, impaired lipid metabolism, and depleted brown fat stores (Tappero, 2021).
- Polycythemia may be observed.

Medical Management

- Identify IUGR during pregnancy and intervene based on the cause.
- Assess for congenital anomalies.
- Suggest oxygen therapy for perinatal depression and respiratory distress.
- Laboratory tests
  - Blood glucose monitoring
  - Hematocrit if polycythemia is suspected
  - Serum calcium levels

Nursing Actions

- Review prenatal and intrapartal records for risk factors.
- Perform a gestational age assessment to determine if the neonate is SGA or preterm.
- Assess for respiratory distress.
- Assess the neonate for gross anomalies.
- Assess the skin for color and signs of meconium staining.
  - Infants with meconium staining have an increased risk of respiratory distress.
- Maintain an NTE.
  - SGA infants have decreased subcutaneous fat and are more susceptible to hypothermia.
- Decrease risk of hypoglycemia.
  - Prevent heat loss and teach the importance of preventing heat loss to parents.
    - SGA infants are at high risk for hypoglycemia due to their decreased amount of subcutaneous fat and thus are at increased risk of cold stress.
  - Assess for signs of hypoglycemia.
  - Monitor blood glucose.

- Provide early and frequent feedings.
  - SGA infants may require higher caloric intake and need gavage feedings due to poor suck or inability to finish feedings due to lack of stamina.
  - Teach parents the importance of frequent feedings.
- Monitor for feeding intolerance.
  - SGA infants are susceptible to NEC due to placental insufficiency.
- Obtain laboratory tests as per orders.
- Monitor for hypocalcemia.
- Weigh daily.
- Monitor vital signs.

LARGE FOR GESTATIONAL AGE

An LGA neonate weighs above the 90th percentile for their gestational age. Characteristically, LGA neonates are macrosomic, defined as birth weight greater that 4,000 g (Fig. 17–7). Maternal diabetes is the leading cause of LGA neonates (Stavis, 2019b) and will be discussed later in the chapter. Infants of diabetic mothers (IDM) typically present with a large body with the head circumference still within normal limits for their gestational age. This is because insulin does not cross the blood-brain barrier (Tappero, 2021).

Risk Factors

- Maternal diabetes (chronic or gestational)
- Multiparity
- Previous macrosomic baby
- Prolonged pregnancy
- Increased maternal weight gain in pregnancy and maternal obesity (Gomella et al., 2020).

Outcomes

LGA fetuses and neonates are at risk for:

- Cesarean or operative vaginal delivery
- Shoulder dystocia
- Birth trauma
- Hypoglycemia
- Polycythemia and hyperbilirubinemia
- Perinatal asphyxia
- Respiratory distress
- Meconium aspiration

Assessment Findings

- Birth trauma associated with LGA
  - Head molding or scalp abrasions
  - Caput succedaneum
  - Fractured clavicle
  - Brachial plexus nerve damage
  - Facial nerve damage
  - Depressed skull fractures

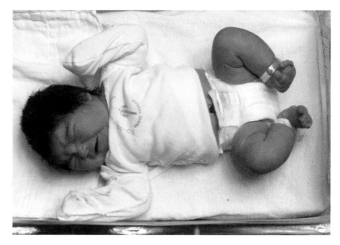

FIGURE 17–7 Large-for-gestational-age neonate.

  - Cephalohematoma
  - Subgaleal hemorrhage
  - Intracranial hemorrhage
  - Asphyxia (Stavis, 2019a)
- Poor feeding behavior
- Hypoglycemia
- Polycythemia in neonates of diabetic mothers related to a decrease in extracellular fluid or fetal hypoxia
- Hyperbilirubinemia that occurs 48 to 72 hours after delivery related to polycythemia, decreased extracellular fluid, or bruising or hemorrhage from birth trauma

Medical Management

- Assessments for birth trauma, hypoglycemia, and respiratory distress
- Laboratory tests:
  - Blood glucose
  - Hematocrit
  - Bilirubin levels when indicated for jaundice

Nursing Actions

- Review prenatal and intrapartal records for risk factors.
- Assess respiratory status.
- Assess neonate for birth traumas such as fractured clavicles, brachial nerve damage, facial nerve damage, and cephalohematoma.
- Obtain and monitor blood glucose per agency protocol.
- Observe for signs of hypoglycemia.
  - LGA neonates have increased risk for hypoglycemia from depletion of glycogen stores.
- Provide early and frequent feedings to decrease risk for hypoglycemia.
  - LGA neonate may feed poorly and require gavage feedings.
- Obtain and monitor hematocrit as per orders.
  - High hematocrit increases the risk for jaundice.
- Assess skin color for signs of polycythemia, which appears as a red, ruddy skin color.
  - IDM are at risk for polycythemia.

- Perform a gestational age assessment.
- Observe for jaundice.
  - LGA neonates are at higher risk for jaundice due to polycythemia.

HYPERBILIRUBINEMIA

Neonatal jaundice is the yellow-orange tint that can be visualized in the sclera and skin of neonates with hyperbilirubinemia (increased bilirubin in the blood). Jaundice affects between 60% and 70% of term and 80% of preterm infants during the first week of life (Gomella et al., 2020). Total serum bilirubin (TSB) is the combination of the two forms of bilirubin: unconjugated (also called indirect) and conjugated (direct). Unbound (unconjugated) bilirubin can deposit into tissue and cross the blood-brain barrier. It cannot be excreted and can settle in tissues, causing jaundice. Conjugated bilirubin is bound to albumin and, once bound, is water-soluble. It is nontoxic and can be excreted through the gastrointestinal tract (Pace et al., 2019). Serum bilirubin cannot be excreted until it is conjugated.

When serum bilirubin levels are greater than 5 mg/dL, neonates will exhibit visible signs of jaundice (Gomella et al., 2020). However, visual assessment of jaundice is not reliable for diagnosis of hyperbilirubinemia. The clinical significance of jaundice is based on the gestational age of the neonate, hours of life, and the TSB level (Kamath-Rayne et al., 2021). Prematurity may result in greater severity of physiological jaundice, and any jaundice among preterm neonates must be evaluated.

A complication of hyperbilirubinemia is acute bilirubin encephalopathy (ABE) and kernicterus, an abnormal and irreversible accumulation of unconjugated bilirubin in the brain cells. Bilirubin accumulates within the brain and becomes toxic to the brain tissue, causing neurological disorders such as deafness, delayed motor skills, hypotonia, and intellectual deficits (Pace et al., 2019). A goal of medical and nursing actions is to prevent kernicterus through early identification and treatment of hyperbilirubinemia.

Hyperbilirubinemia is categorized into physiological jaundice and pathological jaundice.

PHYSIOLOGICAL JAUNDICE

Physiological jaundice results from hyperbilirubinemia that commonly occurs after the first 24 hours of birth and during the first week of life. It is caused by the breakdown of RBCs (hemolysis). Common physiological characteristics of the neonate place it at risk for increased hemolysis and for physiological jaundice:

- Higher RBC mass relative to body weight than adults
- Shorter RBC life span of 70 to 90 days, compared with 120 days in adults
- High bilirubin production (6 to 8 mg/kg/day)
- Neonates reabsorb increased amounts of unconjugated bilirubin in the intestine due to lack of intestinal bacteria, decreased

gastrointestinal motility, and increased beta-glucuronidase (a deconjugating enzyme)
- Decreased hepatic uptake of bilirubin from the plasma due to a deficiency of ligandin, the primary bilirubin binding protein in hepatocytes
- Diminished conjugation of bilirubin in the liver due to decreased glucuronyl transferase activity (Bradshaw, 2021)

Assessment Findings

- Physiological jaundice is typically visible after 24 hours of life.
- TSB levels generally peak on day 3 of life in term neonates and on days 5 or 6 in preterm neonates (Bradshaw, 2021).
- Jaundice is characterized by a yellowish tint to the skin and sclera of the eyes.
- As TSB levels rise, jaundice will progress from the newborn's head down toward the trunk and lower extremities.

PATHOLOGICAL JAUNDICE

Pathological jaundice results when various disorders exacerbate physiological processes that lead to hyperbilirubinemia of the newborn. Such disorders can result in pathological unconjugated or conjugated hyperbilirubinemia. Because conjugated hyperbilirubinemia is always pathological, further investigation must be done to determine its cause (Gomella et al., 2020).

Common causes of conjugated hyperbilirubinemia include:

- Parenteral nutrition (most common cause in the NICU, especially in preterm infants)
- Idiopathic neonatal hepatitis
- Biliary atresia
- Bile duct stenosis
- Metabolic and genetic defects
- Endocrine disorders
- Infection
- Some medications
- Shock
- Hypoxic ischemic liver injury

Causes of pathological unconjugated hyperbilirubinemia include:

- Breastfeeding jaundice (early onset)
- Breast milk jaundice (late onset)
- Rh and ABO incompatibilities
- Glucose-6-phosphate dehydrogenase (G6PD) deficiency
- Hemoglobinopathies
- Blood sequestration (bruising, cephalohematoma, intracranial bleeding)
- Polycythemia
- Metabolic and endocrine disorders
- Gastrointestinal obstruction
- Infection (Gomella et al., 2020)

Assessment Findings

- Criteria to differentiate pathological jaundice from physiological jaundice in a full-term neonate (Kamath-Rayne et al., 2021):
    - Jaundice that occurs within the first 24 hours of life
    - TSB levels that increase by more than 0.2 mg/dL per hour
    - Jaundice lasting more than 2 weeks
    - TSB exceeding the 95th percentile for age in hours
    - A high direct bilirubin (1.5 to 2 mg/dL)
- Risk factors, medical management, and nursing actions are similar for both physiological and pathological jaundice.

Risk Factors for Hyperbilirubinemia

- Maternal factors
    - American Indian, East Asian, or Mediterranean descent
    - ABO incompatibility (e.g., the mother has blood type O and the neonate has blood type A or B)
    - Rh incompatibility (mother is Rh negative and the neonate is Rh positive)
    - Breastfeeding (see Table 17-2)
    - Diabetes
    - Use of oxytocin or bupivacaine during labor
- Neonatal factors
    - Delayed cord clamping, which increases RBC volume (Yang et al., 2019)
    - Hypoxia, asphyxia, acidosis, and temperature instability
    - Delayed or infrequent feedings, or lethargy

- Excessive weight loss after birth
- Bruising or cephalohematoma
- Prematurity
- G6PD deficiency
- Bacterial or viral infection (especially toxoplasmosis, syphilis, varicella-zoster, parvovirus B19, rubella, cytomegalovirus, and herpes [TORCH] infections)
- Previous sibling with hyperbilirubinemia (Gomella et al., 2020)

Medical Management for Hyperbilirubinemia

In 2004, the AAP's subcommittee on hyperbilirubinemia developed clinical practice guidelines for treating hyperbilirubinemia in neonates at 35 or more weeks of gestation (AAP, 2004). These guidelines remain the basis for medical management of hyperbilirubinemia.

Guidelines are based on the Bhutani nomogram (Bhutani et al., 1999), which considers TSB, age in hours, and neurotoxicity risks—isoimmune hemolytic disease, G6PD deficiency, asphyxia, significant lethargy, temperature instability, sepsis, and acidosis—to predict the likelihood of a subsequent bilirubin level to be in the 95th percentile (high risk zone) or greater for that infant (AAP, 2004; Kamath-Rayne et al., 2021).

Depending on the specific infant characteristics, a "threshold" TSB is identified upon which treatment decisions can be based, although individual circumstances may alter clinicians' treatment decisions (AAP, 2004). Tools such as the BiliTool can be accessed online to assist with this process at Bilitool.org.

TABLE 17-2 Hyperbilirubinemia Associated With Breastfeeding: A Comparison of Breastfeeding vs. Breast Milk Jaundice	
BREASTFEEDING-ASSOCIATED JAUNDICE	**BREAST MILK JAUNDICE**
Early onset of jaundice (within the first few days of life).	Late onset (beyond the first week).
It is associated with ineffective breastfeeding.	Gradual increase in bilirubin that peaks at 2 weeks of age.
Dehydration can occur.	Associated with breast milk composition in some women that increases the enterohepatic circulation of bilirubin.
Delayed passage of meconium stool promotes reabsorption of bilirubin in the gut. Expect a slower reduction in serum bilirubin in breastfed compared with bottle-fed babies.	Treatment: Continued breastfeeding in most infants. In some cases where bilirubin levels are excessively high, breastfeeding may be interrupted, and formula feedings are given for several days. This typically results in a decline of the bilirubin level. Breastfeeding is resumed when bilirubin levels decline.
Treatment: Encourage early effective breastfeeding without supplementation of glucose water or other fluids.	If jaundice continues beyond 2 weeks, obtain serum direct and TSB to rule out cholestasis.
Encourage breastfeeding 8 to 12 times per day for the first several days.	
May supplement with pumped breast milk or formula (when breast milk not yet available) if: • Intake inadequate • Weight loss excessive • Dehydration is suspected	

AAP & ACOG, 2017; Bradshaw, 2021; Kamath-Rayne et al., 2021.

- Diagnostic tests
  - TSB, with fractionation of serum bilirubin into direct (conjugated bilirubin) and indirect (unconjugated bilirubin) reacting pigments
  - Antiglobulin (Coombs') test: Used to determine hemolytic disease of the newborn related to Rh or ABO incompatibility
    - Direct antiglobulin (Coombs') test, which can be done on cord blood, is used to detect abnormal in vivo coating of the neonate's RBCs with antibody globulin (maternal antibodies); when present, the test is considered positive.
  - Transcutaneous bilirubinometry (TcB) is a noninvasive method to estimate TSB levels among term and near-term neonates. A bilirubinometer uses reflectance measurements to express the degree of yellowness of the skin. It is used to identify neonates at risk for developing hyperbilirubinemia, and correlates well with TSB.
  - CBC assists in identification of anemia, which could indicate hemolysis and can also evaluate for infection.
  - Reticulocyte count represents immature RBCs, and elevation is indicative of hemolytic disease (Gomella et al., 2020).
- Treatment is determined by the level of bilirubin and the age of the neonate in hours.
- Phototherapy is the most widely used and effective treatment for hyperbilirubinemia.
  - Various types of phototherapy delivery systems are available, including blue lights, white lamps, halogen lamps, fiber-optic blankets, and blue light-emitting diodes (LEDs). The most effective lights are special blue, fluorescent tubes and specially designed LED lights that can produce high-energy output in the blue-green spectrum. These lights are considered "intensive phototherapy" (Kamath-Rayne et al., 2021).
  - Phototherapy results in photoconverting bilirubin molecules to water-soluble isomers that can be excreted in the urine and stool without conjugation in the liver (Bradshaw, 2021).
  - The fiber-optic blanket ("Bili Blanket") is a portable phototherapy device that delivers phototherapy with a fiber-optic light panel. When used in the hospital, it is generally combined with overhead lights, but it can also be used for home phototherapy for less severe cases of hyperbilirubinemia. The infant can be held and fed with the blanket in place, and eye shields are not indicated if used alone.
  - Double phototherapy utilizing fiber-optic and bank overhead lights has been found significantly more effective than single phototherapy, probably due to the increased body surface area in contact with light (Donneborg et al., 2018).
  - TSB levels should drop at a rate of 0.5 to 1 mg/dL per hour, and by 30% to 40% after 24 hours of treatment (Kamath-Rayne et al., 2021).
  - Phototherapy is generally administered continuously, except during feeding times or parental visits, when eye patches are removed to allow for bonding.
- Exchange transfusion is used in cases where phototherapy is not effective or severe hemolytic disease is present (Kamath-Rayne et al., 2021).
  - In this procedure, approximately 85% of the neonate's RBCs are replaced with donor cells, which can reduce serum bilirubin levels by as much as 50% of the pre-exchange level (Gomella et al., 2020).
  - This procedure reduces bilirubin, removes RBCs coated with maternal antibody, corrects anemia, and removes other toxins associated with hemolysis (Kamath-Rayne et al., 2021).
  - Efforts to prevent Rh hemolytic disease with Rh immunoglobulin (RhoGAM) administered to Rh-negative women, along with the use of phototherapy, has diminished the need for exchange transfusion (Kamath-Rayne et al., 2021).
- Intravenous immunoglobulin (IVIG) for hyperbilirubinemia caused by isoimmune hemolysis has been shown to dramatically decrease the need for exchange transfusion (Gomella et al., 2020).
- Neonates discharged before 72 hours of life should be seen for follow-up by a health-care provider within 1 to 2 days to assess the neonate's health status and check for jaundice.
  - Early identification and treatment decrease the risk of bilirubin encephalopathy (Kamath-Rayne et al., 2021).
  - After phototherapy is discontinued, rebound of the TSB level is common. For this reason, the TSB should be re-checked within 24 hours of discontinuation of phototherapy (Kamath-Rayne et al., 2021).

Nursing Actions

See Clinical Judgment: Care of the Infant Receiving Phototherapy for nursing actions for hyperbilirubinemia. Proper nursing care enhances the effectiveness of phototherapy and minimizes complications.

CLINICAL JUDGMENT

Care of the Neonate Receiving Phototherapy

- Review maternal and neonatal record for risk factors.
- Assess degree of jaundice with the use of a transcutaneous meter per unit policy.
- Visually assess degree of jaundice by using a finger to blanch the neonate's skin on the face, upper trunk, abdomen, thigh, and lower leg and feet. The skin will appear yellow after the pressure is released and before skin returns to normal color.
- Document the assessment findings.
  - How rapidly the degree of jaundice progresses guides the method of treatment.
- Notify the physician if jaundice is present.
  - Prompt treatment is essential to preventing bilirubin toxicity.
- Obtain serum bilirubin levels as per orders.
  - Rate of rise of the bilirubin level is critical in determining the treatment needed.
- Ensure adequate hydration by feeding the neonate every 2 to 3 hours to promote excretion of bilirubin in the urine and stool and compensate for insensible water loss due to phototherapy (Gomella et al., 2020).
- Implement phototherapy as ordered.

- Intensive phototherapy lights should be positioned 12 to 16 inches from the infant and 2 inches from the top of an incubator.
  - A photometer should be used to measure irradiance of lamps to facilitate optimal treatment and in intensive phototherapy should measure greater than or equal to 30 microwatts/cm^2/nm (AAP, 2004).
  - Banks of lights should be covered by Plexiglas.
- The neonate should have only a diaper in place for maximal exposure to light.
- Place eye shields on the neonate to protect eyes from the effects of the light and remove every 4 hours for assessment.
  - During feedings, remove eye shields and have the parent or nurse hold the neonate.
- Change the neonate's position frequently to facilitate increased light exposure.
- Vital signs including temperature monitoring should be done per agency protocol.
- Monitor I&O. Phototherapy results in increased insensible fluid loss.
- Assess for side effects of phototherapy:
  - Observe eyes for discharge and tearing.
    - Animal studies have indicated that retinal damage may occur so opaque eye shields must be used to prevent potential eye damage.
    - Assess position of eye shield to ensure it does not occlude nares.
  - Loose stools
  - Dehydration
  - Hyperthermia
  - Lethargy
  - Skin rashes
- For those infants discharged with mild jaundice, provide verbal and written instructions to include measures to assess hydration, excretion of bilirubin, return appointments, and home management of phototherapy lights if applicable, as well as how to identify signs of increasing jaundice and when to notify the physician (Gomella et al., 2020; Kamath-Rayne et al., 2021).

CENTRAL NERVOUS SYSTEM INJURIES

Various types of CNS injuries can occur among term and premature neonates any time in the perinatal or neonatal periods. The location of the injury can be intracranial (such as subdural, subarachnoid, or intracerebral hemorrhage), extracranial (such as subgaleal hemorrhage), or in the spinal cord, plexus, or cranial or peripheral nerves. Perinatal hypoxia and ischemia as well as acute or chronic placental insufficiency can lead to CNS injury (such as hypoxic ischemic encephalopathy). Depending on the extent and location, CNS injuries may result in normal outcomes or serious long-term problems such as seizures, neurological deficits, developmental disability, motor deficits, visual impairments, or death (Hall & Reavey, 2021). See Table 17-3 for types of CNS injuries related to intracranial hemorrhages and the Critical Component boxes for subgaleal hemorrhage and hypoxic ischemic encephalopathy.

Risk Factors for CNS Injuries

- Prematurity
- Birth trauma
- Breech delivery or other malpresentations
- Precipitous labor
- Difficult labor, traumatic delivery, operative delivery
- Hypoxia, asphyxia, hypotension, ischemia, or respiratory distress. Hypoxic events may be related to maternal, placental, or fetal causes (Hall & Reavey, 2021).

Medical Management

- Decrease risk for hypoxia, ischemia, and asphyxia during perinatal and intrapartal periods.
  - Identification and treatment of a compromised fetus may prevent asphyxiation and multiorgan damage (Ditzenberger, 2021).
- Neurological and behavioral evaluation
- Laboratory tests
  - Serum glucose level
  - Electrolyte levels
  - Arterial blood gas, lactate level
  - Blood, urine, CSF cultures
  - CBC with differential
- Computed tomography (CT) scan, ultrasonography, magnetic resonance imaging (MRI), and skull radiographs as indicated
- Lumbar puncture for CSF analysis if clinically indicated
- Electroencephalography to confirm occurrence of seizures and to identify presence and severity of brain damage if clinically indicated
- Neurology consultant as indicated
- Medications to treat seizure activity

Nursing Actions for CNS Injuries

- Review maternal prenatal and intrapartal histories for risk factors.
- Offer delivery room resuscitation.
- Interpret blood gases and laboratory values.
- Monitor vital signs, blood pressure, and perfusion.
- Monitor I&O.
- Administer blood products as ordered.
- Perform physical assessment, including evaluation of tone, reflexes, and behavior.
- Maintain respiratory support as needed.
- Obtain laboratory tests as ordered.
- Ensure that ordered diagnostic tests are completed.
- Assist with diagnostic procedures such as lumbar puncture.
- Administer medications as per order.
- Provide family support and information about the infant's status, treatment, and follow-up.

TABLE 17-3   Types of Central Nervous System Injuries: Intracranial Hemorrhages

	SUBDURAL HEMORRHAGE	SUBARACHNOID HEMORRHAGE	INTRACEREBELLAR HEMORRHAGE
Definition	Tear of the dura overlying the cerebellum or cerebral hemispheres	Intracranial hemorrhage into the CSF-filled space between the pial and arachnoid membranes on the surface of the brain Most common neonatal intracranial hemorrhage	Hemorrhage in the cerebellum from primary bleeding or from extension of intraventricular or subarachnoid hemorrhage into the cerebellum Occurs more commonly in preterm, LBW neonates
Pathophysiology	Excessive molding, stretching, or tearing of the falx and tentorium Stretching or tearing of the vein of Galen or cerebellar bridging veins	May occur because of trauma in a term neonate or hypoxia in a preterm neonate Venous bleeding in the subarachnoid space related to ruptured small vessels in the leptomeningeal plexus or bridging veins in the subarachnoid space	Breech presentation, difficult forceps delivery, external pressure over the occiput History of a hypoxic-ischemic insult Vitamin K deficiency Vascular factors
Manifestations	Symptoms may be delayed for first 24 hours, then: Seizures Decreased level of consciousness Asymmetrical motor function Full fontanel Irritability Lethargy Respiratory abnormalities Facial paralysis	Commonly there are no symptoms. Seizures may occur, starting on day 2 of life. Apnea may occur in preterm neonates.	Manifestations occur within the first 2 days to 3 weeks of life. Apnea Bradycardia Decreasing hematocrit Bloody CSF
Prognosis	Hydrocephalus Mortality rate 45% Hypoxic-ischemic injury	90% of babies with seizures will have normal follow-up. Abnormal outcome is rare.	Poorer outcome in preterm neonates than in term newborns Neurological deficits probable

Ditzenberger, 2021.

CRITICAL COMPONENT

Subgaleal Hemorrhage

Subgaleal hemorrhage is a type of extracranial hemorrhage. Unlike caput succedaneum and cephalohematoma (see Chapter 15), subgaleal hemorrhage can have devastating consequences to the newborn if not promptly recognized and aggressively treated. The subgaleal space is large enough to hold the neonate's entire total blood volume (Hawes et al., 2020). Subgaleal hemorrhage carries a risk of exsanguination, hypovolemic shock, and death.

- Pathophysiology: The condition is associated with vacuum extraction. Bleeding from rupture of the emissary vein causes blood to accumulate in the space between the epicranial aponeurosis and the periosteum. The periosteum is a membrane that wraps around bone. In a cephalohematoma, this membrane acts to enclose bleeding within the suture line, limiting its spread. In contrast, the subgaleal space is located above the periosteum so when bleeding occurs, there is no membrane to contain it.

- Clinical presentation: Firm scalp mass that crosses the suture line. A "fluid wave" may be present, which is a visible movement of fluid under the scalp with palpation. The ears can be displaced anteriorly due to the progressive spreading of edema. Edema can reach the nape of the neck and the orbits of the eyes. Lethargy, pallor, seizures, and shock may occur. Hematocrit level may drop rapidly.

- Assessments: Frequent assessment of heart rate, blood pressure, head circumference, level of consciousness, color, urine output, and capillary refill time. Monitor for presence of seizures by observation or with electroencephalography. Observe closely for signs of shock, kidney or other organ failure, and respiratory distress.

- Laboratory studies: CBC, TSB, and coagulation studies are ordered.
- Treatment: Central blood pressure monitoring, blood products, vasopressors, vitamin K, and phototherapy as indicated are common treatments.
- Outcome: When surviving hypovolemic shock, recovery can occur in 2 to 3 weeks (Ditzenberger, 2021).

CRITICAL COMPONENT

Hypoxic-Ischemic Encephalopathy

Definition: Neurological damage that occurs because of decreased oxygen and inadequate tissue perfusion to the neonatal brain and other organs.

Pathophysiology: Hypoxia or ischemia can be caused by an acute perinatal event such as placental abruption, umbilical cord prolapse, acute blood loss, uterine rupture, infection, cardiac arrest, or hypovolemic shock. Following the hypoxic insult, two phases of neuronal cell death occur. The primary phase occurs within the first 6 hours and is characterized by cellular necrosis. In the secondary phase, occurring between 6 and 15 hours, a complex series of processes occur that exacerbate the original injury. Implementing therapeutic hypothermia (see Evidence-Based Practice: Therapeutic Hypothermia) within the first 6 hours after the insult can reduce the severity of injury that can occur during the secondary phase of hypoxic-ischemic encephalopathy (HIE).

Clinical presentation: The infant is classified into one of three stages: mild, moderate, or severe encephalopathy. This designation is determined by the infant's physical examination including level of consciousness, activity, posture, tone, reflexes, and autonomic responses. The clinical decision to begin therapeutic hypothermia is based on the physical examination; blood gases (umbilical cord and neonatal); presence of seizures; need for respiratory support; and the history, including perinatal compromise, Apgar scores, and resuscitation required.

Laboratory studies: CBC, blood culture, serum electrolytes, glucose, lactate, blood urea nitrogen, creatinine, coagulation panel, and blood gases are often ordered (Gomella et al., 2020).

Evidence-Based Practice

Therapeutic Hypothermia

Jacobs, M., Berg, M., Hunt, R., Tarnow-Mordi, W. O., Inder, T. E., & Davis, P. G. (2013). Cooling for newborns with hypoxic-ischemic encephalopathy. Jacobs, S.E,, Berg M,, Hunt R., Tarnow-Mordi W.O., Inder T.E., & Davis P.G. (2013). Cooling for newborns with hypoxic ischaemic encephalopathy. *Cochrane Database of Systematic Reviews*, 1, 1–88. https://doi:10.1002/14651858.CD003311.pub3.

When oxygen delivery to the fetus or neonate is inadequate, brain metabolism can be compromised leading to HIE of the newborn. Hypoxia and insufficient blood flow can cause decreased tissue perfusion in the brain and other organs. Therapeutic hypothermia is used to treat mild to moderated HIE. In this procedure, the infant's core temperature is reduced to maintain a target of 33.5 degrees centigrade using a cooling blanket (in whole body cooling) or a cooling cap (in selective head cooling). The decision to treat with therapeutic hypothermia must be done within the first 6 hours after occurrence of the hypoxic insult. This decision is based on the physical examination of the infant; blood gases (umbilical cord and neonatal); presence of seizures; need for respiratory support; and history, including perinatal compromise, Apgar scores, and resuscitation required. After 72 hours, gradual rewarming slows the metabolic rate and provides neuroprotection, which reduces cerebral injury and cell death. This can improve outcomes after an HIE.

A Cochrane Review was conducted that analyzed 11 randomized controlled trials (RCTs) that evaluated the effectiveness of therapeutic hypothermia on neonatal outcomes. Therapeutic hypothermia was found to be statistically significant in reducing neonatal mortality and major neurodevelopmental disability and should be used to treat moderate to severe HIE in late preterm and term infants with HIE. The AAP and American College of Obstetricians and Gynecologists (ACOG) (2017) also recommend that based on the available evidence, therapeutic hypothermia should be used to treat neonatal encephalopathy.

INFANTS OF DIABETIC MOTHERS

Diabetes has increased in the United States in recent years in all women, including pregnant women. Up to 2% of pregnant women have type 1 (inability to produce insulin due to pancreatic cell destruction) or type 2 (insulin-resistant) diabetes. Diabetes that develops during pregnancy is called gestational diabetes and affects 6% to 9% of pregnant women (Centers for Disease Control and Prevention [CDC], 2018). Regardless of the type, maternal diabetes during pregnancy is associated with poor outcomes for the fetus and neonate (Armentrout, 2021). IDM may experience complications of high maternal levels of glucose during pregnancy such as:

- Congenital anomalies:
  - Cardiac anomalies, such as transposition of the great vessels, ventricular septal defect, hypertrophic cardiomyopathy, and aortic stenosis (Stavis, 2019b)
  - Skeletal defects, such as sacral agenesis, caudal regression, and neural tube defects
    - These defects occur two to four times more frequently than in the general population, thought to be due to the environment in utero during organ development before recognition of the pregnancy (Armentrout, 2021).
  - Small left colon syndrome and renal anomalies (Stavis, 2019b)
- IUGR, perinatal asphyxia, and SGA due to placental insufficiency (Armentrout, 2021)
- Neurological damage and seizures related to inadequate glucose supply to the brain due to neonatal hyperinsulinism

- Increased risk of juvenile insulin-dependent diabetes (Armentrout, 2021)
- Maternal obesity or gestational diabetes occurring early in pregnancy, which is associated with greater BMI at 1 year of age and increased obesity later in life (Page et al., 2019)

Assessment Findings

- Macrosomia
  - Defined as birth weight greater than or equal to 4,000 g. Increased birth weight is due to fetal exposure to elevated maternal glucose levels. In response to high glucose levels, the fetal pancreas produces insulin. Hyperinsulinemia results in increased fat production and growth (Stavis, 2019b)
- Fractured clavicle or brachial nerve damage
  - Macrosomic neonates are at risk for traumatic deliveries, including shoulder dystocia.
- Hypoglycemia
  - High levels of glucose in maternal circulation cause the fetus to produce increased levels of insulin. Glucose supply drops abruptly at birth while the neonate can continue to produce high levels of insulin resulting in hypoglycemia.
  - Present in up to 40% of IDMs. Incidence is higher in infants with mothers whose blood sugar was not well controlled in pregnancy (Gomella et al., 2020)
- Hypocalcemia and hypomagnesemia
- Polycythemia
  - Fetal hyperinsulinemia increases oxygen consumption, leading to increased RBC production in response to hypoxia (Gomella et al., 2020).
- Hyperbilirubinemia
  - Polycythemia increases the risk of hyperbilirubinemia.
- Low muscle tone, lethargy
- Poor feeding abilities
- Respiratory distress
  - Risk for RDS and transient tachypnea of the newborn (TTN) due to delay in surfactant production related to the high maternal glucose levels and fetal hyperinsulinemia (Armentrout, 2021)

Medical Management

- Assess for complications associated with maternal diabetes.
- Perform laboratory tests such as hematocrit, calcium, and magnesium levels.
- Perform x-ray examinations if clinically indicated for fractures or RDS.
- Perform echocardiogram if cardiac anomalies are suspected.
- Monitor blood glucose with a point of care glucometer. Abnormal results are confirmed by laboratory analysis of plasma glucose (Armentrout, 2021). If the neonate is hypoglycemic, blood glucose levels should be monitored 30 minutes after feeding to evaluate response to treatment.
- Early breastfeeding (by 1 to 2 hours of age) and frequent oral feedings of breast milk or formula is beneficial unless the neonate feeds poorly or is too sick to be fed orally. If oral feedings

are contraindicated or the neonate is hypoglycemic, there are two methods of treatment:

- 40% dextrose gel administered by syringe in the neonate's buccal cavity. A Cochrane Review concluded that 40% dextrose gel should be the first option for neonates with hypoglycemia in the first 48 hours of life (Weston et al., 2016).
- 10% dextrose and water are administered intravenously.

Nursing Actions

- Assess neonate for signs of respiratory distress, birth trauma, congenital anomalies, hypoglycemia, hypocalcemia, polycythemia, and hyperbilirubinemia.
- Monitor blood glucose per agency protocol.
  - May require intravenous fluids along with feedings to maintain adequate blood glucose levels.
- Provide early and frequent feedings to treat and prevent hypoglycemia.
  - May be passive, lethargic, and difficult to arouse.
  - Oral feeding skills must be assessed and supported.
  - Gavage feedings may be indicated.
- Obtain laboratory tests as per orders.
- Maintain an NTE to reduce energy needs.

NEONATAL INFECTION

Infections among neonates are a leading cause of morbidity and mortality (Wright, 2021). The immune system of a neonate is immature, placing the infant at risk for infection during the first several months of life. Table 17-4 lists maternal, neonatal, and environmental factors that predispose a neonate to infection.

Neonatal infections are caused by bacteria, viruses, arboviruses (Zika), fungus, yeast, spirochetes (syphilis), and protozoa. Infections may affect specific organ systems such as respiratory, urinary tract, brain, gastrointestinal tract, and skin, or local sites such as the umbilical stump and eyes. Depending on the type of infection, neonates may be asymptomatic at birth and develop symptoms within a few days of life, or their initial assessment reveals findings related to an infection such as microcephaly (cytomegalovirus [CMV] and Zika) or prominent rashes (chickenpox and rubella).

Neonatal sepsis is a clinical syndrome characterized by systemic illness and bacteremia occurring in the first 28 days of life (Gomella et al., 2020). It can be classified into three categories based on age of onset: early onset, late onset, and very late onset. Early-onset sepsis occurs within the first 7 days of life, or less than 72 hours in an infant less than 1,500 g (Gomella et al., 2020). It is a serious, overwhelming infection that is typically acquired through vertical transmission from the mother (Rudd, 2021). Late-onset sepsis occurs after 7 days of life, or over 72 hours in an infant less than 1,500 g (Gomella et al., 2020). It is associated with a lower mortality rate than early-onset sepsis. Very-late-onset sepsis affects premature and very-LBW babies after 3 months of age. This type of sepsis is related to long-term use of equipment such as indwelling catheters and endotracheal tubes (Rudd, 2021).

TABLE 17-4   Risk Factors for Neonatal Infection

MATERNAL FACTORS	NEONATAL FACTORS	ENVIRONMENTAL FACTORS
Poor prenatal nutrition	Prematurity	Length of stay in hospital
Low socioeconomic status	Birth weight <2,500 g	Invasive procedures
Substance abuse	Difficult delivery	Use of humidification in incubator or ventilatory care
History of sexually transmitted infection	Birth asphyxia	Routine use of broad-spectrum antibiotics
Recurrent abortion	Meconium staining	
Lack of prenatal care	Need for resuscitation	
Prolonged rupture of membranes (>12–18 hours)	Congenital anomalies	
Vaginal GBS colonization	Black neonates	
Chorioamnionitis	Male neonates	
Maternal temperature during labor and delivery	Multiple gestation	
Premature labor		
Difficult or prolonged labor		
Maternal urinary tract infection		
Invasive procedures during labor and delivery		
Maternal or fetal tachycardia		
Fetal scalp electrode use		

Rudd, 2021.

CRITICAL COMPONENT

Congenital Zika Virus

Zika is a virus transmitted through the bite of a mosquito or sexual contact with an infected person (CDC, 2019). Zika can be transmitted from mother to fetus through the placenta. In pregnancies whose mothers tested positive for the Zika virus, 5% to 10% gave birth to infants with birth defects associated with Zika (CDC, 2021).

Outcomes: Infection with Zika during pregnancy can result in a distinct pattern of birth defects called congenital Zika syndrome. The characteristics are severe microcephaly with partially collapsed skull; decreased brain tissue and subcortical calcifications; macular scarring and focal retinal pigmentary mottling; contractures such as clubfoot; and hypertonia. The infant can have cognitive, sensory, and motor disabilities (Moore et al., 2017).

Current recommendations: Initial CDC recommendations have been updated since Zika was first identified. Routine testing of asymptomatic pregnant women is not recommended. Symptomatic pregnant women (fever, rash, headache, joint pain, conjunctivitis, muscle pain) who have traveled recently to areas with a risk of Zika should be tested (CDC, 2019).

Neonates are exposed to infection via vertical or horizontal transmission (Rudd, 2021). Vertical transmission, passing of infection from mother to the baby, can occur in several ways:

- Transplacental transfer: Infection is transmitted to the fetus through the placenta (e.g., syphilis, CMV, and Zika).

- Ascending infection: Infection ascends into the uterus related to prolonged rupture of membranes.
- Intrapartal exposure: The neonate is exposed to infection during the birth process (e.g., herpes virus).
- Horizontal transmission (nosocomial infection) is transmitted from hospital equipment or staff to the neonate (Rudd, 2021).

GROUP B STREPTOCOCCUS

Group B *Streptococcus* (GBS) is the primary cause of neonatal meningitis and sepsis in the United States (ACOG Committee on Obstetric Practice, 2020; Puopolo et al., 2019). Approximately 20% to 30% of all pregnant women are asymptomatic carriers of GBS, found in the urogenital and lower gastrointestinal tract. Evidence supports the use of antibiotics during labor in women who have positive cultures for GBS during pregnancy to reduce vertical transmission of GBS and early-onset GBS sepsis (Puopolo et al., 2019). The CDC, AAP, ACOG, American Society for Microbiology (ASM), American College of Nurse-Midwives, and the American Academy of Family Physicians have collaboratively released new guidelines for the prevention, treatment, and detection of GBS.

- Regardless of planned mode of birth, all pregnant women should undergo antepartum screening for GBS at 36 0/7 to 37 6/7 weeks of gestation, unless intrapartum antibiotic prophylaxis for GBS is indicated because of GBS bacteriuria during the pregnancy or because of a history of a previous GBS-infected newborn.

- All women whose vaginal-rectal cultures at 36 0/7 to 37 6/7 weeks of gestation are positive for GBS should receive appropriate intrapartum antibiotic prophylaxis unless a prelabor cesarean birth is performed in the setting of intact membranes.
- Women with a positive prenatal GBS culture result who undergo a cesarean birth before the onset of labor and with intact membranes do not require GBS antibiotic prophylaxis.
- If the prenatal GBS culture result is unknown when labor starts, intrapartum antibiotic prophylaxis is indicated for women who have risk factors for GBS early-onset disease (EOD). At-risk women include those who present in labor with a substantial risk of preterm birth, who have preterm prelabor rupture of membranes (PPROM) or rupture of membranes for 18 or more hours at term, or who present with intrapartum fever (temperature 100.4°F [38°C] or higher). If intra-amniotic infection is suspected, broad-spectrum antibiotic therapy that provides coverage for polymicrobial infections and GBS should replace the antibiotic that provides specific coverage for GBS prophylaxis.
- If a woman presents in labor at term with unknown GBS colonization status and does not have risk factors that are an indication for intrapartum antibiotic prophylaxis but reports a known history of GBS colonization in a previous pregnancy, the risk of GBS EOD in the neonate is likely to be increased. With this increased risk, it is reasonable to offer intrapartum antibiotic prophylaxis based on the woman's history of colonization.
- Intravenous penicillin remains the agent of choice for intrapartum prophylaxis, with intravenous ampicillin as an acceptable alternative. First-generation cephalosporins (i.e., cefazolin) are recommended for women whose reported penicillin allergy indicates a low risk of anaphylaxis.
- Obstetric interventions, when necessary, should not be delayed solely to provide 4 hours of antibiotic administration before birth (ACOG, 2020).
- Intrapartum antibiotic prophylaxis is only considered adequate if the antibiotics are administered over 4 hours before delivery (Gomella et al., 2020).

Infants with early-onset GBS sepsis become symptomatic by 12 to 24 hours of age.

- Neonates of women who received adequate intrapartum antibiotic prophylaxis do not require routine antibiotic administration unless they exhibit signs of sepsis.
- Neonates born at 35 0/7 weeks' gestation or later may be assessed for risk of early-onset GBS infection using a multivariate model such as the Neonatal Early-Onset Sepsis Calculator (See Evidence-Based Practice: Neonatal Sepsis Calculator) or with enhanced clinical observation.
- Neonates born at 34 6/7 weeks' gestation or sooner are at highest risk for early-onset infection from all causes, including GBS, and may be best approached by using the circumstances of preterm birth to determine management.
- Early-onset GBS is diagnosed by blood and CSF culture. It is not well predicted in asymptomatic neonates by a CBC or C-reactive protein (CRP).

- Evaluation for late-onset GBS disease should be based on clinical signs of illness in the infant. Diagnosis is based on the isolation of GBS from blood, CSF, or other normally sterile sites. Late-onset GBS disease occurs among infants born to mothers who had positive GBS screen results as well as those who had negative screen results during pregnancy. Adequate intrapartum antibiotic prophylaxis does not protect infants from late-onset GBS disease.
- Empirical antibiotic therapy for early-onset and late-onset GBS disease differs by postnatal age at the time of evaluation. Penicillin G is the preferred antibiotic for definitive treatment of GBS disease in infants; ampicillin is an acceptable alternative (Puopolo et al., 2019).
- Neonates at any gestational age who exhibit signs of infection should be immediately and thoroughly evaluated by a provider and have a CBC with a differential, blood cultures,

---

Evidence-Based Practice

Neonatal Sepsis Calculator

Akangire, G., Simpson, E., Weiner, J., Noel-MacDonnell, J., Petrikin, J., & Sheehan, M. (2020). Implementation of the neonatal sepsis calculator in early-onset sepsis and maternal chorioamnionitis. *Advances in Neonatal Care: Official Journal of the National Association of Neonatal Nurses, 20*(1), 25–32. https://doi.org/10.1097/ANC.0000000000000668

Morris, R., Jones, S., Banerjee, S., Collinson, A., Hagan, H., Walsh, H., . . . Matthes, J. (2020). Comparison of the management recommendations of the Kaiser Permanente neonatal early-onset sepsis risk calculator (SRC) with NICE guideline CG149 in infants ≥34 weeks' gestation who developed early-onset sepsis. *Archives of Disease in Childhood. Fetal and Neonatal Edition, 105*(6), 581–586. https://doi:10.1136/archdischild-2019-317165

The use of the neonatal sepsis calculator (NSC) published by Kaiser Permanente and widely available for free online is rapidly increasing (Akangire et al., 2020). The calculator, based on maternal risk factors and physical examination of the neonate, identifies the infection risk level and guides treatment decisions around antibiotic administration. AAP/ACOG guidelines support its use (AAP & ACOG, 2017).

In this quality improvement project, the Plan-Do-Study-Act (PDSA) model was used to study antibiotic and blood culture use in a level III NICU. The rate of antibiotic use before implementation of the PDSA and sepsis calculator was 11% and blood cultures were done on 14.8% of live births. After implementation, the rate of antibiotic use significantly dropped to 5% ($p = .00069$) and blood culture use decreased to 7.6% ($p = .00046$).

The Morris et al. study compared the management decisions guided by the sepsis calculator to the National Institute for Health and Care Excellence (NICE) guidelines. This retrospective multicenter study found that both tools were poor at identifying early-onset sepsis within 4 hours of birth, but NICE was better at identifying asymptomatic cases than NSC. The study recommends that when using the NSC, enhanced nursing observation of the neonate is needed.

It is always important to remember that the use of tools must be supplemented with excellent observation and assessment skills for optimal patient safety.

and a chest x-ray if respiratory symptoms are present (Verklan, 2021). It is possible for infants to have early-onset GBS in the setting of adequate maternal intrapartum antibiotic prophylaxis (Puopolo et al., 2019). Antibiotics (ampicillin and gentamicin) should be started immediately after blood cultures are obtained (Gomella et al., 2020).

Neonates who are term, appear to be healthy, and whose mothers received 4 or more hours of antibiotic prophylaxis can be discharged after 24 hours if they meet all other discharge criteria.

SARS-COV-2

COVID-19 is one of several known coronaviruses. It was first identified in December 2019 in Wuhan, China (CDC, 2021) and is caused by the virus SARS-CoV-2, which is transmitted through respiratory droplets. Symptomatic and asymptomatic individuals, as well as those with mild symptoms, can transmit the virus. Currently it is thought that long-range aerosol transmission, as with tuberculosis and measles, does not occur. Symptoms include fever, chills, cough, dyspnea, fatigue, headache, nasal congestion, rhinorrhea, muscle aches, sore throat, new loss of taste or smell, nausea, vomiting, or diarrhea.

- The incubation period is estimated to be 2 to 14 days. However, it is possible to become infected and remain asymptomatic. Most cases are mild, and most patients, especially children and young adults, will recover without hospitalization.
- As of November 2020, two drugs, remdesivir, an antiviral drug, and baricitinib, used for rheumatoid arthritis, are approved for use in certain COVID-19 patients. Baricitinib received emergency use authorization (EUA) by the FDA for use in combination with remdesivir for hospitalized adult and pediatric patients 2 years and older requiring oxygen, mechanical ventilation, or ECMO. Remdesivir is approved for COVID-19 treatment requiring hospitalization. It remains an EUA for certain hospitalized pediatric patients (U.S. Food and Drug Administration, 2020).
- Maternal newborn care
  - Transmission of the SARS-CoV-2 virus to the neonate is thought to be primarily through droplet exposure during the postnatal period. Vertical transmission appears to be rare, and the clinical significance is unclear (CDC, 2020a).
  - Infections in neonates appear to be uncommon, and of those who are infected, symptoms are either absent or mild. Symptoms of fever, lethargy, rhinorrhea, cough, tachypnea, increased work of breathing, vomiting, diarrhea, and poor feeding have been reported, but it is difficult to determine if they are caused by SARS-CoV-2 or part of other underlying disease processes such as transient tachypnea of the newborn and RDS.
  - Testing of all neonates born to mothers with suspected or confirmed COVID-19 is advised, regardless of the presence or absence of neonatal symptoms (CDC, 2020a). The test performed should be for SARS-CoV2 RNA by reverse transcription polymerase chain reaction (RT-PCR), and can be collected from the nasopharynx, oropharynx, or nasal mucosa. Testing should be performed at 24 hours of age. If the result is negative or not available, it is repeated at 48 hours of age. In asymptomatic neonates who will be discharged before 48 hours of age, one test may be done before discharge at 24 to 48 hours of age.
  - A mother who has tested positive for COVID-19 should be isolated from other mothers and infants. If possible, the mother and her healthy term infant should room together. It is thought that the risk of transmission between mother and infant is low. Furthermore, rooming-in encourages breastfeeding and bonding and promotes family-centered care.
  - Because there is a small potential risk for a COVID-19 positive mother to infect her infant, education of the mother should be aimed at helping her to make an informed decision. Infection control measures must be taught to the mother who isolates with her infant including wearing a mask and practicing excellent hand hygiene. Masks are never to be placed on any child younger than 2 years of age. If the mother elects not to have her infant with her, the hospital's resources and policies will dictate the disposition of the infant.
  - Separation may be necessary if the mother is too ill to care for her infant, or the infant is medically unstable and requires a higher level of care.
  - A negative COVID test is not required for discharge of the infant from the hospital if the infant has otherwise met all criteria for discharge.
  - Close outpatient follow-up is required for neonates who are discharged home with suspected or confirmed COVID-19 infection (CDC, 2020a).

Assessment Findings for Neonatal Infections

- Signs of infection in a newborn are often nonspecific and subtle (Table 17-5).
- Laboratory findings suggestive of infection include:
  - Leukocytosis: An elevated WBC count (greater than 20,000/mm^3)
  - Leukopenia: A low WBC count (lower than 1,750/mm^3)
  - Neutrophilia: Increased neutrophil count
  - Neutropenia: Decreased neutrophil count (less than 1,800/mm^3) is strongly predictive of infection.
  - An immature to total neutrophil ratio (I/T ratio) greater than 0.20, known as a left shift, suggests infection. It indicates an increase in immature neutrophils.
  - Thrombocytopenia: Platelet count below 100,000/mm^3 can be related to viral infection or bacterial sepsis (Rudd, 2021).

Medical Management

- Free online sepsis calculators can be found online by searching "neonatal sepsis calculator" and may be useful in making treatment decisions (Refer to the Evidence-Based Practice: Neonatal Sepsis Calculator feature).

TABLE 17-5   Signs of Neonatal Infection

RESPIRATORY	THERMO-REGULATION	CARDIO-VASCULAR	NEUROLOGICAL	GASTRO-INTESTINAL	SKIN	METABOLIC
Apnea	Hypothermia	Bradycardia	Tremors	Poor feeding	Rash	Glucose instability
Grunting	Fever	Tachycardia	Lethargy	Vomiting	Pustules	Metabolic acidosis
Retractions	Temperature instability	Arrhythmias	Irritability	Diarrhea	Vesicles	
Tachypnea		Hypotension	High-pitched cry	Abdominal distention	Pallor	
Cyanosis		Hypertension	Hypertonia	Enlarged liver or spleen	Jaundice	
		Decreased perfusion	Hypotonia		Petechiae	
			Seizures		Vasomotor instability	
			Bulging fontanels			

Rudd, 2021.

- Laboratory tests to perform if the neonate exhibits signs of infection or is at risk for infection:
  - CBC may be performed, including a differential to evaluate WBC counts.
  - Microbial cultures of the blood, urine, and CSF may be performed.
  - Neonatal sepsis can be diagnosed definitively only with a positive blood culture (Gomella et al., 2020). Urine and CSF cultures may also be obtained when sepsis is suspected. Other cultures are obtained as clinically indicated (e.g., skin).
  - Serial CRP levels may be measured to detect inflammation associated with infection. Two CRP levels are drawn (8 to 24 hours after birth and 24 hours later) (Gomella et al., 2020).
  - Polymerase chain reaction testing for bacterial or viral DNA allows for identification of a specific bacterial or viral gene segment (Gomella et al., 2020).
  - Procalcitonin levels can be drawn. Procalcitonin is released in response to bacterial toxins and can aid detection of neonatal sepsis (Gomella et al., 2020).
- Antibiotic therapy, if indicated for suspected sepsis after cultures are obtained:
  - Antibiotics, such as ampicillin and aminoglycosides (usually gentamicin), that provide broad-spectrum coverage are often started initially (Gomella et al., 2020).
  - If culture results are negative, antibiotics will be stopped after 36 to 48 hours.
  - If sepsis is confirmed, antibiotics continue for 10 to 14 days, and 21 days for meningitis (Gomella et al., 2020).
  - If it is determined the infection is not bacterial in nature, appropriate antiviral or antifungal medications are ordered (Rudd, 2021).
  - The dosage and frequency of medication administration are dependent on the neonate's weight, gestational age, postnatal age, and liver and kidney function.
- Intravenous fluids, as well as parenteral nutrition or feedings
- Monitor glucose and electrolytes.
- Ventilation as indicated

Nursing Actions

- Assess maternal and neonatal histories for factors that may place a neonate at risk for infection, such as maternal GBS status.
- Monitor vital signs, I&O, and weight.
- Assess neonate for signs of infection (see Table 17-5).
  - Notify the physician if the neonate demonstrates signs of infection. Early recognition and treatment of neonatal infection is important in preventing morbidity and mortality.
- Provide respiratory support as needed.
- Monitor glucose and electrolytes.
- Obtain laboratory tests as per order.
- Assist with diagnostic tests such as lumbar puncture for CSF.
  - CSF is obtained and sent to a laboratory for a Gram stain and culture.
  - Holding the infant still in a flexed position is imperative for a successful lumbar puncture.
- Administer antibiotics as per orders.
- Administer feedings, intravenous fluid, and parenteral nutrition as per orders.
- Utilize standard precautions.
  - Wash hands before handling equipment and caring for the neonate.
  - Implement contact, droplet, or enteric precautions depending on diagnosis.
- Provide parents with information about the neonate's status; infection prevention strategies such as hand washing before contact with the baby; and diagnostic tests and treatments as appropriate.

SUBSTANCE ABUSE EXPOSURE

Substance abuse in the United States is a major public health concern. According to the 2019 National Survey on Drug Use and Health, 60.1% of people aged 12 or older self-reported using tobacco, alcohol, kratom, or an illicit drug during the past month (Substance Abuse and Mental Health Services Administration [SAMHSA], 2020). Data suggests that women in the United States account for 40% of the total number of people experiencing a lifetime drug use disorder (Forray, 2016). The use of tobacco, marijuana, prescription pain relievers, or illegal drugs during pregnancy is associated with two to three times the risk of stillbirth (National Institute on Drug Abuse [NIDA], 2020). A recent study by NIDA (2020) indicates that infants of mothers who have used tobacco and alcohol beyond the first trimester of pregnancy had a 12 times greater risk of sudden infant death syndrome (SIDS) than infants who were unexposed or only exposed in the first trimester. It is estimated that 5% of pregnant women use one or more of these substances (NIDA, 2020). Most drugs cross the placenta and affect the fetus (D'Apolito, 2021). Affecting the ability to research and evaluate the impact of maternal factors on neonatal outcomes are many confounding factors.

- Reliance on history obtained from the mother can potentially be inaccurate, and the tendency to withhold information from providers is understandably high.
- Urine drug testing does not provide accurate information about drug use throughout pregnancy.
- It is difficult to study the effects of a single drug, given that many people with substance abuse disorder also use tobacco, alcohol, and are often polydrug users (Gomella et al., 2020). The use of other substances such as tobacco and benzodiazepines in conjunction with an opioid may increase the risk and

severity of withdrawal symptoms experienced by the neonate (Patrick et al., 2020).
- Social and economic factors; systemic racism; maternal physical and mental health; and genetic or epigenetic, nutritional, and environmental factors may play a significant role in determining long- and short-term neonatal outcomes, making it impossible to attribute neonatal outcomes to drug exposure alone (Gomella et al., 2020; Patrick et al., 2020).

An infant born to a mother with a substance use disorder may experience a wide range of neonatal withdrawal symptoms (Gomella et al., 2020). These neonates are referred to as having neonatal abstinence syndrome (NAS) or neonatal opioid withdrawal syndrome (NOWS). Substances that cause NAS are listed on Table 17-6. Symptoms of neonatal abstinence reflect CNS irritability, neurobehavioral disorganization, and abnormal sympathetic activation (Gomella et al., 2020). Ideally, mothers should be screened for substance abuse during their first prenatal visit. Common substances used during pregnancy are as follows:

- Opioids (heroin, methadone, morphine, oxycodone, fentanyl)
  - Marked increase in use and related complications with three times as many opioids prescribed in 2015 than 1999. Heroin and fentanyl use have also increased, and overdoses have grown exponentially since 2011 (Patrick et al., 2020).
  - Widespread opioid use in the general population is mirrored by women during pregnancy. The CDC reports that in 2019, an estimated 14% to 22% of women filled a prescription for opioids during their pregnancy, whereas only

TABLE 17-6   Substances Causing Neonatal Abstinence Syndrome

OPIATES	BARBITURATES	MISCELLANEOUS
Codeine	Butalbital	Alcohol
Heroin	Phenobarbital	Amphetamine
Meperidine	Secobarbital	Chlordiazepoxide
Methadone		Cocaine
Morphine		Desmethylimipramine
Pentazocine		Benzodiazepines
Propoxyphene		Diphenhydramine
		Ethchlorvynol
		Fluphenazine
		Glutethimide
		Hydroxyzine
		Imipramine
		Meprobamate
		Phencyclidine
		Selective serotonin reuptake inhibitors (SSRIs)
		Caffeine

Gomella et al., 2020; NIDA, 2020.

6.6% self-reported opioid use during that time. One in five women who used prescription opioids during pregnancy indicated they misused the medication, and one in four indicated that they wanted or needed to reduce or stop their use (CDC, 2020c).

- Paralleling the rise in maternal opioid use is a higher incidence of NOWS, which increased from 1.2 to 8.8 per 100 hospital births between 2000 and 2016 (Patrick et al., 2020). The rates of opioid-exposed infants increased even more in rural and tribal areas, and in Medicaid patients. American Indian and Alaskan native infants are disproportionately affected by NOWS (Patrick et al., 2020).
- Signs of withdrawal are experienced by 60% to 90% of opiate-exposed infants (Gomella et al., 2020). Most infants display symptoms within 24 to 72 hours of life, but onset may be delayed up to 2 weeks, especially with maternal methadone use (Gomella et al., 2020; Patrick et al., 2020).
- Increased incidence of perinatal distress and fetal growth restriction
  - Lower birth weight and head circumference
  - Reduced incidence of RDS and hyperbilirubinemia
- NOWS is not caused by exposure to opioids around the time of delivery. Drug exposure must be chronic for the infant to exhibit symptoms (Patrick et al., 2020).
- NOWS symptoms vary depending on the type (immediate-release, sustained-release, or maintenance), the timing of the most recent exposure, the mother's metabolism, and use of other substances such as cigarettes, benzodiazepines and gabapentin which can influence the severity of NOWS (Patrick et al., 2020). Symptoms may persist for up to 6 months.
- Cocaine: CNS stimulant and sympathetic activator
  - Causes decreased placental blood flow and fetal hypoxemia.
  - Causes maternal hypertension and decreased cerebral blood flow to the fetus.
  - Associated with increased risk of spontaneous abortion, stillbirth, placental abruption, premature labor, and fetal growth restriction (Gomella et al., 2020).
  - Neonatal symptoms include irritability, tremors, hypotonia, high-pitched cry, hyperreflexia, frantic fist sucking, feeding problems, sneezing, tachypnea, and abnormal sleep patterns (Gomella et al., 2020).
  - Long-term effects can include problems with growth, inhibitory control, attention, language and motor skills, and abstract reasoning (D'Apolito, 2021).
- Alcohol: Considered a teratogen and readily crosses the placenta (AAP & ACOG, 2017). Spontaneous abortion, preterm birth, SGA, and stillbirth can occur. The IQ of children who are born to mothers who have consumed alcohol is variable, with some who exhibit cognitive disabilities and some who do not (D'Apolito, 2021).
  - Fetal alcohol syndrome disorder (FASD) can occur with heavy consumption of alcohol. An estimated 15 out of 10,000 infants born to women who consumed alcohol during pregnancy will have FASD (D'Apolito, 2021).
    - Short-term outcomes include irritability, hypotonia, hypertonia, tremors, twitching, and seizures.

- In preterm infants, intracranial hemorrhage and white matter CNS damage can occur (Gomella et al., 2020).
- Children can exhibit decreased IQ, learning disabilities, speech delay, attention disorders, hyperactivity, poor coordination, and facial dysmorphology including microcephaly, microphthalmos, short palpebral fissures, a poorly developed philtrum, thin upper lip, and hypoplastic maxilla (D'Apolito, 2021).
- Cannabis: Legality of cannabis in many states has posed challenges related to increased accessibility. Smoking marijuana is linked to lower birth weight. Conflicting evidence exists about long-term cognitive and behavioral outcomes in children (National Academies of Sciences, Engineering and Medicine [NAS], 2017).
  - Some research suggests that inhaled cannabis during pregnancy is associated with a negative impact on the fetal brain and adverse outcomes in infants, children, and adolescents (Graves, 2020).
  - Other studies found that children exposed to heavy use during the first trimester had decreased reasoning skills, hyperactivity, impulsivity, decreased attention, and lower scores in reading, math, and spelling (D'Apolito, 2021).
- Methamphetamine. Limited long-term studies are available. Heavy use is associated with anxiety, depression, attention disorders, visual motor processing, and alterations in striatum and frontal lobes of the brain on neuroimaging (Smid et al., 2019).
- Nicotine and smoking: Increased risk of placenta previa, placental abruption, premature rupture of membranes, and preterm birth
  - Infants can be of LBW and have defects of the mouth and lip.
  - SIDS is associated with smoking during pregnancy and in proximity to infant after birth. All members of household are advised to stop smoking (CDC, 2020e).
  - Nicotine use during pregnancy has been linked to altered pulmonary functioning through the first year of life, early menarche in female children, childhood obesity, and possibly lifelong decreased pulmonary function (Crume, 2019).
- SSRIs: Possible effects on children include increased anxiety at 36 months, possible increased risk of autism spectrum disorder (ASD), language difficulties, and alternations in executive functioning (D'Apolito, 2021).

CRITICAL COMPONENT

Signs of Neonatal Withdrawal
- Apnea
- Diarrhea or loose stools
- Excessive crying
- Excoriated skin
- Fever
- High-pitched cry
- Hyperreflexia
- Hypertonia
- Increased rooting reflex, frantic sucking

- Irritability or restlessness
- Lacrimation
- Nasal congestion, sneezing
- Poor feeding—uncoordinated or ineffectual suck and swallow
- Seizures
- Skin mottling
- Sleep problems and wakefulness
- Sneezing
- Sweating
- Tachypnea
- Tremors
- Vomiting or regurgitation
- Weight loss or failure to gain weight
- Yawning, hiccups (Gomella et al., 2020)

Medical Management

- Interdisciplinary approach to obtaining maternal history: Review drug history, trauma and violence, mental health, infectious diseases, and needs of the family.
- Identify neonates at risk.
- Perform physical assessment of the neonate, including observation for physical and behavioral effects of prenatal substance exposure.
- Perform toxicology screening of the neonate.
  - Should be done as soon as possible after birth, as many drugs are quickly metabolized (Patrick et al., 2020).
  - Meconium screening is the optimal method. It can detect drug use from 20 weeks' gestation but does not detect abstinence near delivery (Patrick et al., 2020).
  - Studies suggest that umbilical cord tissue testing may be an effective alternative to meconium testing (Patrick et al., 2020).
- Diagnostic tests such as cranial ultrasound and EEG, if indicated by clinical manifestations of withdrawal symptoms
  - Problems such as infection and hypoglycemia may manifest symptoms similar to those of neonatal withdrawal and should be ruled out by the appropriate diagnostic tests (Patrick et al., 2020).
- Assessment tools are useful to quantify the severity of signs and symptoms and guide treatment; however, more research comparing the efficacy of tools is needed to support evidence-based practice changes. Protocols should be in place to standardize practice within each agency (Patrick et al., 2020).
  - The Finnegan Neonatal Abstinence Scoring System (FNASS) score is the most commonly used system. Points are assigned producing a score that can help with pharmacological treatment decisions. Scores are obtained every 3 to 4 hours. Criticism includes a lack of interrater reliability, need for ongoing training, and subjectivity (Hein et al., 2021).
  - Eat, Sleep, Console (ESC) takes a holistic approach to scoring infants and encourages the parents to participate in much of the care. The tool has three components, which are assessed every 3 to 4 hours. If these conditions are not met, the provider and the caregivers meet to discuss possible pharmacological interventions. A significant decrease in NICU admissions, pharmacotherapy, and length of treatment was found using this method (Grossman et al., 2018).
    - Eat: Can the infant take 1 to 1.5 oz of formula or breast-feed effectively?
    - Sleep: Can the infant sleep for 1 hour (either independently or while being held by the caregiver)?
    - Console: Can the infant be consoled within 10 to 20 minutes?
- Observation of the neonate should be for at least 72 hours and up to 7 days depending on the drug exposure. More research is needed to determine appropriate observation periods (Patrick et al., 2020).
  - NICU is often the setting where observation takes place; however, studies have shown that rooming in with the mother, usually outside of the NICU environment, can decrease pharmacological interventions for NOWS and shorten length of hospital stay (MacMillan et al., 2018).
- Pharmacological therapy is considered for severe withdrawal, in addition to nonpharmacological interventions, to minimize complications such as severe weight loss and dehydration resulting from vomiting and loose stools (Patrick et al., 2020).
  - Morphine is the most common first-line therapy (Patrick et al, 2020).
  - Buprenorphine (Suboxone), methadone, clonidine, and phenobarbital are also used for opioid withdrawal (Patrick et al., 2020).
  - Benzodiazepines are used to treat withdrawal from alcohol.
- Frequent, small feedings with a high calorie formula (22 to 24 calories/oz.) are preferred.
- Monitor feedings, output, and weight daily.
- Engage in patient education regarding substance use and breastfeeding.
- An interdisciplinary team is needed to plan for the safe transition of the infant and family from hospital to home (Patrick et al., 2020). Mothers with substance abuse disorder disproportionately face economic and social challenges. Comprehensive follow-up care for the mother and infant is important to plan before discharge. Infants exposed to substances prenatally often need long-term interdisciplinary physical and developmental care (Patrick et al., 2020).
  - Referrals must be made to the appropriate departments and agencies. Notification of agencies such as Child Protective Services is dependent on the laws of each state, and under certain circumstances, neonates who are positive for prenatal substance exposure are placed in foster care.

Nursing Actions

- Review maternal history, including risk factors of substance use and history of current or past substance use.
- Assess the neonate, including gestational age.
- Assess for congenital anomalies and physical and behavioral signs of withdrawal or NAS.
- Monitor vital signs.

- Obtain toxicology screening as per order.
  - Urine or meconium sample may be ordered.
- Assess for signs of withdrawal on neonates who are at risk for NAS or NOWS:
  - If using the Finnegan scoring tool, notify the provider if the score is outside of what is considered normal.
  - If using the ESC approach, notify the provider if conditions are not met.
  - The provider's decision to treat with medication is based on the neonate's Finnegan score (if using) or ESC evaluation with interdisciplinary team input.

CLINICAL JUDGMENT

Breastfeeding and Substance Abuse Disorder

Breastfeeding is contraindicated in mothers with substance abuse disorder if they are taking illicit drugs, have polydrug abuse, or are infected with HIV (D'Apolito, 2021).

- Methadone and buprenorphine are excreted into human milk in low concentrations and breastfeeding may reduce clinical signs of NOWS. For this reason, breastfeeding is encouraged (Patrick et al., 2020).
- Some SSRIs are safe during breastfeeding. Sertraline (Zoloft) and paroxetine (Paxil) do not readily transfer to the milk. Fluoxetine (Prozac) has been found in high concentrations in breastfed infants of mothers taking the drug, so breastfeeding is discouraged (D'Apolito, 2021).
- The reliability of current research on breastfeeding and cannabis use has been limited due to small sample size, limited follow-up studies, and difficulty separating prenatal use from use during breastfeeding (Gomella et al., 2020; Graves, 2020).
- The primary psychoactive component of cannabis (delta 9-tetrahydrocannabinol or THC) has a long half-life and is stored in fat tissue, including breast milk in variable concentrations (U.S. National Library of Medicine, 2021).
- Research confirms THC stays in breast milk for up to 6 weeks (Wymore et al., 2021).
- Until more research is done regarding the long-term effects on the breastfeeding infant, the recommendation remains for pregnant women and those who intend to become pregnant to avoid both recreational and medicinal use of marijuana (D'Apolito, 2021).
- AAP and ACOG discourage marijuana use while breastfeeding until more substantive evidence can be found to the contrary (AAP & ACOG, 2017).

Substance abuse is a public health crisis and NAS and NOWS are downstream consequences of that crisis (Patrick et al., 2020). It is important to keep in mind that to solve the problem of NAS and NOWS, upstream structural causes, including systemic racism, must be addressed. Access to quality reproductive health care, contraception, public health systems such as prescription drug monitoring programs, and high-quality treatment for substance abuse disorders is needed. Prioritizing the health of our communities will lead to better health outcomes for our babies.

- Care for neonates experiencing NAS or NOWS:
  - Daily weights
  - Skin care, especially in the diaper area where skin can become excoriated from frequent loose stools
  - Provide frequent and small feedings with neonate positioned upright during and after to prevent regurgitation.
    - A higher calorie formula (22 to 24 cal/oz.) can be used to support increased caloric needs.
    - Use a slow flow nipple if the neonate has a strong, frantic suck.
    - Gavage feed if the neonate is unable to organize an effective suck or swallow.
  - Create a gentle, soothing environment for the neonate and caregivers:
    - 1:2 nurse–patient ratio
    - Volunteers to cuddle infants
    - Decreased light and noise
    - Swaddling, pacifier
    - Music therapy
    - Breastfeeding, prone positioning, rooming-in with parents
    - Warm, gentle bathing utilizing swaddling (swaddle-bath)
    - Minimized stress-inducing activities and procedures
    - Acupuncture has been found effective (D'Apolito, 2021).
- Care for the mother of a neonate with NAS and NOWS:
  - Ideally have the mother engage in routine newborn care during hospitalization.
  - Observe maternal-newborn interactions. Involve the mother in newborn care.
  - Provide nonjudgmental, honest, and supportive care, and be aware of potential caregiver implicit bias.
  - Start discharge teaching early and reinforce through hospitalization. Include:
    - Common behaviors (irritability, resistance to being comforted, arching while being held, altered sleep states, poor feeding behavior, easily agitated when stimulated, and difficult transitions from one state to another) and techniques for their management (calm, quiet environment, gentle rocking)
    - Feeding techniques
    - Safe infant sleep education
    - How and when to seek help if the infant's symptoms become unmanageable
    - How and when to seek help for maternal depression, relapse, and respite care

CONGENITAL ABNORMALITIES

Congenital anomalies or birth defects affect 1 in every 33 neonates born in the United States and are the leading cause of infant fatality, accounting for 20% of all infant deaths in the United States (CDC, 2020b). Congenital anomalies are the result of chromosomal abnormalities or environmental factors. Environmental factors include teratogens such as radiation, illicit substances, alcohol, diseases (e.g., diabetes), medications, and infections such as TORCH (see Chapter 7). Abnormalities range from being undetectable at birth to major and life-threatening issues.

Assessment Findings

- Table 17-7 lists common congenital anomalies.
- Table 17-8 lists common cardiac anomalies.
- Table 17-9 lists common metabolic disorders.

Nursing Actions

- Nursing care is determined by the type and severity of the anomaly.
- Genetic disease screening is obtained before discharge of the neonate.
- Provide emotional support for parents and family.
- Provide information on support groups.
- Provide information on the need for follow-up care.

TABLE 17-7 Common Congenital Anomalies

TYPE OF ANOMALY	INCIDENCE	DESCRIPTION	TREATMENT
Esophageal atresia or tracheoesophageal fistula	1 in 1,000–2,500 live births	Interruption in the esophagus Abnormal opening between the trachea and esophagus	Surgical repair
Diaphragmatic hernia	1 in 2,200–3,000 live births	Herniation of abdominal organs through a hole in the diaphragm into the thoracic cavity	Gastric decompression Stabilization Surgical repair
Omphalocele	2.5 in 10,000 live births	Herniation of abdominal contents through the umbilicus, which is covered by the peritoneal sac	Surgical repair Staged surgical repair for large defects (abdominal contents returned gradually)
Gastroschisis	1 in 10,000 live births	Herniation of abdominal contents through a hole in the abdomen, often to the right of the umbilicus	Surgical repair Staged surgical repair for large defects
Cleft lip and cleft palate	Overall, 1 in 500–550 live births	Medial and lateral nasal processes fail to fuse with maxillary process	Surgical repair
Spina bifida: meningocele Myelomeningocele	Overall 2 in 10,000 live births	A sac with meninges and CSF bulge through defect in undeveloped vertebrae A sac with meninges and nerve tissue bulge through a defect in the spinal column	Surgical repair Surgical repair
Anencephaly	1–10 in 1,000 live births	Incomplete formation of the cranium and brain	75% are stillborn and most babies die within a few days of birth
Developmental dysplasia of the hip	1–2 in 1,000 live births	Frank dislocation of the femoral head from the acetabulum	Pavlik harness to promote abduction or flexion to stabilize hip Surgery if Pavlik harness is not successful
Polydactyly	2 in 1,000 live births	Extra digits on the hand or foot	Surgery or ligation
Syndactyly	1 in 2,200 live births	Fusion of digits of hand or foot	Surgery depending on extent of anomaly
Talipes equinovarus	1 in 1,000 live births	Sole of the foot is turned in; the back part of the foot is deformed. Also called "clubfoot," usually bilateral.	Casting or splinting Surgery Treatment depends on severity

Bradshaw, 2021; Ditzenberger, 2021; Lubbers, 2021.

TABLE 17-8   Common Cardiac Anomalies

TYPE OF ANOMALY	INCIDENCE	DESCRIPTION	TREATMENT
Ventricular septal defect (VSD)	2 in 1,000 live births Most common, accounting for 37% of all CHDs	Opening in the septum between the right and left ventricles of the heart	About 90% of small defects close without treatment Treat with digoxin and diuretics if congestive heart failure is present. Surgical repair
Atrial septal defect (ASD)	1 in 5,000 live births	Opening in the septum between the right and left atria	ASDs may close without treatment. Treat congestive heart failure with medication. Surgical repair may be needed.
Coarctation of the aorta	1 in 1,800 live births	Narrowing of the aorta at the transverse aortic arch or near of the ductus arteriosus	Prostaglandin E1 to maintain patency of ductus arteriosus Medical management of congestive heart failure Surgical repair
Tetralogy of Fallot	1 in 5,000 live births	Consists of four defects: VSD Aorta overriding VSD Pulmonary stenosis Hypertrophy of the right ventricle	Medical management includes propranolol for cyanotic infants. Prostaglandin E1 may be administered to maintain a PDA until surgery, for infants with a severe tetralogy of Fallot. Surgical repair
Transposition of great vessels	1 in 5,000 live births	The positions of the great arteries are reversed from the normal position. Aorta emerges from the right ventricle, and the pulmonary artery emerges from the left ventricle.	This defect results in a medical emergency. Stabilization—treat acidosis Administer prostaglandin E1 to maintain a PDA until surgery is performed.

CDC, 2020b; Sadowski & Verklan, 2021.

TABLE 17-9   Common Genetic Disorders of Metabolism

TYPE OF DISORDER	INCIDENCE	DESCRIPTION	TREATMENT
Phenylketonuria	1 in 10,000 live births	Lack of the enzyme needed to convert phenylalanine to tyrosine. If untreated, causes cognitive and physical problems.	Diet that restricts intake of phenylalanine.
Disorders of fatty acid oxidation (e.g., medium chain acyl-CoA-deficiency)	1 in 5,000–10,000 live births	18 disorders identified. Impaired fat metabolism leads to hypoglycemia and organ failure.	Hypoglycemia is treated. Fasting is avoided.
Congenital adrenal hyperplasia	1 in 5,000–15,000 live births	Cortisol production is inhibited. Adrenal hypertrophy results, with excessive production of adrenal androgens. Electrolyte imbalances common, female infants exhibit ambiguous genitalia.	Steroid administration Corrective surgery for ambiguous genitalia.
Maple syrup urine disease	1 in 200,000	Lack of enzymes needed to metabolize leucine, valine, and isoleucine. These amino acids build up in the blood. Disease is fatal if untreated.	Peritoneal dialysis Low-protein diet
Galactosemia	1 in 60,000 live births	Lack of enzyme that converts galactose to glucose. Inability to metabolize lactose. If untreated, results in liver disease, mental retardation, and cataracts.	Lactose-free or soy formula.

Blackburn, 2021; Lubbers, 2021; Merritt et al., 2018.

REGIONAL CENTERS

Women experiencing complications during pregnancy may require transfer to a facility that can provide the appropriate level of care after delivery. Many facilities and communities lack resources to provide care for perinatal complications and critically ill neonates; thus, regional centers were developed to provide such services. Transport of a critically ill neonate to a center with a NICU requires coordination between transferring and receiving hospitals, a highly skilled team, appropriate preparation, and the appropriate equipment (Fig. 17–8).

The following are key considerations of neonatal transport:

- The transport team must be knowledgeable about neonatal complications and have expertise in caring for critically ill neonates (Price-Douglas & Rush, 2021).
  - The neonate is stabilized before transport.
- During transport, thermoregulation is maintained, respiratory support and IV therapy are provided, and the following are monitored:
  - Vital signs, oxygen saturation, blood glucose, the neonate's condition, pain status, and response to transport
- Strategies should be used to provide developmental care during transfer, such as protecting the neonate's eyes from bright lights, using ear protection in noisy vehicles such as helicopters, using a gel mattress to prevent jarring, and using blankets and positioning aids to promote containment.

DISCHARGE PLANNING

Discharge planning for infants with neonatal complications involves many considerations because these neonates often require special care and follow-up after release from the hospital. In some cases, infants require long-term evaluation to monitor health issues, growth, and neurodevelopment. Many neonatal conditions, such as prematurity and related complications, perinatal substance use, and congenital anomalies, have long-term or lifelong physical, cognitive, and behavioral consequences. The

following are critical components of the discharge process for neonates with complications (Hummel & Naber, 2021):

- Planning for discharge begins as the neonate is admitted to the NICU. Parents should be encouraged to be involved with the care of their infant from the time of admission. Care-related teaching with parents should begin as soon after delivery as possible.
- Interdisciplinary teams are often involved in the discharge process. The team may consist of physicians, nurse practitioners, nurses, social workers, occupational therapists, case managers, lactation consultants, respiratory therapists, nutritionists, pharmacists, and home health agency workers and nursing staff.
- The neonate's condition must be stable (e.g., weight gain, temperature stability, able to tolerate feedings, stable respiratory status) (Fig. 17–9).
- All appropriate examinations and screenings are completed, including an eye examination, genetic disease or metabolic disease screening, critical congenital heart disease screening, and a hearing screening.
- Pass the infant car seat challenge. The AAP recommends that all neonates born before 37 weeks undergo and pass an infant car seat challenge before discharge. The preterm neonate can have weaker airways and is thus more susceptible to breathing issues in a semi-reclined position. For a car seat challenge, the neonate:
  - Is secured snugly in an appropriately sized car seat (preferably the infant's own) for at least 90 to 120 minutes or the duration of travel, whichever is longer.
  - Must maintain adequate oxygenation, heart rate, and respiratory rate during trial.
- Family's readiness to take their infant home. The family's willingness and ability to provide care to their infant with special needs is evaluated, as are their financial resources. In addition, the home setting is assessed for safety and adequacy.

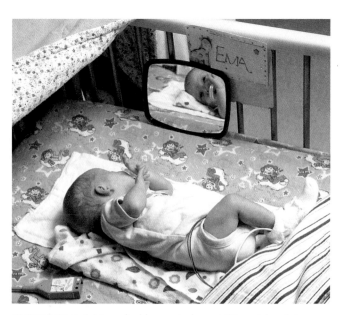

FIGURE 17–9 A 10-week-old neonate, born at 27 weeks' gestation, who will soon be going home.

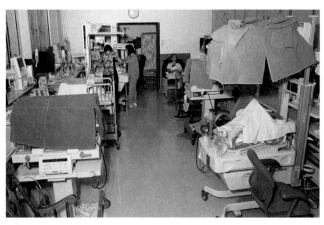

FIGURE 17–8 Neonatal intensive care unit.

- The educational needs of the family are met. Discharge teaching includes:
  - General infant care, such as bathing, feeding, diapering, and skin care
  - Safety issues, such as car seat safety, back to sleep positioning for sleep, infant CPR, babyproofing the house, and shaken baby syndrome prevention
  - Instructions on use of required equipment (e.g., apnea monitoring)
  - Information on treatments (e.g., oxygen, suctioning) and medications ordered
  - Signs of illnesses that must be reported to the primary care provider
  - Infant growth and developmental milestones
  - Follow-up information, including visits with the pediatrician, immunization schedules, and referrals to the appropriate medical and developmental specialists

PSYCHOSOCIAL NEEDS OF PARENTS WITH NEONATES IN THE NICU

The birth of a baby who is premature or has conditions that create risk for illness or death is a significant stressor for the family. Parents may grieve over the loss of an ideal baby and find the experience of having a baby with complications overwhelming. It is devastating for most parents when the mother is discharged and the baby must remain in the hospital.

Common effects on the parents and family are:

- Delay of the attachment process due to the separation of the parent and newborn, which can place the newborn at risk for abuse and neglect
- Guilty feelings by the mother, who may feel she did something wrong to cause her newborn to be ill
- Emotional distancing of parents from their newborn as a protective mechanism due to fear of their child's death
- Anger at the loss of control of having an ill or premature newborn
- Disappointment at not being able to bring their newborn home
- Disruption of family life; parents needing to return to work, caring for other children, and at the same time wanting to spend time in the hospital with their newborn

Nursing Actions

- Orient parents to the NICU environment by explaining equipment used for their newborn.
- Assess parents' comfort level with the NICU environment.
- Provide opportunities for parents to share their concerns and frustrations by developing a trusting rapport with them.
- Provide opportunities for parents to discuss their experiences by asking how they are coping.
- Provide information regarding their neonate's status to parents at an understandable level.

- Inform parents that they should ask any questions they have regarding the condition and care of their neonate.
- Inform parents that they can talk to their neonate's nurse at any time.
- Assess the parents' readiness to care for their neonate and provide opportunities for them to participate in care.
- Encourage parents to touch and hold their child as indicated by the neonate's health status.
- Encourage the mother to pump her breasts and bring the milk to the NICU for feeding.
- Review breast milk storage and provide equipment as needed.
- Provide a private area for the mother to breastfeed when the neonate is able to nurse.
- Encourage parents to take photos to share with their family and friends.
- Praise parents for their involvement in the neonate's care.
- Provide information on support groups for parents of preterm neonates or neonates with disabilities.

LOSS AND GRIEF

When an infant dies, parents must work through profound grief associated with the death of their child and the loss of their hopes and dreams for that child and their family. Grief is an individual process, and members of the family will experience it in different ways and in varied timelines. Signs of grief include sadness and despair, denial, numbness, shock, disbelief, and anger, as well as fatigue and sleep disturbances (Kenner & Boykova, 2021).

Nurses must keep in mind that each person experiences and expresses grief in their own way. Culture, religion, and personal experience and beliefs will impact how individuals and families respond to loss. Nurses can help families that are grieving the death of their newborn with the following measures:

- Allow parents to express their feelings by being present and listening.
- Express empathy and condolences. Avoid trite phrases such as, "At least you are young; you can have another baby."
- Refer to the baby by name if the child has been named.
- Provide information about the grieving process and what to expect physically and emotionally.
- Provide ample opportunity for the parents and family members to spend time with the baby before and after the child dies.
- Provide parents with memorabilia associated with their baby, such as pictures, blankets, a hat, a lock of hair, ID bracelet, footprints, and crib card.
- Offer to contact the hospital chaplain. Encourage the family to contact their own clergy or spiritual leader. Explore the family's desire for baptism or other religious rites.
- Discuss the family's plan for autopsy, a memorial or funeral, and burial or cremation.
- Encourage the family to accept help and support from others.
- Refer parents to community services and support groups that may assist in facilitating the grief process (Kenner & Boykova, 2021).

Clinical Pathway for the Preterm Infant

	Birth to First Hour	1 to 24 Hours of Age	24 Hours of Age to Discharge
Assessments	Review prenatal record to determine projected gestational age.	Complete gestational assessment as per hospital policy.	Assess every 2–4 hours or per hospital policy.
	Obtain Apgar score at 1 and 5 minutes.	Assess every 1–2 hours or per hospital policy.	Weigh the neonate every day or per hospital policy.
	Obtain weight, length, and head circumference.		Obtain length and head circumference weekly or per hospital policy.
	Complete neonatal assessment.		
Thermoregulation	Place neonate on preheated radiant warmer and dry gently immediately after birth.	Prevent heat loss by maintaining an NTE.	Prevent heat loss by maintaining an NTE.
	Cover head with warmed hat.	Assess axillary temperature every 1–2 hours or per hospital policy.	Encourage skin-to-skin contact or kangaroo care when neonate is stable.
	Per hospital policy, wrap in dry, warmed blankets; place in a polyethylene wrap or on a chemical mattress for transport to the NICU.	Assess for cold stress symptoms.	Dress neonate when in an open crib.
		Postpone bathing until neonate is stable.	Assess axillary temperature every 2–4 hours or per hospital policy.
	Place in a preheated radiant warmer or a thermoregulated incubator.		Provide heat source when bathing.
	Assess axillary temperature every 15–30 minutes or per hospital policy.		Assess for cold stress symptoms.
			Teach parents to assess temperature and signs of cold stress.
Respiratory	Clear the nose and mouth of mucus with the use of a bulb syringe.	Assess for signs of respiratory distress: grunting, flaring, and retractions.	Assess for signs of respiratory distress: grunting, flaring, and retractions.
	Immediately after birth, assess the neonate for respiratory effort and provide resuscitation as needed.	Assess lung sounds.	Assess lung sounds.
	Apply pulse oximeter and monitor values.	Provide respiratory support and administer oxygen as needed.	Provide respiratory support and administer oxygen as needed.
	Assess for signs of respiratory distress: grunting, flaring, and retractions.	Monitor pulse oximeter values.	Monitor pulse oximeter values.
	Assess lung sounds.	Obtain chest x-ray and blood gases as ordered.	Obtain chest x-ray and blood gases as ordered.
	Provide respiratory support and administer oxygen as needed.	Monitor I&O.	Monitor I&O.
	Obtain chest x-ray and blood gases as ordered.		Obtain daily weights.
			Teach parents signs and symptoms of respiratory distress.
			Teach parents oxygen management if neonate is to be discharged with oxygen.
Cardiovascular	Assess skin color for cyanosis.	Assess skin color for cyanosis.	Assess skin color for cyanosis.
	Assess heart rate at birth, and at 1 and 5 minutes of age.	Assess heart rate and rhythm every 1–2 hours or per hospital policy.	Assess heart rate and rhythm every 2–4 hours or per hospital policy.
	Assess heart rate and rhythm every 15–30 minutes or per hospital policy thereafter.	Continue on cardiorespiratory monitor for continuous observation.	Continue on cardiorespiratory monitor for continuous observation.
	Place on cardiorespiratory monitor for continuous observation.		Teach parents CPR when neonate is close to discharge.

Clinical Pathway for the Preterm Infant—cont'd

	Birth to First Hour	1 to 24 Hours of Age	24 Hours of Age to Discharge
Nutrition	Obtain and monitor blood glucose levels per hospital policy. Obtain intravenous access and administer parenteral nutrition if ordered.	Obtain and monitor blood glucose levels per hospital policy. Administer parenteral or enteral nutrition as ordered. Encourage mother to begin pumping to supply breast milk for neonate. Encourage kangaroo care to enhance milk supply. Use non-nutritive sucking with tube feedings. Monitor for signs of feeding intolerance. Monitor I&O.	Obtain and monitor blood glucose levels per hospital policy. Administer parenteral or enteral nutrition as ordered. Encourage kangaroo care to enhance milk supply. Use non-nutritive sucking with tube feedings. Monitor for signs of feeding intolerance. As neonate matures, assess for signs of readiness for oral feedings. Monitor I&O. Monitor daily weights. Teach parents proper techniques for breastfeeding or bottle feeding their neonate.
Sepsis	Obtain maternal history for risk factors. Obtain CBC and blood cultures as ordered. Administer antibiotics as ordered. Assess for signs of sepsis.	Assess for signs of sepsis. Administer antibiotics as ordered.	Assess for signs of sepsis. Administer antibiotics as ordered. Teach parents strategies to prevent infection.

CONCEPT MAP

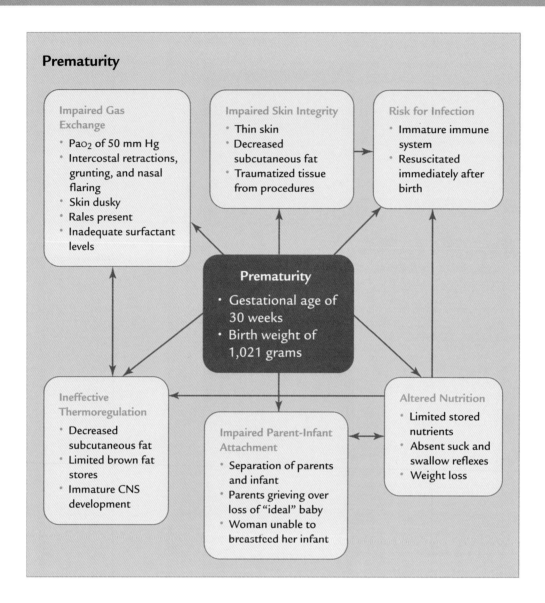

Prematurity

Impaired Gas Exchange
- Pao₂ of 50 mm Hg
- Intercostal retractions, grunting, and nasal flaring
- Skin dusky
- Rales present
- Inadequate surfactant levels

Impaired Skin Integrity
- Thin skin
- Decreased subcutaneous fat
- Traumatized tissue from procedures

Risk for Infection
- Immature immune system
- Resuscitated immediately after birth

Prematurity
- Gestational age of 30 weeks
- Birth weight of 1,021 grams

Ineffective Thermoregulation
- Decreased subcutaneous fat
- Limited brown fat stores
- Immature CNS development

Impaired Parent-Infant Attachment
- Separation of parents and infant
- Parents grieving over loss of "ideal" baby
- Woman unable to breastfeed her infant

Altered Nutrition
- Limited stored nutrients
- Absent suck and swallow reflexes
- Weight loss

CARE PLANS

Problem 1: Impaired gas exchange
Goal: Adequate gas exchange
Outcome: Pao₂ is 60 to 70 mm Hg; Paco₂ is 35 to 45 mm Hg; skin color is pink; lung sounds are clear; and no signs of retractions, grunting, or nasal flaring.

Nursing Actions
1. Monitor vital signs, oxygen saturation, and arterial blood gases.
2. Maintain patent airway.
3. Suction airway as indicated.
4. Administer oxygen as per orders.
5. Maintain an NTE.
6. Cluster nursing activities.
7. Monitor for adverse effects related to surfactant replacement therapy.

Problem 2: Impaired skin integrity
Goal: Intact skin
Outcome: The neonate's skin will be intact and without signs of skin irritation.

Nursing Actions
1. Assess skin for redness, dryness, breakdown, and rashes.
2. Use a neutral pH cleanser and sterile water when bathing.
3. Use adhesives sparingly.
4. Apply emollient to dry areas.
5. Change diapers frequently.
6. Change positions frequently.

Problem 3: Risk of infection

Goal: Be free of infection

Outcome: Neonates will not exhibit signs of infection such as temperature instability, increased apnea, lethargy, feeding intolerance, or purulent drainage.

Nursing Actions

1. Promote hand washing for staff and parents.
2. Assess for signs of infection.
3. Maintain intact skin.
4. Properly prepare sites for invasive procedures.
5. Properly care for invasive lines to maintain sterility.
6. Administer antibiotics as per orders.
7. Encourage use of breast milk for infant feedings.

Problem 4: Ineffective thermoregulation

Goal: Stable temperature within normal range

Outcome: Neonate's temperature will be between 97.7°F and 99.5°F (36.5°C and 37.5°C).

Nursing Actions

1. Keep the neonate dry.
2. Use plastic barriers when indicated.
3. Prewarm all supplies and equipment.
4. Monitor temperature every 2 to 4 hours and adjust environment as needed.
5. Encourage kangaroo care.
6. Keep area free of drafts.
7. Swaddle the neonate when holding outside of warmer or incubator.

Problem 5: Altered nutrition

Goal: Growth and weight gain within normal ranges

Outcome: Neonate will gain 20 to 30 grams per day.

Nursing Actions

1. Administer parenteral nutrition, enteral feedings, or oral feedings as per orders.
2. Encourage use of breast milk.
3. Monitor weight daily.
4. Monitor length and head circumference weekly.
5. Monitor the neonate during feedings for signs of feeding intolerance, such as vomiting, regurgitation, and excessive gastric residual.
6. Encourage breastfeeding when indicated.
7. Monitor I&O.
8. Allow for rest periods between feedings.

Problem 6: Impaired parent–infant attachment

Goal: Positive parent–infant attachment

Outcome: Parents hold the infant close to the body and the infant appears calm and relaxed; parents spend time each day with the infant, participate in care, and respond to infant cues.

Nursing Actions

1. Orient parents to the NICU environment.
2. Provide opportunities for parents to share their concerns and frustrations.
3. Provide opportunities for parents to talk about experiences having a baby in the NICU.
4. Assess parents' readiness to care for their baby and provide opportunities for participation in their baby's care.
5. Instruct parents on neonatal care.
6. Praise parents for their involvement.
7. Encourage the mother to pump her breasts and bring breast milk for infant feeding.
8. Encourage kangaroo holding by both parents.

Case Study

Baby girl Polk is a newly delivered 32 weeks' gestation neonate who is admitted to the NICU. Her mother, Mallory, is a 42-year-old Black single woman. Mallory is a G2 P0 who conceived after three attempts at in vitro fertilization. Mallory was admitted to the birthing unit for preterm labor. She was given magnesium sulfate, ampicillin, and two doses of betamethasone. Her labor continued. When her cervix was 5 cm dilated, a decision was made to discontinue the magnesium sulfate. A few hours after the magnesium sulfate was discontinued, Mallory gave birth spontaneously to a baby girl. The 1- and 5-minute Apgar scores were 7 and 8, respectively. Baby Polk weighed 2,010 g and was assessed at 32 weeks based on the Ballard score.

Detail the aspects of your initial nursing assessment.

List the nursing diagnosis for this neonate.

What are the immediate priorities in the nursing care of Baby Polk?

Discuss the rationale for the selected priorities.

List the anticipated medical care for Baby Polk.

Four hours later:
Baby Polk is on NCPAP. There is an increase in intercostal retractions and expiratory grunting. Results of arterial blood gas tests are P_{CO_2} of 70 and pH of 7.2. CBC indicates increase in WBC.

Medical orders include initial dose of Survanta after intubation, IV of $D_{10}W$, glucose monitoring every 4 hours, ampicillin 50 mg/kg, and gentamicin 4 mg/kg.

Based on this additional information, list the nursing diagnosis for this neonate.

List the anticipated medical care.

Discuss the nursing care for this neonate and mother.

One week later:
Baby Polk is extubated and is placed on an HFNC at 2 L. She is tolerating gavage feedings and gaining weight, experiencing occasional episodes of apnea and bradycardia.

Discuss the criteria for discharge from the NICU.

Describe the discharge teaching for the care of Baby Polk.

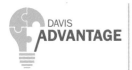

Go to Davis Advantage to complete your learning: strengthen understanding, apply your knowledge, and prepare for the Next Gen NCLEX®.

REFERENCES

Akangire, G., Simpson, E., Weiner, J., Noel-MacDonnell, J., Petrikin, J., & Sheehan, M. (2020). Implementation of the neonatal sepsis calculator in early-onset sepsis and maternal chorioamnionitis. *Advances in Neonatal Care, 20*(1), 25–32. https://doi.org/10.1097/ANC.0000000000000668

Altobelli, E., Angeletti, P. M., Verrotti, A., & Petrocelli, R. (2020). The impact of human milk on necrotizing enterocolitis: A systematic review and meta-analysis. *Nutrients, 12*(5), 1–13. https://doi.org/10.3390/nu12051322

American Academy of Pediatrics. (2004). Management of hyperbilirubinemia in the newborn infant 35 or more weeks of gestation. *Pediatrics, 114*(4), 297–316. https://doi.org/10.1542/peds.114.1.297

American Academy of Pediatrics. (2016). *Textbook of neonatal resuscitation* (7th ed.). American Academy of Pediatrics.

American Academy of Pediatrics & American College of Obstetricians and Gynecologists. (2017). *Guidelines for perinatal care* (8th ed.). American Academy of Pediatrics.

American College of Obstetricians and Gynecologists Committee on Obstetric Practice. (2020). Prevention of group B streptococcal early-onset disease in newborns. Committee Opinion No. 797. *Obstetrics & Gynecology, 135*(2), e51–e72. https://www.acog.org/-/media/project/acog/acogorg/clinical/files/committee-opinion/articles/2020/02/prevention-of-group-b-streptococcal-early-onset-disease-in-newborns.pdf

Armentrout, D. (2021). Glucose management. In M. T. Verklan, M. Walden, & S. Forest (Eds.), *Core curriculum for neonatal intensive care nursing* (6th ed., pp. 144–151). Elsevier.

Balest, A. L. (2019a). *Bronchopulmonary dysplasia (BPD).* Merck Manual Professional Version. https://www.merckmanuals.com/professional/pediatrics/respiratory-problems-in-neonates/bronchopulmonary-dysplasia-bpd

Balest, A. L. (2019b). *Respiratory distress syndrome in neonates.* Merck Manual Professional Version. https://www.merckmanuals.com/professional/pediatrics/respiratory-problems-in-neonates/respiratory-distress-syndrome-in-neonates

Bancalari, E. H., & Walsh, M. C. (2015). Bronchopulmonary dysplasia. In R. J. Martin, A. A. Fanaroff, & M. C. Walsh (Eds.), *Neonatal perinatal medicine: Diseases of the fetus and infant* (10th ed., vol. 2, pp. 1157–1169). Mosby Elsevier.

Beerman, L. B. (2020). *Patent ductus arteriosus (PDA).* Merck Manual Professional Version. https://www.merckmanuals.com/professional/pediatrics/congenital-cardiovascular-anomalies/patent-ductus-arteriosus-pda

Bell, S. G. (2021). Fluid and electrolyte management. In M. T. Verklan, M. Walden, & S. Forest (Eds.), *Core curriculum for neonatal intensive care nursing* (6th ed., pp. 131–143). Elsevier.

Bhutani, V. K., Johnson, L., & Sivieri, E. M. (1999). Predictive ability of a predischarge hour-specific serum bilirubin for subsequent significant hyperbilirubinemia in healthy term and near-term newborns. *Pediatrics, 103*(1), 6–14. https://doi.org/10.1542/peds.103.1.6

Blackburn, S. T. (2021). Endocrine disorders. In M. T. Verklan, M. Walden, & S. Forest (Eds.), *Core curriculum for neonatal intensive care nursing* (6th ed., pp. 543–567). Elsevier.

Bradshaw, W. (2021). Gastrointestinal disorders. In M. T. Verklan, M. Walden, & S. Forest (Eds.), *Core curriculum for neonatal intensive care nursing* (6th ed., pp. 504–542). Elsevier.

Brand, M. C., & Shippey, H. A. (2021). Thermoregulation. In M. T. Verklan, M. Walden, & S. Forest (Eds.), *Core curriculum for neonatal intensive care nursing* (6th ed., pp. 86–98). Elsevier.

Cartwright, J., Atz, T., Newman, S., Mueller, M., & Demirci, J. M. (2017). Integrative review of interventions to promote breastfeeding in the late preterm infant. *Journal of Obstetric, Gynecologic, and Neonatal Nursing, 46*(3), 347–356. https://doi.org/10.1016/j.jogn.2017.01.006

Centers for Disease Control and Prevention. (2018, June 12). *Diabetes during pregnancy.* https://www.cdc.gov/reproductivehealth/maternalinfanthealth/diabetes-during-pregnancy.htm

Centers for Disease Control and Prevention. (2019, December 9). *Zika and dengue testing guidance.* https://www.cdc.gov/zika/hc-providers/testing-guidance.html

Centers for Disease Control and Prevention. (2020a, December 8). *Evaluation and management considerations for neonates at risk for COVID-19.* https://www.cdc.gov/coronavirus/2019-ncov/hcp/caring-for-newborns.html

Centers for Disease Control and Prevention. (2020b, November 17). *Facts about coarctation of the aorta.* https://www.cdc.gov/ncbddd/heartdefects/coarctationofaorta.html

Centers for Disease Control and Prevention. (2020c, July 17). *Prescription opioid pain reliever use during pregnancy.* https://www.cdc.gov/mmwr/volumes/69/wr/mm6928a1.htm

Centers for Disease Control and Prevention. (2020d, June 11). *Prevention guidelines.* https://www.cdc.gov/groupbstrep/guidelines/index.html?CDC_AA_refVal=https%3A%2F%2Fwww.cdc.gov%2Fgroupbstrep%2Fclinicians%2Fqas-obstetric.html

Centers for Disease Control and Prevention. (2020e, July 15). *Substance use during pregnancy.* https://www.cdc.gov/reproductivehealth/maternalinfanthealth/substance-abuse/substance-abuse-during-pregnancy.htm#:~:text=Smoking%20during%20pregnancy%20increases%20the,infant%20death%20syndrome%20(SIDS)

Centers for Disease Control and Prevention. (2021c, February 26). *Overview and infection prevention and control priorities in non-US healthcare settings.* https://www.cdc.gov/coronavirus/2019-ncov/hcp/non-us-settings/overview/index.html

Chowdhury, A. S., Rahman, E. M., Hossain, F., Parvez, A. F. M., Hassan, M. K., Munmun, F., & Begum, P. (2019). Association of serum electrolyte abnormalities in preterm low birthweight infants. *Faridpur Medical College Journal, 14*(1), 31–33.

Churchman, L. (2021). Apnea. In M. T. Verklan, M. Walden, & S. Forest (Eds.), *Core curriculum for neonatal intensive care nursing* (6th ed., pp. 417–424). Elsevier.

Cochran, W. J. (2020). *Necrotizing enterocolitis.* Merck Manual Professional Version. https://www.merckmanuals.com/professional/pediatrics/gastrointestinal-disorders-in-neonates-and-infants/necrotizing-enterocolitis

Crume, T. (2019). Tobacco use during pregnancy. *Clinical Obstetrics & Gynecology, 62*(1), 128–141. https://doi.org/10.1097/GRF.0000000000000413

Curley, M. A. Q., Hasbani, N. R., Quigley, S. M., Stellar, J. J., Pasek, T. A., Shelley, S. S., . . . Wypij, D. (2018). Predicting pressure injury risk in pediatric patients: The Braden QD Scale. *The Journal of Pediatrics, 192u*, 189–195. https://doi.org/10.1016/j.jpeds.2017.09.045

D'Apolito, K. (2021). Perinatal substance abuse. In M. T. Verklan, M. Walden, & S. Forest (Eds.), *Core curriculum for neonatal intensive care nursing* (6th ed., pp. 38–53). Elsevier.

Diehl-Jones, W., & Fraser, D. (2021). Hematologic disorders. In M. T. Verklan, M. Walden, & S. Forest (Eds.), *Core curriculum for neonatal intensive care nursing* (6th ed., pp. 568–587). Elsevier.

Ditzenberger, G. (2021). Neurological disorders. In M. T. Verklan, M. Walden, & S. Forest (Eds.), *Core curriculum for neonatal intensive care nursing* (6th ed., pp. 629–653). Elsevier.

Donneborg, M. L., Vandborg, P. K., Hansen, B. M., Rodrigo-Domingo, M., & Ebbesen, F. (2018). Double versus single intensive phototherapy with LEDs in treatment of neonatal hyperbilirubinemia. *Journal of Perinatology, 38*(2), 154–158. https://doi.org/10.1038/jp.2017.167

Ely, D. M., & Driscoll, A. K. (2020). Infant mortality in the United States, 2018: Data from the period linked birth/infant death file. *National Vital Statistics Reports, 69*(7).

Forest, S. (2021). Care of the extremely low birth weight infant. In M. T. Verklan, M. Walden, & S. Forest (Eds.), *Core curriculum for neonatal intensive care nursing* (6th ed., pp. 377–387). Elsevier.

Forray, A. (2016). Substance use during pregnancy [version 1; peer review: 2 approved]. *F1000 Research, 5*(F1000 Faculty Rev), 887. https://doi.org/10.12688/f1000research.7645.1

Foster, J. P., Psaila, K., & Patterson, T. (2016). Non-nutritive sucking for increasing physiologic stability and nutrition in preterm infants. *Cochrane Database of Systematic Reviews, 10.* https://doi.org/10.1002/14651858.CD001071.pub3

Fraser, D. (2021). Respiratory distress. In M. T. Verklan, M. Walden, & S. Forest (Eds.), *Core curriculum for neonatal intensive care nursing* (6th ed., pp. 394–416). Elsevier.

Goenka, A., Yozawitz, E., Gomes, W. A., & Nafday, S. M. (2020). Selective head versus whole body cooling treatment of hypoxic-ischemic encephalopathy: Comparison of electroencephalogram and magnetic resonance imaging findings. *American Journal of Perinatology, 37*(12), 1264–1270. https://doi.org/10.1055/s-0039-1693466

Gomella, T. L., Eyal, F. G., & Bany-Mohammed, F. (2020). *Gomella's neonatology: Management, procedures, on-call problems, diseases, and drugs* (8th ed.). McGraw-Hill Education.

Graves, L. (2020). Cannabis and breastfeeding. *Paediatrics & Child Health, 25*(Supplement_1), S26–S28. https://doi.org/10.1093/pch/pxaa037

Grossman, M. R., Lipshaw, M. J., Osborn, R. R., & Berkwitt, A. K. (2018). A novel approach to assessing infants with neonatal abstinence syndrome. *Hospital Pediatrics, 8*(1), 1–6. https://doi.org/10.1542/hpeds.2017-0128

Gunatilake, R., & Patil, A. S. (2021, March). *Drugs in pregnancy.* Merck Manual Profession Version. https://www.merckmanuals.com/professional/gynecology-and-obstetrics/drugs-in-pregnancy/drugs-in-pregnancy#v26436779

Hall, A. S., & Reavey, D. A. (2021). In S. L. Gardner, B. S. Carter, M. Enzman-Hines, & S. Niermeyer (Eds.), *Merenstein & Gardner's handbook of neonatal intensive care nursing: An interprofessional approach* (9th ed., pp. 929–968). Elsevier.

Hawes, J., Bernardo, S., & Wilson, D. (2020). The neonatal neurological examination: Improving understanding and performance. *Neonatal Network, (39)*3, 116–127.

Hein, S., Clouser, B., Tamim, M., Lockett, D., Brauer, K., & Cooper, L. (2021). Eat, sleep, console and adjunctive buprenorphine improved outcomes in neonatal opioid withdrawal syndrome. *Advances in Neonatal Care, 21*(1), 41–48. https://doi.org/10.1097/anc.0000000000000824

Hummel, P., & Naber, M. M. (2021). Discharge planning and transition to home. In M. T. Verklan, M. Walden, & S. Forest (Eds.), *Core curriculum for neonatal intensive care nursing* (6th ed., pp. 329–345). Elsevier.

Jacobs, M., Berg, M., Hunt, R., Tarnow-Mordi, W. O., Inder, T. E., & Davis, P. G. (2013). Cooling for newborns with hypoxic ischaemic encephalopathy. *Cochrane Database of Systematic Reviews, 1*, 1–88. https://doi.org/10.1002/14651858.CD003311.pub3

Juliano, G. M., Puchalski, M., & Walsh, S. M. (2019). Implementation of pre-/post-weights to enhance direct breastfeeding in the NICU. *Clinical Lactation, 10*(1), 29–39. https://doi.org/10.1891/2158-0782.10.1.29

Kamath-Rayne, B. D., Froese, P. A., & Thilo, E. H. (2021). Neonatal hyperbilirubinemia. In S. L. Gardner, B. S. Carter, M. Enzman-Hines, & S. Niermeyer (Eds.), *Merenstein & Gardner's handbook of neonatal intensive care nursing: An interprofessional approach* (9th ed., pp. 662–691). Elsevier.

Kaspar, A., & Rubarth, L. B. (2016). Neuroprotection of the preterm infant. *Neonatal Network, 35*(6), 391–395. https://doi.org/10.1891/0730-0832.35.6.391

Kenner, C., & Boykova, M. (2021). Families in crisis. In M. T. Verklan, M. Walden, & S. Forest (Eds.), *Core curriculum for neonatal intensive care nursing* (6th ed., pp. 288–300). Elsevier.

Khazaeni, L. M. (2020). *Retinopathy of prematurity.* Merck Manual Professional Version. https://www.merckmanuals.com/home/children-s-health-issues/eye-disorders-in-children/retinopathy-of-prematurity-rop

Korioth, T. (2020, October 21). Updates to neonatal, pediatric resuscitation guidelines based on new evidence. *AAP News: The Official Newsmagazine of the American Academy of Pediatrics.* https://www.aappublications.org/news/2020/10/21/nrp102120

Lopriore, E. (2019). Updates in red blood cell and platelet transfusions in preterm neonates. *American Journal of Perinatology, 36*(2), 37–40. https://doi.org/10.1055/s-0039-1691775

Lubbers, L. A. (2021). Congenital anomalies. In M. T. Verklan, M. Walden, & S. Forest (Eds.), *Core curriculum for neonatal intensive care nursing* (6th ed., pp. 654–677). Elsevier.

MacMillan, K. L., Rendon C. P., Verma, K., Riblet, N., Washer, D. B., & Holmes, A. V. (2018). Association of rooming-in with outcomes for neonatal abstinence syndrome: A systematic review and meta-analysis. *JAMA Pediatrics, 172*(4), 345–351. http://jamanetwork.com/article.aspx?doi=10.1001/jamapediatrics.2017.5195

Maoz, O., Wainstock, T., Sheiner, E., & Walfisch, A. (2018). Immediate perinatal outcomes of postterm deliveries. *Journal of Maternal-Fetal and Neonatal Medicine, 32*(11), 1847–1852. https://doi.org/10.1080/14767058.2017.1420773

March of Dimes. (2018). *Preterm labor and premature birth: Are you at risk?* https://www.marchofdimes.org/complications/preterm-labor-and-premature-birth-are-you-at-risk.aspx

March of Dimes. (2020). *2020 March of Dimes report card.* https://www.marchofdimes.org/peristats/tools/reportcard.aspx

Martin, J. A., Hamilton, B. E., Osterman, M. J. K., & Driscoll, A. K. (2019). Births: Final data for 2018. *National Vital Statistics Reports, 68*(13).

Massenzi, L., Aufieri, R., Donno, S., Agostino, R., & Dotta, A. (2021). Use of intravenous sodium bicarbonate in neonatal intensive care units in Italy: A nationwide survey. *Italian Journal of Pediatrics, 47*(63). https://doi.org/10.21203/rs.3.rs-48558/v2

Merritt, J. L., Norris, M., & Kanugo, S. (2018). Fatty acid oxidation disorders. *Annals of Translational Medicine, 6*(24), 1–14. https://doi.org/10.21037/atm.2018.10.57

Moldenhauer, J. S. (2020, January). *Postterm pregnancy.* Merck Manual Professional Version. https://www.merckmanuals.com/professional/gynecology-and-obstetrics/abnormalities-and-complications-of-labor-and-delivery/postterm-pregnancy

Montasser, M., & Patel, N. (2021). Pulmonary hypertension in newborn infants: Pathophysiology, clinical assessment, and management. *Paediatrics and Child Health, (31)*1, 32–37. https://doi.org/10.1016/j.paed.2020.10.005

Moore, C. A., Staples, J. E., Dobyns, W. B., Pessoa, A., Ventura, C. V., Borges da Fonseca, E., . . . Rasmussen, S. A. (2017). Characterizing the pattern of anomalies in congenital Zika syndrome for pediatric clinicians. *JAMA Pediatrics, 171*(3), 288–295. https://doi.org/10.1001/jamapediatrics.2016.3982

Morris, R., Jones, S., Banerjee, S., Collinson, A., Hagan, H., Walsh, H., . . . Matthes, J. (2020). Comparison of the management recommendations of the Kaiser Permanente neonatal early-onset sepsis risk calculator (SRC) with NICE guideline CG149 in infants ≥ 34 weeks' gestation who developed early-onset sepsis. *Archives of Disease in Childhood. Fetal and Neonatal Edition, 105*(6), 581–586. https://doi.org/10.1136/archdischild-2019-317165

National Academies of Sciences, Engineering and Medicine. (2017). *The health effects of cannabis and cannabinoids: The current state of evidence and recommendations for research.* The National Academies Press. https://doi.org/10.17226/24625

National Institute on Drug Abuse. (2020, April). *Substance use while pregnant and breastfeeding.* https://www.drugabuse.gov/publications/research-reports/substance-use-in-women/substance-use-while-pregnant-breastfeeding

Ohlsson, A., & Aher, S. M. (2020). Early erythropoiesis-stimulating agents in preterm or low-birth weight infants. *Cochrane Database of Systematic Reviews.* https://doi.org/10.1002/14651858.CD004863.pub6

Pace, E. J., Brown, C. M., & DeGeorge, K. C. (2019). Neonatal hyperbilirubinemia: An evidence-based approach. *Journal of Family Practice, 68*(1), E4–E11. https://cdn.mdedge.com/files/s3fs-public/JFP06801e4.PDF

Page, K. A., Luo, S., Wang, X., Chow, T., Alves, J., Buchanan, T. A., & Xiang, A. H. (2019). Children exposed to maternal obesity or gestational diabetes mellitus during early fetal development have hypothalamic alterations that predict future weight gain. *Diabetes Care, 42*(8), 1473–1480. https://doi.org/10.2337/dc18-2581

Parker, L. A. (2021). Nutritional management. In M. T. Verklan, M. Walden, & S. Forest (Eds.), *Core curriculum for neonatal intensive care nursing* (6th ed., pp. 152–171). Elsevier.

Patrick, S. W., Barfield, W. D., Poindexter, B. B., AAP Committee on Fetus and Newborn, & AAP Committee on Substance Use and Prevention. (2020). Neonatal opioid withdrawal syndrome. *Pediatrics, 146*(5). https://doi.org/10.1542/peds.2020-029074

Pineda, R., Raney, M., & Smith, J. (2019). Supporting and enhancing NICU sensory experiences (SENSE): Defining developmentally-appropriate sensory exposures for high-risk infants. *Early Human Development, 133*, 29–35. https://doi.org/10.1016/j.earlhumdev.2019.04.012

Price-Douglas, W., & Rush, T. (2021). Intrafacility and interfacility neonatal transport. In M. T. Verklan, M. Walden, & S. Forest (Eds.), *Core curriculum for neonatal intensive care nursing* (6th ed., pp. 359–376). Elsevier.

Puopolo, K. M., Lynfield, R., & Cummings, J. J. (2019). Management of infants at risk for group B streptococcal disease. *Pediatrics, 144*(2), 1–17. https://doi.org/10.1542/peds.2019-1881

Radmacher, P. G., & Adamkin, D. H. (2017). Fortification of human milk in preterm infants. *Seminars in Fetal and Neonatal Medicine, 22*(1), 30–35. https://doi.org/10.1016/j.siny.2016.08.004

Rudd, K. M. (2021). Infectious disease in the neonate. In M. T. Verklan, M. Walden, & S. Forest (Eds.), *Core curriculum for neonatal intensive care nursing* (6th ed., pp. 588–616). Elsevier.

Sadowski, S. L., & Verklan, M. T. (2021). Cardiovascular disorders. In M. T. Verklan, M. Walden, & S. Forest (Eds.), *Core curriculum for neonatal intensive care nursing* (6th ed., pp. 460–503). Elsevier.

Seattle Children's. (2019, December). *Hypotension in the neonate*. https://www.google.com/url?sa=t&rct=j&q=&esrc=s&source=web&cd=&ved=2ahUKEwihkO6nz6bvAhX1KX0KHbpbCBQQFjARegQIIxAD&url=https%3A%2F%2Fwww.seattlechildrens.org%2Fglobalassets%2Fdocuments%2Fhealthcare-professionals%2Fneonatal-briefs%2Fhypotension-brief.pdf&usg=AOvVaw13-4b9LSuCrzOhIlqw3fUM

Smid, M. C., Metz, T. D., & Gordon, A. J. (2019). Stimulant use in pregnancy: An under-recognized epidemic among pregnant women. *Clinical Obstetrics & Gynecology, 62*(1), 168–184. https://doi.org/10.1097/GRF.0000000000000418

Spruill, C. T. (2021). Developmental support. In M. T. Verklan, M. Walden, & S. Forest (Eds.), *Core curriculum for neonatal intensive care nursing* (6th ed., pp. 173–190). Elsevier.

Stavis, R. L. (2019a, July). *Birth injuries*. Merck Manual Professional Version. https://www.merckmanuals.com/professional/pediatrics/perinatal-problems/birth-injuries

Stavis, R. L. (2019b, July). *Large for gestational age infants*. Merck Manual Professional Version. https://www.merckmanuals.com/professional/pediatrics/perinatal-problems/large-for-gestational-age-lga-infant

Stavis, R. L. (2019c, July). *Postterm and postmature infants*. Merck Manual Professional Version. https://www.merckmanuals.com/professional/pediatrics/perinatal-problems/posterm-and-postmature-infants

Stavis, R. L. (2019d). *Premature infants*. Merck Manual Professional Version. https://www.merckmanuals.com/professional/pediatrics/perinatal-problems/premature-infants

Stavis, R. L. (2019e, July). *Small for gestational age infants*. Merck Manual Professional Version. https://www.merckmanuals.com/professional/pediatrics/perinatal-problems/small-for-gestational-age-sga-infant

Substance Abuse and Mental Health Services Administration. (2020, September). *Key substance use and mental health indicators in the United States: Results from the 2019 National Survey on Drug Use and Health (HHS Publication No. PEP20-07-01-001, NSDUH Series H-55)*. https://www.samhsa.gov/data/sites/default/files/reports/rpt29393/2019NSDUHFFRPDFWHTML/2019NSDUHFFR090120.htm

Tappero, E. (2021). Physical assessment. In M. T. Verklan, M. Walden, & S. Forest (Eds.), *Core curriculum for neonatal intensive care nursing* (6th ed., pp. 99–130). Elsevier.

Tsakiridis, I., Mamopoulos, A., Athanasiadis, A., & Dagklis, A. (2020). Antenatal corticosteroids and magnesium sulfate for improved preterm neonatal outcomes: A review of guidelines. *Obstetrical and Gynecological Survey, 75*(5), 298–307. https://doi.org/10.1097/OGX.0000000000000778

U.S. Food and Drug Administration. (2020, November 19). *Coronavirus (COVID-19) update: FDA authorizes drug combination for treatment of COVID-19*. https://www.fda.gov/news-events/press-announcements/coronavirus-covid-19-update-fda-authorizes-drug-combination-treatment-covid-19

U.S. National Library of Medicine. (2021). *Drug levels and effects*. U.S. Department of Health and Human Services, National Institutes of Health. https://www.ncbi.nlm.nih.gov/books/NBK501587/

Verklan, M. T. (2021). Adaptation to extrauterine life. In M. T. Verklan, M. Walden, & S. Forest (Eds.), *Core curriculum for neonatal intensive care nursing* (6th ed., pp. 54–68). Elsevier.

Walden, M. (2021). Pain assessment and management. In M. T. Verklan, M. Walden, & S. Forest (Eds.), *Core curriculum for neonatal intensive care nursing* (6th ed., pp. 270–287). Elsevier.

Walter, A. W. (2020, October). *Perinatal polycythemia and hyperviscosity syndrome*. Merck Manual Professional Version. https://www.merckmanuals.com/professional/pediatrics/perinatal-hematologic-disorders/perinatal-polycythemia-and-hyperviscosity-syndrome

Wassink, G., Davidson, J. O., Dhillon, S. K., Zhou, K., Bennet, L., . . . Gunn, A. J. (2019). Therapeutic hypothermia in neonatal hypoxic-ischemic encephalopathy. *Current Neurology Neuroscience Reports, 19*(2). https://doi.org/10.1007/s11910-019-0916-0

Weston, P. J., Harris, D. L., Battin, M., Brown, J., Hegarty, J. E., & Harding, J. E. (2016). Oral dextrose gel for the treatment of hypoglycaemia in newborn infants. *Cochrane Database of Systematic Reviews*. https://doi.org/10.1002/14651858.CD011027.pub2

Wright, K. (2021). Infectious diseases cases. In S. Bellini & M. J Beaulieu (Eds.), *Neonatal advanced practice nursing: A case-based learning approach* (pp. 311–326). Springer.

Wymore, E. M., Palmer, C., Wang, G. S., Metz, T. D., Bourne, D. W. A., Sempio, C., & Bunik, M. (2021). Persistence of Δ-9-tetrahydrocannabinol in human breast milk. *JAMA Pediatrics*. https://doi.org/10.1001/jamapediatrics.2020.6098

Xu, J., Murphy, S. L., Kochanek, K. D., & Arias, E. (2020). Mortality in the United States, 2018. *National Vital Statistics Reports, 355*.

Yang, S., Duffy, J. Y., Johnston, R., Fall, C., & Fitzmaurice, L. E. (2019). Association of a delayed cord-clamping protocol with hyperbilirubinemia in term neonates. *Obstetrics & Gynecology, 133*(4), 754–761. https://doi.org/10.1097/AOG.0000000000003172

Women's Health

Well Women's Health

18

Linda L. Chapman, RN, PhD

HEALTH PROMOTION

Health promotion is defined by the World Health Organization (WHO) as "the process of enabling people to increase control over, and to improve, their health" (WHO, 2017). Throughout women's lives, they will experience both wellness and alterations in their health. Health promotion, a critical component of women's health, focuses on providing women with information and resources that enable them to increase control over and improve their health (Fig. 18–1).

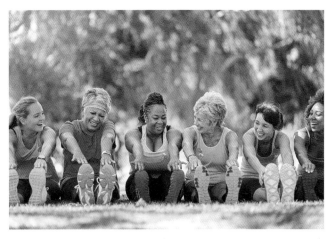

FIGURE 18–1 Health promotion for all ages is a critical component of women's health.

Leading Causes of Death

The following are the leading causes of death in females in the United States (Centers for Disease Control and Prevention [CDC], 2020b):

- Heart disease
- Cancer
- Unintentional injuries and accidents
- Chronic lower respiratory disease
- Stroke
- Alzheimer's disease
- Diabetes
- Kidney disease
- Influenza and pneumonia
- Suicide

CRITICAL COMPONENT

Heart Attack and Stroke Warning Signs

Heart Attack

Symptoms vary among women and differ from those experienced by men. They can include:

- Unusually heavy pressure on the chest
- Sharp upper body pain in the neck, back, and jaw
- Severe shortness of breath
- Cold sweats (not hot flashes from menopause)
- Unusual or unexplained fatigue
- Unfamiliar dizziness or lightheadedness
- Unexplained nausea or vomiting

Stroke

- Sudden onset of numbness or weakness in the face, arm, or leg, especially on one side
- Sudden onset of trouble seeing out of one or both eyes
- Sudden onset of trouble walking, dizziness, loss of balance, or coordination
- Severe headache with no known cause (CDC, 2020f, 2020g)

Risk Reduction

Leading causes of death in females vary by age groups and race (Table 18-1). The risk for these causes of death can be reduced through health promotion and risk reduction actions.

Actions for reducing risks include:

- Eating a healthy diet that is rich in vegetables, fruits, whole grains, fiber, fat-free or low-fat dairy, and fish, and a diet low in foods that are high in saturated fat and sodium (Fig. 18–2). The woman's diet needs to include 3 servings of foods high in calcium such as yogurt, milk, cheese, broccoli, kale, or Chinese cabbage. This helps to decrease the risk of or degree of osteoporosis. Women who cannot get enough calcium in their diets should take a calcium supplement.
- Getting at least 150 minutes of moderate-intensity physical activity per week. This can include brisk walking, swimming, biking, or dancing. Physical activity and weight-bearing exercise improve bone health by slowing bone loss and improving muscle strength and balance. It also helps maintain a healthy weight. Women should consult their health-care providers before starting a new exercise program.

CRITICAL COMPONENT

Physical Activity

Physical activity can lower a woman's risk for:

- Heart disease
- Type 2 diabetes
- Colon cancer
- Breast cancer
- Falls
- Depression

- Receiving the recommended immunization for female adults aged 19 and older. The CDC (2020e) recommends the following:
  - Influenza: Annually
  - COVID-19 vaccine
  - Pneumococcal polysaccharide (PPSV23) for women 65 years or older
  - Pneumococcal conjugate (PCV13) for women with conditions that weaken the immune system or with cerebrospinal fluid leak or cochlear implant
  - Herpes zoster (shingles) vaccine for women 50 years and older
  - Tetanus, diphtheria, and pertussis (Tdap) if not received as an adolescent; then, tetanus and diphtheria (Td) every 10 years
  - Measles, mumps, and rubella vaccine (MMR): 1 dose for adults aged 19 to 59 years; not recommended for adults over age 60 years
  - Varicella (VAR) vaccine: Adults without evidence of immunity to varicella should receive 2 doses of single-antigen VAR 4 to 8 weeks apart.
  - Human papillomavirus (HPV) vaccine: Women aged 19 to 26 years

TABLE 18-1 Top Three Leading Causes of Death in Females by Age Group and Race

AGE	AMERICAN INDIAN OR ALASKA NATIVE	ASIAN OR PACIFIC ISLANDER	BLACK	HISPANIC	WHITE
15–19	• Accidents • Suicide • Homicide	• Suicide • Accidents • Cancers	• Accidents • Homicide • Cancers	• Accidents • Suicide • Cancers	• Accidents • Suicide • Cancers
20–24	• Accidents • Suicide • Homicide	• Accidents • Suicide • Cancers	• Accidents • Homicide • Heart disease	• Accidents • Suicide • Homicide	• Accidents • Suicide • Homicide
25–34	• Accidents • Suicide • Chronic liver disease	• Cancers • Accidents • Suicide	• Heart disease • Accidents • Cancers	• Accidents • Cancers • Suicide	• Accidents • Suicide • Cancers
35–44	• Accidents • Chronic liver disease • Heart disease	• Cancers • Suicide • Accidents	• Cancers • Heart disease • Accidents	• Cancers • Accidents • Heart disease	• Accidents • Cancers • Heart disease
45–54	• Heart disease • Accidents • Cancers	• Cancers • Heart disease • Stroke	• Cancers • Heart disease • Accidents	• Cancers • Heart disease • Accidents	• Cancers • Heart disease • Accidents
55–64	• Cancers • Heart disease • Chronic liver disease	• Cancers • Heart disease • Stroke	• Cancers • Heart disease • Diabetes mellitus	• Cancers • Heart disease • Diabetes mellitus	• Cancers • Heart disease • Accidents
65–74	• Cancers • Heart disease • Diabetes mellitus	• Cancers • Heart disease • Stroke	• Cancers • Heart disease • Stroke	• Cancers • Heart disease • Diabetes mellitus	• Cancers • Heart disease • Chronic lower respiratory diseases
75–84	• Heart disease • Cancers • Chronic lower respiratory disease	• Cancers • Heart disease • Stroke	• Heart disease • Cancers • Stroke	• Heart disease • Cancers • Stroke	• Cancers • Heart disease • Chronic lower respiratory diseases
85	• Heart disease • Cancers • Alzheimer's disease	• Heart disease • Cancers • Stroke	• Heart disease • Cancer • Stroke	• Heart disease • Cancers • Alzheimer's disease	• Heart disease • Cancers • Alzheimer's disease

Kochanek et al., 2016.

CRITICAL COMPONENT

Human Papillomavirus

HPV is the most common sexually transmitted virus in the United States. It is the main cause of cervical cancer and genital warts and can cause cancers of the cervix, vulva, vagina, penis, or anus. It can also cause oropharyngeal cancers, which involve cancer in the back of the throat, base of the tongue, and tonsils.

SAFE AND EFFECTIVE NURSING CARE:
Understanding Medication

HPV Vaccine—Gardasil and Gardasil 9

- Indication: Prevention of cancers of the cervix, vulva, vagina, penis, or anus and prevention of genital warts.
- Action: Formation of antibodies to HPV
- Common side effects: Injection site reaction
- Route and dose: Intramuscular; number of doses varies based on age at administration of first dose.

- Two doses are recommended for a person initiating vaccine before age 15 years. The second dose is given 6 to 12 months after the first dose.
- Three doses are recommended for persons aged 15 and older. The second dose is given 1 to 2 months after the first dose; the third dose is given 6 months after the first dose.

Nursing Actions

- Provide information about the vaccine.
- Explain the importance of completing the entire series.
- Explain the need for continued routine cervical cancer screening.
- Explain that the vaccine does not prevent sexually transmitted infections (STIs).

- Maintaining a healthy weight.
  - Obesity places women at risk for a variety of health problems.
  - 40.3% of women age 20 to 39 are obese.
  - 46.4% of women age 40 to 59 are obese.
  - 42.2% of women 60 and older are obese (Craig et al., 2020).

CRITICAL COMPONENT

Obesity

Obesity has three categories:

- Class 1—Body mass index [BMI] 30 to 35
- Class 2—BMI 35 to 40
- Class 3—BMI greater than 40

Obesity places a woman at higher risk for:

- Hypertension
- Coronary heart disease
- Type 2 diabetes
- Cerebrovascular accident
- Cholecystitis
- Sleep apnea
- Cancer, including endometrial, breast, colon, kidney, gallbladder, and liver
- Osteoarthritis of the knee, hip, and lower back
- Abnormal menstrual cycle and infertility
- High-risk pregnancies related to diabetes and hypertension
- Miscarriage
- Macrosomia (Craig et al., 2020)

- Minimizing exposure to ultraviolet (UV) radiation:
  - UV radiation increases the risk for skin cancer.
  - UV radiation can cause liver spots, actinic keratoses, and solar elastosis.
  - UV radiation can cause premature aging of the skin.
  - The woman can decrease her risk while in the sun by wearing sun-protective clothing, wearing a hat, using sunglasses, applying sunblock with SPF of 15 or greater on exposed skin, and avoiding sun exposure between 10 a.m. to 2 p.m.

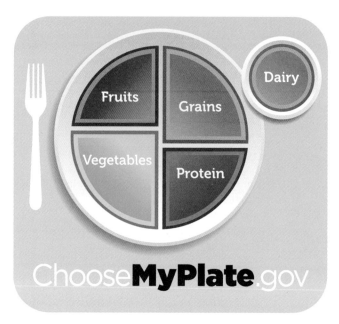

FIGURE 18–2 MyPlate is a tool that can be used when discussing nutrition with a client.

- Avoiding cigarette smoking and secondhand smoke:
  - Tobacco use is a leading cause of heart disease and cancer.
  - Lung cancer is a leading cause of cancer deaths (American Cancer Society, 2021).
  - Tobacco use and secondhand smoke during pregnancy can affect the developing fetus and health of the pregnancy.
    - Increased risk of premature birth
    - Increased risk of low birth weight
    - Increased risk of miscarriages due to increase in CO_2 and decrease in O_2 blood levels
    - Potential damage to fetal lungs and brain development
- Avoiding e-cigarettes
  - May contain nicotine and other harmful chemicals
  - E-cigarettes that contain THC are associated with lung damage (CDC, 2020c)
- Limiting alcohol consumption
  - Those who choose to drink alcohol should do so in moderation, which is one drink per day for women.
  - Drinking during pregnancy increases the risk of:
    - Premature birth
    - Fetal alcohol spectrum disorder
    - Birth defects such as heart defects and hearing and vision impairments
    - Low birth weight
    - Spontaneous abortion
    - Stillbirth
  - Excessive drinking increases a woman's risk for:
    - Infertility
    - Liver disease
    - Diabetes
    - Memory loss and shrinkage of brain
    - Cancer of the mouth, throat, esophagus, liver, colon, and breast
    - Heart damage

- Binge drinking increases the risk for sexual assault (CDC, 2020a).
  - 12% of adult women report binge drinking (five drinks) three times a month.
- Preventing injury from accidents
  - Motor vehicle crashes are a leading cause of death from injury among younger women.
    - Risk reduction: Wear seat belts, follow speed limits, and do not drink alcohol before driving. Do not ride in a car whose driver has been drinking alcohol.
  - Injuries related to falls are the leading cause of injury, death, and disability for women aged 65 years old or older.
    - Risk reduction: Exercise to improve strength and balance, modify home to reduce fall hazards, wear shoes when walking indoors and outside, and conduct medication assessment to minimize side effects such as dizziness.
- Maintaining good sexual health. The WHO defines sexual health as "a state of physical, emotional, mental and social well-being in relationship to sexuality; it is not merely the absence of disease, dysfunction or infirmity. Sexual health requires a positive and respectful approach to sexuality and sexual relationships, as well as the possibility of having pleasurable and safe sexual experiences, free of coercion, discrimination and violence" (CDC, 2019).
- Actions to take to promote sexual health:
  - Discuss sexual health issues with health-care providers (i.e., hypoactive sexual desire, intimate partner violence, and dyspareunia [painful intercourse]).
  - Incorporate methods to prevent STIs and unintentional pregnancies.
  - Discuss with your partner your sexual needs and sexual likes and dislikes.

Routine Screenings

Screening tests assist the woman's health-care provider in identifying potential alterations in health and initiating early interventions. Recommended screenings and immunizations for women are presented in Table 18-2.

Breast Cancer Screening

Early detection of breast cancer when the tumor is small and has not spread provides the best opportunity for successful treatment. Mammograms are recommended for women with average risk for breast cancer; this includes those with no personal or family history of breast cancer and no *BRACA1* or *BRACA2* gene mutation that increases breast cancer risk. MRI screening and mammograms are recommended for women who are at high risk for breast cancer (American Cancer Society, 2020). Women are considered high risk if they have a known *BRACA1* or *BRACA2* gene mutation or a lifetime risk of breast cancer of 20% or greater. Lifetime risk for breast cancer can be calculated using the breast cancer risk assessment tool at cancer.gov. When to start breast cancer screening varies based on a woman's risk for breast cancer. See Table 18-2 for recommended frequency of mammograms. Monthly self-breast examinations are

no longer recommended, but women should be aware of breast changes that need to be reported to her health-care provider (Fig. 18–3).

CRITICAL COMPONENT

Screening Mammograms

A mammogram uses a specially designed low-dose x-ray machine to take an image of the breast to detect abnormal changes. Each breast is placed between the x-ray plate and plastic plate. Pressure is gradually increased to flatten the breast, allowing a clearer picture to be obtained. Women may experience a sense of the breast being squeezed or pinched. The radiologist will compare the present x-ray with previous breast x-rays, looking for changes, lumps or abscesses, and calcifications. When abnormalities are identified on a screening mammogram, further testing is needed; this may include a diagnostic mammogram, ultrasound, MRI, or biopsy. Women with breast implants must inform the mammogram facility, as implants can hide some of the breast tissue. Women should not wear any deodorants, perfume, lotion, or powder under their arms or on their breasts on the day of the appointment. These substances can make shadows on the x-ray.

Cervical Cancer Screening

The American Cancer Society's (2020) cervical cancer screening recommendations are:

- Women older than 65 can stop cervical cancer screening if they have not had any precancerous cells found in the previous 10 years.
- Women who had a total hysterectomy should stop screening, unless hysterectomy was due to cervical precancer or cancer.
- Women who have received HPV vaccine still need to follow the recommended screening for their age group.

See Table 18-2 for recommended frequency of screening.

Intimate Partner Violence Screening

Intimate partner violence (IPV) is abuse or aggression in a romantic relationship. It is a traumatic experience for the victim. One in four women will experience IPV in her lifetime. It occurs in heterosexual and same-sex couples of all races, ages, socioeconomic groups, and religious groups. IPV can include physical violence, sexual violence, psychological aggression, and stalking (CDC, 2020d). Care of women experiencing IPV includes these measures:

- A validated screening tool should be used when screening for IPV and sexual assault.
- Women should be screened for IPV in private during annual examinations, initial prenatal visits, and each trimester and postpartum checkup (American College of Obstetricians and Gynecologists [ACOG], 2012a).

TABLE 18-2   Recommended Screenings and Immunizations for Women Across the Life Span

SCREENING TESTS	AGES 19–39	AGES 40–49	AGES 50–64	AGES 65 AND OLDER
Blood pressure test	Every 1 to 2 years	Every 1 to 2 years	Every 1 to 2 years	Every 1 to 2 years
Cholesterol test	Start at age 20, test regularly if at risk for heart disease.	Test regularly if at risk for heart disease.	Test regularly if at risk for heart disease.	Test regularly if at risk for heart disease.
Dual-energy x-ray absorptiometry (DXA) scan			Frequency is based on health history and risk for osteoporosis.	Frequency is based on health history and risk for osteoporosis.
Type 2 diabetes screening	Yearly if overweight	Yearly if overweight and under 45 years Yearly for individuals over 45	Yearly	Yearly
Mammogram	Discuss with health-care provider.	Discuss with health-care provider.	Discuss with health-care provider.	Discuss with health-care provider.
Cervical cancer screening	Pap test every 3 years for women age 19 to 29 30 and older, a Pap test and HPV test together every 5 years	Pap test and HPV test every 5 years	Pap test and HPV test every 5 years	Frequency is based on health history.
Chlamydia test	If sexually active, yearly until age 24. Yearly ages 25–39, if new partner or multiple partners.	Yearly if new partner or multiple partners	Yearly if new partner or multiple partners	Yearly if new partner or multiple partners
Sexually transmitted infection (STI) tests	Frequency determined by risk for STI. All pregnant women need to be tested for various STIs.	Frequency determined by risk for STI. All pregnant women need to be tested for various STIs.	Frequency determined by risk for STI.	Frequency determined by risk for STI.
Colonoscopy			Every 10 years starting at age 50; more frequently based on risk factors	Every 10 years until age 75; more frequently if at risk for colon cancer
Eye examination	Eye examination if experiencing problems or visual changes	Baseline examination at age 40, then every 2–4 years	Every 2–4 years	Every 1–2 years
Hearing test	Every 10 years	Every 10 years	Every 3 years	Every 3 years
Skin examination	Monthly mole self-examination; every 3 years by health-care provider starting at age 20	Monthly mole self-examination; yearly by health-care provider	Monthly mole self-examination; yearly by health-care provider	Monthly mole self-examination; yearly by health-care provider
Dental and oral cancer examination	Yearly	Yearly	Yearly	Yearly

ACOG, 2018; American Cancer Society, 2020.

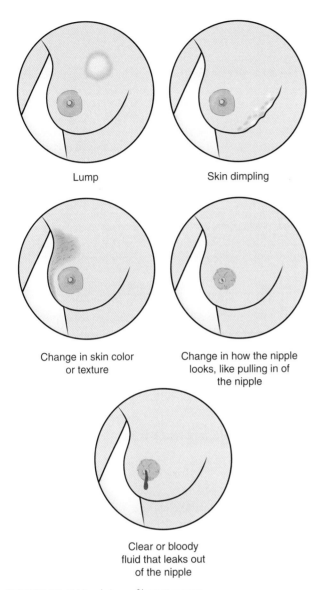

Lump

Skin dimpling

Change in skin color
or texture

Change in how the nipple
looks, like pulling in of
the nipple

Clear or bloody
fluid that leaks out
of the nipple

FIGURE 18–3 Visual signs of breast cancer.

- Women should be asked about their sense of feeling safe in their home and relationship.
- Mandatory reporting laws for IPV vary between states. Health-care providers need to be aware of state IPV laws.
- Women's health-care providers need to be aware of the resources that are available to women who are experiencing IPV.
- A strategy to decrease IPV is to teach safe and healthy relationship skills when people are in their adolescent years (CDC, 2017).

CLINICAL JUDGMENT

Caring for Patients Who Have Experienced Trauma

Often, a nurse is a woman's first point of contact within the health-care system after trauma or the first to recognize somatic or psychological signs that indicate a trauma history

(Bartelson & Sutherland, 2018). Although there is no single definition of trauma, a useful framework recognizes that individual trauma results from an event, series of events, or set of circumstances that is experienced by an individual as physically or emotionally harmful or life threatening and that has lasting adverse effects on the individual's functioning and mental, physical, social, emotional, or spiritual well-being (Substance Abuse and Mental Health Services Administration, 2014). Overall estimates indicate that more than half of all women will experience at least one traumatic event in their lifetimes. Traumatic experiences may be current and ongoing or associated with more remote events of childhood and early life. Traumatic experiences may include IPV; sexual assault and rape, including military sexual trauma; violence perpetrated based on race or sexual orientation; neglect during childhood; combat and service trauma; natural disasters; repeated exposure to community violence; refugee and immigration status; or family separation (ACOG, 2021).

Although trauma spans all races, ages, and socioeconomic statuses, some populations are exposed to trauma at higher rates and with greater frequency of repeated victimization. For example, families struggling with substance use disorder, chronic economic stress and poverty, or homelessness, as well as military families, disproportionately experience trauma.

In addition to affecting physical and mental health, a history of trauma can have a profound effect on attitudes toward medical care (ACOG, 2021). Trauma can induce powerlessness, fear, and hopelessness, while also triggering feelings of shame, guilt, rage, isolation, and disconnection (Substance Abuse and Mental Health Services Administration, 2014).

Experts use the four Rs to describe the key assumptions of any program, organization, or system that is trauma-informed:

- *Realize* the widespread effect of trauma and understand potential paths for recovery.
- *Recognize* the signs and symptoms of trauma in patients and families.
- *Respond* by fully integrating knowledge about trauma into your care and practice.
- *Re-traumatization* should be avoided; seek to actively resist re-traumatization.

Specific strategies include:

- Create a safe physical and emotional environment for patients.
- Note interactions should be patient centered and should be compassionate, with expression of genuine concern and support, and survivors of trauma should be treated with respect and without judgment.
- Offer options during care that can lessen anxiety, such as seeking permission before initiating contact, providing descriptions before and during examinations and procedures, allowing clothing to be shifted rather than removed, and agreeing to halt the examination at any time upon request.

REPRODUCTIVE CHANGES ACROSS THE LIFE SPAN

Throughout a woman's lifetime, her body undergoes physical changes related to hormonal changes. Major reproductive changes occur during puberty and before and after menopause.

Puberty

During puberty, a person becomes sexually mature and capable of reproduction. In girls, the onset of puberty usually occurs between ages 8 and 13, accompanied by accelerated growth of the body that usually begins with the feet and ends with the face. Puberty is triggered by the production of gonadotropin-releasing hormone from the hypothalamus, which stimulates the anterior pituitary to release gonadotropins. Gonadotropins stimulate the ovaries to secrete estrogen (Fig. 18–4). Estrogen is responsible for the development of secondary sex characteristics in females, including:

- Enlargement of breasts: Growth of the duct system of the mammary glands and erection of nipples
- Growth of body hair: Axillary and pubic hair
- Widening of the hips

Menarche, the initial menstrual period, usually occurs 2 to 2.5 years after the beginning of puberty. Puberty is completed when menstruation assumes a regular pattern. For more on the menstrual cycle, see Chapter 3.

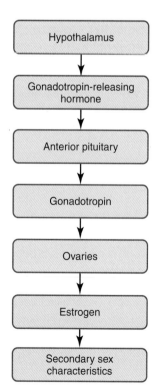

FIGURE 18–4 Hormonal triggers.

Menopause

Menopause is the stage of life that marks the permanent cessation of menstrual activity. This natural biological process usually occurs between ages 40 and 58. Menopause is divided into three stages:

- Perimenopause: Usually in her forties, the woman begins to experience menopausal signs and symptoms that last for 4 to 8 years. During this period of time, the woman experiences irregular menstrual cycles. It is possible for the woman to become pregnant during this stage.
- Menopause: Occurs 12 months after a woman's last menstrual period. Average age in the United States is age 51 with a range of 45 to 55 years of age.
- Postmenopause: Refers to the time after menopause.

As a woman enters her late thirties, the quality and quantity of her ova gradually decline, resulting in a gradual decline in the production of estrogen and progesterone. The woman will begin to experience changes in her body related to the decreasing levels of these hormones. These changes are often referred to as signs and symptoms of menopause. The degree and number of symptoms vary from some women experiencing no symptoms to other women experiencing numerous and severe symptoms.

Signs and Symptoms of Menopause

- Irregular periods may occur.
- The time between cycles may become longer or shorter.
- Menstrual flow may become heavier or lighter.
- Cycles become anovulatory, and the woman is no longer fertile after menopause is complete.
- Hot flashes may occur.
  - Hot flashes are the most common symptom of menopause.
  - This symptom is caused by a vasomotor response to changes in the hormonal levels. This change triggers blood vessels near the surface of the skin to dilate, causing an increase of blood supply and subsequent increase of heat to the skin surface.
  - When a woman experiences a hot flash, she feels a sudden sensation of warmth that spreads through her upper body and face. Her neck and face become red, and she begins to sweat and may feel irritable and exhausted.
  - Warm rooms, alcohol, hot foods, spicy foods, caffeine, and stress can trigger a hot flash.
- Night sweats
  - Night sweats are hot flashes that occur while the woman is sleeping.
  - Women who experience night sweats will wake up with their bed linens and nightwear soaked from sweat.
- Sleep disturbances
  - Women may experience altered sleep patterns related to night sweats and difficulty falling asleep and staying asleep.
- Sexual dysfunction
  - Sexual desire and arousal disorders may occur.
  - Some women experience vaginal atrophy as declining estrogen levels cause vaginal tissue to become thinner and drier.
  - Dyspareunia is also related to vaginal dryness.

- Psychological side effects may include:
  - Mood swings
  - Irritability
  - Anxiety
  - Lethargy
  - Lack of energy
  - Panic attacks
  - Forgetfulness
  - Difficulty coping
  - Depression
- Women may also experience:
  - Thinning of hair or hair loss
  - Food cravings
  - Dry skin and loss of skin elasticity
  - Weight gain, especially around the waist and hips
  - Irregular heartbeat and palpitations

Treating Menopausal Symptoms

There are three approaches for the treatment of menopausal symptoms: lifestyle changes, alternative medicine, and menopause hormone therapy (MHT).

- Lifestyle changes
  - Get 8 hours of sleep per night.
  - Eat a balanced diet.
  - Lose weight if overweight or obese.
  - Exercise.
  - Avoid caffeine and alcohol.
  - Avoid cigarette smoking and secondhand smoke.
- Alternative medicine
  - Herbal supplements
  - Acupuncture
  - Biofeedback
  - Hypnosis
- Menopausal hormone therapy (MHT)
  - There are conflicting research findings on the safety of MHT. Women need to talk with their health-care providers as to the benefits and risks of MHT.
  - Estrogen alone is prescribed for women who do not have a uterus.
    - Types of preparations are oral, transdermal, and vaginal.
  - Estrogen and progesterone therapy are prescribed for women who have a uterus. The use of progesterone with estrogen therapy reduces the risk of endometrial cancer.
    - Types of preparations are oral, transdermal, and progesterone intrauterine devices.
  - Dosage of MHT is based on the severity of symptoms. It is usually started at a low-dose range and increased as needed. The use of transdermal preparation is recommended.
  - Length of use of MHT varies. The woman should take the lowest dose possible that is effective for her. She should continue with routine health monitoring and each year the treatment plan needs to be reevaluated.
  - Estrogen is contraindicated for women who have:
    - Unexplained vaginal bleeding
    - Liver disease
    - Gallbladder disease
    - Blood-clotting disorders
    - Pulmonary embolism
    - Untreated hypertension
    - Uterine cancer
    - Breast cancer

CRITICAL COMPONENT

Menopause and Sexual Well-Being
Physical changes that occur related to declining levels of estrogen can have a negative effect on the women's sexual well-being. As the levels of estrogen decline, the vaginal tissue becomes thinner and vaginal secretions decrease, leading to dryness. These changes can cause dyspareunia. Sleep disturbances, hot flashes, and mood disturbances can also have a negative effect on the woman's sense of sexual well-being.

Treatment for Specific Menopausal Discomforts

- Hot flashes: Avoid alcohol, hot beverages, spicy foods, warm rooms, and smoking; these can trigger hot flashes. Dress in layers, so that the woman can remove clothing as she becomes warm and add clothing as she cools down. Avoid wearing clothing made from wool or synthetics. Use of fans is also helpful.
  - Medications used to treat other conditions that have been shown to decrease hot flashes include low-dose antidepressants such as fluoxetine (Prozac), the antiseizure medication gabapentin (Neurontin), and antihypertensive clonidine (Catapres).
- Night sweats: Sleep in cotton nightwear. Use cotton bed linens. Sleep in a cool room. Sleep with a fan blowing over the body. Take a cool shower before bedtime.
- Sleep disturbances: Establish a regular bedtime pattern. Do not watch TV or use the computer in bed. Keep the bedroom dark, quiet, and cool. Wear loose-fitting, breathable garments. Leave the cell phone in another room at night. Eat dinner early and avoid alcohol and caffeine close to bedtime.
- Sexual dysfunctions related to vaginal dryness: Use water-based lubricants during sexual intercourse. Use vaginal moisturizers. Use estrogen vaginal cream. Soy flour and flaxseeds in the woman's diet may prevent or decrease the degree of vaginal dryness.
- Physiological: Establish a daily physical exercise program. Limit alcohol consumption. Increase exposure to natural light or use a light box to treat seasonal affective disorder.
  - MHT may be prescribed in addition to lifestyle changes.
  - Psychotherapy and medications for depression or anxiety may be used when physiological symptoms have not improved with previously mentioned methods.

Nursing Actions

The focus of nursing is patient education. Topics should include:

- Physiological and emotional changes related to menopause, stressing that menopause is a natural phase of a woman's life.

- Discussion of the individual woman's premenopausal symptoms and methods she uses for relief of these symptoms, including medications, lifestyle changes, and alternative medicines.
- Discussion of the woman's sense of sexual well-being and methods to decrease effects of menopausal changes on her sense of sexual well-being.
- Discussion of additional treatments for specific symptoms, including lifestyle changes, medications, and alternative medicine.

OSTEOPOROSIS

Osteoporosis is the loss of bone mass that occurs when more bone mass is absorbed than the body creates. Bone mass in women usually decreases after age 35. Bone loss accelerates in the first 2 to 3 years after menopause. Osteoporosis affects both men and women, but 80% of Americans diagnosed with osteoporosis are women. Women who experience osteoporosis are at greater risk for vertebral and hip fractures.

Osteoporosis is diagnosed with a dual-energy x-ray absorptiometry (DXA) scan, which measures the bone density in the hip, spine, and forearm. These numbers are compared with the average peak density for those of the same sex and race, assigning a number called a T score:

- A T score of –2.5 or below is indicative of osteoporosis.
- A T score of –1 to –2.5 is indicative of osteopenia, which is lower than normal bone density that puts the person at risk for osteoporosis.

Signs and Symptoms

- Back pain related to a fracture or collapsed vertebrae
- Loss of height related to collapsed vertebrae
- Stooped posture related to collapsed vertebrae
- Bone fractures related to bone weakness

Risk Factors for Osteoporosis

Those at higher risk for developing osteoporosis include:

- White women
- Thin, small-boned women
- Those with a family history of hip fractures
- Current smokers
- Those with an inactive lifestyle
- Those deficient in calcium and vitamin D
  - Vitamin D assists in calcium absorption.
- Those who consume three or more alcohol drinks each day
- Those who take certain medications, including:
  - Corticosteroids for more than 3 months
  - Aromatase inhibitors
  - Proton pump inhibitors
- Those with a BMI less than or equal to 20 (adult weight under 127 pounds)
- Those with a history of eating disorders such as anorexia
- Those who have had weight loss surgery

Risk Reduction

- Maintain a diet high in calcium and vitamin D. This should start around 9 years of age to help form a strong bone matrix and should continue throughout the woman's life based on these guidelines:
  - 1,300 mg of calcium for girls aged 9 to 18 years
  - 1,000 mg of calcium per day for women aged 19 to 50 years
  - 1,200 mg of calcium for women aged 51 years and older
  - 600 to 1,000 IU of vitamin D per day for women 50 years and older
- Engage in weight-bearing exercise.
  - Walking, jogging, dancing, and weight lifting three to four times per week
- Avoid smoking.
  - Avoid both firsthand and secondhand smoke.
- Limit alcohol use.
  - Heavy drinking is linked to lower bone density.

SAFE AND EFFECTIVE NURSING CARE: Patient Education

Calcium Intake

Adequate intake of calcium in a woman's diet is important in decreasing the risk of osteoporosis.

Calcium-Rich Foods

- Canned sardines (3 ounces): 325 mg
- Plain low-fat yogurt (4 ounces): 310 mg
- Cheddar cheese (1.5 ounce): 307 mg
- Orange juice, calcium fortified (8 ounces): 300 mg
- Cheddar cheese (1.5 ounce): 307 mg
- Milk, 2% milk fat (8 ounces): 300 mg
- Almond milk, rice milk, or soy milk (8 ounces): 300 mg
- Salmon (3 ounces): 181 mg
- Kale, frozen (8 ounces): 180 mg

Pharmacotherapy

The ACOG recommends osteoporosis pharmacotherapy for:

- Women who have experienced a fragility or low-impact fracture
- Women with a DXA T score of less than or equal to –2.5
- Women with risk factors and with a DXA T score of less than –1.5 (ACOG, 2012b)

Pharmacotherapy includes the drugs in the following sections.

Bisphosphonates

Action: Inhibits resorption of bone, the process where breakdown of bone and release of minerals occurs with the resulting transfer of calcium from bone fluid to blood. Adverse effects: Musculoskeletal aches and pains, gastrointestinal irritation, and esophageal ulcerations.

- Alendronate (Fosamax)
  - Prevention: 5 mg/day or 35 mg/week
  - Treatment: 10 mg/day or 70 mg/week
- Ibandronate (Boniva)
  - Prevention and treatment: 150 mg/month
  - Treatment: 3 mg every 3 months by IV
- Risedronate (Actonel)
  - Prevention and treatment: 5 mg/day
- Zoledronate (Reclast)
  - Prevention: 5 mg every 2 years by IV
  - Treatment: 5 mg every year by IV

SAFE AND EFFECTIVE NURSING CARE:
Patient Education

Alendronate (Fosamax)

To reduce side effects and to enhance absorption of the oral medication, the woman should:

- Take the medication in the morning on an empty stomach at least 30 minutes before breakfast.
- Take the medication with at least 8 ounces of water (do not take with juice, coffee, or tea, as these can decrease absorption of medication).
- Take the medication in a sitting or standing position to decrease the risk of the pill becoming lodged in the esophagus where it can cause ulcerations and scarring.
- Remain upright for at least 30 minutes to decrease the risk of reflux of the pill into the esophagus (Vallerand & Sanoski, 2021).

Estrogen-Receptor Modulators

Action: Binds with estrogen receptors, producing estrogen-like effects on bone and reducing resorption of bone (Vallerand & Sanoski, 2021)

Adverse effects: Venous thromboembolism, leg cramps, and death from stroke

- Raloxifene (Evista)
  - Prevention and treatment: 60 mg/day

Hormone Therapy

- Conjugated estrogen + medroxyprogesterone acetate (Premphase)
  - Prevention: 0.625 mg of conjugated estrogen once daily on days 1 to 14 and 5 mg medroxyprogesterone acetate once daily on days 15 to 28
  - Prescribed for women who have a uterus
  - Contraindicated for women with known or suspected estrogen-dependent neoplasia
- Conjugated estrogen (Premarin)
  - Prevention: 0.3 to 1.25 mg/day
  - Prescribed for women who do not have a uterus
  - Contraindicated for women with known or suspected estrogen-dependent neoplasia

Other Medications

- Denosumab (Prolia)
- Teriparatide (Forteo)
  - Use with postmenopausal women who are at high risk for fractures; for women with osteoporosis associated with sustained, systemic glucocorticoid
  - Daily subcutaneous injection: 20 mcg

SAFE AND EFFECTIVE NURSING CARE:
Understanding Medication

Denosumab (Prolia)

- Indication: Treatment of osteoporosis in individuals who cannot take bisphosphonates, such as people with reduced kidney function
- Actions: Decreased bone resorption with decreased occurrence of vertebral and hip fractures
- Route and dose: Subcutaneous; 60 mg every 6 months
- Common side effects: Cystitis, hypocalcemia, hypophosphatemia, hypercholesterolemia, back pain, extremity pain, musculoskeletal pain, dyspnea
- Nursing actions: Encourage the woman to have routine dental examinations and care because medication places her at risk for osteonecrosis of the jaw.

Vallerand & Sanoski, 2021.

Nursing Actions

The primary nursing action is patient education. A teaching plan should include the following:

- Discussion of risk factors for osteoporosis and fracture related to osteoporosis
- Information on fall prevention:
  - Remove throw rugs from home.
  - Keep floors clear of objects such as books, paper, or shoes.
  - Ensure stairways are well lit.
  - Install grab bars near the shower, tub, and toilet.
  - Have annual eye examinations and update glasses.
  - Limit alcohol use.
  - Wear shoes inside and outside.
- Reason for bone density assessment and what to expect when having a DXA scan
- Discussion on foods high in calcium and vitamin D
- Discussion on physical activity that can decrease risk for osteoporosis
- Discussion on prescribed medication—explain reason for prescribed medication, dose, route, and side effects
- Discussion, as needed, on avoiding smoking and use of alcohol

SPECIFIC POPULATIONS

Nurses who specialize in health care for women of all ages and sexual orientations should be aware of the needs of these populations.

Adolescent Health

Adolescence, ages 12 to 19 years, is a time of physical, cognitive, and psychosocial development.

- Physical: Biological changes that occur include sexual maturity (development of primary and secondary sex changes), increases in height and weight (adolescent female will grow 2 to 8 inches and gain 15 to 55 pounds), and completion of skeletal growth.
- Cognitive: The adolescent moves from being a concrete thinker to thinking abstractly, using logic to solve problems, using deductive reasoning, and planning for the future. Adolescents begin to be concerned with moral and social issues and compare beliefs with those of peers.
- Psychosocial: The adolescent is working toward role identity—who they are and who they will be in life. They develop personal moral and ethical values and a greater sense of self-esteem and self-worth as well as a satisfactory sexual identity.

Most adolescents are physically healthy but are at risk for health problems. Health problems and issues for female adolescents include:

- Menstrual disorders
- Acne
- Eating disorders—obesity, anorexia, and bulimia
- Sexually transmitted illnesses—chlamydia and gonorrhea are prevalent in adolescents.
- Teen pregnancies—Rates are 16.6 births per 1,000 females aged 15 to 19 and 0.2 births per 1,000 females aged 10 to 14 (Hamilton et al., 2019).
- Issues related to self-esteem—20% of high school students report being electronically bullied, and 23.6% report being bullied on school property (CDC, 2021).
- Mental health issues—46.6% of female high school students reported persistent feelings of sadness and hopelessness (CDC, 2021).
- Unintentional injuries, suicide, and homicides—these are the leading causes of death for females aged 15 to 19 (Heron, 2019).

The 2019 Youth Risk Surveillance surveyed high school students throughout the United States. The survey's questionnaire focused on four categories: sexual behavior, high-risk substance use, experiencing violence, and mental health and suicide. Table 18-3 provides a sample of the results for high school females.

Nursing Actions

Nurses working in the middle school and high school settings are ideally positioned to promote healthy behaviors in adolescents. School nurses are often viewed by youth as safe adults to turn to for issues regarding health or body changes or sexual information. School nurses can provide health information and risk

TABLE 18-3 Youth Risk Behavior Surveillance (Female)—United States 2019

THE PERCENTAGE OF HIGH SCHOOL FEMALE STUDENTS WHO:	
Ever had sex	37.6
Had sex with four or more partners during life	7.2
Are currently sexually active	28.4
Used a condom the last time they had sex	49.6
Used effective hormone birth control the last time they had sex	35.2
Have ever used illicit drugs	14.0
Have ever misused prescription opioids	16.1
Were threatened or injured with a weapon at school	6.5
Did not go to school at least once during the past 30 days because of safety concerns	9.8
Were electronically bullied	20.4
Were bullied on school property	23.6
Were physically forced to have sexual intercourse	11.4
Experienced physical dating violence	9.3
Experienced sexual dating violence	12.6
Had persistent feelings of sadness or hopelessness	46.6
Seriously considered attempting suicide	24.1
Attempted suicide	11.0
Received injuries in suicide attempt	3.3

CDC, 2021.

reduction information to large groups of adolescents based on the needs of their school's population. They can also advocate for the availability of health resources for youth in their school districts.

Older Adult Women's Health

From conception until death, the human body is aging. Early in life, aging is viewed as a process of developing and maturing. Later in life, it can be viewed as a time of decline of health or loss of function. Health promotion is aimed at minimizing the effects of normal aging and maximizing quality of life for older adults.

Age-Related Physiological Changes and Health Promotion

Table 18-4 provides an overview of the common changes that occur in older adults and recommendations for minimizing the effects of these changes.

TABLE 18-4   Age-Related Physiological Changes and Health Promotion

PHYSIOLOGICAL CHANGES	POTENTIAL EFFECT ON OLDER ADULTS	HEALTH PROMOTION
↓ Muscle mass	↓ Strength	• Strength training • Healthy diet
↓ Total body water and ↓ renal tubular secretion and reabsorption	↑ Risk for dehydration	• Minimum fluid intake of 8 glasses; intake spread throughout the day
↓ Smell and ↓ taste	↓ Appetite	• Maintain healthy gums and teeth. • Use "color" in food presentation to make food more interesting.
↓ Metabolism	↑ Body fat and ↓ muscle mass	• ↓ Calorie intake • ↑ Physical activity • Strength training
↓ T-cells	↑ Risk for infections	• Healthy diet • Appropriate hand-washing technique to ↓ risk of infections
↓ Lung tissue elasticity; ↓ Ability to clear the tracheobronchial tree	↑ Risk for pneumonia	• ↑ Physical activity • Healthy diet • Yearly influenza vaccination (PPSV23)
↓ T-cells; ↑ DNA damage with ↓ DNA repair capacity	↑ Risk for cancer	• Cancer screening for early detection of cancers
Loss of high-frequency hearing	↓ Ability to recognize speech	• Hearing evaluation and treatment for hearing loss
↓ Peripheral vision; ↓ depth perception; cataracts	↓ Eyesight	• Eye evaluation and treatment as indicated • Sunglasses when driving in sunlight
↓ Intestinal motility	↑ Incidents of constipation	• Daily exercise • Stay hydrated • Include fruit, vegetables, whole grains, and probiotics in diet
↓ Elasticity of bladder wall; weakening of bladder; urethra blockage due to prolapsed uterus; cystocele	↑ Risk for frequency of urination, urinary incontinence, and cystitis	• Kegel exercises • Maintain ideal weight—obesity can contribute to incontinence • Bladder training—gradually delay urination after getting urge • Double voiding • Timed voiding—urinating on a schedule
Muscle weakness in legs, vertigo, balance difficulties, vision changes, dehydration, hypotension, confusion, foot disorders, arthritis of lower extremities	↑ Risk for falls	• Fall risk evaluation: Develop prevention plan based on evaluation • Home environment: Appropriate lighting; remove loose carpets and floor clutter; install grab bars in bathroom • Adjust medications as indicated • Footwear with flat, nonskid soles • Yearly vision evaluations and appropriate eyeglasses
Osteoporosis	↑ Risk for fractures	• Increase intake of foods high in calcium • Take 600–800 units of vitamin D • Engage in weight-bearing such as walking • Stop smoking
Deposits of lipofuscin, valves thicken, wall of heart thickens, ↑ heart size	↑ Risk for cardiovascular disease ↑ Risk for hypertension ↑ Risk for atrial fibrillation Heart murmurs	• Heart healthy diet • Exercise • Do not smoke • Treatment, as indicated, for diabetes, hypertension, hyperlipidemia

Continued

TABLE 18-4   Age-Related Physiological Changes and Health Promotion—cont'd

PHYSIOLOGICAL CHANGES	POTENTIAL EFFECT ON OLDER ADULTS	HEALTH PROMOTION
↓ Sensitivity of baroreceptors	↑ Risk for orthostatic hypotension	• Slowly rise from sitting or prone positions
Atherosclerosis, cardiovascular diseases, atrial fibrillation	↑ Risk for cerebrovascular accident	• Healthy diet low in saturated fats, trans fats, cholesterol, and sodium • Treat, as indicated, hypertension, diabetes, peripheral artery disease, atrial fibrillation • ↑ Physical activity
↓ Hepatic mass and blood flow, ↓ glomerular filtration	↑ Risk for adverse drug reactions	• Inform health-care provider and pharmacist of all medications—prescribed, over-the-counter, and herbal—that are being taken. • Follow direction for taking medications. • Report any physical or mental changes to health-care provider.
↓ Prefrontal cortex and the hippocampus	Alteration in learning, memory, planning, and other complex mental activities	• Prevention or control of hypertension and diabetes • Take 2.4 mcg of vitamin B$_{12}$; helps the brain, blood, and nervous system • Exercise and physical activity • Healthy diet • Engage in intellectually stimulating activities • Maintain relationships with family, friends, and community

● Dry skin and itching
  ● Causes:
    ● Decreased fluid intake
    ● Decreased humidity
    ● Loss of sweat and oil glands
    ● Increased time in the sun
    ● Smoking
    ● Health problems such as diabetes or kidney disease
  ● Health promotion
    ● Increase fluid intake to 8 or more glasses taken throughout the day.
    ● Apply moisturizers or lotions daily.
    ● Use a humidifier in dry climates.
    ● Use mild soaps and warm water instead of hot water.
    ● Limit time in the sun, use sunscreens, and wear protective clothing when in the sun.
● Nutrition
  ● Diet is a factor in the development of type 2 diabetes, coronary heart disease, atherosclerosis, stroke, and cancer.
  ● Obesity increases the risk for osteoarthritis of the knee, hip, and lower back, which can limit mobility in older adults.
  ● Factors that may affect an older adult's ability to eat well include:
    ● Living alone
    ● Depression—decreased interest in food
    ● Mouth pain
    ● Limited income
    ● Decreased ability to taste food—certain medications can interfere with the ability to taste; gum disease and issues

with dentures can leave a bad taste in the mouth; alcohol and smoking can alter how food tastes.
  ● Health promotion
    ● Take a detailed dietary history that provides information on the woman's eating habits.
    ● Assist the woman in identifying ways to modify diet to enhance her health.
    ● Address medical conditions that may interfere with appetite or ability to taste food or chew.
● Mouth care
  ● Oral health is important to the overall health of older adults.
  ● Healthy teeth and gums facilitate the older adult's ability to eat well and enjoy food.
  ● Health promotion
    ● Brush teeth twice a day with fluoride toothpaste.
    ● Floss once a day.
    ● Receive regular dental checkups every 6 months.
    ● Quit smoking.
    ● Eat a healthy diet and maintain hydration.
● Medications
  ● Older adults are more sensitive to medications, due to slower metabolisms and organ function. The digestive systems, liver, and kidney functions slow as a person ages. These changes affect the degree that drugs are absorbed into the bloodstream, how they react in the organs, and how quickly they are eliminated.
  ● Older people take more medications than younger people, which increases possible drug interactions.

- Health promotion
  - Take medications as directed. Report side effects to the health-care provider.
  - Make a list of all medications (prescribed, over-the-counter, vitamins, and supplements), including name, dose, and reason for taking them. Bring the list to each medical and dental office visit and share the information with health-care providers.
  - Create a file for all medications with all written information that came with the medications.
  - Check expiration dates and take outdated medication to the pharmacy for proper disposal.
- Sexual health
  - Older women are sexually active.
  - Age does not affect the woman's capacity to have an orgasm. The clitoris remains sensitive to stimulation and continues to increase in size when sexually aroused. Intensity of orgasm may decrease as the woman ages.
  - Frequency of sexual intercourse may decrease as a woman ages.
  - Changes related to declining estrogen levels cause vaginal dryness, burning, irritation, itchiness, discharge, and pain on penetration.

SAFE AND EFFECTIVE NURSING CARE: Understanding Medication

Estradiol Cream (Estrace Cream)

- Indication: Management of atrophic vaginitis related to menopause
- Action: Lessens:
  - Dryness and soreness in the vagina
  - Itching, redness, or soreness of the vulva
  - Feeling an urge to urinate more often than is needed or experiencing pain while urinating
  - Pain during sexual intercourse
- Route and dose: Vaginal; 0.5 to 1 g daily for 2 weeks, then twice weekly for maintenance
- Side effects: Breast pain, enlarged breasts, itching of the vagina or genitals, headache, nausea, stinging or redness of the genital areas, and thick, white vaginal discharge without odor or with a mild odor.
- Nursing actions:
  - Provide instruction on proper administration of medications.
  - Recommend use at bedtime to increase effectiveness of absorption.
  - To limit exposure to male sexual partner, do not use just before vaginal intercourse.
  - Check with health-care provider if vaginal estrogen can be used with latex devices such as condoms, diaphragms, and cervical caps (Vallerand & Sanoski, 2021).

- Decreased libido may be related to decreased levels of estrogen and testosterone. Women in their sixties have two times less testosterone than women in their twenties.
- Health promotion
  - Maintain a physically fit state through exercise and healthy diet. This will promote a more energetic life that can create more energy for sex.
  - Local vaginal estrogen applied to the vulva and vagina promotes vaginal health and treats vaginal atrophy and dryness.
  - Encourage open discussion with her partner, sharing feelings about sex and changes that have occurred in her body and her partner's body.
- Driving
  - A person's eyes change and reflexes slow, which can affect the ability to safely drive.
  - Deciding when to give up driving is a difficult decision for older adults because not driving decreases a person's feeling of independence.
  - Health conditions that can interfere with a person's ability to safely drive include:
    - Dementia
    - Visual and hearing changes
    - Stroke
    - Parkinson's disease
    - Arthritis
    - Diabetes
    - Certain medications
  - Health promotion
    - Recommend yearly eye examinations and appropriate visual corrections.
    - Do not drink and drive.
    - Avoid driving at night or in bad weather.
    - Limit distractions while driving: Turn off the radio, avoid conversations with people in the car, and do not text or use a cell phone.
    - Do not drive when taking medications that cause drowsiness or delayed reflexes.
    - Wear sunglasses when driving in sunlight.

Nursing Actions

- Discuss age-related physiological and emotional changes.
- Develop an individualized teaching plan based on the woman's age-related changes.
- Provide health-promotion information based on the woman's assessed needs.

CRITICAL COMPONENT

Signs That Driving Is No Longer Safe
It may be time to limit or stop driving if the person:
- Has trouble seeing or following traffic signals, road signs, and pavement markings.
- Stops at green lights or when there is no stop sign.

- Gets confused by traffic signals.
- Runs stop signs and red lights.
- Gets lost in familiar locations.
- Finds dents and scrapes on the car, fence, mailbox, and garage doors.
- Responds more slowly to unexpected situations.
- Has trouble moving foot from the gas to brake pedal (Colino, 2019).

LGBTQ Health

Lesbian, gay, bisexual, transgender, and queer (LGBTQ) individuals experience health disparities related to societal stigma, discrimination, and denial of civil rights. Lesbians face barriers to quality health care such as lack of health insurance, fear of negative reaction from health-care providers due to sexual orientation, and lack of understanding by health-care providers of lesbian health issues. Due to these barriers, lesbians see their health-care provider less often than do heterosexual women and they seek medical care at a later stage than heterosexual women (Ellis, 2022).

Health issues for lesbians include:

- Cancer: Higher risk for breast, cervical, endometrial, and ovarian cancer due to higher rates of smoking, alcohol use, and obesity than is seen in heterosexual women.
- Obesity: Lesbians tend to have higher body mass than heterosexual women, resulting in higher risk for heart disease and cancer.
- Polycystic ovarian syndrome (PCOS): PCOS is a common hormonal reproductive problem of all women. It appears more frequently in lesbians and increases women's risk for menstrual disorders, infertility, abnormal insulin production, and heart disease.
- Osteoporosis: Higher risk for osteoporosis due to smoking, alcohol, or antidepressant use.
- Heart disease: Higher risk for heart disease due to higher rates of smoking and obesity.
- Tobacco, alcohol, and substance use: Use of these substances is higher in lesbians compared with heterosexual women.
- Domestic violence: Domestic violence also occurs in lesbian relationships. All women need to be screened for domestic violence. There are few agencies that exclusively address domestic violence in lesbian relationships.

Nursing Actions

Nursing actions need to be developed around an understanding of the lesbian culture. To gain this understanding, the nurse needs to develop cultural humility through ongoing self-reflection and education to gain an understanding of one's assumptions and biases about other cultures and how these can affect nursing care (Rudd, 2018). Through cultural humility, the nurse will be able to create a health environment that is welcoming and provides a sense of safety and comfort.

A role of the nurse is to address the psychosocial determinants of health and acknowledge that societal factors play a major role in health issues in the LGBTQ community. Being LGBTQ is not unhealthy; rather, social factors interfere with LGBTQ women having easy access to health care that promotes and supports healthy behaviors.

Patient education is the primary nursing action to assist lesbians in understanding the importance of health promotion. Primary areas of health promotion education include:

- Routine screening and immunization
- Exercise to assist in weight control and bone health
- Healthy diet and weight reduction
- Smoking cessation and avoiding secondhand smoke
- Limiting alcohol use
- Safety planning and resources for women who are experiencing domestic violence
- Risk deduction for osteoporosis

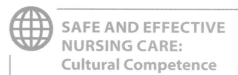

SAFE AND EFFECTIVE NURSING CARE: Cultural Competence

Cultural Humility

In learning to care for a population unfamiliar to the nurse, the nurse needs to develop cultural humility. Cultural competence implies "I am the expert," whereas cultural humility implies "You are the expert" (Rudd, 2018, p. 256).

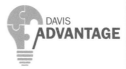

Go to Davis Advantage to complete your learning: strengthen understanding, apply your knowledge, and prepare for the Next Gen NCLEX®.

CONCEPT MAP |

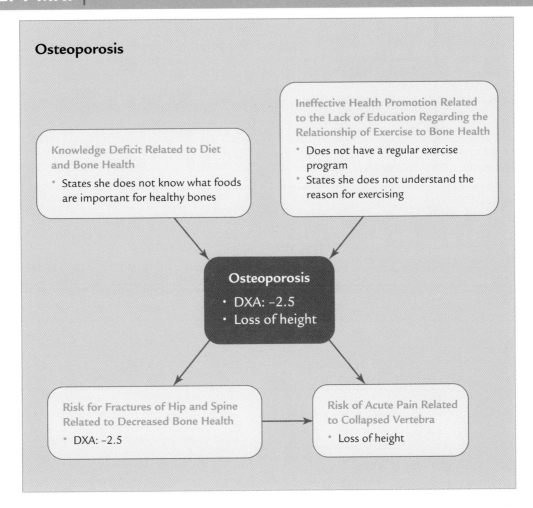

Osteoporosis

Knowledge Deficit Related to Diet and Bone Health
- States she does not know what foods are important for healthy bones

Ineffective Health Promotion Related to the Lack of Education Regarding the Relationship of Exercise to Bone Health
- Does not have a regular exercise program
- States she does not understand the reason for exercising

Osteoporosis
- DXA: –2.5
- Loss of height

Risk for Fractures of Hip and Spine Related to Decreased Bone Health
- DXA: –2.5

Risk of Acute Pain Related to Collapsed Vertebra
- Loss of height

CARE PLANS

Problem 1: Knowledge deficit related to diet and bone health
Goal: Increased knowledge of the relationship between diet and bone health
Outcome: The woman's diet will include foods high in calcium and foods high in vitamin D.
Nursing Actions
1. Assess diet for calcium and vitamin D using a 24-hour food recall.
2. Explain the relationship of calcium and strong bone matrix.
3. Explain that vitamin D helps with calcium absorption.
4. Assist the woman in identifying foods she prefers that are high in calcium and foods that are high in vitamin D.

Problem 2: Ineffective health promotion related to lack of education regarding the relationship of exercise to bone health
Goal: Effective health promotion

Outcome: The woman will develop a regular exercise routine that includes weight-bearing and weight-lifting activities.
Nursing Actions
1. Provide information regarding the causes of osteoporosis.
2. Provide information regarding the relationship of weight-bearing exercise and improved bone mass.
3. Discuss past exercise experiences and identify previous barriers to exercising.
4. Provide information on weight-bearing exercises and weightlifting.
5. Assist the woman in developing an exercise program that reflects her likes and meets the need for improved bone health.

Problem 3: Risk for fractures of hip and spine related to decreased bone health
Goal: Remains free of hip or spine fractures
Outcome: The woman will state three ways to improve bone health.

Continued

Nursing Actions

1. Explain the relationship between osteoporosis and fractures of the hip and spine.
2. Assess the woman's level of knowledge regarding ways to improve bone health.
3. Provide information on nutrition and bone health.
4. Provide information on exercise and bone health.
5. Provide information on prescribed medications for treatment of osteoporosis.

Problem 4: Risk of pain related to collapsed vertebrae
Goal: Does not experience collapsed vertebrae

Outcome: The woman will not experience pain related to osteoporosis.

Nursing Actions

1. Provide information on the benefits of calcium and vitamin D in improving bone health.
2. Provide information on the negative effects of smoking and excessive alcohol consumption on bone health.
3. Provide information on the relationship of osteoporosis and fractures of the spine.
4. Assist the woman in developing an action plan for decreasing her risk for spinal fractures.

Case Study

Kathy is a 65-year-old married woman with three grown children and five young grandchildren. She recently retired from teaching in an elementary school. She is 5 foot 6 inches tall and weighs 170 pounds. Her blood pressure (BP) is 124/96. She has a family history of type 2 diabetes, stroke, and colon cancer. She recently had a DXA that indicated osteopenia. She informs you that she spends most of her day watching TV, sewing, and reading. The nutritional assessment reveals her diet is high in fats and carbohydrates and low in fruits and vegetables. Based on this knowledge and health needs of older women, list the priority learning needs and state the rationale for these selected learning needs.

Describe your teaching plan based on identified priority learning needs. The plan should include:

• Preparation of the learning environment
• Methods to assess her learning needs
• Information that will be shared
• Methods for evaluating the effectiveness of teaching

REFERENCES

Allmen, T. (2016). *Menopause confidential.* HarperCollins.

American Cancer Society. (2020). *American Cancer Society guidelines for the early detection of cancer.* https://www.cancer.org/healthy/find-cancer-early/cancer-screening-guidelines/american-cancer-society-guidelines-for-the-early-detection-of-cancer.html

American Cancer Society. (2021). *Key statistics for lung cancer.* https://www.cancer.org/cancer/lung-cancer/about/key-statistics.html

American College of Obstetricians and Gynecologists. (2012a). Intimate partner violence. Committee Opinion No. 518. *Obstetrics & Gynecology, 119,* 412–417.

American College of Obstetricians and Gynecologists. (2012b). Osteoporosis. *Obstetrics & Gynecology, 120,* 718–733.

American College of Obstetricians and Gynecologists. (2018). *Cervical cancer screening.* https://www.acog.org/womens-health/faqs/cervical-cancer-screening

American College of Obstetricians and Gynecologists. (2021). Caring for patients who have experienced trauma. ACOG Committee Opinion No. 825. *Obstetrics & Gynecology, 137,* e94–e99.

Bartelson, A., & Sutherland, M. (2018). Experiences of trauma and implications for nurses caring for undocumented immigrant women and refugee women. *Nursing for Women's Health, 22,* 411–416. https://doi 10.1016/j.nwh.2018.07.003

Centers for Disease Control and Prevention. (2017). *Preventing intimate partner violence across the lifespan: A technical package of programs, policies and practices.* https://www.cdc.gov/violenceprevention/pdf/ipv-technicalpackages.pdf

Centers for Disease Control. (2019). *Sexual health.* https://www.cdc.gov/sexualhealth/default.html

Centers for Disease Control and Prevention. (2020a). *Excessive alcohol use and risk to women's health.* https://www.cdc.gov/alcohol/fact-sheets/womens-health.htm

Centers for Disease Control and Prevention. (2020b). *Mortality in the United States, 2019.* https://www.cdc.gov/nchs/products/databriefs/db395.htm

Centers for Disease Control and Prevention. (2020c). *Outbreak of lung injuries associated with use of e-cigarettes, or vaping, products.* https://www.cdc.gov/tobacco/basic_information/e-cigarettes/severe-lung-disease.html#overview

Centers for Disease Control and Prevention. (2020d). *Preventing intimate partner violence.* https://www.cdc.gov/violenceprevention/intimatepartnerviolence/fastfact.html

Centers for Disease Control and Prevention. (2020e). *Recommended immunization schedule for adults aged 19 years or older by age group, United States, 2020.* https://www.cdc.gov/vaccines/schedules/hcp/imz/adult-conditions.html

Centers for Disease Control and Prevention. (2020f). *Stroke signs and symptoms.* https://www.cdc.gov/stroke/signs_symptoms.htm

Centers for Disease Control and Prevention. (2020g). *Women and heart disease prevention.* https://www.cdc.gov/heartdisease/women.htm

Centers for Disease Control and Prevention. (2021). *Youth behaviors survey: Data summary & trends 2009–2019.* https://www.cdc.gov/healthyyouth/data/yrbs/pdf/YRBSDataSummaryTrendsReport2019-508.pdf

Colino, S. (2019). *Is it time for your loved one to retire from driving?* https://www.aarp.org/caregiving/basics/info-2019/is-it-time-to-stop-driving.html

Craig, H., Carroll, M., Fryar, C., & Ogden, C. (2020). *Prevalence of obesity and severe obesity among adults: United States, 2017–2018.* https://www.cdc.gov/nchs/products/databriefs/db360.htm

Ellis, S. (2022). Gynecological health care for lesbian, bisexual, and queer women and transgender and nonbinary individuals. In K. Schuiling & F. Likis, *Gynecology health care* (4th ed., pp. 173–201). Jones & Bartlett Learning.

Hamilton, B., Martin, J., & Osterman, J. (2019). *Birth: Provisional data for 2019.* https://www.cdc.gov/nchs/data/nvsr/nvsr68/nvsr68_13-508.pdf

Heron, M. (2019). Deaths: Leading causes for 2017. *National Vital Statistic Reports, 68.* https://www.cdc.gov/healthyyouth/data/yrbs/pdf/YRBSDataSummaryTrendsReport2019-508.pdf

Kochanek, M., Murphy, S., Xu, J., & Tejada-Vera, B. (2016). Deaths: Final data 2014. *National Vital Statistic Reports, 65,* 4.

Rudd, M. (2018). Cultural humility in the care of individuals who are lesbian, gay, bisexual, transgender, or queer. *Nursing for Women's Health, 22,* 255–263. https://doi: 10.1016/j.nwh.2018.03.009

Substance Abuse and Mental Health Services Administration. (2014). *SAMHSA's concept of trauma and guidance for a trauma-informed approach. HHS Publication No. (SMA) 14-4884.* Substance Abuse and Mental Health Services Administration.

Vallerand, A., & Sanoski, C. (2021). *Davis's drug guide for nurses* (17th ed.). F.A. Davis.

World Health Organization. (2017). *Health promotion.* https://www.who.int/topics/health_promotion/en/

Alterations in Women's Health

19

Linda L. Chapman, RN, PhD

LEARNING OUTCOMES

Upon completion of this chapter, the student will be able to:

1. Discuss various causes of abnormal uterine bleeding (AUB).
2. Describe common alterations in women's health, including medical management and nursing actions.
3. Describe potential complications or disorders related to childbirth trauma.
4. Describe the various hysterectomy procedures and the related nursing care.

CONCEPTS

Behaviors
Cellular Regulation
Comfort
Elimination
Growth and Development
Infection
Reproduction and Sexuality
Teaching and Learning

Nursing Diagnosis

- Deficient knowledge related to lack of information regarding chronic pelvic pain (CPP)
- Anxiety related to diagnosis of breast cancer

Nursing Outcomes

- The woman will state methods she can use to decrease her sensation of pain.
- The woman will appear relaxed and report anxiety related to a diagnosis of breast cancer is reduced to a manageable level.

INTRODUCTION

This chapter will address a variety of alterations in women's health including abnormal uterine bleeding (AUB), pelvic pain, infections of the reproductive system, leiomyoma of the uterus, pelvic organ prolapse, breast cancer, and cancers of the reproductive system. Hysterectomy, the most frequent major surgery for women, will be discussed.

MENSTRUAL DISORDERS

Menstrual disorders, one of the most common women's reproductive health problems, include amenorrhea, abnormal uterine bleeding (AUB), dysmenorrhea, and premenstrual syndrome (PMS) (Table 19-1). AUB includes chronic nongestational AUB, acute AUB, and intermenstrual bleeding.

TABLE 19-1   Menstrual Disorders

MENSTRUAL DISORDER	DEFINITIONS, SYMPTOMS, AND SIGNS	PATHOPHYSIOLOGY	MANAGEMENT
Primary amenorrhea	No menses by age 16 and no secondary sex characteristics or no menses by age 13 with secondary sex characteristics	• Body build (e.g., minimal levels of body fat) • Heredity (family history of delayed menses) • Pituitary function (lack of secretion of FSH and LH) • Congenital absence of the vagina	Identify and treat underlying condition (e.g., hormone therapy if related to endocrine dysfunction). Provide emotional support.
Secondary amenorrhea	No menses in 3 months in a woman who has had normal menstrual cycles	• Lack of ovarian production • Pregnancy • PCOS • Nutritional disturbances • Endocrine disturbances • Uncontrolled diabetes • Heavy athletic activity • Emotional distress	Identify and treat underlying condition (e.g., correct nutritional disorder). Explain cause (e.g., heavy athletic activity).
Abnormal uterine bleeding (AUB)	Chronic nongestational AUB: Uterine bleeding that is abnormal in duration, frequency, volume, or regularity for 6 months. Acute AUB: An episode of heavy uterine bleeding that in the opinion of the clinician is of sufficient quantity that it needs immediate intervention. Intermenstrual bleeding: Uterine bleeding between normal menstrual periods	• Polyps • Adenomyosis • Leiomyomas • Malignancy and premalignant • Systemic disorder of hemostasis • Ovulatory disorders • Endometrial cause usually related to inflammation, infection, or disruption of angiogenesis • Iatrogenic such as contraception use	Diagnostic Testing: Ultrasonography, MRI, saline infusion sonohysterography, aspiration biopsy, and dilation and curettage Treatment is aimed at the cause of AUB and ranges from self-management (diet, weight loss, exercise) to hormonal therapy to surgery such as endometrial ablation, uterine artery embolization, and hysterectomy
Primary dysmenorrhea	Painful menstruation: Cramping usually begins 12–24 hours before onset of flow and lasts 12–24 hours. May experience chills, nausea, vomiting, headaches, irritability, and diarrhea.	Excessive endometrial production of prostaglandin; women with primary dysmenorrhea produce 10 times the amount of prostaglandin. Prostaglandin is a myometrial stimulant and vasoconstrictor.	Explain cause. Prostaglandin inhibitors (ibuprofen) Analgesics Heat to back and lower abdomen Warm bath Exercise Oral contraceptives Diet low in fat and meat products may decrease the duration and intensity of the pain. Biofeedback Acupuncture
Secondary dysmenorrhea	Painful menstruation associated with known anatomic factors or pelvic pathology. Pain can be present at any point of the menstrual cycle.	Related to: • Endometriosis • Pelvic adhesions • Inflammatory disease • Cervical stenosis • Uterine fibroids • Adenomyoma	Identify and treat underlying condition. Same symptomatic measures as in primary dysmenorrhea.

TABLE 19-1 Menstrual Disorders—cont'd

MENSTRUAL DISORDER	DEFINITIONS, SYMPTOMS, AND SIGNS	PATHOPHYSIOLOGY	MANAGEMENT
Premenstrual syndrome (PMS)	A combination of emotional and physical symptoms that begin during the luteal phase and diminish after menstruation begins. Symptoms include (but are not limited to) lower abdominal and back pain, bloating, weight gain, breast tenderness, joint and muscle pain, oliguria, diaphoresis, diarrhea, constipation, nausea, vomiting, food cravings, acne, urticaria, headaches, vertigo, fainting, clumsiness, mood swings, depression, irritability, anxiety, lethargy, fatigue, confusion, tension, forgetfulness, sexual arousal, or dysfunction.	Etiology is unknown. PMS might be related to: • Hormonal changes related to the menstrual cycle • Estrogen–progesterone imbalance • Chemical changes in the brain	Healthy, balanced diet Exercise daily. Sleep 8 hours each night. Ibuprofen for physical symptoms such as cramps, backache, and breast tenderness Herbal remedies such as chasteberry Oral contraceptives and selective serotonin reuptake inhibitors (SSRI)

FSH, follicle-stimulating hormone; LH, luteinizing hormone; PCOS, polycystic ovary syndrome.

Alexander et al., 2017; Munro et al., 2018; Schuiling & Likis, 2022.

Uterine bleeding is assessed by frequency, duration, regularity, and flow volume. Normal parameters are:

- Frequency: 24 to 38 days
- Duration: 8 days or less
- Regularity: Shortest to longest cycle variation is 7 to 9 days or less
- Flow volume: Determined by the woman as normal versus light or heavy (Munro et al., 2018)

The hypothalamus, pituitary, and ovaries are the main sites of regulation of the menstrual cycle. Normal menstrual cycles occur when the hormone levels and feedback pathway of the hypothalamus-anterior pituitary-ovaries function appropriately (see Chapter 3 for an overview of the menstrual cycle).

- Hypothalamus: Secretes gonadotropin-releasing hormone (GnRH), also called luteinizing-hormone-releasing hormone, which simulates the anterior pituitary.
- Anterior pituitary: Secretes follicle-stimulating hormone (FSH) and luteinizing hormone (LH) that stimulates the ovaries.
- Ovaries: The ovarian follicles respond to the increase in FSH by producing increasing amounts of estrogen. LH stimulates the ovaries to release the ova and secrete progesterone. Estrogen and progesterone influence the menstrual cycle.

CHRONIC PELVIC PAIN

Chronic pelvic pain (CPP) is defined as pain in the pelvic region that lasts 6 months or longer and results in functional or psychological disabilities. It can affect the woman's physical, emotional, social, and material well-being (International Pelvic Pain Society, 2021). Women with CPP experience a variety of abdominal or pelvic pains:

- Uterine or abdominal cramping
- Sharp pain
- Steady pain
- Intermittent pain
- Pressure or heaviness deep in the pelvis
- Pain during intercourse
- Pain while having a bowel movement

CPP has multiple causes, which can make it difficult to evaluate and treat. Treatment focuses on the underlying cause of pelvic pain. In some cases, the cause of pain is unknown, and treatment focuses on symptom management.

Causes

CPP can stem from:

- Reproductive causes such as pelvic inflammatory disease (PID), leiomyoma, adhesions, endometriosis, and intrauterine contraceptive devices
- Urological causes such as bladder neoplasm, chronic urinary tract infection (UTI), and kidney stones
- Musculoskeletal causes such as compression fracture of lumbar vertebrae, poor posture, and fibromyalgia
- Gastrointestinal causes such as Crohn's disease, celiac disease, colitis, irritable bowel syndrome, and colon cancer

- Neurological causes such as shingles, degenerative joint disease, and herniated disc.
- Psychological causes such as personality disorders, depression, and sleep disorders
- Sexual or physical abuse

Medical Management

Medical management of CPP depends on the cause. It can take several weeks to several months of treatment before the woman will begin to feel better. In some cases, the pain does not completely go away. Treatments may include:

- Pain management, including physical therapy and medications: analgesics (nonsteroidal anti-inflammatory drugs [NSAIDs], acetaminophen, opioids), tricyclic antidepressants, neuroleptics (gabapentin), and muscle relaxants (Flexeril)
- Hormone therapy for pain related to menstrual cycle or endometriosis
- Antibiotics
- Steroids
- Laparoscopy surgery to release adhesions
- Nutrition such as avoiding foods that can increase inflammation of colitis or irritable bowel syndrome
- Psychotherapy to assist the woman in coping with anxiety, depression, and other emotional effects of living with chronic pain
- Alternative medicine

Nursing Actions

- Assess and document the location, characteristic, frequency, and quality of pain.
- Assess the effectiveness of pain interventions.
- Assess the level of knowledge regarding the cause of pain.
- Provide teaching as indicated by knowledge assessment.
- Provide information regarding diagnostic tests or surgeries.
- Provide information on the use of nonpharmacological techniques such as relaxation, guided imagery, heat application, and massage.
- Instruct the woman to use pain-control measures before pain becomes severe.

POLYCYSTIC OVARY SYNDROME

Polycystic ovary syndrome (PCOS) is a hyperandrogenic disorder. The etiology is not fully understood but a current theory is that it has a neuroendocrine origin in which an abnormality in hypothalamic-pituitary function results in excessive androgen production in the ovaries and adrenal glands (Waters et al., 2018). For a PCOS diagnosis, a woman must have two of the following three features:

- Clinical or biochemical androgen excess
- Oligo-ovulation or anovulation
- Polycystic ovarian morphology ultrasound (Fig. 19–1)

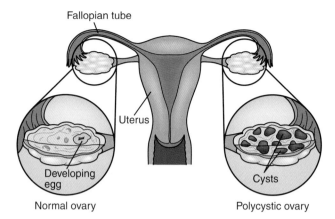

FIGURE 19–1 Polycystic ovary syndrome.

Women with PCOS are at higher risk for:

- Type 2 diabetes: Women with PCOS are at risk for insulin resistance (the body produces insulin but does not use it properly) and hyperinsulinemia (hyperglycemia present despite high levels of insulin). Obesity, common with PCOS, further increases diabetes risk.
- Cardiovascular disease: Insulin resistance and obesity increase the woman's risk for carotid and coronary atherosclerosis; endocrine changes related to PCOS increase the risk for high low-density lipoprotein cholesterol and low high-density lipoprotein.
- Hypertension related to insulin resistance
- Endometrial, ovarian, or breast cancer related to high levels of continuous estrogen
- Dyslipidemia related to endocrine changes
- Infertility: Anovulation related to increased androgen levels and LH and decreased FSH
- Pregnancy and birth complications: Spontaneous abortions, gestational diabetes, preeclampsia, and cesarean sections
- Sleep apnea related to obesity and insulin resistance
- Metabolic syndrome, which affects about one-third of women with PCOS
- Depression, anxiety, and binge eating

CLINICAL JUDGMENT

Metabolic Syndrome

Metabolic syndrome is a group of conditions that increase an individual's risk for heart disease, stroke, and diabetes. To be diagnosed, an individual must have three of the following:

- Abdominal obesity: A waist circumference in women 35 inches or greater
- High triglyceride levels: 150 mg/dL or higher
- Low HDL cholesterol level: 50 mg/dL
- Increased blood pressure: Systolic above 130 mm Hg or diastolic above 85 mm Hg
- Elevated fasting blood glucose: 110 mg/dL or higher (National Heart Lung and Blood Institute, 2016)

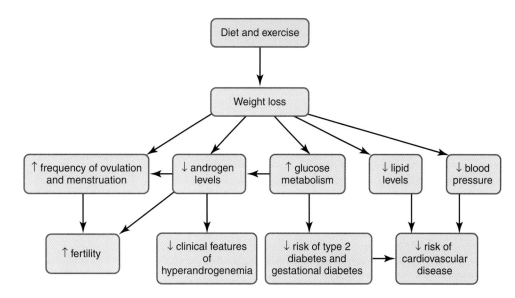

FIGURE 19–2 Effects of weight management in women with PCOS.

Signs and Symptoms

- Infertility: Usually related to anovulatory menstrual cycles
- Menstrual disorders: AUB
- Hirsutism: Increased hair growth on face, chest, stomach, and back
- Ovarian cysts
- Obesity
- Oily skin and acne
- Pelvic pain
- Alopecia

Medical Management

- Diet and exercise to assist in weight loss. It also helps:
  - Reduce risk for type 2 diabetes.
  - Decrease levels of androgens.
  - Improve the frequency of ovulation and menstruation.
  - Reduce risk of cardiovascular disease (Fig. 19–2).
- Hormone therapy
  - Low-dose hormonal contraceptives for women who do not wish to conceive. These contraceptives inhibit LH production, decrease testosterone levels, and reduce degree of acne and hirsutism.
- Anti-androgen medications
  - Reduces scalp hair loss, facial and body hair growth, and acne.
  - Should not be used by women who are pregnant or attempting pregnancy.
- Fertility therapy
  - Medications that induce ovulation, such as Clomid, may be used.
  - Assisted reproductive technology, such as in vitro fertilization, may be used for women who do not respond to medications.
- Diabetic medications
  - Antidiabetic medications are prescribed to lower blood glucose levels. They can also lower testosterone, which reduces the degree of acne, hirsutism, and abdominal obesity and may help regulate the menstrual cycle and treat infertility.

Nursing Actions

PCOS has both physical and psychological effects. Body image can be negatively impacted by changes stemming from PCOS. Women need opportunities to share their concerns about PCOS and receive information on methods to decrease or counteract its effects. Areas to discuss with the woman include:

- Risk factors related to PCOS
- Weight reduction through diet and exercise
  - Explain the benefits of weight loss on PCOS.
  - Provide information on healthy diet and assist in developing a healthy diet plan.
- Treatment options for hirsutism
  - Laser hair removal
  - Eflornithine HCL cream
- Treatment options for acne and oily skin
  - Evaluation and treatment by a dermatologist
- Treatment options for alopecia
  - Evaluation and treatment by a dermatologist
- Infertility issues
- Psychological effects of body changes related to PCOS such as depression and anxiety

SAFE AND EFFECTIVE NURSING CARE:
Understanding Medication

Eflornithine HCL (Vaniqa)

Indication: Reduction of unwanted facial hair in women

Action: Inhibits the enzyme ornithine decarboxylase in skin, which decreases synthesis of polyamines.

Common side effects: Burning, rash, stinging, tingling of skin

Route and dosage: Topical. Apply a thin layer to affected areas of the face and adjacent involved areas under the chin and rub in thoroughly. Do not wash for 4 hours following application. Use twice daily at least 8 hours apart (Vallerand & Sanoski, 2021).

ENDOMETRIOSIS

Endometriosis is a chronic inflammatory disease in which the presence and growth of endometrial tissue is found outside the uterine cavity. The tissue, referred to as endometrial lesions, is usually found in the peritoneal surfaces of reproductive organs and adjacent structures of the pelvis, such as ovaries, fallopian tubes, bladder, bowel, and intestines. Endometrial lesions are estrogen-dependent and most commonly occur during the reproductive years. Lesions respond to the changes in estrogen and progesterone levels of the menstrual cycle; each month they build up, break down, and shed as does the endometrial tissue inside the uterus.

The cause of endometriosis is unknown, though the primary theory attributes it to retrograde menstruation that transports endometrial tissue via the fallopian tubes outside the uterine cavity, where it adheres to surrounding organs. Other theories include genetic predisposition, immunological changes, and hormonal influences.

Signs and Symptoms

One-third of women with endometriosis are asymptomatic. Symptoms vary depending on the location of the lesions. The degree of symptoms does not correlate with the size of lesions.

Pelvic pain and dysmenorrhea usually begin a few days before menses and stop at the end of menstruation. Other symptoms include:

- Low back pain
- Sharp pelvic pain
- Pelvic pressure
- Dyspareunia
- Infertility
- Dysmenorrhea
- AUB
- Diarrhea, pain with defecation, and constipation usually present when there are lesions of the bowel
- Bloody urine and dysuria usually present when there are lesions on the bladder
- Fixed retroverted uterus
- Enlarged and tender ovaries

CRITICAL COMPONENT

Endometriosis

- Abnormal growth of tissue resembling the endometrium is present outside of the uterine cavity.
- Tissue responds to changes in estrogen and progesterone levels.
  - The tissue grows and thickens during the secretory and proliferative stages of the menstrual cycle.
  - Tissue breaks down and bleeds into surrounding tissue during the menstrual phase.

- Bleeding into surrounding tissues causes pain and inflammation.
- Scarring, fibrosis, and adhesions result from continued inflammation.

Emotional Impact

The physical symptoms of endometriosis can affect the woman's mental health. The woman may experience anger and grief related to loss of fertility. The pain related to endometriosis can interfere with her social activities, and dyspareunia can affect intimate relationships.

Medical Management

- Analgesic therapy
  - NSAIDs are commonly used for pain management.
- Hormonal therapy
  - Goal is to suppress menstruation and further growth of lesions.
  - Common medications include:
  - Oral contraceptive pills
  - GnRH agonists such as allopurinol or nafarelin (Synarel)
  - Progestins
  - Danazol (Danocrine)—this drug has adverse effects on developing fetuses and is not recommended for women who are attempting pregnancy.
- Symptoms usually return within 1 to 5 years after medications are stopped.
- Surgical treatment
  - Surgical removal of lesions via laparoscopy procedure and laser treatment is used for women with severe symptoms who are infertile and desire pregnancy. Endometriosis may recur after surgical intervention.
  - Hysterectomy with bilateral salpingo-oophorectomy and removal of adhesions and lesions is used for women with severe symptoms who do not desire pregnancy.

SAFE AND EFFECTIVE NURSING CARE: Understanding Medication

Nafarelin (Synarel)

- Indication: Endometriosis
- Action: A synthetic analogue of GnRH. Prolonged use causes a reduction in serum estrone, E2, testosterone, and androstenedione.
- Side effects: Emotional instability, headaches, vaginal dryness, acne, cessation of menses, impaired fertility, decreased libido, hot flashes
- Route and doses: Intranasal; one spray (200 mcg) in morning in one nostril and one spray (200 mcg) in the other nostril in the evening up to a maximum of 800 mcg/day (Vallerand & Sanoski, 2021)

- Assisted reproduction
  - Ovulation induction with intrauterine insemination or in vitro fertilization may be used for infertile women with endometriosis who have not responded to other therapies for infertility.

Nursing Actions

- Patient education regarding endometriosis
- Patient education regarding pain management
  - NSAIDs
  - Heat therapy
  - Biofeedback
  - Relaxation techniques
- Emotional support
  - Provide opportunities for the woman to explore feelings about living with endometriosis.
- Patient education on prescribed treatment plan
  - Information on medications, including action, side effects, and dosage
  - Information on surgical intervention

INFECTIONS

Infections of the reproductive system and pelvic organs increase a woman's risk for cancer, chronic pain, systemic infections, and infertility. Infections are preventable and treatable. Early interventions decrease the woman's risk for complications related to prolonged or repeated infections of the pelvic region. Infections of the reproductive system and pelvic organs include three types of infections:

- Sexually transmitted infections (STIs)
- Endogenous infections such as bacterial vaginitis
- Iatrogenic infections such as UTI caused by improperly performed medical or nursing procedures

Sexually Transmitted Infections

STIs, also known as sexually transmitted diseases, are infections that are primarily transmitted through vaginal intercourse, anal intercourse, and oral sex. Table 19-2 summarizes the most common STIs. Chlamydia and gonorrhea are the top two reported STIs and are highest in the female adolescent population (CDC, 2021).

Women can have an STI and be asymptomatic. However, women who are asymptomatic are still at risk for infecting their sexual partners. To decrease the risk of reinfection, treatment needs to be directed at both the woman and her partner.

CRITICAL COMPONENT

Sexually Transmitted Infections
Untreated STIs place a woman at risk for:

- Cervical cancer
- Pelvic inflammatory disease
- Infertility due to blocked fallopian tubes
- Ectopic pregnancy due to blocked fallopian tubes
- CPP

Lesbians and bisexual women are at the same risk for STIs depending on partners and practices. They should be offered the same STI screening and assessment as women who identify as heterosexual. The types of sexual behavior that carry a risk for STI between women are:

- Oral-vaginal and vulval contact: Herpes, syphilis, and gonorrhea
- Digital-vaginal contact: Human papillomavirus (HPV), bacterial vaginosis (BV), trichomonas, chlamydia, and gonorrhea
- Oral-anal contact: Syphilis, herpes, and hepatitis A
- Genital–genital and genital–body contact: HPV and herpes
- Insertive sex (sex toys and dildos): Trichomonas, gonorrhea, herpes, and HPV (County of Los Angeles Public Health, 2021)

Nursing Actions

- Provide information on the transmission and treatment of STIs.
- Provide information on methods to decrease the risk of STIs.
  - Be in a monogamous sexual relationship with a partner who has been screened for STIs and is not infected.
  - Use condoms or dental dams correctly every time one is engaged in sexual activity. Dental dams are polyurethane sheets used between the mouth and vagina or anus during oral sex.
  - Talk with the partner about STIs and the use of condoms or dental dams before engaging in sexual activities.
  - Talk with your health-care provider and your sexual partner about any STI you or your partner presently have or have had in the past.
  - Follow current guidelines for frequency of pelvic examinations, Pap tests, and HPV testing.

Vaginitis

The vaginal flora is a delicate ecosystem primarily composed of various lactobacilli, which inhibit the growth of yeast and bacteria. Vaginitis, an inflammation of the vagina, occurs when the vaginal ecosystem is disrupted. Symptoms of vaginitis include vaginal discharge that can be malodorous, depending on the causative agent; burning; irritation; or itching. The two most common types of vaginitis are candida vaginitis and BV.

Candida Vaginitis

Candida vaginitis, also called candidiasis or a yeast infection, is caused by *Candida albicans*. This gram-positive fungus lives on all surfaces of the human body. When the vaginal ecosystem is disturbed, the fungus rapidly grows, causing an infection. Factors that can affect the vaginal ecosystem are:

- Hormonal changes: The presence of candida vaginitis increases before and immediately following the menstrual period due to

TABLE 19-2   Sexually Transmitted Infections

STI	CAUSATIVE AGENT	MANIFESTATION OR SYMPTOMS	TREATMENT
Chlamydia	*Chlamydia trachomatis* (Bacterial)	Most common bacterial in the United States and the leading cause of preventable infertility and ectopic pregnancies. Most infected women are asymptomatic; 30% have a mucopurulent cervical discharge. Other symptoms include spotting, urethritis, lower abdominal pain, nausea, fever, and dyspareunia. Chlamydia is diagnosed via swab test at the infected area or by urine test. Chlamydia can also live in the throat, rectum, and urethra.	Antibiotic therapy: Doxycycline 100 mg orally twice a day for 7 days **or** Azithromycin 1 gm orally given in a single dose. Infected partner needs to be treated to decrease risk of reinfection.
Gonorrhea	*Neisseria gonorrhoeae* (Bacterial)	Women are commonly asymptomatic. Symptoms include vaginal discharge, AUB, postcoital bleeding, low backache, urinary frequency, dysuria, and pain during sexual intercourse. Gonorrhea is diagnosed via swab test of infected area. Home tests are available.	Recommended therapy is single intramuscular (IM) dose of ceftriaxone given in combination with azithromycin or doxycycline. Infected partner should be treated to decrease risk of reinfection.
Syphilis	*Treponema pallidum* (Bacterial)	Syphilis progresses in stages: Primary syphilis symptom is a single, painless ulcer (chancre) in the genital area, mouth, or point of contact. Appears 10–90 days after contact. The chancre lasts 4–6 weeks and usually resolves without treatment. Secondary syphilis symptoms include skin rash, fever, sore throat, lymphadenopathy, muscle aches, weight loss, and fatigue. Appears 6 weeks to 6 months after the appearance of the chancre. If not treated, the symptoms resolve on their own within 2–10 weeks. Tertiary syphilis: Approximately one-third of infected individuals will develop tertiary syphilis. Without treatment, the bacteria can spread throughout the body, and symptoms are related to damage of internal organs. Screening tests include rapid plasma reagin and venereal disease research laboratory.	Doxycycline 100 mg two times a day for 14 days or tetracycline 500 mg four times a day for 14 days Infected partner should be treated to decrease risk of reinfection.
Trichomoniasis	*Trichomonas vaginalis* (Protozoan)	Most women are asymptomatic. Symptoms appear 5–28 days after exposure. Symptoms include profuse frothy gray or yellow-green vaginal discharge with foul odor; erythema, edema, pruritus of the external genitalia, and pain during sexual intercourse. Small, red ulcerations in the vagina or on the cervix may be observed during examination. Diagnosis: Microscopic evaluation to confirm trichomoniasis or rapid trichomoniasis test	Metronidazole (Flagyl) is the medication of choice. It may be administered as a single dose of 2 g orally or 500 mg orally twice a day for 7 days. Partner needs to be treated at the same time and condoms used to prevent future infections. Women should be advised not to drink alcohol for 24 hours after completing metronidazole therapy. The combination of alcohol and medication can cause flushing, nausea, vomiting, headaches, and abdominal cramping.

AUB, abnormal uterine bleeding; STI, sexually transmitted infection.

hormonal changes. High levels of estrogen during pregnancy favor growth of fungus.

- Depressed cell-mediated immunity: Women taking exogenous corticosteroids or who have AIDS are at higher risk for reoccurring candida vaginitis.
- Antibiotic use: Lactobacillus, which inhibits the growth of fungi, is part of the normal vaginal bacteria flora. Certain broad-spectrum antibiotics, such as penicillin and tetracycline, can destroy lactobacillus, allowing the rapid growth of *C. albicans*.

CRITICAL COMPONENT

Prevalence of Candida Vaginitis

Candida vaginitis is common in women of childbearing age. Three out of four women will experience at least one occurrence of candida vaginitis within their lifetime.

Risk Factors

- Suppressed immune system
- Antibiotic therapy
- Steroid therapy
- Diabetes
- Pregnancy
- Menopause

Signs and Symptoms

- Itching and irritation in the vulva and vaginal areas, which are the primary symptoms
- White, cheesy vaginal discharge
- Pain with sexual intercourse
- Burning on urination
- Vaginal pH below 4.5

Medical Management

Most vaginal yeast infections can be treated with over-the-counter (OTC) medications. Women often self-diagnose and self-treat. It is important for women to contact their primary health provider if symptoms continue after treatment or are recurrent.

- Diagnosis with a wet smear of vaginal secretions
- Medication: Fluconazole (Diflucan), an antifungal prescription medication, is given when OTCs are not effective or when there is a severe infection. Treatment is a single oral dose of 150 mg. The safety of use during pregnancy has not been established. It is usually compatible with women who are lactating (Vallerand & Sanoski, 2021). Women with reoccurring candida vaginitis may be treated with a 6-month course of fluconazole.

Nursing Actions

- Teach the woman proper use of OTC medications.
- Instruct the woman to notify her health-care provider if symptoms continue or are recurrent. Women can mistake bacteria vaginosis for candida vaginitis, which has a different treatment plan.
- Instruct the woman to contact her health-care provider if any of the following occur:
  - Bloody discharge
  - Abdominal pain
  - Fever
- Instruct the woman to wear cotton underwear to decrease the risk of recurrent infections.

SAFE AND EFFECTIVE NURSING CARE: Understanding Medication

Use of OTC Medications for Treatment of Candida Vaginitis

- Most vaginal yeast infections can be treated with common OTC remedies:
  - Miconazole (Micon 7, Monistat 3)
  - Tioconazole (Monistat 1, Vagistat-1)
  - Butoconazole (Gynazole-1)
  - Clotrimazole (Mycelex)
- OTCs come in creams and suppositories and are placed in the vagina.
- Length of treatment varies from 1 to 7 days.
- The health-care provider needs to be contacted if symptoms continue for more than a week or if symptoms return.
- Before starting OTC medication, women need to see the health-care provider when:
  - It is their first yeast infection.
  - They are 12 years or younger.
  - They are pregnant or breastfeeding.
  - They have reoccurring yeast infections—more than four per year.
  - They are taking warfarin.
  - They have a suppressed immune system.

Bacterial Vaginosis

BV, the most common vaginal infection, occurs when there is a disruption in the normal vaginal flora that includes a decrease in lactobacilli and an increase in organisms such as genital mycoplasma, *Peptostreptococcus*, and *Gardnerella*.

CRITICAL COMPONENT

Bacterial Vaginosis

- Women who experience abnormal vaginal discharge need to be seen by their health-care providers since symptoms of BV are similar to those of chlamydia, gonorrhea, candidiasis, and trichomoniasis.
- Pregnant women with BV are at greater risk for preterm labor and endometritis.

Risk Factors

- New sexual partner, male or female
- Multiple sexual partners
- Lesbian couples who share sex toys without cleaning them between uses
- Douching, which can alter the normal vaginal flora
- Antibiotic therapy, which can alter the normal vaginal flora

Signs and Symptoms

- Vaginal odor, often described as fishy
- Vaginal discharge that is often thin and white or gray; may also be described as milky

Medical Management

- Microscopic examination of vaginal discharge to rule out other causes such as candidiasis and trichomoniasis
- Gynecological examination to assess the appearance of the vaginal lining and the cervix
- Pharmacological therapy:
  - Metronidazole (Flagyl)—Taken orally as a pill or inserted vaginally in gel form
  - Clindamycin (Cleocin)—Taken orally as a pill or inserted vaginally in gel form
  - Tinidazole (Tindamax)—Taken orally in pill form
- Male partner does not need to be treated.
- Female partner may need treatment.

Nursing Actions

- Provide education on proper administration, actions, and side effects of medications.
- Instruct women who are taking metronidazole (Flagyl) PO to take with meals and avoid drinking alcohol. The combination of metronidazole (Flagyl) and alcohol can cause severe nausea and vomiting, flushing, tachycardia, and shortness of breath.
- Provide information on signs and symptoms of possible recurrence that the woman should report to the health-care provider.
- Provide information of risk factors for BV.

Urinary Tract Infections

A UTI is an infection of the urethra, bladder, ureters, or kidneys. It is more common in women than men because women have a shorter urethra in proximity to the vagina and anus. The two most common UTIs are cystitis and urethritis. UTIs are typically ascending infections. Cystitis is usually related to *Escherichia coli*. Urethritis is usually related to STIs such as chlamydia. Untreated cystitis or urethritis places women at risk for pyelonephritis. Diagnosis of a UTI is usually based on the presenting symptoms and confirmed with a positive urine culture.

Risk Factors

- Young girls and menopausal women related to decreased levels of estrogen

- Suppressed immune system
- Diabetes
- Urinary tract obstructions
- Incomplete or infrequent bladder emptying
- Pregnancy
- Irritation of the urethra during sexual activity, which can cause bacteria to migrate upward into the urinary tract
- Allergic reaction to certain ingredients in soaps, vaginal creams, and bubble baths
- Recent urinary procedures such as urinary surgery or urinary cauterization
- Bowel incontinence

Signs and Symptoms

- Dysuria
- Urinary frequency
- Urgency
- Sensation of bladder fullness
- Suprapubic tenderness
- Cloudy, foul-smelling urine
- Backache and pelvic pain
- Low-grade fever

CLINICAL JUDGMENT

UTI and Older Women
- Older women are more susceptible to UTI due to:
  - Suppressed immune system
  - Weakened muscles that increase risk for incomplete bladder emptying
  - Decreased levels of estrogen, which can alter the normal vaginal flora allowing for growth of *E. coli*, which can spread to the urinary tract
- Older women usually do not present with the common signs of UTI such as fever. When fever does occur, it is related to a serious UTI and needs immediate treatment.
- UTI places stress on the body, and in older women the stress can cause confusion and abrupt changes in behavior.
- Symptoms of UTI in older women can include:
  - Confusion or delirium
  - Agitation
  - Hallucinations
  - Poor motor skills or dizziness
  - Falling

Medical Management

Antibiotic therapy is used for uncomplicated UTI. Medications most commonly used are:

- Trimethoprim or sulfamethoxazole (e.g., Bactrim, Septra).
- Ciprofloxacin (e.g., Cipro).
- Nitrofurantoin macrocrystals (e.g., Macrodantin)
- Fosfomycin (e.g., Monurol)

SAFE AND EFFECTIVE NURSING CARE: Understanding Medication

Trimethoprim or Sulfamethoxazole (Bactrim)

- Indication: UTI (also used for bronchitis, otitis media, pneumonia)
- Action: Inhibits the metabolism of folic acid in bacteria
- Common side effects: Nausea, vomiting, diarrhea, and rashes
- Route and dosage: PO; 160 mg Trimethropin (TMP)/800 mg Sulfamethoxazole (SMX) every 12 hours for 10 to 14 days (recent studies have shown that a 3- to 5-day course is also effective) (Vallerand & Sanoski, 2021).

Nursing Actions

- Teach women to take full course of antibiotic therapy.
- Provide information on strategies to promote bladder health and ways to decrease risk for developing UTI.
  - Drink to thirst and until urine is a clear yellow color. Assess for conditions that require fluid restrictions such as heart disease.
  - Void every 2 to 4 hours; avoid postponing urination. When urine remains in the bladder for prolonged periods, bacteria has increased time to multiply.
  - Empty the bladder before and after intercourse to flush out bacteria in the urethra.
  - Remain hydrated to keep bacteria flushed out of the urinary tract system.
  - Wipe the urethral meatus and perineum from front to back after voiding.
  - Wear cotton underpants and change daily; avoid tight-fitting underwear and pants.
  - Avoid caffeine and alcohol since these can irritate the bladder.
  - Do not douche or use feminine hygiene products that can alter normal vagina flora.
  - Avoid harsh soaps, powders, sprays, and bubble baths.
  - Drinking cranberry juice has no proven evidence that it will prevent UTIs. It should not be taken if the woman takes Coumadin (Vallerand & Sanoski, 2021).
- Teach women about the signs and symptoms of a UTI and to report these to their health-care providers.

LEIOMYOMA OF THE UTERUS

Leiomyomas of the uterus, also referred to as myomas or uterine fibroids, are benign fibrous tumors of the uterine wall. Leiomyomas are the most common tumors in women. They vary in size, number, and location and are estrogen and progesterone sensitive. Growth of leiomyomas is seen during the reproductive years due to increased levels of estrogen and progesterone. Leiomyomas are usually asymptomatic. The severity of symptoms is related to the number, size, and locations of the myomas.

Risk Factors

- Early menarche
- Heredity: Increased risk when mother or sister has myomas
- Race: Black women more likely to have myomas
- Obesity

Signs and Symptoms

- Pelvic pressure from the enlarging mass
- Dysmenorrhea
- AUB
- Pelvic pain, backaches, or leg pain
- Urinary frequency and urgency when myomas are pressing on the bladder
- Palpation of tumor during bimanual pelvic examination

Medical Management

- Pelvic ultrasound is used to confirm diagnosis of tumors and rule out pregnancy.
- Blood transfusions may be needed for severe anemia related to excessive blood loss.
- Treatment for leiomyomas is based on the size and location of the tumors, the degree to which they interfere with the woman's quality of life, and whether the woman desires pregnancy. Most tumors will shrink after menopause. Treatment options include:
  - GnRH agonists are used for 3 months to control bleeding and shrink the tumor.
  - Uterine artery embolization: Polyvinyl alcohol pellets are injected into selected blood vessels to block the blood supply to the tumor and cause it to shrink.
  - Laser surgery: Laser coagulation vaporizes the fibroids and produces necrosis. It can increase the woman's risk for infertility due to uterine scarring.
  - Myomectomy, removal of the tumor, is common for symptomatic women who desire pregnancy.
  - Hysterectomy is recommended for women who do not desire pregnancy and who are experiencing excess bleeding. Leiomyomas are one of the main indicators for hysterectomy.

Nursing Actions

Nursing actions vary based on the method of medical or surgical treatment. Nurses are most likely to care for women being treated for myomas in the inpatient setting following a hysterectomy (see nursing actions following hysterectomy later in this chapter).

OVARIAN CYSTS

Ovarian cysts are enclosed sacs that contain fluid, blood, or cells that develop inside or on the surface of the ovaries. Ovarian cysts are often discovered during routine pelvic examinations.

Most cysts spontaneously disappear either by reabsorption of the fluid within the cyst or by rupturing within 8 weeks (Lobo et al., 2017). Two of the more common types of ovarian cysts are follicular cysts and corpus luteum cysts.

Follicular cysts are the most common type of ovarian cyst. They develop during the follicular phase (first half of the menstrual cycle) when the dominant mature follicle fails to rupture (ovulate) and begins to fill with fluid or when an immature follicle fails to degenerate (Lobo et al., 2017). Follicular cysts are usually asymptomatic. One-quarter of women who have this type of cyst report pain or a heavy, achy feeling in the pelvis.

Corpus luteum cysts form from the corpus luteum during the luteal phase (second half of the menstrual cycle). Normally, the corpus luteum forms after ovulation and gradually degenerates if pregnancy does not occur. Occasionally, the corpus luteum seals and fills with fluid or blood and forms a cyst. The woman may experience acute lower abdominal pain and delayed menses followed by acute AUB.

Some cysts rupture and cause intraperitoneal bleeding. Rupture may be caused by coitus, exercise, lower abdominal trauma, or pelvic examination. The woman with intraperitoneal bleeding will experience sudden and severe abdominal pain and may require surgery and blood transfusions.

Diagnosis is usually based on symptoms and bimanual examination. Ultrasonography may be used to aid in the diagnosis and rule out pregnancy but cannot provide a definitive diagnosis. It is important to rule out ovarian cancer. Additional tests and procedures may be ordered, such as:

- CA 125 test: This measures the amount of CA 125 (cancer antigen 125) in the blood. Elevated levels occur in women with endometriosis, myomas, PID, and ovarian cancer.
- Laparoscopic surgery is used to visualize the ovaries or remove a cyst.

Medical Management

- Since most cysts spontaneously disappear either by reabsorption of the fluid within the cyst or by rupturing within 8 weeks, monitoring the conditions is the treatment of choice when the symptoms are mild.
- NSAIDs are used for pain management.
- Oral contraceptives are prescribed to inhibit ovulation to decrease the risk of developing additional cysts.
- Surgical removal of the cyst is considered when the cyst:
  - Occurs after menopause since postmenopausal women with ovarian cysts have a higher risk for ovarian cancer.
  - Has grown larger.
  - Has an unusual appearance noted on the ultrasound.
  - Causes severe pain.

PELVIC ORGAN PROLAPSE

The pelvic organs are supported by muscles, ligaments, and fascia. When these structures are weakened, pelvic organs can descend into the vagina or against the vaginal wall. This disorder is known as pelvic organ prolapse (POP). POP can affect the bladder, urethra, uterus, and rectum. Common disorders related to POP are uterine prolapse, cystocele, and rectocele (Fig. 19–3). Risk factors for POP are:

- Childbirth trauma related to:
  - Vaginal deliveries
  - Large babies
  - Forceps or vacuum deliveries
  - Poor suturing techniques with repair of episiotomies or lacerations
- Pelvic trauma (i.e., pelvic surgery)
- Stress and strain from heavy lifting, constipation, or violent coughing
- Obesity
- Menopause: Low levels of estrogen weaken the pelvic floor muscles.

Uterine Prolapse

Uterine prolapse occurs when there is a weakening of the pelvic connective tissue, pubococcygeus muscle, and uterine ligaments, allowing the uterus to descend into the vagina. Degrees of prolapse vary from slight prolapse to third-degree prolapse. Also known as complete uterine prolapse, third-degree prolapse occurs when the uterus has descended out of the vagina (see Fig. 19–3).

Assessment Findings

- Protrusion of the uterus into the vagina
- Low backache
- Sensation of heaviness in the pelvis or vagina
- Sensation that the uterus is falling out
- Difficult or painful intercourse

Medical Management

- Vaginal pessary: A rubber- or silicone-based ring placed in the vagina to support the uterus; effective for a mild degree of uterine prolapse (Fig. 19–4)
- Surgery, which may include hysterectomy

Nursing Actions

- Explain the importance of Kegel exercises for improving pelvic muscle strength and teach the woman how to do Kegel exercises.
- Instruct the woman on the treatment and prevention of constipation, such as a high-fiber diet and increased fluid intake. This will help in reducing straining during defecation and decrease stress on existing POP.
- Instruct the woman to avoid heavy lifting to decrease stress on pelvic organs.
- Explain the relationship between increased weight and increased risk of prolapsed uterus and discuss weight-reduction strategies.
- Provide postoperative care for women who have had a hysterectomy.

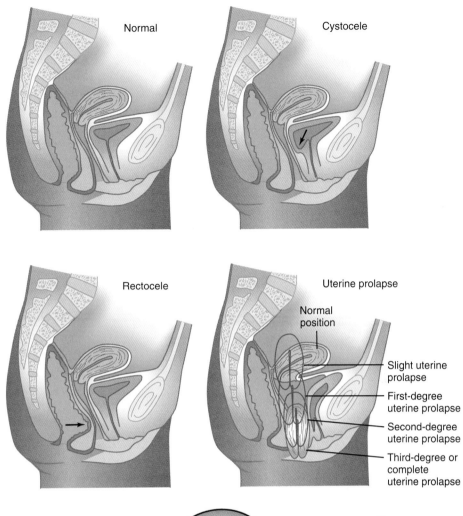

FIGURE 19–3 Cystocele, rectocele, and uterine prolapse.

Cystocele and Rectocele

Cystocele, also known as anterior prolapse, is the bulging of the bladder into the vagina. This occurs when the wall between the vagina and bladder weakens and stretches. Rectocele, also known as posterior prolapse, is the bulging of the rectum into the vagina. This occurs when the wall between the vagina and the rectum weakens and stretches.

Assessment Findings for Cystocele

- Bulging mass in the anterior vaginal wall (see Fig. 19–3)
- Sense of fullness or pressure in the vaginal area
- Degree of bulging increases when straining, coughing, bearing down, lifting, or standing for a prolonged period of time
- Stress incontinence
- Bladder infections
- Urine leakage during intercourse
- Sexual dysfunction such as dyspareunia, vaginal dryness, and irritation

Assessment Findings for Rectocele

- Bulging mass in the posterior vaginal wall (see Fig. 19–3)
- Straining and prolonged standing, which can increase the degree of the bulging

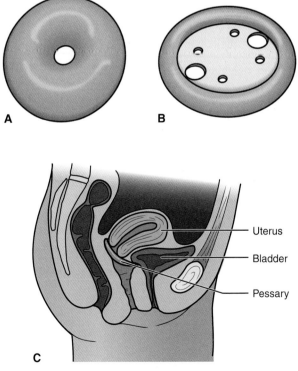

FIGURE 19–4 Vaginal pessary: (A) Doughnut pessary. (B) Ring pessary. (C) Inserted pessary.

- Irritation of the vaginal mucosa
- Constipation

Medical Management

Medical management is based on the degree of bulging, effects on the woman's quality of life, and the woman's overall health. Treatment options include:

- Vaginal pessary to support the bladder
- Estrogen therapy to improve pelvis muscle strength
- Surgical repair of the cystocele or rectocele

Nursing Actions

The primary nursing action is patient education.

- Explain the importance of Kegel exercises for improving pelvic muscle strength and teach the woman how to do Kegel exercises.
- Instruct the woman on the treatment and prevention of constipation, such as a high-fiber diet and increased fluid intake. This will help in reducing straining during defecation and decrease stress on existing POP.
- Instruct the woman to avoid heavy lifting to decrease stress on pelvic organs.
- Explain the relationship between increased weight and increased risk of cystoceles and rectoceles and discuss weight-reduction strategies.

URINARY INCONTINENCE

Urinary incontinence is the loss of bladder control and can range from stress incontinence to a sudden urge to void followed by uncontrolled voiding. Stress incontinence is leakage of urine when there is an increase in intra-abdominal pressure related to coughing, sneezing, or laughing. Urinary incontinence can have a profound effect on the woman's quality of life by limiting her activities due to the embarrassment of uncontrolled urination.

Risk Factors

- Childbirth
- Aging: Leads to a decrease in estrogen and a weakening of muscles, thus decreasing the ability of the urethra to remain closed.
- Obesity: The risk increases for every 5 units of body mass index (BMI) increase (Lobo et al., 2017).
- Smoking: Causes chronic coughing and places stress on the urinary sphincters.

Assessment Findings

- Leakage of urine when coughing, sneezing, laughing, or lifting
- Sudden and intense urge to void followed by uncontrolled voiding

Medical Management

- Treatment is based on the degree of incontinence and the effect it has on quality of life.
- Behavioral techniques
  - Bladder training: Waiting 5 minutes from feeling the urge to void to urinating and gradually increasing the time between urge to voiding
  - Scheduled toilet trips: Developing a schedule for voiding and not waiting to feel the urge to void
  - Limiting alcohol and caffeine use: These act as a bladder stimulant and diuretic.
  - Losing weight
- Pelvic floor exercises
  - Kegel exercises: Improve pelvic floor muscle strength
- Medications
  - Tolterodine (Detrol) and mirabegron (Myrbetriq): Used to treat overactive bladder
  - Estrogen cream applied to the genital tissues: Improves the tone and tissue in the urethral and vaginal areas
- Medical devices
  - Pessary
- Surgery

SAFE AND EFFECTIVE NURSING CARE: Understanding Medication

Tolterodine (Detrol)

- Action: Inhibits cholinergic mediated bladder contractions → decreased urinary frequency, urgency, and urge incontinence
- Common side effects: Dry mouth, headache, and dizziness
- Route and dosage: PO; 2 mg twice daily (Vallerand & Sanoski, 2021)

Nursing Actions

The primary nursing action is patient education.

- Instruct the woman on the importance of Kegel exercises and teach her how to do them.
- Instruct the woman on the treatment and prevention of constipation by increasing fiber in the diet and fluid intake.
- Instruct her to avoid heavy lifting.
- Explain the relationship between increased weight and increased risk of urinary incontinence and discuss weight-reduction strategies.
- Maintain skin integrity by instructing the woman to keep the area clean and dry.
- Encourage the woman to decrease alcohol and caffeine intake, as both cause increased urination.
- Provide strategies for retraining the bladder, such as scheduling toileting times and gradually increasing the wait time after she feels the urge to void.

VAGINAL FISTULAS

Vaginal fistulas are abnormal connections between the vagina and bladder, vagina and urethra, or vagina and rectum. The fistula provides a pathway for fecal material or urine to enter the vagina. Fistulas can develop as a result of trauma to the tissue related to childbirth, trauma from surgery, pelvic radiation damage, weakened pelvic tissue, and violent coitus or sexual abuse.

Assessment Findings

- Leakage of urine or fecal material from the vagina
- Foul vaginal odor
- Irritation of the vaginal mucosa

Medical Management

- Pelvic, rectal, and perineal skin examination are performed to determine the location and severity of the fistula.
- Small fistulas usually resolve on their own if tissue is allowed to rest.
- Larger fistulas may require surgical repair.

Nursing Actions

- Reinforce teaching and clarify information provided by the primary health-care provider.
- Postoperative care:
  - Assess vital signs as per protocol.
  - Assess perineal area for increased bleeding.
  - Assess for pain and use appropriate pain-management techniques.
- Postoperative teaching:
  - Instruct the woman with rectal fistula repair to increase fiber in her diet and increase fluid intake to decrease risk of constipation. Maintaining soft stool decreases trauma to the site and promotes healing.
  - Instruct how to use a sitz bath and explain the importance of sitz baths in promoting healing and comfort.
  - Provide medication information. Antibiotics are usually prescribed.
  - Instruct to notify the surgeon when there is an elevated temperature, increased bleeding, or increased pain.

BREAST DISORDERS

Breast disorders include both benign and malignant changes and diseases. Most breast changes and disorders are benign, but the discovery of a breast mass or changes in the breast still evoke feelings of fear and anxiety. Benign and malignant disorders share similar symptoms, so breast changes must be evaluated by the woman's health-care provider. The use of mammography, ultrasound, and magnetic resonance imaging (MRI) are important in the early detection and treatment of benign and cancerous disorders of the breast. See Chapter 18 for recommended screening and testing. The three most common breast disorder symptoms are:

- Pain: This is usually related to hormonal changes and is most common in perimenopausal women. Pain can also be associated with cysts of the breast. Fewer than 10% of women with breast cancer will present with pain.
- Discharge from the nipple: This is classified as either spontaneous or elicited. Elicited discharge results from nipple compression or stimulation. Elicited discharge from both nipples that is milky in color and non-bloody is considered normal. Spontaneous discharge or elicited discharge from one nipple or discharge that is bloody needs further evaluation. Nipple discharge is not a common symptom of breast cancer.
- Palpable breast masses are common and are usually benign, but all breast masses must be evaluated to rule out malignancy.

Fibrocystic Breasts

Fibrocystic breast is also referred to as benign breast disease or fibrocystic changes. It is common for breasts to develop fibrous tissue and benign cysts. These changes occur in more than 50% of women between the ages of 20 and 50. The cause is unknown but it is believed to be related to imbalance of estrogen and progesterone. The cysts are often tender to touch and fluctuate in size with the menstrual cycle. Caffeine intake may exacerbate the condition.

Signs and Symptoms

- Cyclic bilateral breast pain, usually in the upper, outer quadrants of the breasts
- Increased engorgement and density of the breasts
- Increased nodularity of the breasts
- Fluctuation in the size of the cystic areas

Medical Management

- Differentiate between fibrocystic changes and breast cancer using mammography and ultrasound. The health-care provider may also aspirate the cyst for evaluation of fluid.
- Management centers on symptom relief:
  - Oral contraceptives
  - Use of OTC pain medications such as NSAIDs and acetaminophen
  - Wearing a supportive bra
  - Avoiding caffeine, smoking, and alcohol
  - Applying heat to the breast
- Fine-needle aspiration of the cyst

Nursing Actions

- Instruct the woman to follow recommended breast screenings and notify her health-care provider if she notes changes in her breasts.
- Provide information on methods of symptom relief, such as heat to breast and use of a supportive bra.

Breast Cancer

Breast cancer is the second most common cancer in women in the United States. Black and White women have approximately the same rate of breast cancer, but Black women have a higher fatality rate (Centers for Disease Control and Prevention

[CDC], 2020). Breast cancer prognosis improves with early detection and treatment.

Risk Factors

According to the American Cancer Society (ACS; 2019a) risk factors are:

- Increasing age
- Defects in breast cancer genes *BRCA1* or *BRCA 2*
- Family history of breast cancer
- Dense breasts
- Use of birth control methods that contain hormones
- Women who did not breastfeed
- Personal history of breast cancer in at least one breast
- Exposure to head or chest radiation
- Excess weight
- Exposure to estrogen through early onset of menarche, late menopause, or use of hormone therapy
- Excessive use of alcohol
- Exposure to diethylstilbestrol (DES)

Diagnosis

Screenings and procedures used in the diagnosis of breast cancer include (Fig. 19–5):

- Diagnostic mammograms create images of the area of concern that provide additional information on the size and character of the mass.
- Breast ultrasounds assist in determining if the area of concern is a fluid-filled cyst or solid mass.
- MRI is useful in differentiating benign from malignant tissue, especially in women with dense, fibroglandular breasts; when

scar tissue is present from previous breast surgery; and for new tumors in women who have had previous lumpectomy. Yearly screening MRI and mammogram are recommended for women at high risk for breast cancer.

- Breast biopsy can distinguish between benign and malignant tissue.

Indicators of Disease Prognosis

- Stages of breast cancer indicate the degree of spread. Stages range from stage 0 (ductal carcinoma in situ) to stage IV (the cancer has spread to distant organs).
- Breast cancer grade is based on how much the cancer cells look like normal cells. A low-grade number means the cancer is slow-growing and less likely to spread, whereas a high-grade number means it is fast-growing and more likely to spread.
- Presence of hormone receptor levels: Estrogen and progesterone will attach to these receptors and cause an increase in tumor growth.
- Presence of HER2/neu (human epidermal growth factor receptor 2) in the tumor tissue (ACS, 2019a)

CRITICAL COMPONENT

Breast Cancer Risk Assessment Tool

The breast cancer screening tool developed by the National Cancer Institute (NCI) and National Surgical Adjuvant Breast and Bowel Project estimates a woman's risk of developing invasive breast cancer in 5 years and up to age 90. It considers data such as the woman's age, family history of breast cancer, and previous breast biopsies.

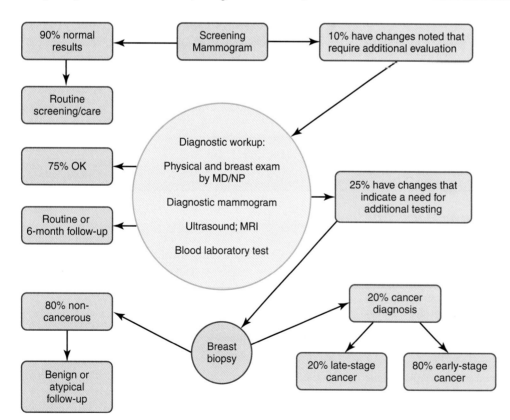

FIGURE 19–5 Breast cancer diagnosis process.

Medical Management

Treatment is determined by the stage of cancer. The breast cancer staging system goes from stage 0 (ductal carcinoma in situ, the earliest form of breast cancer) to stage IV (the cancer has metastasized to distant organs or to distant lymph nodes). Medical management includes:

- Surgical interventions:
  - Lumpectomy: The lump and an area of surrounding normal tissue are removed. This procedure is usually followed by radiation therapy.
  - Partial or segmental mastectomy: The tumor, the surrounding breast tissue, a portion of the lining of the chest wall, and some of the axillary lymph nodes are removed. This procedure is usually followed by radiation therapy.
  - Simple mastectomy: All the breast tissue along with the area surrounding the nipple and areola are removed. This procedure may be followed by radiation therapy, chemotherapy, or hormone therapy.
  - Modified radical mastectomy: The entire breast and several axillary lymph nodes are removed; the chest wall is left intact.
  - Some women who have mastectomies choose to undergo breast reconstruction. Breast reconstruction, when desired, is performed by a plastic surgeon at the same time as the mastectomy.
- Radiation therapy, which usually begins 3 to 4 weeks after surgery
  - External radiation: A radiation therapy machine aims radiation toward the tumor. Treatments are given 5 days a week for 5 to 6 weeks.
  - Internal radiation (mammo site): A radioactive substance sealed in needles, seeds, wires, or a catheter is placed directly into or near the tumor. Treatments are given twice a day for 5 days for a total of 10 sessions.
- Chemotherapy:
  - Oncotype DX test may be performed to determine if the woman is likely to benefit from chemotherapy.
  - Chemotherapy is most commonly used to treat advanced metastatic cancer or to prevent recurrence of cancer.
  - Usually, a combination of two or more drugs is used.
  - Chemotherapy agents may be administered orally or intravenously.
- Hormone therapy:
  - Some breast cancer cells require estrogen to grow and are classified as estrogen-receptor positive. This means that estrogen binds to a protein in these cells.
  - Antiestrogen medications such as tamoxifen (Nolvadex D) bind to these protein receptors, blocking estrogen binding and reducing the influence of estrogen on the tumor.
  - Fulvestrant (Faslodex) may be used to treat hormone receptor (HR)-positive metastatic breast cancer in postmenopausal women with disease progression as well as HR-positive, HER2-negative advanced breast cancer.
  - Aromatase inhibitors such as anastrozole (Arimidex) may be used in postmenopausal women whose cancer is classified as estrogen-receptor positive. Aromatase inhibitors interfere with the amount of estrogen produced by the woman's body tissue (not the ovaries) by blocking the conversion of androgens into estrogens.
- Targeted therapy
  - Trastuzumab (Herceptin), a monoclonal antibody that directly targets the HER2 protein of breast tumors, is a treatment option for women with breast cancer that overproduces HER2.

Nursing Actions

- Provide emotional support to the woman and family, including opportunities for them to share feelings and concerns.
- Provide current, evidence-based information to the woman and family regarding treatment options.
- Encourage the woman to consider all options and seek other opinions or other professionals if she is not comfortable with recommendations.
- Provide information on methods to address treatment side effects (Tables 19-3 and 19-4).
- Provide information on nutrition that promotes healing and enhances the immune system.
- Provide information on complementary modalities such as imagery, journal writing, and hypnosis that can be used to diminish side effects from cancer treatment therapies.

CRITICAL COMPONENT

Oncotype DX Test

- The Oncotype DX test is a genomic assay that assesses the activity of 21 different genes taken from a tissue sample of the cancer tumor. This test assists the health-care provider in determining if the cancer is likely to recur or to benefit from chemotherapy.
- Women with stage I or II, estrogen-receptor-positive (ER+) breast cancer that has not spread to the lymph nodes may benefit from this test in determining type of cancer treatment (ACS, 2021).

SAFE AND EFFECTIVE NURSING CARE: Understanding Medication

Tamoxifen (Nolvadex D)

- Indications: Reduces risk of breast cancer in women who are at increased risk for developing breast cancer; treatment of breast cancer
- Action: Competes with estrogen for binding sites in the breast
- Serious side effects: Pulmonary embolism, stroke, uterine malignancies
- Common side effects: Vaginal dryness, hot flashes, joint pain, leg cramps, nausea
- Route and dose: PO; 10 to 20 mg twice daily or 20 mg once daily for 5 years (Vallerand & Sanoski, 2021).

TABLE 19-3   Management of Radiation Therapy Side Effects

SIDE EFFECT	WAYS TO MANAGE
Diarrhea: Related to damage of healthy cells in large and small intestine	• Drink 8–12 cups of clear liquids; Gatorade or Pedialyte for electrolyte replacement. • Eat small frequent meals; five to six small meals rather than three large meals. • Eat foods that provide nourishment without increasing the risk for diarrhea; foods that are low in fiber, fat, and lactose, such as fresh fruit and cooked vegetables. • Take antidiarrheal medications such as Imodium A-D. • Take care of the rectum; use baby wipes instead of toilet paper. • Take sitz baths.
Fatigue: Related to anemia, depression, infection, and medications	• Get 8 hours of sleep per night; the woman may need more sleep per night than she needed before radiation therapy. • Plan time to rest; take 10- to 15-minute rest breaks throughout the day. • Take several naps during the day. • Decrease daily activities; the woman may not have enough energy for all the activities she used to do. She should select the activities that are most important to her and limit those that are less important. • Exercise; 15–30 minutes of daily exercise improves overall feeling of well-being. • Change work schedule; the client may need to decrease work hours for a few weeks. • Ask family and friends for help at home.
Sexual and fertility changes: Related to damage to healthy tissue of the vagina and ovaries	• Fertility; women desiring future pregnancies need to talk with their health-care provider about ways to preserve fertility, such as preserving eggs for future use. • Sexual difficulties; use water- or mineral-based lubricant if experiencing vaginal dryness. • Vaginal stenosis; discuss use of vaginal dilators with the health-care provider.
Skin changes: Related to damage of healthy tissue	• Skin care; gently wash the area; do not rub, scrub, or scratch. • Avoid heat and cold; wash in lukewarm water. • Do not use heating pads or ice packs. • Wear soft and loose-fitting clothes around the treatment area. • Protect the skin from the sun.
Urinary and bladder changes: Related to damage of healthy cells of the bladder and urinary tract, causing inflammation, ulcers, and infections	• Drink 6–8 cups of fluid per day; avoid coffee, black tea, alcohol, and spices. • Report changes to the health-care provider; may require antibiotic therapy.

Side effects, except for fatigue, are directly related and limited to the site being treated with radiation therapy (e.g., radiation therapy for breast cancer does not cause diarrhea).
ACS, 2017; Cancer Care, 2016.

● Provide information regarding community resources.
  ● Look Good Feel Better is a free program that helps women learn beauty techniques to restore their self-image and cope with appearance-related side effects of cancer treatment. For additional information go to http://lookgoodfeelbetter.org/.
  ● Breast cancer support such as the American Cancer Society Reach to Recovery Program may be beneficial.

GYNECOLOGICAL CANCERS

Gynecological cancer includes cancer of the cervix, uterus (endometrium), ovaries, fallopian tubes, vagina, and vulva. Endometrial cancer is the most common reproductive cancer, followed by cervical and ovarian. Cancers of the fallopian tubes, vagina, and vulva are rare. This section will focus on cervical, endometrial, and ovarian cancers.

Cervical Cancer

Before the routine use of the Papanicolaou (Pap) smear, introduced in the 1950s, cervical cancer was the leading cause of cancer-related deaths in women. It is now ranked as the 21st leading cause of cancer-related deaths (ACS, 2021). This decrease is attributed to the use of Pap smears to detect cervical cancer at an early stage when it can more easily be treated.

HPV, the most common STI, is the primary cause of cervical cancer. Most sexually active people will get the virus at some point.

TABLE 19-4 Management of Chemotherapy Side Effects

Anemia	• Eat high-protein foods such as meat, peanut butter, and eggs. • Eat foods high in iron, such as red meats, leafy greens, and cooked dried beans.
Appetite changes	• Eat five or six small meals per day. • Try new food to keep up interest in foods. • Eat with friends and family. • Eat with plastic forks and spoons and use glass pots if food tastes like metal. • Drink milkshakes or eat soup because these are easier to swallow.
Bleeding problems	• Use electric shaver instead of a razor. • Wear shoes all the time (except when sleeping). • Brush teeth with soft toothbrush. • Avoid being constipated.
Constipation	• Eat high-fiber foods such as whole-grain bread, fruits, and vegetables. • Increase fluid intake. • Exercise 15–30 minutes per day.
Mouth and throat changes	• Brush teeth and tongue with soft toothbrush after each meal. • Rinse mouth with solution prescribed. • Use lip balm. • Choose foods that are soft, wet, and easy to swallow.

Cancer Care, 2016.

Cervical cancer is typically slow-growing and begins with dysplasia, a precancerous condition that is 100% treatable. However, undetected or untreated precancerous changes can develop into cervical cancer that can spread to the bladder, intestines, lungs, and liver.

Pap smear and HPV test are used for cervical cancer screening (see Chapter 18 for recommended screenings and immunizations for women across the life span). Women with abnormal Pap smear or HPV test need further evaluation, since these are screening not diagnostic tests. A colposcopy examination with a biopsy of the abnormal area is done for definitive diagnosis. Most women who are diagnosed with cervical cancer have not had regular Pap testing or have not followed up on abnormal results.

Risk Factors

- HPV infection
- Early onset of sexual activity (before age 16)
- Cigarette smoking
- Weakened immune system
- Multiple sex partners
- In utero exposure to DES
- Use of oral contraception for 5 or more years
- Given birth to three or more children

Risk Reduction

See Chapter 18.

Signs and Symptoms

Early stages of cervical cancer usually do not produce symptoms. Symptoms appear when the cancer is advanced and has invaded nearby tissue.

- Vaginal discharge that may be watery, pink, brown, bloody, or foul-smelling
- Leaking of urine or feces from the vagina
- Abnormal vaginal bleeding between periods, after intercourse, or after menopause
- AUB
- Dyspareunia
- Loss of appetite or weight
- Fatigue
- Pelvic, back, or leg pain

Medical Management

- Cervical cone biopsy
- Testing to determine if cancer is confined to the cervix or has spread to other organs:
  - Computed tomography (CT) scan
  - MRI
  - Positron emission tomography (PET) scan
  - Intravenous pyelography (IVP)
  - Chest x-ray
  - Cystoscopy
  - Blood studies
- Treatment is based on the stage of cancer and the woman's desire for pregnancy.
  - Stages of cervical cancer range from stage 0, abnormal cells are in the epithelium, to stage IVB, cancer has spread to other parts of the body such as the liver, lungs, and bone.
- Treatment options include:
  - Conization
  - Cryosurgery
  - Total hysterectomy and radical hysterectomy
  - Internal or external radiation
  - Removal of lymph nodes
- Chemotherapy is used for cervical cancer that has either metastasized or recurred.
- Angiogenesis inhibitors, such as bevacizumab, are a target drug therapy used with chemotherapy to treat advanced cervical cancer.

Nursing Actions

Patient education and support are critical nursing actions for women with cervical cancer.

- Provide emotional support to the woman and her family.

- Provide information on nutrition that promotes healing and treats or controls side effects from cancer treatments.
- Explain the importance of rest and sleep in the promotion of healing.
- Provide information on community support services.
- Care for women undergoing surgical treatment:
  - Address the woman's and family's questions regarding the surgical procedure.
  - Provide preoperative and postoperative care.
- Care for the woman undergoing radiation therapy:
  - Provide information on ways to manage side effects related to external radiation (see Table 19-3).
  - Teach the importance of skin care in decreasing the risk of tissue breakdown.
  - Instruct the woman to check with her health-care provider regarding types of lotions and creams to use.
  - Instruct the woman to avoid the use of adhesive tape on the treatment area.
  - Recommend exposing the treatment area to air when possible to promote skin integrity.
- Care for the woman undergoing chemotherapy:
  - Administer chemotherapy as per orders.
  - Provide information on the management of side effects related to chemotherapy (see Table 19-4).

CRITICAL COMPONENT

Side Effects: External Radiation for Cervical Cancer

Short-term side effects of external radiation to treat cervical cancer include:

- Fatigue
- Nausea and vomiting
- Diarrhea
- Cystitis
- Bruising
- Anemia
- Skin rash

Long-term side effects include:

- Vaginal stenosis
- Vaginal dryness
- Premature menopause
- Swelling of the legs when pelvic lymph nodes are treated
- Weakened bones—increased risk for hip fractures (ACS, 2020b)

Uterine Cancer

Cancer of the uterus can occur in the endometrium (inner uterine layer) or the myometrium (outer uterine layer). Endometrial carcinoma is the most common uterine cancer. This section will focus on endometrial carcinoma. Diagnosis is established by histological examination of endometrial tissue obtained from an endometrial biopsy.

Risk Factors

- Menopausal hormone therapy: Unopposed estrogen therapy in women with a uterus. This can cause endometrial hyperplasia, an increased number of cells in the lining of the uterus.
- Early menarche or menopause after age 52. These increase the duration of estrogen exposure of the uterus.
- Obesity: Obese women tend to have higher levels of estrogen related to the body making additional estrogen in fatty tissue.
- Tamoxifen: This drug is used to treat breast cancer.
- Nulliparity is a risk factor.
- Diabetes should be considered.

Signs and Symptoms

- Postmenopausal bleeding or AUB (most common symptom)
- Abnormal vaginal discharge
- Difficult or painful urination
- Dyspareunia
- Pelvic pain or pressure

Stages

- Stage 0: Carcinoma in situ; precancerous lesions confined to the surface layer of the endometrium.
- Stage IA: Cancer cells are in the endometrium and have grown less than halfway through the myometrium.
- Stage IB: Cancer cells are in the endometrium and have grown more than halfway through the myometrium; has not spread beyond the uterus.
- Stage II: Cancer cells have invaded cervical stroma but have not extended beyond the uterus.
- Stage III: Tumor has spread outside the uterus but is confined to the pelvis.
- Stage IV: Tumor has spread outside the pelvis or into the mucosa of the bladder or rectum or distant metastasis (ACS, 2019a).

Medical Management

- Treatment is based on the size of the tumor, stage of the tumor, tumor grade, and whether the tumor is affected by estrogen.
- Treatment options
  - Surgery: Hysterectomy, bilateral salpingo-oophorectomy, and pelvic and para-aortic lymph node dissection
  - Radiation therapy
  - Chemotherapy
  - Hormonal therapy (progesterone)
  - Target therapy
    - Lenvatinib and bevacizumab are drugs that interfere with the formation of new blood vessels in the tumor.
    - Pembrolizumab targets PD-1, a protein on T-cells.

Nursing Actions

- Provide emotional support to the woman and her family.
- Provide information on nutrition to promote healing and decrease risk for malnutrition.
- Explain the importance of rest and sleep in the promotion of healing.

- Provide preoperative and postoperative care.
- Administer chemotherapy as per orders.
- Provide information on management of side effects from radiation or chemotherapy as it applies to the woman (see Tables 19-3 and 19-4).

Ovarian Cancer

There are three main types of ovarian cancers: epithelial, germ cell, and stromal. Ovarian cancer mainly occurs in postmenopausal women. Only 25% of ovarian cancer is diagnosed at an early stage. When diagnosed and treated at an early stage, 94% of women live longer than 5 years after diagnosis (ACS, 2020a). Symptoms of ovarian cancer are often vague, making it difficult to diagnose the disease during the early stages. Diagnosis is established by histological examination of the tumor, usually at the time of surgery.

Risk Factors

- Family history of a first-degree relative with ovarian cancer or family history of colorectal or breast cancer
- Personal history of cancer
- Age over 55; risk increases in menopausal women
- Obesity
- First full-term pregnancy after age 35 or never carried pregnancy to full term
- Infertility drugs taken for more than a year
- Tested positive for *BRCA1* or *BRCA2* gene

Signs and Symptoms

Early stages are often asymptomatic or the woman will have vague abdominal, genitourinary, or reproductive symptoms.

- Pressure or pain in the abdomen, pelvis, back, or leg
- Swollen or bloated abdomen
- Urinary urgency and frequency

Stages

- Stage I: Cancer cells are found in one or both ovaries.
- Stage II: Cancer cells have spread to other tissues in the pelvis.
- Stage III: Cancer cells have spread outside the pelvis or to the regional lymph nodes.
- Stage IV: Cancer cells have spread to tissue outside the abdomen and pelvis (ACS, 2020a).

Medical Management

- Tests and procedures
  - CA 125 test
  - Transvaginal ultrasound to identify changes in ovaries
  - CT scan and MRI to confirm presence of pelvic mass
  - PET scan to assess for metastasis to other body organs
  - Barium enema x-ray to determine if there is colon or rectal involvement
- Stage I: Total abdominal hysterectomy and bilateral salpingo-oophorectomy, omentectomy, biopsy of lymph nodes and

other pelvic and abdominal tissues, and chemotherapy when high-grade tumors are present
- Stages II and III: Total abdominal hysterectomy and bilateral salpingo-oophorectomy, omentectomy, and biopsy of lymph nodes and other pelvic and abdominal tissues and chemotherapy with or without radiation therapy
- Stage IV: Surgery to remove as much of the tumor as possible followed by chemotherapy
- Targeted therapy
  - Bevacizumab, an angiogenesis inhibitor
  - Poly (ADP-ribose) polymerase (PARP) inhibitors
  - Larotrectinib—stops proteins made by the abnormal *NTRK* gene (ACS, 2020c)

Nursing Actions

- Provide preoperative and postoperative care.
- Administer chemotherapy as per orders.
- Provide information on management of chemotherapy side effects (see Table 19-4).
- Provide emotional support to the woman and her family.
- Assess for malnutrition and provide nutritional information based on assessment data.

SAFE AND EFFECTIVE NURSING CARE: Patient Education

Nutrition and Cancer Care

Healthy eating habits and good nutrition can help women deal with the effects of cancer and cancer treatments. Protein and calories are essential for healing, fighting infections, and maintaining adequate energy levels. Unfortunately, the side effects of cancer treatments can interfere with women's ability to eat enough food or for their bodies to absorb the nutrients from food, which leads to malnutrition. Suggestions for treating or controlling these side effects are:

- Anorexia: Eat small high-protein and high-calorie meals (i.e., milkshakes, puddings, yogurt, eggs) every 1 to 2 hours versus three large meals.
- Taste changes: Rinse mouth before eating; eat meats with something sweet such as cranberry sauce; use plastic utensils if foods taste metallic; add spice and sauces to foods.
- Nausea: Eat before cancer treatments; rinse mouth before and after eating; eat bland, soft, and easy to digest foods; do not eat in a room that has cooking odors or is very warm.
- Diarrhea: Eat broth, soups, bananas, and canned fruit to replace salt and potassium lost by diarrhea; drink at least 8 cups of fluid per day plus at least 1 cup of fluid after each loose bowel movement; avoid greasy foods, high-fiber foods, milk products, and sugar-free candy until the cause of the diarrhea is identified (National Cancer Institute, 2017).

INTIMATE PARTNER VIOLENCE

According to the CDC, "Intimate partner violence (IPV) includes physical violence, sexual violence, stalking and psychological aggression (including coercive tactics) by a current or former intimate partner, i.e., spouse, boyfriend, girlfriend, dating partner, or ongoing sexual partner" (CDC, 2020, p.8). One in four women in the United States will experience IPV during their lifetime (CDC, 2020). IVP occurs across all socioeconomic, religious, age, and ethnic groups, as well as all sexual orientations.

Physical violence includes but is not limited to slapping, shaking, choking, burning, and use of weapons. Sexual violence includes but is not limited to forcing a partner to engage in sexual activity against her will or to trade sex for food, money, or drugs. Psychological or emotional violence includes but is not limited to humiliating the woman, controlling what she can and cannot do, isolating her from family and friends, and denying access to money.

IPV can have lifelong effects for the woman. These can include:

- Mental health issues such as depression
- Neurological issues such as traumatic brain injury
- Chronic pain from physical injuries
- Sexual and reproductive issues such as vaginal infections, painful intercourse, and unintended pregnancies

Risk Factors

Risk factors for IPV include individual, relationship, community, and societal factors, such as:

- Low self-esteem
- Low academic achievement
- Being an adolescent or young adult
- Alcohol or drug abuse
- Having few friends
- Marital conflict
- Dominance and control of the relationship by one partner over the other (CDC, 2017)

Characteristics of Abusers

- Extreme jealousy
- Possessiveness
- Extremely controlling behavior
- Blaming the partner for anything bad that happens
- Demeaning the partner publicly or privately
- Controlling what the partner wears or how she acts

Nursing Actions

- The American Nurses Association advocates for:
  - Universal screening: All patients are screened for IPV.
  - Documentation of abuse: Documentation is essential for providing a record of abuse and facilitating communication among health professionals.

CRITICAL COMPONENT

Signs of Intimate Partner Violence

- Repeated nonspecific complaints
- Overuse of the health-care system
- Hesitancy, embarrassment, or evasiveness in relating history of injury
- Time lag between injury and presentation for care
- Untreated serious injuries
- Overly solicitous partner who stays close to the woman and attempts to answer questions directed at her
- Injuries of head, neck, face, and areas covered by a one-piece bathing suit; during pregnancy, the breasts and abdomen are particular targets of assault.
- Presence of bruises at various stages of healing

- Reporting IPV: Most states have laws requiring mandatory reporting of IPV.
- Common questions asked in an IPV screening tool are:
  - Do you feel safe in your home?
  - Has your partner ever hit you?
  - Do arguments with your partner result in you feeling bad about yourself?
  - Do you ever feel frightened by what your partner says or does?
  - Do you feel safe in your current relationship?
- When a woman discloses IPV, the nurse should assess to determine urgent safety needs and assist with developing a plan of care, provide information regarding IPV and safe shelters, and assist her in developing strategies to protect herself from harm.

HYSTERECTOMY

Hysterectomy is the surgical removal of the uterus and is one of the most common major surgeries for women. The three most prevalent reasons for hysterectomy are leiomyomas (fibroids), endometriosis, and prolapsed uterus. Other reasons include cancer of the reproductive organs, AUB, and chronic uterine pain.

Types of Hysterectomy Procedures

The type of hysterectomy is determined by the reason for the hysterectomy and the age and health status of the woman. The types are:

- Supracervical hysterectomy or partial hysterectomy: Removal of the uterus (cervix is left in place).
- Total hysterectomy or simple hysterectomy: Removal of the uterus and the cervix.
- Hysterectomy with bilateral salpingo-oophorectomy: Removal of the uterus, cervix, fallopian tubes, and ovaries.
- Radical hysterectomy: Removal of the uterus, cervix, fallopian tubes, ovaries, upper portion of the vagina, and lymph nodes to treat some cases of reproductive cancer.

Surgical and Anesthetic Techniques

- Abdominal hysterectomy: Removal of the uterus and other structures through an abdominal incision. The external incision may be transverse (Pfannenstiel), just above the pubic hairline, or vertical (low midline), below the umbilicus to just above the pubic hairline. Abdominal hysterectomy is usually the preferred technique when the reason for hysterectomy is related to a gynecological cancer. General anesthesia with an endotracheal tube is the preferred anesthetic. When the hysterectomy is for gynecological cancer, in addition to general anesthesia, epidural anesthesia may be used for postoperative pain management.

- Vaginal hysterectomy: The uterus is removed through the vagina. The ovaries and fallopian tubes can also be removed. The woman is placed in a lithotomy position for the operative procedure. A pericervical incision is used. General anesthesia with an endotracheal tube is the preferred anesthetic. Epidural or spinal anesthesia may be used instead of general anesthesia.

- Laparoscope-assisted vaginal hysterectomy (LAVH): The woman is placed in a steep Trendelenburg position. The laparoscope and instruments are inserted through small incisions in the abdomen (Fig. 19–6). The surgeon manually operates the scope and instruments and removes the uterus through the vagina. The hysterectomy is initiated by laparoscopy and subsequent steps are performed vaginally. LAVH carries an increased risk of bladder injury and UTI. General anesthesia with an endotracheal tube is the preferred method due to the CO_2 insufflation required for the laparoscopic procedure and the positioning of the woman during the surgical procedure. CO_2 insufflation causes an increase in intra-abdominal pressure that can cause intraoperative respiratory compromise. The insufflation may also cause cardiovascular compromise from decreased venous return. The steep Trendelenburg position further increases intra-abdominal pressure and may increase the risk of aspiration. The woman needs to be monitored for facial and conjunctival edema. If this occurs, extubation following surgery may need to be postponed due to increased risk of laryngeal edema.

- Robotic-assisted laparoscopic hysterectomy: The woman is placed in a steep Trendelenburg position, and three or four small incisions are made near the umbilicus. A laparoscope and robotic instruments connected to a computer are inserted through the incisions into the abdomen. The surgeon controls the movements of the scope and the instruments from a computer station in the operating room. General anesthesia with an endotracheal tube and with muscle relaxation is the preferred method of anesthesia. The surgeon has limited patient access during robotic surgery because of the bulky equipment placed over the patient. Full muscle relaxation is needed to prevent inadvertent patient movement. Due to the deep Trendelenburg position, the woman needs to be monitored for facial and conjunctival edema. If this occurs, extubation following surgery may need to be postponed due to increased risk of laryngeal edema.

Risks Related to Surgical Procedure

- Complications related to anesthesia
- Injury to ureters, bladder, or bowel
- Hemorrhage
- Infection
- Deep vein thrombosis or venous thromboembolism

Preoperative Care for Abdominal Hysterectomy

To reduce postoperative complications, professional medical organizations recommend the use of checklists developed based on best practice guidelines. One example is the "Safe for Practice" checklist developed by the American College of Surgeons (See Critical Component: Surgical Site Infections Bundles).

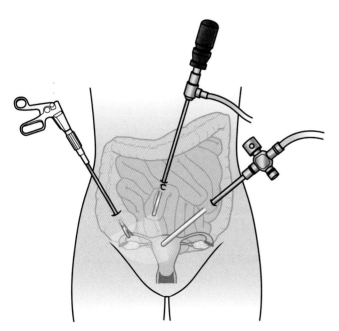

FIGURE 19–6 Laparoscopic hysterectomy.

CRITICAL COMPONENT

Surgical Site Infection Bundles

Strong for Surgery is a public health campaign produced by the American College of Surgeons (2018) to optimize preoperative care before elective surgery to reduce surgical complications. Strong for Surgery recommends preoperative checklists that focus on eight key areas:

- Nutrition
- Glycemic control
- Medication management
- Smoking cessation
- Safe and effective pain management
- Delirium
- Prehabilitation (improving physical well-being before surgery)
- Patient directives (American College of Surgeons, 2018)

The following medical management and nursing actions are performed before an abdominal hysterectomy.

Medical Management

- Physical assessment and health history
- Laboratory tests—complete blood count, type and cross-match, urinalysis
- Electrocardiogram
- NPO 8 hours before surgery
- Informed consent obtained
- Antibiotics when indicated

Nursing Actions

- Complete the appropriate admission assessments and required preoperative forms.
- Ensure that all required documents, such as history and physical, current laboratory reports, and consent forms, are in the woman's chart.
- Verify that the woman has been NPO as directed by her physician.
- Complete the surgical checklist, which includes removal of jewelry, eyeglasses or contact lenses, and dentures.
- Explain to the woman and family or support persons what the woman can expect before surgery and after surgery.
- Start an IV line and IV fluid as per orders.
- Administer antibiotics as per orders.
- Have the woman void or insert a Foley catheter as per orders.
- Provide emotional support for the woman and her family or support persons.
- Address the woman's or family's questions or concerns.

Postoperative Care for Abdominal Hysterectomy

After abdominal hysterectomy, care includes the following:

Medical Management

- IV therapy
- Medications for pain management
- Antibiotic therapy if at risk for infection
- Hormone replacement therapy if ovaries were removed
- Progression of diet within 12 to 24 hours postsurgery
- Foley catheter for 12 to 24 hours postsurgery
- Ambulate once recovered from anesthesia

Nursing Actions

- Monitor vital signs as per protocol.
- Monitor for blood loss—assess for blood on abdominal dressing and perineal pad. The woman will experience small to moderate amounts of vaginal bleeding for several days.
- Monitor level of consciousness and level of sensation and for side effects of anesthesia.

- Assess lung sounds and assist the woman with deep breathing and coughing. Teach the woman to splint her abdomen with a pillow when she coughs.
- Initiate anti-embolism therapy as per orders.
- Assist the woman into a comfortable position and reposition every 2 hours.
- Assess for pain and provide pain relief via prescribed medications, use of relaxation techniques, positioning, or soothing environment.
- Assist the woman with ambulation as per orders. Explain to the woman that ambulation decreases her risk for deep vein thrombosis and facilitates return of intestinal peristalsis, which decreases the amount of gas buildup.
- Monitor intake and output.
- Provide DC IV as per orders.
- Provide DC Foley catheter as per orders.
- Assess bowel sounds and advance to a regular diet as per orders.
- Provide opportunities for the woman to ask questions or share her concerns. She may experience emotional symptoms following surgery related to hormonal changes and loss of fertility.
- Provide discharge teaching:
  - Keep the incision area dry, following the surgeon's instructions for bathing and dressing care.
  - Explain that walking is important in helping the woman to gradually return to her presurgery activity level. The woman needs to follow her surgeon's orders regarding level of activity and heavy lifting.
  - Explain that she may experience light vaginal bleeding for several days.
  - Provide nutritional information—the importance of protein, iron, and vitamin C in the healing process.
  - Provide information on pain management techniques.
  - Instruct the woman not to put anything in the vagina (e.g., do not douche, use tampons, or engage in sexual intercourse) until advised by her surgeon. This will decrease her risk of infections.
  - Instruct the woman to notify her health-care provider if she experiences:
    - Increased pain or pain that is not relieved by medication
    - Drainage, bleeding, redness, or swelling from the incisional site or increased bleeding from the vagina
    - Leg or calf pain, swelling, or redness
    - Fever of 102.2°F (39°C) or higher, or as instructed by the physician

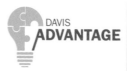

Go to Davis Advantage to complete your learning: strengthen understanding, apply your knowledge, and prepare for the Next Gen NCLEX®.

CONCEPT MAP

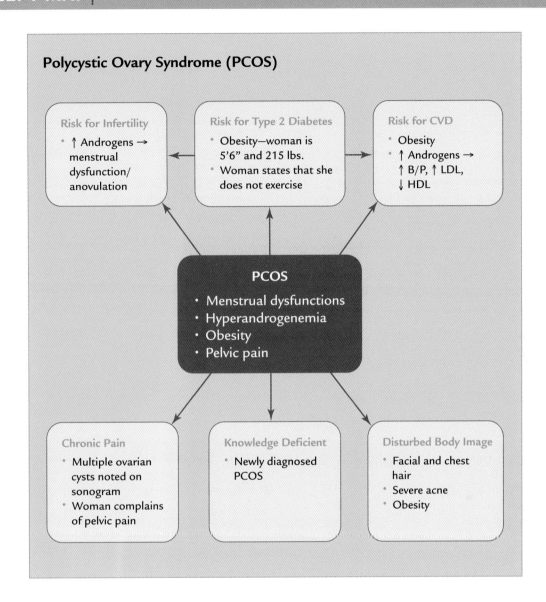

Polycystic Ovary Syndrome (PCOS)

Risk for Infertility
- ↑ Androgens → menstrual dysfunction/ anovulation

Risk for Type 2 Diabetes
- Obesity—woman is 5'6" and 215 lbs.
- Woman states that she does not exercise

Risk for CVD
- Obesity
- ↑ Androgens → ↑ B/P, ↑ LDL, ↓ HDL

PCOS
- Menstrual dysfunctions
- Hyperandrogenemia
- Obesity
- Pelvic pain

Chronic Pain
- Multiple ovarian cysts noted on sonogram
- Woman complains of pelvic pain

Knowledge Deficient
- Newly diagnosed PCOS

Disturbed Body Image
- Facial and chest hair
- Severe acne
- Obesity

CARE PLANS

Problem 1: Risk for infertility

Goal: Increased knowledge regarding relationship of PCOS and infertility

Outcome: The woman verbalizes causes of infertility and methods to improve fertility.

Nursing Actions

1. Provide the woman with information on the causes of infertility related to PCOS—anovulation related to increased androgen levels, increased LH, and decreased FSH.
2. Inform the woman that weight loss can improve fertility— weight loss is the first-line treatment for infertility.
   a. Assist the woman in developing a weight-management program that includes diet and physical activities.

3. Explain medical options for treating infertility.
   a. Treat type 2 diabetes—maintaining normal ranges of serum glucose can regulate the menstrual cycle and increase ovulation rates.
   b. Suggest ovulation-inducing medications.

Problem 2: Risk for type 2 diabetes

Goal: Serum glucose levels within normal ranges

Outcome: The woman exercises 3 days a week for 30 minutes and eats foods low in carbohydrates and fats.

Nursing Actions

1. Explain that weight loss and exercise improve insulin resistance (the body produces insulin but does not use it properly) and hyperinsulinemia (hyperglycemia present despite high levels of insulin).

Continued

2. Explain the other benefits of a weight-management program that includes diet and exercise:
   a. Improves fertility.
   b. Decreases androgen levels.
   c. Decreases lipid levels.
   d. Decreases blood pressure.
3. Assist the woman in developing a weight-management program by:
   a. Asking her to identify the types of physical activities she enjoys and how these can be used in a weight-management program
   b. Asking her to identify the foods she enjoys and incorporate them into a weight-reduction diet
   c. Teaching her food groups important in a healthy diet

Problem 3: Risk for cardiovascular disease (CVD)
Goal: Decrease blood pressure (BP); decrease low-density lipoprotein (LDL), and increase high-density lipoprotein (HDL).
Outcome: The woman exercises 3 days a week for 30 minutes and eats foods low in carbohydrates and fats.

Nursing Actions
1. Explain the importance of weight loss through diet and exercise to decrease CVD risk.
   a. Exercise improves cardiopulmonary function and insulin sensitivity and decreases BMI.
2. Assist the woman in developing a weight-management program with realistic weight loss and exercise goals.
3. Provide information on prescribed medications for decreasing risk of CVD.

Problem 4: Chronic pain
Goal: Decreased pain
Outcome: The woman states her pelvic pain has decreased in frequency and intensity.

Nursing Actions
1. Assess level of pain, location of pain, and frequency of pain.
2. Ask about past pain management techniques and their effectiveness in treating pain related to PCOS.
3. Ask the woman to identify factors that increase or decrease the pain (e.g., lack of sleep, lifting objects).
   a. Discuss ways to decrease factors that increase pain.

4. Assist the woman in developing a pain-management program that includes:
   a. Pain diary: List when pain occurs, intensity of pain, how long it lasted, pain-management measures used, and effectiveness of pain management. Instruct the woman to share this with her health-care provider.
   b. Pharmacological: Take medication at the start of pain and use adequate amounts as prescribed.
   c. Nonpharmacological: Relaxation techniques, massage, and acupressure may be used.

Problem 5: Knowledge deficit
Goal: Increased knowledge regarding PCOS
Outcome: The woman develops a plan of action for living with PCOS.

Nursing Actions
1. Ensure that the environment is conducive for learning—quiet room free of distractions.
2. Assess the woman's level of knowledge regarding PCOS.
3. Assist the woman in identifying priority learning needs and address these needs such as:
   a. Causes of PCOS
   b. Effect of PCOS on her body and mind
   c. Treatment options
   d. Ways to cope with changes related to PCOS
4. Assist the woman in developing a plan of action for living with PCOS.

Problem 6: Disturbed body image
Goal: Improved body image
Outcome: The woman verbalizes methods to decrease degree of acne and methods to decrease facial and chest hair.

Nursing Actions
1. Sit with the woman and, through active listening, encourage her to express her thoughts and concerns regarding facial and chest hair and acne.
2. Provide information on causes of body changes due to PCOS.
3. Provide information on treatment for acne (i.e., dermatological assessment and prescribed medications).
4. Provide information on hair removal.
5. Refer the woman to PCOS support groups.

Case Study

Katherine is a 70-year-old woman who was recently widowed. She retired from the U.S. Postal Service at age 65. She has three grown children; her daughter lives nearby. She weighs 150 lbs. Her height is 5 foot 6 inches; her height at age 50 was 5 foot 8 inches. Her BP is 124/86. She takes Synthroid and a multivitamin each morning. Recent laboratory values are as follows:

Fasting glucose: 110 mg/dL

Hemoglobin: 11.5 g/dL

Hematocrit: 34

Red blood cell: 3.8

White blood cell: 10.5

EKG: Normal.

She is scheduled for a vaginal hysterectomy and repair of cystocele and rectocele. Her admitting diagnosis is pelvic organ prolapse.

What is pelvic prolapse, and what are cystoceles and rectoceles?

What are the priority preoperative nursing actions for Katherine?

What are the postoperative nursing care actions for Katherine?

Develop a discharge teaching plan for Katherine that includes addressing postoperative care and health promotion.

REFERENCES

Alexander, I., Johnson-Mallard, V., Kostas-Polston, E. A., Forgel, C., & Woods, N. (Eds.). (2017). *Women's health care in advanced practice nursing* (2nd ed.). Springer

American Cancer Society. (2017). *Coping with radiation treatment.* https://www.cancer.org/treatment/treatments-and-side-effects/treatment-types/radiation/coping.html

American Cancer Society. (2019a). *Endometrial cancer staging.* https://www.cancer.org/cancer/endometrial-cancer/detection-diagnosis-staging/staging.html

American Cancer Society. (2019b). *Understanding a breast cancer diagnosis.* https://www.cancer.org/cancer/breast-cancer/understanding-a-breast-cancer-diagnosis.html

American Cancer Society. (2020a). *Early detection, diagnosis, and staging.* https://www.cancer.org/cancer/ovarian-cancer/detection-diagnosis-staging/detection.html

American Cancer Society. (2020b). *Radiation therapy for cervical cancer.* https://www.cancer.org/cancer/cervical-cancer/treating/radiation.html

American Cancer Society. (2020c). *Treating ovarian cancer.* https://www.cancer.org/cancer/ovarian-cancer/treating/targeted-therapy.html

American Cancer Society. (2021). *Cancer statistic center.* https://cancerstatisticscenter.cancer.org/#!/

American College of Surgeons. (2018). *Strong for Surgery.* https://www.facs.org/quality-programs/strong-for-surgery/about

American Cancer Society (ACS). (2021). *Breast cancer gene expression tests.* https://www.cancer.org/cancer/breast-cancer/understanding-a-breast-cancer-diagnosis/breast-cancer-gene-expression.html

Cancer Care. (2016). *Understanding and managing chemotherapy side effects.* https://www.cancercare.org/publications/24-understanding_and_managing_chemotherapy_side_effects

Centers for Disease Control and Prevention. (2017). *Genital HPV infection—fact sheet.* https://www.cdc.gov/std/hpv/stdfact-hpv.htm

Centers for Disease Control and Prevention. (2020). *Intimate partner violence.* https://www.cdc.gov/violenceprevention/pdf/ipv/intimatepartnerviolence.pdf

Centers of disease Control and Prevention. (2021). *Sexually transmitted infections treatment guidelines, 2021: Adolescents.* https://www.cdc.gov/std/treatment-guidelines/adolescents.htm

County of Los Angeles Public Health. (2021). *Resources for lesbian and bisexual women.* http://publichealth.lacounty.gov/dhsp/Lesbian-Bisexual.htm

International Pelvic Pain Society. (2021). *Chronic pelvic pain.* https://www.pelvicpain.org/common/Uploaded%20files/Patient%20Handouts/CHRONIC%20PELVIC%20PAIN.pdf

Lobo, R., Gershenson, D., Lentz, G., & Valea, F. (2017). *Comprehensive gynecology* (7th ed.). Elsevier.

Munro, M., Critchley, H., & Fraser, I. (2018). The two FIGO systems for normal and abnormal uterine bleeding symptoms and classification of causes of abnormal uterine bleeding in the reproductive years. *International Journal of Gynecology & Obstetrics, 143,* 393–408.

National Cancer Institute. (2017). *Nutrition in cancer care (PDQ)—patient version.* https://www.cancer.gov/about-cancer/treatment/side-effects/appetite-loss/nutrition-pdq

National Heart Lung and Blood Institute. (2016). *Metabolic syndrome.* https://www.nhlbi.nih.gov/health/health-topics/topics/ms

Schuiling, K., & Likis, F. (2022). *Gynecology health care* (4th ed.). Jones & Bartlett Learning.

Vallerand, A., & Sanoski, C. (2021). *Davis's drug guide for nurses* (17th ed.). F.A. Davis.

Waters, K., Gilchrest, R., Ledger, W., Teede, H., Handelsman, D., & Campbell, R. (2018). New perspectives on the pathogenesis of PCOS: Neuroendocrine origins. *Trends in Endocrinology & Metabolism, 29,* 841–852.

Appendix A Laboratory Values

LABORATORY VALUE	NONPREGNANT	PREGNANT	NEWBORN
Hemoglobin, g/dL	11.7–15.5	First trimester: 11.6–13.9 Second & third trimesters: 9.5–11	15.2–23.6
Hematocrit, %	36–48	First trimester: 35–42 Second & third trimesters: 28–33	46–68
Red blood cell count, 10^6cells/mm^3	3.91–5.11	2.7–4.55 Decreased related to dilutional effects of increased fluid volume	4.51–6.01
White blood cell count, 10^3cells/mm^3	4.5–11.1	5.6–17	9.1–30.1
Platelets, mm^3	140,000–400,000	No significant change	150,000–450,000
Fibrinogen, mg/dL	250–500	↑ levels late in pregnancy	200–500
Total cholesterol, mg/dL	<200	≤350	Rises rapidly after birth, reaching adult levels by day 1
Blood glucose, mg/dL		↓ 10%–20%	Cord blood: 45–96 Premature infant: 20–80 Newborn 2 days–2 yrs: 30–100
Fasting	65–99	≤95	
2-hour postprandial	≤65–139	≤120	
Total bilirubin, mg/dL	0.3–1.2	No significant change	<24 hours: <5.8 1–2 days: <8.2 3–5 days: <11.7

Appendix B Preeclampsia Early Recognition Tool (PERT)

Preeclampsia Early Recognition Tool (PERT)

ASSESS	NORMAL (GREEN)	WORRISOME (YELLOW)	SEVERE (RED)
Awareness	Alert/oriented	• Agitated/confused • Drowsy • Difficulty speaking	• Unresponsive
Headache	None	• Mild headache • Nausea, vomiting	• Unrelieved headache
Vision	None	• Blurred or impaired	• Temporary blindness
Systolic BP (mm HG)	100–139	140–159	≥160
Diastolic BP (mm HG)	50–89	90–105	≥105
HR	61–110	111–129	≥130
Respiration	11–24	25–30	<10 or >30
SOB	Absent	Present	Present
O2 Sat (%)	≥95	91–94	≤90
Pain: Abdomen or Chest	None	• Nausea, vomiting • Chest pain • Abdominal pain	• Nausea, vomiting • Chest pain • Abdominal pain
Fetal Signs	• Category I • Reactive NST	• Category II • IUGR • Non-reactive NST	• Category III
Urine Output (ml/hr)	≥50	30-49	≤30 (in 2 hrs)
Proteinuria (Level of proteinuria is not an accurate predictor of pregnancy outcome)	Trace	• ≥+1** • ≥300 mg/24 hours	
Platelets	>100	50-100	<50
AST/ALT	<70	>70	>70
Creatinine	≤0.8	0.9-1.1	≥1.2
Magnesium Sulfate Toxicity	• DTR +1 • Respiration 16-20	• Depression of patellar reflexes	• Respiration <12

GREEN = NORMAL
Proceed with protocol

YELLOW = WORRISOME
Increase assessment frequency

# Triggers	TO DO
1	• Notify provider
≥2	• Notify charge RN • In-person evaluation • Order labs/tests • Anesthesia consult • Consider magnesium sulfate • Supplemental oxygen

**Physician should be made aware of worsening or new-onset proteinuria

RED = SEVERE
Trigger: one of any type listed below

	TO DO
One of any type	• Immediate evaluation • Transfer to higher acuity level • 1:1 staff ratio
Awareness Headache Visual	• Consider veurology consult • CT scan • R/O SAH/intracranial hemorrhage
BP	• Labetalol/hydralazine in 30 min • In-person evaluation • Magnesium sulfate loading or maintenance infusion
Chest Pain	• Consider CT angiogram
Respiration SOB O2 SAT	• O2 at 10 L per rebreather mask • R/O pulmonary edema • Chest X-ray

Appendix C Cervical Dilation Chart

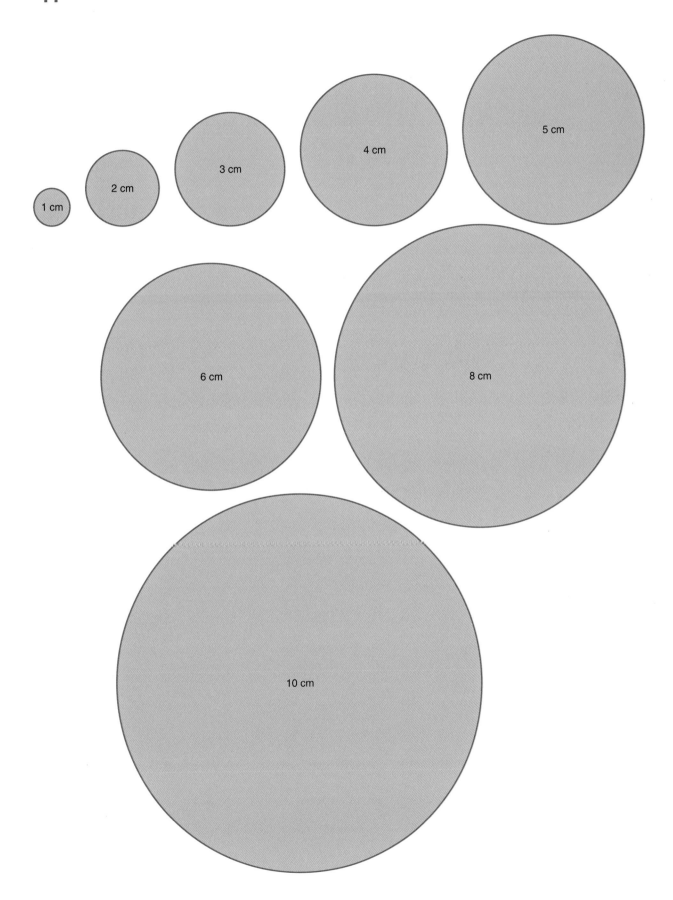

Appendix D Temperature and Weight Conversion Charts

CONVERSIONS:
Approximate Temperature
Equivalents

°C	°F	°C	°F
35.5	95.9	37.8	100.04
35.6	96.08	37.9	100.22
35.7	96.26	38.0	100.4
35.8	96.44	38.1	100.58
35.9	96.62	38.2	100.76
36.0	96.8	38.3	100.94
36.1	96.98	38.4	102.12
36.2	97.16	38.5	101.3
36.3	97.34	38.6	101.48
36.4	97.52	38.7	101.66
36.5	97.7	38.8	101.84
36.6	97.88	38.9	102.02
36.7	98.06	39.0	102.2
36.8	98.24	39.1	102.38
36.9	98.42	39.2	102.56
37.0	98.6	39.3	102.74
37.1	98.78	39.4	102.92
37.2	98.96	39.5	103.1
37.3	99.14	39.6	103.28
37.4	99.32	39.7	103.46
37.5	99.5	39.8	103.64
37.6	99.68	39.9	103.82
37.7	99.86	40.0	104.0

$$°C = (°F - 32) \times 5/9$$

$$°F = (°C \times 1.8) + 32$$

NEWBORN WEIGHT CONVERSION CHART
Pounds and Ounces to Grams

Ounces	Pounds												
	0	1	2	3	4	5	6	7	8	9	10	11	12
0	0	454	907	1361	1814	2268	2722	3175	3629	4082	4536	4990	5443
1	28	482	936	1389	1843	2296	2750	3203	3657	4111	4564	5019	5471
2	57	510	964	1417	1871	2325	2778	3232	3685	4139	4593	5046	5500
3	85	539	992	1446	1899	2353	2807	3260	3714	4167	4621	5075	5528
4	113	567	1021	1474	1928	2381	2835	3289	3742	4196	4649	5103	5557
5	142	595	1049	1503	1956	2410	2863	3317	3770	4224	4678	5131	5585
6	170	624	1077	1531	1984	2438	2892	3345	3799	4252	4706	5160	5613
7	198	652	1106	1559	2013	2466	2920	3374	3827	4281	4734	5188	5642
8	227	680	1134	1588	2041	2495	2949	3402	3856	4309	4763	5216	5670
9	255	709	1162	1616	2070	2523	2977	3430	3884	4337	4791	5245	5698
10	284	737	1191	1644	2098	2551	3005	3459	3912	4366	4819	5273	5727
11	312	765	1219	1673	2126	2580	3034	3487	3941	4394	4848	5301	5755
12	340	794	1247	1701	2155	2608	3062	3515	3969	4423	4876	5330	5783
13	369	822	1276	1729	2183	2637	3091	3544	3997	4451	4904	5358	5812
14	397	850	1304	1758	2211	2665	3119	3572	4026	4479	4933	5386	5840
15	425	879	1332	1786	2240	2693	3147	3600	4054	4508	4961	5415	5868

1 kg = 2.2046 lbs
1 lb = 454 g
1 oz = 28.3 g

Glossary

Abortion (AB)   The spontaneous or induced termination of a pregnancy before 20 weeks' gestation

Abruptio placenta   The separation of the placenta from its site of implantation before delivery

Accelerations   Visually apparent, abrupt increase in fetal heart rate 15 beats above baseline for 15 seconds

Acme phase   The peak of intensity of a contraction

Acrocyanosis   Cyanosis of hands and feet in newborn

Active immunity   Long-term immunity acquired through production of antibodies in response to the presence of antigens

Active phase   Second phase of labor: cervical dilation at 6 or more cm

Advocacy   An action taken in response to our ethical responsibility to intervene on behalf of those in our care

Afterpains   Moderate-to-severe cramp-like pains after birth caused by uterine contractions during the first few postpartum days

Alpha-fetoprotein (AFP)/α_1-fetoprotein/Maternal serum alpha fetoprotein (MSAFP)   A glycoprotein produced by the fetus used for assessing for the levels of AFP in the maternal blood as a screening tool for certain developmental defects in the fetus such as fetal neural tube defects (NTDs) and ventral abdominal wall defects

Amenorrhea   Absence of menstruation

American Nursing Association (ANA) Code of Ethics   Makes explicit the primary goals, values, and obligations of the profession of nursing

Amniocentesis   Diagnostic procedure in which a needle is inserted through the maternal abdominal wall into the uterine cavity to obtain amniotic fluid

Amniotic fluid   Fluid contained within the amniotic sac

Amniotic fluid embolism (AFE)/Anaphylactoid syndrome   A rare, but often fatal complication that occurs during pregnancy, labor and birth, or postpartum in which amniotic fluid, which contains fetal cells, lanugo, and vernix, enters the maternal vascular system and initiates a cascading process that leads to maternal cardiorespiratory collapse and disseminated intravascular coagulation (DIC)

Amniotic fluid index (AFI)   Screening tool that measures the volume of amniotic fluid with ultrasound to assess fetal well-being and placental function

Amniotomy (AROM)   The artificial rupture of membranes

Antepartum/Antepartal   The time period beginning with conception and ending with the onset of labor

Anticipatory guidance   The provision of information and guidance to women and their families that promotes being informed about and prepared for events to come

Apgar score   A rapid assessment of five physiological signs that indicate the physiological status of the newborn at birth

Apnea   Temporary cessation of breathing

Assessment   A systematic, dynamic process by which the nurse, through interaction with women, newborns and families, significant others, and health-care providers, collects, monitors, and analyzes data

Assisted reproductive technologies (ART)   Treatments for infertility that involve surgically removing oocytes and combining them with sperm in a laboratory setting

Asymmetric intrauterine growth restriction   A disproportional reduction in the size of structures and organs; results from maternal or placental conditions that occur later in pregnancy related to impeded placental blood flow

Attachment   Emotional connection that forms between the infant and the child's parents; it is bidirectional from parent to infant and infant to parent

Auscultation   When the Doppler or fetoscope (an audio device) is used to assess the fetal heart rate by listening

Autonomy   Refers to two concepts that operate as a whole; one is the right of self-determination or the right of the individual to make their own choice to accept or reject treatment; the ability to exercise autonomous rights requires and is related to elements in informed consent; the second aspect is concerned with respect of persons, that is, to respect the patient's decision irrespective of the nurses' own values

Babinski reflex   Hyperextension and fanning of neonate's toes in response to stroking the lateral surface of the sole in upward motion

Baby-Friendly Hospital Initiative (BFHI)   A global program that encourages hospitals and birthing centers to support breastfeeding by implementing 10 specific steps to support successful breastfeeding

Ballard Maturational Score (BMS)   Standardized test to calculate the gestational age of the neonate

Ballottement   A technique of feeling for a floating, moveable object in the body; feeling for the rebound of the fetus after a tap from the examiner

Baseline fetal heart rate   The average fetal heart rate (FHR) rounded to increments of five beats per minute (bpm) during a 10-minute segment between uterine contractions, accelerations, or decelerations

Baseline variability   The fluctuations or variations of the fetal heart rate (FHR) of 2 cycles/min or greater during a steady state in the absence of contractions, accelerations, or decelerations

Beneficence   The obligation to do good; beneficence is concerned not only with doing good but also with removing harm and preventing harm

Bilirubin   The yellow pigmentation derived from the breakdown of red blood cells

Biochemical assessment   Involves biological examination and chemical determination

Biophysical profile (BPP)/ Biophysical assessment (BPA) An ultrasound assessment of fetal status along with a non-stress test

Biophysical risk factors Factors that originate from the mother or fetus and impact the development or function of the mother or fetus; these risk factors include genetic, nutritional, medical, and obstetric issues

Biparietal diameter (BPD) The largest transverse measurement and an important indicator of head size; 9.25 cm

Birth rate Number of live births per 1,000 people

Bishop's score An assessment of the cervix to assess cervical ripeness

Blastocyst Stage of embryo development that follows the morula stage; the blastocyst is composed of an inner cell mass, the embryoblast, and an outer cell layer, the trophoblast

Bloody show Brownish or blood-tinged cervical mucus discharge

Body Mass Index (BMI) Measure that relates body weight to height

Bonding Emotional feelings between parent and newborn that begin during pregnancy or shortly after birth; it is unidirectional from parent to newborn

Bradycardia Baseline fetal heart rate of less than 110 bpm lasting for 10 minutes or longer

Braxton-Hicks contractions Intermittent, painless, and physiological uterine contractions occurring in some pregnancies in the second and third trimesters that do not result in cervical change and are associated with false labor

Brazelton Neonatal Behavioral Assessment Scale (BNBAS) Instrument used to assess the neurological and behavioral status of newborns

Breast engorgement Distention of milk glands

Breech presentation Situation in which the presenting part of the fetus is the buttocks or feet

Bronchopulmonary dysplasia (BPD) A chronic lung condition that affects neonates treated with mechanical ventilation and oxygen for problems such as respiratory distress syndrome

Brow presentation When the fetal head presents in a position midway between full flexion and extreme extension

Brown adipose tissue Also referred to as brown fat or non-shivering thermogenesis; a highly dense and vascular adipose tissue that is unique to neonates

Candidiasis Infection caused by fungi *Candida,* most often in the mouth or vagina

Caput succedaneum A localized soft tissue edema of the scalp

Cardinal movements of labor The positional changes that the fetus goes through to best navigate the birth process

Category I fetal heart rate tracings Normal tracings; strongly predictive of a well-oxygenated, nonacidotic fetus with a normal fetal acid–base balance

Category II fetal heart rate tracings Indeterminate tracings; not predictive typically of abnormal fetal acid–base status, yet there is not adequate evidence to classify them as Category I or III; they require evaluation and continued surveillance

Category III fetal heart rate tracings Abnormal tracings; predictive of abnormal fetal acid–base status and require prompt evaluation

Cephalic presentation Situation in which the presenting part is the head

Cephalohematoma Hematoma formation between the periosteum and skull with unilateral swelling

Cephalopelvic disproportion (CPD) A condition in which the size, shape, or position of the fetal head prevents it from passing through the lateral aspect of the maternal pelvis or when the maternal pelvis is of a size or shape that prevents descent of the fetus through the pelvis; the maternal bony pelvis is not large enough or appropriately shaped for fetal descent

Cervical dilation This measurement estimates the dilation of the cervical opening by sweeping the examining finger from the margin of the cervical opening on one side to that on the other

Cervical effacement This measurement estimates the shortening of the cervix from 2 cm to paper thin measured by palpation of cervical length with the fingertips

Cervical insufficiency Describes the inability of the uterine cervix to retain a pregnancy in the absence of the signs and symptoms of clinical contractions, or labor, or both in the second trimester

Cervical os The opening of the cervix that dilates during labor to allow passage of the fetus through the vagina

Cervical ripening The process of physical softening and opening of the cervix in preparation for labor and birth

Cervix The neck or lowest part of the uterus; interfaces with the vagina

Cesarean birth Also referred to as cesarean section or C-section (C/S); an operative procedure in which the fetus is delivered through an incision in the abdominal wall and the uterus

Cesarean delivery on maternal request (CDMR) A cesarean section that is performed at the request of the woman before labor begins and in the absence of a maternal or fetal medical condition that presents a risk for labor

Chadwick's sign Bluish-purple coloration of the vagina and cervix evident in the first trimester of pregnancy

Childbearing and newborn health care A model of care addressing the health promotion, maintenance, and restoration needs of women from the preconception through the postpartum period; and low-risk, high-risk, and critically ill newborns from birth through discharge and follow-up, within the social, political, economic, and environmental context of the mother's, her newborn's, and the family's lives

Chloasma Brownish pigmentation of the skin over the cheeks, nose, and forehead exacerbated by sun exposure; also known as the "mask of pregnancy" or melasma

Cholelithiasis Presence of gallstones in the gallbladder

Chorionic villi Projections from the chorion that embed into the decidua basalis and later form the fetal blood vessels of the placenta

Chorionic villus sampling (CVS) Aspiration of a small amount of placental tissue (chorion) for chromosomal, metabolic, or DNA testing

Chronic pelvic pain (CPP) Pain in the pelvic region that lasts 6 months or longer and results in functional or psychological disabilities or requires treatment or intervention

Circumcision Elective surgical removal of the foreskin of the penis

Circumoral cyanosis A benign localized transient cyanosis around the newborn's mouth

Classical cesarean delivery A vertical midline incision made into the abdominal wall with a vertical incision in the upper segment of the uterus performed for cesarean births

Cleavage Mitotic cell division of the zygote, fertilized oocyte

Clinical pelvimetry Measurements of the dimensions of the bony pelvis during an internal pelvic examination for determination of adequacy of the pelvis for a vaginal birth

Cold stress A term used when there is excessive heat loss that leads to hypothermia and results in the utilization of compensatory mechanisms to maintain the neonate's body temperature

Colic A term used to describe uncontrollable crying in healthy infants under the age of 5 months

Collaborative working relationships Working together with mutual respect for the accountability of each profession to the shared goal of quality patient outcomes

Colostrum Thick, clear to yellowish breast fluid, which precedes milk production; it contains proteins, nutrients, and immune globulins; produced prenatally as early as the second trimester and before lactation in the first days after birth

Combined decelerations A deceleration pattern that has combined features, such as a variable deceleration that is also a late deceleration

Combined spinal epidural analgesia (CSE) Involves the injection of local anesthetic or analgesic into the subarachnoid space

Complete abortion Products of conception are totally expelled from the uterus

Complete breech A fetal presentation where there is complete flexion of the thighs and legs and a buttocks presentation of the fetus

Compound presentation The fetus assumes a unique posture usually with the arm or hand presenting alongside the presenting part

Conception Also known as fertilization; occurs when a sperm nucleus enters the nucleus of the oocyte

Conduction Transfer of heat to cooler surface by direct skin contact such as cold hands of caregivers or cold equipment

Conjugated bilirubin The conjugated form of bilirubin (direct bilirubin), which is soluble and excretable

Continuous positive airway pressure (CPAP) Treatment used for neonates who are at risk for respiratory distress syndrome (RDS) or who have RDS; administered by nasal cannula, nasal mask, nasal prongs, endotracheal tube, or nasopharyngeal route

Contraception Also known as birth control; deliberate use of artificial methods, devices, or techniques to prevent pregnancy

Contraction stress test (CST) Screening tool to assess fetal well-being with electronic fetal monitoring (EFM) in women with nonreactive non-stress test (NST) at term gestation; the purpose of the CST is to identify a fetus that is at risk for compromise through observation of the fetal response to intermittent reduction of in utero placental blood flow associated with stimulated uterine contractions (UCs)

Convection Loss of heat from the neonate's warm body surface to cooler air currents such as air conditioners or oxygen masks

Corpus luteum A temporary hormone-secreting body in the female reproductive system formed on the ovary every month immediately after ovulation

Cotyledons Rounded portions, lobes, of the maternal side of the placenta

Couvade syndrome The occurrence in the mate of a pregnant woman of symptoms related to pregnancy, such as nausea, vomiting, and abdominal pain

Critical congenital heart defect screen (CCHD) Simple pulse oximetry test that compares preductal and postductal oxygen saturation levels as well as the overall oxygenation levels; recommended to be done universally on all neonates after 24 hours of age

Cross-cradle hold Breastfeeding position where the baby is held in the crook of the arm opposite the breast being fed from; an open hand supports the baby's head

Cultural sensitivity Awareness and appreciation that cultural differences or similarities between people exist; acceptance of cultural values, norms, and beliefs that may be different from your own

Cultural stereotyping The practice of making generalizations about a person based on that person's culture

Culturally competent care Providing care to patients and their families that is effective, understandable, and respectful care in a manner that is compatible with their cultural beliefs, practices, and preferred language

Cystitis Infection of the bladder

Cystocele Bulging of the bladder into the vagina

Daily fetal movement count (kick counts) Maternal assessment of fetal movement by counting fetal movements in a period of time to identify a potentially hypoxic fetus

Decidua basalis The portion of the decidua that forms the maternal portion of the placenta

Decrement phase The descending or relaxation of the uterine muscle

Dehiscence The separation of an incision following surgery

Descent The movement of the fetus through the birth canal during the first and second stage of labor

Diabetes mellitus (DM) A chronic metabolic disease characterized by hyperglycemia because of limited or no insulin production

Diagnosis A clinical judgment about the patient's response to actual or potential health conditions or needs; diagnoses provide the basis for determination of a plan of nursing care to achieve expected outcomes

Diaper dermatitis Inflammation of the skin under a diaper

Diaphoresis Profuse sweating postpartum that assists the body in excreting the increased fluid accumulated during pregnancy

Diastasis recti/Diastasis recti abdominis A separation of the two rectus abdominis muscle bands at the midline

Dilation The enlargement or opening of the cervical os

Direct bilirubin Conjugated bilirubin; water-soluble substance that the body can excrete in urine and stool

Direct obstetric death Death of a woman resulting from complications during pregnancy, labor or birth, or postpartum, and from interventions, omission of interventions, or incorrect treatment

Disseminated intravascular coagulation (DIC) Syndrome in which the coagulation pathways are hyperstimulated; occurs when the body is breaking down blood clots faster than it can form a clot, thus quickly depleting the body of clotting factors and leading to hemorrhage

Diversity A quality that encompasses acceptance and respect related to but not limited to age, class, culture, disability, education level, ethnicity, family structure, gender, ideologies, political beliefs, race, religion, sexual orientation, style, and values

Dizygotic twins Twins resulting from fertilization of two eggs

Doula An individual who provides support to women and their partners during labor, birth, and postpartum; the doula does not provide clinical care

Ductus arteriosus Structure in fetal circulation that connects the pulmonary artery with the descending aorta; the majority of the oxygenated blood is shunted to the aorta via the ductus arteriosus with smaller amounts going to the lungs

Ductus venosus Structure in fetal circulation that connects the umbilical vein to the inferior vena cava; this allows the majority of the high levels of oxygenated blood to enter the right atrium

Duration of contractions Length of a contraction measured by counting from the beginning to the end of one contraction and measured in seconds

Dysfunctional labor Abnormal uterine contractions that prevent the normal progress of cervical dilation or descent of the fetus

Dyspnea Difficult or labored breathing; shortness of breath

Dystocia A long, a difficult, or an abnormal labor

Dysuria Painful or difficult urination

Early decelerations A gradual decrease in fetal heart rate, 20 to 30 bpm below baseline; generally the onset, nadir, and the recovery mirror the contraction

Early-term delivery 37 0/7 weeks through 38 6/7 weeks

Eclampsia Preeclampsia with the onset of tonic-clonic seizure or convulsions, which place the mother and fetus at risk for death

Ectoderm The outer layer of cells in the developing embryo

Ectopic pregnancy A pregnancy that develops because of the blastocyst implanting somewhere other than the endometrial lining of the uterus; implantation of a fertilized ovum outside the uterus

Edinburgh Postnatal Depression Scale Screening tool consisting of 10 questions that can indicate whether a parent has symptoms that are common in women with depression and anxiety while pregnant or in the year following birth of a child

Effacement The shortening and thinning of the cervix

Effleurage A massage technique using a very light touch of the fingers in two repetitive circular patterns over the gravid abdomen; done by lightly stroking the abdomen in rhythm with breathing during contractions

Elective abortion (EAB) Termination of pregnancy before viability at the request of the woman but not for reasons of impaired maternal health or fetal disease

Electronic fetal monitoring (EFM) A technique for fetal assessment based on the fact that the fetal heart rate reflects fetal oxygenation

Embryo Term for a developing human from time of implantation through 8 weeks of gestation

Embryoblast The inner cell mass of the blastocyst, which develops into the embryo

Embryonic membranes Two membranes, amnion and chorion, which form the amniotic sac; the chorionic membrane (outer membrane) develops from the trophoblast; the amniotic membrane (inner membrane) develops from the embryoblast; the embryo and amniotic fluid are contained within the amniotic sac

En face Position in which the mother and newborn are face-to-face with eye contact

Endoderm The inner layer of cells in the developing embryo

Endometrial biopsy A biopsy of the endometrial tissue of the uterus to assess for the response of the uterus to hormonal signals that occur during the menstrual cycle

Endometrial cycle Pertains to the changes in the endometrium of the uterus in response to the hormonal changes that occur during the ovarian cycle; this cycle consists of three phases: proliferative phase, secretory phase, and menstrual phase

Endometriosis A chronic inflammatory disease in which the presence and growth of endometrial tissue is found outside the uterine cavity

Endometritis/Metritis An infection of the endometrium that usually starts at the placental site and can spread to encompass the entire endometrium

Endometrium The mucous membrane lining the interior of the uterus

Engagement Occurs when the greatest diameter of the fetal head passes through the pelvic inlet

Engrossment Phenomenon experienced by new fathers who have an intense preoccupation about and interest in their newborn

Entrainment Phenomenon in which the newborn or infant moves the arms and legs in rhythm with the speech patterns of an adult

Environmental risk factors Risks in the workplace or the general environment that impact pregnancy outcomes; various environmental substances can affect fetal development; examples include exposure to chemicals, radiation, and pollutants

Epidural anesthesia Involves the placement of a very small catheter and injection of local anesthesia or analgesia between the fourth and fifth vertebrae into the epidural space

Epidural block An anesthetic injected in the epidural space; located outside the dura mater between the dura and spinal canal via an epidural catheter

Episiotomy An incision in the perineum to provide more space for the fetal presenting part at delivery

Epispadias   An abnormality in which the urethral opening is on the dorsal side of the penis

Epistaxis   Nosebleeds

Epstein's pearls   White, pearl-like epithelial cysts on the neonate's gum margins and palate

Erythema toxicum   A rash with red macules and papules (white to yellowish-white papule in center surrounded by reddened skin), usually affecting the torso; it can appear within 24 hours of birth and up to 2 weeks

Estimated date of delivery (EDD)   The best estimation as to when a full-term infant will be born; also known as estimated date of confinement (EDC)

Estrogen   Hormone produced in the ovaries that promotes the development and maintenance of female characteristics of the body; also produced by the placenta during pregnancy to help maintain a healthy pregnancy

Ethical dilemma   A choice that has the potential to violate ethical principles

Ethnocentrism   The belief that the customs and values of the dominant culture are preferred or superior in some way

Evaluation   The process of determining the patient's progress toward attainment of expected outcomes and the effectiveness of nursing care

Evaporation   Loss of heat that occurs when water on the neonate's skin is converted to vapors such as during bathing or directly after birth

Everted nipple   Protrudes outward from the areola

Evidence-based nursing (EBN)   Combining the best research evidence with clinical expertise while taking into account the patients' preferences and their situation in the context of the available resources part of nursing practice

Evidence-based practice (EBP)   The integration of best research evidence, clinical expertise, and patient values in making decisions about the care of patients

Expulsion   During this cardinal movement, the shoulders and remainder of the infant's body are delivered

Extension   This cardinal movement, which is facilitated by resistance of the pelvic floor, causes the presenting part to pivot beneath the pubic symphysis and the head to be delivered; occurs during the second stage of labor

External rotation   During this cardinal movement, the sagittal suture moves to a transverse diameter and the shoulders align in the anteroposterior diameter; the sagittal suture maintains alignment with the fetal trunk as the trunk navigates through the pelvis

Extremely low birth weight (ELBW)   Less than 1,000 grams at birth

Face presentation   When the fetal head is in extension rather than flexion as it enters the pelvis

Facilitated tucking   A method of soothing premature infants during care; it involves holding the infant's arms and legs in flexed positions close to the midline of the torso

False labor   Irregular contractions with little or no cervical changes

Feeding cues   Subtle cues demonstrated by the newborn to indicate hunger

Ferguson's reflex   A physiological response of the woman, activated when the presenting part of the fetus is at least at +1 station; it is usually accompanied by spontaneous bearing-down efforts

Ferning   When a sample of fluid in the upper vaginal area is obtained, the fluid is placed on a slide and assessed for "ferning pattern" under a microscope to confirm the rupture of membranes

Fertility rate   Total number of live births, regardless of the age of the mother, per 1,000 women of reproductive age, 15 to 44 years

Fetal alcohol syndrome (FAS)   Refers to a wide array and spectrum of physical, cognitive, and behavioral abnormalities associated with maternal alcohol use during pregnancy

Fetal attitude or posture   The relationship of the fetal parts to one another; this is noted by the flexion or extension of the fetal joints

Fetal bradycardia   Baseline fetal heart rate of less than 110 bpm lasting for 10 minutes or longer

Fetal dystocia   May be caused by excessive fetal size, malpresentation, multifetal pregnancy, or fetal anomalies

Fetal fibronectin (fFN)   A protein detected via immunoassay; a positive test is greater than 50 ng/mL

Fetal heart rate accelerations   The visually abrupt, transient increases (onset to peak less than 30 seconds) in the fetal heart rate above the baseline, 15 beats above the baseline; they last from 15 seconds to less than 2 minutes

Fetal heart rate decelerations   Transitory decreases in the fetal heart rate baseline; they are classified as early, variable, or late decelerations

Fetal growth restriction   Condition in which a fetus does not achieve expected growth in utero

Fetal lie   Refers to the long axis (spine) of the fetus in relationship to the long axis (spine) of the woman

Fetal position   Location of the presenting part and specific fetal structures to determine fetal position in relation to the maternal pelvis; relation of the denominator or reference point to the maternal pelvis

Fetal presentation   Determined by the part, or pole, of the fetus that first enters the pelvic inlet

Fetus   Term used for the developing human from 9 weeks' gestation to birth

First-degree laceration   A laceration that involves the perineal skin and vaginal mucous membrane

First stage of labor   Begins with onset of labor and ends with complete cervical dilation

Flexion   When the chin of the fetus moves toward the fetal chest; flexion occurs when the descending head meets resistance from maternal tissues

Folic acid   Water-soluble vitamin belonging to the B-complex group of vitamins; helps the body make healthy new cells

Follicular phase   Part of the ovarian cycle; it begins the first day of menstruation and lasts 12 to 14 days; during this phase, the graafian follicle is maturing

Football hold   Breastfeeding position where the baby is held tucked under the arm as one would hold a football and on the same side that the woman is nursing from

Footling breech   When either one (single footling) or both (double footling) feet of the fetus present first in the pelvis

Foramen ovale   A structure in fetal circulation; it is an opening between the right and left atria; blood high in oxygen is shunted to the left atrium via the foramen ovale

Forceps   An instrument used to assist with delivery of the fetal head, typically done to improve the health of the woman or the fetus

Foremilk   The milk that is produced and stored between feedings and released at the beginning of the feeding session; it has higher water content than typical milk

Fourth-degree laceration   A laceration that extends into the rectal mucosa and exposes the lumen of the rectum

Fourth stage of labor   Begins with the delivery of the placenta and typically ends within 4 hours or with the stabilization of the mother postpartum

Frank breech   A fetal presentation where there is complete flexion of the thighs and the legs extend over the anterior surfaces of the body

Frequency of contractions   Determined by counting the number of contractions in a 10-minute period; counting from the start of one contraction to the start of the next contraction in minutes

Full-term delivery   39 0/7 weeks through 40 6/7 weeks

Functional residual capacity   The volume of air remaining in alveolar sacs at the end of expiration; it helps keep the sacs partially open and decreases the amount of pressure and energy required on inspiration

Fundal height   Measurement of the distance from the pubic bone to the top of the uterus measured in centimeters

Fundus   The upper portion of the uterus

Galactopoiesis   The maintenance of established lactation

Galactosemia   A rare hereditary genetic metabolic disorder affecting how the body processes a simple sugar called galactose that is present in many foods

Gastroenteritis   Inflammation of the stomach and intestines that causes vomiting and diarrhea, typically resulting from bacterial toxins or viral infection

Gate control theory of pain   States that pain sensation is transmitted from the periphery of the body along ascending nerve pathways to the brain; due to the limited number of sensations that can travel along these pathways at any given time, an alternate activity can replace travel of the pain sensation, closing the gate control at the spinal cord and reducing pain impulses traveling to the brain

Gavage   Administration of food or drugs by a tube leading down the throat to the stomach

General anesthesia   The use of IV injection or inhalation of anesthetic agents that render the woman unconscious

Genetic disease screen (GDS)   Blood spot test to screen for infections, genetic diseases, and metabolic disorders; performed on all babies born in the United States

Genital fistulas   An abnormal connection between the vagina and bladder, rectum, or urethra; the fistula provides a pathway for fecal material or urine to enter the vagina

Genome   An organism's complete set of DNA

Genotype   Refers to a person's genetic makeup

Gestation   The period of time between conception and birth

Gestational diabetes mellitus (GDM)   Any degree of glucose intolerance with the onset or first recognition in pregnancy

Gestational hypertension   A relatively benign disorder without underlying physiological changes in the mother; high blood pressure detected for the first time after mid-pregnancy, without proteinuria; diagnosis is made postpartum

Gestational surrogacy   A woman known as a gestational carrier agrees to bear a genetically unrelated child with the help of assisted reproductive technologies for an individual or couple who intend(s) to be the legal and rearing parent(s), referred to as the intended parent(s)

Glans penis   Tip of the penis

Glucosuria   Excess glucose in the urine

Gonadotoxins   Factors, such as drugs, infections, illness, and heat exposure, that can have an adverse effect on spermatogenesis

Goodell's sign   The softening of the cervix in the first trimester of pregnancy

Gravida   A pregnant woman; also, the number of times a woman has been pregnant (Gravida/Para notation)

Group B streptococcus (GBS)   Bacterial infection that can be found in the woman's vagina or rectum; women who test positive for GBS are said to be colonized; can pass from pregnant woman to her fetus during labor

GTPAL   Comprehensive system that gives birth history related to gravida, term, preterm, abortion, and living

Health disparities   Health outcomes occur to a greater or lesser extent among different populations

Hegar's sign   The softening of the lower uterine segment (isthmus) in the first trimester of pregnancy

HELLP syndrome   Acronym for hemolysis, elevated liver enzymes, and low platelets used to designate the variant changes in laboratory values, which is a complication of severe preeclampsia

Hematomas   A collection of blood within the connective tissues; common sites in the postpartum woman are the vagina and perineal areas

Hemorrhoid   Swollen and inflamed vein or group of veins in the anal canal

Hind milk   The milk produced during the feeding session and released at the end of the session; it has a higher fat content than typical milk

Human chorionic gonadotropin   A hormone produced in the human placenta that maintains the corpus luteum during pregnancy

Humoral immunity   Process in which B cells detect antigens and produce specific antibodies against them

Hydatidiform mole   A benign proliferate growth of the trophoblast in which the chorionic villi develop into edematous, cystic, vascular transparent vesicles that hang in grape-like clusters without a viable fetus

Hydrocele   Enlarged scrotum due to excess fluid

Hyperbilirubinemia   Term used for a high level of unconjugated bilirubin in neonatal blood

Hypercoagulation   A condition that causes blood to clot more easily than normally

Hyperemesis gravidarum Vomiting during pregnancy so severe it leads to dehydration, electrolyte and acid-base imbalance, and starvation ketosis

Hyperpigmentation A condition in which patches of skin are darker than surrounding skin

Hyperstimulation Excessive uterine activity

Hypertonic uterine dysfunction Uncoordinated uterine activity

Hypoglycemia Blood glucose level below 40 to 45 mg/dL in the neonate

Hypospadias An abnormality in which the urethral opening is on the ventral surface of the penis

Hypotonic uterine dysfunction Occurs when the pressure of the uterine contractions (UC) is insufficient (less than 25 mm Hg) to promote cervical dilation and effacement

Hypoxic-ischemic encephalopathy (HIE) Neurological damage that occurs because of decreased oxygen and inadequate tissue perfusion to the neonatal brain and other organs

Hysterectomy The surgical removal of the uterus

Hysterosalpingogram A radiological examination that provides information about the endocervical canal, uterine cavity, and the fallopian tubes

Implantation The embedding of the blastocyst into the endometrium of the uterus

Implementation The process of taking action by intervening, delegating, or coordinating; women, newborns, families, significant others, or health-care providers may direct the implementation of interventions within the plan of care

Inadequate expulsive forces Occurs in the second stage of labor when the woman is not able to push or bear down

Incompetent cervix A mechanical defect in the cervix that results in painless cervical dilation and ballooning of the membranes into the vagina followed by expulsion of an immature fetus in the second trimester

Incomplete abortion Fragments of products of conception are expelled and tissue parts are retained in the uterus

Increment phase The ascending or buildup of the contraction that begins in the fundus and spreads throughout the uterus

Indirect bilirubin Unconjugated bilirubin; a fat-soluble substance produced from the breakdown of red blood cells (RBCs)

Indirect obstetrical death Death of a woman due to a preexisting disease or a disease that develops during pregnancy that is not directly related to obstetrical cause but is aggravated by the changes of pregnancy

Induced abortion The medical or surgical termination of pregnancy before viability

Induction The deliberate stimulation of uterine contractions before the onset of spontaneous labor

Inevitable abortion Termination of pregnancy is in progress

Infant mortality Infant death before the first birthday

Infertility The inability to conceive and maintain a pregnancy after 12 months (6 months for women older than 35) of unprotected sexual intercourse

Intensity Strength of the contraction and measure by palpation, or internally by an intrauterine pressure catheter (IUPC) in mm Hg

Interconceptional interval The period of time in between pregnancies

Internal rotation This cardinal movement, the rotation of the fetal head, aligns the long axis of the fetal head with the long axis of the maternal pelvis; occurs mainly during the second stage of labor

Internal uterine pressure catheter (IUPC) This monitoring provides an objective measure of the pressure of contractions expressed as mm Hg

International Board-Certified Lactation Consultant (IBCLC) Professional lactation consultant to assist women with breastfeeding

Intimate partner violence (IPV) Actual or threatened physical or sexual violence or psychological and emotional abuse by a current or former partner or spouse

Intrahepatic cholestasis of pregnancy (ICP) A reversible type of hormonally influenced cholestasis characterized by generalized itching, also known as obstetric cholestasis

Intrapartum period Begins with the onset of regular uterine contractions and lasts until the expulsion of the placenta

Intrauterine growth restriction (IUGR) A decreased rate of fetal growth usually due to a decrease in cell production related to chronic malnutrition; there are two types of IUGR, symmetric and asymmetric

Intraventricular hemorrhage (IVH) Bleeding into the fluid-filled ventricles, surrounded by the brain

Inverted nipple Nipple drawn below the skin surface

Involution The process by which the uterus returns to a pre-pregnant size, shape, and location; and the placental site heals. In relation to breast milk production, it is the last phase of lactation as milk production decreases when there is less demand for breast milk.

Isthmus The narrower, lower segment of the uterus

Jaundice Yellowing of the skin and sclera that can be seen as the bilirubin levels rise

Kangaroo care Practice of placing an infant directly on the mother or caregiver's bare chest; typically dressed only in a diaper with a blanket covering both (skin-to-skin care)

Kegel exercises Exercises performed to strengthen the muscles of the uterus and bladder to prevent urinary incontinence or other pelvic floor problems; involves repetitions of voluntary tightening and relaxing the pelvic floor muscles that control urine flow

Kernicterus An abnormal accumulation of unconjugated bilirubin in the neonate's brain cells

Labor The process in which the fetus, placenta, and membranes are expelled through the uterus

Labor augmentation The stimulation of ineffective uterine contractions after the onset of spontaneous labor to manage labor dystocia

Lacerations Tears in the perineum that may occur at delivery

Lactation The production of breast milk

Lactogenesis The transition from pregnancy to lactation; developing of the alveolar cells into secretory cells to secrete milk; lactogenesis I occurs from pregnancy until postpartum day 2; lactogenesis II occurs from day 3 to 8 following birth

Lanugo   Fine, downy hair that covers the body and limbs of a human fetus or newborn

Large for gestational age (LGA)   Term used for neonates whose weight is above the 90th percentile for gestational age

Last menstrual period (LMP)   First day (onset of bleeding) of the last menstrual period before pregnancy

LATCH assessment   Numerical score given to each of these areas: latch, audible swallowing, type of mother's nipple, comfort, hold or position of newborn at breast

Latching   When the newborn grasps the areola and pulls the breast tissue deep into the mouth

Late deceleration   A visually apparent gradual decrease of fetal heart rate below the baseline; lowest part of the deceleration occurs after the peak of the contraction

Late maternal death   Death of a woman that occurs more than 42 days after termination of pregnancy from a direct or indirect obstetrical cause

Late premature/Late preterm   Neonate born between 34 and 37 completed weeks' gestation

Late-term delivery   41 0/7 weeks through 41 6/7 weeks

Latent phase   First phase of labor; the early and slower part of labor with cervical dilation from 0 to 5 cm

Lecithin/Sphingomyelin ratio (L/S ratio)   Two phospholipids detected in amniotic fluid; method used to assess fetal lung maturity

Leiomyomas of the uterus   Also referred to as myomas or uterine fibroids; benign fibrous tumor of the uterine wall

Leopold's maneuvers   A series of four maneuvers used to palpate a gravid uterus to determine fetal position, presentation, and size

Let-down reflex   Also referred to as milk ejection reflex; results in milk being ejected into and through the lactiferous duct system

Leukorrhea   A white, odorless, physiological vaginal discharge; increases in pregnancy due to increased mucus secretion by cervical glands

LGBTQIA+   Acronym for lesbian, gay, bisexual, transgender, queer or questioning, intersex, asexual

Lightening   Term used to describe the descent of the fetus into the true pelvis, which occurs approximately 2 weeks before term in first-time pregnancies

Linea nigra   Dark vertical line that may appear down the center of the abdomen during pregnancy

Local   An anesthetic injected into the perineum at the episiotomy site

Lochia   Bloody discharge from the uterus that contains sloughed off tissue; it undergoes changes that reflect the healing stages of the uterine placental site

Long-term variability (LTV)   The changes in fetal heart rate (FHR) range or fluctuations in the FHR baseline; this term is no longer used

Lordosis   Abnormal anterior curvature of the lumbar spine

Low birth weight infant (LBW)   1,500 grams to 2,500 grams at birth

Low-lying placenta   Placentas near to but not overlying the os

Luteal phase   Part of the ovarian cycle; it begins after ovulation and lasts approximately 14 days

Macrocephaly   Head circumference greater than the 90th percentile

Macrosomia   Birth weight greater than or equal to 4,000 grams

Mammogenesis   Breast changes that occur during pregnancy in preparation for milk production

Marginal placenta previa   The placenta is at the margin of the internal cervical os

Mastitis   Inflammation or infection of the breast

Maternal death   Death of a woman during pregnancy or within 42 days of termination of pregnancy; the death is related to the pregnancy or aggravated by pregnancy, or management of the pregnancy; it excludes death from accidents or injuries

Maternal tasks of pregnancy   Psychological work done by the pregnant woman toward the development of a positive adaptation to pregnancy and the establishment of a maternal identity

Mature milk   The milk produced in great volume approximately 12 days after birth

Meconium aspiration syndrome (MAS)   When a newborn breathes in a mixture of meconium and amniotic fluid into the lungs around the time of delivery

Meconium-stained amniotic fluid (MSAF)   Meconium stool present in the amniotic fluid occurs with relaxation of the fetus's anal sphincter in utero, usually due to fetal asphyxia

Meconium stool   The first stool eliminated by the neonate; sticky, thick, black, and odorless

Meiosis   A process of two successive cell divisions that produces cells that contain half the number of chromosomes (haploid)

Melasma   Brownish pigmentation of the skin over the cheeks, nose, and forehead exacerbated by sun exposure; also known as the "mask of pregnancy" or chloasma

Mesoderm   The middle layer of cells in the developing embryo

Metritis/Endometritis   An infection of the endometrium that usually starts at the placental site and can spread to encompass the entire endometrium

Microcephaly   Head circumference below the 10th percentile of normal for newborn's gestational age

Milia   White papules on the neonate's face; more frequently seen on the bridge of the nose and chin

Milk expression   Using your hands or a breast pump to rhythmically compress breasts so that milk comes out

Missed abortion   Embryo or fetus dies during first 20 weeks of gestation but is retained in the uterus

Mitotic cell division or mitosis   Occurs when a cell (parent cell) divides and forms two daughter cells that contain the same number of chromosomes as the parent cell

Modified BPP   Combines a non-stress test with an amniotic fluid index (AFI) as an indicator of short-term fetal well-being and AFI as an indicator of long-term placental function to evaluate fetal well-being

Molding   The ability of the fetal head to change shape to fit through the maternal pelvis

Monozygotic twins   Twins from one zygote that divides in the first week of gestation

Moro reflex   Startle reflex present at birth

Morula 16-cell solid sphere that forms 3 days following fertilization because of mitotic cell division of the zygote

Mottling A benign transient pattern of pink and white blotches on the skin

Multigravida A woman who has been pregnant multiple times

Multipara A woman who has given birth after 20 weeks' gestation multiple times

Multiple gestation A pregnancy with more than one fetus

Myomectomy Surgical removal of fibroids

Myometrium The smooth muscle layer of the uterus

Nadir The lowest point of the deceleration; occurs at the peak of the contraction

Naegele's rule The standard formula for calculating an estimated date of birth based on a last menstrual period (LMP) (first day of LMP minus 3 months plus 7 days)

Necrotizing enterocolitis (NEC) A gastrointestinal disease that affects neonates; this disease results in inflammation and necrosis of the bowel, usually at the proximal colon or terminal ileum

Neonatal abstinence syndrome Also referred to as neonatal withdrawal; may result from intrauterine exposure to various substances, including opioids such as heroin, methadone, and oxycodone

Neonatal period The time period from birth through the first 28 days of life

Neural tube defect (NTD) Severe birth defects of the brain and spine

Neutral thermal environment (NTE) Refers to an environment that maintains body temperature with minimal metabolic changes or oxygen consumption

Non-nutritive suck Nonrhythmic sucking that does not effectively transfer milk out of the breast; comfort sucking

Nonreassuring fetal heart rate (FHR) An abnormal FHR pattern that reflects an unfavorable physiological response to the maternal-fetal environment; this term is no longer in common use

Nonshivering thermogenesis Heat production due to brown fat metabolism; unique to neonates

Non-stress test (NST) Screening tool that uses electronic fetal monitoring to assess fetal well-being

Nulligravida A woman who has never been pregnant

Nullipara A woman who has never given birth after 20 weeks' gestation

Nutritive suck Rhythmic suck pattern when baby is sucking and obtaining milk

Obstetrical emergency An urgent clinical situation that places either the maternal or fetal status at risk for increased morbidity and mortality

Occiput posterior When the occiput of the fetus is in the posterior portion of the pelvis rather than the anterior

Occult prolapse When the cord is palpated through the membranes but does not drop into the vagina

Oligohydramnios Decreased amounts of amniotic fluid (less than 500 mL at term or 50% reduction of normal amounts) during pregnancy

Ominous fetal heart rate patterns Fetal heart rates associated with increased risk of fetal acidemia

Oogenesis The formation of a mature ovum (egg)

Open glottis Refers to spontaneous, involuntary bearing down accompanying the forces of the uterine contraction and is usually characterized by expiratory grunting or vocalizations by a woman during pushing

Operative vaginal delivery A vaginal birth that is assisted by a vacuum extraction or forceps

Ophthalmic neonatorum Any conjunctivitis with discharge from the eyes during the first 28 days of life; etiology may be gonococcal or chlamydia trachomatis

Organogenesis The formation and development of body organs that occurs during the first trimester of pregnancy

Orthostatic hypotension A sudden drop in blood pressure when the woman stands up from a sitting or lying position

Otitis media Inflammation of the middle ear

Outcome A measurable individual, family, or community state, behavior, or perception that is responsive to nursing interventions

Ovarian cycle Pertains to the maturation of ova and consists of three phases: follicular phase, ovulatory phase, and luteal phase

Ovulatory phase Part of the ovarian cycle; it begins when estrogen levels peak and ends with the release of the oocyte (egg) from the mature graafian follicle; the release of the oocyte is referred to as ovulation

Oxytocin Hormone released by the pituitary gland; causes uterine contractions in labor; stimulates the ejection of milk into the ducts of the breasts; synthetic oxytocin (Pitocin) is administered after delivery for prophylaxis and treatment of postpartum hemorrhage

Oxytocin induction Pharmacological method for induction of labor with oxytocin

Palmer erythema Redness on the palms of the hands

Palmer grasp Neonate grasps examiner's finger tightly

Papanicolaou smear A screening test used to identify cervical cancer and precancerous conditions of the cervix

Para A woman who has given birth to an infant after 20 weeks' gestation; also, the number of births that occurred after 20 weeks' gestation (Gravida/Para notation)

Partial placenta previa Condition in which the placenta partially covers the internal cervical os

Parturition (or labor) The process in which the fetus, placenta, and membranes are expelled through the uterus

Passage Includes the bony pelvis and the soft tissues of the cervix, pelvic floor, vagina, and introitus (external opening to the vagina)

Passenger The fetus

Passive immunity Short-term immunity resulting from introduction of antibodies from the mother to the fetus through the placenta

Patent ductus arteriosus (PDA) Occurs when the ductus arteriosus remains open or remains open after birth

Paternal postnatal depression (PPND) Some new fathers experience depression during the first 6 months following childbirth

Pathological Jaundice Jaundice of the newborn that occurs within the first 24 hours of life and characterized by a rapid rise in the bilirubin level.

Peak pressure   The maximum uterine pressure during a contraction measured with an IUPC

Pediatric abusive head trauma (PAHT)   Also referred to as abusive head trauma or shaken baby syndrome, a traumatic brain injury that occurs when an infant is violently shaken

Pelvic dystocia   Related to the contraction of one or more of the three planes of the pelvis

Pelvic inflammatory disease (PID)   A general term that refers to an infection of the uterus, fallopian tubes, and other reproductive organs

Pelvic organ prolapse (POP)   The descent of pelvic organs into the vagina or against the vaginal wall

Percutaneous umbilical blood sampling (PUBS)   The removal of fetal blood from the umbilical cord for fetal blood sampling; also referred to as cordocentesis

Perinatal   The time period "around" the birth of a baby; generally refers to the weeks before and after a baby is born, from 28 weeks' gestation to 28 days after birth

Period of reactivity   Neonates transition through two periods of activity, each characterized by predictable behaviors; the initial period of reactivity lasts 30 to 40 minutes; the second period of reactivity lasts 2 to 8 hours after birth

Period of relative inactivity   Period of deep sleep between the initial and second periods of reactivity; begins approximately 30 to 40 minutes after birth and lasts 2 to 4 hours

Periodic and nonperiodic changes   Accelerations or decelerations in the fetal heart rate that are related to uterine contractions and persist over time

Persistent pulmonary hypertension (PPHN)   Results when the normal vasodilation and relaxation of the pulmonary vascular bed does not occur

Pfannenstiel incision or "bikini cut"   A transverse skin incision at the level of the mons pubis with a transverse incision in the lower uterine segment performed for cesarean births

Phenotype   Refers to how the genes are outwardly expressed (i.e., eye color, hair color, height)

Phenylketonuria (PKU)   An inborn error of metabolism that affects the neonate's ability to metabolize phenylalanine, an amino acid commonly found in many foods such as breast milk and formula

Phosphatidylglycerol (PG)   Used as an indicator of fetal lung maturity when present in the amniotic fluid in the last trimester of pregnancy

Phototherapy   The use of a special type of light in the treatment of newborn jaundice

Physiological anemia of pregnancy   A relative anemia in mid to late pregnancy due to physiological hypervolemia without a correspondingly proportionate increase in erythrocytes in the maternal system

Physiological jaundice   Hyperbilirubinemia that commonly occurs after the first 24 hours of birth and during the first week of life; caused by the breakdown of red blood cells

Pica   A craving for and consumption of non-food substances such as starch and clay; can result in toxicity due to ingested substances or malnutrition from replacing nutritious foods with non-food substances

Pilonidal dimple   A small pit or sinus in the sacral area at the top of the crease between the buttocks

Placenta   The temporary fetal organ that develops in the uterus during pregnancy to join the mother and fetus; it provides oxygen and nutrients from the mother to the fetus and provides for removal of waste products from the fetus

Placenta accreta   An abnormality of implantation defined by the degree of invasion into the uterine wall of trophoblast of placenta; invasion of trophoblast beyond the normal boundary

Placenta increta   Invasion of trophoblast that extends into the myometrium

Placenta percreta   Invasion of trophoblast beyond the serosa

Placenta previa   Occurs when the placenta attaches to the lower uterine segment of the uterus, near or over the internal cervical os, instead of in the body or fundus of the uterus; all placentas overlying the os (to any degree) are termed previas and those near to but not overlying the os are termed low-lying

Placental abruption   Separation of the placenta from the wall of the uterus

Placental reserve   Describes the reserve oxygen available to the fetus to withstand the transient changes in blood flow and oxygen during labor

Plantar grasp   Neonate's toes flex tightly down in grasping motion when examiner's thumb placed against the ball of the infant's foot.

Polycystic ovary syndrome (PCOS)   Also known as Stein-Leventhal syndrome, an endocrine disorder that affects 5% to 10% of women of childbearing age that involves multiple follicular cysts on one or both ovaries

Polydactyly   Extra digits of the hands or feet

Polyhydramnios or hydramnios   Increased amounts of amniotic fluid (1,500 to 2,000 mL)

Position   Maternal position during labor and birth

Position of cervix   Relationship of the cervical os to the fetal head; it is characterized as posterior, mid-position, or anterior

Positive signs of pregnancy   Objective signs of pregnancy noted by the examiner that can only be attributed to the fetus

Postpartum   The 6-week period of time following childbirth

Postpartum blues   Also known as baby blues; occurs during the first few weeks postpartum and lasts for a few days; it is a time of heightened maternal emotions with the woman being tearful and irritable with emotional swings

Postpartum chills   Episode of shaking and feeling cold that is experienced by most women during the first few hours following birth

Postpartum depression (PPD)   A mood disorder characterized by severe depression that occurs within the first 6 to 12 months postpartum

Postpartum hemorrhage (PPH)   Blood loss exceeding 500 mL following vaginal birth and 1,000 mL following cesarean birth; primary (early) PPH occurs in the first 24 hours after birth; secondary (late) PPH occurs from 24 hours to 12 weeks postdelivery but is most prevalent during the first 7 to 14 days following birth

Postpartum psychosis (PPP) A variant of bipolar disorder that is the most serious form of postpartum mood disorders

Post-term delivery 42 0/7 weeks and beyond

Post-term pregnancy One that has a gestational period of 42 completed weeks

Powers Refer to the involuntary uterine contractions of labor and the voluntary pushing or bearing down powers that combine to propel and deliver the fetus and placenta from the uterus

Practice standards Standards that help to guide professional nursing practice; they summarize the nursing profession's best judgment and optimal practice based on current research and clinical practice

Precipitous labor Labor that lasts less than 3 hours from onset of labor to birth

Preconception care Well-woman health care focusing on preparation for and anticipation of a pregnancy, including health promotion, risk screening, and implementation of interventions before pregnancy, the goal being to modify risk factors that could negatively impact a pregnancy in order to optimize perinatal outcomes

Preeclampsia Hypertension accompanied by underlying systemic pathology that can have severe maternal and fetal impact; a systemic disease with hypertension accompanied by proteinuria after the 20th week of gestation

Preeclampsia superimposed on chronic hypertension Occurs with hypertensive women who develop new onset proteinuria, proteinuria before the 20th week of gestation, or sudden uncontrolled hypertension

Premature rupture of membranes Rupture of the chorioamniotic membranes before the onset of labor

Prenatal The entire time period during which a woman is pregnant; includes the antepartum or antepartal and the intrapartal periods

Prescriptive behavior Expected behavior of the pregnant woman during the childbearing period

Presenting part The specific fetal structure lying nearest to the cervix

Presumptive signs of pregnancy Physiological changes perceived by the woman; could have other causes other than pregnancy and are not considered diagnostic

Preterm birth Birth between 20 0/7 weeks of gestation and 36 6/7 weeks of gestation

Preterm/Premature neonate Neonate born after 20 weeks' gestation and before 37 weeks' gestation; extremely premature—neonates born less than 28 weeks' gestation; very premature—neonates born between 28 and 31 6/7 weeks' gestation; late premature—neonates born between 34 and 36 6/7 weeks' gestation

Preterm premature rupture of membranes (PPROM) Rupture of membranes with a premature gestation (less than 37 weeks); remote from term is from 24 to 32 weeks' gestation; near term is 31 to 36 weeks' gestation

Previable premature rupture of membranes Rupture of membranes before 23 to 24 weeks

Primary engorgement An increase in the vascular and lymphatic system of the breasts, which precedes the initiation of milk production; the woman's breasts become larger, firm, warm, and tender, and the woman may feel a throbbing pain in the breasts

Primigravida A woman who is pregnant for the first time

Primipara A woman who has given birth after 20 weeks' gestation one time

Probable signs of pregnancy Objective signs of pregnancy including all physiological and anatomical changes that can be perceived by the health-care provider; could have causes other than pregnancy and are not considered diagnostic

Prodromal labor When contractions are frequent and painful in early labor but ineffective in promoting dilation and effacement

Progesterone A female hormone that prepares the uterus to receive and sustain the fertilized ovum and maintain pregnancy

Prolactin The primary hormone responsible for lactation

Prolapse of the umbilical cord When the cord lies below the presenting part of the fetus

Proliferative phase Part of the endometrial cycle; it follows menstruation and ends with ovulation; during this phase the endometrium is preparing for implantation by becoming thicker and more vascular

Prolonged deceleration A visually apparent abrupt decrease in fetal heart rate below baseline that lasts greater than 2 minutes and less than 10 minutes

Prolonged rupture of membranes (PROM) Rupture of membranes longer than 24 hours

Proteinuria Excess protein in the urine

Pruritus Severe itching of the skin

Psychosocial risk factors Maternal behaviors or lifestyles that have a negative response to the mother or fetus; examples include smoking, caffeine, alcohol or drugs, and psychological status

Ptyalism Excessive secretion of saliva

Pudendal block An anesthetic injected in the pudendal nerve (close to the ischial spines) via needle guide known as "trumpet"

Pulmonary surfactant A substance that is composed of 90% phospholipids and 10% proteins that is used in the treatment of respiratory distress syndrome of the neonate

Quad screen Adds inhibin-A to the triple marker screen to increase detection of trisomy 21 to 80%

Quantification of blood loss (QBL) An objective method used to evaluate excessive bleeding by weighing blood-saturated items and blood clots; weight of 1 gram is equal to 1 mL of fluid

Quickening A woman's first awareness or perception of fetal movement within her uterus

Radiation Transfer of heat from neonate to cooler objectives that are not in direct contact with the neonate such as cold walls of isolate or cold equipment near the neonate

Reassuring fetal heart rate (FHR) Normal FHR pattern that reflects a favorable physiological response to maternal-fetal environment; this term is no longer in common use

Rectocele Bulging of the rectum into the vagina

Recurrent abortion Condition in which two or more successive pregnancies have ended in spontaneous abortion

REEDA   Redness, edema, ecchymosis, discharge, approximation of edges of episiotomy or laceration

Relaxin   A hormone produced by the corpus luteum during pregnancy that causes the pelvic ligaments and cervix to relax during pregnancy and delivery

Respect for others   The principle that all persons are equally valued

Respiratory distress syndrome (RDS)   A life-threatening lung disorder that results from underdeveloped and small alveoli, and insufficient levels of pulmonary surfactant

Respiratory syncytial virus   Virus that infects the lungs and breathing passages

Resting tone   The pressure in the uterus between contractions

Restrictive behavior   Activities during the childbearing period that are limited for the woman based on cultural practices

Retinopathy of prematurity   An abnormal growth of vasculature that occurs when tissue grows within the retina or extends into the vitreous body; can lead to blindness

Retracted nipple   Nipple drawn inward but usually easily stimulated to evert

Review of systems (ROS)   A component of the health history that includes systematic questioning about health status by body system, typically in a head-to-toe sequence, in order to gather information about current and past medical experiences

Rh factor   A type of antigen on the surface of red blood cells; if a woman's RBCs have the antigen, she is Rh positive, and if she does not have the antigen, she is Rh negative; this is significant and can cause isoimmunization from blood incompatibility if fetal blood enters the maternal system in an Rh-positive fetus and an Rh-negative mother

Rh isoimmunization   A condition that occurs when an Rh-negative pregnant woman's blood protein is incompatible with her Rh-positive fetus, causing her immune system to develop antibodies against the fetal blood cells

Rights approach   The focus is on the individual's right to choose; includes the right to privacy, to know the truth, and to be free from injury or harm

Risk management   A systems approach to the prevention of litigation; it involves the identification of systems problems, and analysis and treatment of risks before a suit is brought

Rooting reflex   Stimulated by touching the corner of a baby's mouth with a finger or nipple; baby turns head and opens mouth in the direction of the touch

Round ligament   Connective tissue that supports the uterus and stretches as the uterus grows in pregnancy

Rubella   Contagious viral disease (also known as German measles) that can cause fetal malformation if contracted in early pregnancy

Rupture of the uterus   When there is a partial or complete tear in the uterine muscle

Screening test   A test designed to identify those who are not affected by a disease or abnormality

Second-degree laceration   A laceration that involves skin, mucous membrane, and fascia of the perineal body

Second stage of labor   Begins at complete dilation of the cervix and ends with delivery of the neonate

Secretory phase   Part of the endometrial cycle; it begins after ovulation and ends with the onset of menstruation; during this phase the endometrium continues to thicken

Septic abortion   A condition in which products of conception become infected during the abortion process

Short-term variability (STV)   The changes in the fetal heart rate from one beat to the next; is measured with a fetal scalp electrode; this term is no longer used

Shoulder dystocia   Refers to difficulty encountered during delivery of the shoulders after the birth of the head

Shoulder presentation   The presenting part is the shoulder; when the fetal spine is vertical to the maternal pelvis

Skin-to-skin   Practice of placing an infant directly on the mother or caregiver's bare chest; typically dressed only in a diaper with a blanket covering both (Kangaroo care)

Slate gray patches   Flat bluish discolored areas on the lower back or buttock; seen more often in African American, Asian, Latin, and Native American infants; previously called Mongolian spots

Small for gestational age (SGA)   A term used for neonate whose weight is below the 10th percentile for gestational age

Sociodemographic risk factors   Variables that pertain to the woman and her family and place an increased risk to the mother and the fetus; examples include income, access to prenatal care, age, parity, marital status, and ethnicity

Sperm antibodies   An immunological reaction against the sperm that causes a decrease in sperm motility

Spermatogenesis   The process in which mature functional sperm are formed

Spider nevi   Small, dilated blood vessels close to the surface of the skin

Spinal block   An anesthetic injected in the subarachnoid space

Spontaneous abortion (SAB)   Abortion occurring without medical or mechanical means; also called miscarriage

Spontaneous rupture of the membranes (SROM)   Rupture of the membranes that occurs naturally

Standard   An authoritative statement enunciated and promulgated by the profession and by which the quality of practice, service, or education can be judged

Standards of care   Authoritative statements that describe competent clinical nursing practice for women and newborns demonstrated through assessment, diagnosis, outcome identification, planning, implementation, and evaluation

Standards of nursing practice   Authoritative statements that describe the scope of care or performance common to the profession of nursing and by which the quality of nursing practice can be judged; standards of nursing practice for women and newborns include both standards of care and standards of professional performance

Station   The level of the presenting part in the birth canal in relationship to the ischial spines; refers to the relationship of the ischial spines to the presenting part of the fetus and assists in assessing for fetal descent during labor

Stepping reflex   Neonate steps up and down in place when held upright with feed touching flat surface

Striae   A band of depressed tissue most commonly seen on the abdomen, thighs, buttocks, or breasts due to stretching of the skin; synonymous with stretch marks

Stripping the membranes   Digital separation of the chorionic membrane from the wall of the cervix and lower uterine segment during a vaginal examination done by a primary care provider to stimulate labor

Subgaleal hemorrhage   A type of extracranial hemorrhage; the subgaleal space is located above the periosteum so when bleeding occurs there is no membrane to contain it

Subinvolution of the uterus   A term used when the uterus does not decrease in size and does not descend into the pelvis

Suck reflex   Involuntary sucking when the roof of a baby's mouth is touched

Sudden unexplained infant death (SUID)   Term used to describe the sudden and unexpected death of a baby less than 1 year old in which the cause was not obvious before investigation

Supine   Position of lying on the back with face or front upward

Supine hypotensive syndrome   Hypotension resulting from compression of the vena cava when a woman lies supine and the gravid uterus exerts pressure on the inferior vena cava

Supplemental nursing system   A thin tube that attaches to a bottle on one end fastened approximately ¼ inch beyond the mother's nipple to allow the newborn to receive a supplement while nursing

Surfactant   A phospholipid within the alveoli that reduces the surface tension in the lungs and assists in the establishment of respirations; prevents alveoli from collapsing at the end of expiration

Swaddling   To wrap the infant snugly in a blanket to provide warmth and a sense of security that can have a calming effect

Symmetric intrauterine growth restriction   A generalized proportional reduction in the size of all structures and organs except for the heart and brain

Syndactyly   Webbed digits of the hands or feet

Tachycardia   Baseline fetal heart rate of greater than 160 bpm lasting 10 minutes or longer

Tachysystole   Abnormally frequent contractions; five or more contractions in 10 minutes

Teratogens   Any drug, virus, infection, or other exposures that can cause embryo or fetal developmental abnormality

Therapeutic abortion (TAB)   Termination of pregnancy for serious maternal medical indications or serious fetal anomalies

Therapeutic hypothermia   Intentional reduction in a patient's core temperature to treat hypoxic-ischemic encephalopathy

Third-degree laceration   A laceration that involves skin, mucous membrane, or muscle of the perineal body; extends to the rectal sphincter

Third stage of labor   Begins immediately after the delivery of the fetus and involves separation and expulsion of the placenta and membranes

Threatened abortion   Continuation of pregnancy is in doubt as symptoms indicate termination of pregnancy is in progress

Thrombosis   Blood clot within the vascular system

Tocodynamometer   An external uterine monitor to measure contractions

Tonic neck reflex   Neonate "fencing" position with arms and legs extended in direction in which head is turned

TORCH   An acronym that stands for toxoplasmosis, other (hepatitis B), rubella, cytomegalovirus, and herpes simplex virus

Total fertility rate (TFR)   The average number of children that would be born per woman if all women lived to the end of their childbearing years and bore children according to a given fertility rate at each age

Total placenta previa   The placenta completely covers the internal cervical os

Toxoplasma   A protozoan parasite found in cat feces and uncooked or rare beef and lamb

Transcutaneous bilirubinometry (TcB)   Noninvasive method using a bilirubinometer to estimate total serum bilirubin levels among term and near-term neonates

Transepidermal water loss (TEWL)   Water loss that can occur through the neonate's immature skin

Transitional milk   The name for the milk produced after colostrum and before mature milk; about 3 to 6 days after birth

Transitional stool   Neonatal stools that begin around the third day and can continue for 3 or 4 days; the stool transitions from black to greenish black, to greenish brown, to greenish yellow

Transverse presentation   The presenting part is usually the shoulder

Trial of labor after cesarean (TOLAC)   When a trial of labor and vaginal birth is attempted in a woman who has had a prior cesarean birth

Triple marker   A screening that combines all three chemical markers (AFP, hCG, and estriol levels) with maternal age to detect some trisomies and neural tube defects

Trophic feedings   Small-volume enteral feedings that are administered to neonates to stimulate the development of the immature gastrointestinal tract

Trophoblast   Outer cell mass of the blastocyst that assists in implantation and becomes part of the placenta

True labor   Contractions occur at regular intervals and increase in frequency, duration, and intensity; true labor contractions bring about changes in cervical effacement and dilation

Turtle sign   The retraction of the fetal head against the maternal perineum after delivery of the head

Ultrasonography   The use of high-frequency sound waves to produce an image of an organ or tissue

Umbilical artery Doppler flow   Studies assess the rate and volume of blood flow through the placenta and umbilical cord vessels using ultrasound

Umbilical cord   The structure that connects the fetus to the placenta; it consists of two arteries and one vein and is surrounded by Wharton's jelly

Unconjugated bilirubin   A relatively insoluble bilirubin that is mostly bound to albumin; also called indirect bilirubin

Undescended testes   An abnormality in which the testes are not in the scrotum

Universal precautions   Standard set of infection control guidelines to prevent transmission of bloodborne pathogens

Uterine atony   A decreased tone of the uterine muscle postpartum that is the primary cause of immediate postpartum hemorrhage

Uterine hypertonus   An increasing resting tone greater than 20 to 25 mm Hg, peak pressure greater than 80 mm Hg, or Montevideo units greater than 400

Uterine prolapse   Occurs when there is a weakening of the pelvic connective tissue, pubococcygeus muscle, and uterine ligaments, which allows the uterus to descend into the vagina

Uterotonic   A pharmacological agent used to induce contraction of the uterus

Utilitarian approach   This approach suggests that ethical actions are those that provide the greatest balance of good over evil and provide for the greatest good for the greatest number

Utility   The greatest good for the individual or an action that is valued; utility is concerned with the evaluation of risk and benefit or benefit versus burden

Vacuum-assisted delivery   A birth involving the use of a vacuum cup on the fetal head to assist with delivery of the fetal head

Vaginal birth after a cesarean (VBAC)   When a trial of labor and vaginal birth is attempted in a woman who has had a prior cesarean birth

Vaginitis   An inflammation of the vagina

Valsalva maneuver   The method of breath holding, closed-glottis pushing

Variable deceleration   A visually apparent abrupt decrease in the fetal heart rate below baseline; the decrease is 15 bpm or greater lasting 15 seconds or more and less than 2 minutes in duration

Varicosity   Dilated vein that primarily occurs in the lower limbs

Venous thrombosis   Blood clot

Veracity   The obligation to tell the truth

Vernix caseosa   A protective substance secreted from sebaceous glands that covered the fetus during pregnancy

Very low birth weight (VLBW)   1,000 grams to 1,499 grams at birth

Very premature/preterm   Neonate born at less than 32 weeks' gestation

Viability   The threshold for viability is at 25, and rarely fewer, completed weeks' gestation

Vibroacoustic stimulation (VAS)   Screening tool that uses auditory stimulation (using an artificial larynx) to assess fetal well-being with electronic fetal monitoring when a non-stress test is nonreactive

Vitamin K deficiency bleeding   Delayed clotting and hemorrhage of neonate due to temporary vitamin K deficiency after birth

Welcoming and inclusive care   Gender-affirming care to all people, including gender-diverse and transgender individuals

Wharton's jelly   A collagen substance that surrounds the vessels of the umbilical cord and protects the vessels from compression

Zika virus   Virus transmitted by mosquitoes or sexual contact with an infected person; pregnant women can spread to the fetus causing birth defects such as microcephaly, impaired growth, and visual or hearing abnormalities

Zygote   A fertilized oocyte which contains the diploid number of chromosomes (46)

Photo and Illustration Credits

Linda Chapman author photo by Tom Bauer

Chapter 1

Figure 1–1. *Healthy People 2030,* U.S. Department of Health and Human Services, Office of Disease Prevention and Health Promotion. Retrieved July 5, 2021, from https://health.gov/healthypeople/objectives-and-data/social-determinants-health

Chapter 3

Figure 3–1. MedlinePlus, U.S. National Library of Medicine. Cystic fibrosis. Available from https://medlineplus.gov/genetics/condition/cystic-fibrosis/#inheritance

Figure 3–2. MedlinePlus, U.S. National Library of Medicine. Huntington disease. Available from https://medlineplus.gov/genetics/condition/huntington-disease/#inheritance

Figure 3–3. Adapted from MedlinePlus, U.S. National Library of Medicine. Hemophilia. Available from https://medlineplus.gov/genetics/condition/hemophilia/#inheritance

Chapter 5

Figure 5–3. Courtesy of Gwen Ortiz and Randi Willis.

Chapter 6

Figures 6–3 and 6–4. Courtesy of the Allbin family.

Chapter 7

Figure 7–7. Adapted from Gilbert, E. S. (2007). *High-risk pregnancy and delivery* (4th ed.). Mosby Elsevier.

Chapter 8

Concept map created by Sylvia Fisher.

Chapter 10

Figure 10–7. Courtesy of CooperSurgical, Inc.

Figure 10–8. Courtesy of CooperSurgical, Inc.

Chapter 12

Figure 12–5. U.S. Department of Agriculture. www.ChooseMyPlate.gov

Chapter 15

Figure 15–7. Reprinted from Ballard, J. L., Khoury, J. C., Wedig, K. L., Wang, L., Eilers-Walsman, B. L., & Lipp, R. (1991). New Ballard Score, expanded to include extremely premature infants. *The Journal of Pediatrics, 119*(3), 417–423.

Chapter 16

Figure 16–5. Courtesy of Medela Corporation, McHenry, Illinois.

Chapter 17

Figure 17–3. Reproduced with permission from Martha A. Q. Curley; originally published in Curley, M. A. Q., Hasbani, N. R., Quigley, S. M., Stellar, J. J., Pasek, T. A., Shelley, S. S., Kulik, . . . Wypij, D. (2018). Predicting pressure injury risk in pediatric patients: The Braden QD Scale. *Journal of Pediatrics, 192, 189–195*; note that the Braden QD Scale was modified from the Braden Q Scale that was adapted with permission from "Braden Scale for Predicting Pressure Ulcer Risk." Copyright Braden, B., & Bergstrom, N., 1988.

Chapter 18

Figure 18–2. U.S. Department of Agriculture. www.ChooseMyPlate.gov

Figure 18–3. U.S. Department of Health and Human Services, 2012.

Chapter 19

Figure 19–6. Imaginis, 2001.

Appendix B

Adapted from the Improving Health Care Response to Preeclampsia: A California Quality Improvement Toolkit, funded by the California Department of Public Health, 2014; supported by Title V funds.

Index

O